clinical nephrology

Volume 35 – 1991

Dustri Verlag
Dr. Karl Feistle
München-
Deisenhofen

clinical nephrology

Clinical Nephrology appears monthly and publishes reviews, editorials, original papers, case reports, letters, book reviews and current information. The editors reserve the right of selection from submitted manuscripts (after consulting at least two reviewers) and the right to make stylistic changes or abridgements. The manuscripts may not be offered elsewhere for printing or publication; following acceptance the publisher acquires all copyrights. Rejected manuscripts are returned to the authors, the copies being sent under separate cover as printed matter, air mail.

This journal is regularly listed in Current Contents and Index Medicus.

PUBLISHER:
DUSTRI-VERLAG Dr. Karl Feistle,
Bahnhofstraße 9, Postfach 49,
W-8024 München-Deisenhofen, Germany
Telefon München (089) 6135041
Teletex 897156 = DUSTRI
Telefax (089) 6135412

EDITOR-IN-CHIEF (responsible):
Prof. Dr. med. K. M. Koch,
Medizinische Hochschule Hannover,
Zentrum für Innere Medizin,
Konstanty-Gutschow-Straße 8,
W-3000 Hannover 61, Germany

MANAGING EDITOR:
J. Mayer
DUSTRI-VERLAG Dr. Karl Feistle,
Bahnhofstraße 9, Postfach 49,
W-8024 München-Deisenhofen, Germany
Telephone Munich (089) 6135041

Printed in West Germany
by Mayr Miesbach,
Am Windfeld 15,
W-8160 Miesbach, Germany
ISSN 0301-0430

ADVERTISING:
Representatives in USA:
M. J. Mrvica Associates, Inc.
155 S. White Horse Pike
Berlin, NJ 08009, USA
Telephone (609) 768-9360

Germany:
H. P. Eckardt
DUSTRI-VERLAG Dr. Karl Feistle

Volumes 35 and 36 (6 issues per volume) will be published in 1991.
Published monthly.
Subscription price for 1991: DM 312.–, US $ 154.– plus postage (air mail only): Europe: $ 8.50; USA: $ 15.–; Japan/Brazil: $ 24.–; Australia: $ 28.–.
Single copies:
DM 28.–, US $ 15.– plus postage.
Parallel editions in microfiche can be purchased. Prices on order.
Available from all booksellers or direct from the publishers.

Second Class postage rate paid at Jamaica, NY 11431, USA.
U.S. Postmaster: Send address changes to CLINICAL NEPHROLOGY, Publications Expediting Inc., 200 Meacham Avenue, Elmont, NY 11003, USA.
Air freight and mailing in the US by Publications Expediting, Inc.
200 Meacham Ave., Elmont, NY 11003, USA.
Subscriptions are automatically canceled at the end of the year and recommence only with renewal. Prepayment is required on all orders.

Contents for Volume 35

Volume 35 No. 1 1991
January

The prognostic significance of urinary interleukin 6 in IgA nephropathy 1
K. Dohi, M. Iwano, A. Muraguchi, Y. Horii, T. Hirayama, S. Ogawa, H. Shiki, T. Hirano, T. Kishimoto and H. Ishikawa

Resolution of cirrhotic glomerulonephritis following successful liver transplantation 6
N. Ghabra, B. Piraino, A. Greenberg and B. Banner

Changes in the postenteropathic form of the hemolytic uremic syndrome in children 10
N. A. G. Coad, T. Marshall, B. Rowe and C. M. Taylor

Xanthogranulomatous pyelonephritis masquerading as empyema thoracis and later presenting as reno-cutaneous fistula 17
R. Mathur and J. Warren

Intercatheter streptokinase for recurrent peritonitis 20
B. J. Nankivell, N. Lake and A. Gillies

Pneumococcal peritonitis complicating CAPD – was the indwelling intrauterine device to blame? 24
A. Korzets, A. Chagnac, Y. Ori, D. Zevin and J. Levi

Hemodialysis and heparin. Alternative methods of measuring heparin and of detecting activation of coagulation 26
H. A. Ireland, M. D. Boisclair, D. A. Lane, E. Thompson and J. R. Curtis

Echocardiographic findings in hemodialysis patients treated with recombinant human erythropoietin: proposal for a hematocrit most beneficial to hemodynamics 35
H. Tagawa, M. Nagano, H. Saito, M. Umezu and M. Yamakado

Long-term minoxidil treatment in refractory hypertension and renal failure 39
R. Pontremoli, C. Robaudo, A. Gaiter, F. Massarino and G. Deferrari

Letters to the editor 44

Volume 35 No. 2 1991
February

Membranoproliferative glomerulonephritis associated with sickle cell disease in two siblings — 47
S. S. Iskandar, R. G. Morgann, M. C. Browning † and W. B. Lorentz

Oxalate, silicon and vanadium in acquired cystic kidney disease — 52
J. E. Marco-Franco, V. E. Torres, D. E. Nixon, D. M. Wilson, E. M. James, E. J. Bergstralh and J. T. McCarthy

Effects of an acute protein load on urinary albumin excretion in kidney donors — 59
C. Manno, F. D'Elia, M. Mingarelli, M. Stella, M. Cervellati, G. Fornarelli and F. P. Schena

Hyperreninemic hypoaldosteronism due to hepatocellular carcinoma metastatic to the adrenal gland — 66
S. Otabe, S. Muto, Y. Asano, K. Sato, M. Ohtani, C. Kawamoto, K. Ido and K. Kimura

Pharmacokinetics of active vitamins D3, 1 α-hydroxyvitamin D3 and 1 α, 25-dihydroxyvitamin D3 in patients on chronic hemodialysis — 72
Y. Kimura, M. Nakayama, S. Kuriyama, S. Watanabe, Y. Kawaguchi and O. Sakai

The clinical spectrum of renal osteodystrophy in 57 chronic hemodialysis patients: a correlation between biochemical parameters and bone pathology findings — 78
J. A. Chazan, N. P. Libbey, M. R. London, L. Pono and J. G. Abuelo

Letters to the editor — 86

Book reviews — 91

Announcements — 92

Volume 35 No. 3 1991
March

Rheumatoid factors in patients with minimal change nephrotic syndrome — 93
M. Endoh, M. Miyazaki, T. Suga, M. Miura, Y. Nomoto and H. Sakai

Intravenous immunoglobulin therapy of membranous nephropathy: efficacy and safety — 98
R. Palla, C. Cirami, V. Panichi, A. M. Bianchi, M. Parrini and G. Grazi

Acute tubulointerstitial nephritis associated with Yersinia pseudotuberculosis infection — 105
K. Okada, I. Yano, S. Kagami, M. Funai, S. Kawahito, T. Okomoto, A. Imagawa and Y. Kuroda

Acute and chronic renal disease in hospitalized AIDS patients — 110
A. Valeri and A.-J. Neusy

The successful treatment of atypical hemolytic uremic syndrome with plasmapheresis — 119
W. L. M. Robson and A. K. C. Leung

Efficacy of percutaneous renal biopsy in obese patients under computerized tomographic guidance — 123
S.-M. K. Lee, J. King and B. H. Spargo

Correction of hypophosphatemia in patients on hemodialysis using a calcium-free dialyzate with added phosphate — 130
M. Kaye, M. Vasilevsky and E. Barber

Letters to the editor — 133

Announcements — 138

Volume 35 No. 4 1991
April

Wegener's granulomatosis with renal involvement: patient survival and correlations between initial renal function, renal histology, therapy and renal outcome 139
K. Andrassy, A. Erb, J. Koderisch, R. Waldherr and E. Ritz

Renal failure in adult onset hypophosphatemic osteomalacia with Fanconi syndrome: a family study and review of the literature 148
N. A. Harrison, J. M. Bateman, J. G. G. Ledingham and R. Smith

The effect of prostacyclin on intracranial pressure in patients with acute hepatic and renal failure 151
A. Davenport, E. J. Will and A. M. Davison

Effect of osmolar changes on plasma arginine vasopressin (PAVP) in dialysis patients 158
S. J. Rosansky, R. Rhinehart und R. Shade

Influence of erythropoietin treatment on urea kinetic parameters in hemodialysis patients 165
J. A. Van Geelen, M. J. Nubé and P. A. Zuurbier

Acute encephalopathy due to thiamine deficiency (Wernicke's encephalopathy) in a chronic hemodialyzed patient: a case report 171
E. Descombes, C.-A. Dessibourg and G. Fellay

Uremic polyneuropathy: a clinical and electrophysiological study in 135 short- and longterm hemodialyzed patients 176
C. Bazzi, C. Pagani, G. Sorgato, G. Albonico, G. Fellin and G. D'Amico

Letters to the editor 182

Announcements 186

Volume 35 No. 5 1991
May

Progression of a naproxen and amoxicillin induced acute interstitial nephritis with nephrotic syndrome: case report 187
J. Nortier, M. Depierreux, V. Bourgeois, J. Ducobu and P. Dupont

Immunohistochemical detection of renal carbonic anhydrase of patients with recurrent urolithiasis 190
L. Jonas, B. Klein, L. Hoffmann and T. Kumpulainen

Vaccination for prevention of CAPD associated staphylococcal infection: Results of a prospective multicentre clinical trial 198
L. A. Poole-Warren, M. D. Hallett, P. W. Hone, S. H. Burden and P. C. Farrell

Correction of anemia in patients on continuous ambulatory peritoneal dialysis with subcutaneous recombinant erythropoietin twice a week: a long-term study 207
I. K. P. Cheng, C. Cy, M. K. Chan, L. Yu, G. X. Fang and D. Wei

Removal of trace metals by continuous ambulatory peritoneal dialysis after desferrioxamine B chelation therapy 213
J. A. Navarro, V. A. Granadillo, B. Rodríguez-Iturbe, R. García, O. Salgado and R. A. Romero

Vasoactive hormones in uremic patients on continuous ambulatory peritoneal dialysis 218
K. N. Lai, P. K. T. Li, K. S. Woo, S. F. Lui, J. C. K. Leung, E. Law and M. G. Nicholls

Hypersensitivity reactions during hemodialysis related to the use of acetate dialysate. A case report 224
J. T. Papadakis, A. Patrikarea, S. Saradi, K. Papakostas, A. Leondi, A. Kravaritis and S. Vafiadis

Shoulder ultrasound in dialysis related amyloidosis 227
L. P. McMahon, J. Radford and J. K. Dawborn

Letters to the editor 233

Announcements 236

Volume 35 No. 6 1991
June

Effect of dietary proteins and lipids in patients with membranous nephropathy and nephrotic syndrome 237
G. D'Amico, G. Remuzzi, G. Maschio, M. G. Gentile, E. Gotti, L. Oldrizzi, G. Manna, G. Mecca, C. Rugiu and G. Fellin

Crescentic glomerulonephritis in Wegener's granulomatosis: morphology, therapy, outcome 243
W. Grotz, C. Wanner, E. Keller, J. Böhler, H. H. Peter, R. Rohrbach and P. Schollmeyer

Very late recurrence of renal vasculitis 252
A. Innes, R. E. Cotton, P. A. Rowe and R. P. Burden

Glomerular proteinuria as an early sign of renal-transplant rejection 255
J. Steinhoff, A. Feddersen, W. G. Wood, J. Hoyer and K. Sack

Familial juvenile gouty nephropathy with renal urate hypo-excretion preceding renal disease 263
F. Moro, C. S. Ogg, H. A. Simmonds, J. S. Cameron, C. Chantler, M. B. McBride, J. A. Duley and P. M. Davies

Nutritional assessment in anemic hemodialysis patients treated with recombinant human erythropoietin 270
P. Bárány, E. Pettersson, M. Ahlberg, E. Hultman and J. Bergström

Regression of left ventricular hypertrophy after partial correction of anemia with erythropoietin in patients on hemodialysis: a prospective study 280
J. Pascual, J. L. Teruel, J. L. Moya, F. Liaño, M. Jiménez-Mena and J. Ortuño

Letters to the editor 288

Index I

Volume 35,
Supplement No. 1 1991

Cyclosporin A (Sandimmun®) in Nephrotic Syndrome

Guest Editor: Claudio Ponticelli, Milan

Preface S 1

Epidemiology and natural course of idiopathic nephrotic syndrome S 3
N. P. Mallick

Conventional therapy for idiopathic nephrotic syndrome in children S 8
J. Brodehl

Conventional treatment of idiopathic nephrotic syndrome and membranous nephropathy in adults S 16
C. Ponticelli and P. Passerini

Discussion: Summary S 22

Mechanism of action of cyclosporin A and rationale for use in nephrotic syndrome S 23
J. F. Borel

Treatment of idiopathic nephrotic syndrome with cyclosporin A in children S 31
P. Niaudet, M. Broyer and R. Habib

Treatment of adult idiopathic nephrotic syndrome with cyclosporin A
Minimal-change disease and focal-segmental glomerulosclerosis S 37
A. Meyrier, M.-C. Condamin, D. Broneer, and The Collaborative Group of the French Society of Nephrology

Current status of cyclosporin A in the treatment of membranous, IgA and membranoproliferative glomerulonephritis S 43
D. C. Cattran

Safety and tolerability of cyclosporin A (Sandimmun®) in idiopathic nephrotic syndrome S 48
Collaborative Study Group of Sandimmun® in Nephrotic Syndrome

Final Discussion: Summary S 61

Clinical Nephrology, Vol. 35 No. 1 – 1991 (1–5)

The prognostic significance of urinary interleukin 6 in IgA nephropathy

K. Dohi[1], M. Iwano[1], A. Muraguchi[2], Y. Horii[2], T. Hirayama[1], S. Ogawa[1], H. Shiiki[1], T. Hirano[3], T. Kishimoto[2] and H. Ishikawa[1]

[1] *First Department of Internal Medicine, Nara Medical University, 840 Shijo-cho, Kashihara, Nara 634, Japan*
[2] *Division of Immunology, Institute for Molecular and Cellular Biology, Osaka University, 1–3 Yamada-oka, Suita, Osaka 565, Japan*
[3] *Division of Molecular Oncology, Biomedical Research Center, Osaka University Medical School, 4-3-57 Nakanoshima, Kita-ku, Osaka 530, Japan*

Abstract. Our previous study has shown that interleukin 6 (IL-6), a multifunctional cytokine, is closely associated with the pathogenesis of mesangial proliferative glomerulonephritis (mesPGN). To investigate whether urinary IL-6 can be used as an indicator in the prognosis of patients with IgA nephropathy, we monitored IL-6 activity in the urine of patients with IgA nephropathy for 10 months and compared IL-6 activity with clinical data as well as the histological changes of the kidneys obtained from the patients. It was found that among the patients who had continuously high urinary IL-6 activity, histological progression of IgA nephropathy was observed. On the other hand, among the patients whose urinary IL-6 became undetectable during the 10-month follow-up, histological improvement of IgA nephropathy was observed. These data suggest that the measurement of urinary IL-6 is a helpful tool for monitoring the progression of IgA nephropathy.

Key words: interleukin 6 (IL-6) – IgA nephropathy – mesangial cell

Introduction

IgA nephropathy, the most common primary glomerulonephritis in Japan, is histologically characterized by the presence of mesangial IgA deposits and a major entity of mesangial proliferative glomerulonephritis (mesPGN). It is said that about 25% of patients with IgA nephropathy will eventually progress to chronic renal failure. A poor prognosis is associated clinically with nephrotic-range proteinuria, elevated serum creatinine concentration, and hypertension, and on renal biopsy with diffuse crescentic formation, focal and segmental glomerular sclerosis and/or necrosis, interstitial fibrosis and tubular atrophy. However, even without showing the above findings, some patients may progress to chronic renal failure. Thus it is difficult to evaluate the individual prognosis by such conventional laboratory findings [Berger et al. 1969, Clarkson et al. 1977, Kincaid-Smith et al. 1983, Sinniah et al. 1981, Woo et al. 1986, Kusumoto et al. 1987, Dohi et al. 1987]. IL-6 is closely associated with the pathogenesis of mesPGN. [Horii et al. 1989, Suematsu et al. 1989]. In our previous study [Horii et al. 1989], 19 out of 38 urine samples of mesPGN patients (34 IgA nephropathy and 4 non-IgA nephropathy) were found to contain significant IL-6 activity, whereas none of the urine samples of 27 minimal change nephrotic syndrome (MCNS) and 20 healthy volunteers had detectable IL-6 activity. Only 2 samples from 27 cases of membranous nephropathy (MN) showed significant IL-6 activity. In addition, there is a correlation between the levels of urinary IL-6 and the pathological stage of mesPGN.

These data have suggested that the measurement of IL-6 activity in patient urine is useful not only for the differential diagnosis of the primary glomerulonephritis but also for evaluating the pathological stage of mesPGN.

In this study, we addressed the question of whether the activity of urinary IL-6 can be used as an indicator to evaluate the prognosis in IgA nephropathy, and whether measurement of urinary IL-6 can be used to partly replace renal biopsy.

Received July 9, 1990; in revised form October 5, 1990.
Reprint requests to K. Dohi.

Patients and Methods

Patients

A total of 52 patients with IgA nephropathy followed by the First Department of Internal Medicine, Nara Medical University, were studied. These patients were diagnosed as IgA nephropathy by light and immunofluorescence microscopies. Patients who had systemic disease such as Schoenlein-Henoch purpura, liver disease, renal dysfunction (endogenous creatinine clearance was less than 70 ml/min) or idiopathic crescentic glomerulonephritis on renal biopsy were excluded. None of the patients received any immunosuppressive drugs but all the patients received anti-platelet drugs. According to the degree of mesangial proliferation on renal biopsy as described previously, the remaining 32 patients were divided into two groups, IgA nephropathy with mild mesangial proliferation (group I) and with moderate mesangial proliferation of more than 50% of the glomeruli (group II) [Pirani et al. 1968, Dohi et al. 1987]. In group II, focal accentuation of glomeruli such as segmental sclerosis and small crescent formation, were also observed in less than 20% of the glomeruli. In all cases, less than 30% of the cortex was involved by interstitial fibrosis and cellular infiltrates. All biopsy specimens contained at least ten glomeruli. IL-6 activity in urine samples obtained from these 32 patients was measured. Ten of 32 urine samples were found to contain significant IL-6 activity. Thus, these 10 patients were selected for follow-up study. All patients were normotensive during follow-up and the urinary protein excretion ranged from 180 mg to 3,000 mg per day. The first biopsy was performed between March 1987 and December 1988. The second biopsy was performed on group II (5 patients) between September 1989 and December 1989.

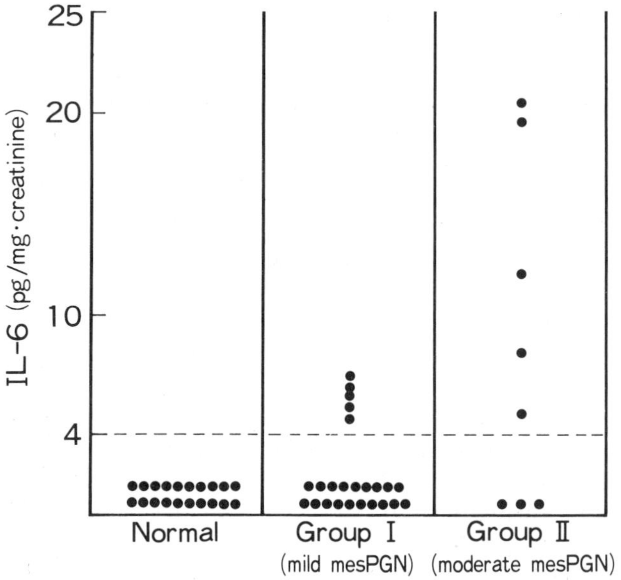

Fig. 1 IL-6 activity in urine samples from patients with IgA nephropathy. A correlation between IL-6 activity and the pathological stage of IgA nephropathy is observed. Urinary IL-6 levels were measured, utilizing frozen urine samples at time of renal biopsy.

Light microscopic findings

The tissue specimens for light microscopy were fixed in 10% neutral phosphate-buffered formalin, then embedded in paraffin and cut at 3 μm in thickness. The sections were stained with periodic acid Schiff.

Urine samples

Urine samples were collected every five months. Fresh urine samples collected into 15 ml centrifuge tubes were centrifuged at 1000 g for 5 min at 4° C, passed through a 0.45 μm filter and dialyzed twice against phosphate-buffered saline (pH 7.2) for 2 hours and once against RPMI 1640 for 2 hours at 4° C. Samples were harvested from the dialyzing tubes and frozen at −20° C until use.

IL-6 assay

IL-6 activity was measured by using an IL-6 dependent murine hybridoma clone, MH60.BSF2. as described previously [Matsuda et al. 1988]. IL-6 activity was expressed in a value corrected by the urinary creatinine concentration.

Results

Detection of IL-6 activity in urine samples from the patients with IgA nephropathy

IL-6 activity was examined in 32 urine samples from patients with IgA nephropathy as well as 20 normal healthy volunteers. As shown in Figure 1, 5 of 24 urine samples in group I and 5 of 8 urine samples in group II were found to contain significant IL-6 activity (ranging from 4.2 to 20.8 pg/mg creatinine). None of the urine samples obtained from healthy volunteers had detectable IL-6 activity. The urinary IL-6 level in group II was significantly higher than that in group I. These data are compatible with the previous data [Horii et al. 1989], showing that urinary IL-6 correlates well with the degree of mesangial

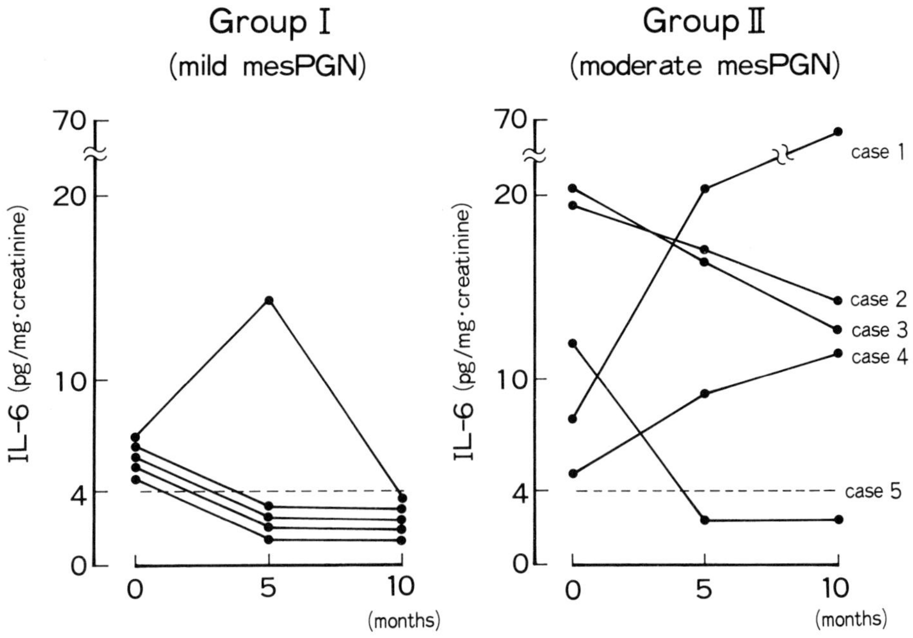

Fig. 2 Time course of urinary IL-6 activity. Group I; IgA nephropathy with mild mesangial proliferation. Group II; IgA nephropathy with moderate mesangial proliferation.

proliferation. The activity of IL-6 in urine samples was neutralized by the addition of anti-IL-6 antibody, thus indicating its specific identity (data not shown). No significant correlation between IgG or IgA level in serum, the number of episodes of gross hematuria or recurrent upper respiratory tract infections and urinary IL-6 was observed in the patients studied.

Time course of urinary IL-6 activity

In group I, urinary IL-6 activity became undetectable (less than 4 pg/mg creatinine) in all patients during follow-up as shown in Figure 2. All patients in this group showed microscopic hematuria, recurrent gross hematuria and/or modest proteinuria (24-hour protein excretion, 230 to 640 mg), at the time of the first percutaneous renal biopsy. During the about one year follow-up, both gross hematuria and proteinuria in these patients had disappeared. These data clearly show that urinary IL-6 and clinical findings are correlated in this group.

In group II, the time course of IL-6 activity assumed three patterns as shown in Figure 2: Case 1: IL-6 activity was remarkably elevated during follow-up. Cases 2, 3, 4: IL-6 activity was continuously detectable during follow-up. Case 5: IL-6 activity became undetectable during follow-up.

Pathological and clinical changes in group II

A second biopsy was performed in all patients belonging to group II and pathological changes were evaluated and compared with the findings of the first biopsy.

Case 1: In this case, IL-6 activity was markedly elevated from 7.0 to 69.5 pg/ml creatinine during follow-up, whereas clinical data, such as the 24-hour protein excretion and the 24-hour endogenous creatinine clearance (Ccr), remained stable. A massive urinary protein excretion (between 2.0 g/day and 3.0 g/day) was detected and Ccr was always more than 70 ml/min during follow-up. Histological findings showed, however, that IgA nephropathy had progressed considerably in all microscopic aspects, when compared with the first biopsy specimen, as shown in Figure 3 A, B. Case 2, 3, 4: In these cases, IL-6 activity was continuously detectable. In these cases, a substantial urinary protein excretion (between 0.8 g/day and 1.5 g/day) was detected and Ccr was always more than 70 ml/min during follow-up. Other clinical data, such as BUN and serum creatinine, were also stable. Pathological study from renal biopsy showed that IgA nephropathy had progressed in these cases. Active lesions such as segmental sclerosis and foci of tubular fibrosis, which were not observed in the first biopsy, were present.

Case 5: In this case, IL-6 activity became undetectable during follow-up. Clinical data were also stable. A slight urinary protein excretion (between 0.5 g/day and 0.8 g/day) was detected and Ccr was always more than 70 mg/min during follow-up. Pathological findings revealed remission of IgA nephropathy as shown in Figure 4 A, B. However, we cannot completely deny the possibility that these histological changes were due to sampling problems in biopsy specimens.

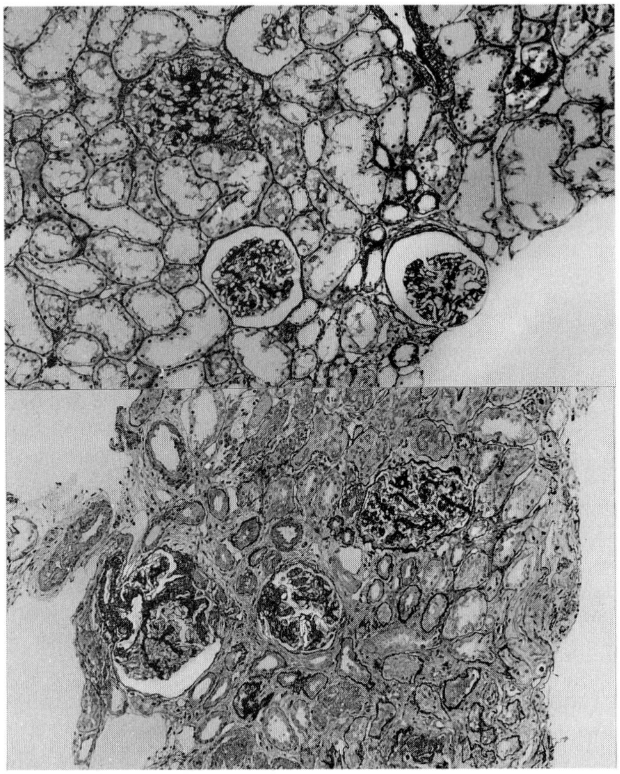

Fig. 3 Light microscopy of case 1. Histological progression is observed, comparing the second biopsy (*B*) with the first biopsy (*A*). Adhesion to Bowman's capsule in all glomeruli and tubular involvement are observed on the second biopsy. (×80)

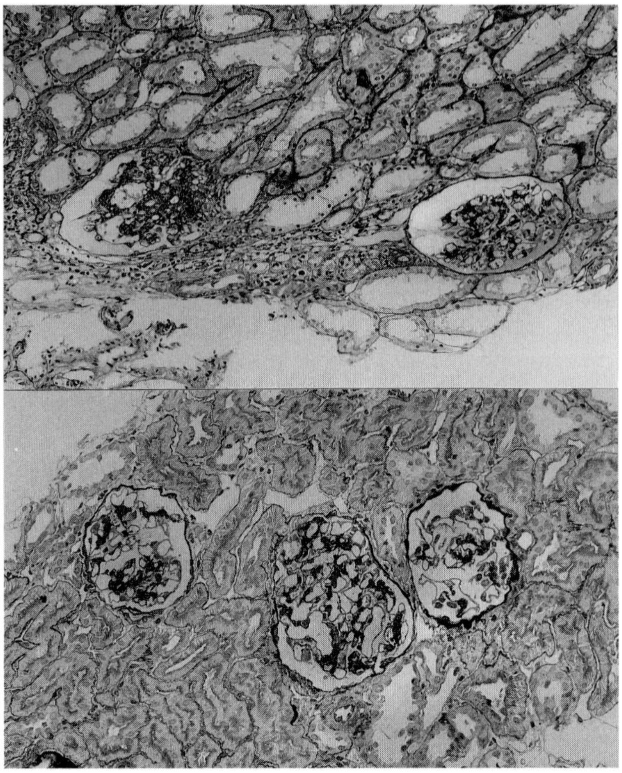

Fig. 4 Light microscopy of case 5. Histological regression is observed, comparing the second biopsy (*A*) with the first biopsy (*B*). One glomerulus showed severe mesangial proliferation on the first biopsy. On the other hand, the second biopsy revealed only minor changes in the mesangium. (× 100)

Discussion

Several cytokines have been recently found to be involved in the pathogenesis of glomerulonephritis by inducing the proliferation of mesangial cells (MC) and mesangial matrix synthesis [Lovett et al. 1983, 1986, Melcion et al. 1982, MacCarthy et al. 1985, Tranqui et al. 1985, Sterzel et al. 1986, Striker et al. 1985, Border et al. 1990]. Overexpression of some cytokines such as tumor necrosis factor (TNF) and interleukin 1 (IL-1) are demonstrated in the renal cortex of immune-complex mediated glomerulonephritis such as NZB/WF1 mice [Boswell et al. 1988, Tomosugi et al. 1989]. In a previous study, we have demonstrated that IL-6 is a possible autocrine growth factor for rat MC, and unregulated production of IL-6 in human MC may be involved in the pathological proliferation of MC in mesPGN. Mesangial areas in biopsy specimens of Case 1, Case 2 and Case 3 in this report were stained with anti-IL-6 antibody as it has been shown previously. Thus, mesangial cells are most likely to be responsible for an increased urinary IL-6 production in patients with IgA nephropathy. However, we cannot completely deny the possibility that crescent forming cells or interstitial infiltrating cells such as monocytes are responsible for urinary IL-6 production. As we have previously shown, crescent formation may be associated with high IL-6 level, and infiltrating cells have the potentiality to procedure IL-6.

In this report, we demonstrated that urinary IL-6 activity correlated well with the degree of mesangial proliferation in IgA nephropathy. However, 3 out of 8 urine samples in group II were not found to contain IL-6 activity. Probably, in such cases, mesangial cells do not always produce IL-6. Furthermore, we demonstrated that there is a correlation between time course of urinary IL-6 activity and pathological change of IgA nephropathy: 1) among the patients who had continuously high IL-6 activity during a 10-month follow-up, pathological progression of IgA nephropathy was observed, 2) among the patients whose urinary IL-6 became undetectable during the follow-up, pathological improvement of IgA nephropathy was observed. The clinical management of patients with IgA nephropathy is difficult because of the lack of definite criteria that permit identification of those individuals who are likely to progress. While the renal pathological changes were considered to be the most useful prognostic indicator of IgA nephropathy, the prognostic significance of proteinuria and hematuria remains controversial [Kincaid-Smith et al. 1983]. There are no non-invasive laboratory methods to assess the degree of mesangial proliferation. In this study, we indicated that a better correlation between urinary IL-6 and the morphological data was observed, compared to other clinical data such as proteinuria or hematuria in group II, suggesting that urinary IL-6 may reveal the pathological changes more sensitively than proteinuria and hematuria. However, we have no evidence that increased urinary IL-6 is detectable even before morphologic or conventional laboratory parameters indicate more rapid progression. We must carry out follow-up studies on the same patients for more than five years in order to elucidate this important point.

To the best of our knowledge, this is the first clinical study that demonstrates that the time course of urinary IL-6 activity may directly reflect the mesangial proliferation in IgA nephropathy. The results of the present study indicate that the measurement of urinary IL-6 is a helpful tool for monitoring the progression of IgA nephropathy and it can be used to partly replace the renal biopsy.

Acknowledgements

This study was supported by a Research Grant for "Progressive renal disease" from "Specially selected diseases by the Ministry of Health and Welfare Research Project", Ministry of Health and Welfare, Japan, and Program Project Grant of Health and Welfare of Japan.

REFERENCES

Berger J 1969 IgA glomerular deposits in renal disease. Transplant Proc *1:* 939

Border WA, Okuda S, Languino LR, Ruoslahti E 1990 Transforming growth factor-β regulates production of proteoglycans by mesangial cells. Kidney Int *37:* 689

Boswell JM, Yui MA, Burt DW, Kelley VE 1988 Increased tumor necrosis factor and IL-1 β gene expression in the kidneys of mice with lupus nephritis. J Immunol *141:* 3050

Boswell JM, Yui MA, Endres S, Burt SW, Kelley VE 1988 Novel and enhanced Il-1 gene expression in autoimmune mice with lupus. J Immunol *141:* 118

Brennan DC, Yui MA, Wuthrich RP, Kelley VE 1989 Tumor necrosis factor and Il-1 in New Zealand Black/White mice. J Immunol *143:* 3470

Clarkson AR, Seymour AE, Thompnson AJ, Haynes WD, Chan YL, Jackson B 1977 IgA nephropathy: a syndrome of uniform morphology, diverse clinical features, and uncertain prognosis. Clin Nephrol *8:* 459

Dohi K, Nakamoto Y, Ishikawa H 1987 Mesangial proliferative glomerulonephritis. Natural history and effects of Dextran sulfate. Jpn J Med *26:* 50

Horii Y, Muraguchi A, Iwano M, Matsuda T, Hirayama H, Fujii Y, Dohi K, Ishikawa H, Ohmoto Y, Yoshizaki K, Hirano T, Kishimoto T 1989 Involvement of interleukin 6 in mesangial proliferative glomerulonephritis. J Immunol *143:* 3949

Jacob CO, McDevitt HO 1988 Tumor necrosis factor-α in murine autoimmune lupus nephritis. Nature *331:* 356

Kincaid-Smith P, Nicholls K 1983 Mesangial IgA nephropathy. Am J Kid Dis *3:* 90

Kusumoto Y, Takebayashi S, Taguchi T, Harada T, Naito S 1987 Long-term prognosis and prognostic indices of IgA nephrophathy in juvenile and in adult Japanese. Clin Nephrol *28:* 118

Lovett DH, Ryan JL, Sterzel RB 1983 Stimulation of rat mesangial cell proliferation by macrophage interleukin 1. J Immunol *131:* 2830

Lovett DH, Szamel M, Ryan JL, Sterzel RB, Gemsa D, Resch K 1986 Interleukin 1 and the glomerular mesangium. I. Purification and characterization of a mesangial cell-derived autogrowth factor. J Immunol *136:* 3700

Lovett DH, Sterzel RB 1986 Cell culture approaches to the analysis of glomerular inflammation. Kidney Int 30: 246

MacCarthy EP, Hsu A, Ooi YM, Ooi BS 1985 Modulation of mouse mesangial cell proliferation by macrophage products. Immunology *56:* 695

Matsuda T, Hirano T, Kishimoto T 1988 Establishment of an interleukin 6 (IL-6)/B cell stimulatory factor 2 (BSF-2)-dependent cell line and preparation of anti-IL-6/BSF-2 monoclonal antidodies. Eur J Immunol *18:* 951

Melcion C, Lachman L, Killen PD, Morel-Maroger L, Striker GE 1982 Mesangial cells, effect of monocyte products on proliferation and matrix synthesis. Transplant proc *14:* 559

Pirani CL, Salinas-Madrigal L 1968 Evaluation of percutaneous renal biopsy. Pathol A *3:* 249

Sinniah R, Javier AR, Ku G 1981 The pathology of mesangial IgA nephritis with clinical correlation. Histopathology *5:* 469

Sterzel, B, Lovett DH, Foellmer HG, Perfetto M, Biemesderfer D, Kashgarian M 1986 Mesangial cell hillocks: nodular foci of exaggerated growth of cells and matrix in prolonged culture. Am J Pathol *125:* 130

Striker GE, Striker LJ 1985 Biology of disease. Glomerular cell culture. Lab Invest *53:* 123

Suematsu S, Matsuda T, Aozasa K, Akira S, Nakano N, Ohno S, Miyazaki J, Yamamura K, Hirano T, Kishimoto T 1989 IgG1 plasmacytosis in interleukin 6 transgenic mice. Proc Natl Acad Sci USA *86:* 7547

Tomosugi NI, Cashman SJ, Hay H, Pusey CD, Evans DJ, Shaw A, Rees AJ 1989 Modulation of antibody-mediated glomerular injury in vivo by bacterial lipopolysaccharide, tumor necrosis factor, and IL-1. J Immunol *142:*3083

Tranqui I, Duperray A, Chenais F, Alix JL, Cordonnier D 1985 Influence of human platelet factors on the proliferation of rat mesangial glomerular cells. Tromb Res *38:* 245

Woo KT, Edmondson RPF, Wu AYT, Chiagn GSC, Pwee HS, Lim CH 1986 The natural history of IgA neprhitis in Singapore. Clin Neprhol *25:* 15

Clinical Nephrology, Vol. 35 No. 1 – 1991 (6–9)

Resolution of cirrhotic glomerulonephritis following successful liver transplantation

N. Ghabra[1], B. Piraino[1], A. Greenberg[1] and B. Banner[2]

[1]*Renal-Electrolyte Division, Department of Medicine and* [2]*Department of Pathology, University of Pittsburgh, School of Medicine, Pittsburgh, PA, USA*

Abstract. A 38-year-old man with liver failure due to Laennec's cirrhosis developed nephrotic range proteinuria and hematuria. Renal biopsy showed membranoproliferative glomerulonephritis with 2+ staining for IgA and complement consistent with cirrhotic glomerulonephritis. After orthotopic liver transplantation, proteinuria and hematuria rapidly resolved. This case indicates that glomerulonephritis associated with cirrhosis may be successfully treated with hepatic transplantation. Whether the improvement in glomerular abnormalities resulted from immunosuppression therapy or from restoration of normal hepatic function is unknown.

Key words: glomerulonephritis – cirrhosis – liver transplantation – IgA

Glomerulonephritis is a well described complication of cirrhosis associated with hepatitis B surface antigen or alcohol excess [Baxter 1946, Fisher 1959, Sakagushi 1968, Nochy 1976, Morzycka 1979, Takeda 1988, Callard 1975]. Its pathogenesis is not well understood, but the frequent presence of immunoglobulin, particularly IgA, in the glomeruli provides evidence for an immunological basis [Callard 1975, Newell 1987]. Cirrhotic glomerulonephritis is usually asymptomatic [Nochy 1984]. However, it can be associated with significant proteinuria or hematuria and, on occasion, renal failure [Nochy 1976]. Little is known about the prognosis of cirrhotic glomerulonephritis, as the patient's liver disease typically overshadows the renal disease. The patient presented in this report had biopsy proven glomerulonephritis associated with end-stage liver disease. Proteinuria and hematuria resolved following successful orthotopic liver transplant.

Case report

A 38-year-old man with anasarca was admitted to Presbyterian Unversity Hospital on July 24, 1988 for evaluation for possible liver transplantation. He had been a heavy alcohol abuser for more than 12 years. Portal hypertension was first diagnosed in 1972 when pancytopenia in association with splenomegaly and gastroesophageal varices were noted. A splenectomy and splenorenal shunt were performed. Subsequently, the patient required numerous admissions for treatment of anasarca and hepatic encephalopathy. In 1985 proteinuria was detected and quantitated at 0.5 g/d. There was a history of hepatitis A at age 12 years. The patient had received blood transfusions in 1983. There was no history of intravenous drug use. Medications at the time of admission were furosemide, spironolactone, potassium chloride, folic acid, and oral neomycin.

The blood pressure was 140/86. Spider angiomata, gynecomastia, a right pleural effusion, ascites, hepatomegaly, 4+ edema of the lower extremities and asterixis were present.

Laboratory data are shown in Table 1. The serum ammonia level was 103 μmol/l. A urinalysis disclosed 100 mg/dl protein, moderate blood, too numerous to count RBCs and WBCs and occasional red blood cell casts. The C3 was 51 mg/dl and the C4 6 mg/dl. Hepatitis B surface antigen and antibody levels were negative. The serum protein electrophoresis showed decreased total protein and albumin, a polyclonal gammopathy, and immune complexes. Urine protein electrophoresis was consistent with a glomerular pattern. The IgG level was 1,570 mg/dl, the IgA level 965 mg/dl, and the IgM level 155 mg/dl. An ultrasound of the kidneys showed the right kidney to be 13 cm and the left kidney 12.9 cm in length.

The patient was treated with infusions of salt poor albumin with simultaneous administration of

Received September 13, 1990; in revised form October 31, 1990.

Reprint requests to Dr. B. Piraino, 11431 Presbyterian University Hospital, Pittsburgh, PA 15213, USA.

Table 1 Laboratory results before and after liver transplantation

	Pre-transplant	11 d post-transplant	18 mo post-transplant
BUN, mg/dl	9	20	26
creatinine, mg/dl	0.6	1.0	1.5
alkaline phosphatase, IU/l	173	69	39
SGOT, IU/l	250	38	24
SGPT, IU/l	93	23	24
bilirubin, total, mg/dl	0.4	1.5	1.2
albumin, g/dl	<1.0		4.2
prothrombin time, s	15.9	12.0	12.0
urinary protein, g/24 h	4.3	0.16*	0.20
creatinine clearance, ml/min	79	103*	62

* done 6 d post-transplant, serum creatinine 0.9 mg/dl

furosemide, vitamin K, and lactulose. His weight fell 10 kg and his serum albumin rose to 2.4 mg/dl. He was discharged, but readmitted 10 days later with encephalopathy, having discontinued his lactulose the previous week. The ammonia level was 135 µmol/l. Lactulose was reinstituted. Urinalysis again showed an active sediment. An open right renal biopsy was done after administration of fresh frozen plasma to correct the coagulopathy.

The patient underwent orthotopic liver transplantation 9 days later which had immediate excellent function. As initial immunosuppressive therapy he received 240 mg methylprednisolone and 5 mg/kg cyclosporine by intravenous infusion. The day following, his urine was dipstick negative for both blood and protein.

Eighteen months after the transplant his urinalysis was unremarkable, without blood or protein by dipstick, and no cellular elements or casts on microscopic examination. His liver function tests were normal (Table 1). His immunosuppressive medications were prednisone, 15 mg each day, and cyclosporine, 150 mg twice a day.

Histology

The wedge biopsy of the kidney showed membranoproliferative glomerulonephritis consistent with chronic liver disease. Over fifty glomeruli were present, and only one was sclerotic. The others all exhibited expansion of the mesangium, which appeared fibrillar on the PAS stain (Figure 1). Capillary walls were thickened, and tram tracks and reduplicated basement membrane were apparent on the silver stain (Figure 2). Mesangial cellularity was mildly increased. There were no segmental lesions or crescents and no significant interstitial fibrosis. Arteriolar sclerosis was minimal. Over forty glomeruli were present in the section taken for immunofluorescence. There was 2+ IgM, IgA, C1Q, and C3, 1+ IgG, and trace properdin in mesangium and around the capillary loops. Ultrastructurally, there was expansion of the mesangium by increased matrix, cell processes, and deposits (Figure 3). The capillary walls were irregularly thickened by subendothelial deposits often mixed mesangial cell processes and reduplicated basement membrane.

The native liver removed at the time of the transplant showed cirrhosis. Regenerative nodules were surrounded by bands of fibrosis containing a sparse inflammatory infiltrate indicative of minimal activity. There were no morphologic indicators as to etiology, except for diffuse steatosis and Mallory's hyaline consistent with the history of alcohol abuse.

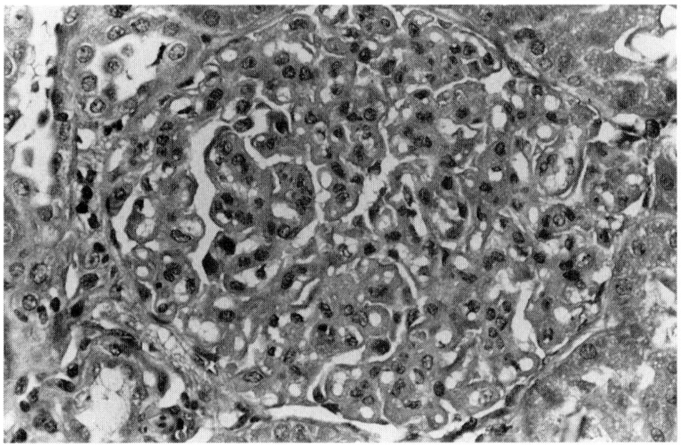

Fig. 1 Glomerulus showing measangial expansion and mild hypercellularity (HE × 100)

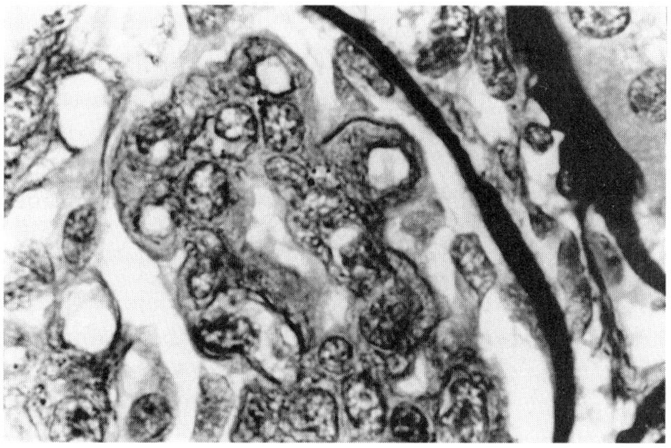

Fig. 2 Portion of a glomerulus showing tram tracks in several capillary loops (Jones × 400)

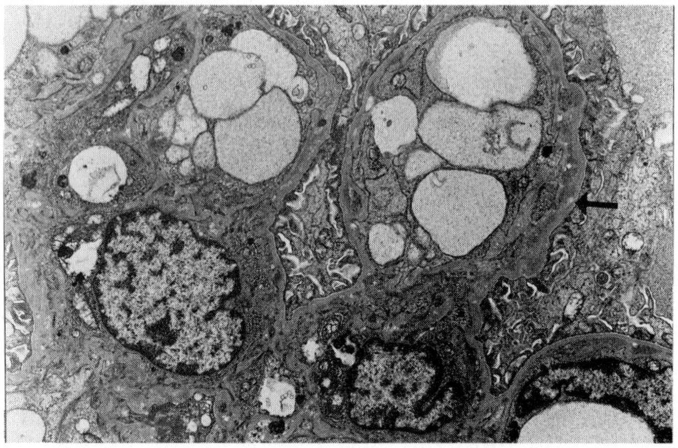

Fig. 3 Electron micrograph showing two capillaries and mesangium. There is reduplication of basement membrane around both capillary loops, with scattered small trapped electron dense deposits. Mesangial interposition is present (arrow). Capillary lumens are filled with swollen cell processes (× 10,400)

Discussion

Although sodium and fluid retention, electrolyte abnormalities and hepatorenal syndrome are the most common and conspicuous effects of hepatic dysfunction on the kidneys, cirrhosis-associated glomerular abnormalities have been noted for more than 40 years [Baxter 1946, Horn 1942]. The reported incidence of glomerular abnormalities in cirrhotic patients varies from 25 to 100% [Fisher 1959, Sakagushi 1968, Takeda 1988]. Although early studies noted a variety of lesions, more recent studies note principally membranoproliferative or mesangial proliferative glomerulonephritis with mesangial expansion or sclerosis. Mesangial IgA deposition is noted in most [Masugi 1979, Newell 1987], but not all cases [Montoliu 1986]. IgM, IgG, and C3 may also be present, but they tend to occur with lesser frequency [Nochy 1976, Newell 1987]. Electron microscopy may show mesangial lucencies with or without deposits as well as the mesangial cell interposition characteristic of membranoproliferative glomerulonephritis [Callard 1975, Nochy 1984]. The case presented here is consistent with these previous descriptions, in that the renal biopsy demonstrated mesangial expansion and hypercellularity, reduplication of the basement membrane and immunofluorescence positive for IgA, IgM, and C3.

Most cases of cirrhotic glomerulonephritis are clinically silent [Nochy 1984]. In a combined biopsy and autopsy series, eighty-nine of 202 (44%) patients with chronic liver disease had overt signs of glomerular disease [Nochy 1984]. Patients with cirrhotic glomerulonephritis may have microscopic or macroscopic hematuria, proteinuria of varying degree, and renal failure [Fisher 1959, Nochy 1976, Newell 1987, Nochy 1984]. Nephrotic syndrome has been noted in up to 14% of patients with cirrhosis who had a renal biopsy performed [Eknoyan 1983]. However, in a large series of consecutive patients with cirrhosis, only 1.6% were observed to have nephrotic range proteinuria [Nakamoto 1981]. Thus, the present patient, who had hematuria and nephrotic range proteinuria, represents the more severe end of the spectrum seen in cirrhotic patients.

The pathogenesis of cirrhotic glomerulonephritis is poorly understood. The finding of IgA-containing immune complexes in the kidney and serum, as in our patient, is consistent with an immune mediated glomerulonephritis. IgA in the glomeruli of cirrhotic patients with glomerulonephritis is predominantly of subclass IgA2 [Andre 1980]. The presence of this subclass, which is produced by plasma cells in respiratory or digestive endothelium, is evidence for a gastrointestinal source. Since the Kupffer cells clear immune complexes of dietary origin from the portal circulation, liver dysfunction or portacaval shunting may lead to circulating immune complexes [Rifai 1984, Sinniah 1984]. Their subsequent deposition in the kidney may then result in glomerular damage [Andre 1980, Woodroffe 1981].

Treatment for cirrhotic glomerulonephritis has not been established. In one preliminary report, prednisolone was used with success [Genin 1984]. Corticosteroid treatment of chronic active hepatitis associated with hematuria resulted in resolution of both the liver and kidney disease in one case [Case records 1981]. In another patient with chronic active hepatitis, treatment with alpha interferon led to an improvement in liver histology and a decrease in proteinuria [Lisker-Melman 1989]. The present report is the first description of a patient with cirrhosis and associated glomerulonephritis successfully treated for both conditions with orthotopic liver transplantation. Here, the response was striking with an almost immediate disappearance of proteinuria and hematuria. As liver transplantation was accompanied by administration of methylprednisolone and cyclosporine, it is impossible to determine whether the improvement was due to restoration of hepatic function or to immunosuppression. Modest renal dysfunction 18 months after the transplant was most likely due to cyclosporine nephrotoxicity. Although repeat renal biopsy was not performed, the absence of hematuria and proteinuria and the disappearance of the cellular casts suggest that the glomerular lesion remitted. Thus, we conclude that glomerulonephritis associated with cirrhosis is not a contraindication to liver transplantation. Indeed, hepatic transplantation may well provide a means of treatment for severe and progressive cases.

Acknowledgement

We appreciate the assistance of Dr. Francis C. Imbarrato in providing follow-up data on the patient.

REFERENCES

Andre C, Berthoux FC, Andre F, Gillon J, Genin C, Sabatier JC 1980 Prevalence of IgA2 deposits in IgA nephropathies. N Engl J Med *303:* 1343–1346

Baxter JH, Ashworth CT Renal lesions in portal cirrhosis. Arch Path *41:* 476–477

Callard P, Feldmann G, Prandi D, Belair MF, Mandet C, Weiss Y, Druet P, Benhamou JP, Bariety J 1975 Immune complex type glomerulonephritis in cirrhosis of liver. Am J Path *80:* 329–340

Case Records of Masachusetts General Hospital (Case 7–1983) 1983 N Engl J Med *308:* 382–389

Eknoyan G 1983 Glomerular abnormalities in liver disease. In: *Epstein M* (ed) The kidney in liver disease. Elsevier, NY, pp 119–145

Fisher ER, Hellstrom HR 1959 The membranous and proliferative glomerulonephritis of hepatic cirrhosis. Am J Clin Path *32:* 48–55

Genin C, Sabatier JC, Laurent B, Laurent P, Gonthier R, Berthoy F 1984 The membranoproliferative glomerulonephritis associated with cirrhosis: good evaluation after steroids and plasma exchange therapy (abstract). Kidney Int *26:* 497

Horn RC Jr, Smetana H 1942 Intercapillary glomerulosclerosis. Am J Path *18:* 93–100

Lisker-Melman M, Webb D, Di Bisceglie AM, Kassianides C, Martin P, Rustgi V, Waggoner JG, Park V, Hoofnagle JH 1989 Glomerulonephritis caused by chronic hepatitis B Virus infection: treatment with recombinant human alpha-interferon. Ann Intern Med *111:* 479–483

Masugi Y, Ishizaki M, Fukuda Y, Sano J, Kogoshi T, Maekawa A, Sugisaki Y 1979 Immunopathologic studies of renal glomerular change in liver cirrhosis with special reference to its pathogenesis. Acta Path Jap *29 (4):* 571–583

Montoliu J, Darnell A, Torras A, Revert L 1986 Glomerular disease in cirrhosis of the liver: low frequency IgA deposits. Am J Nephrol *6:* 199–205

Morzycka M, Slusarczk J 1979 Kidney glomerular pathology in various forms of acute and chronic hepatitis 1979. Arch Path Lab Med *103:* 38–41

Nakamoto Y, Iida H, Kobayashi K, Dohi K, Kida H, Hattori N, Takeuchi J 1981 Hepatic glomerulonephritis: characteristics of hepatic IgA glomerulonephritis as the major part. Virchows Arch (Path Anat) *392:* 45–54

Newell GC 1987 Cirrhotic glomerulonephritis: incidence, morphology, clinical features, and pathogenesis. Am J Kid Dis *9:* 183–190

Nochy D, Callard P, Bellon B, Bariety J, Druet P 1976 Association of overt glomerulonephritis and liver disease: a study of 34 patients. Clin Neph *6:* 422–427

Nochy D, Druet P, Bariety J 1984 IgA nephropathy in chronic liver disease. Contr Nephrol *40:* 268–275

Rifai A, Mannik M 1984 Clearance of circulating IgA immune complexes is mediated by a specific receptor on Kupffer cells in mice. J Exp Med *160:* 125–137

Sakagushi N, 1968 Hepatic glomerulosclerosis – light microscopic study of autopsy cases. Acta Path J *18:* 407–415

Sinniah R 1984 Heterogeneous IgA glomerulonephropathy in liver cirrhosis. Histopathology *18:* 947–962

Takeda S, Kida H, Katagiri M, Yokoyama H, Abe T, Hattori N 1988 Characteristics of glomerular lesions in hepatitis B virus infection. Am J Kid Dis *11:* 57–62

Woodroffe AJ 1981 IgA, glomerulonephritis and liver disease. Aust NZ J Med *11:* 109–111

Clinical Nephrology, Vol. 35 No. 1 – 1991 (10–16)

Changes in the postenteropathic form of the hemolytic uremic syndrome in children

N. A. G. Coad[1], T. Marshall[2], B. Rowe[3] and C. M. Taylor[1]

[1] *Department of Nephrology, The Children's Hospital, Birmingham B16 8ET, UK*
[2] *Department of Social Medicine, The Medical School, Birmingham B15, UK*
[3] *Division of Enteric Pathogens, Public Health Laboratory, Colindale, London, UK*

Abstract. An analysis was made of clinical and laboratory findings in children with the diarrheal form of the hemolytic uremic syndrome (HUS) treated at The Children's Hospital, Birmingham between 1970 und 1987. From 1982 the rate of referral increased, the prodromal illness more often consisted of bloody diarrhea, and the mean age at presentation doubled from 2 to 4 years. For patients with a good outcome there was an excess of males in the period 1970–81, and females in the period 1982–87. Moreover, in the years 1982–87 the disorder was distinguished from that of the earlier time by a positive correlation between adverse outcome and both neutrophil leukocytosis and a higher hemoglobin concentration at presentation. Prognostic scores obtained by logistic regression analysis were specific for each period. From July 1983 stool samples were analyzed for verocytotoxin-producing *Escherichia coli* (VTEC) and neutralizable verotoxin. Positive results were obtained in 39% of cases. The nature of HUS has changed and the new form of the disorder is associated with VTEC infection.

Key words: hemolytic uremic syndrome – neutrophil count – prognosis – verocytotoxin-producing *Escherichiae coli*

Introduction

The hemolytic uremic syndrome (HUS) consists of a heterogeneous group of disorders which in clinical practice is usefully divided into diarrhea-associated and non-prodromal types. The former is common and the enteropathic prodrome points to an infective cause. By contrast, in the latter group a relapsing course and sometimes familial nature of the disease suggests that intrinsic biological defects underlie the rarer and more serious type [Levin and Barratt 1984]. Some authors have attempted to take this classification further and subdivide the diarrhea-associated "extrinsic" group [Drummond 1985].

In the report of an outbreak of HUS in the West Midlands it was suggested that a change had occurred in the nature of the postenteropathic form [Taylor et al. 1986]. To clarify this we have reviewed clinical and laboratory data from cases of HUS treated at the Children's Hospital, Birmingham from 1970 to 1987.

Received September 21, 1989; in revised form June 13, 1990.
Reprint requests to Dr. C. M. Taylor.

Patients and methods

All children with HUS who presented between January 1970 and December 1987 were reviewed. The diagnostic criteria of acute renal impairment and microangiopathic hemolytic anemia in the absence of other causes, particularly septicemia were met in all patients.

The hemoglobin, total white cell count, differential and platelet counts were obtained for the day of presentation and daily when available for the next 14 days. Fecal specimens were obtained as soon as possible and cultured for *Salmonella, Shigella* and *Campylobacter* species. From July 1983 fecal samples were sent to the Division of Enteric Pathogens, Central Public Health Laboratory where DNA probes were used to detect verocytotoxin-producing *Escherichia coli* (VTEC), which were isolated by culture and serotyped. Stool samples were further examined for the presence of neutralizable fecal verocytotoxin (VT).

Renal outcome was determined on latest follow up, which in all cases was >12 months from onset using the following scheme: Good outcome patients had normal blood pressure for age, and a normal plasma creatinine concentration for body height (height : creatinine ratio greater than 2 cm/μmol/l). Mild isolated proteinuria was permitted up to an arbitrary limit of 50 mg protein/mmol creatinine on an early morning urine sample; normal range <20 mg/mmol [Elises et al. 1988].

Poor outcome patients were those with hypertension, glomerular filtration rate (GFR) <75 ml/min/1.73 m^2 body surface area (as estimated from the formula: height(cm)/plasma creatinine (μmol/l) × 40, end-stage renal failure or death.

Statistical methods

Change in the annual admissions of patients with HUS was analyzed using the Cumulative Sum (Cusum) technique [Chaput de Saintonge and Vere 1974] and Wilcoxon's Rank Sum test. The Cusum technique is applied to sequential data to detect movement away from a previously observed average and the timing of such an event. Differences between the good and poor outcome groups were tested using the t-test for numerical variables and χ^2 with Yate's correction for categorical variables. Factors at presentation predictive for a good or poor outcome were explored by logistic regression analysis using a GLIM statistical package on an Apricot Xen-i microcomputer. By this means for any chosen variable (V), a coefficient (C) is derived and the probability (P) of a poor outcome is given by the equation:

$$1n(P/1 - P) = constant + (V^1C^1) + (V^2C^2) + (V^3C^3)... etc$$

If the variables corresponding to any individual are inserted into this equation the result (x) is converted to the probability of a poor outcome (P) by calculating $e^x/e^x + 1$. For patients predicted to have a poor outcome P approaches 1, whereas for those with a good prognosis P approaches zero.

Results

Seventy-nine children were referred with HUS of whom 5 were excluded; 4 non-enteropathic or familial cases and one child who returned from abroad in the recovery phase of the illness. This left 33 boys and 41 girls with postenteropathic HUS whose mean age at onset was 3.5 years (range 4 months to 13 years). The number of patients referred in each year is shown in Figure 1. Cusum analysis showed that an abrupt increase in referrals occurred between 1981 and 1982, and the data were therefore divided at this point for further analysis. Nineteen patients presented between 1970 and 1981 compared to 55 in the period 1982–87, a significant increase in the later period (Wilcoxon's

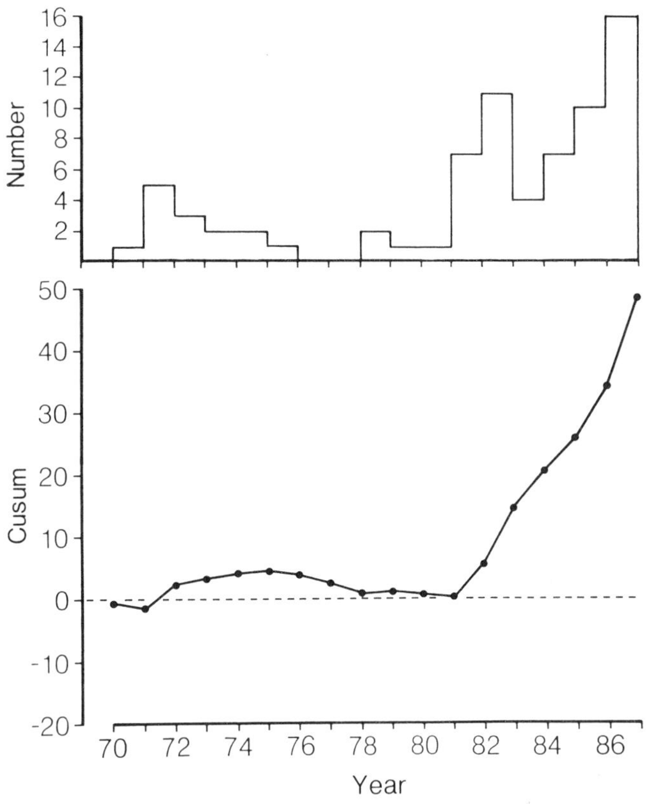

Fig. 1 Referrals and Cusum analysis by year

Rank Sum test p <0.01). Further analysis showed significant differences between these periods with regard to age, prodromal features, clinical complications, and outcome (Table 1).

The 1970–81 group was significantly younger (mean age ± SEM 23.8 ± 6.4 months) than the 1982–87 group (mean age ± SEM 48.3 ± 5.1 months; t = 2.47 p <0.02). Although no significant difference in sex ratio was observed between the two periods, unvariate analysis showed that amongst good outcome patients there was an excess of males in the period 1970–81 (males 8, females 2), whereas in the years 1982–87 there was an excess of females (males 16, females 28; χ^2 4.6, p <0.05). In the earlier period patients presented at a steady rate throughout the seasons. However from 1982 more cases presented in the months April–September with a peak in July.

From 1982 diarrhea was macroscopically bloody in a higher proportion of cases (p <0.02), but there was no significant change in either the duration of diarrhea or the incidence of prodromal vomiting, abdominal pain or respiratory symptoms. As in the 1970–81 period there was no correlation between the duration of prodrome and outcome. In the later period three patients had major abdominal complications (intussusception 1 and intestinal perforation 2),

Table 1 Clinical features

	1970–81	1982–87	p
Number	19	55	<0.001
Mean age (months)	23.8	48.3	<0.02
Sex (M/F)	11/8	22/33	NS
Season (April–September)	10 (53%)	39 (71%)	NS
Prodromal features			
Bloody diarrhoea	7 (37%)	39 (71%)	<0.02
Vomiting	19 (100%)	41 (74%)	NS
Abdominal pain	1 (5%)	13 (24%)	NS
Seizures	5 (26%)	10 (18%)	NS
Hypertension	9 (47%)	14 (25%)	NS
Dialysis	17 (89%)	27 (49%)	<0.01
Extrarenal manifestations			
Seizures	11 (58%)	11 (20%)	<0.01
Major CNS complications	6 (32%)	5 (9%)	<0.05
Cardiac	2	1	NS
Abdominal surgical complication	0	3	NS

two developed insulin dependent diabetes mellitus and a further girl developed cardiomyopathy associated with congestive cardiac failure 8 weeks after the onset of her illness.

Convulsions were the most frequent extra-renal manifestation and were usually related to hyponatremia. They were significantly more common in the earlier period ($p < 0.01$) as were major CNS manifestations such as hemiplegia and coma when assessed together ($p < 0.05$). However, neither seizures nor other neurological complications were predictive of renal outcome. Hypertension was noted in 9 (47%) children from 1970–81 and 14 (25%) from 1982–87 (not significant). No correlation was found between hypertension, identified at presentation or developing during the acute phase of the illness, and outcome in either period.

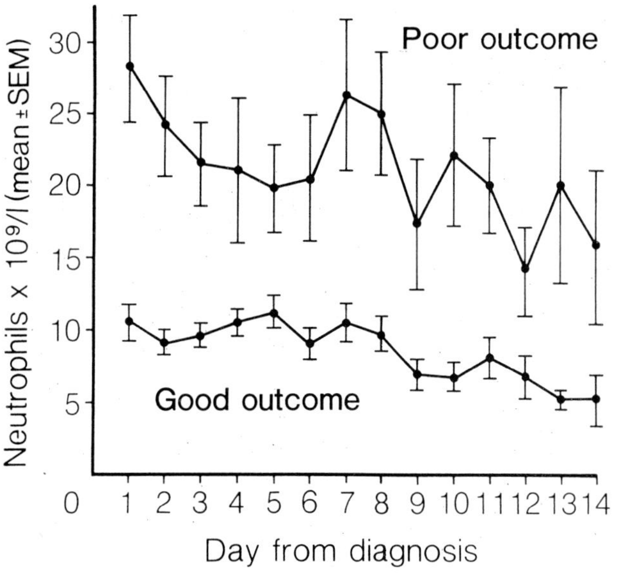

Fig. 2 Neutrophil count from the day of diagnosis: patients from 1982–87

Peritoneal dialysis was performed in 17 (89%) of the 1970–81, and 27 (49%) of the 1982–87 patients ($p < 0.01$). There was a correlation between dialysis of more than 14 days duration and poor prognosis (dialysis >14 days; good outcome 4 of 54, poor outcome 11 of 16 patients; χ^2 24.5, $p < 0.001$). This did not achieve significance within the earlier period alone where numbers were small.

Outcome

No child in this series changed outcome group between 1 year from onset, the least follow-up period, and their latest assessment. Good renal outcome occurred in 10 (53%) of the 19 children from 1970–81 compared to 44 (80%) of the later period ($p < 0.05$). Urinary protein excretion was normal in all but four, three from 1970–81 and one from 1982–87, who had mild isolated proteinuria (early morning urine protein/creatinine 20–50 mg/mmol).

A poor outcome occurred in 9 of the 19 children from 1970–81. Five died, all but one in the acute phase of the illness, one was successfully transplanted, two have stable chronic renal failure (GFR 55 ml/min/1.73 m^2 in each) and a further child has hypertension and persistent heavy proteinuria. Between 1982–87 11 children (20%) had a poor outcome. Four died, 2 in the acute phase, three are in end-stage renal failure and four have impaired renal function (GFR 33–60 ml/min/1.73 m^2) with hypertension.

Laboratory investigations

Since 1983 acute stool samples from 38 patients were examined for verocytotoxin-producing *E. coli* (VTEC) and neutralizable free verotoxin (VT). VTEC were detected in 13 cases (serotypes 0157 11 cases, 0163 and 0165 one case each) and neutralizable fecal VT in the absence of VTEC in a further two, indicating infection in 39% of recent patients. VTEC or VT was found in 2 of 9 poor outcome and 13 of 29 good outcome patients (not significant). In addition *Campylobacter* was found in the stools of one patient and an *Adenovirus* in another, neither of whom had laboratory evidence of VTEC infection.

Table 2 Laboratory investigations at presentation (mean ± SEM)

	Good outcome	Poor outcome	p
1970–81			
Hb (g/dl)	6.4 ± 1.1	7.8 ± 0.7	NS
WCC (× 10^9/l)	16.0 ± 1.9	17.0 ± 2.5	NS
Neutrophils	9.1 ± 1.5	12.1 ± 2.4	NS
Lymphocytes	6.9 ± 1.2	6.4 ± 1.6	NS
Platelets	50.5 ± 8.2	91.5 ± 20.4	NS
1982–87			
Hb (g/dl)	7.8 ± 0.3	10.9 ± 0.9	<0.001
WCC (× 10^9/l)	17.9 ± 1.4	31.5 ± 3.4	<0.001
Neutrophils	10.6 ± 1.0	24.9 ± 2.5	<0.001
Lymphocytes	5.5 ± 0.8	5.4 ± 1.1	NS
Monocytes	1.0 ± 0.2	1.8 ± 0.2	<0.01
Platelets	88.8 ± 13.9	133 ± 33.7	NS

Table 3 Logistic regression analysis for the probability of a poor outcome

Variable	Coefficient	SE
1970–81		
Constant	− 70.73	301.1
Platelet count (10^9/l)	+ 2.374	1.76
Sex (male = 1, female = 0)	−141.9	334.7
Season (Apr–Sep = 1, Oct–Mar = 0)	− 65.83	297.4
1982–87		
Constant	− 10.86	3.88
Hemoglobin (g/dl)	+ 0.455	0.248
Neutrophils (10^9/l)	+ 0.326	0.126
Lymphocytes (10^9/l)	− 0.185	0.159
Sex (male = 1, female = 0)	+ 1.469	1.323

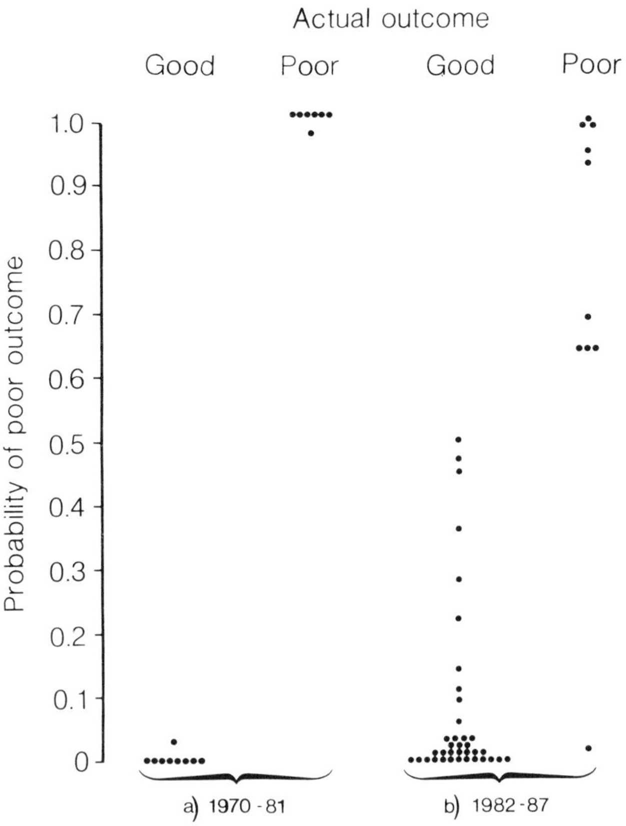

Fig. 3 Actual and predicted outcome: (a) 1970–81, (b) 1982–87

Table 2 shows the hematological parameters at diagnosis and their relationship to outcome within each time period. For 1970–81 there was no significant difference between outcome groups for any of these observations. However, for 1982–7 the poor outcome patients had significantly higher hemoglobin concentrations, total white cell, neutrophil and monocyte counts compared to those with good outcome, the difference in total white count being made up primarily of the neutrophil component. Figure 2 shows that the difference in mean neutrophil count was maintained throughout the first 2 weeks, but was greatest at the time of diagnosis. Using the initial neutrophil count alone the best separation of outcome groups was obtained with a cut off value of 20 × 10^9/l. Ninety-three percent of patients with a neutrophil count <20 × 10^9/l had a good outcome compared with 33% of those with a neutrophil count ≥20 × 10^9/l ($p < 0.001$).

Prognostic variables at presentation

Following the univariate analysis above, the prognostic value of the following variables was analyzed by logistic regression: age, sex, season, hemoglobin, total white cell, lymphocyte, neutrophil and platelet counts. For the 1970–81 period complete data sets, which are essential for this analysis, were available in 16 cases, 9 good and 7 poor outcome. Total white cell, neutrophil and lymphocyte counts contributed nothing to the discrimination between outcome groups, the most important factor being the platelet count. The best equation was produced by combining the variables platelet count, sex and season; a high platelet count, female sex and winter presentation contributed to an adverse outcome (Table 3). The large standard errors, a consequence of convergence within the GLIM package, arise because of the small number of observations and high inter-correlations between the predictor variables and outcome in this period. Nevertheless, there was excellent discrimination between good and poor outcome groups (Figure 3a).

For the 1982–87 patients complete data were available on 37 good and 10 bad outcome cases. Analysis showed that platelet count, the strongest discriminating factor for pre-1982 cases, made no contribution and an entirely different equation was derived. The neutrophil count, which had been of no value in the 1970–81 cases, became the most important variable, half the variance of outcome being explained by this factor alone. Hemoglobin also contributed, higher values indicating a worse outcome. The addition of lymphocyte count improved the discrimination a little, but season contributed nothing. In contrast to the earlier period male sex was associated with a poorer outcome. The predictive equation produced a clear separation of actual outcome categories (Figure 3b), with the exception of one boy who was incorrectly predicted to do well. He made a good initial recovery and was discharged from hospital with near normal renal function. Nine months later he developed acute renal failure without evidence of microangiopathy and died; the nature of the subsequent illness is not known.

Discussion

This retrospective analysis indicates that the nature of postenteropathic HUS has changed. The recent form of the disease appears to be more common, the prodrome more often consists of a bloody diarrhea, the age at onset is greater and girls tend to have better outcome. It is further distinguished by a strongly positive correlation between neutrophilia and poor outcome.

Attempts to identify the causes of HUS have focused on investigation of the prodromal enteropathy. A variety of pathogens have been reported in this context but until recently proof of a causal relationship was often lacking [Drummond 1985]. The association with VTEC was first reported by Karmali et al. in 1983 and was later estimated to pertain in 75% of cases [Karmali et al. 1985]. In our patients studied from the latter part of 1983 onwards either VTEC or VT were identified in the feces of 39% of patients. However excretion of VTEC may be brief so that this figure may be an under estimate of the true association [Wells et al. 1983, Milford et al. 1990], and precludes an analysis between VTEC infection and prognosis in our data. Without similar bacteriological studies on patients from the earlier period, the change in disease pattern cannot be attributed with certainty to the arrival of VTEC. Nevertheless the doubling of the percentage of HUS patients presenting with bloody diarrhea after 1982 is consistent with an increase of infection by this organism. It is noteworthy that extensive retrospective analyses of fecal *E. coli* stored prior to the 1980s have, with rare exceptions, failed to identify verotoxin producing organisms [Wells et al. 1985, Day et al. 1983] whereas VTEC 0157/H7 is now frequently associated with hemorrhagic colitis in man [Smith et al. 1987].

An increased admission rate of less severely affected cases is weak evidence of a change in etiology and may simply imply a greater awareness and referral by regional pediatricians, especially after the publicity surrounding the Wolverhampton outbreak of July 1983 [Taylor et al. 1986]. However, the Cusum analysis demonstrated an abrupt increase before this and for the purposes of further enquiry it was logical to divide the data between 1981 and 1982.

It is widely accepted that part of the improvement in outcome in HUS is due to greater expertise in supportive care, while interventional treatments have not been shown by controlled studies to affect prognosis. A possible exception to the latter is the use of plasma infusion [Loirat et al. 1988], but this multicenter study was criticized for not distinguishing between diarrhea-associated and non-prodromal forms of the syndrome [Cole 1988]. Heparin or thrombolytic agents were frequently used in the 1970s [Stuart et al. 1974], followed in the early 1980s by treatments aimed at correcting a supposed deficiency in prostacyclin, either by the infusion of fresh frozen plasma [Remuzzi et al. 1979] or treatment with vitamin E [Powell et al. 1984]. Typically, acute renal failure is well established by the time the diagnosis of HUS is made, and the brunt of the renal damage has already occurred. Since 1984, therefore, we have used supportive management only, except in the rare patients with cerebro-vascular involvement when prostacyclin infusion was used. We have not adopted a policy of elective early dialysis for HUS. It seems unlikely to us that changes in interventional treatment explain the improved prognosis of later years. Improved supportive care may be relevant, but an alternative explanation is that the better outcome of recent patients reflects a change in etiology.

A stronger argument for a change in the nature of the disease is that clinical and laboratory parameters at presentation exhibit distinctive correlations with outcome at different times. These parameters have the advantage that they are unlikely to have been affected by therapy and are close in time to the infective prodrome. Trompeter et al. [1983] analyzed prognostic variables by logistic regression in patients from the south-east of England between 1969 and 1980. Although a principal finding was that enteropathic and non-prodromal forms of the syndrome behave differently, they observed that young males presenting in the summer months with diarrhea fared better. Our data from the same period supports this. However, their prognostic score did not apply to West Midlands patients in 1982–83 [Taylor et al. 1986] or subsequently. During the 1970s it was widely accepted that older children with HUS had a worse outcome. However, from 1982 onwards the mean age of our patients at diagnosis was twice that of former years and yet the renal outcome improved. Moreover, in the United Kingdom national survey 1985–88 older subjects, especially females >10 years of age, had a more favorable outcome [Milford et al. 1990], a finding in keeping with our data for 1982–87. Our experience, therefore, resembles that of other parts of the United Kingdom. The prognostic indices from the two periods 1970–81 and 1982–87 clearly separated the data from which they derived (Figure 3), but each failed to apply to the other period.

Other authors have explored the relationship between clinical findings and outcome [Loirat et al. 1984, Proesmans and Eeckels 1989]. Unlike them we were unable to find an association between either hypertension or duration of prodrome and adverse renal outcome. However, we do confirm a positive correlation of poor outcome and the severity of renal failure as indicated by the duration of dialysis. Former studies have correlated outcome with clinical and laboratory features which develop or become apparent later in the course of the acute illness. We attempted to circumvent the possibility that these parameters may be influenced by treatment by concentrating on information available at diagnosis.

The association between neutrophilia and poor outcome was first shown by Walters et al. [1989] in British children presenting between 1980 and 1986. Our logistic regression analysis confirmed this for children presenting after 1982 in whom as much as half of the variance of outcome was attributable to the neutrophil count alone at the time of diagnosis. Here there are parallels with *Shigella*-induced HUS in which a leukamoid response is associated with immune complex formation, exposure to endotoxin and poor outcome [Koster et al. 1978]. Moreover, both verotoxins are biologically similar to, and VT 1 probably identical with Shiga toxin [O'Brien and Holmes 1987, Smith and Scotland 1987]. The role of neutrophils and monocytes in the pathogenesis of HUS induced by either VTEC or *Shigella* has yet to be evaluated. However, it is noteworthy that granulocytes have a pivotal role in the Shwartzman reaction in rabbits, which in some respects resembles the human disorder [Bohn and Muller-Berghaus 1976, Butler et al. 1985].

In the later period a small contribution to adverse outcome was made by higher hemoglobin, lower lymphocyte count and male sex. Current understanding of the pathogenesis offers no simple explanation for these findings. The association between higher hemoglobin and poor prognosis may relate to hypovolemia accentuating acute renal failure [Walters et al. 1989], but one would have expected it to apply equally to patients prior to 1982.

The changes in the postenteropathic form of HUS appear to date from 1981–2, since when a strong association between HUS and VTEC has been recognized. A reciprocal deduction is that before this date other unidentified agents were responsible. This change from an earlier VTEC-unrelated to a later VTEC-related type is unlikely to be absolute and clinicians probably still encounter occasional patients with the earlier form of the disease among the now common VTEC-related cases. This heterogeneity within the postenteropathic subgroup of HUS, and the significance of neutrophilia in contemporary cases deserves recognition. We conclude that the change in clinical features reflects altered etiology and has implications for the use of prognostic scores, both for present day clinical decision making and the scientific evaluation of treatment trials.

Acknowledgements

The authors are grateful to their colleagues Professor R. H. R. White and Dr. M. H. Winterborn for permission to report their patients. This study was supported in part by the National Kidney Research Fund and the Renal Research Fund of The Children's Hospital, Birmingham.

REFERENCES

Bohn E, Muller-Berghaus G 1976 The effect of leukocyte and platelet transfusion on the activation of intravascular coagulation by endotoxin in granulocytopenic and thrombocytopenic rabbits. Am J Path *84:* 239–268

Butler T, Hamidur R, Al-Mahmud KA, Islam M, Bardhan P, Kabir I, Rahman MM 1985 An animal model of haemolytic-uraemic syndrome in shigellosis; lipopolysaccharides of *Shigella dysenteriae 1* and *S. flexneri* produce leucocyte-mediated renal cortical necrosis in rabbits. Br J Exp Pathol *66:* 7–15

Chaput de Saintonge DM, Vere DW 1974 Why don't doctors use cusums? Lancet *1:* 120–121

Cole BR 1988 Plasma infusion therapy in hemolytic uremic syndrome: is it warrented? Pediatr Nephrol *2:* 286–287

Day NP, Scotland SM, Cheasty T, Rowe B 1983 Escherichia coli 0157:H7 associated with human infection in the United Kingdom. Lancet *1:* 825

Drummond KN 1985 Hemolytic uremic syndrome – then and now. N Engl J Med *312:* 116–118

Elises JS, Griffiths PD, Hocking MD, Taylor CM, White RHR 1988 Simplified quantification of urinary protein excretion in children. Clin Nephrol *30:* 225–229

Karmali MA, Petric M, Lim C, Flemming PC, Arbus GS, Lior H 1985 The association between idiopathic hemolytic uremic syndrome and infection by verotoxin-producing Escherichia coli. J Infect Dis *151:* 775–782

Karmali MA, Steele BT, Petric M, Lim C 1983 Sporadic cases of haemolytic-uraemic syndrome associated with fecal cytotoxin and cytotoxin-producing Escherichia coli in stools. Lancet *1:* 619–620

Koster F, Levin J, Walker L, Tung KSK, Gilman RH 1978 Hemolytic uremic syndrome after Shigellosis: Relation to endotoxemia and circulating immune complexes. N Engl J Med *298:* 927–933

Levin M, Barratt TM 1984 Hemolytic uremic syndrome. Arch Dis Childh *59:* 397–400

Loirat C, Sonsino E, Varga Moreno A, Pillion G, Mercier JC, Beaufils F, Mathieu H 1984 Hemolytic-uremic syndrome: an analysis of the natural history and prognostic features. Acta Paediatr Scand *73:* 505–514

Loirat C, Sonsino E, Hinglais N, Jais JP, Landais P, Fermanian J 1988 Treatment of the childhood haemolytic uraemic syndrome with plasma. Pediatr Nephrol *2:* 279–285

Milford DV, Taylor CM, Guttridge B, Rowe B, Klearhous H 1990 Haemolytic uraemic syndromes in the British Isles 1985–88: association with verocytotoxin producing Escherichia coli. Part 1: clinical and epidemiological aspects. Arch Dis Childh *65:* 716–721

O'Brien AD, Holmes RK 1987 Shiga and Shiga-like toxins. Microbiological Reviews *51:* 206–220

Powell HR, McCredie, Taylor CM, Burke JR, Walker RG 1984 Vitamin E treatment of haemolytic uraemic syndrome. Arch Dis Childh *59:* 401–404

Proesmans W, Eeckels R 1989 The hemolytic uremic syndromes. Ergeb Inn Med Kinderheilkd *58:* 55–82

Remuzzi G, Misiani R, Marchesi D, Livio M, Mecca G, de Gaetaro C, Donati MB 1979 Treatment of the hemolytic uremic syndrome with plasma. Clin Nephrol *19:* 279–284

Smith HR, Rowe B, Gross RJ, Fry NK, Scotland SM 1987 Haemorrhagic colitis and verocytotoxin-producing Escherichia coli in England and Wales. Lancet *1:* 1062–1065

Smith HR, Scotland SM 1988 Verocytotoxin-producing strains of Escherichia coli. J Med Microbiol *26:* 77–85

Stuart J, Winterborn MH, White RHR 1974 Thrombolytic therapy in haemolytic-uraemic syndrome. Br Med J *2:* 217–221

Taylor CM, White RHR, Winterborn MH, Rowe B 1986 Haemolytic-uraemic syndrome: clinical experience of an outbreak in the West Midlands. Br Med J *292:* 1513–1516

Trompeter RS, Schwartz R, Chantler C, Dillon MJ, Haycock GB, Kay R, Barratt TM 1983 Haemolytic-uraemic syndrome: an analysis of prognostic features. Arch Dis Childh *58:* 101–105

Walters MDS, Matthei U, Kay R, Dillon MJ, Barratt MT 1987 The polymorphonuclear leucocyte count in childhood haemolytic uraemic syndrome. Pediatr Nephrol *3:* 130–134

Wells JG, Davis BR, Wachsmith IK, Riley LW, Remis RS, Sokolow R, Morris GK 1983 Laboratory investigation of hemorrhagic colitis outbreaks associated with a rare Escherichia coli serotype. J Clin Microbiol *18:* 512–520

Clinical Nephrology, Vol. 35 No. 1 – 1991 (17–19)

Xanthogranulomatous pyelonephritis masquerading as empyema thoracis and later presenting as reno-cutaneous fistula

R. Mathur and J. Warren

St. Margaret's Hospital, Epping, Essex CM16 6TN, UK

Abstract. A case of xanthogranulomatous pyelonephritis presenting as empyema thoracis on one occasion and later with a persistent reno-cutaneous fistula.

Key words: xanthogranulomatous pyelonephritis – reno-cutaneous fistula – empyema thoracis

Introduction

Xanthogranulomatous pyelonephritis is a rare disease accounting for 0.6% of all cases of chronic pyelonephritis [Kierce et al. 1985]. Pleural empyema and reno-cutaneous fistula are unusual features of this condition. It should be suspected in any patient who is systemically unwell and has an obstructed infected, non-functioning and enlarged kidney. Should a reno-cutaneous fistula develop in this setting, the diagnosis is practically certain [Braun et al. 1985].

Case report

A 62-year-old woman was admitted with severe pleuritic left lateral chest pain of three weeks' duration. This was accompanied by cough with mucopurulent expectoration and streaky hemoptysis. There was no history of flank pain, dysuria or hematuria.

She had two episodes of left ureteric colic four years ago. An intravenous urography and ultrasound at that time showed multiple left renal calculi with mild hydronephrosis. Her blood urea then was 4.8 mmols/l and creatinine was 67.6 μmols/l. A few months later she spontaneously passed a calculus composed of uric acid and calcium phosphate.

Next year she had an episode of symptomatic urinary tract infection which was treated with antibiotics. There was no history of diabetes mellitus, hypertension or any lipid abnormality.

On examination she had a temperature of 38° C and pulse of 120 per minute. There was a moderate size left pleural effusion. She had mild diffuse abdominal tenderness. The liver was non-palpable and both the flanks were normal.

A chest X-ray confirmed left pleural effusion. Her white cell count was 12.3×10^9/l. A diagnostic left pleural tap aspirated 25 ml of thick pus which grew *Proteus* and *Bacteroides.* Blood and urine cultures were sterile and urinalysis was unhelpful.

She was started on parenteral antibiotics with a diagnosis of pleural empyema. An intercostal tube drained a total of 200 ml pus over the next 2–3 days.

She improved remarkably over the next few days and several subsequent chest X-rays and chest ultrasounds confirmed that pus in the pleural cavity had been completely evacuated. A fibroptic bronchoscopy was normal and she was discharged home.

She was seen again two months later with a 1-week history of persistent discharge from the back of her chest. Examination revealed a draining sinus at the site of previous thoracostomy. Repeat X-rays and chest ultrasound showed no effusion and the sinus pus grew coliforms. Sinogram revealed that the tract was extrapleural and communicating with the left kidney and ureter (Figure 1). Abdominal ultrasound showed left hydronephrosis with a calculus at upper pole. No perinephric or subphrenic collections were found. Urinalysis revealed sterile pyuria. Hemoglobin was 11.7 g% microcytic, hypochromic red cells and white cell count 12.6×10^9/l. Iron studies pointed to iron reutilization defect. Albumin was 30 g/l but other liver functions were normal. Cystourethroscopy and retrograde pyelography confirmed obstruction due to calculus with possible pyonephrosis above. Intravenous urography and isotope renal scan confirmed non-functioning left kidney. The other kidney and ureter were normal and so was overall renal function with urea of 4.6 mmol/l and creatinine 90 mmol/l.

Received June 27, 1990; in revised form September 4, 1990.

Reprint requests to Dr. J. Warren.

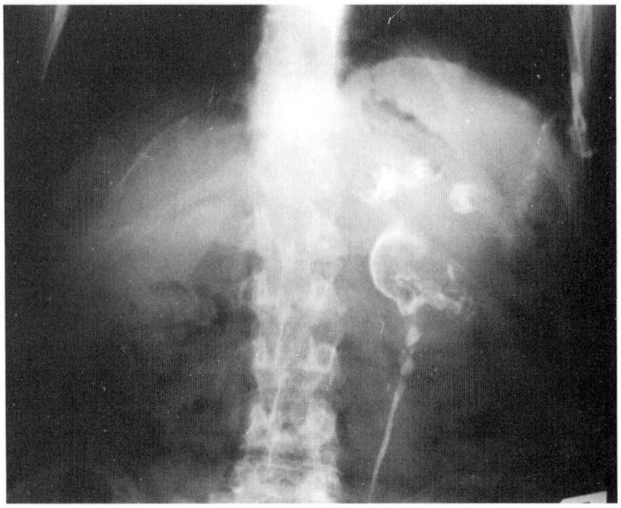

Fig. 1 Sinogram showing an extrapleural tract communicating with left kidney and ureter

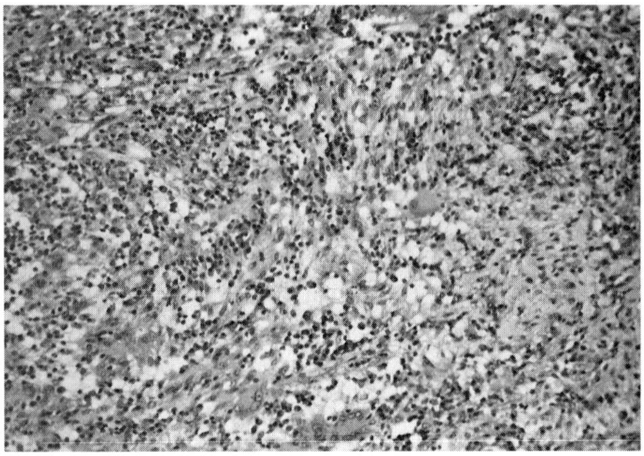

Fig. 2 Photomicrograph of kidney showing xanthoma cells, multinucleate giant cells and chronic inflammatory infiltrate

The patient was accepted for exploration with a diagnosis of left pyonephrosis and nephrolithiasis. At surgery, extensive adhesions were found across the left kidney fixing it to descending colon. These were released and nephrectomy performed.

The kidney weighed 202 grammes and the calyces were dilated with a yellow scalloped lining. The cortex was narrow, scarred and pale. Microscopy revealed calyces to be replaced by actively inflamed granulation tissue rich in foam cells, neutrophils, lymphocytes and plasma cells (Figure 2). Cortex was extensively scarred and glomeruli hyalinized. There was no evidence of malignancy but cultures from resected kidney were unavailable.

Postoperatively the patient made good recovery and the fistula drainage ceased. Her overall renal functions remain normal.

Discussion

Xanthogranulomatous pyelonephritis (XGP) is an unusual form of chronic renal suppuration and obstruction seen mostly in middle-aged women although all ages and sexes may be affected. Gram negative organisms are usually present and *Proteus mirabilis* is the commonest offending organism. Common symptoms are renal pain, recurrent urinary infections, urolithiasis with colic and systemic features like fever, malaise, anorexia and weight loss. Significant physical findings include renal mass (62%), hypertension (31%) and hepatomegaly (27%) [Malek and Elder 1978].

Only 4–8% cases have a draining flank sinus [Godman et al 1979]. Pleural effusion and empyema are extremely uncommon and there is no report of a patient with XGP having both pleural empyema and reno-cutaneous fistula. It may, however, mimic other renal diseases like hypernephroma, hydronephrosis, pyonephrosis with or without calculi, renal carbuncle, tuberculosis or other specific granulomas [Cohen 1986, Montgomerie and Guze 1977].

Investigations typically show reversible hepatic dysfunction and an enlarged non-functioning hypovascular kidney with lithiasis and chronic sepsis. The renal involvement may be segmental or diffuse and may extend into pararenal tissue producing dense adhesions. The kidney is enlarged and shows bright yellow masses in the parenchyma. These masses microscopically show central necrosis and foamy macrophages whose cytoplasm is laden with cholesterol and neutral lipids from necrotic purulent material [Goodman et al. 1979]. These xanthoma cells may form multinucleate giant cells and may be confused with clear cell type of hypernephroma. The granulomas also have large numbers of neutrophils, lymphocytes and plasma cells and are surrounded by prolifering fibroblasts and capillaries. The renal parenchyma elsewhere shows chronic inflammation and effects of obstruction.

Several causative factors have been postulated for pathogenesis of XGP. These include calculi, urinary obstruction, ineffectively treated urosepsis, renal ischemia, lymphatic blockage and alterations in lipid metabolism [Malek and Elder 1978]. Antonakopoules et al. believe that a defect exists in the lysosomal procession of bacteria by host macrophages [Antonakopoules et al. 1988]. There are case reports of cold agglutinins and leukocyte specific antinuclear antibodies in patients with XGP. These antibodies may interfere with neutrophil chemotaxis, requiring macrophages to produce a xanthogranulomatous reaction to bacterial invasion.

The treatment is nephrectomy and the disease does not recur after surgery even though the lesion has been partially excised [Anhalt et al. 1971].

REFERENCES

Anhalt MA, Cawood CD, Scott R Jr 1971 Xanthogranulomatous pyelonephritis: a comprehensive review with report of 4 additional cases. J Urol *105:* 10–17

Antonakopoulos GN, Chapple CR, Newman J 1988 Xanthogranulomatous pyelonephritis: a reappraisal and immunohistochemical study. Arch Pathol Lab Med *122:* 275–281

Braun G, Moussali L, Blanxar JL 1985 Xanthogranulomatous pyelonephritis in children. J Urol *133:* 236–239

Cohen MS 1986 Urological clinics of North America, Vol. 13, No. 4, November

Godman M, Curry T, Russell T 1979 Xanthogranulomatous pyelonephritis: a local disease with systemic manifestations: report of 23 patients and review of literature. Medicine (Baltimore) *58:* 171–184

Kierce F, Carrol R, Guiney EJ 1985 Xanthogranulomatous pyelonephritis in childhood. Br J Urol *57:* 261–264

Malek RS, Elder JS 1978 Xanthogranulomatous pyelonephritis: a critical analysis of 26 cases and of the literature. J Urol *119:* 589–593

Montgomerie J, Guze L 1977 The renal response to infection. In: The Kidney Vol. 2, WB Saunders Co. Philadelphia, pp 1079–1112

Intracatheter streptokinase for recurrent peritonitis in CAPD

B. J. Nankivell[1], N. Lake[2] and A. Gillies[2]

[1]Department of Renal Medicine, Westmead Hospital, Westmead 2145, Australia
[2]Department of Nephrology, Royal Newcastle Hospital, Newcastle 2300, Australia

Abstract. Intracatheter streptokinase (SK) is advocated as effective treatment with minimal adverse effects in both recurrent bacterial peritonitis and catheter fibrin blockage in continuous ambulatory peritoneal dialysis (CAPD) patients. We reviewed 35 instillations in 20 patients noting a high (86%) side effect profile consisting of fever, onset of turbid dialysis effluent and/or abdominal pain. SK probably releases fibrin clot containing bacteria, leukocytes and debris from the colonized catheter into the peritoneal cavity causing a "peritonitis-like syndrome" of 1 to 3 days duration. Fungal peritonitis occurred after SK in 2 patients. Failure of SK therapy was encountered in *Staphylococcus epidermidis* infection ($p < 0.05$ versus other organisms), which may be related to its protective capsular polysaccharide slime and ability to adhere to plastic prosthetic devices. SK, in this study, was useful treatment in relapsing bacterial peritonitis (50% overall cure) but failed to correct catheter malfunction.

Key words: recurrent bacterial peritonitis – staphylococcus epidermidis – continuous ambulatory peritoneal dialysis – streptokinase

Introduction

Recurrent bacterial peritonitis and catheter malfunction due to outflow obstruction are two major problems in CAPD treatment for which streptokinase (SK) has been advocated. SK lyses the fibrin clots in the catheter lumen that serve as sanctuary sites for bacteria that relapse after antibiotic treatment for peritonitis is completed. In the case of catheter malfunction SK may dissolve the obstructing fibrin plugs. Previous papers have reported success in small numbers of patients with minimal side effects. This contradicts our clinical experience with the drug used for both recurrent peritonitis and catheter malfunction.

Methods

Twenty patients, aged 21–74 years old maintained on CAPD in Royal Newcastle and Westmead Hospitals, who received intracatheter streptokinase from 1986 to 1989, were retrospectively analyzed. Twenty-one Tenckhoff catheters were involved and a total of 35 instillations of SK given. Indications for usage were recurrent peritonitis and catheter malfunction. Recurrent bacterial peritonitis was defined as clinical and microbiological evidence of bacterial peritonitis recurring within 10 days after antibiotic cessation. Treatment relapse, due to catheter microbiological colonizations was assumed if the recurrent peritonitis was caused by the same bacterial organism and treatment failure due to antibiotic resistance or catheter tunnel infection had been excluded.

Streptokinase (Streptase® Behring Institute) was given as previously described [Palacios et al. 1982] (750,000 units in 100 ml of normal saline), instilled in 30 ml boluses, with the catheter clamped for 24 hours. All treatments of streptokinase were performed during resolving peritonitis and were followed by an additional 10 days of intraperitoneal antibiotics as appropriate for the recurring organism. Vancomycin was used in 8/9 instances of *Staphylococcus epidermidis* infection. The procedure was repeated in 10–14 days, in the case of relapsing peritonitis and as required for catheter malfunction. Treatment success was defined as no further peritonitis due to the same organism in the 6 weeks following, or normalization of dialysis outflow in the cases of catheter malfunction.

Side effects were derived from analysis of medical and nursing notes, temperature charts and peritoneal dialysate records for each separate SK instillation.

Received September 28, 1990.
Reprint requests to Dr. B. J. Nankivell.

Maximal temperatures in the 24-h period before and after the beginning of SK instillation were recorded and compared. Fever was designated as an increase of 1° C or more in temperature. The onset of abdominal pain, tenderness, analgesics given and turbid (cloudy) dialysate bags subsequent to SK were noted, and two or more of these features were designated as "peritonitis like syndrome".

All data is presented as means ± standard error of mean, comparisons via paired t-test and Fisher's exact test where appropriate. Values of $p < 0.05$ are considered significant.

Results

Twenty patients (21 Tenckhoff catheters) received 35 instillations of SK (see Table 1). Sixteen patients received SK for relapsing peritonitis (cases 1–16) with 8 successes, 7 failures (of which 6 were *Staphylococcus epidermidis* colonization) and 1 unknown result. Treatment failed for all 5 catheters with catheter malfunction (3 were related to catheter malposition or omental wrapping).

Side effects of SK instillations were frequent. Fever was seen in 21 treatments, abdominal pain in 27 (16 of whom received narcotic analgesia) and the new onset of turbid dialysate effluent noted following 17 uses of SK. Transient, mildly blood stained effluent was returned in 3 instances. A peritonitis like syndrome composed of cloudy bags and fever or abdominal pain occurred in 19 instances (54%). This syndrome occurred more commonly when SK was administered soon after a recent episode of peritonitis. The interval between SK administration and most recent peritonitis was short (8.1 ± 1.5 days) in patients who encountered the syndrome compared with those who remained symptom free (21.7 ±

Table 1

Patient	Age/Sex	Disease	Indication for SK	No SK	Result	Temp	Pain	Turbid effluent	Catheter removal
1	65/F	GN	*S. epidermidis*	2	recur		×		×
2	51/M	Diabetes	*S. epidermidis*	2	recur	×	×	×	×
3	49/F	GN	*S. epidermidis*	1	recur		×	×	×[a]
4	53/M	PAN	*S. epidermidis*	2	recur	×	×	×	×
5	63/F	AN	*S. epidermidis*	1	recur	×	×	×	×
6	56/F	AN	*S. epidermidis*	1	fungal	×			×
7	M	GN	*S. epidermidis*	1	unknown	×			[b]
8	73/F	AN	*S. epidermidis*	2	clear	×			
9	68/M	Calculus disease	*S. epidermidis*	2	clear			×	×[c]
10	70/F	AN	*Pseudomonas Maltophilia*	2	clear	×	×	×	
11	51/F	GN	*Citrobacter*	3	clear	×	×	×	
12	58/F	AN	*Acinetobacter*	2	clear	×	×	×	
13	57/M	AN	*Acinetobacter*	2	clear	×	×	×	×[d]
14	56/F	Diabetes	*diptheroids*	2	clear	×	×	×	×
15	63/F	AN	*S. aureus*	2	clear	×	×		
16	69/F	AN	*B. licheniformis*	2	recur		×	×	×
17	69/F	CIN	catheter malfunction	1	fungal				×
18	21/M	GN	catheter malfunction	1	fail				×[e]
19[a]	49/F	CIN	catheter malfunction	1	fail	×	×	×	×[f]
19[b]	49/F	CIN	catheter malfunction	2	fail	×	×	×	×
20	74/F	Un-diagnosed	catheter malfunction	1	fail				×

[a] Purpuric rash developed on arms and legs 2 days after SK use.
[b] Patient died at home 1 week after receiving SK.
[c] Removal due to poor urea clearance.
[d] SK cleared *Acinetobacter* but 5 weeks later recurrent peritonitis with new *Staphylococcus epidermis* began.
[e] Catheter repositioned but not removed.
[f] Catheter placed 9 months previously and capped after partial renal recovery and restarted with drainage impeded by fibrin strands.

7.5 days, p = NS). The peritonitis-like syndrome occurred in 59% of instillations given within 2 weeks of peritonitis. It was also noted in 3 out of 5 uses of SK to clear postoperative catheter malfunction. Abdominal pain occurred more frequently if SK was used soon after active peritonitis. Instillations of SK producing pain occurred 7.1 ± 1.3 days after peritonitis compared with pain free instillations occurring 32 ± 10.1 days, $p < 0.05$. Average peak temperature increased significantly from 36.9 ± 0.06° C to 37.6 ± 0.2° C ($p < 0.001$) giving an average rise of 0.7 ± 0.13° C. Operative intervention was undertaken with 14 catheter removals and 1 repositioning. Only 6 out of 21 catheters remained. When analyzed according to infecting organism only 2/7 *S. epidermidis* infections were cleared (excluding unknown cases 6 and 7) compared with 6/7 cures of other organismus (Fisher's exact test, $p < 0.05$). The most serious side effect was the occurrence of fungal peritonitis, occurring 5 days after the first SK instillation (cases 6 and 17). In one case a *Paecilomyces* fungal intraluminal cast causing poor drainage was aspirated subsequent to SK, and in another case *Candida albicans* was cultured. Both catheters were removed under amphotericin cover and in one patient peritoneal fungal sepsis precluded further catheter insertion. In case 20 a new diphtheroid peritonitis was encountered in 2 days after SK use. In case 13 recurrent *Acinetobacter* peritonitis was cleared by streptokinase but 5 weeks later recurrent *S. epidermidis* peritonitis developed. This may represent recolonization of a partially cleared fibrin layer.

Discussion

Streptokinase, a purified protein derived from Group C hemolytic streptococci, is a powerful fibrinolytic enzyme in humans, acting via the streptokinase-plasminogen activator complex generating plasmin which hydrolyzes fibrin and fibrinogen [Brogden et al. 1973].

In recurrent bacterial peritonitis, unresponsive to repeated courses of appropriate antibiotics, bacterial colonization in the fibrin attached to the peritoneal catheter has been demonstrated by scanning electron microscopy [Schuenemann et al. 1981]. Relapse after antibiotic cessation is thought to result from colonies in sanctuary sites within the fibrin layer. Streptokinase, by destroying this layer, has been successfully employed in the treatment of recurrent peritonitis [Block et al. 1983, Norris et al. 1987]. Clearly, this therapy would not be of benefit in peritonitis due to resistant bacteria, catheter tunnel infection or external reinfection secondary to poor sterile technique.

Previous papers on SK usage have reported resolution of relapsing peritonitis [Block et al. 1983, Norris et al. 1987] or catheter malfunction [Palacios et al. 1982, Bergstein et al. 1988, Weigmann et al. 1985] with minimal or no adverse reactions. Our study demonstrated a 50% cure rate in relapsing peritonitis, although only 2 of the 9 patients with *Staphylococcus epidermidis* were cleared. This disproportionate number of treatment failures may be related to the ability of *Staphylococcus epidermidis* to adhere to plastic or metal prosthetic devices [Peters et al. 1982]. It can produce an alcian blue staining mucoid material, "slime" [Bayston et al. 1982] of which a galactose rich capsular polysaccharide mediates adhesion to polyethylene and other plastics [Ludwicka et al. 1984]. Electron microscopy of peritoneal dialysis catheters has demonstrated *Staphyloccus epidermidis* adherent to dialysis catheter biofilms. These matted colonies are extremely resistant to antiseptic agents and biocides. Antibiotic penetrance is of importance. Vancomycin was shown to be useful in reducing the number of colonizing *S. epidermidis* organisms of cannulae [Elliot 1988] although another study showed a 50% reduction at 24 hours of bacterial colony counts in a latex model of catheter biofilms treated with vancomycin at 20 mg/l. Streptokinase may be enzymatically effective against catheter fibrin but not on the *S. epidermidis* polysaccharide slime. Further research should be directed to developing dialysis catheter capable of preventing adherence of fibrin and slime producing microorganisms.

Catheter malfunction, with outflow obstruction, especially if postoperative or related to catheter omental wrapping, responded poorly to SK, in keeping with other reports [Wiegmann et al. 1985]. SK treatment avoided operative intervention in only 7 out of 21 catheters.

In contrast to previous papers, a high incidence of side effects was noted including fever (55%), abdominal pain or tenderness (71%) which required narcotic analgesia (60%) and the onset of turbid dialysis bags (45%), occurring after SK instillation. The intended action of streptokinase in relapsing peritonitis is dissolution of the intra-catheter fibrin layer which, along with its bacterial inflammatory cells and microbiological debris, is washed into the peritoneal cavity by the next dialysis influx. This is the likely pathophysiology of the peritonitis-like syndrome observed in 54% of instillations. A high rate of reactions associated with streptokinase given early was noted; however, the issue of further delaying the streptokinase treatment to reduce the incidence of side effects is unproven. Most serious was the occurrence of 2 cases of fungal peritonitis 5 days after SK administration, suggesting co-existent catheter colonization with fungi within the intra-catheter fibrin layer, and release into the peritoneal cavity.

In balance, despite the high side effect profile of SK, it remains a useful tool in the treatment of relapsing bacterial peritonitis occurring within 10 days after antibiotic cessation, in which catheter tunnel infection and antibiotic resistance has been excluded. A trial of streptokinase may preclude the need for catheter withdrawal.

REFERENCES

Bayston R, Penny SR 1972 Excessive production of a mucoid substance in staphylococcus S11A: a possible factor in colonisation of Holfer shunts. Dev Med Child Neurol *14* (suppl): 25–28

Bergstein JM, Andreoli SP, West KW, Grosfield JL 1988 Streptokinase therapy for occluded Tenckhoff catheters in children on CAPD. Perit Dial Bull *8:* 137–139

Block RA, Taylor B, Frederick B 1983 Intraperitoneal infusion of streptokinase in the treatment of recurrent peritonitis. Perit Dial Bull *3:* 162

Brogden RN, Speight TM, Avery MS 1973 Streptokinase. A review of its clinical pharmacology, mechanism of action and therapeutic uses. Drugs *5:* 357–445

Elliot TSJ 1988 Plastic devices: new fields for old microbes. Lancet *1:* 365–366

Ludwicka A, Uhlenbruck G, Peters G, Seng PN, Gray ED, Jeljaszewicz, Pulverer G 1984 Investigation on extracellular slime substance produced by staphyloccus epidermidis. Zentralbl Bakteriol Mikrobio Hyg [A] *258:* 256–267

Norris KC, Shinaberger JH, Reyes GD, Kraut JA 1987 The use of intra-catheter instillation of streptokinase in the treatment of recurrent bacterial peritonitis in continuous ambulatory peritoneal dialysis. Am J Kid Dis *10:* 10, 62–65

Palacios M, Schley W, Dougherty JC 1982 Use of streptokinase to clear peritoneal catheters. Dial Transplant *11:* 172–174

Peters G, Locci R, Pulverer G 1982 Adherence and growth of coagulase – negative staphylococci on surfaces of intravenous catheters. J Inf Dis *146:* 479–482

Schuenemann B, Schwartz P, Mergerian H 1981 Fibrin coating of the peritoneal catheter as a cause of recurrent peritonitis. In: *Gohl GM, Kessel M, Nolph KD* (eds). Advances in peritoneal dialysis. Proceedings of the second International Symposium on peritoneal dialysis Berlin (West), June 16–19, 1981. Amsterdam, Excerpta Medical, pp 296–298

Wiegmann TB, Stveive B, Duncan KA 1985 Effective use of streptokinase for peritoneal catheter failure. Am J Kid Dis *6,2:* 119–128

Clinical Nephrology, Vol. 35 No. 1 – 1991 (24–25)

Pneumococcal peritonitis complicating CAPD – was the indwelling intrauterine device to blame?

A. Korzets, A. Chagnac, Y. Ori, D. Zevin and J. Levi

Department of Nephrology, Hasharon Hospital, Petach-Tikva, Israel
(Affiliated with the Sackler School of Medicine, Tel-Aviv University, Israel)

Abstract. A 45-year-old woman on CAPD developed pneumococcal peritonitis. This is the second such case of *Streptococcus pneumoniae* peritonitis complicating CAPD. The role of an indwelling intrauterine device (IUD) in producing ascending infection into the peritoneum is discussed, especially in women with evidence of retrograde menstruation. A review of the literature concerning pneumococcal peritonitis associated with IUD is given. Possible contraception to women on CAPD is briefly mentioned.

Key words: CAPD – pneumococcal peritonitis – intrauterine device

Introduction

Pneumococcal peritonitis is a known complication in patients, especially children, with the nephrotic syndrome [Gorensek et al. 1988] and in cirrhotics [Epstein et al. 1968]. Pneumococcal peritonitis has also received attention recently as a complication of indwelling intrauterine devices [Goldman et al. 1986, Lucas and Brook 1987]. However, although bacterial peritonitis remains the major problem in CAPD, pneumococcal peritonitis has been previously described only once in this population. We hereby detail such a case and focus on a possible pathogenesis.

Case report

A 45-year-old Jewess, married and mother of 2 children, entered a chronic CAPD program in 1986 because of end-stage renal failure. The underlying renal disease was membranoproliferative glomerulonephritis. An IUD (Lippes loop) had been inserted in 1985. CAPD peritonitis was infrequent (3 episodes in 4 years: *Staphylococcus albus, Streptococcus viridans, Pseudomonas aeruginosa*). In 1987–1988 bloody peritoneal effluent, related directly to menstruation, was noted on 3 separate occasions. Ultrasound examination of the pelvis did not reveal ovarian cysts. The patient was never hypoalbuminemic.

Received July 26, 1990; in revised form October 2, 1990.

Reprint requests to Prof. J. Levi, Department of Nephrology, 7 Keren Kayemet Street, P.O. Box 121, Petah-Tikva, Israel.

In April 1990 the patient developed abdominal pain and a cloudy effluent (460 WBC/mm^3). Intraperitoneal vancomycin and aztreonam were commenced. The patient responded quickly with dialysate effluent turning clear after three days of treatment. Dialysate cultures grew *Streptococcus pneumoniae.* All blood cultures were sterile. Intramuscular procaine penicillin was added on the 7th day of treatment. A gynecological examination, performed 5 days after abdominal pain was first complained of, was normal. The IUD was removed and *Eschericia coli* was subsequently cultured from the IUD itself. The patient remains free of further peritonitis 3 months after all antibiotics were ceased. Her serum progesterone level (on day 21 of her regular period) is 19 ng/ml. Current contraception used by the patient is oral “Logynon” (levonorgestral 0.05 mg, 0.075 mg, 0.125 mg; ethinylestradiol 0.03 mg, 0.04 mg, 0.03 mg). A liver-spleen scan is normal, as are serum IgG, IgM and IgA levels.

Discussion

To the best of our knowledge only one previous case of pneumococcal peritonitis has been previously documented in a CAPD patient [Fenton et al. 1981]. On the other hand, pneumococcal peritonitis in females is not uncommon and a suggested pathogenesis in these women includes ascending infection of the peritoneum from an infected genital tract [McCartney and Fraser 1922]. IUD can cause inflammatory pelvic disease and at times severe infectious disease [Rowland 1971]. Furthermore, at least five reports have documented seven cases of pneumococcal peritonitis complicating indwelling IUD [Herbert and Mortimer 1974, Gruer et al. 1983, Ron-El et al. 1985, Goldman et al. 1986, Lucas and Brook 1987]. We feel that our patient may have also developed peritonitis secondary to an infected IUD. Although *S. pneumoniae* was not cultured from the IUD, this is also the case in most of the previous reports. Indeed growth of *E. coli* on the IUD in our patient only serves to demonstrate the possible infectivity of the IUD. Of the seven reported patients five had their IUD removed. All five women recovered. The only death was in a 46-year-old woman whose IUD was not removed.

Only one case of peritonitis secondary to an IUD in a patient on CAPD has been previously described [Stuck et al. 1986]. This patient presented with acute pelvic inflammatory disease, peritonitis and Enterococcus was cultured from the IUD. Noteworthy is that both this patient and our patient had prior episodes of bloody dialysate effluent, indicating retrograde menstruation between the genital tract and the peritoneal cavity.

In conclusion we recommend a very cautious use of IUD in CAPD patients, especially in those women with a history of retrograde menstruation. Periodic testing of ovulation should be carried out to see if contraception is indeed warranted, and in this day and age the use of local barriers or low dose estrogen contraceptives seems a reasonable approach in these patients. Deep vein thrombosis and hypertension occur in only a small percentage of women on these new oral agents [Peterson and Lee 1989]. Furthermore, if one regards the uremic patient as immunosuppressed, then it is of interest to know that immunosuppressed women have an increased incidence of IUD-related pelvic inflammatory disease [O'Donnell et al. 1985].

Finally, any female CAPD patient with an indwelling IUD who presents with peritonitis should have an immediate gynecological examination performed. Vaginal smears and cultures should be taken promptly and removal of the IUD seriously considered if pneumococcal peritonitis is subsequently confirmed.

REFERENCES

Epstein M, Calia FM, Cabuzda GJ 1968 Pneumococcal peritonitis in patients with postnecrotic cirrhosis. N Engl J Med *278:* 69–71

Fenton S, Wu G, Cattran D, Wadgymar A, Allen AF 1981 Clinical aspects of peritonitis in patients on CAPD. Perit Dial Bull *1:* 54–57

Goldman JA, Yeshaya A, Peleg D, Dekel A, Dicker D 1986 Severe pneumococcal peritonitis complicating IUD: case report and review of the literature. Obst Gyn Survey *41:* 672–674

Gorensek MJ, Lebel MH, Nelson JD 1988 Peritonitis in children with nephrotic syndrome. Pediatrics *81:* 849–856

Gruer LD, Collingham KE, Edwards CW 1983 Pneumococcal peritonitis associated with an IUCD. Lancet *2:* 677

Herbert TJ, Mortimer PP 1974 Recurrent pneumococcal peritonitis associated with an intra-uterine contraceptive device. Br J Surg *61:* 901–992

Lucas RE, Brook MG 1987 Pneumococcal peritonitis related to an intrauterine device. J Infection *15:* 280–281

McCartney JE, Fraser J 1922 Pneumococcal peritonitis. Br J Surg *9:* 479–489

O'Donnell D, Jamieson J, Botha JR 1985 Peritonitis in the immunosuppressed female – possible role of the IUCD. South Afr Med J *68:* 136–137

Peterson HB, Lee NC 1989 The health effect of oral contraceptives: misperceptions, controversies and continuing good news. In: *Pitken RM* (ed). Clinical obstetrics and gynaecology. J. B. Lippincott Co., Philadelphia, 339–355

Ron-El R, Bukovski I, Kharasch J, Letcoy Y, Caspi E 1985 Pneumococcal peritonitis with the presence of an intrauterine contraceptive device. Int J Gynaecol Obstet *23:* 339–341

Rowland TC 1971 Severe peritonitis complicating an intrauterine contraceptive device. Am J Obstet Gynec *110:* 786–787

Stuck A, Seiler A, Frey FJ 1986 Peritonitis due to an intrauterine device in a patient on CAPD. Perit Dial Bull *6:* 158–159

Clinical Nephrology, Vol. 35 No. 1 – 1991 (26–34)

Hemodialysis and heparin. Alternative methods of measuring heparin and of detecting activation of coagulation

H. A. Ireland, M. D. Boisclair, D. A. Lane, E. Thompson and J. R. Curtis

Departments of Haematology and Medicine, Charing Cross and Westminster Medical School, London, W6 8RP, UK

Abstract. A bolus dose of heparin was administered pre-dialysis to patients (n = 6) undergoing regular maintenance hemodialysis with cuprophane flat plate and hollow fiber membranes. Blood samples were withdrawn at hourly intervals for measurement of a) heparin and b) activation markers of coagulation, fibrinolysis and platelets. Two assay methods for heparin were employed; amidolytic assay of anti-factor Xa activity in plasma and a simple whole blood clotting time based upon factor Xa inhibition (Heptest). Results from these heparin assays correlated well with each other (r = 0.89) and both showed similar negative correlations (r = −0.72, amidolytic and r = −0.66, Heptest) with levels of a marker of fibrin clot formation, fibrinopeptide A (FPA). Large differences in levels of FPA were observed during dialysis with the two dialyzer types, when similar levels of heparin were present. Heparin levels declined from 1–5-h dialysis and were associated with rises in plasma levels of FPA, thrombin-antithrombin complex (TAT) and β thromboglobulin (BTG), but not of D-dimer. Regression analysis revealed the best correlation was between FPA and TAT (r = 0.94), followed by FPA and BTG (r = 0.81). FPA and D-dimer exhibited significant, but lower (r = 0.42), correlation. TAT levels, like FPA levels, showed good correlation with heparin (r >0.65). It is concluded that the Heptest assay may be a useful bedside measurement of heparin levels and the TAT assay may be a simplified means of evaluating coagulation system activation during dialysis.

Key words: hemodialysis – fibrinopeptide A – thrombin-antithrombin complex – heparin measurement – β thromboglobulin – fibrin degradation products

Introduction

In our experience, measurement of fibrinopeptide A (FPA) has proved to be a valuable test for monitoring adequacy of heparinization during hemodialysis using cuprophane flat plate membranes. As heparin levels are progressively reduced, there is an associated rise in FPA levels, reflecting increased activation of coagulation. FPA measurement has enabled an objective assessment of coagulation system activation within the dialysis circuit during dose ranging studies of heparin [Ireland et al. 1984], low molecular weight heparins [Lane et al. 1986a, b, Ireland et al. 1988] and related compounds [Ireland et al. 1986]. Similar conclusions regarding the utility of FPA measurement have been drawn by others [Wilhelmsson et al. 1981, Ljunberg 1985, Ljunberg et al. 1987].

Recently, other assays have been developed which have potential application in the measurement of activation of coagulation and/or fibrinolysis: these are the ELISAs to crosslinked fibrin fragment D-dimer [Rylatt et al. 1983] and to thrombin-antithrombin complex (TAT) [Pelzer et al. 1988].

The assay for D-dimer enables fibrin degradation products rather than those of fibrinogen to be detected. The assays can be performed on plasma rather than on serum. In many clinical situations, good correlations have been found between measurements of plasma D-dimer and more conventional FDP assays, such as the latex agglutination test for serum FDPs and radioimmunoassay to serum fibrinogen fragment E [Wilde et al. 1989, Boisclair et al. 1990]. However, in renal failure, levels of some of the fragments measured by conventional serum FDP tests are increased because of their reduced renal clearance, rather than due to increased activation of the coagula-

Received February 8, 1990; in revised form October 23, 1990.
Reprint requests to Dr. H. Ireland.

tion/fibrinolytic systems. In contrast, levels of D-dimer in the majority of patients with renal failure are not increased above normal controls and show no correlation with creatinine clearance, indicating that results obtained with this assay are not artifactually elevated in renal disease [Gordge et al. 1989]. This indicates a potential use for the D-dimer assay in the investigation of imbalanced hemostasis in these patients during hemodialysis.

TAT is formed as thrombin is rapidly inactivated by the plasma proteinase inhibitor, antithrombin. Assay of TAT has not yet been subjected to as many clinical investigations as that of D-dimer. It is certain that thrombin generation occurs during hemodialysis if heparinization is inadequate, as this leads to the cleavage of FPA from fibrinogen. Inevitably, some of the thrombin will be inactivated by antithrombin. However, whether an assay to TAT is sensitive enough to be able to detect the presence of thrombin generation and inhibition due to inadequate heparin has not been established.

Commonly used tests for measurement of heparin in plasma are based upon the kaolin cephalin clotting time. However, these tests are not sensitive to low molecular weight heparins and heparinoids, which may be used with increasing frequency in dialysis in the near future. Amidolytic assays for measurement of heparin, low molecular weight heparins and heparinoids are, however, now well established. In the course of studies of several heparin-related compounds [Ireland et al. 1986, 1988, Lane et al. 1986a and b], the different heparins used were always measured by amidolytic anti-factor Xa assay, but on occasions anti-factor IIa assays were also used [Tew et al. 1988]. No significant correlation was achieved when the anti-factor IIa activities of a low molecular weight heparin were compared with FPA levels by linear regression analysis [Tew et al. 1988]. A significant correlation was, however, achieved between the FPA levels and anti-factor Xa activities, suggesting that assays based on inhibition of added factor Xa are preferable to those based on thrombin inhibition when these compounds are being monitored. For heparin monitoring during hemodialysis to be of clinical value, the optimum level which adequately suppresses clot formation must be determined. Furthermore, the method of heparin measurement must be applicable to individual test samples and allow rapid output of results. While chromogenic substrate assays have proved useful in retrospective analysis, they do not allow "bedside control". A recently developed commercial clotting test (Heptest), based upon the inhibition of added factor Xa, would seem a potential alternative method of measurement of these compounds, particularly as whole blood measurements can be made.

The aims of the present study were therefore two-fold: firstly, the newly developed simple factor Xa-based whole blood clotting assay (Heptest) was compared with an established anti-factor Xa amidolytic assay, in patients undergoing hemodialysis. Secondly, D-dimer and TAT levels were compared to those of FPA and heparin. Could these assays provide equally effective and more convenient means of monitoring heparin levels and assessing coagulation activation? We have also re-evaluated the measurement of the platelet release protein, BTG, as a marker of activation.

Materials and methods

Study design

In past dose finding studies we have almost exclusively studied patients during dialysis with cuprophane flat plate membranes. The Renal Unit at Charing Cross Hospital has recently changed to the use of cuprophane hollow fiber membranes. As we had no experience of measuring levels of activation markers during dialysis with hollow fiber membranes, for this study we have made measurements using both membrane types.

Six patients with chronic renal failure, undergoing regular maintenance haemodialysis in the Renal Unit at Charing Cross Hospital, were randomly selected for study and consented to participate after the details of the study had been fully explained. Each patient was studied on 2 occasions, once during dialysis with cuprophane flat plate and once with hollow fiber dialysis membranes. On the first occasion three patients were studied using flat plate and the other three using hollow fiber membranes. Gambro AK proportionating machines were used with dialysis fluid flow rates of 500 ml/min. The hollow fiber and flat plate membranes were matched for their rate of clearance of various toxins and for blood flow rates. Gambro GF 120H hollow fiber membranes were matched with 5N flat plate membranes (2 patients) and GF 120N hollow fiber membranes were matched with 3H flat plate membranes (4 patients). A bolus dose of 4000 iu heparin (Leo Laboratories) was administered prior to each dialysis to provide anticoagulant cover. This dose was chosen, as it was known that it would be able to completely suppress activation of coagulation only at the beginning of dialysis.

Blood samples were collected pre-dialysis and at hourly intervals (up to 6 h) during dialysis for measurement of FPA, D-dimer, TAT, BTG and heparin. No allowance was made for the possible changing hematocrit in the proportion of anticoagulant used in the blood collection tubes. The bubble trap of the

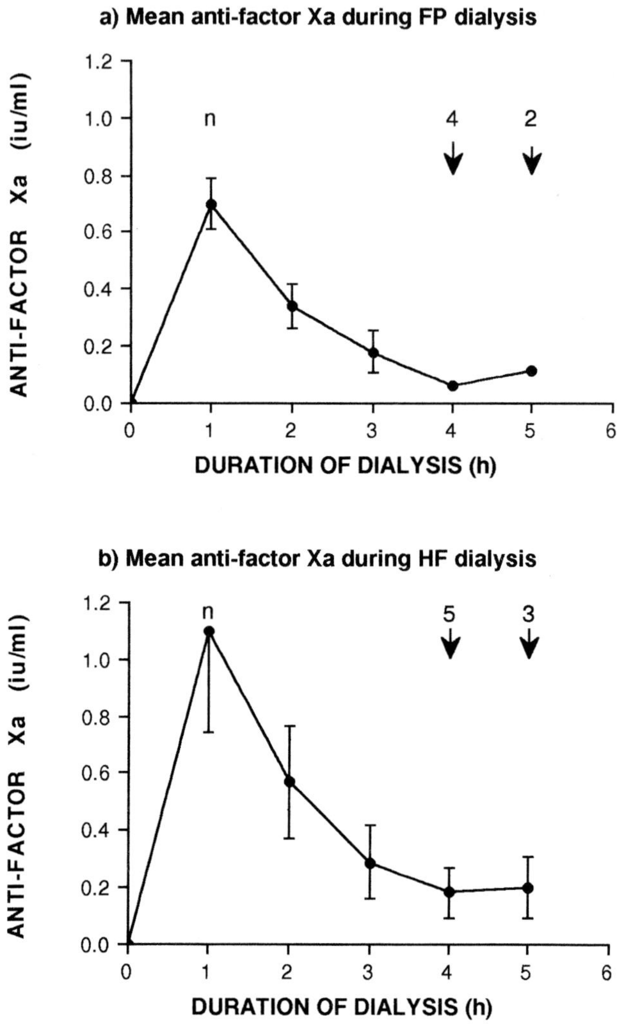

Fig. 1 Mean (± sem) heparin levels (measured by anti-factor Xa amidolytic assay) during 5-h dialysis using a) flat plate (FP, n = 6) and b) hollow fiber (HF, n = 6) membranes. (The numbers of patients available for study were reduced towards the end of dialysis due to excessive clotting at the dialyzer bubble trap, requiring additional heparin administration for the continuance of dialysis)

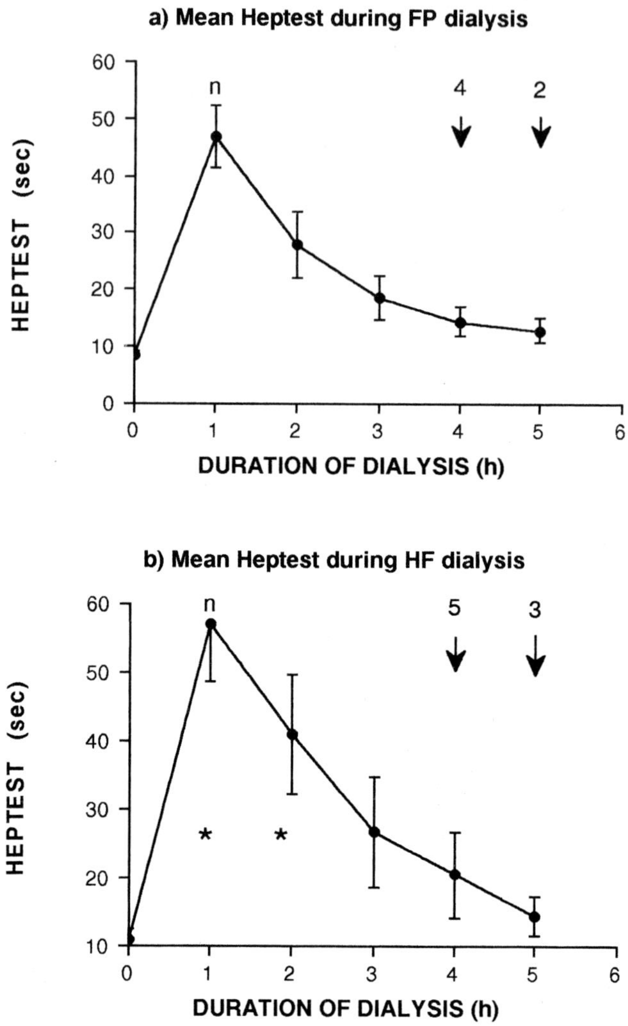

Fig. 2 Mean (± sem) Heptest during 5-h dialysis using a) flat plate (FP, n = 6) and b) hollow fiber (HF, n = 6) membranes, * denotes statistically significant elevation above corresponding hours during FP dialysis

dialyzer was monitored for signs of clot formation. If considered to be excessive, extra heparin was administered and no further samples were collected.

Measurement of heparin

Anti-factor Xa activity was measured as described for the "Coatest" method, Kabi Vitrum, Stockholm, Sweden. Plasma was stored frozen at −20° C prior to assay. Reagents for the whole blood Heptest-Hi were obtained from Haemachem Inc., St. Louis, USA. Whole blood Heptest was performed within 5 min of blood collection. For the test, 100 µl of factor Xa was added to 100 µl of whole blood at 37° C and continually stirred for 30 sec. 100 µl of Recalmix was immediately added at 30 sec and the time of clot formation recorded. The test was performed using a Fibrintimer, Coadata 1000, Labor, Hamburg.

Measurement of activation markers

FPA (Imco) and BTG (reagents supplied by Dr. D. Pepper, Scottish National Blood Transfusion Service, Edinburgh) levels were measured by radioimmunoassay as described previously [Lane et al. 1982].

Plasma D-dimer (Agen, USA) and TAT (Behring, West Germany) were measured by ELISA following the manufacturers' instructions. Blood samples were collected into 3.2% tri-sodium citrate for plasma D-dimer and into EDTA (collected as for BTG) for TAT.

Statistical analysis of results

Assay results at each hour were usually compared to pre-dialysis levels by Wilcoxon matched pairs analysis. For FPA however, pre-dialysis values are high due to in part reduced clearance of the peptide [Ireland et al. 1984]. FPA levels at subsequent hours were therefore compared to the 1-h values. Log-transformed levels for all assays from 1–6 h of dialysis were compared also by regression analysis. Results of the two heparin assays were compared in this way to FPA levels, as were results of the other activation marker assays.

Results

The heparin levels determined by both methods of measurement showed a similar decline from 1 to 5-h dialysis using each membrane type (Figures 1, 2). A difference was observed between levels of heparin measured by anti-factor Xa activity (amidolytic) during flat plate compared with hollow fiber dialysis, although this was not statistically significant. Significantly lower levels of the whole blood Heptest were obtained using flat plate membranes at 1 and 2 h ($p < 0.05$). Regression analysis of all results with both types of membrane revealed a correlation coefficient (r) for whole blood Heptest with amidolytic anti-factor Xa activity of 0.89 (n = 49).

FPA levels during dialysis with hollow fiber membranes showed a small but significant elevation ($p < 0.05$) at 4-h dialysis compared to the 1-h levels (Figure 3). Dialysis using flat plate membranes caused a much larger rise in FPA earlier in dialysis (2 and 3 h, $p < 0.03$) (Figure 3). At these times the FPA levels were also significantly higher than at corresponding times during dialysis with hollow fiber membranes ($p < 0.03$). The higher FPA levels during dialysis with flat plate membranes may have been caused in part by the lower level of heparin. However, the levels of heparin measured at 3 h using hollow fiber were similar to those measured at 2 h using flat plate membranes. This level of heparin was associated with a significant rise in FPA during flat plate dialysis but not during hollow fiber dialysis. It seems unlikely, therefore, that the difference in heparin levels alone could be responsible for the differences in FPA levels. The lower FPA levels during hollow fiber dialysis may be explained by either improved biocompatability of this membrane or its increased clearance through the membrane: additional studies are required to clarify and distinguish these alternatives.

When logarithmic regression analysis was performed between results of both heparin measurements (Heptest and amidolytic assay) and FPA levels at all hours during dialysis, statistically significant correlations were obtained. Correlation coefficients (r) of > -0.63 ($p < 0.01$) were obtained for whole blood Heptest and anti-factor Xa activity for both dialysis membranes analyzed separately (Figure 4, 5).

At 1 h dialysis using hollow fiber membranes, when heparinization was adequate (FPA levels low)

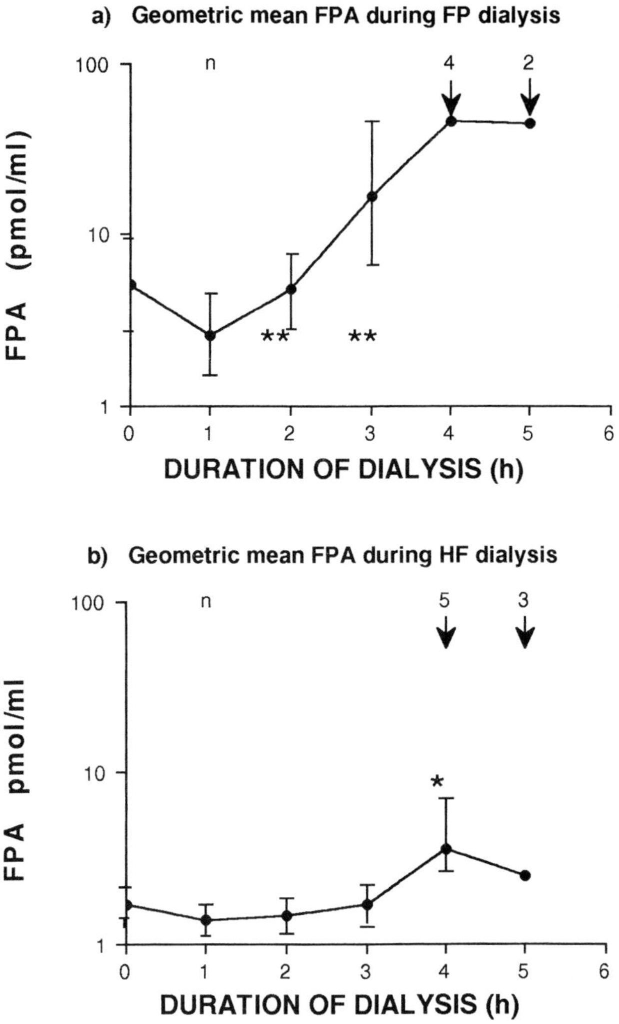

Fig.3 Geometric mean FPA levels during 5-h dialysis using a) flat plate (FP, n = 6) and b) hollow fiber (HF, n = 6) membranes. *denotes statistically significant elevation above 1 h values ($p < 0.05$). **denotes significant elevation above 1 h values ($p < 0.03$) and also above corresponding times during hollow fiber dialysis ($p < 0.03$)

no significant elevation in TAT levels was observed (Figure 6). Furthermore, as the heparin level fell progressively there was an associated rise in both FPA and TAT levels in dialysis conducted with both membranes, although both markers showed much higher levels during dialysis with flat plate membranes. Regression analysis using log-transformed data revealed a good correlation between FPA and TAT levels, when all results from 1–6 h were analyzed regardless of membrane type ($n = 48$, $r = 0.94$, $p < 0.01$, Figure 7). BTG levels also increased towards the end of dialysis, but showed an additional small elevation at 1 h for both membrane types which may have been due to a direct effect of the dialysis membrane on platelets (Figure 8). A good correlation was also observed between log-transformed FPA and BTG levels for all results during both dialyses ($n = 49$, $r = 0.81$, $p < 0.01$, Figure 9). No significant elevations in D-dimer were observed during either flat plate or hollow fiber dialysis (Figure 10). D-dimer however showed a weak correlation with FPA using log-transformed data ($n = 51$, $r = 0.42$, $p < 0.03$, Figure 11).

TAT levels were negatively correlated with heparin levels measured by anti-factor Xa assay using log-transformed data, hollow fiber and flat plate membranes analyzed separately, $r = -0.65$ to -0.75 ($n = 22$, $p < 0.01$). BTG and anti-factor Xa showed a correlation only for flat plate dialysis and D-dimer with anti-factor Xa showed a just significant correlation during hollow fiber dialysis, $r = -0.43$ ($n = 27$, $p < 0.05$).

Discussion

There is considerable variation in the perceived heparin requirements for routine hemodialysis for chronic renal failure. In a recent survey of anticoagu-

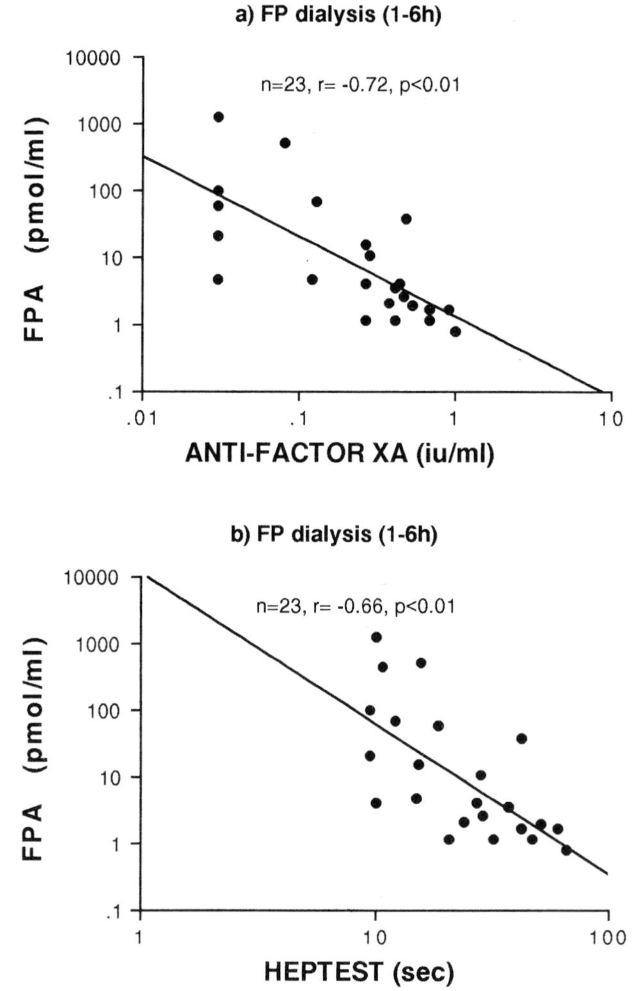

Fig. 4 Scattergram of FPA against a) anti-factor Xa levels and b) Heptest, during flat plate (FP) dialysis

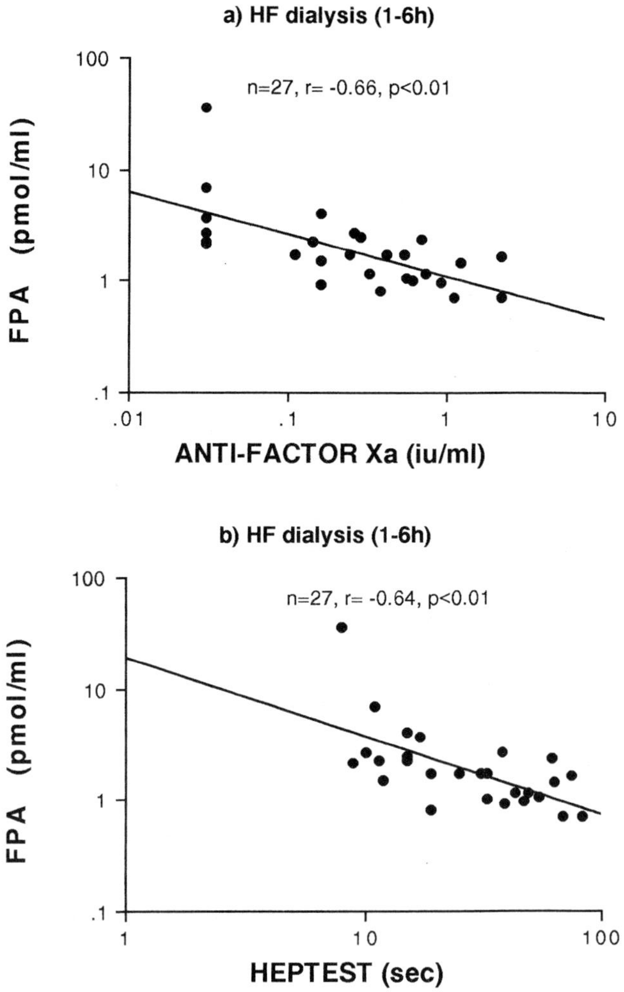

Fig. 5 Scattergram of FPA against a) anti-factor Xa levels and b) Heptest, during hollow fiber (HF) dialysis

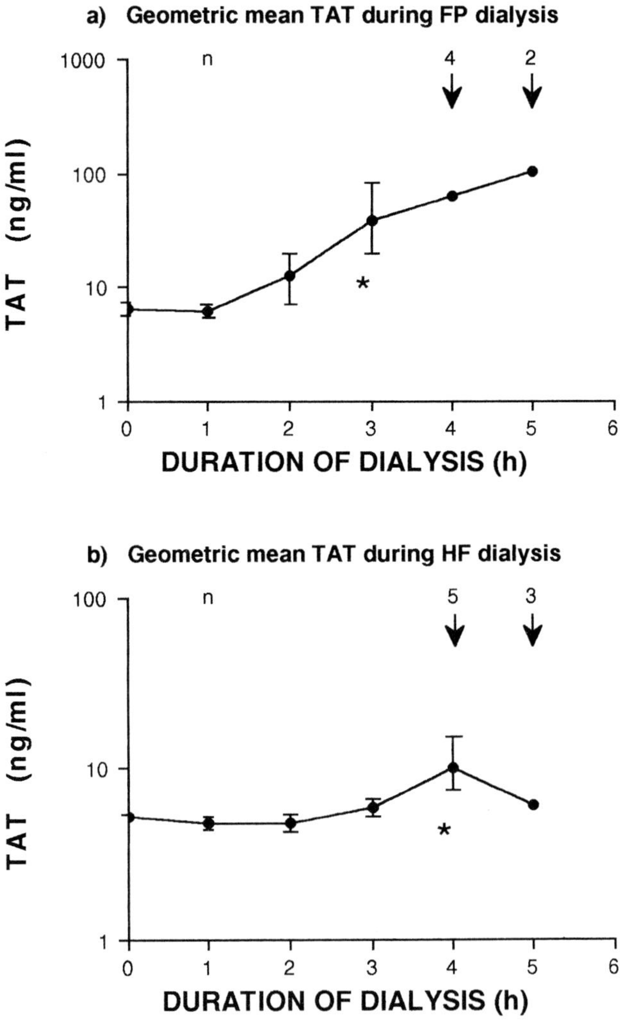

Fig. 6 Geometric mean TAT during dialysis with a) flat plate (FP) membranes and b) hollow fiber (HF) membranes. *denotes a statistically significant elevation above pre-dialysis or 1 h values within each dialysis (p <0.05)

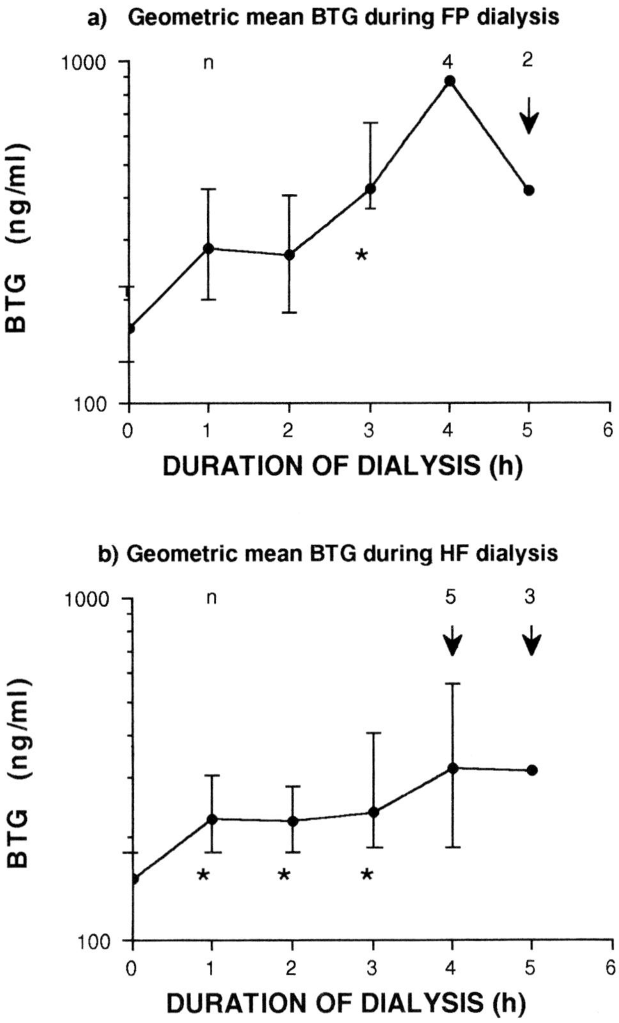

Fig. 8 Geometric mean BTG during dialysis with a) flat plate (FP) and b) hollow fiber (HF) membranes. *denotes statistically significant elevations above pre-dialysis values within each dialysis

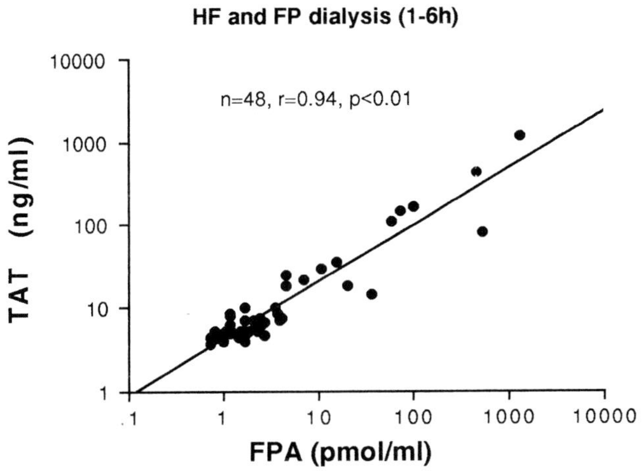

Fig. 7 Scattergram of FPA against TAT levels during both hollow fiber (HF) and flat plate (FP) dialysis

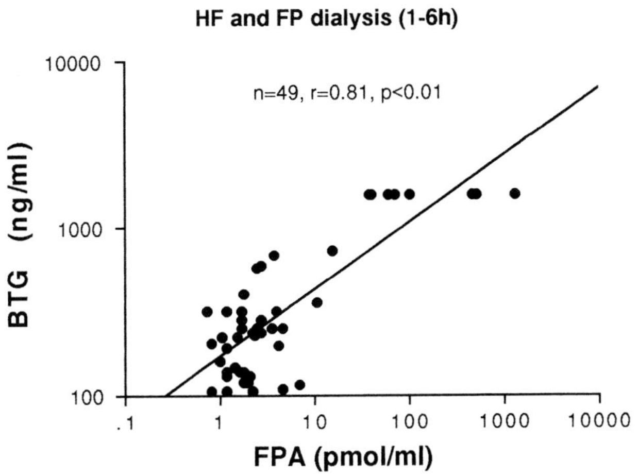

Fig. 9 Scattergram of FPA against BTG levels during both hollow fiber and flat plate dialysis

lant usage in the UK it was found that different Renal Units routinely administer heparin in doses that differ as much as 4-fold [Ireland et al. 1989]. Part of this variability is due to the problems of assessing both the actual level of heparin and its anticoagulant effects during dialysis. In this paper, we evaluate a simplified means of measuring heparin levels in whole blood, Heptest and compare it to an established plasma amidolytic method. We conclude that the whole blood Heptest provides a useful alternative to an amidolytic assay of anti-factor Xa activity during hemodialysis. The former test has the advantage that a result could be obtained minutes after blood collection. However, it should be stressed that the level of heparin alone does not necessarily provide an unambiguous guide to the suppression of blood coagulation activation in these patients: for the same heparin level different amounts of FPA generation and possibly clot formation can be obtained, depending on the type of dialysis membrane used.

We have shown previously in a series of studies that the FPA assay provides an objective means of detecting activation of coagulation during dialysis. Decreasing the dose of administered heparin produces decreasing plasma heparin levels and results in a progressive increase in FPA levels. Using the FPA assay, we have been able to compare the anticoagulant effects of heparin with those of low MW heparins and related compounds. However, there are a number of problems associated with the use of the FPA assay that have hindered its widespread adoption for this purpose. Firstly, meticulous attention has to be paid to blood collection and the processing procedures, in order that artifacts can be avoided. Secondly, a radioactive tracer has to be prepared and used. Finally, the minimum time required for assay is several hours, and optimum sensitivity can only be obtained if an overnight incubation step is included. Clearly, an assay that provides similar information, but that did not have these disadvantages might enjoy more widespread use.

In this paper we have compared the performance characteristics of two commercial assays used as markers for activated coagulation and presented as ELISAs, with those of the FPA assay (radioimmunoassay). We have also compared the characteristics of a platelet release marker (BTG) with FPA. Both ELISAs can be performed using citrated plasma (although blood collected into EDTA was used for this study) within 2 h and neither uses radioactive tracers. The results indicate that the FPA and TAT assays both respond similarly when the coagulation system is activated. FPA is generated when thrombin is generated, while TAT results from the inactivation

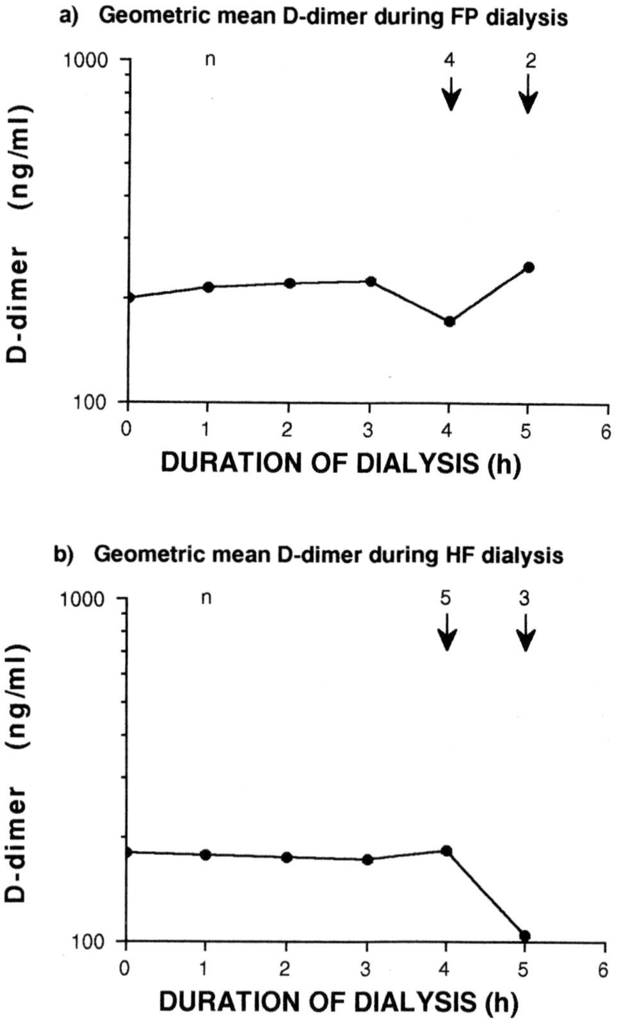

Fig. 10 Geometric mean D-dimer during dialysis with a) flat plate (FP) and b) hollow fiber (HF) dialysis

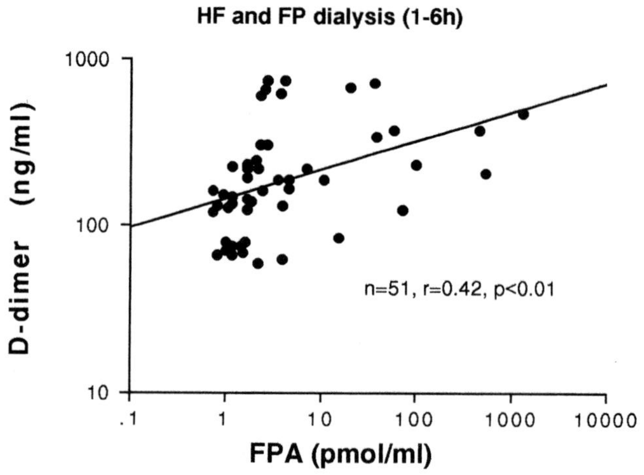

Fig. 11 Scattergram of FPA against D-dimer levels during both hollow fiber and flat plate dialysis

of thrombin by antithrombin. The present results suggest that in a situation in which heparin is limited and coagulation is stimulated, these two processes of proteolysis by thrombin and its inactivation are temporally related. The results further suggest that assay of TAT will provide a more readily available means of detecting activation of coagulation during hemodialysis.

In order that crosslinked fibrin fragments containing the D-dimer antigen be generated from clotting blood, both factor XIII and the fibrinolytic systems have to be activated. Previous studies using a low molecular weight marker of fibrinolytic system activation, fibrinogen fragment β1–42, suggested that during the time of hemodialysis (up to 6 h), in which fibrin had been generated (FPA was elevated), there was no simultaneous activation of fibrinolysis [Ireland et al. 1984]. This observation provides an explanation for the poor performance of the D-dimer assay in the present study; it appears that the fibrinolytic system may take considerable time to become activated sufficiently to generate D-dimer fragments from the fibrin that is rapidly formed during inadequate heparinization. Clearly, the D-dimer assay cannot be used to monitor activation of the coagulation/fibrinolytic system over the time period of a single dialysis session.

The final marker of hemostatic system imbalance investigated in this study is the platelet activation marker BTG, which was included here for completeness. Previous studies have suggested that the BTG assay can be used to monitor enhanced platelet release during hemodialysis, but that it does not respond to heparin inadequacy as well as the FPA assay. The present results confirm that BTG is a poorer marker than FPA and TAT. While both of these latter markers show a high negative correlation with the amount of heparin in plasma, BTG is less well correlated with anti-factor Xa levels during flat plate dialysis and not significantly correlated during hollow fiber dialysis. Elevated BTG levels first occur at the beginning of dialysis, when heparin levels are high, FPA and TAT levels low. BTG generation at this time may be caused by a direct effect of the dialysis membranes on platelets rather than by thrombin activity. BTG levels towards the end of dialysis with both membrane types follow more closely thrombin generation observed by FPA and TAT measurements. These elevations in BTG at 1-h dialysis can explain the lower correlations with heparin measurements (compared with FPA and TAT levels).

Acknowledgement

This work was supported by a grant from the Wellcome Trust to DAL.

REFERENCES

Boisclair MD, Lane DA, Wilde JT, Ireland H, Preston FE, Ofosu FA 1990 A comparative evaluation of assays for markers of activated coagulation and/or fibrinolysis: thrombin-antithrombin complex, D-dimer and fibrinogen/fibrin fragment E antigen. British Journal of Haematology *74:* 471

Gordge MP, Faint RW, Rylance PB, Ireland H, Lane DA, Neild GH 1989 Plasma D dimer: a useful marker of fibrin breakdown in renal failure. Thrombosis and Haemostasis *61* (3): 522

Ireland H, Lane DA, Curtis JR 1984 Objective assessment of heparin requirements for haemodialysis in humans. Journal of Laboratory and Clinical Medicine *103:* 643

Ireland H, Lane DA, Flynn A, Anastassiades E, Curtis JR 1986 The anticoagulant effect of heparinoid Org 10172 during haemodialysis: an objective assessment. Thrombosis and haemostasis *55:* 2271

Ireland H, Lane DA, Flynn A, Pegrum AC, Curtis JR 1988 Low molecular weight heparin in haemodialysis for chronic renal failure: dose finding study of CY222. Thrombosis and haemostasis *59:* 2240

Ireland H, Kesterven P, Rylance P 1989 Heparin as an anticoagulant during extracorporeal circulation. In: *Lane DA, Lindahl U* (eds). Heparin: chemical and biological properties, clinical applications. Edward Arnold, London, p 549

Lane DA, Ireland H, Flynn A, Anastassiades E, Curtis JR 1986a Haemodialysis with low MW heparin: dosage requirements for the elimination of extracorporeal fibrin formation. Nephrology Dialysis Transplantation *1:* 179

Lane DA, Ireland H, Wolff S, Grant R, Jennings S, Allen-Mersh T 1982 Plasma concentrations of fibrinopeptide A, fibrinogen fragment BB1–42 and B-thromboglobulin following total hip replacement. Thrombosis Research *26:* 111

Lane DA, Flynn A, Ireland H, Anastassiades E, Curtis JR 1986b On the evaluation of heparin and low molecular weight heparin in haemodialysis for chronic renal failure. Haemostasis *16* (suppl. 2): 38

Ljunberg B 1985 A low molecular weight fragment as an anticoagulant during haemodialysis. Clinical Nephrology *24:* 15

Ljunberg B, Blomback M, Johnsson H, Lins L-E 1987 A single dose of a low molecular weight fragment for anticoagulation during haemodialysis. Clinical Nephrology *27:* 31

Pelzer H, Schwarz A, Heimburger N 1988 Determination of human thrombin-antithrombin III complex in plasma with an enzyme-linked immunosorbent assay. Thrombosis and Haemostasis *59:* 101–106

Rylatt DB, Blake AS, Cottis LE, Massingham DA, Fletcher WA, Masci PP, Whitaker An, Elms M, Bunce I, Webber AJ, Wyatt D, Bundseden PG 1983 An immunoassaý for human D dimer using monoclonal antibodies. Thrombosis Research *31:* 767

Tew CJ, Lane DA, Thompson E, Ireland H, Curtis JR 1988 Relationship between proteinase (factor Xa and thrombin) assays and in vivo anticoagulant effect of very low MW heparin CY222. British Journal of Haematology *70:* 335

Wilde JT, Kitchen S, Kinsey S, Greaves M, Preston FE 1989 Plasma D-dimer levels and their relationship to serum fibrinogen/ fibrin degradation products in hypercoagulable states. British Journal of Haematology *71:* 65

Wilhemsson S, Kockum K, Ivermark C, Kudryk KB, Robinson D, Biberfeld P 1983 Thrombin activity during haemodialysis evaluated by the fibrinopeptide A assay. A comparison between a high and a low dose heparin regime. Thrombosis Research *31:* 685

Clinical Nephrology, Vol. 35 No. 1 – 1991 (35–38)

Echocardiographic findings in hemodialysis patients treated with recombinant human erythropoietin: proposal for a hematocrit most beneficial to hemodynamics

H. TAGAWA, M. NAGANO, H. SAITO, M. UMEZU AND M. YAMAKADO

Department of Internal Medicine, Mitsui Memorial Hospital, Kanda Izumicho, Tokyo 101, Japan

Abstract. We investigated the hemodynamic effects of the correction of anemia with recombinant human erythropoietin (rHuEPO) in 28 hemodialysis patients with severe anemia. Echocardiograms were recorded before the administration of rHuEPO (period I) with a hematocrit of 19.2 ± 1.5% (mean ± SD) and repeated twice (periods II and III) when the hematocrit was increased to 25.7 ± 1.1% and to 30.0 ± 1.0%. Left ventricular end-diastolic dimension (LVDd) decreased from 51.0 ± 6.1 to 48.8 ± 5.8 and to 48.3 ± 7.1 mm, but no changes were observed in left ventricular end-systolic dimension. Cardiac output (CO) decreased from 5.89 ± 1.46 to 5.00 ± 1.44 and to 4.67 ± 1.33 l/min. The thickness of the interventricular septum and the left ventricular posterior wall remained unchanged. Blood pressure was kept rather constant, although antihypertensive therapy needed to be adjusted to prevent the occurrence or aggravation of hypertension. Total peripheral resistance increased from 1481 ± 359 to 1832 ± 487 and to 1946 ± 493 dynes · sec/cm^5. The decreases in LVDd and CO were significant between periods I and II, without further changes between periods II and III. More antihypertensive therapy was needed in period III than in period II. Similar echocardiographic results were observed in 10 patients in whom antihypertensive therapy was not required throughout the study. In conclusion, an increase in hematocrit to 25% would be appropriate in order to obtain an effective hemodynamic improvement with rHuEPO therapy in dialysis patients although a higher hematocrit level might be desirable in order to improve working capacity.

Key words: echocardiography – hemodialysis – hemodynamics – hypertension – recombinant human erythropoietin

Introduction

Blood erythropoietin levels in dialysis patients are inappropriately low for the severity of anemia [Tagawa et al. 1990] and numerous clinical studies have confirmed that recombinant human erythropoietin (rHuEPO) remarkably improves anemia [Winearls et al. 1986, Eschbach et al. 1987, Akizawa et al. 1988] which is the major cause of the symptoms that limit the quality of life and preclude full rehabilitation.

Echocardiographic evaluations have revealed that left ventricular hypertrophy and dilatation are predominant features in patients with chronic renal failure [Cohen et al. 1979, Miach et al. 1981, Mehta et al. 1983] and that the enlargement of the left ventricle is closely related to the extent of anemia [London et al. 1987]. It is therefore expected that the correction of anemia with rHuEPO could normalize cardiac function, although the increase in blood pressure frequently observed with the therapy may oppose the beneficial hemodynamic effects [Eschbach and Adamson 1988, Samtleben et al. 1988]. In the present study, we investigated the hemodynamic effects of rHuEPO therapy using echocardiography and proposed the most appropriate hematocrit level to obtain the most efficient hemodynamic benefits.

Patients and methods

The study was performed in 28 hemodialysis patients (15 males and 13 females) with severe renal

Received June 18, 1990; in revised form November 12, 1990.
Reprint requests to Dr. H. Tagawa.

Table 1 Comparison of hematocrit and hemodynamic parameters for all 28 patients

	period I	period II	period III
hematocrit (%)	19.2 ± 1.5	25.7 ± 1.1[a]	30.0 ± 1.0[a,d]
body weight (kg)	49.0 ± 8.6	48.9 ± 8.7	48.9 ± 9.1
LVDd (mm)	51.0 ± 6.1	48.8 ± 5.8[b]	48.3 ± 7.1[b]
LVDs (mm)	32.7 ± 6.9	31.9 ± 6.5	32.2 ± 8.4
IVST (mm)	12.2 ± 2.0	12.5 ± 2.4	12.6 ± 3.1
PWT (mm)	11.0 ± 2.4	11.4 ± 1.9	11.3 ± 1.7
ET (sec)	0.36 ± 0.03	0.35 ± 0.04	0.35 ± 0.04
HR (beats/min)	71.5 ± 10.5	70.1 ± 9.9	70.3 ± 8.6
SV (ml/beat)	83.1 ± 19.8	71.5 ± 17.7[a]	67.2 ± 19.6[a]
CO (l/min)	5.89 ± 1.46	5.00 ± 1.44[a]	4.67 ± 1.33[a]
EF (%)	68.3 ± 9.5	66.5 ± 9.1	65.3 ± 11.9[b]
mVcf (circle/sec)	1.04 ± 0.24	1.02 ± 0.24	0.99 ± 0.30
SBP (mmHg)	151.4 ± 18.6	154.7 ± 20.6	152.4 ± 19.9
DBP (mmHg)	79.6 ± 10.5	84.7 ± 11.1[c]	84.8 ± 12.7
MBP (mmHg)	103.6 ± 12.4	108.0 ± 13.3	107.3 ± 14.0
TPR (dynes · sec/cm^5)	1481 ± 359	1832 ± 487[a]	1946 ± 493[a]

Values are expressed as means ± SD.
[a]p <0.001, [b]p <0.01, [c]p <0.05 compared to period I.
[d]p <0.001 compared to period II.
Abbreviations are defined in the text.

anemia having a mean hematocrit of 19.2%. Their ages ranged from 19 to 70 years (mean of 46). They were undergoing regular hemodialysis for 4 to 4.5 hours three times a week using a hollow fiber dialyzer for periods between 2 to 156 months (mean of 62). Antihypertensive drugs had been administered in 15 patients. No patients had any apparent cardiac symptoms.

Patients were treated by intravenous administration of rHuEPO (Chugai Pharmaceutical Co., Ltd., Tokyo) at the end of each hemodialysis. The starting dose was 1,500 units and the dose was doubled to 3,000 or 6,000 units to maintain the steady increase in the hematocrit.

Echocardiograms were recorded before rHuEPO therapy (period I) and repeated twice when the hematocrit was increased by 5% to approximately 25% (period II) after treatment for between 4 and 24 weeks (mean of 9) and 30% (period III) after treatment for between 7 and 42 weeks (mean of 18). Echocardiographic studies were performed on the day after hemodialysis using a Toshiba Sonolayer SSH-65A with a probe Toshiba PSB-37R for M-mode and two-dimensional measurements. The ultrasonic beam was directed to traverse the left ventricular chamber at the level of the edges of mitral valve leaflets or the chordae. Left ventricular end-diastolic diameter (LVDd) and end-systolic diameter (LVDs), interventricular septal thickness (IVST), left ventricular posterior wall thickness (PWT) and ejection time (ET) were measured by the same observer following the recommendations of the American Society of Echocardiography [Sahn et al. 1978]. Data were derived from an average of at least 3 consecutive cardiac cycles. Stroke volume (SV) and ejection fraction (EF) were calculated from a regression equation described by Teicholz et al. [1976]. The mean velocity of circumferential fiber shortening (mVcf) was estimated using the method of Cooper et al. [1972]. Cardiac output (CO) and total peripheral resistance (TPR) were calculated according to the following formulae:

$$CO = SV \times HR \text{ (heart rate)},$$
$$TPR = (MBP/CO) \times 80,$$

where MBP (mean blood pressure) = DBP + (SBP − DBP) / 3; DBP = diastolic blood pressure, and SBP = systolic blood pressure.

The paired t-test was used to determine p values for statistical significance.

Results

Data concerning the hematocrit and the hemodynamic parameters are shown in Table 1. The hematocrit rose significantly from 19.2 ± 1.5% (period I; mean ± SD) to 25.7 ± 1.1% (period II) and 30.0 ± 1.0% (period III).

Correction of anemia induced a significant decrease in LVDd between periods I and II, but no further decrease was observed between periods II and III. No changes were observed in LVDs, IVST or PWT with an increase in hematocrit. HR remained fairly constant. SV and CO decreased with a correction of anemia; statistically significant differences were seen between periods I and II. EF decreased but mVcf did not change with an increase in hematocrit.

Blood pressure appeared to remain rather constant except for an increase in DBP between periods I and II. However, out of 15 patients who had received antihypertensive drugs, the doses were increased in 2 patients during period II and in 4 other patients during period III, while they decreased in only 1 and 2 other patients, respectively. Out of 13 patients who had not received antihypertensive drugs, antihypertensive therapy was initiated in 2 patients during period II and in another patient during period III. They consisted of calcium channel antagonists, converting enzyme inhibitors, beta-blockers and alpha$_1$-blockers. The need for initiating or intensifying antihypertensive therapy was related neither to the duration for the improvement of anemia nor to the dosage

Table 2 Comparison of hematocrit and hemodynamic parameters in 10 patients in whom antihypertensive drugs were not administered throughout the study

	period I	period II	period III
hematocrit (%)	19.1 ± 0.9	25.9 ± 1.2[a]	30.5 ± 0.5[a,c]
body weight (kg)	49.4 ± 9.6	49.6 ± 9.9	49.4 ± 10.2
LVDd (mm)	47.7 ± 2.9	45.2 ± 4.0[b]	44.0 ± 3.6[b]
LVDs (mm)	29.4 ± 3.9	28.3 ± 3.2	27.5 ± 4.0
IVST (mm)	11.6 ± 1.6	11.4 ± 1.3	11.7 ± 1.9
PWT (mm)	9.5 ± 1.6	10.7 ± 1.3	10.6 ± 1.8
ET (sec)	0.36 ± 0.03	0.35 ± 0.04	0.35 ± 0.03
HR (beats/min)	66.4 ± 9.7	65.8 ± 11.9	69.6 ± 11.1
SV (ml/beat)	74.6 ± 12.9	62.9 ± 12.6[b]	57.5 ± 12.9[b]
CO (l/min)	4.89 ± 0.68	4.04 ± 0.64[b]	3.90 ± 0.60[a]
EF (%)	71.5 ± 9.0	70.2 ± 4.2	69.5 ± 8.6
mVcf (circle/sec)	1.06 ± 0.15	1.08 ± 0.16	1.09 ± 0.22
SBP (mmHg)	147.6 ± 18.2	148.7 ± 22.1	141.1 ± 20.0
DBP (mmHg)	79.4 ± 12.4	81.5 ± 10.8	79.4 ± 12.3
MBP (mmHg)	102.2 ± 14.0	103.9 ± 13.7	100.0 ± 14.3
TPR (dynes · sec/cm^5)	1700 ± 303	2136 ± 604[b]	2097 ± 442[b]

Values are expressed as means ± SD.
[a] $p < 0.001$, [b] $p < 0.01$ compared to period I.
[c] $p < 0.001$ compared to period II.
Abbreviations are defined in the text.

of rHuEPO. Correction of anemia induced a marked rise in TPR with a statistically significant difference between periods I and II.

Table 2 shows the data for 10 patients in whom antihypertensive drugs were not administered throughout the study. The results were virtually identical to those mentioned above except for the absence of the changes in blood pressure.

Discussion

The present study indicates that the correction of anemia with rHuEPO in dialysis patients decreased left ventricular dimension and cardiac output and increases total peripheral resistance with the increase in hematocrit, although we have to admit there are unavoidable errors based on echocardiographic measurements and calculations.

It has been reported that hypertension frequently develops or becomes aggravated during rHuEPO therapy [Eschbach and Adamson 1988, Samtleben et al. 1988]. Total peripheral resistance increases with a rise in hematocrit; statistical significance was observed between hematocrits of 20% and 30%. This may be due to an increase in whole blood viscosity, better tissue oxygenation with suppression of hypoxic vasodilation, or possibly a direct vascular effect of erythropoietin. Blood pressure remained rather constant with the increase in hematocrit in the present study; however, antihypertensive therapy needed to be adjusted to maintain close control of blood pressure in some patients. The results might not be influenced by the change or initiation of antihypertensive drugs because a similar increase in peripheral resistance was also observed in patients in whom antihypertensive therapy was not required nor intensified throughout the study.

Myocardial hypertrophy has been reported to prevail in dialysis patients mainly because of earlier hypertension. We failed to show a regression of myocardial hypertrophy after the correction of anemia with rHuEPO. This may be due to the persistence or aggravation of hypertension and possibly from a short observation period. It has been reported that the left ventricular mass decreased with a rise in hematocrit in spite of the constancy of myocardial thicknes [London et al. 1989]. The apparent discrepancy of findings could be due to the formula employed by the previous investigators where reduction of the left ventricular dimension would overestimate the left ventricular mass decrease.

A decrease in ejection fraction was observed with the correction of anemia. This may not indicate the worsening of cardiac function, but could result from a reduction in the left ventricular dimension because no change in the velocity of circumferential fiber shortening was observed. Investigations have shown partially contradictory results with respect to myocardial contractility. It was indicated that the improved myocardial contractility was obtained by an elevation of ejection fraction and the velocity of circumferential fiber shortening, although a decrease in left ventricular fraction was observed in some cases [Löw et al. 1989]. Other investigators have observed an absence of significant changes in ejection fraction and the velocity of circumferential fiber shortening [London et al. 1989]. The discrepancy in the findings may result from previous differences in heart size or myocardial impairment due to hypertension, fluid imbalance, calcification or uremic toxins.

An enlargement of the left ventricular cavities accompanied by an increase in cardiac output has been observed in dialysis patients. This may be mainly attributed to chronic flow overload and to decreased vascular resistance due to renal anemia and a dialysis fistula in the absence of overt fluid retention. The present observation that left ventricular dimension and cardiac output decreased in parallel with the correction of anemia with rHuEPO has also been observed in previous studies [Löw et al. 1989, London et al. 1989]. Although heart size and cardiac output decreased with a rise in hematocrit from 20% to 25%, further improvements were not observed for a hematocrit of 30% in patients as a whole and more antihypertensive therapy was required in some patients with a hematocrit of 30% than in those with one of 25%. Similar echocardiographic results were obtained in patients who were normotensive without antihypertensive therapy throughout the study. It is therefore proposed that an increase in hematocrit to 25% may be beneficial in order to obtain efficient hemodynamic improvement although a higher hematocrit level would be desirable for improving working capacity.

Acknowledgements

The authors are greatly indebted to Dr. Tadahiro Nishi of Nishi Clinic, Dr. Kyosuke Nishio of Shin-Koiwa Clinic, Dr. Richiko Sato of Keiyo Hospital, Dr. Kimihiko Haida of Hanzomon Hospital, Dr. Akiko Ogura of Higashi-Kanda Clinic and Dr. Noriko Kimura of Izumi Clinic for entering their patients in the study, and to Chugai Pharmaceutical Co., Ltd. for supplying the rHuEPO.

REFERENCES

Akizawa T, Koshikawa S, Takaku F, Urabe A, Akiyama N, Mimura N, Otsubo O, Nihei H, Suzuki Y, Kawaguchi Y, Ota K, Kubo K, Marumo F, Maeda T 1988 Clinical effect of recombinant human erythropoietin on anemia associated with chronic renal failure. A multi-institutional study in Japan. Int J Artif Organs *11:* 19

Cohen MV, Diaz P, Scheuer J 1979 Echocardiographic assessment of left ventricular function in patients with chronic uremia. Clin Nephrol *12:* 156

Copper RH, O'Rourke RA, Karliner JS, Peterson KL, Leopold GR 1972 Comparison of ultrasound and cineangiographic measurements of the mean heart rate of circumferential fiber shortening. Circulation *46:* 914

Eschbach JW, Adamson JW 1988 Recombinant human erythropoietin: implications for nephrology. Am J Kid Dis *11:* 203

Eschbach JW, Egrie JC, Downing MR, Browne JK, Adamson JW 1987 Correction of the anemia of end-stage renal disease with recombinant human erythropoietin. Results of a combined phase I and II clinical trial. N Engl J Med *316:* 73

London GM, Fabiani F, Marchais SJ, De Vernejoul MCh, Guerin AP, Safar ME, Metivier F, Llach F 1987 Uremic cardiomyopathy: an inadequate left ventricular hypertrophy. Kidney Int *31:* 973

London GM, Zins B, Pannier B, Naret C, Berthelot J-M, Jacquot C, Safar M, Drueke TB 1989 Vascular changes in hemodialysis patients in response to recombinant human erythropoietin. Kid Int *36:* 878

Löw I, Grützmacher P, Bergmann M, Schoeppe W 1989 Echocardiographic findings in patients on maintenance hemodialysis substituted with recombinant human erythropoietin. Clin Nephrol *31:* 26

Mehta BR, Ireland MA, Shiu MF 1983 Echocardiographic evaluation of cardiac size and function in dialysis patients. Clin Nephrol *20:* 61

Miach PJ, Dawborn JK, Louis WJ, McDonald IG 1981 Left ventricular function in uremia: echocardiographic assessment in patients on maintenance dialysis. Clin Nephrol *15:* 259

Sahn DJ, De Maria A, Kisslo J, Weyman A 1978 Recommendations regarding quantitation in M-mode echocardiographic measurements. Circulation *58:* 1072

Samtleben W, Baldamus CA, Bommer J, Fassbinder W, Nonnast-Daniel B, Gurland HJ 1988 Blood pressure changes during treatment with recombinant erythropoietin. Contrib Nephrol *66:* 114

Tagawa H, Umezu M, Saito T, Yamakado M, Nagano M, Urabe A, Takaku F 1990 Regulatory mechanisms of erythropoietin levels in dialysis patients. Jpn J Nephrol *32:* 297

Teicholz LE, Kreulen T, Herman MV, Gorlin R 1976 Problems in echocardiographic volume determinations. Echocardiographic-angiographic correlations in the presence or absence of asynergy. Am J Cardiol *37:* 7

Winearls CG, Oliver DO, Pippard MJ, Reid C, Downing MR, Cotes PM 1986 Effects of human erythropoietin derived from recombinant DNA on the anaemia of patients maintained by chronic haemodialysis. Lancet *2:* 1175

Clinical Nephrology, Vol. 35 No. 1 – 1991 (39–43)

Long-term minoxidil treatment in refractory hypertension and renal failure

R. Pontremoli[1], C. Robaudo[1], A. Gaiter[2], F. Massarino[1] and G. Deferrari[1]

[1] *Divisions of Nephrology and of Clinical Methodology, University of Genoa, Italy*
[2] *Present address: Division of Nephrology, Aosta Hospital, Italy*

Abstract. Twenty-two patients with severe or accelerated hypertension refractory to conventional hypotensive therapy have been treated with minoxidil for an extended period. Patients were divided in three groups according to different degrees of renal function or the presence of accelerated hypertension. In the first group (8 patients with normal or slightly decreased renal function) BP fell from 197 ± 11/118 ± 3 before minoxidil therapy to 157 ± 7/98 ± 2 after six months ($p < 0.001$), and remained steady during the following eighteen months. In the second group (9 patients with creatinine clearance of 30 ± 3 ml/min · 1.73 m^2) BP decreased from 192 ± 9/119 ± 4 to 147 ± 6/91 ± 4 at six months ($p < 0.001$); renal function did not show any significant modification during the eighteen months of the study. In the third group (5 patients with accelerated hypertension) BP fell from 243 ± 14/137 ± 6 to 166 ± 13/99 ± 7 at six months ($p < 0.01$). Seven patients, four in the first and three in the second group, were followed for more than six years; these patients, with mild renal insufficiency (creatinine clearance 50 ± 4 ml/min) before minoxidil therapy, were on a protein unrestricted diet for the entire length of the study. In this group of patients BP fell from 182 ± 9/115 ± 3 to 150 ± 6/96 ± 2 after one year ($p < 0.01$) and remained well controlled for the following six years or more. Renal function did not show any significant worsening over the years (monthly decrement in creatinine clearance 0.08 ml/min). In conclusion minoxidil proved to be highly effective in the management of severe hypertension both in patients with normal renal function and with different degrees of renal insufficiency; the control of blood pressure values obtained with minoxidil therapy is associated with a slow down in the progression of renal failure.

Key words: minoxidil – severe hypertension – accelerated hypertension – renal failure progression

Introduction

Minoxidil (6-amino-1,2-dihydroxyl-1-hydroxy-2-imino-4-piperidinopyrimidine) is an orally active potent vasodilator drug which acts directly on the arteriolar smooth muscle [DuCharme and Zins 1980, Lowenthal and Affrime 1980]. Like other vasodilators, it causes reflex tachycardia and fluid retention. These side effects can be effectively overcome with the use of diuretics and beta blockers or clonidine [Gilmore et al. 1970, DuCharme et al. 1973, DuCharme and Zins 1980]. Earlier studies have shown the effectiveness of minoxidil in the treatment of severe hypertension or hypertension refractory to common hypotensive agents [Gottlieb et al. 1972, Larochelle et al. 1980]. Furthermore, in the short term, minoxidil therapy has been shown to preserve glomerular filtration rate in patients with severe hypertension and decreased renal function [Gilmore et al. 1970, Gottlieb et al. 1972, Grim et al. 1979, Larochelle et al. 1980]. However, the effects of minoxidil on renal function during long-term treatment are not well known [Dargie et al. 1977, Andersson and Sivertsson 1980, Kern et al. 1980, Mitchell and Pettinger 1980, Taverner et al. 1983]. The purpose of this study is to report the effects of minoxidil on blood pressure and renal function in patients with severe or accelerated hypertension, both in the short period and after several years follow-up.

Received February 20, 1990; in revised form November 12, 1990.

Reprint requests to Dr. R. Pontremoli, Dipartimento Medicina Interna, Division of Nephrology, Viale Benedetto XV, 6, I-16132 Genova, Italy.

Patients and methods

Patients

From January 1978 up to the present date, we have studied 22 patients with severe or accelerated hypertension. Major clinical

Table 1 Clinical data before minoxidil therapy

	Group I	Group II	Group III
Patients	8	9	5
Age (years)	54± 3	46±5	44± 2
History of hypertension (years)	8± 4	7±1	4± 2
GFR (ml/min · 1.73 m^2)	73± 8	30±3	6.0± 1.7*
Blood pressure (mmHg)	S 197±11	S 192±9	S 243±13
	D 118± 3	D 119±4	D 137± 6
Heart rate (beats/min)	72± 3	73±5	70± 3
Retinal lesions**	0–II	0–II	II–IV
ECG pattern	normal – –LVH+strain	normal – –LVH+strain	normal – –LVH+strain

* Serum creatinine values; ** According to Keith-Wagener-Barker classification

characteristics of the patients are reported in Table 1. Patients were divided into three groups according to different degrees of renal function or the presence of accelerated hypertension. The first group included 8 patients (4 men and 4 women) with glomerular filtration rate normal or slightly decreased before minoxidil treatment. Three had renovascular hypertension, two nephroangiosclerosis, one essential hypertension, one chronic pyelonephritis and one chronic glomerulonephritis. The second group included 9 patients (8 men and 1 woman) with mild to moderate renal failure (creatinine clearance between 20 and 50 ml/min × 1.73 m^2). Five had nephroangiosclerosis, two chronic pyelonephritis, one renovascular hypertension and one chronic glomerulonephritis. Finally the third group was composed of 5 men with accelerated hypertension (one with renovascular hypertension, and four with essential hypertension).

All patients were on a low sodium, protein-unrestricted diet during previous antihypertensive treatment and continued so during the entire study. At the beginning of minoxidil therapy, no patient showed evidence of chronic heart failure or renal failure on a prerenal basis. Criteria to start minoxidil therapy were: ineffective blood pressure control after three months of therapy with various combinations of common antihypertensive agents, or side effects unacceptable to patients.

Medication given to patients before minoxidil therapy was gradually withdrawn except for beta blockers and diuretics. Monoxidil was started at a 2.5 mg/day dose and increased periodically as well as beta blockers and diuretics to counteract fluid retention and tachycardia. All patients were aware of possible side effects of the drug and gave informed consent prior to initiation of therapy with minoxidil.

Before minoxidil treatment was started, blood pressure and heart rate, ECG, eyeground and common laboratory tests were evaluated. Renal function was evaluated during the study using creatinine clearance in patients of group 1, and serum creatinine in patients of group 2 and 3. Patients in the first and second group were seen at intervals of three months after the beginning of therapy and followed up to 18 months. Patients in the third group were followed only for twelve months. Seven patients, four in the first group (creatinine clearance 57.5 ± 2.0 ml/min × 1.73 m^2), two with renovascular hypertension, one with nephroangiosclerosis, one with chronic pyelonephritis, and three in the second group (creatinine clearance 42.0 ± 3.5 ml/min × 1.73 m^2), two with nephroangiosclerosis and one with renovascular hypertension, were seen every six months and followed up for more than six years (97 ± 9 months).

Methods

Clinical examination, including body weight estimation, blood pressure measurements, blood and urinary tests and urinalysis were performed at the time of each visit. Blood pressure was determined after a ten-minute rest in supine position with a Riva Rocci sphygmomanometer using the fifth phase of Korotkoff sounds to determine the diastolic pressure. The average of three consecutive readings was calculated and considered the blood pressure reading for that visit. Serum and urine creatinine concentrations were determined according to Hare's method, based on colorimetric reaction of Jaffé [Hare 1950]. Urinary urea was determined enzymatically [Chaney and Marbasch 1962]. Statistical analysis was performed by analysis of variance by using a completely randomized design. A randomized block design was applied to the analysis of variance of the paired data [Snedecor and Cochran 1967]. Results are given as mean ± SEM.

Results

Table 1 shows the results of minoxidil therapy on blood pressure and renal function in the patients of groups 1 and 2. In group 1 patients after 3 months of minoxidil therapy systolic blood pressure fell from 197 ± 11 to 160 ± 8 mmHg ($p < 0.001$) and remained steady during the following months. Diastolic blood pressure fell from 118 ± 3 to 100 ± 3 after 3 months ($p < 0.001$) and further decreased significantly to 96 ± 4 at 18 months. Creatinine clearance did not show any significant change in these patients during the period of the study. In the patients of the second group systolic blood pressure fell from 192 ± 9 to 157 ± 6 after 3 months ($p < 0.001$) and remained significantly lower than basal value after 18 months (150 ± 8). Diastolic blood pressure fell to 98 ± 4 after 3 months from a basal value of 119 ± 4 ($p < 0.01$) and was 90 ± 5 ($p < 0.001$) at 18 months. Serum creatinine did not show any significant modification in the meantime. Figure 1 shows the effects of minoxidil on blood pressure and serum creatinine in 5 patients with accelerated hypertension. Systolic blood pressure fell significantly from 243 ± 13 to 173 ± 12 ($p < 0.001$) and diastolic blood pressure from 137 ± 6 to 98 ± 5 ($p < 0.01$) after 3 months. Values remained steady during the following months for the entire period of study. As indicated by the course of renal function in these patients, 2 out of 5 had a remarkable improvement of serum creatinine after blood pressure control was achieved. Three patients showed progressive worsening of their renal function over a period of 12 months despite a good control of blood pressure.

After 18 months of therapy, minoxidil was given at a daily dosage of 15 ± 3 mg in patients of group 1 and 10 ± 1 mg in group 2. Furosemide dosage was 115 ± 31 mg/day and 140 ± 64 mg/day, respectively in the first and second group. In patients of the third group, the mean daily dosage of minoxidil was 18 ± 5 mg after 12 months and furosemide 344 ± 101 mg/day (Table 3). Body weight was not significantly modified during minoxidil treatment.

The results of minoxidil therapy in 7 patients followed up for a very long time (97 ± 9 months, range 72–136) are reported in Figure 2. This figure shows the course of blood pressure and renal function during a six-year period. Five of these patients were followed up for an even longer period of time and the latest available data are also reported in the figure. Systolic blood pressure after a fall from 182 ± 9 to 150 ± 6 ($p < 0.01$) during the first year remained steady throughout the study and was 141 ± 5 after 6 years. Diastolic blood pressure fell from 115 ± 3 to 96 ± 2 ($p < 0.001$) after one year and was 90 ± 3 after 6 years of therapy. Creatinine clearance was unchanged over the years of the study (50 ± 4 ml/min × 1.73 m^2 before minoxidil therapy and 49 ± 8 after six years). Urinary urea was 280 ± 35 mmol/24 h and was consistent with an average protein intake of 0.93 ± 0.10 g/kg body wt/day, as calculated by applying the formula proposed by Mitch [Mitch 1988]. In this group of patients, after six years, minoxidil and

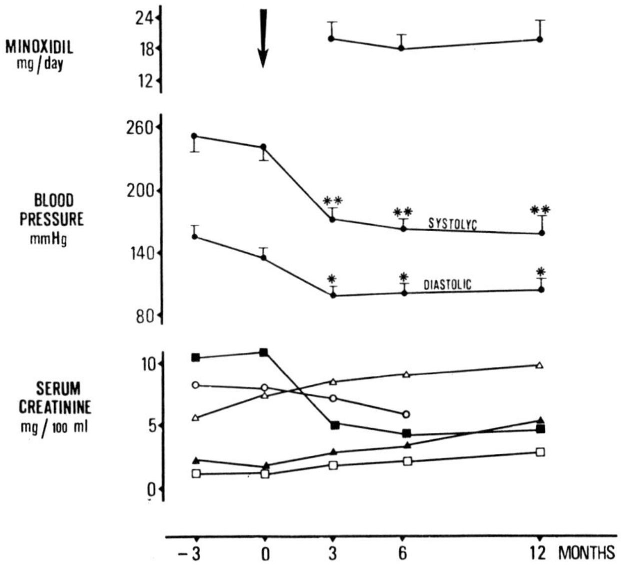

Fig. 1 Effects of minoxidil therapy on blood pressure and individual plasma creatinine values during twelve months follow up in group 3 patients. Significance of difference from basal values (0 time): * = $p < 0.01$, ** = $p < 0.001$

Table 2 Effects of minoxidil therapy on blood pressure and renal function during eighteen months follow up in patient group 1 and 2

	Basal values				3 months of minoxidil therapy					6 months of minoxidil therapy				
	SBP mmHg	DBP mmHg	Serum creat. mg%	Creatinine clearance ml/min· 1.73 m²	SBP mmHg	DBP mmHg	Serum creat. mg%	Creatinine clearance ml/min· 1.73 m²	Minoxidil dosage mg/day	SBP mmHg	DBP mmHg	Serum creat. mg%	Creatinine clearance ml/min· 1.73 m²	Minoxidil dosage mg/day
Group 1	197±11	118±3	1.2±0.1	73±8	160±8^c	100±3^c	1.3±0.2	79±10	9±2	157± 7^c	98±2^c	1.4±0.2	76±11	12±3
Group 2	192± 9	119±4	3.0±0.4	30±3	157±6^c	98±4^b	3.1±0.4	-	10±2	147± 6^c	91±4^c	3.1±0.4	-	11±2
					12 months of minoxidil therapy					18 months of minoxidil therapy				
Group 1	197±11	118±3	1.2±0.1	73±8	152±7^c	94±1^c	1.4±0.2	77±10	13±3	155±10^c	96±4^c	1.3±0.2	79± 8	15±3
Group 2	192± 9	119±4	3.0±0.4	30±3	149±6^c	91±3^c	3.3±0.4	-	12±2	150± 8^a	90±5^c	2.9±0.4	-	10±1

Basal values refer to data obtained on maximal therapy before minoxidil institution. Abbreviations used: SBP = systolic blood pressure; DBP = diastolic blood pressure. Significance of difference from basal values: a = $p < 0.025$; b = $p < 0.01$; c = $p < 0.001$. Data are reported as mean ± SEM.

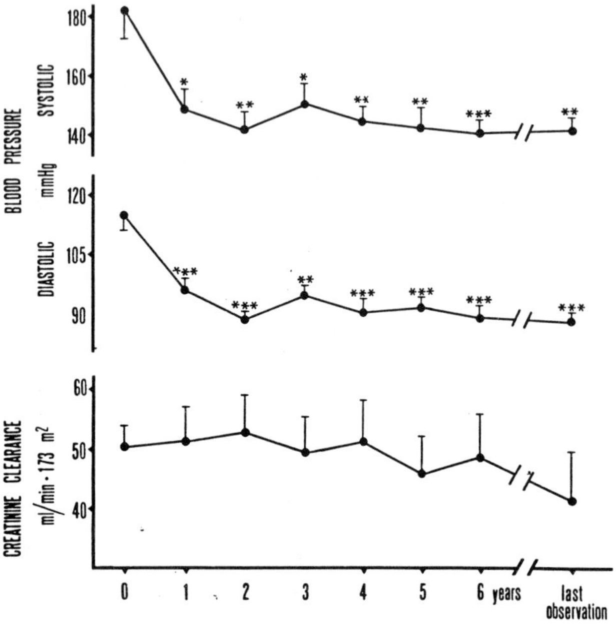

Fig. 2 Effects of minoxidil therapy on blood pressure and creatinine clearance in seven patients followed up for more than six years. Significance of difference from basal values (0 time): * = $p < 0.05$, ** = $p < 0.005$, *** = $p < 0.001$

Table 3 Antihypertensive therapy after 18 months of treatment (mg/day)

	Group I	Group II	Group III*
Minoxidil	15± 3	10± 1	18± 5
Blockers			
Propranolol	150±34	160±80	200±40
Pindolol	14± 8	–	–
Atenolol	100	75±14	100
Acebutolol	–	200	–
Nadolol	–	40	–
Furosemide	115±31	140±64	344±101

* Values at 12 months

furosemide dosage was 10 ± 2 mg/day and 125 ± 53 mg/day, respectively.

Discussion

Minoxidil was generally well tolerated. Side effects have been few and reasonable in the context of adequate blood pressure control. Hypertrichosis of various degrees was common in men as well as in women but was considered bothersome only by the women. No patients developed clinical or electrocardiographic signs assignable to heart ischemia following institution of the minoxidil regimen. ECG was performed at each outpatient visit and did not show any significant changes after the beginning of minoxidil therapy. Generally headache decreased or disappeared after reduction of arterial blood pressure with minoxidil and in no case increased. Tachycardia and fluid retention were fairly well controlled by using beta blockers and furosemide. Neither orthostatic hypotension nor severe hypokalemia was observed in any patient, even when large doses of furosemide were given. We did not observe tolerance to the drug during the study, and in no case did minoxidil therapy have to be stopped. Patients found the minoxidil regimen easier than their previous complicated therapy and therefore full compliance was achieved.

In our experience, as proven by many other reports [Gilmore et al. 1970, Pettinger and Mitchell 1973, Zacest et al. 1976, Dargie and Dolleri 1977, Devine et al. 1977, Keušch et al. 1978, Andersson and Sivertsson 1979, Grim et al. 1979], minoxidil was a very useful drug in patients where other antihypertensive drugs were poorly effective. Most patients achieved good blood pressure control. Remarkable results were obtained in patients with renal insufficiency. It is noteworthy that the blood pressure response was not related to the degree of renal functional impairment. In fact the average percentage of systolic and diastolic decrements were similar in patients of group 1 (21% systolic and 19% diastolic) and 2 (22% systolic and 25% diastolic). Renal function did not change significantly in patients of groups 1 and 2 during minoxidil treatment. Satisfactory blood pressure control was achieved even in patients with accelerated hypertension and two out of five patients showed an improvement of their renal function after control of their markedly elevated blood pressure.

It is worthy to note that in our patients with moderate renal failure (creatinine clearance between 36 and 65 ml/min × 1.73 m^2) on an unrestricted diet, followed up for more than six years with good control of blood pressure, creatinine clearance did not show any significant change: the monthly decline in creatinine clearance was 0.08 ml/min. A similar progression rate of renal insufficiency has been claimed in studies which evaluated for 16–20 months the role of hypoproteic diets on the decline of renal function in patients with creatinine clearance between 30 and 60 ml/min at the beginning of observation. In the study of Barsotti et al. [1984] patients with chronic renal failure and well controlled arterial blood pressure showed a monthly decline in creatinine clearance of 0.53 ml/min on a low protein diet, whereas a smaller decrement (0.07 ml/min/mo) was observed on a low-phosphorus, low-nitrogen diet. In the study of Rosman et al. [1986] patients allocated to a free diet group had a monthly decrease of creatinine clearance of 0.29 ml/min, while those treated with a low protein diet demonstrated a significantly better trend (mean decline in creatinine clearance 0.13 ml/min/mo). In this last study blood pressure values were comparable between the two groups, but it was not clear if they were well controlled. Accordingly, the role of arterial blood pressure in the progression of renal damage was not taken into account. When our results are compared with those reported in the above mentioned studies, it appears that good blood pressure control obtained through minoxidil, even in the absence of dietary restriction, slows down the worsening of renal function in patients with chronic renal failure. It has to be pointed out, however, that different degrees of renal impairment at the beginning of the study, as well as the presence of dissimilar nephropathies may have influenced in a different fashion the progression of renal insufficiency. In any case, the very long follow-up of our study, even in the presence of a small number of patients, suggests stimulating conclusions. Our data seem to indicate that blood pressure control, independent of dietary management, plays a role in slowing down the progression of renal failure, confirming other observations [Alvestrand et al. 1988, Brazy et al. 1989, Brazy and Fitzwilliam 1990]. A specific role of minoxidil per se in influencing the course of renal damage is so far unknown. In conclusion, minoxidil is highly effective in the management of severe hypertension both in patients with normal renal function and with different degrees of renal insufficiency. Minoxidil proved to be safe and well tolerated. On the basis of our results, a broader use of this drug in patients with severe hypertension and renal failure is strongly suggested. Whether minoxidil may exert a specific beneficial effect on renal hemodynamics deserves further study.

Acknowledgement

We gratefully acknowledge the help of Bioindustria Farmaceutici s. p. a. (Novi Ligure, Italy) for the supply of minoxidil.

REFERENCES

Alvestrand A, Gutierrez A, Bucht H, Bergstrom J 1988 Reduction of blood pressure retards the progression of chronic renal failure in man. Nephrol Dial Transplant *3:* 624

Andersson O, Sivertsson R 1979 Minoxidil in refractory hypertension. Acta Med Scand *205:* 213

Andersson O, Sivertsson R 1980 Renal function and vascular resistance during long-term minoxidil treatment of severe hypertension. J Cardiovasc Pharmacol *2:* S123

Barsotti G, Giannoni A, Morelli E, Lazzeri M, Vlamis I, Baldi R, Giovannetti S 1984 The decline of renal function slowed by very low phosphorus intake in chronic renal patients following a low nitrogen diet. Clin Nephrol *21:* 54

Brazy PC, Stead WN, Fitzwilliam JF 1989 Progression of renal insufficiency: role of blood pressure. Kidney Int *35:* 670

Brazy PC, Fitzwilliam JF 1990 Progression renal disease: role of race and antihypertensive medications. Kidney Int *37:* 1113

Chaney AL, Marbach PE 1962 Modified reagents for determination of urea and ammonia. Clin Chem *8:* 130

Dargie HJ, Dolleri CT, Daniel J 1977 Minoxidil in resistant hypertension. Lancet *2:* 515

Devine BL, Fife R, Trust PM 1977 Minoxidil for severe hypertension after failure of other hypotensive drugs. Br Med J *2:* 667

DuCharme DW, Freyburger WA, Graham BE, Carlson RG 1973 Pharmacologic properties of minoxidil: a new hypotensive agent. J Pharmacol Exp Ther *184:* 662

DuCharme DW, Zins GR 1980 Minoxidil. In: Pharmacology of antihypertensive drugs. *Scriabine A* (ed), New York, p 415

Gilmore E, Weil J, Chidsey C 1970 Treatment of essential hypertension with a new vasodilator in combination with beta-adrenergic blockade. N Eng J Med *282:* 521

Gottlieb TB, Katz FH, Chidsy C 1972 Combined therapy with vasodilator drugs and beta-adrenergic blockade in hypertension. Circulation *45:* 571

Grim CE, Luft FC, Grim CM, Klotman PE, Van Huysse JW, Weinberger MH 1979 Rapid blood pressure control with Minoxidil. Arch Intern Med *139:* 529

Hare RS 1950 Endogenous creatinine in serum and urine. Proc Soc Experiment Biol Med *74:* 148

Kern T, DeQuattro V, Bornheimer JF, DeQuattro E, Kolloch RE 1980 Longterm effects of minoxidil therapy on renal function of patients with refractory hypertension: the significance of albuminuria. J Cardiovasc Pharmacol *2:* S156

Keusch GW, Weidmann P, Campese V, Lee DBN, Upham AT, Massry SG 1978 Minoxidil therapy in refractory hypertension. Analysis of 155 patients. Nephron *21:* 1

Larochelle P, Beroniade V, Hamet P, Kuchel O 1980 Treatment of refractory hypertension with minoxidil. J Cardiovasc Pharmacol *2:* S107

Lowenthal DT, Affrime MB 1980 Pharmacology and pharmacokinetics of minoxidil. J Cardiovasc Pharmacol *2:* S93

Mitch WE 1988 Nutritional therapy and the progression of renal insufficiency. In: *Mitch WE, Klahr S* (eds) Nutrition and the kidney. Little, Brown and Company, Boston, p 154

Mitchell HE, Pettinger WA 1980 Renal function in long-term minoxidil-treated patients. J Cardiovasc Pharmacol *2:* S163

Pettinger WA, Mitchell HC 1973 Minoxidil – An alternative to nephrectomy for refractory hypertension. N Eng J Med *289:* 167

Rosman JB, Donker AJM, Meijer S, Sluiter WJ, Piers-Becht TPM, van der Hem GK 1986 Two years' experience with protein restriction in chronic renal failure. Contr Nephrol *53:* 109

Snedecor GW, Cochran WG 1967 Statistical methods. Ames: Iowa State University Press

Taverner D, Bing RF, Heagerty A, Russel GI, Pohl JEF, Swales JD, Thurston H 1983 Improvement of renal function during long-term treatment of severe hypertension with minoxidil. Quart J Med *206:* 280

Zacest R, Frewin DB, Robinson MA, Wilson LL, Lawrence JR, Clarkson AR, Jackson B 1976 Clinical and haemodynamic effects of minoxidil in refractory hypertension. Drugs *11:* 177

LETTERS TO THE EDITOR

Platelet factor 4 in IgA nephritis

Sir, – Increased in-vivo platelet activity has been demonstrated in various forms of glomerulonephritis and may play a role in the pathogenesis of IgA nephritis. We have previously shown that plasma β-thromboglobulin levels are increased in IgA nephritis and correlated with the degree of glomerular sclerosis [Woo et al. 1981 Throm Res *24:* 259–262]. Others have shown the presence of glomerular platelet aggregates in patients with glomerulonephritis [Kincaid-Smith 1983, Glomerulonephritis, 871–890] and intra-glomerular deposition of coagulation-fibrinolysis factors and platelet related antigens in IgA nephritis [Deguchi et al. 1989, Nephron *51:* 377–383]. This suggests that platelets are involved in progressive glomerular lesions.

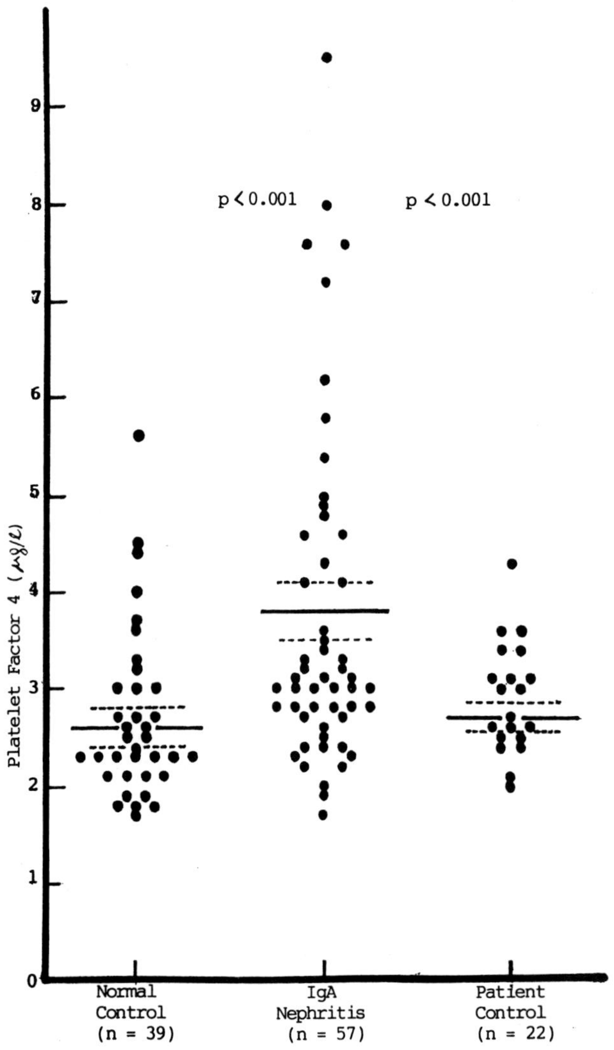

Fig. 1 Plasma platelet factor 4 concentrations in IgA nephritis, non-IgA nephritis and normal controls. Mean ± SEM shown. The platelet factor 4 concentrations were higher in IgA nephritis than those of non-IgA nephritis ($p < 0.001$) and normal controls ($p < 0.001$).

Platelet factor 4 (PF4) is a platelet specific protein that is released by the α-granule during platelet aggregation. It can thus be used as an index of in-vivo platelet aggregation. We measured plasma PF4 levels in patients with IgA nephritis and studied correlations with serum creatinine, proteinuria and histological parameters.

Plasma PF4 levels were determined using an enzyme immunoassay (Enzygnost Platelet Factor 4, Behringwerke AG, Marburg, Germany) in 57 patients with biopsy-proven IgA nephritis with serum creatinine ranging from 0.6 mg/dl to 1.6 mg/dl (1.1 mg/dl ± 0.04, mean ± SEM). PF4 levels were also determined in 39 patients with non-IgA nephritis and 22 normal healthy controls. The coefficient of variation for the PF4 assay was 9.7%.

Results are expressed as mean ± SEM. One-way analysis of variance and the Student's t-test were used to compare differences between the three groups, and Pearson's and Spearmann's correlations were used to study correlations between PF4 and various parameters.

The mean plasma PF4 levels in IgA patients (3.8 μg/l ± 0.26) was significantly elevated above the normal controls (2.63 μg/l ± 0.18, $p < 0.001$) and patient controls (2.7 μg/l ± 0.14, $p < 0.001$) (Figure 1). PF4 levels did not correlate with serum creatinine, proteinuria or histological parameters (percentage of sclerosis, arteriolar hyperplasia, crescents, fibrin deposits and intensity of mesangial IgA staining on immunofluorescence).

The present data suggest that in-vivo platelet activation is present in IgA nephritis although the actual site and mechanism of the platelet activity remains speculative. This evidence of increased platelet activity in IgA nephritis may form the basis for treatment regimens that include antiplatelet agents in this form of glomerulonephritis [Lee et al. 1989 Clin Nephrol *31:* 276, Woo et al. 1987 Clin Nephrol *27:* 56–64].

G. S. L. Lee, Y. K. Lau, K. T. Woo
Department of Renal Medicine, Singapore General Hospital, Singapore 0316

Reduced duration of bed rest after percutaneous renal biopsy*

Sir, – The period of bed rest employed after percutaneous renal biopsy in order to minimize hemorrhagic complications is usually 24 hours [Rosenbaum et al. 1978 Kidney Int 14: 87–92, Proesmans et al. 1982 Clin Nephrol 18: 257–262] but the optimum duration of bed rest has not been evaluated. It has been our impression that hemorrhage after percutaneous renal biopsy usually is apparent clinically within a few hours of the procedure, and a study we have carried out is consistent with this hypothesis.

* Supported by the Quality Assurance Project Grants Scheme of the Department of Health, NSW Government.

Table 1 Perirenal hematoma measurements (cm)

	TS L	W	A	C	LS L	W	A	C
6 h*	3.01 ± 1.10	0.79 ± 0.62	2.16 ± 2.91	7.22 ± 3.16	4.68 ± 2.03	0.78 ± 0.71	2.73 ± 2.22	10.62 ± 4.29
24 h*	2.73 ± 1.23	0.64 ± 0.53	1.56 ± 1.92	6.49 ± 3.09	4.19 ± 2.59	0.66 ± 0.69	2.20 ± 2.49	9.21 ± 5.28
p	<0.01	<0.001	<0.01	<0.01	<0.05	<0.01	<0.02	<0.01

Abbreviations:
TS transverse section, LS longitudinal section, L length, W width, A area, C circumference. Results are mean ± SD, n = 93.
* Signifies after percutaneous renal biopsy. p signifies p value by Student's t-test for paired data.

Consecutive patients having elective percutaneous renal biopsy followed by bed rest for 24 hours were studied. Biopsy was performed with fluoroscopic guidance using either a Tru-Cut disposable or a Franklin modified Vim-Silverman biopsy needle. Renal ultrasonography, principally with 3.5-MHz transducer, was performed by a single observer (M. P.) approximately 6 hours and 24 hours after biopsy using a real-time scanner (Diasonic DRF 400), and measurements of post biopsy hematoma size were made, the measurements at 24 hours being made without access to records of measurements at 6 hours. Maximum length and width of hematoma were measured in longitudinal and transverse planes, and area and circumference were calculated in the same planes using a computer digitization of hematoma outline. Clinical complications of biopsy were detected by scrutiny of medical records soon after discharge, and details confirmed by interview of attending medical and nursing staff. Perirenal hemorrhage was diagnosed clinically if manifest as loin pain requiring narcotic analgesia, which was ordered by house staff who were unaware of the study.

During a 14-month period 137 biopsies, of which 128 yielded renal tissue, were carried out on 127 normotensive adult patients whose serum creatinine was 0.13 ± 0.22 mmol/l (mean ± SD). Clinical complications developed after 9 biopsies. There was 1 case of perirenal hemorrhage and 8 cases of macroscopic hematuria. Bleeding became apparent within 6 hours of biopsy except for 3 cases of macroscopic hematuria when no urine was passed until after this time. However, in these 3 cases the first urine sample, passed between 7 and 12 hours after biopsy, contained macroscopic blood. Ultrasonography was achieved after 98 biopsies, but was precluded in the remainder due to organizational factors. Hematoma measurements are shown in Table 1.

Thus, 6 of 9 clinical complications were diagnosed within 6 hours of biopsy, and although the time of onset of the other 3 is not definite, the circumstances are consistent with development of bleeding within the first 6 hours. The changes in hematoma measurements by ultrasound show a strong trend for lessening of hematoma size between 6 and 24 hours after biopsy, compatible with cessation of bleeding by 6 hours after biopsy. Hematoma volume was not estimated but the several measurements in two opposite planes would necessarily reflect any changes in volume. Evidence indicates that changes in echogenicity of blood between 6 and 24 hours after clotting begins [Alanen and Kormano 1985 J Ultrasound Med 4: 421–425] should not cause underestimation of hematoma size 24 hours after biopsy.

Although commonly practiced, the need for bed rest for 24 hours after percutaneous renal biopsy has not been evaluated and thus may be unnecessary, resulting in inefficient use of hospital resources. This study favors the proposition that, in patients having 24-h bed rest after percutaneous renal biopsy, hemorrhagic complications manifest clinically within 6 hours of the procedure.

A study in patients undergoing percutaneous liver biopsy showed a similar frequency of hematoma formation in those having 6 hours of bed rest compared to 24-h bed rest [Minuk et al. 1987 Gastroenterology 92: 290–293], and further studies to evaluate the safety of mobilization 6 hours after percutaneous renal biopsy are warranted.

B. Jones, M. Puvaneswary, R. Nanra, P. Trevillian, S. Carney, A. Gillies
Departments of Nephrology and Radiology, Royal Newcastle Hospital, Newcastle NSW 2300, Australia

Mycobacterial avium-intracellulare infection of a renal allograft

Sir, – Renal allograft recipients are susceptible to a wide variety of infections with both common and opportunistic agents. Pathogens that rarely cause serious infection in normal hosts such as fungi and viruses frequently cause problems in renal allograft recipients. Though uncommon [Lichtenstein and MacGregor 1983], mycobacterial infections remain a serious problem among renal transplant recipients. By far the most frequent species is mycobacterial tuberculosis. Mycobacterial avium-intracellulare (MAI) infection is rare with involvement of the renal allograft not being heretofore described.

A 35-year-old asymptomatic HIV seropositive male recipient of a cadaveric renal transplant, with end-stage renal disease secondary to focal segmental glomerulosclerosis, presented with fever, acute allograft dysfunction and sterile pyuria 12 months postengraftment. Initial immunosuppression consisted of cyclosporine 5 mg/kg/day, prednisone 0.5 mg/kg/day and azathioprine 3 mg/kg/day. Early post-transplant course was remarkable for delayed graft function, one acute rejection episode successfully treated with methylprednisolone succinate and a stable serum creatinine of 185 μmol/l (2.1 mg/dl). Renal allograft biopsy revealed numerous beaded acid-fast bacilli both in granulomatous foci and focal area of suppurative inflammation involving both glomeruli and tubules. Biopsy culture grew MAI. There was no other evidence of mycobacterial infection with a normal chest roentgenogram, a negative tuberculin test and urine, sputum and bone marrow all negative for acid-fast bacilli. Anti-mycobacterial chemotherapy with isoniazid, rifampin and ethambutol was begun, and immunosuppressants were tapered. Fever subsided but renal function continued to deteriorate. Renal biopsy 2 weeks later showed partial resolution of granulomata with disappearance of acid-fast bacilli. A transplant nephrectomy performed 3 months later for recurrent fever and tender graft did not reveal acid fast bacilli or granulomata, but instead showed acute and chronic rejection with heavy interstitial infiltrates and intimal fibrosis with tubular atrophy.

Transplant recipients require treatment with corticosteroids in conjunction with other immunosuppressants which include azathioprine, cyclosporine, monoclonal and polyclonal antilymphocyte globulins, all of which interfere with cell-mediated immunity and thus predispose to mycobacterial disease, as shown by Lichtenstein and MacGregor [Lichtenstein and MacGregor 1983] who noted a high percentage (34%) of nontuberculous mycobacterial infections and an increased frequency of disseminated infection (43.5%) among renal transplant recipients. In addition, the propensity of HIV seropositive patients to develop symptomatic extrapulmonary mycobacterial disease is well known.

MAI is a ubiquitous and commonly identified environmental organism with a low virulence in normal hosts, though chronic pulmonary infection in patients with previous pulmonary damage has been described [Rosenzweig and Schlueter 1981]. Disseminated MAI, however, is being increasingly recognized in patients with AIDS or immunosuppression for hematologic malignancies [Greene et al. 1982, Guarda et al. 1984]. Organs involved include lung, lymph nodes, bone marrow, liver and gastrointestinal tract with involvement of brain, spleen and adrenals being described in AIDS patients at autopsy.

Whether the cause for MAI infection in our patient was related to HIV disease, pharmacologic immunosuppression or both, remains to be determined. Either way it represents a previously unrecognized cause of renal dysfunction in a renal allograft recipient.

N. Sumrani, V. Delaney, J. H. Hong, B. G. Sommer
Department of Surgery and Medicine, Division of Transplantation, State University of New York Health Science Center at Brooklyn, 450 Clarkson Ave, Box 40, Brooklyn NY 11203, USA

REFERENCES

Greene JB, Sidhu GS, Lewin S, Levine JF, Masur H, Simberkoff MS, Nicholas P, Good RC, Zolla-Pazner SB, Pollock AA, Tapper ML 1982 Mycobacterium avium-intracellulare: a cause of disseminated life threatening infection in homosexuals and drug abusers. Ann Intern Med *97:* 539–546

Guarda LA, Luna MA, Smith JL, Mansell PWA, Gyorkey F, Roca AN 1984 Acquired immunodeficiency syndrome: postmortem findings. Am J Clin Pathol *81:* 549–557

Lichtenstein IH, MacGregor RR 1983 Mycobacterial infections in renal transplant recipients: report of five cases and review of the literature. Rev Infect Dis *5:* 216–222

Rosenzweig DY, Schlueter DP 1981 Spectrum of clinical disease in pulmonary infection with mycobacterium avium-intracellulare. Rev Infect Dis *3:* 1046–1501

Clinical Nephrology, Vol. 35 No. 2 – 1991 (47 – 51)

Membranoproliferative glomerulonephritis associated with sickle cell disease in two siblings

S. S. Iskandar, R. G. Morgann, M. C. Browning† and W. B. Lorentz

Departments of Pathology and Pediatrics, The Bowman Gray School of Medicine, Wake Forest University, Winston Salem, North Carolina, USA

Abstract. The cases of two brothers with sickle-cell anemia complicated by the nephrotic syndrome and membranoproliferative glomerulonephritis are presented. The literature related to this infrequent association is reviewed and possible explanations for the occurrence of the latter in two brothers are discussed.

Key words: membranoproliferative glomerulonephritis – mesangiocapillary glomerulonephritis – immune-complexes – sickle cell disease – nephrotic syndrome

Introduction

In 1958 Berman and Schreiner published what was probably the first case report of sickle cell disease (SDC)-associated nephrotic syndrome. Since then, 55 additional SCD patients with clinical evidence of glomerular disease, other than poststreptococcal glomerulonephritis, have been reported [Berman and Tublin 1959, Sweeney et al. 1962, Barnett and Bernstein 1968, McCoy 1969, Walker et al. 1971, Antonovytch 1972, Strom et al. 1972, Elfenbein et al. 1974, Pardo et al. 1975, Bakir et al. 1987]. The morphologic lesions most frequently identified in these cases appear to be membranoproliferative glomerulonephritis (MPGN), and focal glomerulosclerosis (FGS). We present here the cases of two brothers with sickle-cell anemia who developed the nephrotic syndrome within 2 weeks of each other due to biopsy-proven MPGN. We also critically review the pathologic data available in the 55 other cases of SCD-associated nephropathy unrelated to streptococcal infection identified in the literature.

Case reports

Case 1

WG is a 17-year-old black male sickle cell anemia patient who presented to his local physician with a 3-day history of abdominal fullness, swollen ankles, facial swelling, and shortness of breath. On physical examination, his blood pressure was 150/78 mmHg, and periorbital and pretibial edema was present accompanied by ascites. There was proteinuria of >3 g/l, 4–6 RBC/HPF, numerous leukocytes and 0–2 fine granular casts/HPF. Total serum protein was 41 g/l, albumin 18 g/l, plasma cholesterol 7.06 mmol/l, and triglycerides 248 mg/dl.

Urine protein was 12.8 g/24 h and the creatinine clearance was 1.53 ml/s/m^2. Serum streptozyme level was 400 IU/ml. ANA was negative, as was a screen for circulating immune complexes. C3 was 0.47 g/l (normal 0.55–1.20 g/l). The hemoglobin level was 49 g/l and the hematocrit was 0.14. The white blood cell count was 23 × 10^9/l. Serum liver enzyme levels were unremarkable.

The patient received a blood transfusion and a renal biopsy was performed.

Case 2

KG is the 15-year-old brother of WG. He presented to his local physician, 2 weeks after the onset of his brother's illness complaining of facial and ankle swelling, and abdominal distension. Hemoglobin electrophoresis revealed sickle-cell anemia. On physical examination at North Carolina Baptist Hospital he weighed 129 lb. Blood pressure was 130/80 mmHg. Serum electrolytes were normal. Serum creatinine was 141 µmol/l and BUN 24 mmol/l. Serum protein, albumin, and cholesterol were 45 g/l, 21 g/l and 8.04 mmol/l respectively. Urinalysis revealed proteinuria of 3 g/l, 10–15 RBC/HPF, 1–3 WBC/HPF and few bacteria. His hemoglobin was 84 g/l and the hematocrit was 0.23. The white blood cell and differential counts were within normal limits. A 12-hour urine collection revealed a creatinine

Received August 17, 1990; in revised form November 12, 1990.

Reprint requests to Dr. S. S. Iskandar, Department of Pathology, The Bowman Gray School of Medicine, 300 S. Hawthorne Road, Winston Salem, NC 27103, USA.

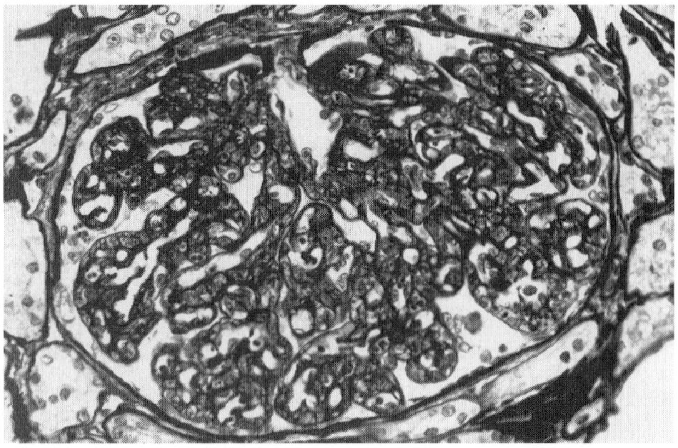

Fig. 1 Glomerulus in biopsy of case 1. Note the global thickening of capillary walls due to apparent duplication of glomerular basement membrane. Neutrophils are conspicuous. (PAMS, 339×)

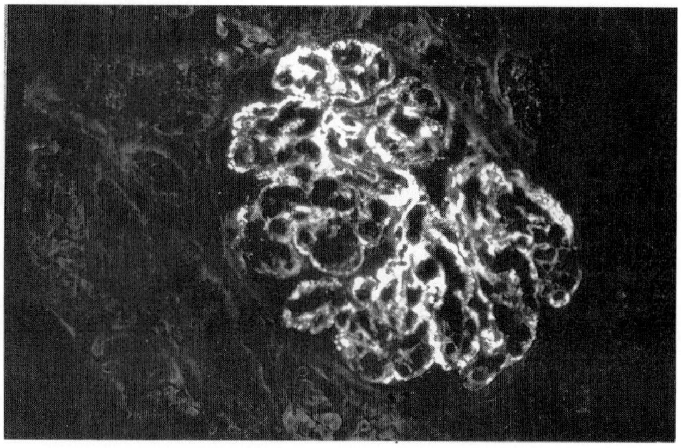

Fig. 2 Frozen section of case 1. Note the granular mesangial and peripheral capillary wall deposition pattern. (Fluoresceinated goat anti-human IgG, 138×)

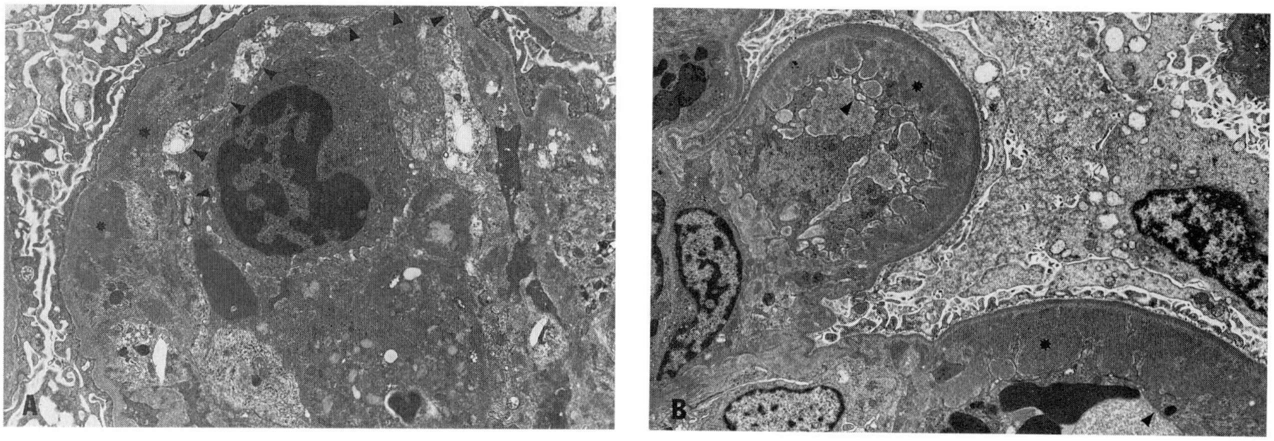

Fig. 3 Electronmicrographs of glomeruli from biopsies of case 1 (*A*) and case 2 (*B*). Note circumferential mesangial interposition (*A*) and subendothelial electron-dense deposits (star). Arrow-heads point to endothelium. (Lead citrate-uranyl acetate, *A:* 7640×, *B:* 5800×)

clearance of 0.93 ml/s/m^2 and a protein excretion rate of 10.52 g/d. ANA was negative, and the serum streptozyme level was 300 IU/ml. Serum C3 level was 0.07 g/l (normal range 0.55–1.2 g/l). Serum liver enzyme levels were within normal ranges. Percutaneous renal biopsy was performed.

Renal biopsies

Case 1

Twenty-six glomeruli were available for light microscopy. All were markedly hypercellular with a neutrophilic contribution (Figure 1). Exaggerated lobulation was evident, and 20% of glomeruli had crescents. Most glomeruli were hyperemic. Increased mesangial matrix and "tram-tracking" of the peripheral capillary walls were apparent on the periodic acid-Schiff (PAS) and periodic acid-methenamine silver (PAMS) stains. Moderate, patchy tubular atrophy and interstitial fibrosis were noted. Hemosiderin granules were present in the tubular epithelium.

On immunofluorescence microscopy (IF), capillary wall and mesangial deposits of IgG (4+) (Figure 2), IgA (4+), IgM (3+), C3 (4+), Clq (1+), and fibrin (2+) were identified.

Electron microscopy (EM) confirmed the presence of mesangial expansion and peripheral mesangial interposition (Figure 3A). Numerous subendothelial and mesangial, and scattered subepithelial electron-dense deposits were present. Endothelial microtubular inclusions were absent.

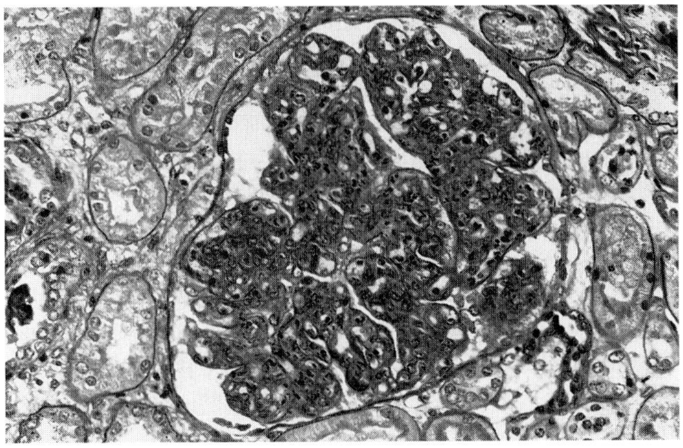

Fig. 4 Glomerulus in biopsy of case 2. The glomerular tuft has features similar to those illustrated in Figure 1. (PAS, 347×)

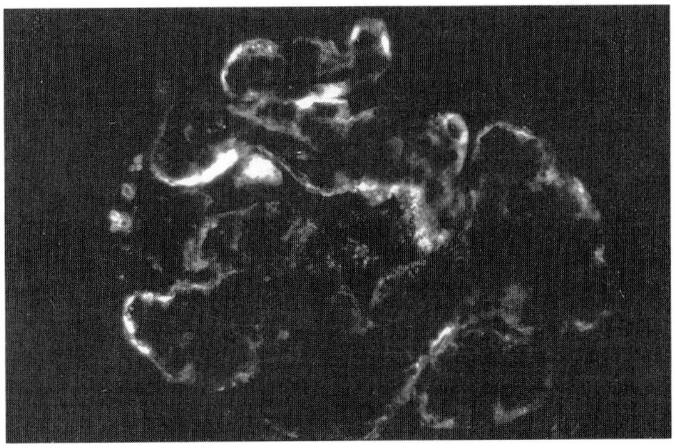

Fig. 5 Frozen section of case 2. Note the distinctive pattern of deposits outlining the glomerular lobules. (Fluoresceinated rabbit anti-human Clq, 245×)

Case 2

The specimen included at least 32 glomeruli, four of them obsolescent. The remaining glomeruli were enlarged and globally hypercellular with a prominent neutrophilic component (Figure 4). The PAS and PAMS stains brought out the "reduplication" of the peripheral capillary wall characteristic of MPGN. Patchy tubular atrophy and interstitial fibrosis were present. IF revealed diffuse global capillary wall and mesangial deposits of IgG (2+), IgA (2+), IgM (0.5+), C3 (4+) and Clq (1+) (Figure 5). EM (Figure 3 B) revealed prominent peripheral mesangial interposition and subendothelial deposits.

Indirect immunofluorescence search for antibodies to renal tubular antigen in the patients' sera was performed by overlaying cryostat sections with serial dilutions of the patients' sera for 30 minutes. Following 3 ten-minute washes in phosphate-buffered saline, the slides were overlayed with fluoresceinated goat anti-human immunoglobulin diluted 1:8 in phosphate-buffered saline. Following 3 additional washes and mounting, the slides were viewed on a Zeiss microscope (Carl Zeiss, Federal Republic of Germany). The result of this study was negative.

Clinical follow up

In the months following biopsy, both patients had urine specific gravities exceeding 1.020 on several occasions, indicating preserved concentrating ability.

WG has moderate sickle cell disease. His spleen is not palpable but he experiences 1 to 2 pain crises or episodes of pneumonia a year, and requires blood transfusion every 6 to 8 months. Since first seen at North Carolina Baptist Hospital he has suffered a stroke and is now in end-stage renal disease. Serologic studies for hepatitis A and B before initiation of hemodialysis were negative. KG has mild disease. He has experienced one pain crisis in the last two years, and has required transfusion only once during the same period. He has persistent proteinuria, but still has normal renal function.

Because of previous evidence that the occurrence of MPGN in siblings is linked to a common MHC haplotype [Welch et al. 1986], HLA typing was performed. WG's phenotype is A23, A28; B49, Bw53; Cw7, Cw-; DR2, DR4; DQwl, DQw3. KG's phenotype is A10, A28; Bw53, Bw57; Cw7, Cw-; DR2, DR3; DQwl, DQw4.

Complement profile studies two years after presentation revealed that patient WG had levels of C3, Factor B and B1H below normal range with normal or elevated levels of the other components; patient KG had normal or elevated levels of all complement proteins.

Discussion

Our two patients had features diagnostic of MPGN type I as defined by Habib and Levy [Levy and Habib 1979, Habib and Levy 1983]. These features include: 1) mesangial expansion with hypercellularity and peripheral interposition; 2) immunofluorescent deposits of immunoglobulins, C3 and frequently Clq; and 3) subendothelial immune-complex-type electron-dense deposits.

Review of the literature has identified only 10 other cases of sickle cell anemia-associated glomerulopathy with demonstrated immune complex deposition [Antonovytch 1972, Strom et al. 1972, Pardo et al. 1975] among 55 sickle cell anemia patients with glomerular disease unrelated to streptococcal infection [Berman et al. 1959, Sweeny et al. 1962, Barnett et al. 1968, McCoy 1969, Walker et al. 1971, Antonovytch 1972, Strom et al. 1972, Elfenbein et al. 1974, Pardo et al. 1975, Markenson et al. 1978, Tejani et al. 1985, Bakir et al. 1987]. Nine of these were cases of MPGN [Antonovytch 1972, Pardo et al. 1975], and one was a case of membranous glomerulopathy [Strom et al. 1972]. Other forms of glomerulopathy reported include minimal change disease [Barnett et al. 1968, Markenson et al. 1978], focal and segmental glomerulosclerosis [Markenson et al. 1978, Tejani et al. 1985] and a MPGN-like glomerulopathy without immune-complex deposits [McCoy 1969, Elfenbein et al. 1974, Bakir et al. 1978]. Strauss et al. [1975] were the first to draw attention to the contribution of immune-complex deposition to the pathogenesis of certain cases of SCD-associated glomerulopathy. They presented evidence incriminating a renal tubular antigen. We were unable to identify antibodies to such an antigen in our patients' sera in an indirect immunofluorescence assay. Still, such antibodies may have been present at levels below the sensitivity of the assay. Because MPGN was diagnosed in the two brothers within 2 weeks of each other, the possibility of a common environmental factor arises. One notable possibility is hepatitis B antigenemia [Venkataseshan et al. 1990]. As indicated above, hepatitis B serology in WG was negative, ruling out this as a shared etiologic agent. The streptozyme values were consistent with previous exposure to streptococcus; however there was no recent history of sore throat or of skin infections. In addition, the biopsy findings of massive subendothelial electron-dense deposits and circumferential mesangial interposition with lack of subepithelial humps were clearly those of MPGN and not those of poststreptococcal glomerulonephritis. No other common predisposing environmental factor is known to have been shared by the two brothers. There was no serological evidence to suggest systemic lupus erythematosus. The occurrence of MPGN in siblings has previously been reported [Berry et al. 1981]. Underlying this may be the sharing of a common major histocompatibility-complex haplotype [Welch et al. 1986], or of an inherited complement deficiency [Coleman et al. 1983]. Neither of these associations applies to the subjects of this report. The two brothers were haploidentical but both phenotypes were different from that reported by Welch et al. [1986]. In a series of 22 MPGN cases reported by Mandelenakis et al. [1971], not a single patient was black, at variance with the demographic profile of the population served by that particular medical center. The fact that our patients and similarly reported cases are blacks thus suggests a causal association between SCD and MPGN. In addition to deposition of immune-complexes for which accepted presumptive evidence is present in these two cases, i.e. IF identification of immunoglobulins and complement components and EM detection of electron-dense deposits; accessory mechanisms may include intraglomerular sickling and sludging of erythrocytes and hypercoagulability. We would like again to emphasize that the lesion in these two brothers is presumed to be immune-complex mediated and as such is different from the lesion described by McCoy [1969] and Bakir et al. [1987] which resembles MPGN by light microscopy but lacks IF and EM evidence of glomerular immune-complex deposition.

REFERENCES

Antonovytch T 1972 Ultrastructural changes in glomeruli of patients with sickle cell disease and the nephrotic syndrome (abstract). Proc Vth Ann Meet Am Soc Nephrol, Washington, DC, p 3

Bakir AA, Hathiwala SC, Ainis H, Hryhorczuk DO, Rhee HL, Levy PS, Dunea G 1987 Prognosis of the nephrotic syndrome in sickle cell glomerulopathy. Am J Nephrol *7:* 110–115

Barnett HL, Bernstein J 1968 Clinical pathological conference. J Ped *73:* 936–941

Berman LB, Schreiner GE 1958 Clinical and histologic spectrum of the nephrotic syndrome. Am J Med *24:* 249–267

Berman LB, Tublin I 1959 The nephropathies of sickle cell disease. Arch Intern Med *103:* 602–606

Berry, McEnery PT, McAdams AJ 1981 Membranoproliferative glomerulonephritis in two sibships. Clin Nephrol *16:* 101–106

Coleman TH, Forristal J, Kosaka T 1983 Inherited complement component deficiencies in membranoproliferative glomerulonephritis. Kidney Int *24:* 681–690

Elfenbein IB, Patchefsky A, Schwartz W 1974 Pathology of the glomerulus in sickle cell disease with and without the nephrotic syndrome. Am J Pathol *77:* 357–374

Mandenelakis N, Mendoza N, Pirani CL 1971 Lobular glomerulonephritis. A clinical and pathologic study based on renal biopsies. Medicine (Baltimore) *50:* 319–355

Markenson AL, Chandra M, Lewy JG, Miller DN 1978 Sickle cell anemia, the nephrotic syndrome, and hypoplastic crisis in a sibship. Am J Med *64:* 719–723

McCoy 1969 Ultrastructural alterations in the kidney of patients with sickle cell disease and the nephrotic syndrome. Lab Invest *21:* 85–95

Pardo V, Strauss J, Kramer H 1975 Nephropathy associated with sickle cell anemia: An autologous immune complex nephritis. II. Clinicopathologic study of seven patients. Am J Med *59:* 650–659

Strauss J, Pardo V, Koss MN 1975 Nephropathy associated with sickle cell anemia: An autologous immune complex nephritis. I. Studies on nature of glomerular bound antibody and antigen identification in a patient with sickle cell disease and immune deposit glomerulonephritis. Am J Med *58:* 382–387

Strom T, Muehrcke RC, Smith RD 1972 Sickle cell anemia with the nephrotic syndrome and renal vein obstruction. Arch Intern Med *129:* 104–107

Sweeney MJ, Dobins WT, Etteldorf JN 1962 Renal disease with elements of the nephrotic syndrome associated with sickle cell anemia. J Pediatr *60:* 42–51

Tejani A, Phadke K, Adamson O 1985 Renal lesions in sickle cell nephropathy in children. Nephron *39:* 352–355

Venkataseshan VS, Lieberman K, Kim DU 1990 Hepatitis-B-associated glomerulonephritis: Pathology, pathogenesis, and clinical course. Medicine (Baltimore) *69:* 200–216

Walker BR, Alexander F, Birsdall TR 1971 Glomerular lesions in sickle cell nephropathy. JAMA *215:* 437–440

Welch TR, Beischel L, Balakrishnan K 1986 Major-histocompatibility-complex extended haplotypes in membranoproliferative glomerulonephritis. N Engl J Med *314:* 1476–1481

Clinical Nephrology, Vol. 35 No. 2 – 1991 (52–58)

Oxalate, silicon and vanadium in acquired cystic kidney disease

J. E. Marco-Franco, V. E. Torres, D. E. Nixon, D. M. Wilson, E. M. James, E. J. Bergstralh and J. T. McCarthy

Division of Nephrology and Internal Medicine, Departments of Laboratory Medicine and Pathology, Diagnostic Radiology, and Health Sciences Research, Section of Biostatistics, Mayo Clinic and Mayo Foundation, Rochester, MN, USA

Abstract. We have investigated the importance of several clinical and laboratory parameters on the development of acquired cystic kidney disease (ACKD) as detected by ultrasonography in 19 patients who had received dialysis therapy for at least three years. We were particularly interested on the possible effect of the serum levels of oxalate and silicon, which can produce tubular obstruction, and that of vanadium, which can affect cell proliferation. The severity of ACKD increased with the duration of dialysis and was greater in men than in women. Positive correlations were observed between the grades of ACKD and the levels of hemoglobin, hematocrit, and parathyroid hormone, while there was a negative correlation between ACKD and serum ferritin levels. The serum levels of oxalate, silicon, and vanadium, pre- and postdialysis, were markedly and significantly higher than those in normal controls, but there was no significant correlation between these levels and the duration of dialysis therapy or severity of ACKD. The pre- and postdialysis levels of vanadium were not significantly different, while the levels of oxalate and silicon were significantly lower in the postdialysis samples. No significant correlations were detected between ACKD and age of the patients, blood pressure, protein catabolic rate, efficiency of dialysis index, or the serum levels of iron, sodium, potassium, calcium, phosphorus, aluminum, and β_2-microglobulin.

Key words: acquired cystic kidney disease – dialysis – oxalate – silicon – vanadium

Introduction

The acquired renal cystic disease (ACKD) associated with uremia and its potential for malignant transformation have been recognized since the description by Dunnill in 1977 [Dunnill et al. 1977, Ishikawa et al. 1980, Fayemi and Ali 1980, Feiner et al. 1981, Levine et al. 1984, Mickisch et al. 1984, Gehrig et al. 1985, Bretan et al. 1986, Hughson et al. 1986, MacDougall et al. 1987, Katz et al. 1987, Jabour et al. 1987, Truong et al. 1988]. The pathogenesis is not known. Several possible mechanisms have been proposed, including tubular obstruction, stimulation of renal tubular cell proliferation by uremic toxins and renal ischemia [Dunnill et al. 1977, Ishikawa et al. 1980, Fayemi and Alli 1980, Feiner et al. 1981, Levine et al. 1984, Mickisch et al. 1984, Gehrig et al. 1985, Bretan et al. 1986, Hughson et al. 1986, MacDougall et al. 1987, Katz et al. 1987, Jabour et al. 1987, Truong et al. 1988]. We have attempted to assess the importance of some of these mechanisms by correlating certain pertinent clinical and laboratory parameters with the severity of ACKD in a group of 19 patients who had received dialysis treatment for three or more years. In addition, we have studied the possibility that vanadium, a trace element which accumulates in the kidney [Phillips et al. 1983] and has an effect on cell proliferation [Klarlund 1985], might play a role in the pathogenesis of this disorder.

Received August 15, 1990; in revised form November 12, 1990.

Reprint requests to Dr. V. E. Torres, Division of Nephrology, Mayo Clinic, 200 First Street, SW, Rochester, MN 55905, USA.

Material and methods

Nineteen patients who had received dialysis therapy at the Mayo Clinic for at least three years and had never been transplanted agreed to participate in the study. Seventeen were treated by hemodialysis and two by chronic ambulatory peritoneal dialysis. None had been treated with erythropoietin.

Renal ultrasounds and pre- and postdialysis serum levels of silicon, oxalate, and vanadium were

Table 1 Grading scale for ACKD on ultrasound examination

Grade	Number of cysts	Renal size
0	0	–
1	1–5	–
2	>5	<10 cm
3	>5	≥10 cm

Table 2 Distribution of patients according to ACKD grades*

Grade	Number of patients
0	3
1	2
2	4
3	1
4	5
5	1
6	3
	19

* ACKD grades for patient result from adding the grades for each kidney.

obtained for the purpose of the study. The remaining clinical and laboratory data were obtained from a computerized data system (Computing Clinical Ltd., London, England) and a review of the clinical records. This information included age, gender, number of months on dialysis, and the average value during the year preceding the study for the following parameters: systolic blood pressure, diastolic blood pressure, hemoglobin, hematocrit, iron, ferritin, sodium, potassium, calcium, phosphorus, immunoreactive parathyroid hormone (iPTH), aluminum, and β_2-, microglobulin. In addition, the protein catabolic rate (PCR) and an efficiency of dialysis index expressed as the product of dialyzer urea clearance (K) and treatment time (T) divided by the body urea distribution volume (V), or Kt/V [Sargent and Gotch 1980], during one and three years prior to the study, were abstracted from the computerized data system.

The patients were examined with commercially available real-time ultrasound instruments utilizing transducer frequencies of 3.5 or 5 MHz. Each kidney was assessed for size, number of cysts, and presence of solid masses and assigned a grade according to the scale shown in Table 1. A grade was assigned to each patient by adding up the grades of the kidneys.

Oxalate was determined in serum pre- and postdialysis. Determinations of oxalate were performed by an immobilized oxalate oxidase method [Kasidas and Rose, 1985, Kasidas and Rose 1986]. At present, there are no certified reference control sera with normal physiological concentrations of oxalate, but ultrafiltrates of previously analyzed sera were run with our samples. In addition, certified reference control urines (Sigma Chemical Company, St. Louis, MO) with normal and elevated oxalate concentrations are run daily in our laboratory. The normal serum oxalate range (mean ± 2 SD) in our laboratory is 2.0 – 4.2 µmol/l.

Vanadium and silicon were measured in serum pre- and postdialysis and in the dialysis solution. Acid-washed polypropylene containers for trace metals and special collection procedures were utilized in order to avoid contamination [McCarthy et al. 1986]. The vanadium analyses were performed on a Perkin-Elmer Model 3030 Zeeman Corrected Graphite Furnace Atomic Absorption Spectrophotometer, equipped with a model HGA-600 graphite furnace and AS-60 autosampler (Ishida et al. 1989]. Silicon was determined by inductively coupled plasma emission spectroscopy [Nixon et al. 1986]. At present, no certified reference control sera exist with concentrations of vanadium and silicon certified at normal physiological concentrations. For our analysis of vanadium, instrument response calibration was performed by adding known quantities of a certified vanadium atomic absorption standard solution to pooled normal sera. Consistently low reagent blank values (0.000 A·s) and consistent calibration curve slopes have reassured us that the analyses are correct. For silicon analyses, an inductively coupled plasma (ICP) emission spectrometer was calibrated with aqueous silicon standards prepared from a certified atomic absorption standard. To assure that background interferences were absent, the analyses were performed by simple dilution with comparison to the aqueous response curve and by the method of standard additions. Identical results were obtained by both techniques. The normal serum vanadium range in our laboratory is 0–0.24 ng/ml. The normal serum silicon range in our laboratory is 0.01–0.25 µg/ml. Our normal values for vanadium and for silicon are similar to those reported by others [Ishida et al. 1989, Mauras et al. 1980].

The remaining biochemical determinations were performed routinely in our clinical laboratories. The samples for serum aluminum determinations were collected in special acid-washed polypropylene syringes using special precautions and measured using flameless electrothermal atomization atomic absorption spectroscopy with a L'Vov platform and Zeeman background correction [McCarthy et al. 1986]. iPTH levels were determined by a radioimmunoassay that primarily measures carboxy terminal fragments along with some intact hormone [Kao et al. 1982].

Differences between groups of patients were analyzed using a rank-sum test. Student's t-test for

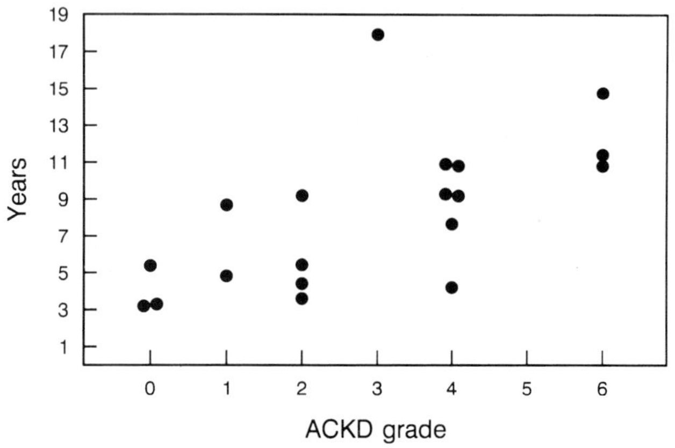

Fig. 1 ACKD grades according to duration of dialysis therapy in years

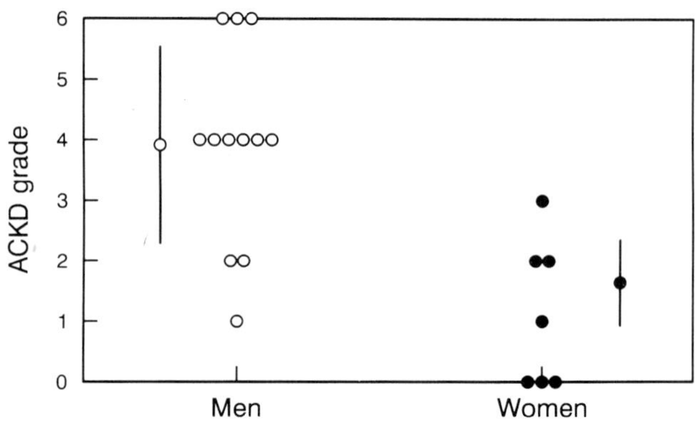

Fig. 2 ACKD grades in men and women who have received dialysis treatment for three or more years

paired observations was used to analyze changes between pre- and postdialysis values. Spearman's correlation coefficient was used to assess associations between continuous or ordinal parameters. All p values reported are two-tailed. The level of significance was taken to be 0.05.

Results

Sixteen of the 19 patients had cysts. Two patients had less than five cysts limited to one kidney only. The distribution of the patients according to the grades of cystic disease is shown in Table 2. No solid masses were detected.

The extent of the cystic disease increased with the duration of dialysis (Figure 1) and was greater in men than in women (Figure 2). Men had been on dialysis longer than women (median of 9.3 years versus 5.0 years, $p = 0.057$). However, the extent of cystic disease remained higher in men ($p = 0.004$) even when adjusting for dialysis duration using multiple regression.

Positive correlations were observed between the grades of ACKD and the levels of hemoglobin ($r = 0.46$, $p = 0.05$), hematocrit ($r = 0.49$, $p = 0.03$), and PTH ($r = 0.46$, $p = 0.05$), while there was a negative correlation between the grades of ACKD and serum ferritin levels ($r = 0.55$, $p = 0.01$). No significant correlations were detected for grade of ACKD with age of the patients, systolic and diastolic blood pressures, PCR, KT/V, iron, sodium, potassium, calcium, phosphorus, aluminum, and β_2-microglobulin.

Silicon and vanadium were undetectable in the dialysis solution. The pre- and postdialysis levels of oxalate, silicon, and vanadium were markedly and significantly higher than normal controls (Figure 3). The serum levels of oxalate and silicon were significantly lower in the post-dialysis samples than in the pre-dialysis samples (Figure 3). On the other hand, the pre- and postdialysis levels of vanadium were not significantly different. There was no significant correlation between the serum levels of oxalate, silicon, and vanadium and the duration of dialysis therapy or the severity of ACKD.

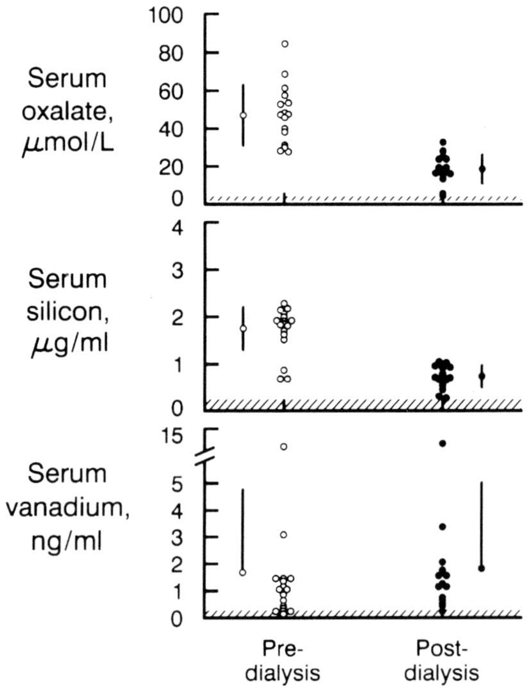

Fig. 3 Pre- and postdialysis serum concentrations of oxalate, silicon, and vanadium. Bars detect mean ± 1 SD. Dashed area indicates the normal range (mean ± 2 SD)

Discussion

The cystic transformation of end-stage kidneys and its potential for malignant degeneration have received considerable attention since the initial description by Dunnill in 1977 [Dunnill et al. 1977, Ishikawa et al. 1980, Fayemi and Ali 1980, Feiner et al. 1981, Levine et al. 1984, Mickisch et al. 1984, Gehrig et al. 1985, Bretan et al. 1986, Hughson et al. 1986, MacDougall et al. 1987, Katz et al. 1987, Jabour et al. 1987, Truong et al. 1988]. The frequencies of ACKD among dialysis patients and of associated neoplasms and carcinomas depend largely on the criteria used to define these entities and on the sensitivity of the techniques used for their detection. For example, 80% of patients who have been on dialysis for more than three years have multiple renal cysts detectable by computed tomography [Ishikawa et al. 1980]. It has been estimated that 20% of these patients will progress to renal tumors and 1% to metastatic disease [Bretan et al. 1986].

Our data confirm previous observations that the cystic transformation of the kidneys increases with the duration of dialysis [Dunnill et al. 1977, Ishikawa et al. 1980, Fayemi and Ali 1980, Feiner et al. 1981, Levine et al. 1984, Mickisch et al. 1984, Gehrig et al. 1985, Bretan et al. 1986, Hughson et al. 1986, MacDougall et al. 1987, Katz et al. 1987, Jabour et al. 1987, Truong et al. 1988] and that this process is more severe in men than in women [Fayemi and Ali 1980]. The weak, but significant, correlation between ACKD and serum iPTH levels is probably explained by the increasing severity of secondary hyperparathyroidism with the duration of dialysis. Nevertheless, the possibility that the high circulating levels of parathryoid hormone might contribute to the development of ACKD by a mechanism linked to the intracellular generation of cyclic AMP cannot be excluded [Mangoo-Karim et al. 1989]. Our results also confirm previous studies in which a correlation between hematocrit and severity of ACKD was found [Goldsmith et al. 1982, Shalhoub et al. 1982].

The pathogenesis of ACKD is not well understood. Although initially described in association with long-term hemodialysis, it is also observed in peritoneal dialysis patients [Katz et al. 1987, Jabour et al. 1987, Truong et al. 1988] and in uremic patients who have never been dialyzed [Mickisch et al. 1984]. Therefore, it seems unlikely that phthalate, a plasticizer in the dialysis tubing, or any other factor unique to hemodialysis is the cause of this disease [Crocker and Safe 1984]. The role of uremia or uremia-related factor in its pathogenesis is supported by the reported regression of cysts following successful renal transplantation [Ishikawa et al. 1983].

Obliterative intimal fibrosis of the renal blood vessels is characteristic of the end-stage kidney in dialysis patients [Tolnai et al. 1969]. A role for ischemia in cyst formation is often mentioned in review articles of ACKD [Dunnill et al. 1977, Ishikawa et al. 1980, Fayemi and Ali 1980, Feiner et al. 1981, Levine et al. 1984, Mickisch et al. 1984, Gehrig et al. 1985, Bretan et al. 1986, Hughson et al. 1986, MacDougall et al. 1987, Katz et al. 1987, Jabour et al. 1987, Truong et al. 1988] and has received recent attention [Torres et al. 1988, Cohen and Elliott 1990]. The association of renal ischemia and renal cysts or adenomas was well recognized in early pathology studies [Trinkle 1936, Budin and McDonnell 1984]. Epithelial cell growth proliferation and cyst formation in ischemia could be stimulated by acidosis, intrarenal generation of angiotensin II, or other undetermined factors [Torres et al. 1988, Cohen and Elliott 1990]. Nevertheless, it seems unlikely that these irreversible vascular changes alone are responsible for the development of the cysts, since ACKD can reverse following renal transplantation [Ishikawa et al. 1983].

Other proposed mechanisms include tubular obstruction by interstitial fibrosis, oxalate [Fayemi et al. 1979, Ono 1986, Ono et al. 1987, Ono et al. 1989], silicon [Dobbie and Smith 1986, Dobbie et al. 1990], or β_2-microglobulin [Bommer et al. 1985] and stimulation of renal tubular cell proliferation caused by accumulation of mitogenic polyamines [Bagdade et al. 1979], growth factors, or other substances in the uremic milieu.

Our data do not support nor disprove any of these pathogenetic mechanisms, since we assessed only indirectly some of the hypotheses. For example, serum oxalate levels do not necessarily reflect the severity of deposition of oxalate in the kidney. While the deposition of oxalate in the kidney increases with the duration of dialysis therapy [Fayemi et al. 1979], there are conflicting results on whether the serum oxalate levels correlate with the duration of this treatment [Ono et al. 1987, Ono 1986]. Yet, Ono et al. reported a significant correlation between serum oxalate levels and kidney size in a series of 51 hemodialysis patients [Ono et al. 1987]. Experimental studies on the effect on vitamin C and oxalate supplemented diets on the development of renal cysts in the five-sixths nephrectomized rat model have been inconclusive [Ono et al. 1989].

The kidney is the main organ engaged in the elimination of absorbed silicon. Silicon accumulates in renal failure especially in patients dialyzed against solutions with a high silicon content [Dobbie and Smith 1986, Dobbie et al. 1990, Mauras et al. 1980, Hershey et al. 1983]. It has been known for some time that the administration of silicon to experimental animals can result in tubular epithelial damage and tubular dilatation [Policard and Collet 1954, Policard et al. 1960]. Recently, silicon has been added to the list of possible pathogenetic factors in ACKD [Dobbie et al. 1990]. The intraperitoneal injection of silicon to rats that results in serum silicon levels similar to those in dialysis patients causes a lesion resembling ACKD in these animals [Dobbie et al. 1990]. As in the case of oxalate, our results provide no support for, but do not disprove this hypothesis.

One of the main goals of our study was to investigate the possibility that accumulation of vanadium might be important in the pathogenesis of ACKD. Vanadium is one of the more abundant trace elements in nature, is principally eliminated in the urine, and accumulates in the kidney, primarily in the renal cortex [Phillips et al. 1983]. Vanadium can induce natriuresis and diuresis by inhibiting the sodium potassium ATPase in the proximal tubules [Day et al. 1980, Higashi and Bello-Reuss 1980]. In addition, vanadium can 1) inhibit several ATPase [Bond and Hudgins 1979, Grantham and Glynn 1979, Cantley et al. 1977, O'Neal et al. 1979] and phosphatases [Klarlund 1985, Swarup et al. 1982] and activate adenylcyclase [Schwabe et al. 1979, Grupp et al. 1979, Lichtstein et al. 1982], 2) modulate the function of many oncogene products and growth factor receptors associated with tyrosine kinase activity by inhibiting phosphotyrosine phosphatase [Klarlund 1985, Swarup et al. 1982], 3) mimic or potentiate the effects of growth factors such as epidermal growth factor [Carpenter 1981], fibroblast growth factor [Carpenter 1981], insulin [Dubyak and Kleinzeller 1980], estrogens [Sato et al. 1987], and interleukin-3 [Tojo et al. 1987], 4) stimulate cell division and block cell differentiation in cell culture systems [Carpenter 1981, Dubyak and Kleinzeller 1980, Sato et al. 1987, Tojo et al. 1987, Hori and Oka 1980, Smith 1983, English et al. 1983], and 5) increase thymidine incorporation in the colon of animals treated with the carcinogen dimethylhydrazine and ammonium metavanadate [Kinksnorth et al. 1986]. At higher concentrations, vanadium can also be toxic to cells in culture [Paris et al. 1987] and cause cellular necrosis in the kidney and liver [Domingo et al. 1986]. Given the main sites of accumulation and action of vanadium in the kidney and its potential effects on cell proliferation in many systems, it seems reasonable to speculate that, if vanadium accumulates in renal failure, it could play an important role in the pathogenesis of ACKD, a disorder characterized by cysts originating mainly from the proximal tubules [Feiner et al. 1981, Ishikawa 1985, Ishikawa et al. 1989, Ishikawa et al. 1989] and involving predominantly the renal cortex [Dunnill et al. 1977, Ishikawa et al. 1980, Fayemi and Ali 1980, Feiner et al. 1981, Levine et al. 1984, Mickisch et al. 1984, Gehrig et al. 1985, Bretan et al. 1986, Hughson et al. 1986, MacDougall et al. 1987, Katz et al. 1987, Jabour et al. 1987, Truong et al. 1988].

There is little information on the blood or tissue levels of vanadium and its consequences in renal failure. Recently, Tajiri and Hirasawa have found that the blood vanadium levels are markedly higher in uremic patients than in healthy subjects and that the blood vanadium concentration correlates with the level of serum creatinine [Tajiri and Hirasawa 1985]. They also found that the blood vanadium concentration is higher in postdialysis than in predialysis blood samples. In our study, there was no significant difference between pre- and postdialysis serum vanadium levels, in marked contrast to the silicon and oxalate levels which decreased significantly during dialysis. The likely explanation for this difference is that the transport of vanadium in the blood is in the lipid fraction [Schroeder et al. 1963]. Since vanadium is not removed by dialysis, it seems likely that it accumulates in the tissues in renal failure and that it might contribute to the morbidity of uremia including the increased risk for malignancy [Matas et al. 1975, Miach et al. 1976, Sutherland et al. 1977] and the development of ACKD. Our results, however, do not provide support for this hypothesis.

In conclusion, there are multiple hypotheses to explain the development of cysts in end-stage kidneys, but their validity remains unproven and the pathogenesis of ACKD remains unknown. We have not found any correlations between the serum levels of oxalate, silicon, or vanadium and the presence or severity of ACKD. However, any attempt to interpret this information is limited by the fact that these serum values may not be reflective of total body stores or renal content. Future studies measuring total body stores or renal content of these substances may draw different conclusions.

REFERENCES

Bagdade JD, Subbaiah PV, Bartos D, Bartos F, Campbell RA 1979 Polyamines: an unrecognized cardiovascular risk factor in chronic dialysis? Lancet *1:* 412

Bommer J, Waldherr R, Ritz E 1985 Kidney lesions in uraemic patients and β-microglobulin derived amyloid. Lancet *2:* 1437

Bond GH, Hudgins PM 1979 Kinetics of inhibition of NaK-ATPase by MG(2^+), K^+, and vanadate. Biochemistry *18:* 325

Bretan PN Jr, Busch MP, Hricak H, Williams RD 1986 Chronic renal failure: a significant risk factor in the development of acquired renal cysts and renal cell carcinoma. Cancer *57:* 1871

Budin RE, McDonnell PJ 1985 Renal cell neoplasms: their relationship to arteriolonephrosclerosis. Arch Pathol Lab Med *108:* 138

Cantley LC Jr, Josephson L, Warner R, Yanagisawa M, Lechene C, Guidotti G 1977 Vanadate is a potent (Na,K)-ATPase inhibitor found in ATP derived from muscle. J Biol Chem *252:* 7421

Carpenter G 1981 Vanadate, epidermal growth factor and the stimulation of DNA synthesis. Biochem Biophys Res Commun *102:* 1115

Cohen EP, Elliott WC Jr 1990 The role of ischemia in acquired cystic kidney disease. Am J Kidney Dis *15:* 55

Crocker JFS, Safe SH 1984 Animal model of hemodialysis induced polycystic kidney disease (PKD). Kidney Int *25:* 183

Day H, Middendorf D, Lukert B, Heinz A, Grantham J 1980 The renal response to intravenous vanadate in rats. J Lab Clin Med *96:* 382

Dobbie JW, Abdullah AA, Smith MJB 1990 Silica-induced polycystic kidney disease, In: *Carone FA, Dobbie JW* (eds) Advances in the Pathogenesis of Polycystic Kidney Disease. Baxter Healthcare Corporation/TP & T, Chicago (in press)

Dobbie JW, Smith MJB 1986 Urinary and serum silicon in normal and uraemic individuals. Ciba Found Symp *121:* 194

Domingo JL, Liobet JM, Tomas JM, Corbella J 1986 Influence of chelating agents on the toxicity, distribution and excretion of vanadium in mice. J Appl Toxicol *6:* 337

Dubyak GR, Kleinzeller A 1980 The insulin-mimetic effect of vanadate in isolated rat adipocytes: dissociation from effects of vanadate as a (Na^+-K^+)ATPase inhibitor. J Biol Chem *255:* 5306

Dunnill MS, Millard PR, Oliver D 1977 Acquired cystic disease of the kidneys: a hazard of long-term intermittent maintenance haemodialysis. J Clin Path *30:* 868

English LH, Macara IG, Cantley LC 1983 Vanadium stimulate the (Na^+-K^+) pump in Friend erythroleukemia cells and blocks erythropoiesis. J Cell Biol *97:* 1299

Fayemi AO, Ali M 1980 Acquired renal cysts and tumors superimposed on chronic primary kidney diseases. Path Res Pract *168:* 73

Fayemi AO, Ali M, Braun EV 1979 Oxalosis in hemodialysis patients: A pathologic study of 80 cases. Arch Pathol Lab Med *103:* 58

Feiner HD, Katz LA, Gallo GR 1981 Acquired cystic disease of kidney in chronic dialysis patients. Urology *17:* 260

Gehrig JJ, Gottheiner TI, Swenson RS 1985 Acquired cystic disease of the end-stage kidney. Am J Med *79:* 609

Goldsmith HJ, Ahmad R, Raichura N, Lal SM, McConnell CA, Gould DA, Gyde OHB, Green J 1982 Association between haemoglobin concentration and renal cyst formation in patients on long-term regular haemodialysis treatment. Proc Eur Dial Transplant Assoc *19:* 313

Grantham JJ, Glynn IM 1979 Renal NA,K-ATPase: determinants of inhibition by vanadium. Am J Physiol *236:* F530

Grupp G, Grupp I, Johnson CL, Wallick ET, Schwartz A 1979 Effect of vanadate on cardiac contraction and adenylate cyclase. Biochem Biophys Res Commun *88:* 440

Hershey CO, Ricanati ES, Hershey LA, Varnes AW, Lavin PJM, Strain WH 1983 Silicon as a potential uremic neurotoxin: trace element analysis in patients with renal failure. Neurology *33:* 786

Higashi Y, Bello-Reuss E 1980 Effects of sodium orthovanadate on whole kidney and single nephron function. Kidney Int *18:* 302

Hori C, Oka T 1980 Vanadate enhances the stimulatory action of insulin on DNA synthesis in cultured mouse mammary gland. Biochem Biophys Acta *610:* 235

Hughson MD, Buchwald D, Fox M 1986 Renal neoplasia and acquired cystic kidney disease in patients receiving long-term dialysis. Arch Pathol Lab Med *10:* 592

Ishida O, Kihira K, Tsukamoto Y, Marumo F 1989 Improved determination of vanadium in biological fluids by electrothermal atomic absorption spectrometry. Clin Chem *35:* 127

Ishikawa I 1985 Unusual composition of cyst fluid in acquired cystic disease of the end-stage kidney. Nephron *41:* 373

Ishikawa I, Horiguchi T, Shikura N 1989 Lectin peroxidase conjugate reactivity in acquired cystic disease of the kidney. Nephron *51:* 211

Ishikawa I, Saito Y, Onouchi Z, Kitada H, Suzuki S, Kurihara S, Yuri T, Shinoda A 1980 Development of acquired cystic disease and adenocarcinoma of the kidney in glomerulonephritic chronic hemodialysis patients. Clin Nephrol *14:* 1

Ishikawa I, Saito Y, Shikura N, Yuri T, Shinoda A, Shiraiwa K, Tsugawa R 1989 Excretion of hippuran into acquired renal cysts in chronic hemodialysis patient. Nephron *52:* 110

Ishikawa I, Yuri T, Kitada H, Shinoda A 1983 Regression of acquired cystic disease of the kidney after successful renal transplantation. Am J Nephrol *3:* 310

Jabour BA, Ralls PW, Tang WW, Boswell WD Jr, Colletti PM, Feinstein EI, Massry SG 1987 Acquired cystic disease of the kidneys: computed tomography and ultrasonography appraisal in patients on peritoneal and hemodialysis. Invest Radiol *22:* 728

Kao PC, Jiang N-S, Klee GG, Purnell DC 1982 Development and validation of a new radioimmunoassay for parathyrin (PTH). Clin Chem *28:* 69

Kasidas GP, Rose GA 1985 Continuous flow assay for urine oxalate using immobilized oxalate oxidase. Ann Clin Biochem *22:* 412

Kasidas GP, Rose GA 1986 Measurement of plasma oxalate in healthy subjects and in patients with chronic renal failure using immobilized oxalate oxidase. Clin Chem Acta *154:* 49

Katz A, Sombolos K, Oreopoulos DG 1987 Acquired cystic disease of the kidney in association with chronic ambulatory peritoneal dialysis. Am J Kidney Dis *9:* 426

Kinksnorth AN, LaMuraglia GM, Ross JS, Malt RA 1986 Vanadate supplements and 1,2-dimethylhydrazine induced colon cancer in mice: Increased thymidine incorporation without enhanced carcinogenesis. Br J Cancer *53:* 683

Klarlund JK 1985 Transformation of cells by an inhibitor of phosphatases acting on phosphotyrosine in proteins. Cell *41:* 707

Levine E, Grantham JJ, Slusher SL, Greathouse JL, Krohn BP 1984 CT of acquired cystic kidney disease and renal tumors in long-term dialysis patients. AJR *142:* 125

Lichtstein D, Mullikin-Kilpatrick D, Blume AJ 1982 Modification of neuroblastoma X glioma hybrid NG108-15 adenylate cyclase by vanadium ions. Biochem Biophys Res Commun *105:* 1157

MacDougall ML, Welling LW, Wiegmann TB 1987 renal adenocarcinoma and acquired cystic disease in chronic hemodialysis patients. Am J Kidney Dis *9:* 166

Mangoo-Karim R, Uchic ME, Grant M, Schumate WA, Calvet JP, Park CH, Grantham JJ 1989 Renal epithelial fluid secretion and cyst growth: The role of cyclic AMP. FASEB J *3:* 2629

Matas AJ, Simmons RL, Kjellstrand CM, Buselmeier TJ, Najarian JS 1975 Increased incidence of malignancy during chronic renal failure. Lancet *1:* 883

Mauras Y, Riberi P, Cartier F, Allain P 1980 Increase in blood silicon concentration in patients with renal failure. Biomedicine *33:* 228

McCarthy JT, Milliner DS, Kurtz SB, Johnson WJ, Moyer TP 1986 Interpretation of serum aluminum values in dialysis patients. J Clin Pathol *86:* 629

Miach PJ, Dawborn JK, Xipell J 1976 Neoplasia in patients with chronic renal failure on long-term dialysis. Clin Nephrol *5:* 101

Mickisch O, Bommer J, Bachmann S, Waldheer R, Mann JFE, Ritz E 1984 Multicystic transformation of kidneys in chronic renal failure. Nephron *38:* 93

Nixon DE, Moyer TP, Johnson P, McCall JT, Ness AB, Fjerstad WH, Wehde MB 1986 Routine measurement of calcium, magnesium, copper, zinc, and iron in urine and serum by inductively coupled plasma emission spectroscopy. Clin Chem *32:* 1660

O'Neal SG, Rhoads DB, Racker E 1979 Vanadate inhibitor of sarcoplasmic reticulum Ca^{2+}-ATPase and other ATPases. Biochem Biphys Res Commun *89:* 845

Ono K 1986 Secondary hyperoxalemia caused by vitamin C supplementation in regular hemodialysis patients. Clin Nephrol *26:* 239

Ono K, Ono H, Ono T, Kikawa K, Oh Y 1989 Acquired renal cysts in five-sixths nephrectomized rats: the roles of oxalate deposits in renal tubules and a renotropic factor. Nephron *51:* 393

Ono K, Yasukohchi A, Kikawa K 1987 Pathogenesis of acquired renal cysts in hemodialysis patients: the role of oxalate crystal deposition in renal tubules. Trans Am Soc Artif Intern Organs *33:* 245

Paris S, Chambard J-C, Pouysségur J 1987 Coupling between phosphoinositide breakdown and early mitogenic events in fibroblasts. J Biol Chem *262:* 1977

Phillips TD, Nechay BR, Heidelbaugh ND 1983 Vanadium: Chemistry and the kidney. Federation Proc *42:* 2969

Policard A, Collet A 1954 Étude expérimental des lésions rénales provoquées par élimination de la silice. J d Urol Med Chir *60:* 164

Policard A, Collet A, Daniel-Moussard H, Pregermain S 1960 Cytopathologie infrastructurale. Dépôt de silice dans les mitochondries du tube urinaire. Rôle dans l'épuration rénale. Compt Rend Acad Sci *251:* 314

Sargent JA, Gotch FA 1980 Mathematical modeling of dialysis therapy. Kidney Int *18:* 510

Sato B, Miyashita Y, Maeda Y, Noma K, Kishimoto S, Matsumoto K 1987 Effects of estrogen and vanadate on the proliferation of newly established transformed mouse Leydig cell line in vitro. Endocrinology *120:* 1112

Schroeder HA, Balassa JJ, Tipton IH 1963 Abnormal trace metals in man-chromium. J Chron Dis *16:* 1047

Schwabe U, Puchstein C, Hannemann H, Sochtig E 1979 Activation of adenylate cyclase by vanadate. Nature (London) *277:* 143

Shalhoub RJ, Rajan U, Kim VV, Goldwasser E, Kark JA, Antoniou LD 1982 Erythrocytosis in patients on long-term hemodialysis. Ann Intern Med *97:* 686

Smith JB 1983 Vanadium ions stimulate DNA synthesis in Swiss mouse 3T3 and 3T6 cells. Proc Natl Acad Sci USA *80:* 6162

Sutherland GA, Glass J, Gabriell R 1977 Increased incidence of malignancy in chronic renal failure. Nephron 18: *182*

Swarup G, Cohen S, Garbers DL 1982 Inhibitor of membrane phosphotyrosyl-protein phosphatase activity by vanadate. Biochem Biophys Res Commun *107:* 1104

Tajiri M, Hirasawa Y 1985 Vanadium retention and its possible toxic effects on membrane transport in uremic patients. Nippon Jinzo Gakkai Shi *27:* 499

Tojo A, Kasuga M, Urabe A, Takaku F 1987 Vanadate can replace interleukin 3 for transient growth of factor-dependent cells. Exp Cell Res *171:* 16

Tolnai G, Sarkar K, Jaworski ZF, Irvine AH 1969 Obliterative intimal fibrosis in kidneys of dialyzed patients. Can Med Assoc J *100:* 116

Torres VE, Berndt TJ, Okamura M, Nesbit JW, Holley KE, Carone JA, Knox FG, Romero JC 1988 Mechanisms affecting the development of renal cystic disease induced by diphenylthiazole. Kidney Int *33:* 1130

Trinkle AJ 1936 The origin and development of renal adenomas and their relation to carcinoma of the renal cortex (hypernephroma). Am J Cancer *27:* 676

Truong LD, Ansari Q, Ansari J, Wheeler TM, Mattioli CM, Gillum D 1988 Acquired cystic kidney disease: occurrence in patients on chronic peritoneal dialysis. Am J Kidney Dias *11:* 192

Clinical Nephrology, Vol. 35 No. 2 – 1991 (59–65)

Effects of an acute protein load on urinary albumin excretion in kidney donors

C. Manno[1], F. D'Elia[1], M. Mingarelli[1], M. Stella[1], M. Cervellati[1], G. Fornarelli[1] and F. P. Schena[2]

[1] *'S. Rita' Nephrology and Dialysis Center, Bari and* [2] *Chair of Nephrology, University of Bari, Bari, Italy*

Abstract. In six kidney donors with normal baseline urinary albumin excretion (UAE) we studied the behavior of the UAE after 150 g of a meat protein meal and after a carbohydrate meal of equal caloric (1,370 kcal), water (1 liter) and sodium content (51 mEq). The mean creatinine clearance (C_{cr}) increased significantly after a protein load at the first ($p < 0.01$) and second hour ($p < 0.05$), while it did not change after the carbohydrate meal. The mean UAE increased significantly after the protein meal at the first ($p < 0.05$) and second hour ($p < 0.05$), while after the carbohydrate meal the mean values were increased at the first ($p < 0.05$), second ($p < 0.05$) and third hour ($p < 0.05$). Furthermore, the mean values of UAE after the protein meal were significantly higher ($p < 0.05$) than those found at the same time after the carbohydrate meal. Diuresis and natriuresis increased significantly after both meals. These findings show that the increased UAE after the protein meal may be due to a further increase in C_{cr} in the hyperfiltering remaining kidney, while the smaller increase in the UAE observed after the carbohydrate meal may be due to water load and increased urine flow, which impairs albumin tubular reabsorption. The prognostic importance of microalbuminuria after either meal is therefore uncertain.

Key words: microalbuminuria – kidney donors – glomerular hyperfiltration

Introduction

Experimental studies in animal models have shown that an extensive reduction in nephron mass induces hemodynamic variations, resulting in glomerular hypertension and hyperfiltration [Brenner et al. 1982, Hostetter et al. 1986a]; subsequently, glomerular sclerosis, proteinuria, arterial hypertension and progressive impairment of renal function appear [Olson et al. 1982]. Hostetter et al. [1986 b] have also demonstrated that an even less extensive reduction of renal mass, i.e. uninephrectomy, may trigger off the same compensatory mechanisms in glomerular hemodynamics.

Prior to unilateral nephrectomy, living-related kidney donors are carefully selected for normal renal function and the absence of systemic diseases. They provide an excellent human model for studying the clinical consequences of chronic hyperfiltration in the solitary kidney.

Received June 15, 1990; in revised form October 16, 1990.

Reprint requests to Dr. C. Manno, Via Cagnazzi 34, I-70124 Bari, Italy.

Long-term studies on kidney donors have given contradictory results as regards the clinical consequences of sustained hyperfiltration on the remaining kidney. Some investigators have demonstrated a high prevalence of arterial hypertension [Hakim et al. 1984, Tapson et al. 1984, Talseth et al. 1986, Mathillas et al. 1988] and/or an increased urinary protein excretion (Vincenti et al. 1984, Miller et al. 1985, Fehrman et al. 1986, Williams et al. 1986]. However, most reports have shown no correlation between increased protein excretion and hypertension or the degree of renal function [Hakim et al. 1984, Vincenti et al. 1984, Miller et al. 1985, Anderson et al. 1985, Williams et al. 1986]. It can, thus, be concluded that, despite these mild and sporadic abnormalities, long-standing hyperfiltration does not seems to have any detectable adverse effect on kidney function [Swainson and Smith 1989].

In order to determine the nature of the proteinuria, some studies have measured urinary albumin excretion (UAE) as a marker for glomerular origin. UAE was found to be normal after uninephrectomy by several investigators [Tapson et al. 1984, Vincenti et al. 1984, Bertolatus et al. 1985], but moderately increased by others [Fehrman et al. 1986, Talseth et al. 1986, Mathillas et al. 1988, Watnik et al. 1988]. Since an increased UAE is considered to be an early sign of glomerular hyperfiltration in diabetic patients who subsequently develop nephropathy [Mogensen 1987], measurement of the UAE may be useful for studying the effects of glomerular hyperfiltration in the remaining kidney.

The entity of glomerular hyperfiltration can be explored by the renal functional reserve, i. e. the renal capacity to acutely increase the glomerular filtration rate (GFR) in response to various stimuli [Bosch et al. 1983, Ter Wee et al. 1985, 1986]. It has been demonstrated that an acute protein load induces a transient increase in the GFR [Bosch et al. 1983] and can be useful for measuring the renal functional reserve, which is proportional to the number of normal-functioning glomeruli and inversely correlated to the resting level of GFR. In a recent study [Amore et al. 1988] carried out in six patients nephrectomized for renal lithiasis and reduced renal functional reserve, the acute protein load may amplify the effects of hyperfiltration on permselective properties of the glomerular membrane, leading to a further increase of the already existing microalbuminuria.

On the basis of these findings we studied the effects of an acute protein load on the UAE only in kidney donors, who were ascertained to be healthy subjects with two-normal kidneys at the time of donation and selected for normal UAE at the time of entry to this study.

Methods

Patients

We evaluated 6 subjects who had donated a kidney. The study group comprised 2 men and 4 women with a mean age at donation of 50.5 ± 5.0 years and 51.8 ± 4.9 years at follow-up. The average follow-up period after kidney donation was 16.7 ± 4.8 months. The subjects were selected carefully prior to donation for normality of renal function and the absence of systemic diseases. Their mean body weight was 78.0 ± 6.3 kg, while their mean body surface area was 1.78 ± 0.05 m^2. Each subject had a normal urinary sediment, a negative Albustix test, a daily proteinuria less than 150 mg and normal blood pressure (<140/90 mmHg). Their diet was not controlled or restricted in any way. Their estimated mean protein intake was evaluated by dietary interviews and urea nitrogen appearance and urinary urea excretion [Maroni et al. 1985]. It was 1.07 ± 0.03 g/kg body weight/day. The mean sodium intake, evaluated by daily urinary sodium excretion, was 137.6 ± 12.6 mEq/day. No drugs were given to any subject. The UAE was evaluated, firstly, under basal conditions, and then, before and after an acute protein load. Informed consent was obtained from all subjects.

Acute oral protein load

All kidney donors were studied before and after an acute protein load. The meal consisted of 700 g of cooked red meat weighed and prepared at a special diet unit, which corresponded to 150 g of animal protein (2 g/kg body weight).

In control studies, carried out after 15 days, the same subjects received a carbohydrate meal of equal caloric (1,370 kcal) and sodium content (51 mEq). The carbohydrate meal contained 6 g of animal protein.

During the two days of study the subjects were admitted to our Center at 8.00 a. m. after an overnight fast. The basal UAE, creatinine clearance (C_{cr}), fractional albumin excretion ($C_{alb}/C_{cr} \times 10^{-6}$) and urinary sodium excretion were measured. At noon the subjects ate the meals in 30 min with a simultaneous water load of 1 liter. The water diuresis was carried out in order to minimize potential errors due to incomplete bladder emptying. Urine samples were collected at voluntary voiding under direct supervision. After the

Table 1 Clinical baseline findings in six kidney donors

	n	C_{cr} ml/min/1.73 m^2	Ratio[a] %	ΔC_{cr}[b] ml/min/1.73 m^2	MAP[c] mmHg	UAE µg/min
Preoperative	6	97.8 ± 13.9	80.2 ± 5.9	28.7 ± 2.3	97.0 ± 1.3	3.1 ± 0.7
Current	6	77.5 ± 7.9[d]			93.2 ± 4.0	3.0 ± 0.6

Values are expressed as mean ± SEM.

[a] Current C_{cr} as a percentage of preoperative C_{cr}.

[b] Increase in C_{cr} in the remnant kidney, calculated as current C_{cr} – ½ preoperative C_{cr}.

[c] Mean arterial pressure.

Comparisons were made between the current and preoperative values: [d] $p < 0.05$.

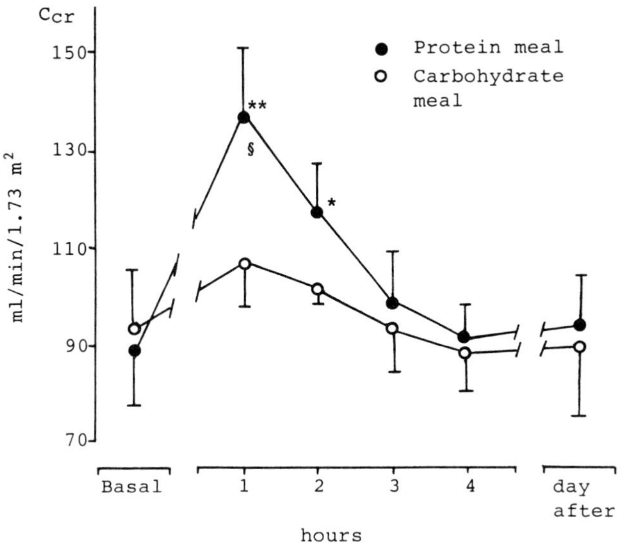

Fig. 1 Behavior of C_{cr} in six kidney donors before and after different meals. The values are expressed as mean ± SEM. The data were analyzed by analysis of variance. Comparisons between test and basal values: * p <0.05, ** p <0.01. Comparisons between protein and carbohydrate meal: § p <0.01

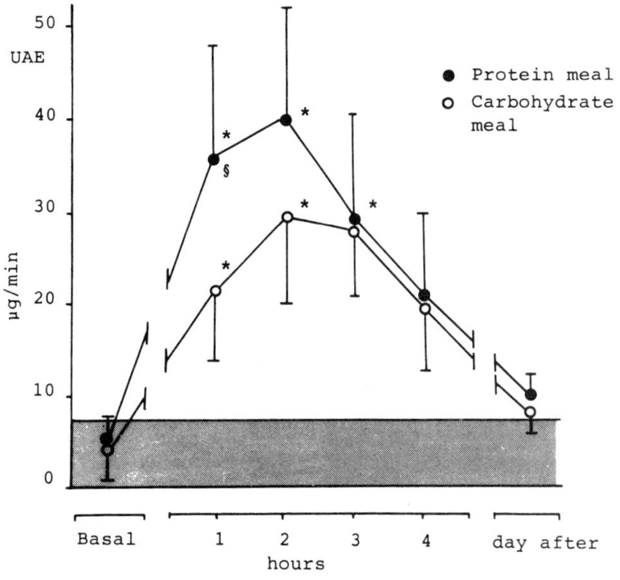

Fig. 2 Behavior of UAE in six kidney donors before and after different meals. The values are expressed as mean ± SEM. The data were analyzed by analysis of variance. Comparisons between test and basal values: * p <0.05. Comparisons between protein and carbohydrate meal: § p <0.05

meals, blood and urine samples were collected every 60 min for an additional 4 hours. The UAE, C_{cr}, fractional albumin excretion and urinary sodium excretion were determined. On the following day, the same assays were evaluated after an overnight fast.

UAE measurement

Overnight urine collections were used for the measurement of UAE by a radioimmunoassay kit (Sclavo, Siena, Italy). Urine samples were stored at −20°C for 4 weeks; cloudy samples were centrifuged before testing. 25 µl of urine were used for each individual determination. In every tube 100 µl of ^{125}I-albumin, 100 µl of rabbit anti-albumin serum and 100 µl of goat anti-rabbit-γ-globulins were added. The tubes were incubated for 1 hour at room temperature, and a further 2 ml of PEG were added to all tubes. After centrifugation for 10 min (at 1500 g) at room temperature the supernatant was aspired and discarded. The radioactivity was then determined with

Table 2 Behavior of the diuresis, natriuresis and FE_{Na} in 6 kidney donors before and after protein (PM) and carbohydrate (CM) meals

Time		Baseline	1 h	2 h	3 h	4 h	Following day
Diuresis (ml/min)	PM	1.42 ± 0.20	1.98 ± 0.17[a]	2.35 ± 0.35[a]	2.40 ± 0.36[a]	2.45 ± 0.43[a]	1.48 ± 0.16
	CM	1.50 ± 0.16	1.70 ± 0.20	2.34 ± 0.33[a]	2.55 ± 0.43[a]	2.26 ± 0.42	1.58 ± 0.16
Natriuresis (µEq/min)	PM	125.5 ± 11.8	224.0 ± 30.5[b]	216.8 ± 29.9[a]	185.5 ± 24.4	155.8 ± 31.1	113.1 ± 14.4
	CM	127.3 ± 12.7	143.3 ± 23.7[c]	201.3 ± 29.8[a]	196.6 ± 33.0	175.8 ± 37.1	118.8 ± 20.1
FE_{Na}	PM	1.06 ± 0.16	1.18 ± 0.16	1.32 ± 0.17	1.48 ± 0.30	1.22 ± 0.22	0.85 ± 0.11
	CM	1.02 ± 0.16	0.97 ± 0.11	1.42 ± 0.27	1.16 ± 0.16	1.20 ± 0.24	1.06 ± 0.29

Values are expressed as mean ± SEM. The data were analyzed by analysis of variance.
Comparisons were made between the test values and basal values: [a] p <0.05, [b] p <0.02.
Comparisons were made between protein and carbohydrate load: [c] p <0.05.

a gamma-counter (Packard Instruments, Zurich, Switzerland). The standard curve was constructed and the unknown concentration of albumin was determined by interpolation from the graph. The mean value obtained from normal subjects was 3.5 ± 1.9 µg/min (± SD).

Statistical analysis

Results were expressed as mean ± SEM, unless otherwise stated. The responses to protein and carbohydrate meals were analyzed by two-way analysis of variance; when variance analysis demonstrated statistical significance ($p < 0.05$), Student's t-test and Wilcoxon's test for paired data were used to compare data of each period to basal values. The latter were furthermore used to compare the same periods during two meals.

Results

The current mean level of serum creatinine in 6 kidney donors was 1.01 ± 0.09 mg/dl and did not differ from that measured before uninephrectomy (1.02 ± 0.07 mg/dl). No donor showed a serum creatinine greater than 1.5 mg/dl. The whole GFR, expressed by the C_{cr}, was reduced significantly from 97.8 ± 13.9 ml/min/1.73 m^2 to 77.5 ± 7.9 ml/min/1.73 m^2 ($p < 0.001$). The mean ratio between the current and the preoperative C_{cr} was 80.2 ± 5.9% (Table 1). No donor had a current C_{cr} value less than 50% of his preoperative value. The absolute mean increase in the C_{cr} in the remaining kidney, calculated from current C_{cr} – ½ preoperative C_{cr} and expressed as ΔC_{cr}, was 28.7 ± 2.3 ml/min/1.73 m^2 (Table 1).

The mean arterial pressure did not differ before (97.0 ± 1.3 mmHg) and after (93.2 ± 4.0) uninephrectomy.

The current mean value for UAE was 3.0 ± 0.6 µg/min and did not differ from the preoperative mean value (3.1 ± 0.7 µg/min) nor from the mean value found in normal subjects. No donor showed a UAE of more than 7.3 µg/min, i.e. two standard deviations from the mean value found in normal subjects (Table 1).

Acute oral protein load

The hemodynamic renal response to the meals showed a significant ($p < 0.005$) increase in the C_{cr} only after the protein load (Figure 1). The basal mean C_{cr} before the two different loads did not differ significantly (89.2 ± 10.2 and 94.2 ± 11.9 ml/min/1.73 m^2, respectively). It increased significantly in the first hour after the protein load (137.3 ± 14.1 ml/min/1.73 m^2; $p < 0.01$) and remained higher at the second hour ($p < 0.05$), returning to baseline values at the fourth hour. The difference between the increase in the C_{cr} at the first hour after the protein load (stimulated) and the baseline C_{cr} (unstimulated) was considered to be an index of the renal functional reserve. The mean value of the renal functional reserve was 51.3 ± 6.8 ml/min/1.73 m^2, corresponding to an increment of 61.8 ± 10.9%.

After the carbohydrate meal the mean C_{cr} did not change significantly, even though a mild increase was observed at the first hour. Furthermore, at that time, the mean value after the protein meal was significantly higher than that obtained after the carbohydrate meal ($p < 0.01$), while the levels did not differ on the following days.

The behavior of UAE showed a significant increase after the protein ($p < 0.005$) and the carbohydrate ($p < 0.005$) meal. The basal mean value of the UAE before the two meals did not differ. The mean level of UAE increased significantly after the protein load at the first (36.7 ± 12.3 µg/min; $p < 0.05$) and second hour (40.4 ± 13.9 µg/min; $p < 0.05$). It had declined slowly at the third and fourth hour, reaching the basal level on the next day. The mean value of the UAE after the carbohydrate meal was significantly increased at the first (23.7 ± 7.7 µg/min; $p < 0.05$), second (29.4 ± 9.0 µg/min; $p < 0.05$) and third hour (27.3 ± 7.3 µg/min; $p < 0.05$) and returned to the basal value in the following day. Furthermore, the mean value of the UAE at the first hour after the protein load was significantly ($p < 0.05$) higher than that found at the same period after the carbohydrate meal. The fractional albumin excretion ($C_{alb}/C_{cr} \times 10^{-6}$) increased significantly both after protein ($p < 0.01$) and carbohydrate ($p < 0.005$) meals. The mean value rose significantly from 1.72 ± 0.47 to 7.25 ± 2.35 ($p < 0.05$) after the protein meal and from 1.52 ± 0.42 to 6.59 ± 2.08 ($p < 0.05$) after the carbohydrate meal. No difference was seen between the two experiments.

Table 2 shows the behavior of diuresis, natriuresis and fractional sodium excretion (FE_{Na}) on the experimental and the control days. The mean basal levels of each parameter before the two meals did not differ significantly. The diuresis increased significantly after the protein ($p < 0.005$) and carbohydrate ($p < 0.005$) load. The increase was significant at the first ($p < 0.05$), second ($p < 0.05$), third ($p < 0.05$) and fourth hour ($p < 0.05$) after the protein load and at the second ($p < 0.05$) and third hour ($p < 0.05$) after the carbohydrate meal. No difference was found between the two meals at the same hours. The urinary sodium excretion increased significantly after both meals:

p <0.001 for protein and p <0.025 for carbohydrate meal, respectively. However, after the protein load, the natriuresis increased rapidly and significantly at the first (p <0.02) and the second hour (p <0.05), while on the control day the rise was significant only after the second hour (p <0.05). Furthermore, at the first hour, coincidental with the highest GFR value, the mean value of natriuresis after the protein load (224.0 ± 30.5 μEq/min) was higher (p <0.05) than that found at the same period on the control day (143.3 ± 23.7 μEq/min).

The FE_{Na} did not change significantly after either meal even though a moderate increase was observed at the second and third hour after the protein load and at the second hour after the carbohydrate meal. No difference was seen between the two meals at the same period.

Discussion

This short-term follow-up study did not show any adverse effects of glomerular hyperfiltration in the remaining kidney of kidney donors. No increase in arterial blood pressure, urinary protein excretion or progressive renal failure was observed. A compensatory increase in the GFR (as expressed by the C_{cr}) in the remaining kidney of our kidney donors was found under basal conditions and regular protein intake. However, we did not find the microalbuminuria, confirming what has been reported by others [Tapson et al. 1984, Vincenti et al. 1984, Weiland et al. 1984]. On the other hand Bertolatus et al. [1985] demonstrated a transient increase in the UAE one week after uninephrectomy that returned to preoperative values during the first month. The length of the follow-up was similar to our period of observation and the presence of microalbuminuria was not found. The absence of microalbuminuria in our subjects may have been due to the regular protein intake, since it has been demonstrated that the persistent [Brenner et al. 1982, Hostetter et al. 1986a] or acute [Hostetter 1986c] modifications in dietary protein intake may influence the GFR. We have not examined the long-term effects of dietary protein modifications on the GFR and the UAE in kidney donors. However, a recent study in patients with a single kidney and an augmented UAE under basal conditions has demonstrated a change in the UAE with a different protein intake [Coppo et al. 1988]. Nevertheless, most of the patients differed from our subjects, because they underwent uninephrectomy mainly for chronic renal diseases and therefore had microalbuminuria even with a regular protein intake; although tubular function was shown to be normal, it was not possible to exclude the presence of glomerular damage.

In addition to a regular, high protein intake, it has been demonstrated that an acute protein load may transiently increase the GFR [Hostetter 1986c] and may be useful for measuring the renal functional reserve [Bosch et al. 1983], which was found to be normal in kidney donors by some investigators [Tapson et al. 1986], but reduced [Rodríguez-Iturbe et al. 1985, Ter Wee et al. 1987] or absent [Wheeler et al. 1987] by others.

Our results demonstrated that, despite the high level of chronic hyperfiltration, the remaining kidney is still able to increase the GFR rapidly when acutely stimulated by a protein meal. Even though the C_{cr} may overestimate the GFR in acute studies, it has been demonstrated that the accuracy is improved by the use of early and frequent blood and urine sampling; furthermore the first clearance peak must be utilized to measure the renal functional reserve [Laville et al. 1989]. Other investigators [Bosch et al. 1984, Rodríguez-Iturbe et al. 1985, Molina et al. 1988] have found that C_{cr} and inulin clearance after a protein load gave similar results and concluded that C_{cr} may be a reliable indicator of the GFR changes when the renal function is within normal limits.

The acute increase in the GFR in our kidney donors was associated with a rapid increase in the UAE. To the best of our knowledge this is the first study which examines the acute effects of a protein load on the UAE in kidney donors. A similar study [Amore et al. 1988], carried out on patients nephrectomized for renal lithiasis and high mean baseline UAE, observed an ulterior increase on the UAE after protein load; this study concluded that the increasing UAE may be due to a pre-existing loss of glomerular permselectivity and thus could be a subclinical sign of renal disease. On the other hand, our study was carried out in kidney donors who had two normal kidneys at donation and normal baseline UAE before the acute protein load. It is not easy to explain the increased UAE after the protein load, since an increased UAE was also found after the carbohydrate meal, even though the rise was slower and less pronounced. The increased diuresis and natriuresis after both meals suggest that the increased UAE after protein load may be due in part to the glomerular hyperfiltration and in part to the increased urine flow, while the increase in the UAE after the carbohydrate meal may be due to the water load. Some studies on healthy subjects with two normal kidneys have reported a slight increase in the UAE both after protein load and after water load [Amore et al. 1988, Viberti et al. 1982]. Since the tubular reabsorption of filtered albumin operates at maximal capacity under normal conditions [Bertolatus et al. 1985], an increased urine flow may give rise to a tubular washout of the increased filtered albumin resulting from glomerular hyperfiltration [Viberti et al. 1982].

Finally, despite the fact that the glomerular hyperfiltration may increase the filtered albumin, the tubular reabsorption under basal conditions may mask the presence of microalbuminuria. During a protein load the additional increase in the GFR and the filtered albumin, associated with water and sodium diuresis, gives rise to microalbuminuria at a level greater than that found after a carbohydrate load, when only the water and sodium load were present. At this point it is not possible to conclude whether the appearance of the microalbuminuria after a protein meal has a prognostic importance or if it is a physiological response to hormonal and hemodynamic variations.

Acknowledgements

Part of this work was presented at the 2nd Roma Nephrology Conference, September 22–23, 1989, Fiuggi, Italy. The authors express their gratitude to Dr. Justine Claudatus and Dr. Michele Carbone for their excellent collaboration, Miss Alessandra Di Falco and Miss Lidia Vulpi for their contribution as dieticians and Mr. Giovanni Carlucci for assisting in typing the manuscript.

REFERENCES

Amore A, Coppo R, Roccatello D, Martina G, Rollino C, Basolo B, Novelli F, Amprimo MC, Cavalli G, Piccoli G 1988 Single kidney function: Effect of acute protein and water loading on microalbuminuria. Am J Med *84:* 711

Anderson CF, Velosa JA, Frohnert PP, Torres VE, Offord KP, Vogel JP, Donadio JVJ, Wilson DM 1985 The risks of unilateral nephrectomy: status of kidney donors 10 to 20 years postoperatively. Mayo Clin Proc *60:* 367

Bertolatus JA, Friedlander MA, Scheidt C, Hunsicker LG 1985 Urinary albumin excretion after donor nephrectomy. Am J Kidney Dis *5:* 165

Bosch JP, Saccaggi A, Lauer A, Ronco C, Belledonne M, Glabman S 1983 Renal functional reserve in humans. Effect of protein intake on glomerular filtration rate. Am J Med *75:* 943

Bosch JP, Lauer A, Glabman S 1984 Short-term protein loading in assessment of patients with renal disease. Am J Med *77:* 873

Brenner BM, Meyer TW, Hostetter TH 1982 Dietary protein intake and the progressive nature of renal disease: the role of haemodynamically mediated glomerular injury in the pathogenesis of progressive glomerular sclerosis in aging, renal ablation and intrinsic renal disease. N Engl J Med *307:* 352

Coppo R, Amore A, Roccatello D, Martina G, Rollino C, Basolo B, Piccoli G 1988 Microalbuminuria in single kidney patients: relationship with protein intake. Clin Nephrol *29:* 219

Fehrman I, Widstam U, Lundgren G 1986 Long-term consequences of renal donation in humans. Transplant Proc *18:* 102

Hakim RM, Goldszer RC, Brenner BM 1984 Hypertension and proteinuria: Long-term sequelae of uninephrectomy in humans. Kidney Int *25:* 930

Hostetter TH, Olson JL, Rennke HG, Venkatachalam MA, Brenner BM 1986a Hyperfiltration in remnant nephrons: a potentially adverse response to renal ablation. Am J Physiol *241:* F85

Hostetter TH, Meyer TW, Rennke HG, Brenner BM 1986b Chronic effects of dietary protein in the rat with intact and reduced renal mass. Kidney Int *30:* 509

Hostetter TH 1986c Renal hemodynamic response to a meat meal in humans. Am J Physiol *250:* F613

Laville M, Hadj-Aissa A, Pozet N, Le Bras JH, Labeeuw M, Zech P 1989 Restrictions on use of creatinine clearance for measurement of renal functional reserve. Nephron *51:* 233

Maroni BJ, Steinman TI, Mitch WE 1985 A method for estimating nitrogen intake of patients with chronic renal failure. Kidney Int *27:* 58

Mathillas Ö, Attman PO, Aurell M, Bryngel H 1988 Glomerular filtration rate, hypertension and proteinuria after renal ablation: a long-term follow-up study in kidney donors. Scand J Urol Nephrol (Suppl 108): *49*

Miller IJ, Suthanthiran M, Riggio RR, Williams JW, Riehle RA, Vaughan ED, Stubenbord WT, Mouradian J, Cheigh JS, Stenzel KH 1985 Impact of renal donation. Am J Med *79:* 201

Mogensen CE 1987 Microalbuminuria as a predictor of clinical diabetic nephropathy. Kidney Int *31:* 673

Molina E, Herrera J, Rodríguez-Iturbe B 1988 The renal functional reserve in health and renal disease in school age children. Kidney Int *34:* 809

Olson JL, Hostetter TH, Rennke HG, Brenner BM, Venkatachalam MA 1982 Altered glomerular permselectivity and progressive sclerosis following extreme ablation of renal mass. Kidney Int *22:* 112

Rodríguez-Iturbe B, Herrera J, García R 1985 Response to acute protein load in kidney donors and in apparently normal post-acute glomerulonephritis patients: evidence for glomerular hyperfiltration. Lancet *2:* 461

Swainson CP, Smith C 1989 The long-term risks of unilateral nephrectomy in man: A case control study. (abstract) Kidney Int *35:* 233

Talseth T, Fauchald P, Skrede S, Djøseland O, Berg JK, Stenstrøm J, Heilo A, Brodwall EK, Flatmark A 1986 Long-term blood pressure and renal function in kidney donors. Kidney Int *29:* 1072

Tapson JS, Marshall SM, Tisdall SR, Wilkinson R, Ward MK, Kerr DNS 1984 Renal function and blood pressure after donor nephrectomy. Proc EDTA-ERA *21:* 520

Tapson JS, Mansy H, Marshall SM, Tisdall SR, Wilkinson R 1986 Renal functional reserve in kidney donors. Q J Med *231:* 725

Ter Wee PM, Geerlings W, Rosman JB, Sluiter WJ, Van Der Geest S, Donker AJM 1985 Testing renal reserve filtration capacity with an amino acid solution. Nephron *41:* 193

Ter Wee PM, Rosman JB, Van Der Geest S, Sluiter WJ, Donker AJM 1986 Renal haemodynamics during separate and combined infusion of amino acids and dopamine. Kidney Int *29:* 870

Ter Wee PM, Tegzess AM, Donker AJM 1987 The effect of low-dose dopamine on renal function in uninephrectomized patients: special emphasis on kidney donors before and after nephrectomy. Clin Nephrol *28:* 211

Viberti GC, Mogensen CE, Keen H, Jacobsen FK, Jarret RJ, Christensen CK 1982 Urinary excretion of albumin in normal man: the effect of water loading. Scand J Clin Lab Invest *42:* 147

Vincenti F, Amend WJC, Kaysen G, Feduska N, Birnbaum J, Duca R, Salviterra O 1984 Long-term renal function in kidney donors. Transplantation *36:* 626

Watnik TJ, Jenkins RR, Rackoff P, Baumgarten A, Bia MJ 1988 Microalbuminuria and hypertension in long-term renal donors. Transplantation *45:* 59

Weiland D, Sutherland DER, Chavers B, Simmons RL, Asher NL, Najarian JS 1984 Information on 628 living-related kidney donors at a single institution, with long-term follow-up in 472 cases. Transplantation Proc *16:* 5

Wheeler DC, Cosgriff PS, Bennet SE, Walls J 1987 Measurement of renal functional reserve on the single kidney in man. Clin Nephrol *28:* 87

Williams SL, Oler J, Jorkasky DK 1986 Long-term renal function in kidney donors: A comparison of donors and their siblings. Ann Int Med *105:* 1

Clinical Nephrology, Vol. 35 No. 2 – 1991 (66–71)

Hyperreninemic hypoaldosteronism due to hepatocellular carcinoma metastatic to the adrenal gland

S. Otabe[1], S. Muto[2], Y. Asano[2], K. Sato[1], M. Ohtani[1], C. Kawamoto[1], K. Ido[1] and K. Kimura[1]

Departments of Gastroenterology[1] and Nephrology[2], Jichi Medical School, Tochigi, Japan

Abstract. Metastases to the adrenal glands are common in patients with cancer, but among those affected, hyperreninemic hypoaldosteronism is noted very rarely. A case of hyperreninemic hypoaldosteronism secondary to metastatic hepatocellular carcinoma is reported. Laboratory data revealed selective aldosterone deficiency with hyperreninemia. Biopsy documented replacement of the adrenal glands with metastatic hepatocellular carcinoma. A review of the literature disclosed that the present case was an extremely rare one of its kind.

Key words: hyperreninemic hypoaldosteronism – hepatocellular carcinoma

Introduction

Rare cases of hyperreninemic hypoaldosteronism have been described recently. The underlying or associated disorders included idiopathic hypoparathyroidism [Marieb et al. 1974, Saenger et al. 1982], diabetes mellitus [Morimoto et al. 1979], critical illness [Zipser et al. 1981, Davenport and Zipser, 1983], amyloidosis [Silver et al. 1982], heparin administration [O'Kelly et al. 1983], deficiency of angiotensin converting enzyme [Findling et al. 1987], and postulated deficiency of angiotensin II receptors [Williams et al. 1983]. Despite the frequency with which the adrenal glands are affected by metastases in patients with cancer, neoplastic destruction of these organs is an extremely rare cause of hyperreninemic hypoaldosteronism. There has been only one reported case of selective aldosterone deficiency caused by metastatic squamous cell lung cancer [Taylor et al. 1988]. In a review of the literature, we were unable to find any report of hepatocellular carcinoma associated with liver cirrhosis being responsible for selective hypoaldosteronism. Here, we describe a patient who had hyperreninemic hypoaldosteronism and in whom both adrenal glands were destroyed by metastases from a hepatocellular carcinoma.

Received March 3, 1990; in revised form November 12, 1990.

Reprint requests to Dr. S. Otabe, Division of Endocrinology & Metabolism, Department of Medicine, Kurume University, School of Medicine, Kurume-Shi, Fukuoka-Ken, 830 Japan

Case report

A 56-year-old Japanese man was admitted to our hospital as an ambulatory patient on February 8, 1989, with numbness of the right shoulder, a poor appetite and difficulty in raising the right arm. Past history revealed multiple hepatocellular carcinoma (Edmondson grade II) with severe liver cirrhosis with negative serological markers for hepatitis B, and metastasis of the carcinoma to the right adrenal gland, which was diagnosed by laparoscopic needle biopsy in August 1987 (Figures 1 and 2). Thereafter, transaortic embolization and intraaortic mitomycin C injection were performed. Fluorouracil was also given orally at a dose of 150 mg three times daily.

On admission, the patient was alert; the temperature was 35.5° C, pulse, 88/min, blood pressure, 138/80 mmHg in a recumbent position, height, 154 cm, weight 53.5 kg. He was built average and fairly well nourished. His skin was dry with no obvious pigmentation. Heart sounds were clear and rhythm was regular without audible murmurs or rhonchi. Examination of the abdomen revealed a large, smooth and hard mass in the right upper quadrant. No signs of ascitic fluid were found. There was no peripheral edema in the extremities. Neurological examinations showed the cranial nerves to be intact. Examination of motor function disclosed difficulty in elevation of the right deltoid and suprascapular abduction. Neither the biceps nor triceps reflex on the right was demonstrable. There were no pathological reflexes. Examination of sensory function revealed numbness in the right segmental C4 area.

Examination of the blood on admission revealed: RBC 295 × $10^4/mm^3$, Hb 12.6 g/dl, Ht 36.7%, platelet 25.2 × 10^4/mm^3, WBC 4.6 × 10^3/mm^3 with 63% segmented neutrophils, 4% band forms, 1% myelocytes, 1% eosinophils, 28% lymphocytes, and 3% monocytes. The sedimentation rate was 46 mm/h. Blood chemistry showed: T-Bil 5.1 mg/dl, D-Bil 2.5 mg/dl, thymol turbidity test 62 KU. U, zinc turbidity test 22.4 KU. U, GOT 228 mU/ml, GPT 232 mU/ml, LDH 1,708 mU/ml, choline-esterase 0.25 ΔpH, total cholesterol 346 mg/dl, triglyceride 272 mg/dl, BUN 24 mg/dl, creatinine 0.9 mg/dl, and total protein 6.2 g/dl including albumin 48.4%, α_1-globulin 4.1%, α_2-globulin 4.8%, β-globulin 15.9%, and γ-globulin 26.8%. Coagulation time, 10.4 s (control, 11.4 s); thrombotest, 58.0%; serum fibrinogen was 207 mg/dl. Serum electrolytes were as follows: sodium 140 mEq/l, potassium 3.8 mEq/l, chloride 103 mEq/l. The fasting blood glucose level was normal. Serologic tests revealed: C-reactive protein 0.165 mg/dl, α_1-fetoprotein 129,400 ng/ml, CA 19-9 3 U/ml. Urinalysis showed a specific gravity of 1.015 and a positive test result for urobilinogen without glucose or protein. Microscopic examination of urinary sediment revealed 1 to 2 white blood cells and 1 to 2 phosphate crystals per high-power field.

X-ray examination of the cervical spine showed extensive destruction of the body of the fourth cervical vertebra probably due to metastatic hepatocellular carcinoma, and compression on the right side. A barium esophagogram and endoscopy demonstrated large varices involving the lower two-thirds of the esophagus. Abdominal ultrasonography demonstrated multiple space-occupying lesions in the atrophic liver and large low-echoic lesions on the bilateral adrenals without ascites. A computed tomographic scan of the abdomen also revealed the space-occupying lesions in the atrophic liver and a 16 × 15-cm mass in the right adrenal and a 6 × 6-cm mass in the left adrenal (Figure 3). From these histological as well as radiological findings, adrenal insufficiency secondary to metastasis of the hepatocellular carcinoma to the bilateral adrenal glands was suspected. At this point, several studies were carried out to evaluate the adrenocortical function.

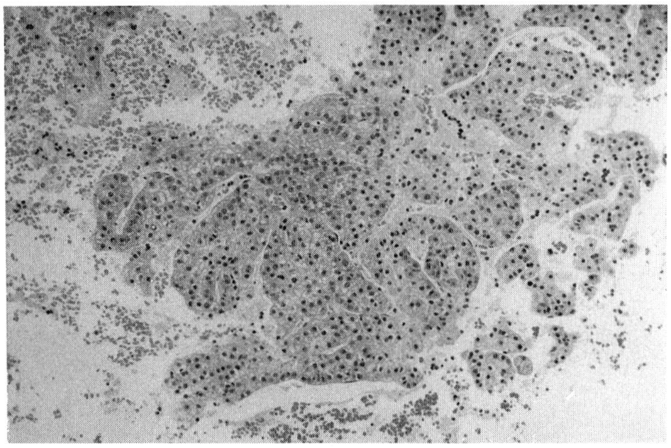

Fig. 1 Photomicrograph of liver showing hepatocellular carcinoma associated with liver cirrhosis (Hematoxylin and eosin stain, ×50).

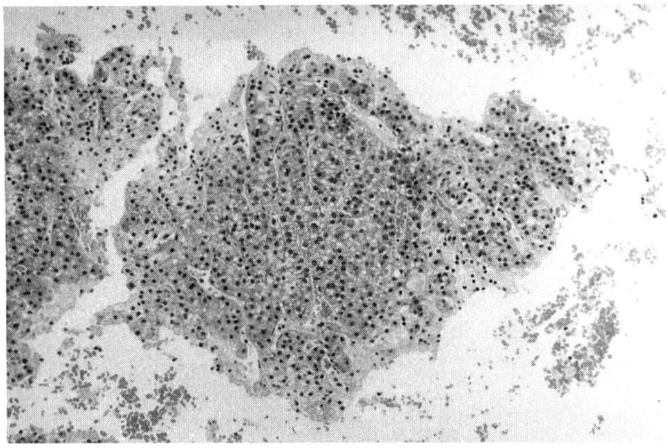

Fig. 2 Photomicrograph of right adrenal gland showing complete replacement by hepatocellular carcinoma with a similar histological picture to that seen in Figure 1 (Hematoxylin and eosin stain, ×50).

Methods

Serum aldosterone [Ogihara et al. 1977], plasma renin activity [Ikeda et al. 1982] and serum cortisol [Rudder et al. 1972] were measured according to previously described methods. Specific radioimmunoassay was used to measure serum adrenocorticotropic hormone (ACTH) (ACTH kit; Nippon DPC Corporation, Tokyo, Japan). Plasma angiotensin I, angiotensin II, serum angiotensin converting enzyme and atrial natriuretic peptide were measured by radioimmunoassay at Special Reference Laboratories (Tokyo, Japan).

Administration of angiotensin II, ACTH or furosemide was started at 0800:0900 h after an overnight-fast and with the patient supine.

Angiotensin II amide (Hypertension, Ciba Pharmaceutical Co., Summit, NJ, USA) was infused intravenously at a rate of 40 ng/kg/min for 30 min, and supine blood pressure wasa measured at 2-min intervals throughout the infusion. Blood samples were drawn before and 30 min after angiotensin II administration for determination of serum aldosterone and plasma renin activity.

A rapid ACTH stimulation test was performed in the following manner: After blood samples had been taken for baseline cortisol and aldosterone, 250 µg of soluble ACTH (1–24) (Cortrosyn, Organon) was injected intravenously, and blood samples for deter-

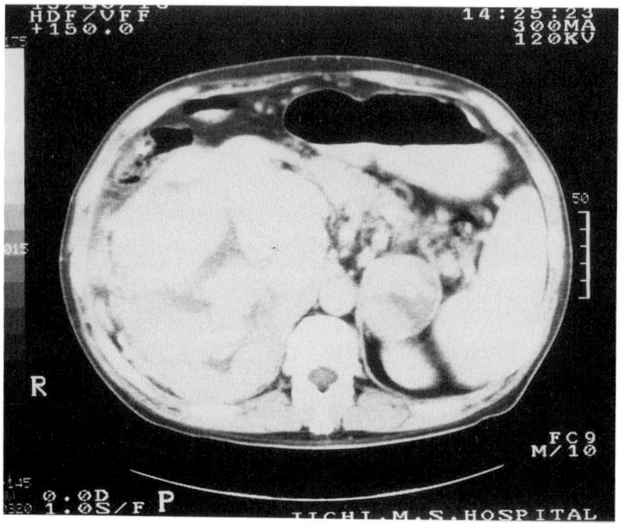

Fig. 3 Computed tomography of abdomen showing massive adrenal glands with nodular masses.

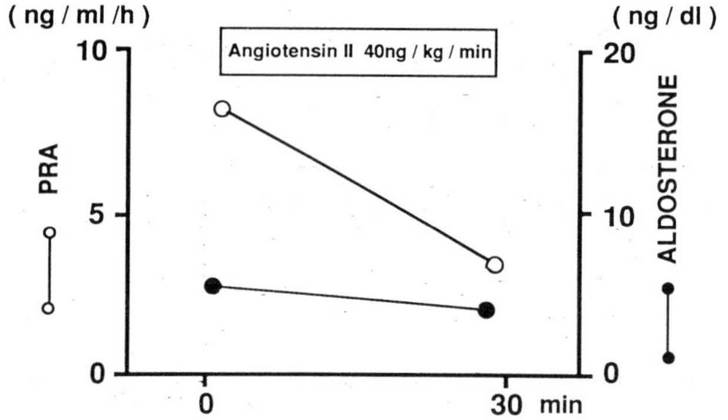

Fig. 4 Effects of angiotensin II on plasma renin activity and serum aldosterone level. PRA: Plasma renin activity.

mination of stimulated cortisol and aldosterone were drawn 30 min and 60 min after this injection.

Furosemide (Lasix, Hoechst), 40 mg, was injected intravenously, and the patient was kept recumbent for 2 hours. Blood samples for determination of baseline and stimulated renin and aldosterone levels were drawn.

Results

The basal morning serum aldosterone level was less than 0.5 ng/dl (normal, 5.0–15.0 ng/dl), which was markedly suppressed, despite extremely high plasma renin activity 15.7 ng/ml/h (normal, 1.17 ± 0.9 ng/ml/h). The basal morning cortisol level was 11.5 μg/dl (normal, 4.0–12.0 μg/dl) and the early evening cortisol level 7.8 μg/dl. The urinary excretion of 17-hydroxycorticosteroids and 17-ketogenic steroids was 2.7 mg/g creatinine/day (normal, 1.6–6.7 mg/g creatinine/day) and 2.7 mg/g creatinine/day (normal, 2.0–7.6 mg/g creatinine/day), respectively. In addition, the basal morning ACTH level was 19.1 pg/ml (normal, 20–40 pg/ml) and the plasma natriuretic peptide level 40 pg/ml (normal, 33–80 pg/ml). Plasma angiotensin I and II concentrations were 390 pg/ml (normal, less than 250 pg/ml) and 7 pg/ml (normal, less than 25 pg/ml), respectively. Serum angiotensin converting enzyme activity was 14.1 IU/l/37° C (normal, 8.3–21.4 IU/l/37° C).

Figure 4 shows the effects of angiotensin II on plasma renin activity and serum aldosterone level. After the administration of angiotensin II at a dose of 40 ng/kg/min, the blood pressure was adequately increased from 107/60 to 139/89 mmHg and plasma renin activity was sufficiently suppressed from 7.85 to

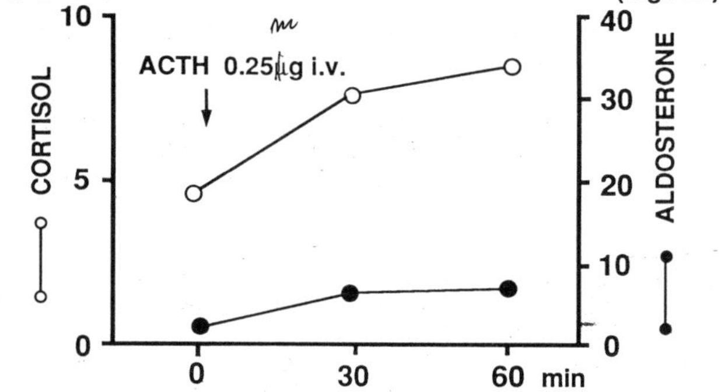

Fig. 5 Effects of rapid ACTH administration on serum cortisol and aldosterone levels.

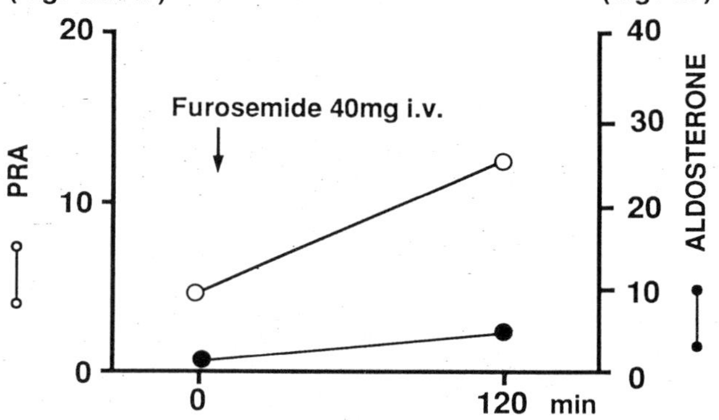

Fig. 6 Effects of furosemide injection on plasma renin activity and serum aldosterone level. PRA: Plasma renin activity.

3.50 ng/ml/h, with no increase in serum aldosterone (from 5.4 to 4.1 ng/dl).

Figure 5 shows the effects of rapid ACTH administration on serum cortisol and aldosterone levels. Basal serum aldosterone level (2.9 ng/dl) was low. After ACTH administration, the serum aldosterone level was increased to 7.6 ng/dl although the peak value of the serum aldosterone was in the normal range of the basal level. On the other hand, the serum cortisol level was increased from 4.8 to 8.6 µg/dl.

Figure 6 shows the effects of furosemide injection on plasma renin activity and serum aldosterone level. Basal serum aldosterone concentration (2.7 ng/dl) was low despite the extremely high plasma renin activity (7.0 ng/ml/h). Furosemide administration produced a definite increase of serum aldosterone to 6.9 ng/dl although this peak value was at the lower limit of the normal basal range.

Discussion

The present diagnosis of hepatocellular carcinoma causing primary selective hyperreninemic hypoaldosteronism secondary to metastases to the adrenal glands was supported by the following data: (1) a very low basal morning level of serum aldosterone; (2) impaired response of serum aldosterone levels to independent stimulation with angiotensin II, ACTH, and furosemide; (3) elevation of plasma renin activity; (4) normal fasting plasma ACTH and serum cortisol levels; (5) normal levels of urinary 17-hydroxysteroids and 17-ketogenic steroids; (6) circadian rhythm of serum cortisol. We believe our data are most consistent with variable degrees of depression of steroid synthesis in association with the tumor replacing the entire right adrenal gland and sparing only minimal zonae fasciculata and reticularis of the left adrenal gland. However, we cannot exclude the possibility of a subtle defect in the zona fasciculata, because the maximum increment of serum cortisol level after ACTH administration appeared somewhat blunted. Thus, the isolated aldosterone deficiency in the present patient seems most likely to be a milder form or an early state of Addison's disease. The acquired nature of the defect was confirmed by a needle aspiration biopsy of the right adrenal gland on laparoscopy, which showed near total destruction of the gland by hepatocellular carcinoma. Additional causes of hyperreninemic hypoaldosteronism such as diabetes mellitus, hypoparathyroidism, critical illness, amyloidosis and heparin administration did not appear to be relevant in our patient.

The adrenal gland is a common site of metastasis from various neoplasmas. Reports from autopsy studies show that as many as 16% of stomach cancers [Cedermark et al. 1977], 42% of lung cancers [Willis 1953], 58% of breast cancers [Glomset 1938], and 14% of colorectal cancers [Cedermark et al. 1977] metastasize to the adrenal glands. Other reports have described adrenal metastasis in 28–42% of lung primaries and 12–34% of breast primaries [Bullock and Hirst 1953, Sahagian-Edwards and Holland 1954]. Although metastasis to the adrenal glands is a common finding, few well documented reports of adrenal insufficiency involving selective hypoaldosteronism, associated with adrenal metastasis, have been published. Only 28 cases in which both laboratory and histologic evidence was obtained for adrenal insufficiency secondary to metastatic carcinoma have appeared in the literature (Table 1). Other reported cases lacked either chemical or microscopic documentation.

The case we present here is unique in several aspects. Documented selective hypoaldosteronism resulting from metastatic hepatocellular carcinoma has

Table 1 Functional adrenal insufficiency in cancer patients with histologically confirmed adrenal metastases

Site of primary tumor	No. of cases	References
Lung	13	Wallach & Scharfman (1952)
		Sahagian-Edwards & Holland (1954)
		MacKenzie (1955)
		Hill & Wheeler (1965)
		Schambelan et al. (1969)
		Weber & Murphy (1971)
		Vieweg et al. (1973)
		Seidenwurm et al. (1984)
Lymphoma	5	Case Report (1967)
		Sparagana (1970)
		Feinmann et al. (1976)
		Schnitzer et al. (1986)
		Carey et al. (1986)
Colon	3	Black et al. (1981)
		Seidenwurm et al. (1984)
		Omoigui et al. (1987)
Stomach	2	Leary & Masters (1957)
		Ezio & Francesco (1964)
Breast	2	Alpers et al. (1962)
		Sparagana (1970)
Testis	1	Heuson (1966)
Pancreas	1	Hagtuet (1963)
Bladder	1	Kennedy et al. (1987)

not been reported previously. Only one case of selective hypoaldosteronism caused by metastasis of squamous cell carcinoma to the adrenal glands was recently reported by Taylor et al. [1988]. They described a 56-year-old white man with squamous cell carcinoma who showed low serum aldosterone and high plasma renin activity. At autopsy, near total destruction of both adrenal glands by the metastatic tumor was demonstrated. The true incidence of adrenal insufficiency in patients with carcinoma metastatic to both adrenal glands is not known. Sporadic cases of adrenal hypofunction secondary to adrenal metastasis have been reported since Addison's first description of adrenal insufficiency [Addison 1855]. Most of these reports have been single case reports usually diagnosed retrospectively and based on clinical presentation unconfirmed by endocrinologic tests [Sahagian-Edwards and Holland 1954, Wallach and Scharfman 1952, Leary and Masters 1957, Alpers et al. 1962, Hill and Wheeler 1965, Galloway and Perloff 1960]. However, the incidence of selective hypoaldosteronism in our present patient was disclosed prospectively at the time of diagnosis of bilateral adrenal gland metastasis, and was confirmed by radiologic, histologic and endocrinologic tests.

Clinical findings of dehydration and orthostatic hypotension, and laboratory findings of hyponatremia and intermittent hyperkalemia in the setting of urinary salt-wasting are characteristic of aldosterone deficiency. However, such abnormalities were not demonstrated in our patient, and the underlying mechanisms were not known. The absence of the typical features of selective aldosterone deficiency may possible be explained by the limited residual adrenocortical function, because clinical symptoms do not occur in most patients until more than 80% of the adrenal mass is destroyed [Bondy 1985].

In summary, we have described a patient with metastatic hepatocellular carcinoma causing hyperreninemic hypoaldosteronism, confirmed by radiologic, histologic and endocrinologic tests.

Acknowledgement

We are grateful to Miss H. Shimada for her excellent secretarial work in preparing the manuscript.

REFERENCES

Addison T 1855 On the constitutional and local effects of disease of the suprarenal capsules. London: Samuel Highley

Alpers DH, Engelman K, Foley FD 1962 Addison's disease secondary to carcinoma of the breast. Ann Int Med *57:* 464

Black RM, Daniels GH, Coggins CH, Mueller PR, Data RE, Lichtenstein N 1981 Adrenal insufficiency from metastatic colonic carcinoma masquerading as isolated aldosterone deficiency. Report of a case and review of the literature. Acta Endocrinol *98:* 586

Bondy PK 1985 Disorders of the adrenal cortex. In: Textbook of Endocrinology, 7th ed., ed. by *Wilson JD* and *Foster DN,* 852

Bullock WK, Hirst AE 1953 Metastatic carcinoma of the adrenal cortex. Am J Med Sci *226:* 521

Carey RW, Harris N, Kliman B 1987 Addison's disease secondary to lymphomatous infiltration of the adrenal glands. Recovery of adrenocortical function after chemotherapy. Cancer *59:* 1087

Case Report 1967 Unexplained Addison's disease. Postgrad Med *42:* 339

Cedermark BJ, Blumenson LE, Pickren JW, Holyoke DE, Elias EG 1977 The significance of metastasis to the adrenal glands in adenocarcinoma of the colon and rectum. Surg Gynecol Obstet *144:* 537

Cedermark BJ, Blumenson LE, Pickren JW, Elias EG 1977 The significance of metastasis to the adrenal glands from carcinoma of the stomach and esophagus. Surg Gynecol Obstet *145:* 41

Davenport WK, Zipser RD 1983 Association of hypotension with hyperreninemic hypoaldosteronism in the critically ill patient. Arch Intern Med *143:* 735

Ezio C, Francesco G 1964 Acute adrenal insufficiency caused by bilateral massive metastases of gastric carcinoma. Osped Maggiore *59:* 442

Feinmann C, Gillett R, Irving MH 1976 Hodgkin's disease presenting with hypoaldosteronism. Br Med J *2:* 455

Findling JW, Adams AH, Raff H 1987 Selective hypoaldosteronism due to an endogenous impairment in angiotensin II production. New Engl J Med *316:* 1632

Galloway JA, Perloff WH 1960 Addison's disease secondary to adrenocortical destruction by metastatic carcinoma of the breast. Am J Med *28:* 156

Glomset DA 1938 The incidence of metastasis of malignant tumors to the adrenals. Am J Cancer *32:* 57

Hagtuet J 1963 Adrenocortical insufficiency due to metastatic infiltration of the adrenal glands. Acta Med Scand *174:* 1

Heuson JC 1966 Addison's disease secondary to occult metastatic seminoma. Infarction of the adrenals as the probable mechanism of their destruction. Cancer *19:* 1754

Hill GJ, Wheeler HW 1965 Adrenal insufficiency due to metastatic carcinoma of the lung. Cancer *18:* 1467

Ikeda I, Iinuma K, Takai M, Yanagawa Y, Kurata K, Ogihara T, Kumahara Y 1982 Measurement of plasma renin activity by a simple solid phase radioimmunoassay. J Clin Endocrinol Metab *54:* 423

Kennedy RL, Ball RY, Dixon AK, ApSimon AT 1987 Metastatic transitional cell carcinoma of the bladder causing Addison's disease. J Urol *137:* 986

Leary OC, Masters J 1957 Adrenal insufficiency produced by metastases from gastric carcinoma. Ann Int Med *46:* 1161

MacKenzie DH 1955 Fatal suprarenal hemorrhage in an adult due to metastases from a bronchial carcinoma. J Pathol Bact *69:* 333

Marieb NJ, Melby JC, Lyall SS 1974 Isolated hypoaldosteronism associated with idiopathic hypoparathyroidism. Arch Int Med *134:* 424

Morimoto S, Kyung SK, Yamamoto I, Uchida K, Takeda R, Kornel L 1979 Selective hypoaldosteronism with hyperreninemia in a diabetic patient. J Clin Endocrinol Metab *49:* 742

Ogihara T, Iinuma K, Nishi K, Arakawa Y, Takagi A, Kurata K, Miyai K, Kumahara Y 1977 A non-chromatographic non-extraction radioimmunoassay for serum aldosterone. J Clin Endocrinol Metab *45:* 726

O'Kelley R, Magee F, McKenna JJ 1983 Routine heparin therapy inhibits adrenal aldosterone production. J Clin Endocrinol Metab *56:* 108

Omoigui NA, Cave WT Jr, Chang AYC 1987 Adrenal insufficiency. A rare initial sign of metastatic colon carcinoma. J Clin Gastroenterol *9:* 470

Rudder HJ, Guy RL, Lipsett MB 1972 A radioimmunoassay for cortisol in plasma and urine. J Clin Endocrinol Metab *35:* 219

Saenger P, Levine LS, Irvine WJ, Gottesdiener K, Rauh W, Sonino N, Chow D, New MI 1982 Progressive adrenal failure in polyglandular autoimmune disease. J Clin Endocrinol Metab *54:* 863

Sahagian-Edwards A, Holland JF 1954 Metastatic carcinoma to the adrenal glands with cortisol hypofunction. Cancer *7:* 1242

Schambelan M, Slaton PE Jr, Murray JF, Biglieri EG 1969 Adrenal insufficiency and inappropriate secretion of antidiuretic hormone. Arch Int Med *124:* 197

Schnitzer B, Smid D, Lloyd RV 1986 Primary T-cell lymphoma of the adrenal glands with adrenal insufficiency. Human Pathol *17:* 634

Seidenwurm DJ, Elmer EB, Kaplan LM, Williams EK, Morris DG, Hoffman AR 1984 Metastases to the adrenal glands and the development of Addison's disease. Cancer *54:* 552

Silver J, Rosler A, Friedlander M, Poportzer MM 1982 Unmasking of isolated hypoaldosteronism after renal allotransplantation in familial Mediterranean fever. Israel J Med Sci *18:* 495

Sparagana M 1970 Addison's disease due to reticulum cell sarcoma apparently confined to the adrenals. J Am Geriatr Soc *18:* 550

Taylor HC, Shah B, Pillay I, Mayes DM 1988 Isolated hyperreninemic hypoaldosteronism due to carcinoma metastatic to the adrenal gland. Am J Med *85:* 441

Vieweg MVR, Reitz RE, Weinstein RL 1973 Addison's disease secondary to metastatic carcinoma: an example of adrenocortical and adrenomedullary insufficiency. Cancer *31:* 1240

Wallach JB, Scharfman WB 1952 Addison's disease due to metastatic bronchogenic carcinoma. J Am Med Assoc *148:* 729

Weber CL, Murphy ML 1971 Adrenal hypofunction secondary to adrenocortical destruction by metastatic carcinoma of the lung. J Arkansas Med Soc *68:* 181

Williams FA Jr, Schambelan M, Biglieri EG, Carey RM 1983 Acquired primary hypoaldosteronism due to an isolated zona glomerulosa defect. New Engl M Med *309:* 1623

Willis RA 1953 Pathology of Tumors. St. Louis: C. V. Mosby, 178 *Zipser RD, Davenport MW, Martin KL, Tuck ML, Warner NE, Swinney*

Willis RA 1953 Pathology of Tumors. St. Louis: C. V. Mosby, 178

Zipser RD, Davenport MW, Martin KL, Tuck ML, Warner NE, Swinney RR, Davis CL, Horton R 1981 Hyperreninemic hypoaldosteronism in the critically ill: a new entity. J Clin Endocrinol Metab *53:* 867

Clinical Nephrology, Vol. 35 No. 2 – 1991 (72–77)

Pharmacokinetics of active vitamins D3, 1 α-hydroxyvitamin D3 and 1 α, 25-dihydroxyvitamin D3 in patients on chronic hemodialysis

Y. Kimura[1], M. Nakayama[2], S. Kuriyama[2], S. Watanabe[1], Y. Kawaguchi[2] and O. Sakai[2]

[1]*Department of Internal Medicine, Jikei University School of Medicine, Kashiwa Hospital, Chiba, Japan*
[2]*Second Department of Internal Medicine, Jikei University School of Medicine, Tokyo, Japan*

Abstract. Two active forms of vitamin D3, 1α, 25-dihydroxyvitamin D3 (1α, 25 [OH] 2D3) and 1α-hydroxyvitamin D3 (1α, [OH] D3) are widely used for treating osteodystrophy in patients with chronic renal failure. Since the pharmacokinetics of these agents during long-term oral administration are unclear, we measured the circulating concentrations of 1α, 25 (OH) 2D before and after their long-term oral administration in patients receiving maintenance hemodialysis.
After 12 weeks of treatment with a daily dose of 1α, (OH) D3 (0.5 μg), the administration of a single dose (2 μg) of 1α, (OH) D3 showed that the area under the curve over 24 h (AUC) was increased significantly compared with day 1 of therapy. In contrast, after the teatment with a daily dose of 1α, 25 (OH) 2D3 (0.25 μg), a single dose of 1α, 25 (OH) 2D3 (1 μg) did not exhibit this effect on the AUC. A single dose of each agent produced no significant change in either the peak increment above basal values or the elimination half-time (T1/2) of circulating plasma 1α, 25 (OH) 2D. The overall basal concentration of 1α, 25 (OH) 2D achieved by 1α, (OH) D3 after 12 weeks of administration was cumulative, but this effect was not observed in patients on 1α, 25 (OH) 2D3.
These data indicate that the pharmacokinetics of the two forms of active vitamin D3 did not differ as to peak increment and T1/2 except for the AUC, even after long-term dosage. It is suggested that 1α, (OH) D3 may be more effective in maintaining a consistent circulating level of 1α, 25 (OH) 2D in patients on chronic hemodialysis.

Key words: pharmacokinetics – vitamin D3 – chronic hemodialysis

Introduction

Two forms of active vitamin D3, 1α, (OH) D3 and 1α, 25 (OH) 2D3 are being widely used for treating renal osteodystrophy in patients with chronic renal failure on chronic hemodialysis. These patients presumably have a deficiency in the endogenous production of active vitamin D3. It is well known that drug therapy is effective in supplying vitamin D3 to these patients. Both 1α, (OH) D3 and 1α, 25 (OH) 2D3 have been shown to be useful clinically for maintaining serum calcium levels and thus preventing secondary hyperparathyroidism [Henderson et al. 1974, Slatopolsky et al. 1984]. It is noteworthy that 1α, 25 (OH) 2D3 is the final active hormone, whereas 1α, (OH) D3 must be hydroxylated to yield 1α, 25 (OH) 2D3 in the liver. In this context, it is important to consider any differences between these two agents to ensure their effective clinical use.

Although the circulating concentrations of 1α, 25 (OH) 2D following a single oral administration of 1α, 25 (OH) 2D3 as well as of 1α, (OH) D3 have been previously reported [Mason et al. 1980, Seino et al. 1987, Papapoulos et al. 1982], little is known of their pharmacokinetics after preloaded daily administrations. Considering the plethora of clinical data on the effects of oral vitamin D3 on bone and mineral metabolism in patients with renal osteodystrophy, a comparative pharmacokinetic evaluation of these agents was indicated.

Received July 16, 1990; in revised form November 4, 1990.

Reprint requests to S. Kuriyama M. D. Second Department of Internal Medicine, Jikei University School of Medicine, 3–25–8, Nishi-shinbashi, Minato-ku, Tokyo, 105 Japan.

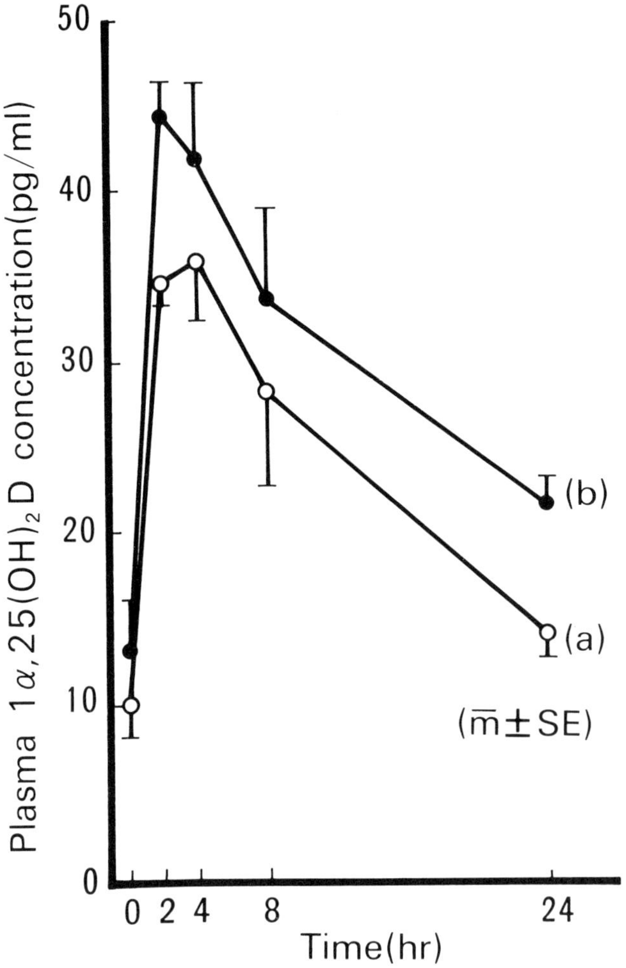

Fig. 1 Changes in plasma 1α, 25 (OH) 2D concentration following a single oral dose of 1α, 25 (OH) 2D3, 1.0 μg under the condition of high plasma 1α, 25 (OH) 2D levels (Study 2).

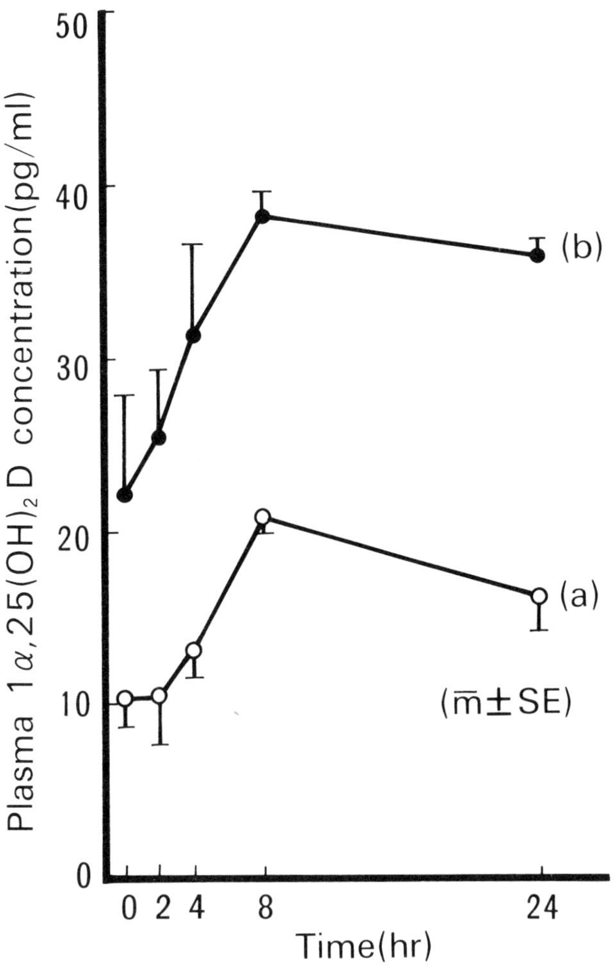

Fig. 2 Changes in plasma 1α, 25 (OH) 2D concentrations following a single oral dose of 1α, (OH) D3, 2.0 μg (Study 1, Group B). *(a)* Open circles denote plasma concentrations at 0 week. *(b)* Closed circles denote plasma concentrations at 12 weeks.

We therefore studied the long-term pharmacokinetic effects of each agent in patients on chronic hemodialysis, administrating them for 12 weeks.

Materials and methods

Enrolled in this study were six females with renal failure due to chronic glomerulonephritis (mean age 42.8 ± 3.8 years old), who were receiving maintenance hemodialysis (HD) for five hours three times a week. Their residual renal function was estimated to be less than 3.0 ml/min with daily urine volumes less than 100 ml. The dialysis system employed a 1.2 m cupurophane membrane. The dialysate consisted of Na 132 mEq/l, Ca 3.5 mEq/l and HCO3- 35 mEq/l. They were in good condition without symptomatic complications. To participate in the study, the patients had to be on HD for at least six months before the study. The mean dry body weight of these patients was 43.4 ± 1.2 kg, which was kept constant throughout the study. The patients ate their regular meals ad libitum during the study, although they were given general advice regarding intake of fluid and salt restriction. Patients were divided into two groups. Group A was placed 1α, 25 (OH) 2D3 on a daily dose of 0.25 μg and group B on 1α, (OH) D3 (0.5 μg/day). The groups were comparable with respect to age, body mass index, blood pressure and duration of HD. At least 4 weeks before the study, the administration of active vitamin D3 was discontinued. Calcium carbonate was administered with the meals (1.5 to 3.0 g/day) during the trial. Dosage was adjusted arbitrarily to keep the serum phosphate levels below 5.5 mg/dl and serum calcium levels below 10.5 mg/dl.

Table 1 Pharmacokinetic parameters for plasma 1α, 25 (OH) 2D in two groups of dialyzed patients (Group A and B). Half-life: elimination half-life of circulating plasma 1α, 25 (OH) 2D after drug administration. AUC: area under the curve over a 24-hour period following drug administration.

Group		peak increment above basal values (pg/ml)	half-time (h)	AUC 24 h (pg/ml)
A: 1α, 25 $(OH)_2D_3$	0 w	31.9 + 6.9	12.8 + 2.3	589 + 119
	12 w	26.9 + 6.1	18.4 + 7.0	710 + 49
(p-value)		ns	ns	ns
B: 1α, (OH) D_3	0 w	10.6 + 3.0	36.0 + 11.1	409 + 50
	12 w	16.4 + 6.7	43.2 + 7.5	822 + 64
(p-value)		ns	ns	$p < 0.05$

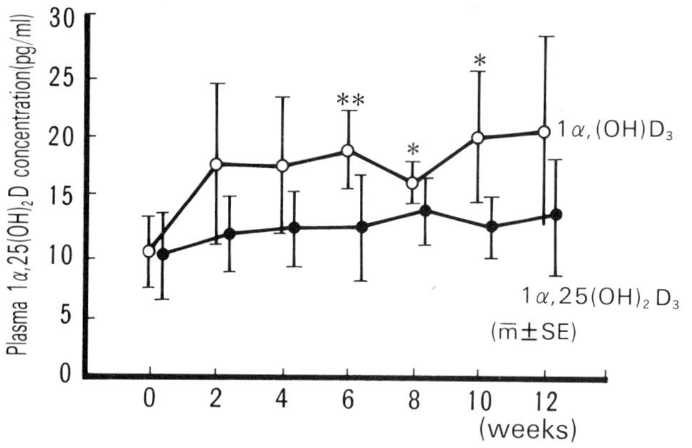

Fig. 3 Changes in basal plasma 1α, 25 (OH) 2D concentrations in patients on 1α, (OH) D3 and on 1α, 25 (OH) 2D3 during the study (Study 1, Group A and B). Open circles denote the mean basal plasma concentrations in patients on 1α, (OH) D3, 0.5 μg daily. Closed circles denote the mean basal plasma concentrations in patients on 1α, 25 (OH) 2D3, 0.25 μg daily. Asterisks indicate a significant difference compared to the values in the 1α, 25 (OH) 2D3 group.

Study 1

A control blood sample was drawn from each patient to measure the plasma concentration of 1α, 25 (OH) 2D on a HD-free day following an overnight fast. Immediately thereafter, three patients received 1 μg of 1α, 25 (OH) 2D3 orally (group A) and another three patients, 2 μg of 1α, (OH) D3 (group B). Blood was then sampled at 0, 2, 4, 8 and 24 h. Curves were constructed to yield the peak increment above basal level (peak increment), elimination half-life (T1/2) and the area under the curve (AUC). Thereafter, the patients in group A received 0.25 μg of 1α, 25 (OH) 2D3 and those in group B, 0.5 μg of 1α, (OH) D3 for 12 weeks. Drugs were administered orally before breakfast. During this period the plasma concentration of 1α, 25 (OH) 2D was measured before starting the drug (basal plasma level) and again every two weeks. At the 12th week, the same baseline pharmacokinetic evaluation was repeated. Maintenance dose of 1α, 25 (OH) 2D3 was one half that of 1α, (OH) D3 conventionally. Also, since the effect of 1α, 25 (OH) 2D3 on the serum calcium levels is reportedly more pronounced than that of 1α, (OH) D3, one can safely assume that the effective dose of 1α, 25 (OH) 2D3 is less than that of 1α, (OH) D3 [Ohno et al. 1982].

Study 2

To explore the possible influences of markedly elevated plasma concentration of 1α, 25 (OH) 2D on the bioavailability of orally dosed 1α, 25 (OH) 2D3, two patients in group A were admininstered a loading dose of 4.0 μg of this agent before initiating the study at the 24th week. Pharmacokinetics of the orally administered single dose of 1α, 25 (OH) 2D3 1 μg were then evaluated.

Blood specimens were centrifuged and the plasma was stored at −30 °C until analysis. The levels of circulating 1α, 25 (OH) 2D were then determined by a specific radioimmunoassay.

Statistical analysis employed paired and unpaired t-tests as appropriate. The statistical significance was given at $p < 0.05$. Data are expressed as mean ± SD unless otherwise indicated.

Results

1. Pharmacokinetic parameters on chronic 1α, 25 (OH) 2D3 (Study 1, group A)

Figure 1 depicts the circulating plasma level of 1α, 25 (OH) 2D in group A following a single oral dose of 1.0 μg of 1α, 25 (OH) 2D3. At baseline and at 12 weeks, in both studies, the pattern is characterized by a sharp increase in plasma 1α, 25 (OH) 2D levels within 2 h followed by an exponential decrease over 24 h. As shown in Table 1, there were no significant differences between the two time course studies either in basal plasma levels or the peak increment over basal values. The half-life of circulating plasma 1α, 25 (OH) 2D did not differ significantly at 0 week vs 12 weeks. No significant difference was found in the area under the curve (AUC) at pretherapy as compared with that obtained at the 12th week.

2. Pharmacokinetic parameters on chronic 1α, (OH) D3 (Study 1, group B)

Figure 2 depicts the increase in the plasma level of 1α, 25 (OH) 2D following a single oral dose of 2.0 μg of 1α, (OH) D3 at baseline and again at 12th week. At both times, the pattern was characterized by a continuous slow elevation of circulating 1α, 25 (OH) 2D levels within 8 h and a grandual decline over 24 h. As shown in Table 1, the pharmacokinetic parameters of 1α, (OH) D3 differed significantly from those of 1α, 25 (OH) 2D3. The AUC on the 12th week was much greater than that at the first day (409 ± 50 pg/ml vs 822 ± 64 pg/ml, $p<0.05$) (Table 1). In contrast, no significant difference was found with respect to the peak increment above basal values or the plasma half-life of circulating 1α, 25 (OH) 2D.

3. Basal plasma levels of 1α, 25 (OH) 2D during the 12-week study, chronic effects of orally administered 1α, 25 (OH) 2D3 (Study 1, Group A and B)

Changes in the mean basal 1α, 25 (OH) 2D plasma levels in groups A and B are shown in Figure 3. In patients placed on 1α, (OH) D3, significant elevations of the plasma level of 1α, 25 (OH) 2D were found at the 6th week (18.8 ± 3.2 pg/ml; $p<0.01$); the 8th week (16.0 ± 1.8 pg/ml; $p<0.05$) and the 10th week (20.0 ± 5.4 pg/ml; $p<0.05$) as compared to day 1 (10.1 ± 1.5 pg/ml). In contrast, the daily administration of 1α, 25 (OH) 2D3 did not induce any apparent elevations of the plasma levels of 1α, 25 (OH) 2D throughout the study.

4. Pharmacokinetics of 1α, 25 (OH) 2D3 after a loading dose of 4 μg (Study 2)

Figure 4 shows the results of the second study. Plasma levels of 1α, 25 (OH) 2D just before a single dose administration of 1.0 μg of 1α, 25 (OH) 2D3 (time 0) were 77.0 and 98.2 pg/ml, respectively, which is extremely high as compared with those of normal subjects. In both patients tested, substantial increase in the plasma 1α, 25 (OH) 2D level occurred within 2 h of the oral intake of 1.0 μg of the indicated agents, reaching peak levels, 81.2 and 116.6 pg/ml, respectively followed by an exponential decrease over 24 h.

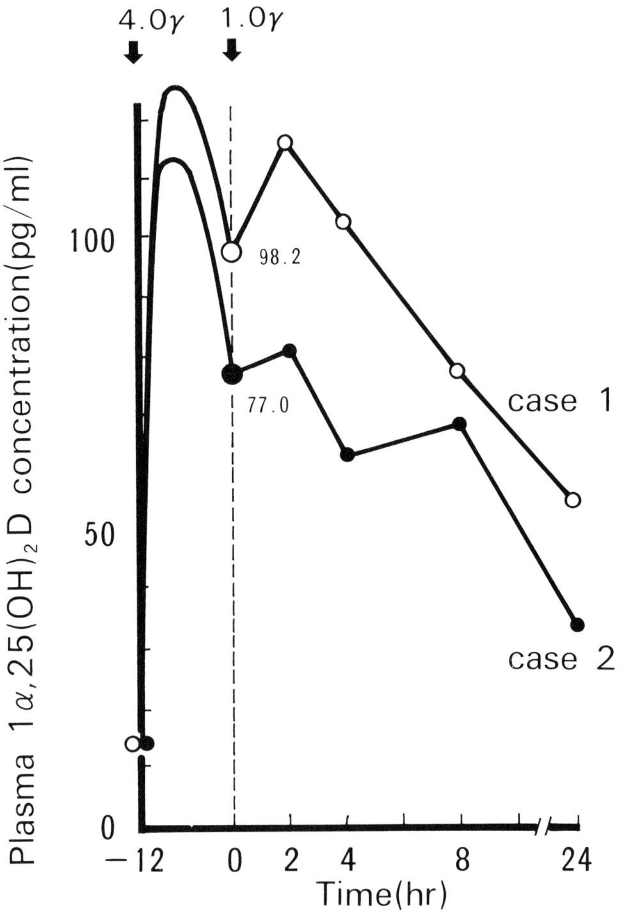

Fig. 4 Changes in plasma 1α, 25 (OH) 2D concentrations following a single oral dose 1α, 25 (OH) 2D3, 1.0 μg (Study 1, Group A). *(a)* Open circles denote plasma concentrations at 0 week. *(b)* Closed circles denote concentrations at 12 weeks.

No side effect with the indicated two agents was observed throughout all study periods in both groups.

Discussion

While the circulating plasma levels of 1α, 25 (OH) 2D following a single oral dose of 1α, 25 (OH) D3 have previously been reported in the patients on chronic HD [Papapoulos et al. 1982], little was known about the effects of their repeated oral administration. It has been suggested that the pharmacokinetics of these agents may differ after long-term oral administration. For example, the oral administration of 1α, 25 (OH) 2D3 to rats proved much less effective than intravenous administration in terms of mobilizing calcium from bone and in stimulating intestinal calcium absorption, suggesting that this agent given orally is rapidly destroyed by the intestine; it may even induce its own destruction [Tanaka et al. 1972]. An increased rate of both the disappearance of 1α, 25 (OH) 2D3 and the appearance of its metabolites in the intestine has been demonstrated in rats administered daily with oral doses of this agent [Frolik et al. 1973]. Initial dose was set as 0.25 μg/day of 1α, 25 (OH) 2D3 and 0.5 μg/day of 1α, (OH) 3D, since it has been demonstrated that the effect of one mole of the former is approximately the same as two moles of the latter in terms of changes in blood Ca levels and serum level of circulating 1α, 25 (OH) 2D [Ohno et al. 1982].

The present study in humans showed no differences in several pharmacokinetic parameters following long-term dosage of 1α, 25 (OH) 2D3 and 1α, (OH) D3 except for a change in AUC in patients receiving 1α, (OH) D3, which is inconsistent with the previously postulated hypothesis. Our results support the suggestion that the repeated oral administration of the two active forms of vitamin D3 do not facilitate the degradation of 1α, 25 (OH) 2D3 in the intestine, at least, not at a daily dose of 0.25 μg of that agent or a dose of 0.5 μg of 1α, (OH) D3. It seems clear that increased AUC in the patients taking 1α, (OH) D3 was elicited from the elevated basal plasma levels of 1α, 25 (OH) 2D. As shown in Figure 3, the basal levels of this substance in plasma in the group taking 1α, (OH) D3 increased gradually throughout the study until the 12th week, in contrast to the group on 1α, 25 (OH) 2D3, which showed no significant elevation in the basal level of 1α, 25 (OH) 2D during the trial. This increase in basal level after repeated 1α, (OH) D3 administration may account for the larger AUC in those patients. It may also suggest the accumulation of 1α, 25 (OH) 2D in plasma. Brickman et al. [1976] reported a progressive increase in the intestinal absorption of calcium in uremic patients receiving 1α, (OH) D3 which may explain our results. Therefore, we feel that the oral administration of 1α, (OH) D3 may be more effective than 1α, 25 (OH) 2D3 in maintaining consistent plasma levels of 1α, 25 (OH) 2D. An additional study conducted to explore the possible interference of the intestinal absorption of 1α, 25 (OH) 2D3 showed that even with markedly elevated plasma levels of 1α, 25 (OH) 2D, a further increase in plasma level occurred following the single oral dose of 1α, 25 (OH) 2D3, 1.0 μg (Figure 4). Recent advances in the treatment of secondary hyperparathyroidism include the administration of vitamin D3. Slatoplosky et al. [1984] reported that an intravenous infusion of active vitamin D3 was required to suppress PTH, whereas orally administered 1α, 25 (OH) 2D3 failed to increase the plasma concentration of 1α, 25 (OH) 2D. In this regard, it was of particular interest to examine the pharmacokinetics of a high dose 1α, 25 (OH) 2D in patients with renal osteodystrophy. We found that even after achieving a high circulating concentration of 1α, 25 (OH) 2D, a loading dose of 1α, 25 (OH) 2D3 significantly increased the plasma levels of 1α, 25 (OH) 2D. It is not clear which fraction of 1α, 25 (OH) 2D3 was taken up by the intestinal epithelial cells. Further investigation is required in this respect with each active vitamin D3.

In conclusion, this pharmacodynamic study demonstrated a steep elevation of 1α, 25 (OH) 2D in response to a single dose of 1α, (OH) 2D3 and a mild increase in plasma 1α, 25 (OH) 2D in response to a single dose of 1α, (OH) D3, effects observed even after long-term (12 weeks) treatment with those agents. In addition, it is suggested that the chronic administration of 1α, (OH) D3 may more effectively maintain a stable plasma level of α, 25 (OH) 2D as compared to 1α, 25 (OH) 2D3.

Acknowledgements

We are grateful to the staff of the Chugai Pharmaceutical Co. for their technical assistance in determining plasma levels of 1α, 25 (OH) 2D. Dr. S. Kuriyama is the recipient of a grant from the Japanese Ministry of Education.

REFERENCES

Brickman AS, Coburn JW, Friedman GR, Okamura WH, Massry SG, Norman AW 1976 Comparison of effects of 1α-hydroxy-vitamin D3 and 1,25-dihydroxy-vitamin D3 in man. J Clin Invest *57:* 1540–1547

Frolic CA, DeLuca HF 1973 The stimulation of 1,25-dihydroxychole-calciferol metabolism in vitamin D-deficient rats by 1,25-dihydroxycholecalciferol treatment. J Clin Invest *52:* 543–548

Henderson RG, Russell RGG, Ledingham JGG, Smith R, Oliver DO, Walton RJ, Small DG, Preston C, Warner GT 1974 Effects of 1,25-dihydroxycholecalciferol on calcium absorption, muscle weakness, and bone disease in chronic renal failure. Lancet *1:* 379–384

Holick MF, Kasten-Schraufrogel P, Tavela J, DeLuca HF 1975 Biological activity of 1α-hydroxyvitamin D3 in the rat. Arch Biochem Biophys *166:* 63–66

Mason RS, Lisser D, Posen S, Norman AW 1980 Blood concentrations of dihydroxylated vitamin D metabolites after an oral dose. Br Med J *280:* 449–450

Ohno J, Kubota M, Hirasawa Y, Suzuki M, Mimura N, Minamikata T 1982 Clinical evaluation of 1α-hydroxy-cholecalciferol and 1α, 25-dihydroxycholecalciferol in the treatment of renal osteodystrophy. In: *Norman AM, Schaefer K, Herrath Dv, Grigoleit H-G* (eds) Vitamin D Chemical, Biochemical and Clinical Endocrinology of Calcium Metabolism. Walter de Gruyter, Berlin, New York, pp 847–852

Papapoulos SE, Clements TL, Sandler LM, Fraher LJ, Winer J, O'Riordan JLH 1982 The effect of renal function on changes in circulating concentrations of 1,25-dihydroxycholecalciferol after an oral dose. Clin Science *62:* 427–429

Seino Y, Tanaka H, Yamaoka K, Yabuuchi H 1987 Circulating 1α, 25-dihydroxyvitamin D levels after a single dose of 1α, 25-dihydroxy-vitamin D3 or 1α-hydroxyvitamin D3 in normal men. Bone and Mineral *2:* 479–485

Slatopolsky E, Weert C, Thielan J, Horsat R, Harter H, Martin KJ 1984 Marked suppression of secondary hyperparathyroidism by intravenous administration of 1,25-dihydroxycholecalciferol in uremic patients. J Clin Invest *74:* 2136–2134

Tanaka Y, Frank H, DeLuca HF 1972 Role of 1,25-dihydroxy-cholecalciferol in calcification of bone and maintenance of serum calcium concentration in the rat. J Clin Nutr *102:* 1569–1578

Clinical Nephrology, Vol. 35 No. 2 – 1991 (78–85)

The clinical spectrum of renal osteodystrophy in 57 chronic hemodialysis patients: a correlation between biochemical parameters and bone pathology findings

J. A. Chazan[1], N. P. Libbey[2], M. R. London[1], L. Pono[3] and J. G. Abuelo[1]

[1] *Department of Medicine, Division of Renal Diseases, Rhode Island Hospital; Division of Biological and Medical Sciences, Brown University, Providence, RI 02903, USA*
[2] *Roger Williams General Hospital, Department of Pathology, Providence, RI 02908, USA*
[3] *Artificial Kidney Center of Rhode Island, East Providence, RI 02914, USA*

Abstract. Fifty-nine chronic hemodialysis patients who had been on dialysis for an average of 77 months underwent bone biopsies and the pathologic findings were correlated with biochemical and demographic data. All but two had evidence of renal osteodystrophy, 23 with osteitis fibrosa (OF), 19 with osteomalacia and/or adynamic disease (OM/AD), and 15 with mixed osteodystrophy (MOD). Patients in each group were similar with regard to age, sex distribution, duration of dialysis, unstimulated serum aluminum, calcium and phosphorus. Patients with osteitis fibrosa (OF) had statistically higher DFO stimulated aluminum, alkaline phosphatase and PTHC levels than the other two groups although there was marked individual variation. The bone biopsies were also evaluated for the amount of aluminum deposited in the osteoid seam. All 23 of the patients with OF and 11 of the 15 patients with MOD had no, mild, or minimal aluminum deposition but 12 of the 19 patients with OM/AD had moderate to marked aluminum deposition. Patients with minimal to mild aluminum deposition were similar in age, duration of dialysis, sex distribution, unstimulated and DFO stimulated aluminum levels, calcium, phosphorus, alkaline phosphatase to those with moderate to marked deposition but had significantly higher parathormone levels. All patients had been treated in a similar fashion regarding diet, oral phosphate binders and vitamin D; therefore, the observed differences in bone pathology were not readily explicable. However, patients who were found to have osteitis fibrosa and those with minimal to mild aluminum deposition had significantly higher parathormone levels when compared with patients in the other groups at the inception of dialysis.

Key words: renal osteodystrophy – bone pathology – biochemical parameters in chronic hemodialysis patients

Introduction

Renal osteodystrophy is a common problem among patients with chronic renal failure and frequently results in a wide range of musculoskeletal symptoms [Alvarez-Ude et al. 1978, Coburn et al. 1986, Cushner and Adams 1986, Nebeker et al. 1986, Slatopolsky 1987, Stanbury and Lumb 1962, Stanbury and Lumb 1966]. The commonly recognized forms of renal osteodystrophy include osteitis fibrosa, osteomalacia, mixed osteodystrophy (elements of both osteitis fibrosa and osteomalacia) and aplastic bone disease [Sherrard 1986, Sherrard et al. 1983]. The observed bone lesion is thought to be the result of the interplay between the abnormalities in vitamin D metabolism and secondary hyperparathyroidism [Coburn 1983, Kleeman et al. 1987, Mayor et al. 1977]. In addition, aluminum overload is an important etiologic and/or contributing factor in the development of bone disease, particularly aplastic bone disease, and osteomalacia [Slatopolsky 1987, Sherrard 1986, Cournot-Witmer et al. 1981, Quarles et al. 1985, Quarles et al. 1986, Ott et al. 1982, Malluche et al. 1986].

The purpose of this study was to correlate the pathologic findings on bone biopsy in 57 relatively asymptomatic chronic hemodialysis patients with var-

Received August 2, 1990; in revised form November 2, 1990.

Reprint requests to Dr. J. A. Chazan, Division of Renal Diseases, Rhode Island Hospital, Providence, RI 02903, USA.

ious demographic, clinical, and biochemical data. There was such a large variation in biochemical findings that it was not possible to predict the nature of the bone pathology from the laboratory findings alone. In patients who may require deferoxamine therapy or parathyroidectomy, bone biopsy should be performed prior to specific therapy.

Methods

All patients (236 patients were evaluated) were chronic hemodialysis patients who had received virtually all of their outpatient dialysis at the Artificial Kidney Center of Rhode Island, a facility where water used for dialysate has always been treated by reverse osmosis and consistently has had aluminum levels <10 μg/l. All patients were encouraged to have a bone biopsy and informed consent was obtained. Biopsies were performed between November 1986 and September 1988. Clinical evaluation, laboratory data and skeletal X-rays were obtained at the time of the biopsy. Unstimulated and deferoxamine (DFO) stimulated plasma aluminum levels were obtained in the manner previously described (normal unstimulated aluminum <10 μg/l, stimulated levels vary with time on dialysis) [Chazan et al. 1988]. C terminal middle molecule parathormone levels (normal values 61–315 μg/l) were performed by Lifechem, Rockleigh, NJ.

Patients had been treated with varying amounts of aluminum and calcium phosphate binders with or without vitamin D but it was not possible to accurately assess compliance. Prior to the biopsy the patients were given in vivo tetracycline labels by administering declomycin 150 mg two times a day for 3 days, no drug for 14 days, and then oxytetracycline HCl 250 mg two times a day for 3 days. A transiliac bone biopsy was performed under local anesthesia one to three days after completion of the second antibiotic using a 5 mm Bordier trephine (Ecole Professionnelle de Dessin Industriel, Paris).

The specimen was immediately fixed in 10% neutral buffered formalin, dehydrated in acetone and embedded in methyl methacrylate according to standard technique [Recker 1983]. Multiple 4 μm sections were taken at 20 μm intervals on a Reichert-Jung Polycut microtome for modified Gomori trichrome, hematoxylin and eosin, von Kossa, toluidine blue and Aluminom stains [Ott et al. 1982]. Unstained sections were cut at 15 μm and examined for tetracycline labeling using a Leitz orthoplan fluorescent microscope with an HBO 200 W mercury lamp and a BG 38 filter.

All of the biopsies were examined by one of the authors (N. L.) without knowledge of the biochemical or clinical findings. A quantitative histomorphometry was performed on 49 specimens by a standard point and intersect counting method using a Merz-Schenk reticule [Chazan et al. 1988] at 100 or 250× for surface and volume measurement and a linear micrometer at 400× for distance measurements. An average of 162 microscopic fields or 99.3 mm^2 tissue area was examined for each biopsy to determine static parameters. In addition, an average of 924 and 1793 surface intersects was counted for each biopsy to determine respectively the extent of surface tetracycline labeling and surface aluminum deposition. Eight biopsies were not suitable for complete quantitative histomorphometry and were evaluated qualitatively and semiquantitatively for the same parameters. Biopsies of 19 age-matched patients without evidence of renal disease, abnormal parathyroid function or osteomalacia, evaluated because of osteopenia (OP) (8 normal bone and 11 osteoporosis), were selected for comparison.

Each biopsy was characterized as to its predominant pattern of renal osteodystrophy based on its morphological and morphometric findings, according to the most explicit definitions of these patterns [Sherrard 1986]. Because significant overlap in generally used morphometric parameters occurred, the mineralization lag time (Mlt), which reflects both mineralization and bone formation, previously not specified as a discriminating parameter, was used as an index to separate osteitis fibrosa and osteomalacia from mixed osteodystrophy [Libbey et al. 1990]. The patterns identified include:

1. Osteitis fibrosa (OF) characterized by increased bone remodeling with high osteoblastic and osteoclastic surfaces, peritrabecular fibrosis and normal mineralization as indicated by increased tetracycline labeled surface and relatively short mineralization lag time (<35 days). Also included in this category are cases with little or no fibrosis which correspond to what has been identified as mild hyperparathyroidism or early osteitis fibrosa [Sherrard 1986, Sherrard et al. 1983].
2. Mixed osteodystrophy (MOD) characterized by increased bone remodeling, variable peritrabecular fibrosis and impaired mineralization as indicated by a normal to slightly decreased tetracycline labeled surface and a moderately prolonged mineralization lag time (35 to 100 days).
3. Osteomalacia (OM) characterized by markedly increased osteoid surface and volume and markedly impaired mineralization as indicated by markedly decreased or absent tetracycline labeling and markedly prolonged mineralization lag time (>100 days).

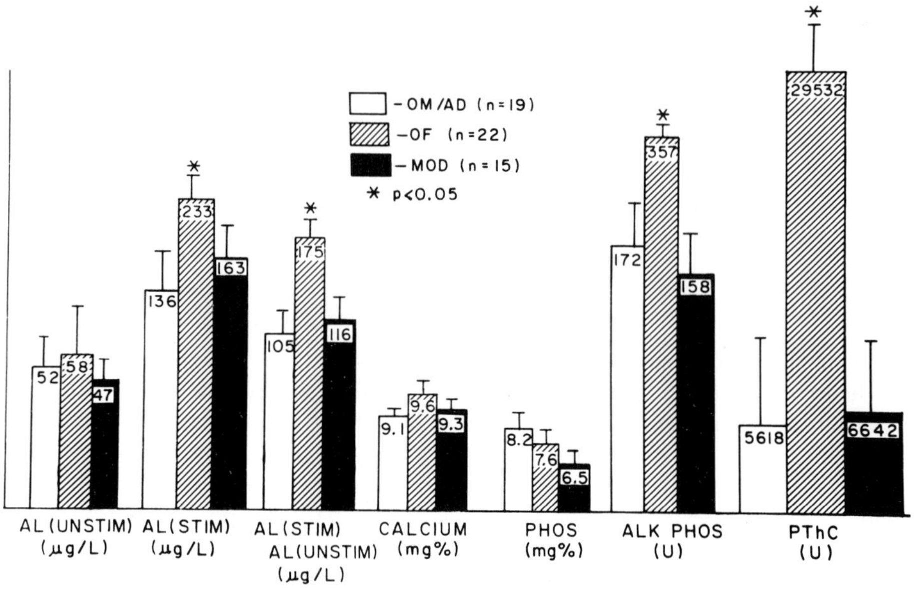

Fig. 1 The serum aluminum (unstimulated, stimulated and the differences between stimulated and unstimulated), calcium, phosphorus, alkaline phosphatase and C terminal middle molecule parathormone levels for all 57 biopsies are shown (mean values ± SD). Patients with osteitis fibrosa had statistically higher alkaline phosphatase when compared with the other two groups and statistically higher DFO stimulated aluminum levels when compared to the OM/AD group only.

4. Aplastic bone disease (AD) characterized by decreased bone remodeling with low osteoblastic and osteoclastic surfaces, mildly to moderately increased osteoid surface with narrow osteoid seams, and decreased tetracycline labeled surface. Because of the small amount of labeled surface mineralization lag times were prolonged paralleling those of the OM group.

All biopsies were graded according to the extent of aluminum deposition at the osteoid mineralized bone interface: no or minimal aluminum (<10%), mild (>10% but less than 33%), moderate (>33% and <67%) and marked (>67%).

The data base stored in a computer was analyzed using ANOVA, χ^2, and simple regression. Significance was determined by t-tests, Fisher exact tests and F statistics where appropriate. P = 0.05 or less was considered statistically significant. All data are shown with standard deviation.

Results

Fifty-nine patients had bone biopsies performed. Two showed only osteoporosis without evidence of renal osteodystrophy and were not included in the subsequent analysis. The 57 patients whose biopsies were evaluated consisted of 20 males and 37 females ranging in age from 26–87 years (mean 56 years) who had been on hemodialysis for 3–186 months (mean 77 months). None of the patients had evidence of seizures, dementia or bone fractures, but many had non-specific musculoskeletal complaints such as aches and pains in joints and muscles along with generalized weakness. In an attempt to assess whether the patients biopsied were representative of the general dialysis population, we compared the demography of this group of 57 patients with the 236 patients who had been on dialysis at the Center during 1987. There were more females (65% compared to 51%) in the biopsied group and the study group had been on dialysis longer (average of 77 months compared to 38 months) than the remainder of the dialysis population. There were no changes in the unstimulated aluminum, serum phosphorus, or parathormone levels between the two groups. Patients who were biopsied had higher serum calcium (9.3 vs 9.0 mEq/l) and alkaline phosphatase (243 vs 152 units) and lower stimulated aluminum (182 vs 107 µg/l) all with p <0.01 levels than the total dialysis population. These differences could be explained by the disparity of time on dialysis between the two groups [Chazan et al. 1989a].

We also compared the 57 biopsied patients with 57 patients from the dialysis population matched for sex, age and duration of dialysis to see if the biochemical parameters in the biopsied group were similar to those not biopsied. The unstimulated serum aluminum, deferoxamine stimulated aluminum, phosphorus, alkaline phosphatase and parathormone levels were similar in both groups. Although the differences in serum calcium were statistically different (9.3 mEq/l vs. 9.0 mEq/l p <0.05) this difference does not appear to be of clinical importance. It thus appears that the patients who were biopsied had similar biochemical findings when compared with their peers who chose not to have a bone biopsy.

Based on the morphologic and morphometric findings on bone biopsy, 23 patients were identified as having osteitis fibrosa (OF) (normal mineralization lag time <35 days), including 4 with mild hyperparathyroidism; 15 had mixed osteodystrophy (MOD) (moderately prolonged mineralization lag time 35–100 days); and 19 had markedly prolonged mineralization lag time >100 days, 16 having osteomalacia (OM) and 3 having aplastic disease (AD) [Parfitt et al. 1987]. All but three of the osteomalacic biopsies showed low osteoblastic and osteoclastic surfaces and moderately thickened osteoid seams (adynamic osteomalacia) and thus showed significant morphologic overlap with the aplastic group. The patients with OM/AD had similar morphologic findings without significant differences in the laboratory studies or clinical findings and therefore the two groups are presented together.

The sex distribution (25–40% males), mean age (55–58 years) and mean duration of dialysis (75–78 months) were comparable in all three groups. The laboratory data obtained at the time of biopsy are shown in Figure 1. Patients with osteitis fibrosa had statistically higher alkaline phosphatase ($p < 0.05$) when compared with the other two groups and statistically higher deferoxamine stimulated aluminum levels ($p < 0.05$) when compared with the OM/AD group only. There was no statistical difference in unstimulated aluminum, calcium or phosphorus or the presence of demineralization among the groups. There were no statistical differences in the occurrence of demineralization or subperiosteal elevation among the three groups. Parathyroidectomy had been performed in 3 patients with OM/AD (8–10 years previously), 1 patient with OF (6 years previously) and 2 patients with MOD (2–7 years previously).

The 57 biopsies were quantitatively evaluated for aluminum deposition in the osteoid seam and were then divided into four groups based on the amount of aluminum deposited in the osteoid seam (see Methods). All 23 of the patients with OF, 12 of the 15 patients with MOD and 7 of the 19 patients with OM/AD were categorized as no or only minimal to mild aluminum deposition. The patients were similar in sex distribution (25–40% M), mean age (56 years) and mean duration of dialysis (74–82 months). The biochemical parameters are shown in Figure 2. The mean unstimulated and stimulated aluminum levels, serum calcium and phosphorus were not statistically different. However, the C terminal PTH level was higher ($p < 0.01$) among the patients with minimal to mild aluminum deposition when compared to patients with moderate to marked aluminum deposition (Figure 4). The patients with moderate to marked aluminum deposition tended to be on dialysis longer and have lower alkaline phosphatase although these differences did not reach statistical significance. When patients with OF were excluded from the comparison and patients with either OM/AD or MOD were divided into minimal and mild aluminum deposition (18 patients) compared to those with moderate and

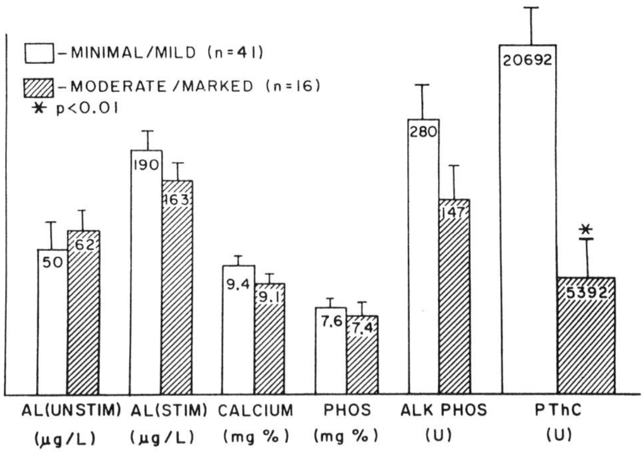

Fig. 2 The serum aluminum (unstimulated and stimulated), calcium, phosphorus, alkaline phosphatase and C terminal middle molecule PTH levels (mean values ± SD) for the 57 patients' bone biopsies classified by the amount of the percent of osteoid seam stained with aluminum; no or minimal aluminum less than 10%, mild 10–32%, moderate 33–66% and marked 67% or greater. The biochemical parameters were not statistically different except the parathormone levels which were significantly lower for the group with moderate to marked aluminum deposition.

marked aluminum deposition (16 patients), there was no statistical difference between the two groups either biochemically or demographically except that the patients with moderate to marked aluminum deposition had significantly higher unstimulated aluminum levels, 62 μg/l compared to 38 μg/l ($p < 0.05$).

We were unable to retrospectively quantitate the amounts of phosphate binders and vitamin D taken by the patients because no data concerning compliance could be documented. However, there was no difference in the amount of those medications which had been prescribed and there was no reason to believe that there was a systematic bias among the study population. We evaluated the calcium, phosphorus, alkaline phosphatase and parathormone levels obtained near the inception of the dialysis to see if they were predictive of the bone pathology that was subsequently found at the time of bone biopsy some years later. Serum aluminum levels were not done routinely until 1985 and therefore were not included in the analysis. On initiation of dialysis, patients who later proved to have OF on biopsy had significantly higher parathormone levels than those with OM/AD or MOD although there were no differences in the other biochemical parameters (Figure 3). Also on initiation of dialysis, patients who subsequently had mild to no aluminum deposition had significantly higher parathormone levels than patients with moderate to marked aluminum deposition (Figure 4).

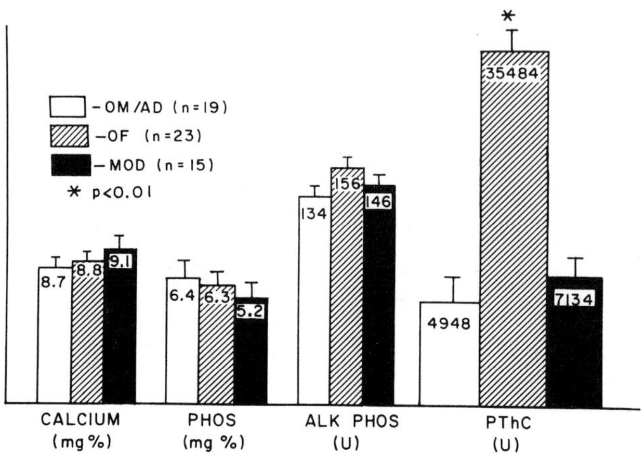

Fig. 3 The initial serum calcium, phosphorus, alkaline phosphatase and C terminal middle molecule parathormone levels (mean values ± SD) in the 57 patients who underwent bone biopsy classifed by the type of bone disease found years later at the time of the biopsy. Blood values were obtained as close to the inception of dialysis as possible; however, because of differences in methodology used over the years, there was occasionally a hiatus of several years between inception of dialysis and the first PTH determination. As can be seen, the only statistical difference is that the initial C terminal middle molecule PTH was significantly higher in the patients who subsequently were found to have osteitis fibrosa.

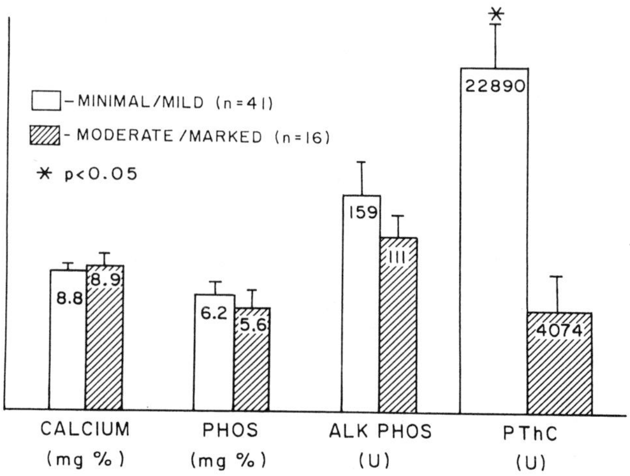

Fig. 4 The initial serum calcium, phosphorus, alkaline phosphatase and C terminal middle molecule parathormone levels (mean values ± SD) in all 57 patients who had bone biopsies classified by the amount of aluminum deposited in the osteoid seam. Blood values were obtained as close to the inception of dialysis as possible. However, because of differences in methodology used over the years, there was occasionally a hiatus of several years between inception of dialysis and the first PTH determination. Initial parathormone levels were significantly lower in patients with moderate to marked aluminum deposition.

Discussion

Renal osteodystrophy occurs in virtually all patients who have had chronic renal failure for a prolonged period of time [Alvarez-Ude et al. 1978, Coburn et al. 1986, Cushner and Adams 1986, Nebeker et al. 1986, Slatopolsky 1987, Stanbury and Lumb 1962, Stanbury and Lumb 1966]. The causes for the development of this abnormality relate to the interplay between abnormalities in vitamin D metabolism and factors that stimulate hyperfunction of the parathyroid glands [Coburn 1983, Kleeman et al. 1987, Mayor et al. 1977]. The interplay between these two abnormalities results in the development in one of three types of bone disease: 1) osteomalacia (OM) (markedly prolonged mineralization lag time >100 days), 2) osteitis fibrosa (OF) (normal mineralization lag time <35 days), or 3) a combination of these two abnormalities, mixed osteodystrophy (MOD) (moderately prolonged mineralization lag time 35–100 days). The pathogenesis of aplastic disease (AD), or more commonly observed adynamic osteomalacia (AOM), is not completely understood but has been related to aluminum overload and bone aluminum deposition resulting in possible suppression of osteoblastic and parathyroid function in symptomatic patients [Coburn et al. 1986, Sherrard 1986, Ott et al. 1982, Parisien et al. 1988, Andress et al. 1987, Goodman 1987, Heaf et al. 1987, Moriniere et al. 1989].

Bone biopsy has proven to be a safe, reliable, relatively simple diagnostic procedure which has allowed one to quantify and specify the static and dynamic features of bone disease in a given patient. Most previous studies had a small or selected patient population and, therefore, the prevalence of the various forms of osteodystrophy in a large chronic hemodialysis population is not well documented.

In this study we asked all of our patients to undergo a bone biopsy and during an 18-month period of time, 59 patients agreed to have the procedure performed. Two patients showed only osteoporosis, thus 57 patients were evaluated in detail and formed the basis of this study. The biochemical values between the biopsied patients and the general dialysis population were different but the differences could be explained by the difference in the duration of dialysis between the two groups [Chazan et al. 1989a]. Therefore, we chose a subset of the dialysis population matched for sex, age, and duration of dialysis and compared their biochemical findings with the patients who had had bone biopsies. In this comparison, the biochemical findings were quite similar between the groups leading us to conclude that the patients who chose to be biopsied were representative of their peers and that the extrapolation of these findings to the general hemodialysis population is reasonable.

It is interesting to note that osteitis fibrosa (23 patients) (mineralization lag time <35 days), mixed osteodystrophy (15 patients) (mineralization lag time 35–100 days), and osteomalacia and adynamic bone diseases (mineralization lag time >100 days) considered together (19 patients, 3 aplastic disease, 13 adynamic osteomalacia and 3 osteomalacia) occurred with nearly equal frequency. There was no clinical difference among these patients since most had nonspecific musculoskeletal symptoms and none had myopathy or active central nervous system disease. The patients in each group were comparable in age, sex distribution, duration of dialysis, and serum calcium and phosphorus concentrations and they had been treated in a similar fashion regarding diet, oral phosphate binders, and vitamin D therapy, and all patients were dialyzed in the same facility for virtually all of their treatments. Therefore, we could not identify what role if any was played by modifications of dietary or therapeutic interventions.

Patients with osteitis fibrosa (mineralization lag time <35 days) had higher alkaline phosphatase ($p < 0.05$) and parathormone levels ($p < 0.02$) than the patients in the other two groups, which is certainly consistent with the pathophysiology of hyperparathyroidism. Again, the overlap between the groups is quite large and no individual laboratory test was both specific and sensitive. The parathormone level >5000 units had a 90% sensitivity but only a 50% specificity for osteitis fibrosa (mineralization lag time <35 days) and a parathormone level of >20,000 had a specificity of 95% but a sensitivity of only 60%. It is conceivable, however, that the intact PTH molecule assay (IRMA) may prove to be of greater predictive value and needs to be studied further.

The role of aluminum

The syndrome of aluminum toxicity described in the early 1980s characterized by osteomalacia, bone and joint pain, muscle weakness, stuttering speech, seizures, dementia and microcytic hypochromic anemia [Alfrey 1986, Alfrey 1983, Drueke et al. 1986, Hodsman et al. 1982, Ihle et al. 1982, Ihle et al. 1986, Ott 1983, Pierides et al. 1980, Prior et al. 1982, Wills and Savory 1983, Ward et al. 1978] has now become rare [Chazan et al. 1988, Chazan et al. 1989a]. The prevention of this syndrome has occurred because the role of aluminum is now well recognized, and aluminum has been removed from water used to make the dialysate and the use of oral aluminum salts has virtually ceased. However, patients who have been on dialysis for some years have had a large exposure to aluminum and may well have increases in total body aluminum even without the development of signs or symptoms of toxicity [Ott et al. 1982, Chazan et al. 1988, Moriniere et al. 1989, Charhon et al. 1985].

The role that aluminum plays in the development of renal osteodystrophy is somewhat complicated. It is felt that aluminum deposition in the osteoid seam results in osteomalacia. However, osteomalacia was well documented in uremic patients long before these patients were exposed to either large amounts of aluminum or even chronic hemodialysis [Alvarez-Ude et al. 1978, Stanbury and Lumb 1962, Stanbury and Lumb 1966]. Whether this osteomalacia (MLt >100 days) was of an adynamic type which is seen more commonly in our study or the type classically described in vitamin D deficiency, seen in only three of our patients, is not known. In addition, most but not all patients with adynamic osteomalacia or aplastic disease have evidence of aluminum deposition in their bone (12 of 16) and only one of three patients with apparently classic osteomalacia had significant bone aluminum deposition. It is not clear whether the bone aluminum deposition is the cause or the consequence of the adynamic state [Slatopolsky 1987, Sherrard 1986, Cournot-Witmer et al. 1981, Quarles et al. 1985, Quarles et al. 1986, Ott et al. 1982, Malluche et al. 1986, Hodsman et al. 1985].

In patients with osteitis fibrosa, there was mild to no aluminum deposited but in 12 of 19 patients with aplastic disease or osteomalacia and in 4 of 15 patients with mixed osteodystrophy the aluminum deposition was moderate to marked. There were no clinical differences and no differences in serum values of unstimulated or stimulated aluminum, calcium, phosphorus, and alkaline phosphatase between groups with small or large amounts of aluminum deposition. Only the parathormone levels were significantly higher among the patients who had minimal to mild deposition when compared to those with moderate to marked aluminum deposition ($p < 0.01$) (Figure 2).

It is of interest that there is no difference in the unstimulated plasma aluminum levels in the three groups. However, the deferoxamine stimulated aluminum levels were significantly higher in the group with osteitis fibrosa when compared to the group with adynamic osteomalacia (Figure 1). Studies have shown that the higher DFO stimulated plasma aluminum levels are associated with aluminum bone disease; however, these studies were performed on a selected population of symptomatic chronic hemodialysis patients [Coburn et al. 1986, Nebeker et al. 1986, Coburn and Norris 1986, Milliner et al. 1984]. Our findings along with those of others [DeVernejoul et al. 1989, Turner et al. 1988, von Herrath et al. 1986] do not support these observations and cast serious doubt on the usefulness of this test in evaluating asymptomatic chronic hemodialysis patients for aluminum bone disease. It could be considered paradoxical that patients with osteitis fibrosa who have little or no aluminum stainable in their bone have higher stimulated aluminum levels. However, since these patients have been exposed to similar amounts of oral aluminum as patients in the other two groups, it is reasonable to assume that their total body aluminum is also similar. The aluminum may be deposited in tissues other than bone and may be in a pool which is more available for chelation [Hakim et al. 1987].

Elevated serum aluminum levels have been shown to be associated with increased morbidity and mortality [Chazan et al. 1988, Chazan et al. 1989b, Llach et al. 1986, Starkey 1987]. Therefore, elevated serum aluminum levels per se should be considered evidence of increased body aluminum and should be treated by decreasing oral ingested aluminum [Chazan et al. 1989a, Finch et al. 1986, Iwamoto et al. 1986] with or without deferoxamine therapy [Chazan et al. 1989a, Andress et al. 1987, Charhon et al. 1987].

In an attempt to ascertain whether the biochemical findings observed at or near the inception of dialysis might predict the nature of the bone disease that is present or developed subsequently, we looked at the patients' calcium, phosphorus, alkaline phosphatase and parathormone levels as close to the inception of dialysis as possible (Figures 3 and 4). It appears that patients who subsequently had evidence of osteitis fibrosa and minimal to mild aluminum deposition years later, had statistically higher parathormone levels initially. Those with statistically lower parathormone levels were more likely to develop adynamic osteomalacia with moderate to marked aluminum deposition. These observations require further evaluation and might be confirmed by correlation of the biochemical parameters with the findings of bone biopsies near the inception of dialysis.

Acknowledgements

To Audrey Gagne and Marian Poisson for preparing bone specimens and to Kathy Cote for invaluable assistance in data collection and manuscript preparation.

REFERENCES

Alfrey AC 1986 Dialysis encephalopathy. Kidney Int *29:* S53

Alfrey AC 1983 The toxicity of the aluminum burden. Semin Nephrol *3:* 329

Alvarez-Ude F, Feest TG, Ward MK, Pierides AM, Ellis HA, Peart KM, Simpson W, Weightman D, Kerr DNS 1978 Hemodialysis bone disease: correlation between clinical, histologic, and other findings. Kidney Int *14:* 68

Andress DL, Nebeker HG, Ott SM, Endres DB, Alfrey AC, Slatopolsky EA, Coburn JW, Sherrard DJ 1987 Bone histologic response to deferoxamine in aluminum-related bone disease. Kidney Int *31:* 1344

Charhon SA, Chavassieux P, Boivin G, Parisien M, Chapuy MC, Traeger J, Meunier PJ 1987 Deferoxamine-induced bone changes in haemodialysis patients: a histomorphometric study. Clin Sci *73:* 227

Charhon SA, Chavassieux PM, Meunier PJ, Accominotti M 1985 Serum aluminum concentration and aluminum deposits in bone in patients receiving haemodialysis. Brit Med J *290:* 1613

Chazan JA, Blonsky SL, Abuelo JG, Pezzullo JC 1988 Increased body aluminum. An independent risk factor in patients undergoing long-term hemodialysis? Arch Intern Med *148:* 1817

Chazan JA, Abuelo JG, Blonsky SL 1989a Plasma aluminum levels (unstimulated and stimulated): clinical and biochemical findings in 185 patients undergoing chronic hemodialysis for 4 to 95 months. Am J Kidney Diseases *13:* 284

Chazan JA, Leu N, Lowrie E 1989b Increased serum aluminum: an independent risk factor for mortality in chronic hemodialysis patients. (Abstract) Am Soc Nephrol, Dec. 1989, Washington, DC

Coburn JW, Norris KC, Nebeker HG 1986 Osteomalacia and bone disease arising from aluminum. Seminars in Nephrology *6:* 68

Coburn JW, Norris KC 1986 Diagnosis of aluminum-related bone disease and treatment of aluminum toxicity with deferoxamine. Seminars in Nephrology *6:* 12

Coburn JW 1983 Introduction and overview of bone disease in uremia. In: *Frame B, Potts J* (eds) Clinical disorders of bone and mineral metabolism. Excerpta Medica, Amsterdam – Oxford – Princeton, pp. 249–253

Cournot-Witmer G, Zingraff J, Plachot JJ, Escaig F, Lefevre R, Boumati P, Bourdeau A, Garabedian M 1981 Aluminum localization in bone from hemodialyzed patients: relationship to matrix mineralization. Kidney Int *20:* 375

Cushner HM, Adams ND 1986 Review: renal osteodystrophy – pathogenesis and treatment. Am J Med Sci *4:* 264

De Vernejoul MC, Marchais S, London G, Bielakoff J, Chappuis P, Morieux C, Llach F 1989 Deferoxamine test and bone disease in dialysis patients with mild aluminum accumulation. Am J Kidney Diseases *14:* 124

Drueke TB, Lacour B, Touam M, Drueke TB, Lacoun B, Touam M, Jucquel J-P, Plachot J-J, Cournot-Witmer G, Galle P 1986 Effect of aluminum on hematopoiesis. Kidney Int *29:* S 45

Finch JL, Bergfeld M, Martin KJ, Chan YL, Teitelbaum S, Slatopolsky E 1986 The effects of discontinuation of aluminum exposure on aluminum-induced osteomalacia. Kidney Int *30:* 318

Goodman WG 1987 Thyroparathyroidectomy modifies the skeletal response to aluminum loading in the rat. Kidney Int *31:* 923

Hakim RM, Stivelman JC, Schulman G, Fosburg M, Wolfe L, Imber MJ, Lazarus JM 1987 Iron overload and mobilization in long-term hemodialysis patients. Am J Kidney Dis *10:* 293

Heaf JG, Joffe P, Podenphant J, Andersen JR 1987 Noninvasive diagnosis of uremic osteodystrophy: uses and limitations. Am J Nephrol *7:* 203

Hodsman AB, Hood SA, Brown P, Cordy PE 1985 Do serum aluminum levels reflect underlying skeletal aluminum accumulation and bone histology before or after chelation by deferoxamine? J Lab Clin Med *106:* 674

Hodsman AB, Sherrard DJ, Alfrey AC, Ott S, Brickman AS, Miller NL, Maloney NA, Coburn JW 1982 Bone aluminum and histomorphometric features of renal osteodystrophy. J Clin Endocrinol Metab *54:* 539

Ihle B, Buchanan M, Stevens B, Marshal A, Plomley R, d'Apice A, Kincaid-Smith P 1982 Aluminum associated bone disease: Clinico-pathologic correlation. Am J Kidney Dis *2:* 255

Ihle BU, Becker GJ, Kincaid-Smith PS 1986 Clinical and biochemical features of aluminum-related bone disease. Kidney Int *29:* S80

Iwamoto N, Ono T, Yamazaki S, Fukuda T, Kondo M, Yamamoto N, Hiratake Y, Masugi Y, Kubo Y, Hino M, Shigeno C, Yamamoto I 1986 Clinical features of aluminum-associated bone disease in long-term hemodialysis patients. Nephron *42:* 204

Kleeman CR, Norris K, Coburn JW 1987 Is the clinical expression of primary hyperparathyroidism a function of the long-term vitamin D status of the patient? Mineral Electrolyte Metab *13:* 305

Libbey NP, Chazan JA, London MR, Pono L, Abuelo JG 1990 The relevance of mineralization lag time in the evaluation of histologic changes in renal osteodystrophy. J Bone & Mineral Res *5:* S-106

Llach F, Felsenfeld AJ, Coleman MD, Keveney JJ Jr, Pederson JA, Medlock TR 1986. The natural course of dialysis osteomalacia. Kidney Int *29:* S-74

Malluche HH, Faugere MC, Smith AJ Jr, Friedler RM 1986 Aluminum intoxication of bone in renal failure – fact or fiction? Kidney Int *29:* S-70

Mayor GH, Keiser JA, Makdani D, Ku PK 1977 Aluminum absorption and distribution: effect of parathyroid hormone. Science *197:* 1187

Milliner DS Nebeker HG, Ott SM, Andress DL, Sherrard DJ, Alfrey AC, Slatopolsky EA, Coburn JW 1984 Use of the deferoxamine infusion test in the diagnosis of aluminum-related osteodystrophy. Ann Intern Med *101:* 775

Moriniere P, Cohen-Solal M, Belbrik S, Boudailliez B, Marie A, Westell PF, Renaud H, Fievet P, Lalau JD, Sebert JL, Fournier A 1989 Disappearance of aluminic bone disease in a long term asymptomatic dialysis population restricting $Al(OH)_3$ intake: emergence of an idiopathic adynamic bone disease not related to aluminum. Nephron *53:* 93

Nebeker HG, Andress DL, Milliner DS, Ott SM, Alfrey AC, Slatopolsky EA, Sherrard DJ, Coburn JW 1986 Indirect methods for the diagnosis of aluminum bone disease: plasma aluminum, the desferrioxamine infusion test, and serum iPTH. Kidney Int *29:* S 96

Ott SM, Maloney NA, Coburn JW, Alfrey AC, Sherrard DJ 1982 The prevalence of bone aluminum deposition in renal osteodystrophy and its relation to the response to calcitriol therapy. N Engl J Med *307:* 709

Ott SM 1983 Aluminum related osteomalacia. Int J Artif Organs *6:* 173

Parfitt AM, Drezner MR, Glorieux FH, Kanis JA, Malluche H, Meunier PJ, Ott SM, Recker RR 1987 Bone histomorphometry: standardization of nomenclature, symbols and units. J Bone Min Res *2:* 595

Parisien M, Charhon SA, Arlot M, Mainetti E, Chavassieux P, Chapuy MC, Meunier PJ 1988 Evidence for a toxic effect of aluminum on osteoblasts: a histomorphometric study on hemodialysis patients with aplastic bone disease. J Bone Min Res *3:* 259

Pierides AM, Edwards WG Jr, Cullum UX Jr, McCall JT, Ellis HA 1980 Hemodialysis encephalopathy with osteomalacic fractures and muscle weakness. Kidney Int *18:* 115

Prior JC, Cameron EC, Knickerbocker WJ, Sweeney VP, Suchowersky O 1982 Dialysis encephalopathy and osteomalacic bone disease. Am J Med *72:* 33

Quarles LD, Dennis VW, Gitelman HJ, Harrelson JM, Drezner MK 1985 Aluminum deposition at the osteoid-bone interface. J Clin Invest *75:* 1441

Quarles LD, Gitelman HJ, Drezner MK 1986 Aluminum: culprit or accessory in the genesis of renal osteodystrophy. Seminars in Nephrology *6:* 90

Recker RR (ed) 1983 Bone histomorphometry: techniques and interpretation, CRC Press, Boca Raton, FL.

Sherrard D, Ott S, Maloney N, Andress D, Coburn J 1983 Uremic osteodystrophy: classification, cause and treatment. In: *Frame B, Potts J* (eds) Clinical Disorders of Bone and Mineral Metabolism. Excerpta Medica, Amsterdam – Oxford – Princeton, pp. 254–259

Sherrard DJ 1986 Aluminum in renal osteodystrophy. Seminars in Nephrology (suppl) *6:* 5–11

Slatopolsky E 1987 The interaction of parathyroid hormone and aluminum in renal osteodystrophy. Kidney Int *31:* 842

Stanbury SW, Lumb GA 1962 Metabolic studies of renal osteodystrophy. Medicine *41:* 1

Stanbury SW, Lumb GA 1966 Parathyroid function in chronic renal failure. Quart J Med *25:* 1

Starkey BJ 1987 Aluminium in renal disease: current knowledge and future developments. Ann Clin Biochem *24:* 337

Turner MW, Ardla M, Hutchinson T, Prichard S, Barre PE, Beauvais J, Kaye M 1988 Sporadic aluminum osteomalacia: identification of patients at risk. Am J Kidney Dis *11:* 51

von Herrath D, Asmus G, Pauls A, Delling G, Schaefer K 1986 Renal osteodystrophy in asymptomatic hemodialysis patients: evidence of a sex-dependent distribution and predictive value of serum aluminum measurements. Am J Kidney Dis *8:* 430

Ward MK, Feest TG, Ellis HA, Parkinson IS, Kerr DNS 1978 Osteomalacic dialysis osteodystrophy: evidence for a water-borne aetiological agent, probably aluminium. Lancet *1:* 841

Wills MR, Savory J 1983 Aluminum poisoning: dialysis encephalopathy, osteomalacia and anemia. Lancet *2:* 29

LETTERS TO THE EDITOR

Cholelithiasis associated with hemolytic uremic syndrome

Sir, – Cholelithiasis is an extremely unusual complication of hemolytic uremic syndrome (HUS), though it is a well recognized complication of hemolytic disease [Schweighofer et al. 1980]. We report on a patient who presented with jaundice and right upper quadrant abdominal pain, three months after recovery from HUS, and her abdominal ultrasound examination revealed gallstones.

Case report

A 15-year-old girl, previously well, presented with a history of bloody diarrhea, vomiting and oliguria of 1-week duration. On admission, the only clinical finding was that of pallor, and abdominal examination was normal. Investigations revealed a plasma creatinine of 2172 μmol/l, hemoglobin 6.9 g/dl and platelet count of 90×10^9/l. Peripheral blood smear showed marked anisocytosis and poikilocytosis with abundant fragmented red blood cells. Her liver function tests were normal and abdominal ultrasound examination revealed normal kidneys and gallbladder. She was treated with acute peritoneal dialysis for 6 days and during this period she received packed cell transfusion. Following satisfactory clinical and biochemical improvement, she was discharged 14 days after admission.

At 2 months following admission, she was normotensive and her creatinine clearance was 130 mls/min/1.73 m^2. Three months following admission, she presented with a 5-day history of vomiting and intermittent colicky right upper quadrant abdominal pain. On examination, she was mildly icteric but abdominal examination was normal. Investigation revealed a plasma total bilirubin of 77 μmol/l (conjugated 51 μmol/l), ALT 202 U/l, AST 130 U/l. Routine urinalysis showed bilirubinemia but no urobilinogen. Abdominal ultrasound examination revealed a thickened gallbladder, pericholecystic lucent halo and 2 gallstones of 8 mm and 5 mm size within the fundus of the gallbladder (Figure 1). The pancreas, spleen and both kidneys were normal.

She was treated conservatively with analgesics and intravenous fluids. She made a complete recovery and was discharged 5 days later.

On follow-up 6 weeks later, she remained asymptomatic and repeat abdominal ultrasound showed normal gallbladder with no calculi.

Discussion

Cholelithiasis is uncommon in childhood and adolescence [Sleisenger and Fordtran 1978] and the female preponderance observed in the adult population is not as marked [Silverman and Roy 1988]. It is well recognized as a complication of hemolytic disease, but has been reported on only one occasion, in association with HUS [Schweighofer et al. 1980].

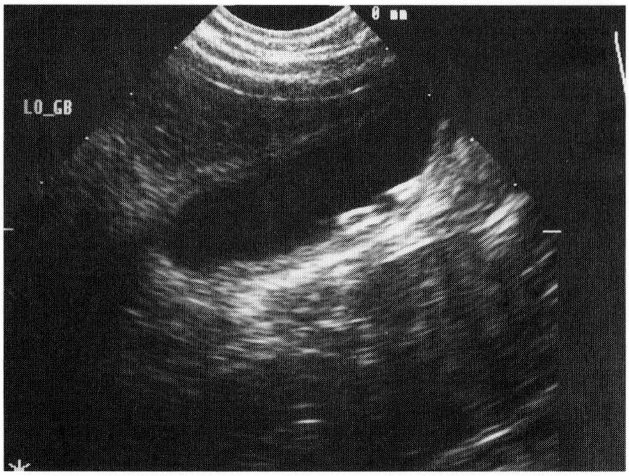

Fig. 1. Sagittal ultrasonic section through the gallbladder demonstrates 2 gallstones with acoustic shadowing, gallbladder wall thickening and an echo-free halo around the gallbladder wall.

In this patient the gastrointestinal symptoms persisted after improvement in the renal and hematological manifestations of HUS. In the present case, however there was an interim asymptomatic period of 3 months between the acute illness and the subsequent presentation with cholelithiasis.

Although HUS has not been included in the list of cases with gallstones in several recent reviews [Whitington et al. 1979, Liebermann 1982, Giamantonio 1978], one should consider this possibility in a patient presenting with suggestive symptoms following HUS. An abdominal ultrasound examination would easily and readily confirm the diagnosis.

S. K. Parida[1], *A. S. Hollman*[2], *T. J. Beattie*[1]
[1]Department of Nephrology and [2]Radiology, Royal Hospital for Sick Children, Yorkhill, Glasgow

REFERENCES

Giamantonio CA 1978 Haemolytic uraemic syndrome. In: *Edelmann LM Jr* (ed) Pediatric kidney disease. Little Brown and Co, Boston, pp 724–736

Liebermann E 1972 Hemolytic uraemic syndrome. J Pediatr *80:* p 1–16

Schweighofer S, Primack WA, Stovis TL, Hight DW, Fleischmann LE 1980 Cholelithiasis associated with haemolytic uraemic syndrome. Am J Dis Child *134:* 622

Silverman A, Roy CC 1983 Pediatric Clinical Gastroenterology. CV Molby Co, p 799

Sleisenger MH, Fordtran JS 1978 Gastrointestinal disease: pathophysiology. Diagnosis. Management. WB Saunders Co, Philadelphia, pp 1248–1263

Whitington PF, Friedman AL, Chesney RW 1979 Gastrointestinal disease in the haemolytic uraemic syndrome. Gastroenterology *76:* 728–733

Sodium ferric gluconate complex given intravenously for iron deficiency in hemodialysis

Sir, – Iron deficiency is an increasing complication in hemodialysis (HD) patients and frequently oral supplementation is not enough for adequate repletion of iron stores [MacDougall et al. 1989 Br Med J 299: 157–158]. On the other hand, an excess of oral iron could interfere with other medications such as phosphate binders. Iron dextran has usually been given intravenously for iron deficiency treatment [Hamstra et al. 1980 JAMA 243: 1726–1731]. However, this form of therapy is accompanied by an excess of adverse reactions, including fatal or life-threatening anaphylactoid ones [Hamstra et al. 1980, Becker et al. 1966 Ann Intern Med 65: 745, Lane 1964 Lancet 1: 852]. We have administered sodium ferric gluconate complex (Nattermann, Cologne, Germany), 1 g divided into 8 doses after HD sessions (slow injection) to 19 HD patients (8 males), aged 50 ± 15 years, distributed in 3 groups: I) 8 patients with renal anemia and iron deficiency, II) 6 patients with renal anemia, iron deficiency and concomitant treatment with nandrolone decanoate i.m. (200 mg weekly), III) 5 patients with iron deficiency associated with poor response to treatment of renal anemia with erythropoietin. All patients had been taking oral ferrous glutamate 600 mg/day before parenteral administration, with a poor response of hematological parameters. Significant rises in hemoglobin concentration were obvious after 1 month in all groups and they were maintained after 3 and 6 months (Table 1). Serum ferritin levels also had risen within 1 month and slowly declined from month 3 to 6. A total of 152 infusions were performed, and there were no immediate or delayed reactions or adverse effects. Our data support that i.v. ferric gluconate is safe and efficient in treating severe iron deficiency.

Iron deficiency will become an increasing problem as erythropoietin is used more widely unless prophylactic iron is administered i.v. when serum ferritin falls below adequate levels.

J. Pascual[1], J. L. Teruel[1], F. Liaño[1], A. Sureda[2], J. Ortuño[1]
Departments of Nephrology[1] and Hematology[2], Hospital Ramón y Cajal, Madrid, Spain

Table 1. Evolution of hemoglobin (Hb) and serum ferritin (SF) concentrations

Group		Before i.v. iron	After i.v. iron***: 1 month	3 months	6 months
I	Hb (g/dl)*	7.7 ± 0.6	8.4 ± 0.9	8.9 ± 1.3	8.6 ± 1.3
	SF (μg/l)**	23 (14–48)	149 (67–263)	163 (107–561)	111 (98–329)
II	Hb (g/dl)*	8.4 ± 1.6	8.8 ± 0.8	9.3 ± 2.4	9.6 ± 1.3
	SF (μg/l)**	28 (17–37)	130 (45–464)	231 (174–370)	199 (151–392)
III	Hb (g/dl)*	8.5 ± 1.4	10.7 ± 2.5	11.2 ± 1.6	10.3 ± 2.7
	SF (μg/l)**	26 (20–39)	193 (58–1040)	213 (80–298)	154 (115–927)

* = Arithmetic mean ± SD, ** = Geometric means (range), *** = All values higher with respect to basal ones ($p < 0.05$, paired t-test)

Sterile pyuria

Sir, – We have recently reported a technique for identifying nonsquamous nucleated cells and cellular casts in urine using a panel of commercially available monoclonal antibodies and an immunoperoxidase technique [Segasothy et al. 1988] and by quantifying these cells it was possible to determine the urine cell profiles in various renal diseases [Segasothy et al. 1989, in press] and in renal allograft recipients [Segasothy et al. 1989]. These profiles summarized in Tables 1 and 2 indicate that in acute interstitial nephritis, analgesic nephropathy, polycystic kidney disease, medullary sponge kidney disease, allograft rejection and early post-transplant acute tubular necrosis, granulocytes account for 82–95% of cells present in urine, and in nontransplant acute tubular necrosis, crescentic glomerulonephritis and noncrescentic glomerulonephritis, granulocytes constitute 24–32% of cells present in urine. No growth of aerobic, anaerobic or fastidious organisms was recorded in 127 of the 133 urine specimens, thus excluding urinary tract infection as a cause of pyuria. The presence of large numbers of granulocytes in urine in these conditions suggest that they may have a pathogenetic role.

M. Segasothy[1], K. F. Fairley[2], D. F. Birch[3], P. Kincaid-Smith[2]
Department of Medicine[1], University Kebangsaan Malaysia, Jalan Raja Muda, Kuala Lumpur 50300, Malaysia
Department of Medicine[2], University of Melbourne,
Department of Nephrology[3], Royal Melbourne Hospital, Australia

REFERENCES

Segasothy M, Birch DF, Fairley KF, Kincaid-Smith P 1989 Monoclonal antibody identification of nucleated cells in urine: diagnosis of allograft rejection. Transplant Proc *21:* 1879

Table 1. Cell viability and percentages of different cell* types in renal disease

Parameter	ATN (n = 30)	CN (n = 20)	NCN (n = 12)	AIN (n = 10)
Viability	43 ± 4	58 ± 5	59 ± 7	68 ± 5
Total cell number**	61000 ± 9000	104000 ± 27000	20000 ± 3000	530000 ± 150000
Granulocytes	23.8 ± 3.8	28.9 ± 4.0	31.8 ± 5.5	82.3 ± 6.1
Monocytes	2.2 ± 0.7	12.2 ± 1.3	7.3 ± 1.5	4.0 ±1.6
Lymphocytes	0.2 ± 0.1	9.8 ± 0.8	6.2 ± 1.6	2.2 ± 1.4
Eosinophils	0.2 ± 0.1	2.3 ± 0.3	1.3 ± 0.4	2.9 ± 0.7
Tubular cells	72.7 ± 4.1	58.6 ± 4.8	55.8 ± 6.2	13.0 ± 3.5

* All values are expressed as mean ± SEM. The number of patients per group is in parentheses. ** Total cell number is expressed per ml of urine, ATN = Acute tubular necrosis, CN = Crescentic glomerulonephritis, NCN = Noncrescentic glomerulonephritis, AIN = Acute interstitial nephritis

Table 2. Cell viability and percentages of different cell* types in renal disease and in renal allograft recipients

Parameter	AN (n = 9)	PCKD (n = 13)	MSKD (n = 3)	AR (n = 21)	T_x ATN (n = 12)
Viability	73 ± 5	83 ± 5	85 ± 4	73 ± 6	85 ± 5
Total cell number**	23000 ± 5000	27000 ± 6000	39000 ± 12000	910000 ± 290000	590000 ± 260000
Granulocytes	86.2 ± 2.9	86.2 ± 3.6	84.5 ± 8.6	82.7 ± 30.5	94.9 ± 42.9
Monocytes	1.3 ± 0.6	3.1 ± 1.0	1.2 ± 1.0	4.2 ± 1.2	2.9 ± 1.2
Lymphocytes	0	0	0	4.2 ± 0.5	1.0 ± 0.3
Eosinophils	2.1 ± 0.8	2.6 ± 0.4	2.5 ± 1.4	ND	ND
Tubular cells	12.5 ± 2.4	8.9 ± 1.5	8.1 ± 2.2	26.8 ± 4.2	13.1 ± 3.9

* All values are expressed as mean ± SEM. The number of patients per group is in parentheses. ** Total cell number is expressed per ml of urine. AN = Analgesic nephropathy, PCKD = Polycystic kidney disease, MSKD = Medullary sponge kidney disease, AR = Renal allograft rejection, T_x ATN = Posttransplant acute tubular necrosis, ND = Not done

Segasothy M, Birch DF, Fairley KF, Kincaid-Smith P 1989 Urine cytologic profile in renal allograft recipients determined by monoclonal antibodies: diagnosis of allograft rejection. Transplantation *47:* 482

Segasothy M, Fairley KF, Birch DF, Kincaid-Smith P 1989 Immunoperoxidase identification of nucleated cells in urine in glomerular and acute tubular disorders. Clin Nephrol *31:* 281

Segasothy M, Fairley KF, Birch DF, Kincaid-Smith P 1990 The use of monoclonal antibodies in microscopic urinalysis in analgesic nephropathy, polycystic kidney disease and medullary sponge kidney disease. Nephron (in press)

Segasothy M, Kincaid-Smith P, Birch DF, Fairley KF 1988 Monoclonal antibodies: use in urine sediment examinatioin. In: *Haber MH, Corwin HL* (eds) Clinics in Laboratory Medicine. WB Saunders Co, Philadelphia, vol 8, p 483

Segasothy M, Lau TM, Birch DF, Fairley KF, Kincaid-Smith P 1988 Immunocytologic dissection of the urine sediment using monoclonal antibodies. Am J Clin Pathol *90:* 51

Renal transplant patients' knowledge concerning cyclosporine treatment

Cyclosporine (Sandimmun®, Sandoz Pharmaceuticals) is widely used in organ transplant programs. Formulations for oral use include capsules and a liquid which requires dosage measurement by a pump.

Patient information leaflets are included as a package insert, but it is unknown whether patients treated with cyclosporine understand this material. Patient compliance is enhanced by an increased knowledge about their medication [Meichenbaum and Turk 1987] and is critical for cyclosporine where specific knowledge and instruction may greatly influence therapeutic outcome [Rovelli et al. 1989]. We investigated the knowledge of renal transplant patients about cyclosporine dosing, administration and indication, the reasons for blood tests and monitoring, and patients' experiences with side effects and missed doses.

A questionnaire was designed and piloted in 6 randomly selected renal transplant patients from our institution, and amended appropriately to exclude ambiguities.

All renal transplant patients over the age of 18 years who were currently taking cyclosporine were eligible for recruitment into the study. Patients must have been taking cyclosporine for at least 3 months prior to the study. Patients who were unable to communicate or those who could not self-administer their medications because of disability were excluded. Patients who had reading difficulties were included.

Eligible patients gave informed consent and completed the questionnaire while attending the monthly outpatient clinic, in private and in a confidential manner.

All such patients undergoing renal transplantation had been routinely entered into a teaching program according to unit policy.

Responses to items on the questionnaire were scored and entered on a data base system. Data were assessed in terms of percent response. No attempt was made to correlate responses with serum or blood cyclosporine concentrations.

Of 65 eligible patients, 55 were approached to complete the questionnaire. Ten were excluded because of clinic scheduling difficulties, and 5 declined to participate. Fifty (32 males, mean ± SD age 42 ± 15 years) were successfully recruited. Patients were taking 4.3 ± 1.9 drugs and 311 ± 125 mg cyclosporine per day. Forty-five patients knew the indication for cyclosporine, but only 39% knew why they had regular blood tests and 21% knew the meaning of immunosuppression.

Nineteen and 27 patients took the drug on an empty or full stomach, respectively. Thirty-seven patients correctly took the cyclosporine liquid with a cold drink to improve palatability, although 23 claimed the palatability remained unacceptable. All patients had experienced taking both formulations, but 31 preferred capsules. Only 7 patients understood the necessity to accurately measure the dose of liquid cyclosporine using the dosage pump provided.

Most patients (42) knew that they should take a missed dose as soon as they remembered, but 7 gave inappropriate responses such as they would omit that dose. Most patients experienced common side effects such as hirsutism (43), trembling hands (30) and persistent gastrointestinal upset (9) and said they would inform their doctor. Ten said they would not tell their doctor if they had a fever, sore throat or signs of infection and 29 felt it was permissible to drink alcohol while taking cyclosporine.

Forty-three patients felt the package insert was adequate to very good and 46 felt it was comprehensible. Twelve patients said they received too little medication information from their doctor or pharmacist.

A recent study highlighted non-compliance with medication as a major cause of organ rejection [Rovelli et al. 1989], although this may not be universally accepted. Patients must have a clear understanding of the need for good compliance, since failure to comply with cyclosporine could result in a rejection episode, loss of the graft and a return to maintenance dialysis.

There is cause for concern regarding our patients' potential inaccuracy in dosing and their methods of administration. The package insert describes how to use and store the dosage pump but does not adequately cover the measuring of a dose or the need for accuracy. An illustration of the barrel of the pump highlighting the dosage increments may be useful. Most of our patients preferred the capsule formulation, and extensive use of capsules could minimize these problems.

In our patient population and despite our teaching program, there remains a deficit of knowledge in crucial areas such as dose administration and measurement. It is unknown whether these data can be extrapolated to other centers. This issue requires further effort to ensure maximal benefit from cyclosporine therapy.

M. Malone[1], *J. Hemingway*[2], *P. Wiffen*[2] and *G. R. Bailie*[3]
[1]Regional Pharmaceutical Service, Oxford, England, UK
[2]Department of Pharmacy, Churchill Hospital, Oxford, England, UK
[3]Albany College of Pharmacy, 106 New Scotland Avenue, Albany, New York 12208, USA

REFERENCES

Meichenbaum D, Turk DC 1987 In: *Meichenbaum D, Turk DC* (eds) Facilitiating treatment adherence. Plenum Press, New York

Rovelli M, Palmeri D, Vossler E et al. 1989 Non compliance in organ transplant recipients. Transplant Proc *21:* 833–834

Hemolytic anemia due to G6PD deficiency and urate oxidase in a kidney-transplant patient

The authors report the observation in a kidney-transplant patient where the appearance of hemolytic anemia after administration of urate oxidase revealed a deficiency in glucose-6-phosphate dehydrogenase (G6PD).

Mr. PE, born in 1924 in Italy presented with, in 1983, an inferior myocardial necrosis requiring aortocoronarian bypass of the anterior interventricular artery and the first marginal artery. In April 1985 he began periodic hemodialysis in Novare, Italy. On November 23, 1988, he underwent kidney transplantation in Marseille. On November 30, 1988, the patient presented with a digestive hemorrhage. Endoscopic examination revealed a duodenal ulcer causing massive diminution in the number of red blood cells (RBC 2.30 × 10^6/mm^3, Hb 6 g/100 ml). Four units of pure erythrocytes were transfused. A gastroenterostomy was performed and the patient received on the same day for a hyperuricemia of 500 µmol/l, an i. v. injection of one ampoule of 1,000 units of urate oxidase. Hepatic activity was strictly normal. Three days later, bilirubinemia was at 40 µmol/l. On December 15, 1988, renal function was normal (creatininemia 120 µmol/l) as was liver function (total bilirubin 10 µmol/l). Red cells were at 3.33 × 10^6/mm^3 with hemoglobin at 9.8 g/100 ml. At the beginning of 1989 the patient returned to Italy. On February 3, 1989, he presented a hyperuricemia at 520 µmol/l and was treated with urate oxidase: an intramuscular injection (i. m.) of 1,000 units was given every other day up to and including October 15, 1989, for a total of 127,000 units. The biological exams regularly performed during this treatment revealed a uricemia that was constantly superior to 450 µmol/l and total bilirubin was always inferior to 10 µmol/l.

On October 16, 1989, Mr. PE was readmitted to the Clinique de la Résidence du Parc for a coronary angiography after an episode of left cardiovascular failure during a fibrillo flutter arrhythmia. Creatininemia was at 243 µmol/l, red cell count at 3.30 × 10^6/mm^3, 9 g/100 ml of hemoglobin, and uricemia was at 700 µmol/l. Liver function was normal (total bilirubin 9 µmol/l). Before performing the angiography, 1 ampoule (i. v.) of 1,000 units of urate oxidase per 24 hours was injected for 3 consecutive days. On October 20, 1989, the patient presented a conjunctival subicterus that became generalized and complete the next day and was accompanied by anginal pain at rest, orthopnea, and reddish urine. The biological exam confirmed hemolytic anemia: red cell count 2.10 × 10^6/mm^3, with anisocytosis, anisochromia, Hb 7 g/100 ml, total bilirubinemia 131 µmol/l, low haptoglobin 0.2 g/l, 17% reticulocytes with rare schizocytes, and 22% erythroblasts. Folates (radioimmunologic dosage) were normal at 25.01 nmol/l. G6PD had fallen to 0.60 U/g Hb (normal values: 3.5 to 5.5 U/g Hb) (enzymatic kinetic). Pyruvate kinase was elevated at 16.86 U/g Hb (enzymatic kinetic at 25° C). Hemoglobin electrophoresis was normal. At the same time, kidney function was very altered: azotemia 63 µmol/l, carbon dioxide content 14 mmol/l, kaliemia 3.8 mmol/l, and uricemia 5 µmol/l. Other immunological tests revealed no abnormalities. Six units of pure erythrocytes associated with one hemodialysis session were required. Two days (48 h) later, bilirubin was at 44 µmol/l, creatinine at 300 µmol/l, and red cells were at $3.15 \times 10^6/mm^3$ with 10 g/100 ml of hemoglobin. On November 8, 1989, liver function was normal, creatininemia was at 250 µmol/l, and uricemia at 662 µmol/l. A coronary angiography was performed and revealed total occlusion of the aortocoronary bypass. On the same day, the rate of G6PD was verified and confirmed the deficiency at 1.4 U/g Hb.

By transforming uric acid into allantoin, urate oxidase, a protein enzyme of fungic origin, brings about the formation of an oxidizing agent H_2O_2 [Laboureur and Langlois 1968] and consequently can cause hemolytic anemia in patients with G6PD deficiency. Only one other case has been observed and it was not reported in the literature. This was the case of a child presenting with pleuropulmonary metastases from a right nephroblastoma who had received urate oxidase during a course of chemotherapy in November 1978 at the Institut Gustave Roussy.

In our observation, the first i.v. injection of urate oxidase 8 days after the transplantation very probably triggered a hemolytic crisis that clinically went unnoticed. The elevation of total bilirubin was parallel to the blood transfusions and was very rapidly normalized. Despite their repetition and prolonged prescription, i.m. injections of urate oxidase did not bring about clinical or biological hemolytic crises. However, the various studies by Royer et al. [1967] then Brogard et al. [1973] demonstrated that the efficacy of this product was identical by both i.m. or i.v. routes. On the other hand, it is known that at more or less long term in certain cases, there is the possibility of progressive depletion of its efficacy. This is probably due to an immunological mechanism that is secondary to the appearance of anti-urate-oxidase antibodies [Mourad et al. 1984, Sibony et al. 1984]. This hypothesis would not seem to apply in the present observation insofar as the uricemia in our patient was reduced only once to 450 µmol/l (otherwise, it remained between 535 and 600 µmol/l). This is due to an absence of efficacy of the product for which the enzymatic activity is dependent on the temperature and is inversely proportional to the degree of acidity of the medium [Desprey et al. 1976]. The pH for optimal activity is 8.5 [Laboureur and Langlois 1968]. The inactivity of the product when injected intramuscularly can be explained by the dilution of this lyophilized agent in a slightly acid solution: xylocaine to diminish the pain during injection of the product.

Finally, it was only after a series of three i.v. injections of urate oxidase that the diagnosis of G6PD deficiency was made in our patient. Indeed, after the massive liberation of H_2O_2, he was not able to maintain a normal level of reduced glutathion in the erythrocytes and although the hemolytic crisis was severe, it was rapidly reversible after treatment was discontinued.

The ethnic origin of our patient makes it possible to classify his G6PD deficiency in one of the GD (−) B Mediterranean variables.

It seemed of interest to report this observation which adds urate oxidase to the long list of products responsible for hemolysis during congenital dificiencies of G6PD. Indeed, this molecule is very frequently prescribed for kidney-transplant patients in whom immunosuppression treatment does not permit the use of uric acid synthesis inhibitors.

J. Ducros[1], S. Saingra[1], M. Rampal[2], C. Coulange[2], M.-C. Barbe[3], G. Verzetti[3]

[1]Service de Néphrologie Clinique de la Résidence du Parc, Rue Gaston Berger, F-13010 Marseille, France

[2]Service de Chirurgie Urologique et Transplantation Rénale, Hôpital de la Timone, Bd. Jean Moulin, F-13005 Marseille, France

[3]Unità Socio Sanitaria Locale 51, Ospedale Maggiori, Novara, Italy

REFERENCES

Brogard J-M, Frankhauser J, Stahl A 1973 Application de l'uricolyse enzymatique au traitement des hyperuricemies d'origine rénale. Schweiz Med Wschr *103:* 404–410

Desprey Th, Plouvier B, Devulder B, Tacquet A 1976 Etudes in vitro des facteurs modifiants l'activité de l'urate oxydase. Lille Médical *21* (5): 433–436

Laboureur P, Langlois C 1968 Urate oxydase d'aspergillus flavus. 1. Obtention, purification, propriétés; 2. Métabolisme, inhibitions, spécificité. Bulletin de la Société de Chimie organique *50* (4): 811–825; *50* (4): 827–841

Mourad G, Cristol J-P, Chong G, Andary M, Mion C 1984 Rôle d'anticorps précipitants anti-urate oxydase dans l'hyperuricémie résistante à l'urate oxydase. La Presse Médicale *13* (42): 2585

Royer R, Lamarche M, Kissel P 1967 Etude de l'action d'une urate oxydase fongique sur l'uricémie et l'excrétion de l'azote urique chez l'homme. Thérapie *22:* 1113, 1125

Sibony G, North M-L, Bergerat J-P, Lang J-M, Oberling F 1984 Hyperuricémie résistante à l'urate oxydase. Rôle d'anticorps précipitants antiurate oxydase sériques. La Presse Médicale *13* (7): 443

BOOK REVIEWS

Peritoneal Dialysis: New Concepts and Applications. Contemporary Issues in Nephrology, Vol. 22. *Twardowski Z. J., K. D. Nolph, R. Khanna* (eds). Churchill Livingstone, New York, 1990. 266 pages, $ 59.

Because some excellent monographs on peritoneal dialysis appeared recently including a comprehensive book by one of these authors in 1989, it may seem surprising that Twardowski, Nolph and Khanna have edited another treatise on the subject at this time. The implicit aim of the editors of Peritoneal Dialysis appears to be a review of some important contemporary issues related to the procedure. They have achieved this quite well, largely with chapters by the University of Missouri faculty supplemented by the writings of a few international experts. Clearly this Nephrology Division is among the most expert in the field of peritoneal dialysis and it can be most useful for those less experienced to learn their views. The reader must accept that authoritative groups tend toward, "Our results distinctly demonstrate" and "Our neighbor's data may possibly show, pending verification", and they may exhibit a parochialism in reference citations. Nevertheless, a unified message emerges which is quite valuable.

The book has 11 chapters beginning with a scholarly review of peritoneal anatomy by the Israeli experts Gotloib and Shostak. Mactier nicely reviews osmotic ultrafiltration and lymphatic absorption. In this and the next two chapters, however, idealized curves are presented without acknowledgement of error. This makes the text appear to be a simplified instruction when it is a rather detailed exposition. Lal and Nolph cleverly address a few specific methods of pharmacological acceleration of fluid and mass transfer rates. Twardowski astutely presents an abundant potpourri of information on dialysis techniques and prescriptions promoting the evaluations and methods they have previously championed. In the next chapter Khanna cogently and practically discusses catheters for access to the peritoneum. A further discussion of the results of the US CAPD registry and comparison with data from other sources are provided by Nolph. Peritonitis is sagely discussed by Everett who includes practical prophylactic, diagnostic and therapeutic pointers. A lucid discussion of the Y connector system is then given by the Italian experts Maiorca and Cancarini. A scholarly, informative discussion of renal osteodystrophy with particular reference to CAPD follows by Delmez. The final chapters describe the special circumstances of CAPD for management of diabetic and of pediatric patients.

The book is authoritative and extensively referenced. It is not a text for beginners in the field and presents little hands-on practical information. It does not present two sides of controversy so the reader can follow the logic easily. Although much of the data reported here may be found in earlier reports, the chapters are very nice syntheses of current information.

There is some redundancy and overlap of tables among chapters, but this is offset by each representing a comprehensive treatise on its own subtopic. Finally, the reader should not be bothered by the multiple errors of type, misspellings, split infinitives, or other grammatical aberrations. The wealth of information that this book contains should override any nonmedical inaccuracy. Those with a serious interest in peritoneal dialysis should find this monograph most useful. Even those already familiar with many of their data should appreciate the assembly of information into a single volume.

J. F. Maher, Bethesda, Maryland

Textbook of Hemodialysis for Patient Care Personnel. *Mark A. Newberry* 1989, Charles C. Thomas, Springfield, Illinois, 606 pages, $ 80.75.

This book is intended for hemodialysis' nurses and technicians, but it can also be of great benefit to trainees in nephrology. Dr. Newberry provides useful information necessary for understanding and performing hemodialysis, and he does so by describing the development of hemodialysis, current concepts of renal anatomy and physiology, and then modern hemodialysis systems and technology. His approach to an expanding and complex topic is well-organized and succinctly written.

The text is divided into eleven chapters. The first chapter is a historical overview including the epidmiology and the economics of end-stage renal disease. The next several chapters address renal and electrolyte physiology, renal anatomy, acute and chronic renal failure, and conditions leading to end-stage renal disease. This sets the stage for the major emphasis of the text, hemodialysis. The description of the principles of hemodialysis starts with basic definitions and includes functional characteristics of the hemodialyzer. He discusses, in detail, the types of dialyzers available, with a description of dialyzer specifications, and explains the advantages and disadvantages of each. He also describes the various dialysis membranes in use today. Dialysis tubing, dialysate delivery systems, and water treatment systems are reviewed. Chapter nine outlines types of vascular access available for both acute and chronic therapy. Chapters ten and eleven discuss hemodialysis technique and maintenance hemodialysis respectively, and are helpful in regard to daily patient management. The author also discusses muscle cramping, pruritis, dialysis disequilibrium syndrome, and acetate intolerance, all of which are common problems in the dialysis population. He includes an impressive number of references, tables, and illustrations, which enhance the usefulness of the text. I highly recommend this text to dialysis nurses and technicians as well as those physicians who are new to the field of hemodialysis. It provides much needed information in a concise, readable format.

Maria V. DeVita

New York, New York

ANNOUNCEMENTS

The **Arbeitsgemeinschaft für Klinische Nephrologie e. V.** would be pleased to receive submission of papers from candidates for the Nils-Alwall-Prize- This Prize is awarded to young scientists engaged in clinical research in German speaking regions in the field of nephrology, with particular emphasis on activities involving dialysis or similar methods of extracorporeal elimination or kidney transplants.

The award comprises the Nils-Alwall Medal, a certificate and prize money of DM 15000,–.

The prize may be awarded to up to three nominees.

Candidates up to 45 years of age are required to submit either non-published work, work published up to one year before submission or a summary of original extended research work (but not a habilitation thesis).

If this work involved patients it must explicitly confirm that all relevant ethical principles have been observed (Helsinki Agreement 1964, Tokyo Agreement 1975).

A total of six copies of the paper submitted are required. These are to be in anonymous form and accompanied by a short curriculum vitae and information regarding the candidates present professional activities. These documents are to reach the Chairman of the Prize Committee, Professor Dr. G. A. Jutzler, former Director of the Department of Nephrology *not later than April 15, 1991,* at the following address:

Am Brunnen 2
W-6650 Homburg/Saar, Germany

The **Fourth International Course on Peritoneal Dialysis** will be held in Vicenza, Italy, from May 21–24, 1991. English will be the official language but English-Italian simultaneous translations will be provided.

For further information please write to Dr. M. Feriani, Secretariat of the 4th International Course on Peritoneal Dialysis, Department of Nephrology, St. Bortolo Hospital, I-36100 Vicenza, Italy.

The **International Workshop on Alport Syndrome** will take place August 23–24, 1991 in Oulu, Finland. The objective of this workshop is to give a concise picture of the clinical aspects of Alport syndrome. The workshop will also cover the new available approaches for diagnosis. It will be of interest to nephrologists, pathologists, clinical geneticists and to molecular biologists specializing in kidney disease and basement membranes.

Deadline for application is July 1, 1991. Please contact Secretariat, International Workshop on Alport Syndrome, Biocenter and Department of Biochemistry, University of Oulu, SF-90570 Oulu, Finland, Tel: 358–81–352355, Fax: 358–81–352356.

The **VIth International Congress on Nutrition and Metabolism in Renal Disease** will be held August 26–30, 1991 in Harrogate, UK. Topics will include all aspects of nutrition and metabolism in relation to acute and chronic renal disease, with State of the Art lectures, free communications, posters and debates.

For further information, contact Dr. A. Meguid El Nahas (UK Organizing Secretary), Sheffield Kidney Institute, Northern General Hospital, Herries Road, Sheffield S5 7AU, UK. Tel.: 0742-434343 (ext 4017), Fax: 0742-560472.

The **XXVIIIth Congress of the European Dialysis and Transplant Association – European Renal Association** (EDTA/ERA) will be held in Belgrade, Yugoslavia from September 1 to 4, 1991.

For further information, contact the Organizing Secretariat: Yugotours, Congress, Incentive & Exhibition Department, Djure Djakovića 31, Y-11000 Belgrade, Yugoslavia. Tel.: 3811/763-028, 764-622; Telex: 11000, 12902; Fax: 3811/766-447.

A **Festakt in honor of Priscilla Kincaid-Smith** will be held on November 5–8th, 1991 in Melbourne, Australia. Events will include state of the art lectures and symposia.

For further information contact The Festschrift Organizing Committee, c/o Department of Nephrology, The Royal Melbourne Hospital, Victoria 3050, Australia.

The **IIIrd International Conference on SLE** will be held in the Queen Elizabeth II Conference Centre, Westminster, London, April 13–15, 1992.

For further details, please contact Dr. Graham Hughes or Mrs. Denzil Fletcher, Rheumatology Department, St. Thomas' Hospital, London SE1 7EH. Tel. and Fax: 016339422.

The **Third Symposium on Uroradiology** (Imaging and Intervention) will take place August 24–27, 1992 at Herlev Hospital, University of Copenhagen, Denmark.

For further information, please contact Dr. Henrik S. Thomsen, Department of Diagnostic Radiology 54E2, Herlev Hospital, Herlev Ringvej 75, DK-2730 Herlev, Denmark. Tel.: 4544/535300, Ext. 278; Fax: 4544/535332.

Clinical Nephrology, Vol. 35 No. 3 – 1991 (93–97)

Rheumatoid factors in patients with minimal change nephrotic syndrome

M. Endoh, M. Miyazaki, T. Suga, M. Miura, Y. Nomoto and H. Sakai

Department of Internal Medicine, School of Medicine, Tokai University, Japan

Abstract. Several immunological aberrations, especially T-cell abnormalities, have been shown to be involved in the development of the minimal change nephrotic syndrome (MCNS) although the responsible factors have not been identified. We studied rheumatoid factors (RF), thought to be a consequence of polyclonal B-cell hyperactivation, in sera from patients with MCNS using a sensitive fluorescence immunoassay (FIA). Significant increases of IgG and IgM RFs and marginal increase of IgA RF were observed during the nephrotic stages. Some patients still showed high titers of IgM RF in the early remission phases. The levels of RFs were normalized during complete remission. It was suggested that polyclonal B cell activation might be involved in the development of this disorder along with T cell abnormalities.

Key words: rheumatoid factor – MCNS – nephrotic syndrome

Introduction

The pathogenic mechanism of minimal change nephrotic syndrome (MCNS) is not understood. The negative charge barrier of the glomerular basement membrane may be impaired by some factor which may cause a massive leak of serum albumin into the urine. Some investigators recently proposed that an unknown lymphokine produced by the patient's T cells might be a factor responsible for alteration of glomerular permeability and thus a major pathogenic factor in this disease [Lagrue et al. 1975, Tomizawa et al. 1985, Heslan et al. 1986, Bakker et al. 1988, Yoshizawa et al. 1989].

Elevated levels of serum IgE have also been observed in over half of the patients with MCNS [Lagrue et al. 1984, Shu et al. 1988], which suggests involvement of hyper B cell activity as well as an allergic mechanism in the pathogenesis of this disorder [Yap et al. 1983]. In fact, increases of peripheral IgG bearing B cells [Dall'Aglio et al. 1984, Yokoyama et al. 1985] and spontaneous in vitro production of immunoglobulins [Beale et al. 1983] were reported in patients with MCNS.

We have developed a sensitive assay for three Ig class rheumatoid factors (RFs), studied the possibility of increases of RFs in sera from patients with MCNS, and evaluated their clinical significance in these patients.

Received September 11, 1990; in revised form November 20, 1990

Reprint requests to Dr. M. Endoh, Department of Internal Medicine, School of Medicine, Tokai University, Isehara, Kanagawa 259-11, Japan

Materials and methods

Patients

Twenty patients (twelve males and eight females) with minimal change nephrotic syndrome (MCNS; eight in the nephrotic state, eight in remission with steroids and four in complete remission without steroids) were studied. Mean age of the patients was 23 (16–34). Duration of the disease was one month to five years. The majority of patients was studied in the initial phase of the disease except for two in the relapse phase. All patients were diagnosed by open renal biopsy evaluated by light microscopy, electron microscopy and immunofluorescent staining. No patients with renal insufficiency were included in this study. Ten patients with rheumatoid arthritis (RA) and 30 healthy adults were studied as positive and negative controls, respectively.

Assay system

A solid-phase fluorescence immunoassay was employed to determine rheumatoid factors. Polyacrylamide beads (Immunobeads Reagent Coupling Kit, Bio-Rad Laboratories, Richmond, CA) were coupled covalently with rabbit IgG fraction (Cappel Laboratories, Cochranvielle, PA) according to the instructions. Briefly, 200 mg of polyacrylamide beads

(5–10 μm in diameter) were mixed with 10 mg of rabbit IgG and 40 mg of 1-ethyl, 3-dimethyl aminopropyl carbodiimide (EDAC) in 0.003 M phosphate buffer (pH 6.3) at 4° C overnight. These beads were then washed with phosphate buffered saline (PBS, pH 7.2) three times, followed by 1.4 M NaCl-PBS three times, and finally by PBS three times. These reagents were stored in 20 ml of 0.005 M phosphate/1% bovine serum albumin (BSA) buffer at 4° C.

These immunobead reagents were reconstituted at a concentration of 1 mg/ml in 0.1% Tween in PBS (PBS-Tween) prior to use. Duplicate samples of 1.0 ml of immunobeads and 20 μl of sera were mixed in a 17 × 100 mm plastic tube (Nissui, Tokyo) and incubated at 37° C for 2 h with occasional mixing by a vortex mixer. After incubation, each tube was centrifuged at 1,700 g for 10 min, insoluble reagents were washed three times with PBS-Tween, and then 50 μl of FITC-conjugated heavy chain specific rabbit anti-human IgG, IgA or IgM antiserum (Cappel Lab.) was added. These antisera were previously diluted five-fold with PBS, and centrifuged at 105,000 g for 30 min to remove aggregates. After incubation with antisera for 2 h at 37° C, immunobeads were washed three times with PBS-Tween. The precipitate was resuspended in 2.0 ml of PBS and the fluorescence intensity of each sample was determined by a fluorescence spectrophotometer (Hitachi MPF-4, Tokyo) using filters at an excitation wavelength of 485 nm and emission wavelength of 525 nm. The value of corrected relative fluorescence indicates the value of the sample minus that of a reagent blank. The specificity of this assay was tested by absorbing the sera from RA patients with aggregated rabbit IgG (Cappel Lab.).

Routine serological tests for rheumatoid factors such as the latex fixation test (RA test) and sensitized erythrocyte agglutination test (RAHA test) were performed in the central laboratory of our hospital.

The Mann-Whitney U-test was used for statistical analysis.

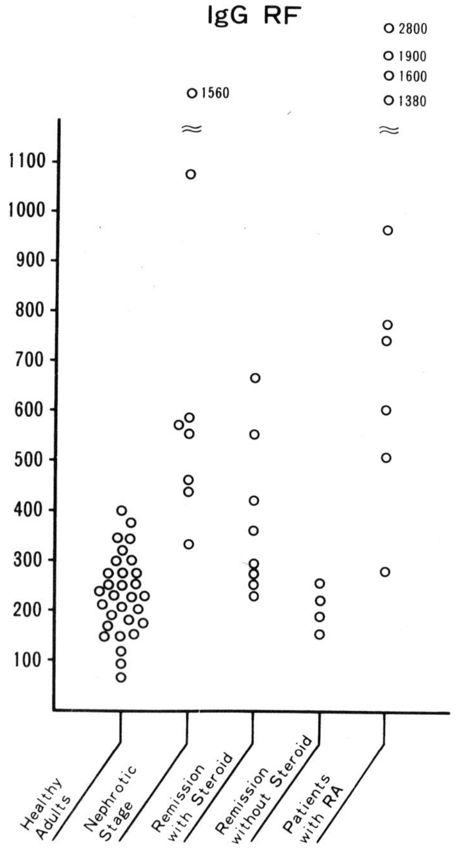

Fig. 1 IgG RF in patients with minimal change nephrotic syndrome (MCNS) and those with rheumatoid arthritis (RA). A significant increase was observed in patients with MCNS during the nephrotic stage. Patients in complete remission without steroid showed normal IgG RF levels.

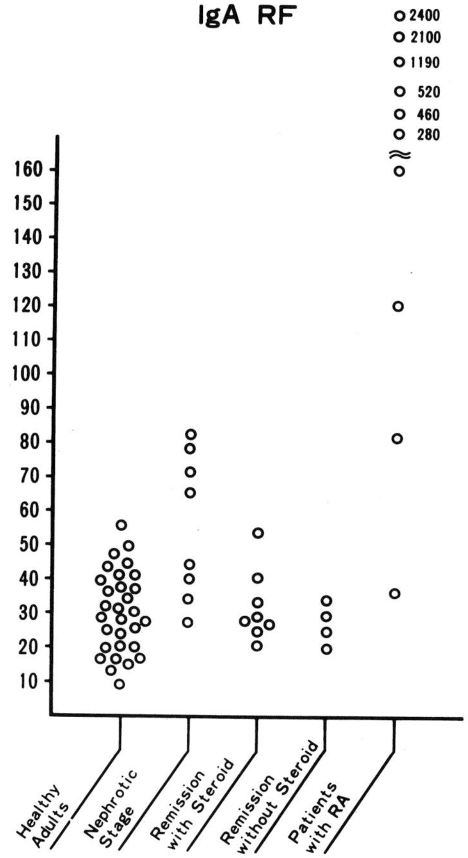

Fig. 2 IgA RF in patients with MCNS. A marginal increase was observed only in the nephrotic stage.

Results

All sera from patients with minimal change nephrotic syndrome (MCNS) were negative for the routine rheumatoid factor tests, i.e. RA test and RAHA test, whereas sera from patients with rheumatoid arthritis (RA) were strongly positive.

Serum titers of IgG, IgA and IgM rheumatoid factors (RF) are shown in Figures 1 through 3. Levels of IgG RF and IgM RF in patients with MCNS were significantly increased during the active stage (nephrotic stage). Some patients still showed high titers of IgG RF and/or IgM RF in the early phase of remission with steroid therapy. In the phase of complete remission, in which steroid was not required, all patients showed normal serum titers for the three classes of RFs. IgA RF was not increased in patients with MCNS, except for marginal increases in the nephrotic stage in some patients. No significant influence of RF titers was observed according to the duration of disease or sex. There was no significant correlation between the values of creatine clearance and the levels of RFs. Nine out of 10 patients with rheumatoid arthritis showed significant increases of all Ig class RFs in their sera, which were much greater than those in MCNS. The specificity of this assay was assured by normalization of RF titers after absorbing RA sera with aggregated rabbit IgG.

Figure 4 illustrates a typical patient with MCNS whose serum RF levels were serially studied. Both IgG and IgA RFs became normal after the administration of predonisolone in conjunction with the reduc-

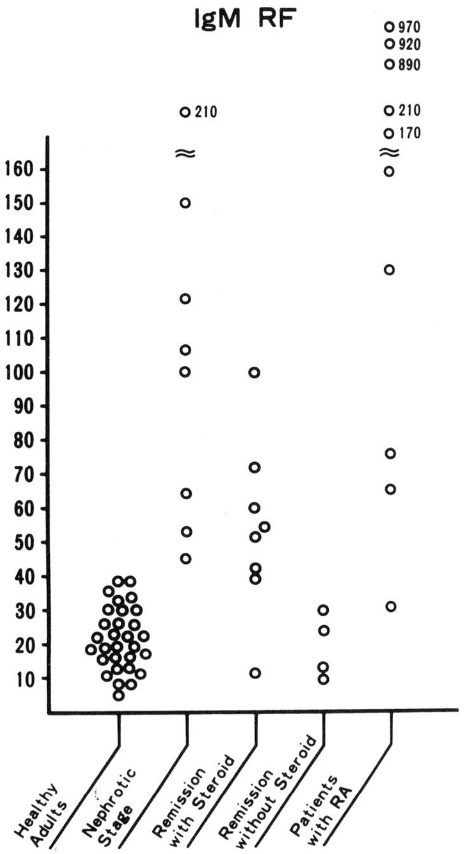

Fig. 3 IgM RF in patients with MCNS. A significant increase was observed in the nephrotic stage and in early remission with steroid therapy. Patients in complete remission without steroid showed normal IgM RF levels.

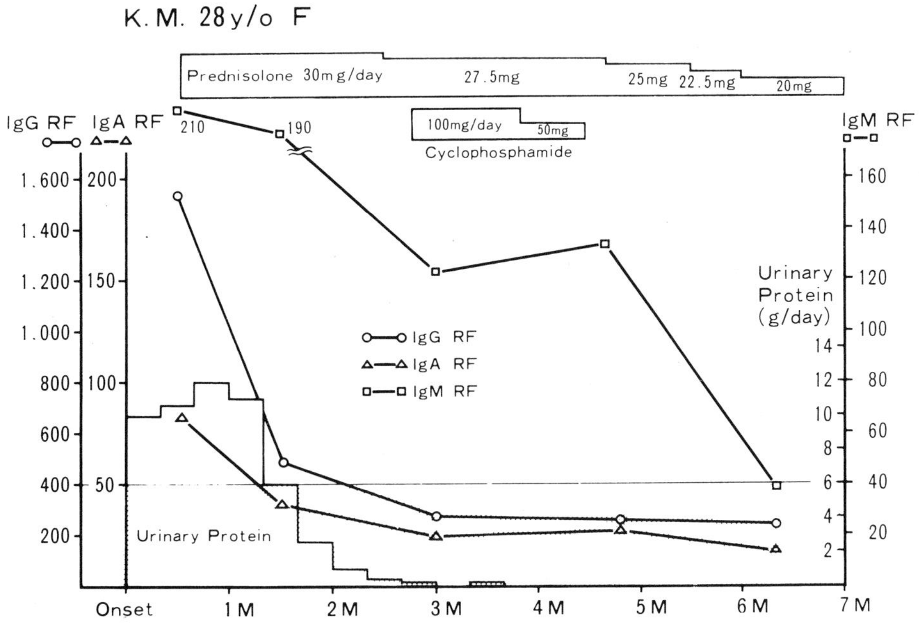

Fig. 4 Serial study of serum levels of RFs in patients with MCNS. Levels of IgM RF remained high during incomplete remission. The normal level (mean + 2 SD) of each RF is shown by the horizontal line.

tion of proteinuria. However, IgM RF was still positive during incomplete remission, i.e. while minimal levels of proteinuria were occasionally observed. After the administration of cyclophosphamide, complete remission of the nephrotic syndrome was achieved together with normalization of the serum IgM RF level.

Discussion

Immunological abnormalities have been suggested in the development of the minimal change nephrotic syndrome (MCNS) although the precise mechanism is unknown. Recent studies by Levin et al. [1985, 1989] demonstrated a charge neutralizing factor in plasma and urine from patients with MCNS. T lymphocytes might be responsible for such factors. Tomizawa et al. [1985] and Heslan et al. [1986] showed a vascular permeability factor in the culture supernatant of T lymphocytes from patients in the nephrotic stage using the skin window technique. Yoshizawa et al. [1989] also demonstrated a glomerular permeability factor in Con A stimulated culture supernatants using an in vivo technique. These observations suggested a deep involvement of T cells in this disorder. Hyporesponsiveness of peripheral blood mononuclear cells to mitogens [Schnaper and Aune 1985, Matsumoto 1989] and certain antigens in vivo [Garin and Barrett 1988] were reported, as well as impaired lymphocyte function such as natural killer activity [Dohi et al. 1988] and delayed type hypersensitivity [Matsumoto et al. 1984]. This hyporesponsiveness might be a consequence of in vivo activation of these cells since spontaneous in vitro production of vascular permeability factor [Tomizawa et al. 1985] and β2 microglobulin [Robeva et al. 1988] by peripheral blood lymphocytes was observed in active stage patients.

Occasional increase of serum IgE observed in active MCNS [Lagrue et al. 1984, Shu et al. 1988] suggested the presence of hyper-B-cell function. Dall'Aglio et al. [1984] and Yokoyama et al. [1985] reported an increase of IgG bearing B cell in peripheral blood from patients with MCNS in the nephrotic stage. Beale et al. [1983] also demonstrated that spontaneous immunoglobulin production by PBMC in vitro was significantly increased in nephrotic patients with MCNS.

We developed a sensitive assay for three Ig classes of RF, thought to be a factor reflecting polyclonal B-cell activation, using a fluorescence immunoassay (FIA). This method has the advantage of a wider measurable range with a linear standard curve than the ELISA system. We reported increases of RFs in sera from patients with various types of glomerulonephritis [Endoh et al. 1985] and its significance as a component of immune complexes, especially in patients with diffuse proliferative lupus nephritis [Miyazaki et al. 1990].

In this study, we measured RFs in sera from patients with MCNS. Increases of RFs in the nephrotic stage and normalization in complete remission were observed. In a serial study of one case, IgM RF remained at a high level even in the remission phase, and did not become normal until several weeks after remission. It was suggested B cell activation might be sustained during the early remission phase in patients with MCNS.

Immunoglobulin deposition is not seen in the glomeruli of patients with MCNS so the RFs do not have a direct pathogenic role. RFs might participate in the formation of immune complexes and influence the charge of the glomerular basement membrane without accumulation in the glomeruli. Another possible mechanism of increases of RFs is a phenomenon associated with other lymphocyte activation such as vascular permeable factor production by T cells. Prolonged high expression of IgM RF might be related to the active immunological state in vivo even in the remission stage because the majority of patients still showed high titers of IgM RF in the initial phase of remission. Therefore, this assay may be useful for monitoring the immunological activity of patients with MCNS during steroid or immunosuppressive therapy.

It is concluded that there are significant increases of RFs in patients with MCNS, and that monitoring of RFs may be useful for evaluation of disease activity and treatment of these patients.

REFERENCES

Bakker WW, van Luijk WHJ, Hene RJ, Desmit EM, van der Hem GK, Vos JTWM 1988 Loss of glomerular polyanion in vitro induced by mononuclear blood cells from patients with minimal-change nephrotic syndrome. Am J Nephrol *6:* 107–111

Beale MG, Nash GS, Bertovich MJ, MacDermott RP 1983 Immunoglobulin synthesis by peripheral blood mononuclear cells in minimal change nephrotic syndrome. Kidney Int *23:* 380–386

Dall'Aglio P, Meroni PL, Barcellini W, Brigati C, Chizzolini C, De Bartolo G, Migone L, Zanussi C 1984 Altered expression of B lymphocyte surface immunoglobulins in minimal change nephrotic syndrome and focal glomerulosclerosis. Nephron *37:* 224–228

Dohi K, Yamada H, Takai M, Fujii Y, Ishikawa H 1987 Natural killer activity and antibody-dependent cell-mediated cytotoxity in primary glomerular diseases. Clin Nephrol *2:* 11–14

Endoh M, Suga T, Sakai H 1985 IgG, IgA and IgM rheumatoid factors in patients with glomerulonephritis. Nephron *39:* 330–335

Garin EH, Barrett DJ 1988 Pneumococcal polysaccharide immunization in patients with active nephrotic syndrome. Nephron *50:* 383–388

Heslan J-M, Branellec A, Laurent J, Lagrue G 1986 The vascular permeability factor is a T lymphocyte product. Nephron *42:* 187–188

Lagrue G, Xheneumont S, Branallec A, Hirbec G, Weil BA 1975 A vascular permeability factor elaborated from lymphocytes. I. Demonstration in patients with nephrotic syndrome. Biomed. *23:* 37–40

Lagrue G, Laurent J, Hirbec G, Ansquer JC, Noirot C, Laurent G, Nebout T, Kestenbaum S 1984 Serum IgE in primary glomerular diseases. Nephron *36:* 5–9

Levin M, Smith C, Walters MPS, Gascoine P, Barratt TM 1985 Steroid-responsive nephrotic syndrome. A generalized disorder of membrane negative charge. Lancet *ii:* 239–242

Levin M, Gascoine P, Turner MW, Barratt TM 1989 A highly cationic protein in plasma and urine of children with steroid responsive nephrotic syndrome. Kidney Int. *36:* 867–877

Matsumoto K, Osakabe K, Katayama H, Okano K, Watanabe S, Hatano M 1984 Impaired delayed hypersensitivity in lipoid nephrosis. Nephron *37:* 273–275

Matsumoto K 1989 Decreased production of interleukin-1 by monocytes from patients with lipoid nephrosis. Clin Nephrol *31:* 292–296

Miyazaki M, Endoh M, Suga T, Yano N, Kuramoto T, Matsumoto Y, Eguchi K, Yagame M, Miura M, Nomoto Y, Sakai H 1990 Rheumatoid factors and glomerulonephritis. Clin exp Immunol *81:* 250–255

Robeva R, Heslan JM, Branllec A, Kaurebt J, Lagrue G 1988 Enhanced β2-microglobulin levels in lymphocyte culture supernatants from patients with idiopathic nephrotic syndrome. Inhibition of lymphocyte activation by cyclosporine. Clin Nephrol *30:* 211–215

Schnaper HW, Aune TM 1985 Identification of the lymphokine soluble immune response suppressor in urine of nephrotic children. J Clin Invest *76:* 341–349

Shu KH, Lian JD, Yang YF, Lu YS, Wang JY 1988 Serum IgE in primary glomerular disease and its clinical significance. Nephron *49:* 24–28

Tomizawa S, Maruyama K, Nagasawa N, Suzuki S, Kuroume T 1985 Studies of vascular permeability factor derived from T lymphocytes and inhibitory effect of plasma on its production in minimal change nephrotic syndrome. Nephron *41:* 157–160.

Yap HK, Yip WC, Lee BW, Ho TF, Teo J, Aw SE, Tay JS 1983 The incidence of atopy in steroid-responsive nephrotic syndrome. Clinical and immunological parameters. Ann Allergy *51:* 590–594

Yokoyama H, Kida H, Tani Y, Abe T, Tomosugi N, Koshino Y, Hattori N 1985 Immunodynamics of minimal change nephrotic syndrome in adults T and B lymphocyte subsets and serum immunoglobulin levels. Clin exp Immunol *61:* 601–607

Yoshizawa M, Kusumi Y, Matsumoto K, Oshima S, Takeuchi A, Kawamura O, Kubota T, Kondo S, Niwa H 1989 Studies of a glomerular permeability factor in patients with minimal-change nephrotic syndrome. Nephron *51:* 370–376

Intravenous immunoglobulin therapy of membranous nephropathy: efficacy and safety

R. Palla, C. Cirami, V. Panichi, A. M. Bianchi, M. Parrini and G. Grazi

2nd Medical Clinic Institute, University of Pisa, Pisa, Italy

Abstract. Preliminary results of the efficacy of high-dose intravenous human IgG in patients with biopsy-confirmed idiopathic membranous nephropathy (IMGN) were reported. Five patients with normal renal function (creatinine clearance 125.2 ± 16 ml/min/1.73 m^2 BSA) (Group A) and 4 patients with moderate renal insufficiency (creatinine clearance 65.5 ± 8.3 ml/min/1.73 m^2 BSA) (Group B) received pulse doses of IgG (0.4 g/kg BW) for 3 consecutive days; these 3-day boli were repeated 3 times at 21-day intervals; since then for a 10-month period one bolus once every 3 weeks has been administered. Five responder patients at the end of the trial received a new renal biopsy. In 4 Group A patients complete remission of proteinuria (daily proteinuria <0.2 g) was observed, whereas 1 patient showed partial remission (proteinuria 2 g/day). In Group B patients, 1 showed complete remission and 2 partial remission; in 1 patient no variation of proteinuria was noted. In responder patients clinical and biological findings of the nephrotic syndrome disappeared and a statistically significant increase of creatinine clearance was observed. In control biopsies at the end of the trial the immunofluorescence staining failed to find immunodeposits and recovery of glomerular lesions at light microscopy. In conclusion, IgG therapy seems to be of benefit to patients with IMGN but a randomized clinical trial to confirm this preliminary report is needed.

Key words: human IgG – membranous nephropathy – nephrotic syndrome therapy

Introduction

Glomerular lesions of membranous nephropathy in humans are mediated by humoral immunologic mechanisms as suggested by immunohistochemical and electron-microscope patterns [Zollinger and Mihatsch 1978].

These peculiar immunopathologic findings may be explained by: 1) glomerular deposition of circulating immune complexes composed of low-affinity antibody and an oligovalent exogenous or endogenous antigen [Germuth et al. 1979]; 2) in situ subepithelial immune complex formation with glomerular antigens [Couser and Salant 1980]; 3) glomerular assembly of immune complexes for the reaction of antibodies to an antigen or antigens which have been "planted" in subepithelial space by virtue of biochemical or electrostatic affinity for certain glomerular components [Adler et al. 1983]. These subepithelial immune complex deposits induce a marked increase in glomerular capillary permeability by activating the complement system. Experimentally, C5b-9 membrane attack complex seems to be essential to induce proteinuria [Couser et al. 1985, Adler et al. 1984].

According to the pathogenetic mechanisms, several lines of therapeutic intervention have been suggested: immunosuppressive drug therapy and steroids may affect antibody synthesis and deposition [Ponticelli et al. 1989].

Cyclosporin A has recently been proposed for membranous nephropathy treatment [De Santo et al. 1987]. Finally the use of polycations may have therapeutic rationale, but results are reported only in animals [Adler et al. 1983, Adler et al. 1985]. Monoclonal antibody or chimeric toxins may represent other therapeutic lines to block autoimmunity selectively, especially in animals. These new high technological approaches seem to mark the way in the near future in the treatment of glomerulopathy in man [Strom and Kelley 1989].

Intravenous infusions of immunoglobulin (IVGG) were first reported to increase the platelet count in patients with idiopathic thrombocytopenic purpura, a well defined autoimmune disease [Imbach et al. 1981].

In other autoimmune diseases such as immune neutropenia [Pollach et al. 1982], myasthenia gravis [Gajdos et al. 1984], Kawasaki disease [Funusho et al. 1984], pure antibody mediated red-cell aplasia

Received February 27, 1990; in revised form July 3, 1990.

Reprint request to Dr. C. Cirami, Istituto Clinica Medica II, Università di Pisa, Via Roma 67, 56100 Pisa, Italy.

Table 1 Demographic and clinical data of patients.

Name	Sex/Age	Group	CCr	Cr	UPE	NSA	R	RB
CL	F/27	A	109	61.9	4	8	Y	Y
MG	F/49	A	99	53	4.2	8	Y	Y
BA	M/20	A	179	97.2	6.8	59	Y	Y
VL	M/45	A	109	88.4	10.2	6	Y	Y
BA	M/25	A	130	97.2	11.5	7	Y	N
RG	M/44	B	76	106.1	9.9	12	Y	N
CA	M/60	B	79	114.9	4	12	Y	Y
NM	M/65	B	61	114.9	4.8	7	N	N
TG	F/54	B	54	114.9	8	10	Y	N

CCr = Creatinine clearance (ml/min/1.73 m^2 BSA); Cr = plasma creatinine (μmol/l); UPE = urinary protein excretion (g/day); NSA = nephrotic syndrome age (months); R = responder patients; RB = rebiopsied patients.

Table 2 Histological stage (HS) and tubular-interstitial infiltrate (TII) in renal specimens of complete remission (CR), partial remission (PR) and non-responder (NR) patients.

Name	Group	HS	TII	AT
CL	A	II	–	CR
MG	A	II	–	CR
BA	A	II	–	CR
VL	A	III	+–	CR
BA	A	II	–	PR
RG	B	II	–	PR
CA	B	III	–	CR
NM	B	III	++	NR
TG	B	II	–	PR

– = no TII; +– = one TII in all renal specimens; ++ = four or more TII areas in all renal specimens. AT = after therapy.

[McGuire et al. 1987], anti-idiotypic autoantibodies production [Sultan et al. 1984], IVGG has been used as an immunomodulator. In this paper we report our preliminary results in patients with idiopathic membranous nephropathy treated with intravenous high dose human gamma-globulins.

Methods

Patients

We studied 9 patients with a biopsy-established diagnosis of membranous nephropathy and nephrotic syndrome. All secondary causes of MN after complete clinical and biological screening were excluded. In particular, we carefully searched for S. L. E., diabetes mellitus, amyloid, drug addiction or chronic hepatitis.

Biopsy renal specimens were processed for immunofluorescence and light microscopy as described by Zollinger [Zollinger and Mihatsch 1978].

In vitro other serial 4 μm cryostat sections of the same renal specimens were incubated for 4 hours at 37° C with human IgG solution (6 mg/ml) (the same used for IgG infusion) prior to FITC antisera staining procedure [Cirami et al. 1989]. To detect IgG and C3c deposits on glomerular structures, fluorescein-conjugated anti-human IgG (IgG/F[ab]2-fragment) and anti-human C3c antibodies from rabbits (Behringwerke AG, Marburg, Germany) were used.

At the end of the study period five patients were rebiopsied to control the glomerular pattern of deposits.

Group A

In this group there were 5 patients (3 males, 2 females; mean age 33.2, range 20–49 years) with normal renal function (mean creatinine clearance 125.2 ± 16 ml/min/1.73 m^2). The nephrotic syndrome had been present for 17.6 ± 10 months. Daily protein urinary excretion was 7.2 ± 1.7 g. One patient was treated with methylprednisone (1 mg/day for 3 months, then tapered in the next month) and cyclophosphamide (2 mg/kg/day for 6 months) 12 months prior to our trial.

Histological glomerular patterns revealed: stage 2 in 4 patients and stage 3 in 1 patient and a slight tubular-interstitial infiltrate in one patient (Table 2).

Group B

This group consisted of 4 patients (3 males, 1 female; mean age 55.7, range 44–65 years) with moderate renal insufficiency (mean creatinine clearance 65.5 ± 8.8 ml/min/1.73 m^2). The nephrotic syndrome had been present for 10.2 ± 1.1 months. Daily proteinuria was 6.4 ± 2 g. None of them had steroid or cytostatic treatment.

Histological glomerular features showed: stage 2 in 2 patients and stage 3 in the other 2 patients; a heavy and important (more than 4-area) tubular-interstitial infiltrate was observed (Table 2).

All patients received a diet with 2 g of Na and 1 g of total protein per kg body wt per day.

In Table 1 the summary of demographic and clinical data of patients is reported.

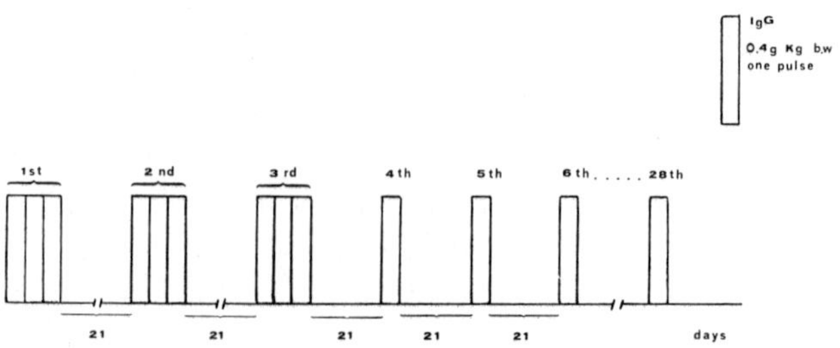

Fig. 1 Schematic outline of IgG infusion.

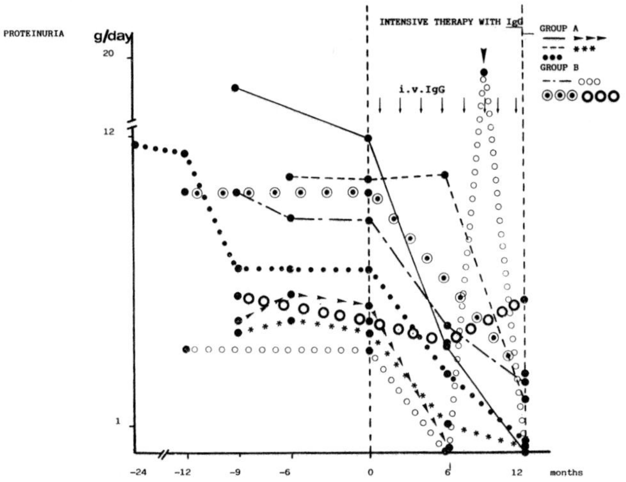

Fig. 2 Time course of daily proteinuria of every patient before and during therapy.

Patient assessment

The following parameters were evaluated every month: creatinine clearance, daily proteinuria, serum albumin, total protein and electrophoretic pattern, plasma cholesterol, triglycerides and fibrinogen, plasma immunoglobulins, complement factors level and function, circulating immunocomplexes (CIC).

Laboratory: plasma and urine creatinine were evaluated by autoanalyzer; proteinuria was assessed by Red-Ponceau colorimetric method; total protein by biuret method and serum albumin by electrophoresis; immunoglobulins, C3c and C4 were assessed by laser-nephelometry; C3a-desarg and C5a-desarg by RIA (Upjohn); CH50 by hemolytic method.

CIC were detected by ELISA-C1q and Conglutinin solid phase (Immunomedics).

Definitions: we arbitrarily defined the criteria of outcome as follows: 1) partial remission (daily proteinuria >0.2 to 3.5 g), 2) complete remission (daily proteinuria <0.2 g) (1 + 2 = responders).

Statistics: paired Student's t-test was applied to evaluate statistical differences between baseline and values during and at the end of treatment; results are expressed as ± standard error of mean (SEM).

Treatment

For 6 months prior to treatment, all patients received diuretics and human albumin as required to control the nephrotic syndrome; afterwards they received pulse doses of IgG (0.4 g/kg body wt) for three consecutive days; this three-day dose was repeated three times at 21-day intervals (intensive cycle). Since then, for a ten-month period one pulse once every three weeks was administered (Figure 1). In 3 patients, between the third and sixth month of therapy, the pulses were repeated every two weeks to maintain plasma IgG about 800 mg/dl. We used human IgG obtained from Cohn F II, PEG treated and IgA selectively eliminated by ion-exchange chromatography (Endobulin-Immuno AG, Wien).

Table 3 Patient data before (BE) and after (AF) therapy

Group	CCr (B = BE)	CCr (A = AF)	Cr (B = BE)	Cr (A = AF)	UPE (B = BE)	UPE (A = AF)
A	125 ± 16	160 ± 14	79.5 ± 9	70.7 ± 8	7.5 ± 3.5	0.7 ± 0.9
	p <0.05		n.s.		p <0.001	
B	65 ± 15	83 ± 29	113 ± 2	117 ± 15	6.2 ± 3.5	2.8 ± 2.8
	n.s.		n.s.		p <0.05	

SA(B)	SA(A = AF)	PT(B = BE)	PT(A = AF)	PC(B = BE)	PC(A = AF)	PF(B = BE)	PF(A = AF)
3.1 ± 0.4	4 ± 0.24	170 ± 44	146 ± 29	284 ± 77	209 ± 37	404 ± 80	312 ± 54
p <0.001		n.s.		p <0.01		p <0.01	
2.8 ± 0.2	3.2 ± 0.3	193 ± 36	218 ± 34	342 ± 78	285 ± 61	435 ± 59	362 ± 48
p <0.01		n.s.		p <0.01		p<0.01	

CCr = Creatinine clearance (ml/min/1.73 m^2 BSA); Cr = plasma creatinine (μmol/l); UPE = urinary protein excretion g/day; S = serum albumin (g/dl); PT = plasma triglycerides (mg/dl); PC = plasma cholesterol (mg/dl); PF = plasma fibrinogen (mg/dl).

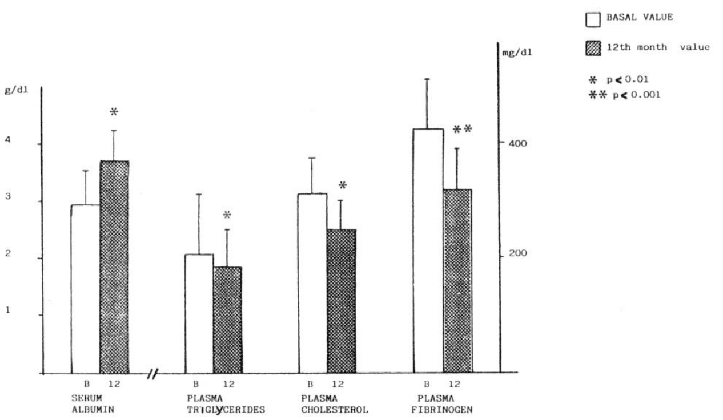

Fig. 3 Serum indices of nephrotic syndrome.

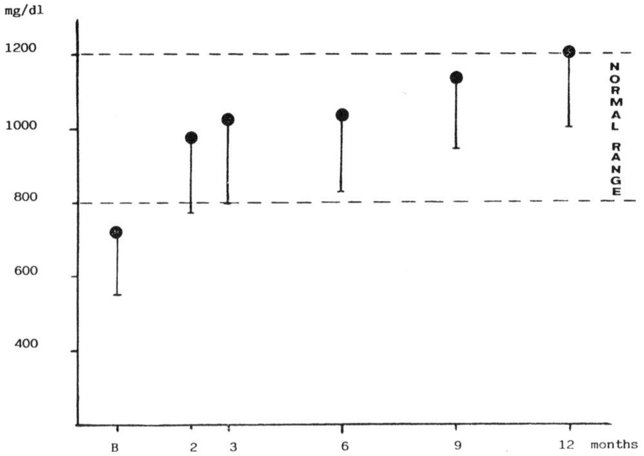

Fig. 4 IgG plasma level during treatment.

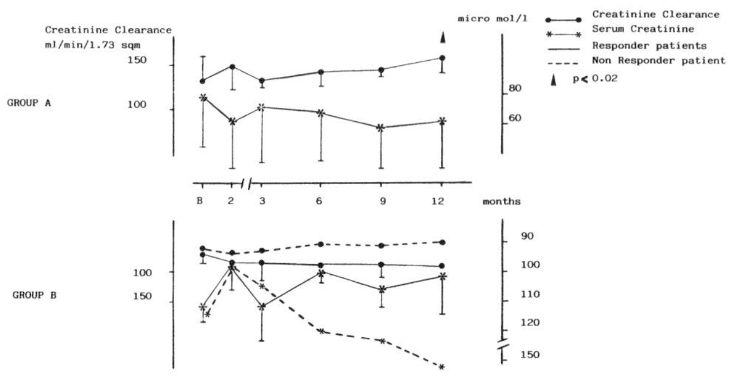

Fig. 5 Renal function in Group A and Group B patients.

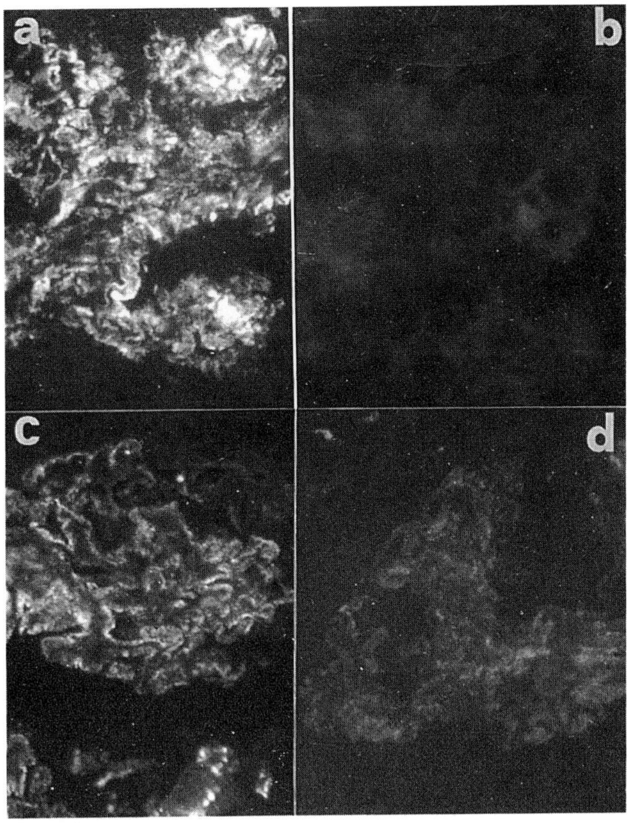

Fig. 6 Disappearance of immune deposits at glomerular level after in vitro incubation with IgG solution [FITC conjugated anti-human IgG before (a) and (b), C3c before (c) and after (d) incubation].

Results

In Group A patients, 4 patients showed complete remission of proteinuria, 1 showed partial remission (mean daily proteinuria 2 g versus 10 g prior treatment) (Figure 2 and Table 3). The reduction of proteinuria was observed after variable time since the beginning of therapy. Proteinuria decreased to a non-nephrotic range after 3 months in 3 patients and after 6 months in others. Then in the complete remission group patients in the following 2–3 months proteinuria progressively decreased until disappearance. Complete remission group patients included a patient who had received in the past treatment with steroids and cyclophosphamide.

In Group B patients, 1 patient had complete remission, 2 had partial remission, 1 did not respond to therapy (Figure 2 and Table 3). After nine months of treatment the Group B patient in complete remission showed a relapse of the nephrotic syndrome (daily proteinuria: 17 g). He received a new intensive cycle of therapy as at the beginning of the trial and after two months the patient was again in complete remission. In this last group proteinuria decrement began during the 3 to 6-month period of therapy; then it progressively decreased to a non-nephrotic range or it disappeared.

In Group A patients serum albumin increased from 3.1 ± 0.4 g/dl to 4 ± 0.24 g/dl (p <0.001), plasma fibrinogen decreased from 404 ± 80 mg/dl to 312 ± 54 mg/dl (p <0.01), plasma cholesterol from 284 ± 77 mg/dl to 209 ± 37 mg/dl (p <0.01) and trigylcerides from 170 ± 44 mg/dl to 146 ± 29 mg/dl.

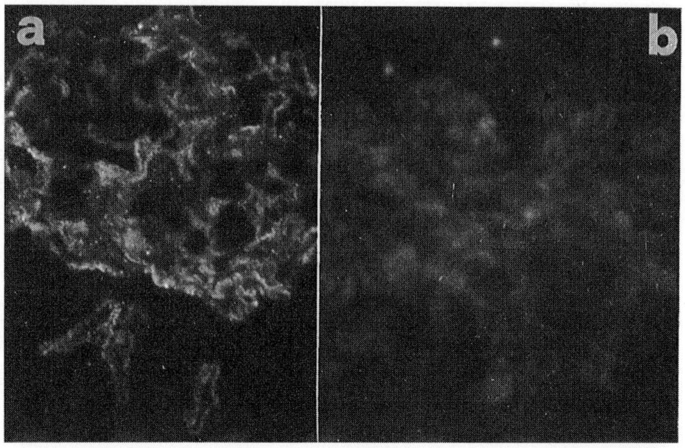

Fig. 7 Disappearance of IgG deposits at glomerular level in the rebiopsy of complete remission patient. FITC conjugated anti-human IgG before (a) and after (b) treatment.

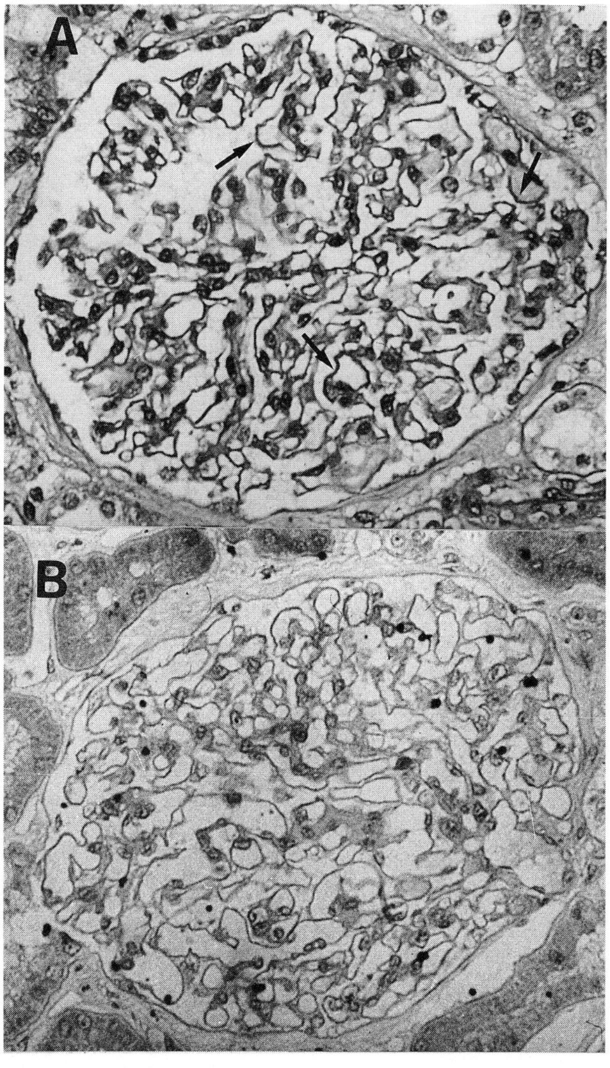

Fig. 8 Silver Methenamine staining of renal specimens. In basal biopsy (A) a typical basal membrane thickening is evident (stage II) (arrows). In rebiopsy (B) of the same patient (performed after complete remission of proteinuria) basal membrane appears normal.

IgG augmented from 568 ± 188 mg/dl to 1,235 ± 157.5 mg/dl.

In Group B patients serum albumin increased from 2.8 ± 0.2 g/dl to 3.2 ± 0.3 g/dl ($p < 0.01$) and plasma IgG from 930 ± 236 mg/dl to 1,241 ± 271 mg/dl, plasma fibrinogen diminished from 435 ± 59 mg/dl to 362 ± 48 mg/dl ($p < 0.01$), cholesterol from 342 ± 78 mg/dl to 285 ± 61 mg/dl ($p < 0.01$); triglycerides changed from 193 ± 36 mg/dl to 218 ± 34 mg/dl.

In summary in responder patient's serum albumin rose stepwise from 2.93 ± 0.21 to 3.69 ± 0.21 g/dl ($p < 0.01$); plasma fibrinogen decreased from 423 ± 30 to 320 ± 25 mg/dl ($p < 0.001$).

Plasma cholesterol decreased from 321 ± 39 to 253 ± 35 mg/dl ($p < 0.01$) and triglycerides from 209 ± 41.7 to 184 ± 24.6 mg/dl ($p < 0.01$) (Figure 3).

IgG increased from 729 ± 138 to 1020 ± 132 mg/dl during the first semester of treatment, then remained in the normal range (Figure 4); IgA and IgM remained unchanged for the whole period of treatment time. Complement factors C3c, C4, CH50 and C3a, C5a remained in the normal range during the trial.

No variation of serum albumin (from 2.76 g/dl to 2.78 g/dl), fibrinogen (from 380 mg/dl to 400 mg/dl) or triglycerides (from 125 mg/dl to 127 mg/dl) in non-responder patient was observed. However we noted a slight decline of cholesterol from 223 mg/dl to 158 mg/dl.

Creatinine clearance in Group A patients increased from 125 ± 16 to 160 ± 14 ml/min/1.73 m^2 ($p < 0.05$) (Table 3); in Group B responder patients increased from 65 ± 8.3 to 83 ± 16 ml/min/1.73 m^2; in the non-responder patient creatinine clearance decreased from 61 to 53 ml/min/1.73 m^2 (Figure 5).

CIC were detected only in one Group A patient, but after 2 months of therapy were undetectable.

The study of in vitro solubilization of IgG and C3c glomerular deposits showed disappearance in all patients but one (the same clinically non-responder patient) (Figure 6). At the rebiopsy of responder patients we observed at immunofluorescence staining no depositions of IgG and C3c in all cases (Figure 7), whereas light microscopy showed regression from stage II to stage I in two patients and complete histological pattern resolution but some sclerotic glomeruli in others (Figure 8).

Discussion

Membranous nephropathy is characterized by dense deposits in the subepithelial space representing antigen antibody complexes. Based on an immunologic pathogenesis, many attempts have been made with steroids alone [Cattran et al. 1989] or in combination with alkylating agents to treat this glomerular disease. In evaluating the results of therapy there are two major problems:

1. It is not possible to predict the natural history of this disease accurately because the outcome of idiopathic MGN is variable: spontaneous remission occurs in some patients.

2. The response to therapy is slow: the renal function may remain unmodified for years despite persistent proteinuria. In a percentage of patients (about 20%) [Donadio et al. 1988] there is a rapid evolution to end stage renal failure, when proteinuria is very heavy. Bearing in mind these limitations, our preliminary and uncontrolled results may open up new horizons in the treatment of MGN. In fact, with high dose IgG we obtained 4 total remissions and 1 partial remission in Group A patients and 1 total remission and 2 partial remissions in Group B patients; the non-responder patient had the worse renal function (creatinine clearance 61 ml/min/ 1.73 m^2 BSA). This high therapeutic success seems to indicate not a chance result but a real impact on the management of glomerular derangement. To support this view there are the results obtained with repeated biopsies of responder patients and in vitro studies of the immunofluorescence pattern of renal tissue before and after incubation with high dose IgG.

In all responder patients the creatinine clearance increased stepwise during treatment and at the end of the trial was increased by 28% in group A and by 31% in Group B; in the non-responder patient the creatinine clearance declined from 61 to 53 ml/min (–13%) in the year of observation. These results are well compatible with complete control of the nephrotic syndrome and with the recovery of glomerular lesions.

The side effects of IgG infusion were of minor significance and only after the first dose: asthenia in 3 patients, fever inferior to 38° C in 4 patients, lethargy in 1 and headache in 1. These side effects are prevented by a very slow infusion of IgG (more than 3 h). All patients invariably refer to well-being during the trial. On the contrary, the drug regimens designed for MGN treatment are very dangerous: diabetes mellitus, hypertension and osteoporosis are the main side effects of steroids; the inhibition of spermatogenesis, myelosuppression and cancerogenesis those of alkylating agents.

The mechanisms of the action of IgG in the treatment of MGN are speculative: they could dissociate the IC deposed at the glomerular level. To support this hypothesis we found a complete solubilization of immune deposits in vitro after incubation of renal biopsy specimen with high-dose IgG-containing Fc fragment (an effect not obtained with low-dose IgG).

We observed that the effects on proteinuria and other markers of the nephrotic syndrome were obtained when the plasma levels of IgG were maintained in a normal range for a 3/6-month period. These observations may also indicate an inhibition of anti-idiotypic antibody activity in vivo, as described in vitro [Abdou et al. 1981]. Finally, IgG may block macrophage and B-cell Fc receptors inhibiting the anti-idiotypic antibody synthesis from B-lymphocytes [Durandy et al. 1981].

These preliminary results prompt us to begin a controlled randomized clinical trial to confirm the effectiveness of IgG in treating IMGN.

Acknowledgements

The authors wish to thank Mrs Martha M. Eibl, professor of Immunology of the University of Wien, for her main advice and for the revision of this paper. We also thank Miss Maria Elisa Mariani for her valuable collaboration and Mr Leonardo Casarosa for technical assistance.

REFERENCES

Abdou JL, Wall H, Lindsey HD, Halsey JF, Suzuki T 1981 Network theory on autoimmunity. In vitro suppression of serum anti-DNA antibody binding to DNA by anti-idiotypic antibody in systemic Lupus Erythematosus. J Clin Invest *67:* 1297–1304

Adler S, Baker P, Pritzl P, Couser WG 1985 Effect of alterations in glomerular charge on deposition of cationic and anionic antibodies to fixed glomerular antigens in the rats. J Lab Clin Med *106:* 1–11

Adler SG, Baker PJ, Pritzl PM, Couser WG 1984 Presence of terminal complement components in complement-dependent experimental glomerulonephritis. Kidney Int *26:* 830–837

Adler SG, Wang H, Ward HJ, Cohen AH, Border WA 1983 Electrical charge. Its role in the pathogenesis and prevention of experimental membranous nephropathy in the rabbit. J Clin Invest *71:* 487–499

Cattran DC, Delmore T, Roscoe J, Cole E, Cardella C, Charron R, Ritchie S 1989 A randomized controlled trial of prednisone in patients with idiopathic membranous nephropathy. N Eng J Med *320:* 210–215

Cirami C, Casarosa L, Panichi V, Bianchi AM, Parrini M, Grazi G, Baronti A, Cominotto R, Palla R 1989 In vitro solubilization of glomerular IgG, IgA and C3 deposits after incubation with high concentration human IgG solution. Kidney Int *35:* 755

Couser WG, Baker PJ, Adler S 1985 Complement and the direct mediation of immune glomerular injury: a new perspective. Kidney Int *28:* 879–890

Couser WG, Salant DJ 1980 In-situ immune complex formation and glomerular injury. Kidney Int *17:* 1–5

DeSanto NG, Capodicasa G, Giordano C 1987 Treatment of idiopathic membranous nephropathy unresponsive to methylprednisolone and chlorambucin with cyclosporin. Am J Nephrol *7:* 74–76

Donadio JV Jr., Torres VE, Velosa JA, Wagoner RD, Holley KE, Okamura M, Ilstrup DM, Chu CP 1988 Idiopathic membranous nephropathy: the natural history of untreated patients. Kidney Int *33:* 708–715

Durandy A, Fischer A, Griscelli C 1981 Dysfunction of pokeweed mitogen-stimulated T and B lymphocyte responses induced by gamma-globulin therapy. J Clin Invest *67:* 867–877

Furusho K, Nakano H, Kamiya T 1984 High-dose intravenous gammaglobulin for Kawasaki disease. Lancet *II:* 1055–1058

Gajdos PH, Outin H, Elkharrat D, Bruneld O, Rohan-Chabot P, Raphael JC, Goulon M, Goulon-Goeau C, Morell E 1984 High-dose intravenous gammaglobulin for myasthenia gravis. Lancet *I:* 406

Germuth FG Jr, Rodriguez E, Korelle CA 1979 Passive immune complex glomerulonephritis in mice: models for various lesions found in human disease. II. Low avidity complexes and diffuse proliferative glomerulonephrithis with subepithelial deposits. Lab Invest *41:* 366–371

Imbach P, D'Apuzzo V, Irth A 1981 High-dose intravenous gammaglobulin for idiopathic thrombocytopenic purpura in childhood. Lancet *I:* 1228

McGuire WA, Yang HH, Bruno E, Brandt J, Briddell R, Coates TD, Hoffman R 1987 Treatment of antibody-mediated pure red-cell aplasia with high-dose intravenous gamma-globulin. N Eng J Med *317:* 1004–1008

Pollach S, Cunningham-Rundles C, Smithwich EM, Barandun S, Good RA 1982 High-dose intravenous gammaglobulin for auto-immune neutropenia. N Eng J Med *307:* 253–255

Ponticelli C, Zucchelli P, Passerini P, Cagnoli L, Cesano B, Pozzi C, Pasquali S, Imbasciati E, Grassi C, Radaelli B, Sasdelli M, Locatelli F 1989 A randomized trial of methylprednisolone and chlorambucil in idiopathic membranous nephropathy. N Eng J Med *320:* 8–13

Strom TB, Kelley VE 1989 Toward more selective therapies to block undesired immune responses. Kidney Int *35:* 1026–1033

Sultan Y, Maisonneuve P, Kazatchkine MD, Nydegger UE 1984 Anti-idiotypic suppression of autoantibodies to Factor VIII (anti-haemophilic factor) by high-dose intravenous gammaglobulin. Lancet *II:* 765–768

Zollinger HU, Mihatsch MJ 1978 Renal Pathology in Biopsy, pp. 252–281, Springer-Verlag, Berlin – Heidelberg – New York

Clinical Nephrology, Vol. 35 No. 3 – 1991 (105–109)

Acute tubulointerstitial nephritis associated with Yersinia pseudotuberculosis infection

K. Okada[1], I. Yano[2], S. Kagami[1], M. Funai[1], S. Kawahito[3], T. Okamoto[3], A. Imagawa[3], and Y. Kuroda[1]

[1] *Department of Pediatrics, School of Medicine, University of Tokushima, Kuramoto-cho 3-chome Tokushima 770, Japan*
[2] *Department of Pediatrics, Ritsurin Social Insurance Hospital, Ritsurin-cho 3-chome Takamatsu 760, Japan*
[3] *Department of Pediatrics and Urology, Takamatsu Red Cross Hospital, Ban-cho 4-chome Takamatsu 760, Japan*

Abstract. Two siblings infected with Yersinia pseudotuberculosis suffered from acute renal failure about 2 weeks after the onset of the disease. Renal histology in both siblings showed acute tubulointerstitial nephritis. Yersinia pseudotuberculosis type VB was isolated from feces of one of them, antibodies to Yersinia pseudotuberculosis type VB in their sera were elevated. The results of the present study suggest that acute renal failure complicating infections with Yersinia pseudotuberculosis is due to acute tubulointerstitial nephritis.

Key words: acute renal failure – tubulointerstitial nephritis – Yersinia pseudotuberculosis

Introduction

Infections with Yersinia pseudotuberculosis (Y. pst.) and Yersinia enterocolitica (Y. ent.) have been recognized in a worldwide distribution [Anonymous 1984]. Clinical features of yersinosis are fever, abdominal pain, diarrhea, arthritis and erythema nodosum [Ahvohnen 1972]. Renal complications which have been reported are acute glomerulonephritis in infections with Y. ent. [Leino and Kalliomäki 1974, Forsström et al. 1977, Friedberg et al. 1978, 1981, Denneberg et al. 1981] and acute renal failure (ARF) following Y. pst. septicemia in adults [Davenport et al. 1987]. However, there is little information about ARF following Y. pst. infection in childhood.

In this study, we report two siblings with ARF due to acute tubulointerstitial nephritis (TIN) in Y. pst. infection.

Reports

Case 1

On 4 April 1986, a nine-year-old Japanese girl was admitted to Takamatsu Red Cross Hospital because of persistent fever, sore throat and diarrhea. She had had high fever and facial exanthema and had been diagnosed as having exanthema infectiosum on 28 March 1986. There were no particular findings in her family history. She had been drinking well water.

On admission, her weight was 36 kg, height 140 cm, body temperature 39.2° C, blood pressure 100/60 mmHg and her pulse was 136/min and regular. Her throat was infected and tonsils were swollen. Conjunctivae palpaebrae were not anemic nor hyperemic. No abnormalities were found in the chest nor abdomen.

Laboratory findings are shown in Table 1. Mild leukocytosis was seen in the peripheral blood and erythrocyte sedimentation rate increased to 60 mm per hour. C reactive protein (CRP) was strongly positive and serum IgM was increased to 348 mg/dl. Titer of antistreptolysin O (ASO) and serum complement level was normal. Blood urea nitrogen (BUN) was 12.9 mg/dl, and serum creatinine was 0.7 mg/dl. Urinalysis showed mild proteinuria and 10 leucocytes per high-power field. No pathogenic organisms were isolated from throat culture.

She was intravenously administered a dosage of 60 mg/kg of Latamoxef sodium, but diarrhea persisted and small amounts of bloody stool were occasionally seen. On April 8, fever decreased but she felt general malaise with a decrease of urinary volume on the next day. On April 10, she became oliguric although she was receiving rehydration therapy and

Received April 4, 1990; in revised form November 26, 1990.

Table 1 Laboratory findings of case 1 on admission

ESR	60 mm/h	GOT	26 IU/l
		GPT	16 IU/l
Peripheral blood		BUN	12.9 mg/dl
WBC	10800/mm^3	s-Cr	0.7 mg/dl
RBC	407×10^4/mm^3	C_3	104 mg/dl
Hb.	11.3 g/dl	C_4	60 mg/dl
Ht.	33.7%	CH-50	43.2 U/ml
Plat.	29.2×10^4/mm^3	IgG	1200 mg/dl
WBC classification		IgA	198 mg/dl
st.	3.0%	IgM	348 mg/dl
seg.	74.0%	Urinalysis	
lymph.	22.0%	Protein	(+)
mono.	0.5%	Glucose	(−)
baso.	0.5%	Sediments	RBC 1/hpf
CRP	6+		WBC 10/hpf
ASO	<100 T. U.		Casts (−)

Table 2 Laboratory findings of case 2 on admission

ESR	62 mm/h	GOT	37 IU/l
		GPT	27 IU/l
Peripheral blood		BUN	8.6 mg/dl
WBC	13100/mm^3	s-Cr	0.6 mg/dl
RBC	406×10^4/mm^3		
Hb.	11.6 g/dl	C_3	100 mg/dl
Ht.	35.1%	C_4	48 mg/dl
Plat.	35.0×10^4/mm^3	CH-50	42.6 IU/ml
WBC classification			
st.	1.5%	IgG	1320 mg/dl
seg.	73.0%	IgA	166 mg/dl
lymph.	22.5%	IgM	372 mg/dl
mono.	2.5%		
baso.	0.5%	Urinalysis	
CRP	5+	Protein	(2+)
ASO	<100 T. U.	Glucose	(−)
Na	131 mEq/l	Sediments	RBC 10/hpf
K	3.7 mEq/l		WBC 15/hpf
C1	101 mEq/l		Casts (+)

diuretics. On April 11, BUN was 113.5 mg/dl, serum creatinine was 10.3 mg/dl, and urinalysis showed glucosuria, hematuria and cylinduria in addition to proteinuria and leucocyturia. No bacteria were seen in the urine or isolated from the urine culture. As shown in Table 3, urinary sodium concentration was 72 mEq/l and fractional excretion of sodium [FENa] was 30.3%, the urine to plasma creatinine ratio was 2.0, and the urine to plasma osmolality ratio was 1.0. These results indicated ARF due to renal parenchymal damage. Renal needle biopsy was carried out and peritoneal dialysis began on April 11. Serum creatinine and BUN gradually decreased followed by increase in volume of urine with improvement of her clinical state. The indices of renal function were also improved by April 19, in association with an improvement of the urinary findings (Table 3). On April 24, renal function was completely restored to normal; BUN 14.9 mg/dl, serum creatinine 0.7 mg/dl, creatinine clearance 100 ml/min. Peritoneal dialysis was stopped and she was discharged on May 2 and thereafter she has been followed as an outpatient. She has been well, and renal function and urinary findings have stayed normal. Hypertension or edema was not seen throughout the period of the disease.

No pathogenic organisms were isolated from the culture of feces. Serum titer of antibody to Y. pst. type VB, measured by hemoagglutination test, was ×160 on April 11 and elevated to ×1280 on April 22, which indicated that the disease was due to Y. pst. infection.

Case 2

The patient was seven years old, a younger sister of the patient in case 1. On 28 March 1986, she had fever and exanthema in her face, and she was diagnosed a having erythema infectiosum. On April 3, abdominal pain and diarrhea appeared with persistent fever. She was admitted to Takamatsu Red Cross Hospital with the diagnosis of acute enterocolitis. She had been drinking well water.

On admission, her weight was 28 kg, height 125 cm, body temperature 39.6° C, blood pressure 96/50 mmHg and her pulse was 120/min and regular. Conjunctivae palpaebrae were not anemic nor hyperemic. Her throat was not infected and no abnormal findings were found in the chest. She had tenderness without muscular defense in the right lower quadrant of the abdomen but hepatosplenomegaly was not found.

Laboratory findings (Table 2): Erythrocyte sedimentation rate increased to 62 mm per hour and leucocytosis (13100/mm^3) was seen in the peripheral blood. The cell counts of erythrocytes and platelets were normal. CRP was strongly positive and serum IgM was increased to 372 mg/dl. The titer of ASO and serum complement level were normal. Serum creatinine was 0.6 mg/dl and BUN was 8.6 mg/dl. Urinalysis showed proteinuria (2+), microhematuria (10 erythrocytes per high-power field) and leukocyturia (15 per high-power field) with urinary casts. Glucosuria was not seen.

She was administered Fosfomycin in a dosage of 70 mg/kg/day. Fever had decreased to normal by April 8 but diarrhea with abdominal pain and vomiting persisted. Then, the volume of urine decreased to an oliguric level. On April 11, serum creatinine was

Table 3 Indices of renal function

	Case 1		Case 2	
	Oliguric (4/11)	Recovering (4/19)	Oliguric (4/11)	Recovering (4/11)
BUN (mg/dl)	113.5	12.5	87.0	17.1
s-Cr (mg/dl)	10.3	0.6	8.2	0.7
UNa (mEq/l)	72	5	105	4
U/P-Cr	2.0	46.8	2.0	35.0
U/P-Osm	1.0	1.5	1.0	1.8
UOsm (mOsm/l)	289	442	293	548
FENa (%)	30.3	0.1	39.5	0.1

U/P-Osm = ratio of urinary to plasma osmotic pressure

8.2 mg/dl and BUN was 87.0 mg/dl despite management with rehydration and use of diuretics. Urinalysis showed glucosuria. leucocyturia and cylinduria. Urinary sodium concentration and FENa were high and urinary to serum creatinine ratio and ratio of urinary to plasma osmotic pressure were low as shown in Table 3, which indicated ARF due ro renal tubular damage. She received a needle renal biopsy and therapy by peritoneal dialysis. Serum creatinine and BUN were decreased and her clinical state improved.

Urinary volume increased and the indices of renal function were improved by April 19. On April 24, peritoneal dialysis was stopped because renal function was almost restored to normal: BUN 16.8 mg/dl, serum creatinine 0.6 mg/dl, creatinine clearance 79 ml/min. She was discharged on May 2 because urinary findings had recovered to normal and thereafter she has been well.

Y. pst. serotype VB was isolated from the culture of her feces. The titers of antibody against Y. pst. type VB were elevated to ×160 on April 11 and ×1280 on April 22.

Renal histological study

For light microscopy, renal tissue was fixed in 10% buffered formalin (pH 7.4), embedded in paraffin, sectioned at 3 μm and stained with hematoxylin and eosin, periodic acid-Shiff, periodic acid

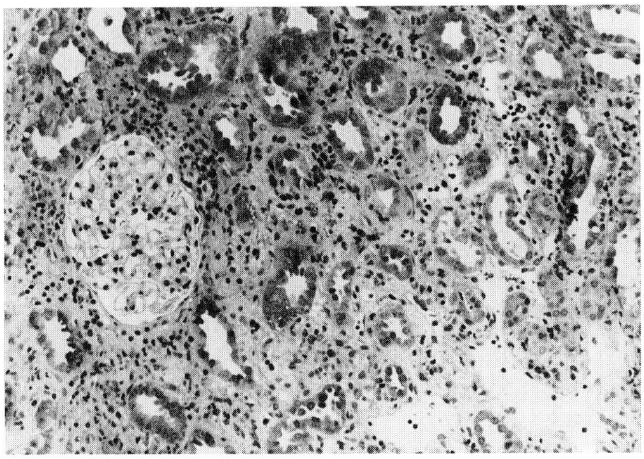

Fig. 1 A light microscopic photograph of kidney from case 1. Extensive tubular atrophy and interstitial widening with infiltrates of monouclear cells are seen. The glomerulus shows minimal change (hematoxylin eosin stain, ×760).

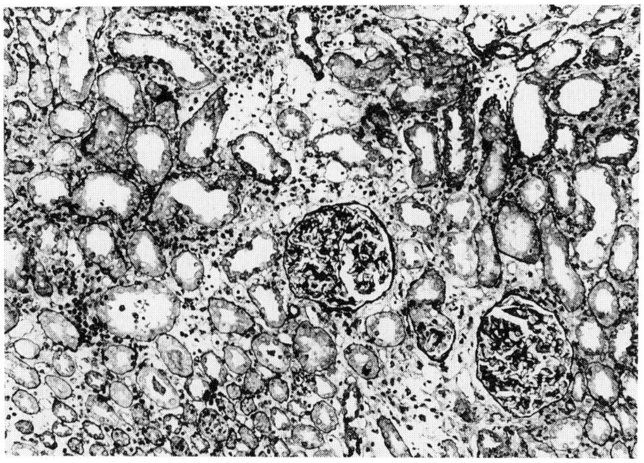

Fig. 2 A light microscopic photograph of kidney from case 2. Interstitial edema and widening are seen in association with infiltrate of mononuclear cells and extensive tubular atrophy (periodic acid silver methenamin stain, ×550).

methenamine silver and azan. For electron microscopy, the tissue was fixed in 2% glutaraldehyde in PBS (pH 7.4), rinsed with PBS, and then postfixed with 1% osmium tetroxide. The tissue was dehydrated in a graded alcohol series and embedded in epon. Ultrathin sections were stained with uranyl acetate and lead citrate and examined in a Hitachi (H-S 12) electron microscope.

Histological findings

Histological changes of the kidneys in both cases showed acute TIN.

On light microscopy, extensive tubular atrophy with tubular epithelial degeneration was found but the glomeruli had only minimal lesions (Figures 1 and 2). Edematous changes and widening of the interstitium were seen in association with infiltrates of mononuclear cells, lymphocyte, polymorphonuclear leukocyte and plasma cells. Eosinophilic granulocytes were rarely seen.

On electron microscopy, electron dense deposits were not seen in the glomerulus nor in the tubular basement membrane. In the glomeruli, small amounts of fibrillar structures were found in the subendothelial space and partly in the mesangium. Degenerative changes of the tubular epithelium were seen in the proximal and the distal nephrons. Infiltrates of phagocytosed cells, mononuclear cells and lymphocytes were seen in the interstitium.

Discussion

Yersiniosis, infections with Y. pst. or Y. ent., produces various clinical features including fever, abdominal pain, diarrhea, arthritis and erythema nodosum [Ahvonen 1972]. In Y. pst. infection, glomerulonephritis has been reported as one complication of this disease [Leino and Kalliomäki 1974, Forsström et al. 1977, Friedberg et al. 1978, 1981, Denneberg et al. 1981]. Friedberg et al. [1981] showed that 12 of 17 patients with Y. ent. infection had proliferative and 4 patients had epimembranous glomerulonephritis. In the glomerulus of these patients, deposits of complement, IgG, and almost always IgM and IgA were seen and Y. ent. antigens were also found by immunofluorescence, which strongly suggested immune complex-mediated renal disease. However, only little information is available on the renal complications with Y. pst. infection. Prober et al. [1979] reported Y. pst. septicemia and postdiarrheal hemolytic uremic syndrome in a 15-month-old boy who ingested unpasteurized goat's milk. Renal histology was not examined in this case. Recently, Davenport et al. [1987] reported two adult patients with ARF following Y. pst. (type IV) septicemia, whose renal lesions were acute tubular necrosis with widespread intra-renal thrombosis.

In the present study, we report two siblings infected with Y. pst. and complicated by ARF about 2 weeks after the onset of the disease. The titres of Y. pst. type VB were significantly elevated in their sera and the organism type VB was isolated from the culture of one patient. Renal lesions in both cases showed acute TIN but intra-renal thrombosis was not seen. The results of our study suggest that ARF can be associated with Y. pst. infection and is based on acute TIN.

Yersinia in human beings has been presumed to be transmitted by contaminated food, or contact with human or animal carriers of Y. pst. or Y. ent. [Knapp 1968, Mollaret 1971]. Two siblings with yersiniosis in this study had been drinking well water. Thus, Y. pst. in our cases might have been aquired via infected well water and it may be helpful for early diagnosis of yersiniosis to note a history of drinking well water.

Previous cases of renal involvement in infections with Y. ent. have shown immune complex mediated glomerulonephritis [Forsström et al. 1977, Friedberg et al. 1978, 1981, Denneberg et al. 1981]. It is therefore remarkable that TIN without glomerular involvement was found in our cases. Etiologic agents of acute TIN are various [Churg et al. 1985]. Many patients with TIN due to drug hypersensitivity have fever, rash, eosinophilia, and tubular dysfunction with eosinophilia casts may aid in the diagnosis [Henrich et al. 1978]. The patients in this study received Latamoxef sodium or Fosfomycin for treatment of yersiniosis and simultaneously suffered from ARF about 2 weeks after the onset of the disease. The lack of a skin rash or eosinophilia in connection with the development of ARF does not exclude a drug-induced renal lesion which started well in advance of ARF but makes it less likely. To our knowledge, there are no reports of ARF caused by Fosfomycin or Latamoxef sodium except one case showing transient elevation of serum creatinine in 63 patients treated with Moxalactam [Mogabgab et al. 1983]. Our patients received different drugs, which also makes it likely that TIN was due to yersiniosis. The facts that dehydration was slight in both patients on admission and FENa in the acute phase of ARF was over 2.0 denies a prerenal origin of ARF. Acute TIN has also occurred following systemic infections such as Group A streptococcal infection, diphtheria, toxoplasmosis, Legionnaire's disease and Brucellosis [Churg et al. 1985]. Therefore, ARF due to acute TIN in both cases might be closely related to Y. pst. infection, like other systemic infections.

The results of this study are a warning to us that Y. pst. infection can be complicated with ARF due to TIN in childhood.

REFERENCES

Ahvohnen P 1972 Human yersiniosis in Finland. II. Clinical features. Ann Clin Res *4:* 39–48

Anonymous 1984 Yersiniosis today (Editorial). Lancet *1:* 84–85

Churg J, Cotran RS, Sinniah R, Sakaguchi H, Sobin LH 1985 Introduction and classification of tubulointerstitial diseases. In: *Churg J, Cotran RS, Sinniah R, Sakaguchi H, Sobin LH (eds)* Renal Disease, *Igaku Shoin,* Tokyo–New York, p 1–3

Davenport A, O'Conner B, Finn R 1987 Acute renal failure following Yersinia pseudotuberculosis septicaemia. Postgrad Med J *63:* 815–816

Denneberg T, Friedberg T, Samuelsson T, Winblad S: 1981 Glomerulonephritis infections with Yersinia enterocolitica O-serotype 3. Acta Med Scand *209:*97–101

Forsström J, Viander M, Lehtonen A, Ekfors T 1977 Yersinia enterocolitica infection complicated by glomerulonephritis. Scand J Infect Dis *9:* 253–256

Friedberg M, Larsen S, Denneberg T 1978 Yersinia enterocolitica and glomerulonephritis. Lancet *1:* 498–499

Friedberg M, Denneberg T, Brun C, Hannover Larsen J, Larsen S: 1981 Glomerulonephritis in infections with Yersinia enterocolitica O-serotype 3. II. The incidence and immunological features of Yersinia infection in a consecutive glomerulonephritis population. Acta Med Scand *209:* 103–110

Henrich WL, Anderson RJ, Shrier RW 1978 Drugs and renal failure. In: *Straus J (ed)* Pediatric nephrology vol. 4; Renal failure. Current concepts in diagnosis and management. Garland STPM Press, New York & London, p 45–57

Knapp W 1968 Die Pseudotuberculose des Menschen. Klinik, Diagnose, Therapie und Epidemiologie. Ther Umsch *25:* 195–200

Leino R, Kalliomäki JL 1974 Yersiniosis as an international disease. Ann Intern Med *81:* 458–461

Mogabgab WJ, Bauman DC, LaCorte WF, Pollock B, Pauling B, Beville RB, Holmes BJ 1983 Moxalactam therapy of difficult infections in patients with serious underlying conditions. J Int Med Res *11:* 269–278

Mollaret HH 1971 L'infection humaine á "Yersinia enterocolitica" en 1970, á la lumiére de 642 cas récents. Aspects cliniques et perspectives épidémiologigues. Pathol Biol (Paris) *19:* 189–205

Prober CG, Tune B, Hoder L 1979 Yersinia pseudotuberculosis septicemia. Am J Dis Child *133:* 623–624

Clinical Nephrology, Vol. 35 No. 3 – 1991 (110–118)

Acute and chronic renal disease in hospitalized AIDS patients

A. Valeri and A.-J. Neusy

Department of Medicine, New York University Medical Center, N. Y., N. Y., USA

Abstract. We performed a retrospective chart analysis on 449 AIDS patients admitted to Bellevue Hospital Center from 1983–1986 to characterize the etiologies and clinical course of acute renal failure (ARF) and to define the incidence and clinical course of AIDS-associated nephropathy (AAN) in an unselected hospitalized AIDS population. Defining ARF as a rise from baseline serum creatinine of at least 2.0 mg%, we found 88 cases (a prevalence of almost 20%) or 14.5 cases per 100 admissions. Volume depletion was the most common etiology and was as severe a cause of ARF as other etiologies. There were 21 cases of ARF in 17 patients with a peak serum creatinine ≥6.0 mg%. Volume depletion accounted for 7/21 of these cases. Baseline renal insufficiency existed in 9/17 patients (12/21 cases) and volume depletion was the cause of ARF in 3 of these cases. Only 4 cases required dialysis. There were 34 patients (prevalence of 7.6% or 3.0 cases per 100 patient-years) with otherwise unexplained chronic renal insufficiency and/or persistent qualitative or quantitative proteinuria and thus were defined on clinical grounds to have AIDS-associated nephropathy. Thirty-two of these patients (94%) had evidence of AAN at or within 1 year of presentation. Eleven patients (32%) reached ESRD (serum creatinine ≥6.0 mg%); 9 patients did so within 1 year of presentation and 3 required dialysis. In those with adequate follow-up (9 cases), the mean survival from time of ESRD was 25.5 days and all cases died within 6 months of reaching ESRD. By life table analysis, there was a significantly shorter median survival time in those with AAN compared to all other AIDS patients in this study (9.5 months vs 12.25 months, $p < 0.05$ by chi-square analysis).

Key words: AIDS – AIDS-associated nephropathy – acute renal failure

Introduction

The AIDS (Acquired Immunodeficiency Syndrome) epidemic has put a heavy demand on health resources in many cities in the United States. These patients often have prolonged hospitalizations related to multiple and severe opportunistic infections with exposure to many forms of nephrotoxic insults. Thus, acute renal failure is a potentially significant complication during the hospitalization of these patients [Gardenswartz et al. 1984, Pardo et al. 1984, Vaziri et al 1985, Rao et al. 1987]. In addition, many centers have reported the development of a chronic glomerular disease, appearing as a focal and segmental or globally collapsed form of glomerulosclerosis which can progress to ESRD, in patients with HIV-1 (Human Immunodeficiency Virus-1) infection [Rao et al. 1984, Gardenswartz et al. 1984, Pardo et al. 1984 and 1987, Bourgoigne et al. 1988, Cohen and Nast, 1988, Carbone et al. 1989, Langs et al. 1990]. Other centers have not found the association of AIDS with chronic renal disease [Welch et al. 1984, Humphreys and Schoenfeld (ed), 1987, Humphreys and Schoenfeld 1987]. In addition, the incidence of AIDS-associated nephropathy (AAN) has been variable in reports from different centers. While east coast centers in the United States, particularly from New York and Miami, find a significant incidence of chronic renal disease related to AIDS [Gardenswartz et al. 1984, Pardo et al. 1984, Rao et al. 1985, Humphreys and Schoenfeld 1987, Bourgoigne et al. 1988], west coast centers do not concur and have speculated that this may be due to the differing demographics of patients from these centers with the former centers having a higher percentage of intravenous drug users (IVDU) and black and Hispanic patients [Humphreys and

Received October 3, 1990; in revised form December 13, 1990.

Reprint requests to Dr. Anthony Valeri, NYU Medical Center, Rm TH-440, 550 First Avenue, New York, New York 10016.

Material contained herein has appeared in abstract form at the annual meeting of the American Society of Nephrology in December 1988.

Schoenfeld (ed), 1987]. Rao et al. and others have used the clinical course, histology and occurrence of FSGS in non-IVDU AIDS patients as evidence for a separate and unique glomerulopathy related to AIDS [Pardo et al. 1984, Cohen and Nast, 1988, Carbone et al. 1989, Langs et al. 1990]. Many studies encompass a selective review of patients (e.g., renal biopsy cases only or renal consultation cases only) and thus may tend to underestimate the true incidence of AIDS-associated nephropathy because of incomplete retrieval of affected patients [Gardenswartz et al. 1984, Pardo et al. 1984, Rao et al. 1983, Bourgoigne et al. 1988]. This is especially true since AIDS-associated nephropathy may not present with overt nephrotic syndrome [Gardenswartz et al. 1984, Cabone et al. 1989, Langs et al. 1990].

Because of the large volume of AIDS patients who are cared for at Bellevue Hospital Center, a large municipal hospital in New York City, we undertook a retrospective analysis of AIDS patients admitted to our institution over a period of approximately two-and-one-half years for the following purpose: (1) to catalogue the etiologies, course and outcome of acute renal failure in AIDS patients, and (2) to determine the incidence, clinical course and outcome of AIDS-associated nephropathy in an unselected group of hospitalized AIDS patients.

Methods

All available charts of patients admitted to Bellevue Hospital Center from August 1983 to December 1986 with either a primary or secondary diagnosis of AIDS were reviewed. Charts of patients with the following clinical abnormalities were selected for in-depth review:

(1) Acute Renal Failure (ARF) subgroup – all patients with an acute but reversible rise in serum creatinine >0.3 mg%, and

(2) AAN subgroup – all patients with otherwise unexplained chronic renal insufficiency with a serum creatinine >1.3 mg% and/or persistent qualitative (30 mg% or greater by random urine dipstick measurement) or quantitative (≥500 mg protein/24 h) proteinuria. All patients with an antecedent history of renal disease or edema (present for more than 2 years before clinical presentation of HIV infection), diabetes, secondary amyloidosis (due to IVDU or "skin-popper's" amyloidosis), acute glomerulonephritis or a family history of inheritable renal disease were excluded from analysis as well as patients with residual chronic renal insufficiency due to drug toxicity (e.g., from amphotericin B, pentamidine, etc.) or those whose proteinuria was not documented to be persistent over the course of available follow-up.

AIDS was defined by CDC criteria.

For uniformity, the following additional definitions were used:

(1) duration of ARF – defined as the length of time from the day of first elevation in serum creatinine until the first day of return of serum creatinine to within 0.3 mg% of the previously established baseline

Table 1 Patient demographics (in 246 patients with 1 or more episodes of ARF)

Characteristic:	
Age (mean, in years)	35.7
Gender, male: female (ratio)	9:1
Race/Ethnicity	
Caucasian	27%
Black	31%
Hispanic	41%
Other	0%
AIDS risk factor	
IVDU	47%
Homosexual	41%
IVDU/Homosexual	6%
Other/Unknown	6%
Outcome at last follow-up (% alive)	54%

Table 2 Opportunistic infections and malignancies (in 246 patients with 1 or more episodes of ARF)

	Number of cases (percent)
Infections:	
Pneumocystis carinii pneumonia (PCP)	180 (73%)
Cryptococcal meningitis	15 (6%)
CNS toxoplasmosis	30 (12%)
Mycobacteriosis (disseminated M. tuberculosis or MAI)	71 (29%)
Esophageal/Candidiasis	46 (19%)
Salmonellosis	9 (4%)
Disseminated CMV	22 (9%)
Cryptosporidiosis	10 (3%)
Disseminated histoplasmosis	8 (3%)
Herpes infection (disseminated H. Varicella-Zoster or Simplex)	13 (5%)
Primary/Bacteremia (no obvious source)	28 (11%)
Malignancies:	
Epidemic Kaposi's sarcoma	53 (22%)
Diffuse/Histiocytic lymphoma or Burkitt's lymphoma	6 (2%)

Table 3 Etiologies of ARF (n = 425 episodes) in 449 AIDS patients

	Number of cases (percent)
Volume depletion	160 (38%)
Bactrim AIN	38 (9%)
Pentamidine nephrotoxicity	74 (17%)
Aminoglycoside nephrotoxicity	10 (2%)
Other drug-related nephrotoxicity	5 (1%)
Contrast nephrotoxicity	16 (4%)
Bactrim and/or pentamidine nephrotoxicity	4 (1%)
Pentamidine and/or aminoglycoside nephrotoxicity	2 (0.5%)
Amphotericin nephrotoxicity	48 (11%)
Volume depletion with superimposed	
contrast use	1 (<0.5%)
Bactrim use	1 (<0.5%)
rhabdomyolysis	1 (<0.5%)
Urinary retention/obstruction	1 (<0.5%)
Acute glomerulonephritis	1 (<0.5%)
Unknown	30 (7%)
Hemodynamically mediated ARF	
Sepsis	12 (3%)
Shock (systolic BP <90)	12 (3%)
Sepsis + shock	9 (2%)

or stabilization of 3 successive daily values to within 0.3 mg% of each other;

(2) Bactrim acute interstitial nephritis (AIN) – defined as an acute rise in serum creatinine associated with high dose Bactrim therapy for proven or suspected PCP with associated new onset microscopic hematuria (≥5 RBCs per HPF) and/or pyuria (≥5 WBCs per HPF) or with evidence of acute tubular dysfunction (i. e., hyperkalemia or Type IV RTA) out of proportion to the severity of the resulting renal dysfunction;

(3) residual chronic renal insufficiency – defined as the stabilization of the serum creatinine to more than 0.3 mg% above previously established baseline values after recovery from an episode of ARF; and

(4) hemodynamically-mediated ARF – defined as that episode of ARF occurring in temporal relationship to shock of any etiology (systolic BP <90 mmHg) or sepsis (positive blood cultures) in the absence of overt shock.

Results

From August 1983 to December 1986, there were 607 patients encompassing 923 admissions to Bellevue Hospital Center with either a primary or secondary

Table 4 Clinical characteristics of ARF (n = 425 episodes) in 449 AIDS patients

Cause (number of cases)	Contributing hemodynamic factors (shock and/or sepsis)	Average peak creatinine (mg%)	Average maximal rise in creatinine (mg%)	Average duration of ARF (days)
Volume depletion (160)	11 (7%)	2.3	1.2	5.5
Bactrim (38)	1 (3%)	2.1	1.1	9.0
Pentamidine (74)	3 (4%)	2.3	1.3	11.6
Amphotericin B (48)	6 (13%)	2.4	1.3	21.2
Aminoglycosides (10)	2 (20%)	3.3	2.0	14.4
Contrast (16)	0	2.6	1.4	6.8
Bactrim and/or Pentamidine (4)	0	2.5	1.5	8.5
Pentamidine and/or an aminoglycoside (2)	0	3.5	2.2	14.0
Other drug (5)	1 (20%)	2.9	1.9	13.4
Acute glomerulonephritis (1)	0	5.0	3.7	38.0
Hemodynamic ARF (33)	33 (100%)	3.7	2.4	7.6
Urinary retention (1)	0	4.1	2.4	8.0
Unknown (30)	3 (10%)	3.1	1.6	9.2
Volume depletion superimposed on:				
Contrast (1)	1 (100%)	1.4	0.7	3.0
Bactrim (1)	0	4.6	3.7	4.0
Pentamidine	–	–	–	–
Rhaddomyolysis (1)	0	3.4	2.4	1.0

Table 4 A Clinical outcome of 425 episodes of ARF in 449 AIDS patients

Cause (number of cases)	Recovered	Residual renal insufficiency	Died
Volume depletion (160)	145 (90%)	2 (1%)	13 (8%)
Bactrim (38)	32 (84%)	1 (3%)	5 (13%)
Pentamidine (74)	60 (81%)	5 (7%)	9 (12%)
Amphotericin B (48)	34 (71%)	10 (21%)	4 (8%)
Aminoglycosides (10)	4 (40%)	1 (10%)	5 (50%)
Contrast (16)	15 (94%)	0 (–)	1 (6%)
Bactrim and/or Pentamidine (4)	4 (100%)	0 (–)	0 (–)
Pentamidine and/or an aminoglycoside (2)	1 (50%)	0 (–)	1 (50%)
Other drug (5)	4 (80%)	0 (–)	1 (20%)
Acute glomerulonephritis (1)	1 (100%)	0 (–)	0 (–)
Hemodynamic ARF (33)	8 (27%)	1 (3%)	24 (70%)
Urinary retention (1)	1 (100%)	0 (–)	0 (–)
Unknown (30)	22 (73%)	2 (7%)	6 (20%)
Volume depletion superimposed on:			
Contrast (1)	1 (100%)	0 (–)	0 (–)
Bactrim (1)	1 (100%)	0 (–)	0 (–)
Pentamidine (0)	0 (–)	0 (–)	0 (–)
Rhabdomyolysis (1)	0 (–)	0 (–)	1 (100%)

Table 5 Subgroup analysis of clinical course of ARF (n = 425 episodes) in 449 AIDS patients

Cause	Average peak creatinine (in mg%)		Average maximal rise in creatinine (in mg%)		Average duration of ARF (in days)	
Total	≥2.0 (n = 225)	≥6.0 (n = 21)	≥2.0 (n = 88)	≥6.0 (n = 7)	≥5 (n = 264)	≥10 (n = 126)
Volume depletion	70 (31%)	7 (33%)	26 (30%)	2 (29%)	61 (23%)	13 (10%)
Bactrim	12 (5%)	1 (5%)	4 (5%)	1 (14%)	32 (12%)	13 (10%)
Pentamidine	33 (15%)	5 (24%)	11 (13%)	1 (14%)	61 (23%)	36 (29%)
Amphotericin B	37 (16%)	0 (–)	8 (9%)	0 (–)	41 (16%)	29 (23%)
Aminoglycosides	8 (4%)	0 (–)	3 (3%)	0 (–)	9 (3%)	6 (5%)
Contrast	13 (6%)	0 (–)	5 (6%)	0 (–)	9 (3%)	3 (2%)
Bactrim and/or Pentamidine	3 (1%)	0 (–)	1 (1%)	0 (–)	3 (1%)	2 (2%)
Pentamidine and/or aminoglycoside	2 (1%)	0 (–)	1 (1%)	0 (–)	2 (1%)	2 (2%)
Other drug	3 (1%)	0 (–)	2 (2%)	0 (–)	5 (2%)	1 (1%)
Acute glomerulonephritis	1 (<1%)	0 (–)	1 (1%)	0 (–)	1 (1%)	1 (1%)
Hemodynamic ARF	24 (11%)	5 (24%)	15 (17%)	2 (29%)	18 (7%)	12 (10%)
Urinary retention	1 (<1%)	0 (–)	1 (1%)	0 (–)	1 (1%)	0 (–)
Unknown	16 (7%)	3 (14%)	8 (9%)	1 (14%)	21 (8%)	8 (6%)
Volume depletion superimposed on:						
Contrast	0 (–)	0 (–)	0 (–)	0 (–)	0 (–)	0 (–)
Bactrim	1 (<1%)	0 (–)	1 (1%)	0 (–)	0 (–)	0 (–)
Pentamidine	–	–	–	–	–	–
Rhabdomyolysis	1 (<1%)	0 (–)	1 (1%)	0 (–)	0 (–)	0 (–)

diagnosis of the acquired immunodeficiency syndrome (AIDS). Of these, 449 patient charts (74%) covering 608 admissions (66%) were available for review and formed the basis of this retrospective analysis.

Of these patients, 246 (55%) had one or more episodes of acute renal failure (ARF) for a total of 425 episodes, defined as a sustained but reversible rise in serum creatinine >0.3 mg% and 34 (7.6%) had evidence of AIDS-associated nephropathy (AAN), defined as otherwise unexplained abnormal and persistent qualitative or quantitative proteinuria and/or chronic renal insufficiency. These patient charts were then reviewed in detail.

The demographic characteristics of these patients are shown in Table 1. The opportunistic infections and malignancies which these patients incurred are shown in Table 2.

Acute renal failure

The identifiable etiologies of ARF in these 246 patients are shown in Table 3. Volume depletion represented the most common etiology for a reversible cause of ARF, followed by a variety of drug-induced insults (both nephrotoxic and due to allergic interstitial nephritis). The relative frequencies of the different drug-related insults probably reflect both the inherent nephrotoxicity of the agent as well as the frequency of use of the particular drug. For example, the high incidence of toxicity from Bactrim and Pentamidine is not surprising since PCP was the most common infection to be treated in this population; whereas the inherent nephrotoxicity of amphotericin B lead to a significant incidence of ARF despite the relatively lower rate of use of the agent.

The clinical features, course and outcome of these episodes are shown in Tables 4, 4 A and 5. Among the most frequent causes of ARF (volume depletion, Bactrim, Pentamidine, Amphotericin B, aminoglycosides and hemodynamically-mediated ARF), aminoglycosides and hemodynamic ARF tended to produce a slightly higher peak creatinine and a higher change in creatinine compared to the other causes. In addition, volume depletion and contrast nephrotoxicity were the quickest to reverse once treated, while the drug-related causes of ARF all produced a longer duration of ARF with Amphotericin B producing the longest duration. Duration of ARF in excess of 3 weeks occurred with greatest frequency with amphotericin B (21/37 cases, 44%), aminoglycosides (2/8 cases, 20%) and pentamidine (11/74 cases, 15%). Volume depletion, because of ongoing profuse infectious diarrhea of a resistant nature, produced 4/160 episodes (6%) where ARF lasted in excess of 3 weeks. The frequency distribution of the peak serum creatinine and the maximal rise in creatinine reveals that volume depletion was as significant a cause of ARF as that due to Bactrim and Pentamidine.

There were 21 cases of ARF occurring in 17 patients in which the peak serum creatinine was ≥6.0 mg%. In 7 of these 21 cases, volume depletion was the cause for the acute deterioration in renal function. In 12 of the 21 cases (encompassing 9 patients), there was pre-existent or baseline renal insufficiency and volume depletion was the superimposed insult leading to ARF in 3 of these cases. Four of the 17 patients required dialysis. Nine of the 17 patients died.

It should be noted that the clinical course for Amophotericin B-related nephrotoxicity is affected by the pattern of its use in that the drug is administered unless the serum creatinine rises >2.0 mg% at which time it is held and then resumed when the creatinine falls below this critical value.

In the surviving patients, recovery of renal function was essentially complete except for that related to the aminoglycosides and Amphotericin B. The latter may be related to the standard of care in effect at the time at Bellevue Hospital Center where patients with cryptococcal meningitis were placed on "maintenance" Amphotericin B therapy to try to prevent relapse. The greatest mortality was seen in association with hemodynamically-mediated ARF (i. e., sepsis and/or shock) and the aminoglycosides (probably more a manifestation of the underlying or associated medical problems).

Table 6 Demographics of patients with AIDS-associated nephropathy (n = 34 patients)

Characteristic:	
Age (average, in years)	35.5
Gender, male: female (ratio)	10 : 1
Race/Ethnicity	
Caucasian	18%
Black	47%
Hispanic	35%
Other	0%
AIDS risk factor	
IVDU	56%
Homosexual	35%
IVDU/Homosexual	6%
Other/Unknown	3%

AIDS-associated nephropathy (AAN)

There were 34 patients with unexplained chronic renal insufficiency and/or persistent qualitative or quantitative proteinuria who were defined as having AIDS-associated nephropathy (AAN). Their demographics are given in Table 6. There were an additional 49 patients with either transient proteinuria or proteinuria documented on only a single occasion without sufficient follow-up evaluation that were excluded from analysis. Compared to the study group as a whole, the patients with AAN had the same age and gender distribution but tended to have a higher percentage of black patients (47% in those with AAN compared to 28% in those without AAN, $X^2 = 4.82$, $0.05 < p < 0.10$) and patients with a history of IVDU (56% in those with AAN compared to 46% in those without AAN, $X^2 = 1.56$, p = NS), which has been noted by others in studying the epidemiology of AAN.

Clinical features of the renal disease at the time of presentation to Bellevue Hospital Center with manifestations of HIV infection (ARC or AIDS) and during subsequent follow-up are given in Table 7. Thirty-five percent of patients with AAN already had chronic renal insufficiency (serum creatinine >1.3 mg%) at the time of presentation with HIV infection to the hospital. Quantitative proteinuria was available in 17 of the 34 patients. Of these 17 patients, 12 patients (71%) had at least 3.5 g of proteinuria on a 24-hour urine collection. The average 24-hour urine protein excretion for these 17 patients was 7.0 g. By the time of last available follow-up, only 35% of these patients were still alive.

Nineteen of the 34 patients had evidence of AAN at the time of presentation, and an additional 13 had evidence of AAN within 1 year of presentation (total of 32/34). Eleven of the 34 patients reached ESRD (serum creatinine ≥6.0 mg%) during the course of follow-up. No patient had ESRD at the time of first presentation (though this has been reported by many other workers), but 9 of 11 patients reached ESRD within 1 year of follow-up. Three of these 9 patients received dialysis. From the time of reaching ESRD, the mean survival time was 25.5 days for the 9 patients with adequate follow-up. All 9 patients died within 6 months of reaching ESRD.

Table 7 Characteristics of AAN at presentation and during follow-up for HIV infection (n = 34 patients)

	At presentation	At follow-up
Azotemia:		
% with renal insufficiency (creatinine >1.3 mg%)	35%	82%
% with ESRD (creatinine ≥6.0 mg%)	0%	32%
Urinanalysis abnormalities:		
% with proteinuria (30 mg% or greater by dipstick)	79%	97%
% with hematuria (≥5 RBC/HPF)	6%	3%
% with pyuria (≥5 WBC/HPF)	24%	21%
Other clinical features:		
% with hypertension	9%	12%
% with edema	15%	35%
% with serum albumin ≤3.5 mg%	82%	91%
% with serum albumin ≤2.5 mg%	29%	41%
% with serum cholesterol >250 mg%	2.3%	2.3%
% alive at last follow-up		35%

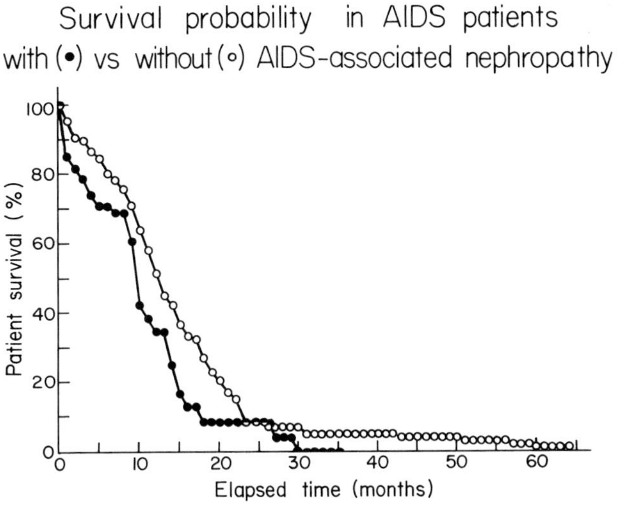

Fig. 1 Survival curve for patients with AIDS-associated nephropathy (●), n = 34, compared to those without AAN (○), n = 112, measured from the time of clinical diagnosis of symptomatic HIV infection, ARC or AIDS ($p < 0.05$ by chi square analysis)

By life-table analysis (Figure 1), there was a significantly shorter survival time in patients with AAN compared to the other AIDS patients examined in this study (a median survival of 9.5 months, N = 34, in patients with AAN measured from the time of diagnosis of clinical HIV infection, i.e., ARC or AIDS, compared to 12.25 months, N = 212, in all other AIDS study patients reviewed, $X^2 = 5.33$, $p < 0.05$). This was also true if survival was measured from the time of first opportunistic infection (9 months, N = 33, in patients with AAN compared to 10.5 months, N = 204, in all other study patients, $X^2 = 3.98$, $p < 0.05$). Sub-group analysis of patients initially presenting with ARC showed no difference in survival (median of 13.25 months, N = 11, in those with AAN compared to 15 months, N = 26, in those without AAN, $X^2 = 0.54$, p = NS) (graphs not shown).

Discussion

ARF in hospitalized patients adds significantly to the morbidity, mortality and health costs sustained by these patients. Because of the severity of the chronic and inter-current acute illnesses sustained by patients with AIDS, we undertook a retrospective assessment of the etiology, course and outcome of ARF in hospitalized AIDS patients. In addition, the incidence of AAN is disputed from various centers, and in many cases, the size of the population from which cases are drawn is unknown. We undertook to estimate the incidence of AAN in hospitalized AIDS patients via a nonselective chart review of all cases admitted to Bellevue Hospital Center over a defined period of time.

Acute renal failure

From the period of August 1983 to December 1986, there were 607 patients admitted to Bellevue Hospital Center with either a primary or secondary diagnosis of AIDS of which 449 patient charts (74%) were available for review. This covered 608 hospital admissions during this time period. Of this group, 246 patients (55%) had a total of 425 episodes of ARF. The demographics of these AIDS patients is similar to the case mix of AIDS patients seen at Bellevue Hospital Center being young adults, predominantly male, predominantly black and Hispanic and having IVDU (intravenous drug use) and homosexuality as their major AIDS risk factors [Siegler and Holzmann, 1989]. Using a more restrictive criteria for ARF such as a rise in serum creatinine of ≥2.0 mg%, the incidence of ARF was 88 cases in 449 patients (20%). This is considerably greater than the 4.9% (37 cases out of 762 patients) reported by a recent study in a general non-AIDS hospital population using similar criteria [Schusterman et al. 1987].

In this group of patients with ARF, PCP was the most common infection occurring one or more times in 73% of these patients followed by disseminated mycobacterial infection, Esophageal Candidiasis and CNS Toxoplasmosis. Again, this is similar to that seen in the general AIDS population at Bellevue Hospital over this time [Siegler and Holzman, 1989]. Approximately one-fifth of these patients had the epidemic form of Kaposi's sarcoma.

The most common cause of ARF was volume depletion accounting for 38% of all recorded episodes, followed by pentamidine nephrotoxicity, amphotericin B nephrotoxicity and trimethoprim-sulfisoxazole-induced allergic interstitial nephritis. Seven percent of all cases went undiagnosed in terms of etiology of ARF. The frequency of these drugrelated episodes of nephrotoxicity reflect in all probability the inherent degree of toxicity of these agents and their relative frequency of use. Hemodynamically-mediated ARF or ATN (septic shock, sepsis without shock, and shock of unknown etiology) accounted for 8% of all episodes of ARF. These findings are similar to those in the study of Schusterman et al. [1989] which found volume depletion, congestive heart failure (CHF), aminoglycosides, contrast and septic shock to be the main independent risk factors for ARF. The demographics of the AIDS population and the types of infections sustained accounts for the absence of CHF and the lower incidence of aminoglycoside toxicity as risk factors for ARF in our population.

Most episodes of ARF due to volume depletion, TMP/SMX and pentamidine were mild. For example, less than 1/2–2/3 of all cases of ARF in these 3 categories had a peak serum creatinine ≥2.0 mg%. Amphotericin B, aminoglycosides and hemodynamically mediated ARF tended to be associated with the more severe episodes of ARF and be of the greatest duration. Volume depletion and contrast ATN were the most rapidly reversed form of ARF; TMP/SMX and pentamidine toxicity were intermediate in duration.

Our very general definition of ARF (i. e., an acute and reversible rise in serum creatinine >0.3 mg%) led to what appears to be a rather high incidence of ARF, many of which were mild. Of 425 episodes, only about one-half (225 cases) had peak serum creatinines ≥2.0 mg% and only 21 cases had peak serum creatinines ≥6.0 mg%. Further, in only 88 of the 425 episodes did the serum creatinine rise 2.0 mg% or more from its baseline. Some would question whether our very broad definition has led to the inclusion of spurious laboratory errors as cases of ARF. Even using a more restrictive definition as suggested by others (a rise in serum creatinine of >1.9 mg% from baseline), we would still find an incidence of 88 cases in 449 patients (almost 20%) over 608 admissions (about 14.5 cases per 100 admissions). This raises the issue as to whether AIDS patients are in some way more susceptible to ARF. We cannot answer this question from our data as we would need a control group of non-AIDS hospitalized patients exposed to the same frequency and degree of nephrotoxic insults. This would require a careful case control study.

Dialysis was infrequently required in management, as only 4 cases received such therapy, one with pentamidine nephrotoxicity and 3 with hemodynamically-mediated ARF secondary to sepsis and/or shock. The mild degree of renal insufficiency in many of the drug-related causes of toxicity probably reflects the keen awareness of the medical staff of the nephrotoxicity of these agents and the close monitoring of these patients for signs of toxicity to allow for prompt withdrawal of the drug and/or dosage adjustment (particularly in the case of amphotericin B and pentamidine).

Outcome was, in general, very good with the majority of patients recovering fully. Significant residual renal insufficiency was low (<10% in all groups) except in the case of amphotericin B toxicity. This was probably related to the continuing use of amphotericin B as a maintenance form of therapy with dose titration if the serum creatinine went >2.0 mg% after completing a 1.5–2.0 g course of therapy for cryptococcal meningitis.

Mortality during episodes of ARF was low (<15%) in all forms of ARF, probably related to the inclusion of very mild forms of ARF, except for those episodes related to aminoglycoside toxicity and hemodynamically mediated ARF. This latter finding probably relates to the severity of the underlying disease in those cases.

AIDS-associated nephropathy

Of the 449 patients available for review, there were 34 cases (7.6% or 3.0 cases per 100 patient-years) of unexplained chronic renal insufficiency and/or persistent qualitative or quantitative proteinuria which were clinically classified as AAN. Unfortunately, most of these cases were not confirmed by renal biopsy.

The demographics of this group of hospitalized AIDS patients differed from the general AIDS population at Bellevue Hospital Center. While these patients were predominantly young adult males, there was a greater percentage of black patients and a greater percentage of these patients had IVDU as their underlying AIDS risk factors. Clearly, there was also a significant percentage (35%) of these patients without a history of IVDU. This has also been described by other workers.

As only one patient had a confirmatory renal biopsy, our diagnosis of AAN was often a clinical and not a pathologic one (and often a diagnosis of exclusion); and thus we cannot exclude that a patient with chronic glomerulonephritis or some other form of previously undiagnosed chronic renal disease (which was clinically silent until discovered coincidentally at the time of presentation of clinical HIV infection) has not been inadvertently included in our case identification. But the similarity of the demographics, clinical presentation, course and outcome of our group to what has been described in the literature from other centers suggests that our AAN case definition is a reasonable one. Because of the problems inherent in a retrospective chart review, especially in terms of incomplete patient evaluation and data retrieval, a prospective study would still be of benefit to more fully characterize and define the incidence and clinical course of AAN.

At initial presentation of AIDS to Bellevue Hospital Center, 35% of these cases already had renal insufficiency and 79% had proteinuria. Nineteen of the 34 patients had some evidence of AAN at presentation. The remainder developed AAN within 1 year of initial presentation. Hypertension and clinical nephrotic syndrome were rare features. One-half of the patients had quantitative 24-h urine protein measurements. Of these cases, 71% had nephrotic range proteinuria (≥3.5 g/24 h).

During the course of available follow-up, 47% developed renal insufficiency (total of 82% with renal insufficiency at last available follow-up) and 11 patients (32%) reached ESRD (serum creatinine ≥6.0 mg%). ESRD was achieved in 9/11 patients within 1 year of follow-up, and in these 11 cases, 9 patients died within 6 months of reaching ESRD (mean of 25.5 days).

By life table analysis, the median time from clinical diagnosis of HIV infection, i.e., ARC or AIDS, to ESRD in these 34 patients was 12 months, from first clinical renal abnormality to ESRD was 9.25 months, from ESRD to death was <1 month and from clinical diagnosis of HIV infection to death was 9.5 months. There was a significantly shorter survival time in those patients with AAN compared to other AIDS patients reviewed in this study (median survival time of 9.5 vs 12.25 months, $p < 0.05$ by Chi-square analysis, Figure 1). This was also true if the initial or entry point for analysis of survival data was taken as the time of diagnosis of first opportunistic infection (9 months in those with AAN compared to 10.5 months in those without AAN, $p < 0.05$, graph not shown). No difference in survival is seen if ARC is used as the entry point for survival analysis but this represented only a small subgroup of the study population (15%) who first presented in this fashion. These results in patients without AAN are also comparable with the median survival of 330 days (approximately 11 months) reported by Siegler and Holzman [1989] in 213 hospitalized AIDS patients seen at Bellevue Hospital over a similar period of time (1982–1985). The significantly shorter survival time in hospitalized AIDS patients with AIDS-associated nephropathy may relate to the higher risk of ARF in patients with pre-existent or baseline renal insufficiency, as about 57% (12 out of 21) of our cases of ARF with peak serum creatinine ≥6.0 mg% occurred in patients with pre-existent renal insufficiency, usually AAN. As reported by others, the life span of AIDS patients with ESRD and active opportunistic infections appears short.

REFERENCES

Bourgoigne JJ, Meneses R, Ortiz C, Jaffe D, Pardo V 1988 a The Clinical Spectrum of Renal Disease Associated with Human Immunodeficiency Virus. AJKD *12(2):* 131–137

Bourgoigne JJ, Meneses R, Pardo V 1988 b The Nephropathy related to AIDS. Adv Nephrol *17:* 113–126

Carbone L, D'Agati V, Cheng JT, Appel GB 1989 Course and prognosis of human immunodeficiency virus-associated Nephropathy. Am J Med *87:* 389–395

Cohen AH, Nast CC 1988 HIV-Associated Nephropathy: A unique combined glomerular, tubular and interstitial lesion. Modern Pathology *1(2):* 87–97

Gardenswartz MH, Lerner CW, Seligson GR, Zebetakis PM, Rotterdam H, Tapper ML, Michelis MF, Bruno MS 1984 Renal disease in patients with AIDS: A Clinicopathologic study. Clin Nephrol *21(4):* 197–204

Humphreys MH, Schoenfeld PY 1987 Renal complications in patients with the acquired immune deficiency syndrome (AIDS). Am J Nephrol *7:* 1–7

Humphreys MH, Schoenfeld PY 1987 AIDS and Renal Disease. The kidney *20(2):* 7–12

Langs C, Gallo GR, Schacht RG, Sidhu G, Baldwin DS 1990 Rapid renal failure in AIDS-associated focal glomerulosclerosis. Arch Int Med *150:* 287–292

Ortiz C, Meneses R, Jaffe D, Fernandez JA, Perez G, Bourgoigne JJ 1988 Outcome of patients with human immunodeficiency virus on maintenance hemodialysis. KI *34:* 248–253

Pardo V, Aldana M, Colton RM, Fischl MA, Jaffe D, Moskowitz L, Hensley GT, Bourgoigne JJ 1984 Glomerular lesions in the acquired immunodeficiency syndrome. Ann Int Med *101:* 429–434

Pardo V, Meneses R, Orsa L, Jaffe DJ, Strauss J, Roth D, Bourgoigne JJ 1987 AIDS-Related Glomerulopathy: occurrence in specific risk groups. KI *31:* 1167–1173

Rao TKS, Fillippone EJ, Nicastri AD, Landesman SH, Frank E, Chen CK, Friedman EA 1984 Associated focal and segmental glomerulosclerosis in the acquired immunodeficiency syndrome. NEJM *310(11):* 669–673

Rao TKS, Friedman EA, Nicastri AD 1987 The types of renal disease in the acquired immunodeficiency syndrome. NEJM *316(17):* 1062–1068

Shusterman N, Strom BL, Murray TG, Morrison G, West SL, Maislin G 1987 Risk factors and outcome of hospital-acquired acture renal failure: clinical epidemiologic study. Am J Med *83:* 65–76

Siegler EL, Holzman RS 1989 The spectrum of illness in the acquired immunodeficiency syndrome: The Bellevue Experience, 1980–1985. Medical Rounds *2(5):* 207–222

Vaziri ND, Barbari A, Licorish K, Cesario T, Gupta S 1985 spectrum of renal abnormalities in the acquired immune-deficiency syndrome. J Nat Med Assoc *77(5):* 369–375

Welch K, Finkbeiner W, Alpers CE, Blumenfeld W, Davis RL, Smuckler EA, Beckstead JH 1984 Autopsy findings in the acquired immune deficiency syndrome. JAMA *252:* 1152–1159

Clinical Nephrology, Vol. 35 No. 3 – 1991 (119–122)

The successful treatment of atypical hemolytic uremic syndrome with plasmapheresis

W. L. M. Robson and A. K. C. Leung

Department of Pediatrics, University of Calgary and Alberta Children's Hospital, Calgary, Alberta, Canada

Abstract. A seven and a half-year-old boy presented with idiopathic atypical hemolytic uremic syndrome (HUS). He initially appeared to respond to plasma infusions. When he became refractory to plasma infusion, plasmapheresis was initiated. The treatment with plasmapheresis dramatically reversed the deterioration in glomerular filtration rate and platelet count. The use of plasma infusion and plasmapheresis in HUS is discussed. The authors advise the use of plasmapheresis in idiopathic atypical HUS.

Key words: hemolytic uremic syndrome (HUS) – plasmapheresis – acute renal failure – thrombocytopenia

The use of intravenous plasma infusion or plasmapheresis (plasma exchange) in the management of children with typical post diarrheal hemolytic uremic syndrome (HUS) is controversial [Cole 1988]. Plasma infusion and plasmapheresis, however, may be of benefit in children with atypical HUS. We report a seven and a half-year-old boy who developed rapidly progressive renal failure due to atypical HUS and who responded dramatically to plasmapheresis.

Case Report

A seven and a half-year-old Egyptian boy presented in the month of March with a petechial rash. The boy had an upper respiratory infection two weeks prior to the rash. There was no history of diarrhea. On examination, there was a generalized petechial rash, blood pressure (BP) was 120/90 mm Hg, and weight was 30.6 kg. The admission laboratory results and the subsequent changes over time in hemoglobin, platelet count, creatinine, and urea are summarized in Table 1. The typical laboratory features of hemolytic uremic syndrome were present, including a microangiopathic hemolytic anemia, thrombocytopenia, and acute renal failure. The urinalysis revealed red cells too numerous to count, 10–15 granular casts per high powered field, and 4+ protein by dipstick. The urine output was normal. He was treated with daily intravenous plasma, 10 ml/kg/day, and daily vitamin E, 1 gm/m^2/day. Over a period of several days, the platelet count improved significantly. Several weeks later, a new petechial rash developed in association with vomiting, fever, and cough. An examination revealed a temperature of 39.3° C, a BP of 130/60 mm Hg, a heart rate of 140 beats per minute, and a generalized petechial rash. The laboratory investigations revealed deterioration in platelet count and in glomerular filtration rate (GFR). He was treated with daily intravenous plasma and vitamin E. Within several days, the platelet count improved and he was discharged on daily vitamin E. Several weeks later a new petechial rash developed, notwithstanding a platelet count of 169 × 10^9/l. He was treated with daily intravenous plasma and vitamin E was continued. The BP required treatment with both captopril and propranolol. The platelet count improved and biweekly prophylactic intravenous plasma infusions were administered for two weeks. Notwithstanding the infusions, the GFR progressively declined and the platelet count continued to fall (Table 1). A renal biopsy showed a glomerular and arterial thrombotic microangiopathy consistent with hemolytic uremic syndrome. The interlobular arteries and the medium and small sized arterioles showed complete obstruction due to intimal proliferation and swelling. There were small granular fibrin deposits sporadically in the vessels. The more proximal portions of the interlobular arteries were largely uninvolved. Approximately 50% of the glomeruli showed extrinsic compression of the glomerular capillary loops secondary to solidification of the tuft by a dense eosinophilic material resembling mesangial matrix. There was mild hyper-

Received August 29, 1990; in revised form December 10, 1990.

Reprint requests to Dr. W. L. M. Robson, #300, 10601 Southport Road SW Calgary, Alberta T2W 3M6, Canada

Table 1 Laboratory results in a boy with idiopathic atypical hemolytic uremic syndrome treated with plasmapheresis

								P		P	P	P	P	P					
Number of days since presentation	1	6	25	39	42	49	68	76	77	78	81	83	85	91	93	171	355	704	1190
Creatinine μmole/l	99	137	168	154	147	172	311	555	569	538	425	403	285	143	114	106	77	60	60
Urea mmole/l	17.0	18.6	19.4	16.3	14.6	16.5	18.4	26.7	25.8	24.5	22.2	21.1	15.6	11.6	8.8	9.2	8.4	5.1	4.8
Hemoglobin g/l	82	54	78	81	68	67	61	69	71	73	72	67	65	63	58	109	122	119	125
Platelets × 10^9/l	45	116	91	369	198	136	111	77	119	140	407	392	442	421	336	592	400	345	312

P = plasmapheresis

cellularity of the mesangium. The tubules showed atrophic changes. The interstitium contained a mononuclear cell infiltrate and numerous plasma cells. A diffuse interstitial fibrosis was present. The child was treated with plasmapheresis on six occasions over the next two weeks. From 817 to 1405 ml of plasma were used with each plasmapheresis. There was an immediate and dramatic response to plasmapheresis (Figure 1). The platelet count increased and creatinine and urea, which had been progressively deteriorating, leveled off, and then showed a progressive improvement. One week following the discontinuation of the plasmapheresis, he was started on prednisone 50 mg qd (1.5 mg/kg/day). Prednisone was maintained at this dosage for two months, was then reduced to 25 mg qd (0.75 mg/kg/day) and was subsequently slowly tapered and eventually discontinued fourteen months later.

The boy has been followed for four years since the original episode and has not developed another recurrence of HUS. At his four year follow-up, his GFR was normal, he was taking captopril 0.25 mg/kg/day for control of mild hypertension, and he had 5–7 red blood cells per high-powered field in his urinalysis.

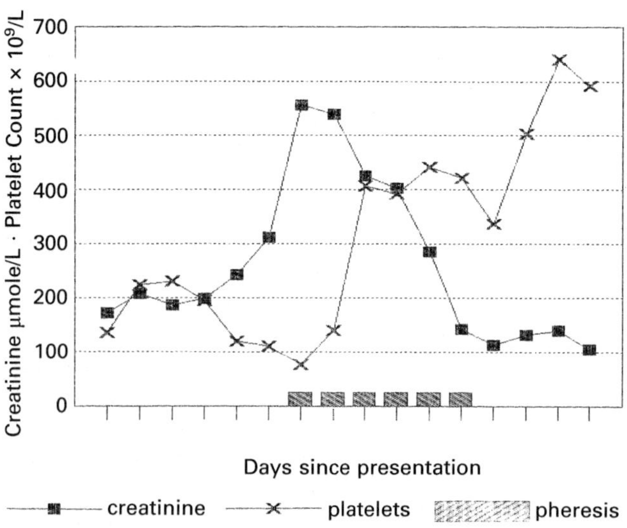

Fig. 1 The change in serum creatinine and platelet count with plasmapheresis in a boy with idiopathic atypical hemolytic uremic syndrome.

Discussion

The majority of children with HUS present with typical HUS. Typical HUS presents in the warmer spring and summer months, follows a diarrheal prodrome, and has a relatively good prognosis. This boy presented with atypical HUS. The atypical features in this boy included his presentation in the month of March, the absence of a diarrheal prodrome and the recurrence of episodes. Atypical HUS usually has a poor prognosis.

The child we report initially appeared to respond to plasma infusions but then became refractory to further infusions of plasma. When his GFR showed a progressive and rapid deterioration, plasmapheresis was initiated. No other therapeutic intervention was made at the time of the plasmapheresis. The dramatic reversal of the deterioration in his GFR and the improvement in his platelet count are likely due to the effects of the plasmapheresis.

The mechanism by which plasmapheresis improved the GFR and the platelet count in this boy is not clear. Several authors have suggested the presence of a circulating factor that either promotes or inhibits the pathophysiological process of HUS. Prostacyclin (PGI_2) production by endothelial tissue has been implicated in the pathogenesis of HUS [Remuzzi et al. 1978]. PGI_2 is a prostaglandin which acts as a vasodilator and also as an inhibitor of platelet aggregation. The deficiency of a plasma factor that stimulates PGI_2 production, the presence of an inhibitor of PGI_2 production, or very rapid degradation of PGI_2, have been suggested as possible causes of HUS [Remuzzi et al. 1978].

Since intravenous plasma infusions initially appeared to improve the situation, it may be that plasmapheresis added a factor to the blood. Any factor that was added could have either acted directly, or indirectly by stimulating the production of an endogenous substance. Improvement in PGI_2 supporting capacity has been noted after the infusion of fresh frozen plasma [Remuzzi et al. 1979] and after the ex-vivo mixing of normal serum with HUS serum [Siegler 1987]. These observations have lead to the "missing factor" hypothesis and to speculation that the infusion of fresh frozen plasma replaces the missing factor. It is also possible that a factor was added inhibiting an endogenous substance that was causing the HUS. The boy we report appeared to respond, during his first two admissions, to plasma infusions with 10 ml of plasma per kg body weight per day. On his third admission, he did not demonstrate an improvement with intravenous plasma infusion. Plasmapheresis was performed using from 817 ml to 1405 ml (26.7 ml/kg to 45.9 ml/kg) of plasma and he demonstrated a dramatic improvement. It may be that the larger volume of plasma with the plasmapheresis was responsible for the therapeutic effects.

Alternatively, since the HUS has not recurred subsequent to plasmapheresis, it is possible that a factor causing the HUS was removed during plasmapheresis. Had the improvement been due to the addition of a factor, and presuming that the factor would eventually have been metabolized or otherwise cleared from circulation, a recurrence would be theoretically possible. Levin et al. [1983] have shown that an inhibitor of PGI_2 production is present in the plasma of patients with atypical HUS and that plasmapheresis is capable of removing such an inhibitor. Plasmapheresis may also work by removing a platelet agglutinating factor, damaged red blood cell membranes, or the products of platelet and white cell secretion.

The use of plasma infusion or plasmapheresis in HUS is controversial [Cole 1988]. Rizzoni et al. [1988] reported on a controlled trial of 32 children with HUS, 17 of whom received plasma infusions. After 16 months of follow-up, they did not find any difference in creatinine clearance, blood pressure, proteinuria, or hematuria. Misiani et al. [1982] reported on 10 children and 7 adults with HUS who were treated with plasma infusions. Sixteen of the patients appeared to improve. The one patient who did not improve with plasma infusion eventually did improve with plasmapheresis. Loirat et al. [1988] reported on a prospective study of 79 children with HUS, 39 of whom received plasma infusions. They reported a higher serum creatinine in the control group at both three months and at six months after the acute episode, but not at twelve months. Diffuse cortical necrosis was present in 7 children in the control group but in none of the plasma treated children. Sheth et al. [1988] reported on 12 children with HUS who received plasma infusions and compared these children to 31 historical controls. They did not find any difference between the two groups in the acute resolution of HUS or in the long term sequelae of HUS. Eddy et al. [1989] reported on two children with typical HUS who had a prolongation of the duration of acute renal failure due to hyperproteinemia associated with excessive plasma infusion therapy. They speculated that the hyperproteinemia either altered the colloid osmotic pressure or aggravated the tubulo-interstitial injury and prolonged the duration of acute renal failure. Vickers et al. [1989] reported a nine month old girl who developed HUS notwithstanding prophylactic plasma infusions that were administered during the prodrome of hemorrhagic colitis. In the reports by Sheth et al. [1988], Vickers et al. [1989], and Eddy et al. [1989], the children all had typical HUS. The children in the studies by Rizzoni et al. [1988], Misiani et al. [1982], and Loirat et al. [1988] were not separated into typical or atypical HUS and their studies may have contained children with both typical and atypical HUS.

Plasmapheresis has been helpful in the management of some patients with thrombotic thrombocytopenic purpura (TTP) [Bukowski et al. 1977], a disease with many similarities to HUS. Bukowski et al. [1977] reported complete recovery in two patients with TTP treated with plasmapheresis. Ansell et al. [1978], however, did not find any improvement with plasmapheresis in a patient with TTP.

Powell et al. [1984] reported that vitamin E was beneficial in children with HUS. The improvement was speculated to be due to the antioxidant effects of vitamin E. Vitamin E did not appear to be of any benefit in the present study.

Prednisone has been used in patients with TTP [Moake et al. 1985, Rossi et al. 1974]. Improvement related to the prednisone was speculated to be due to the inhibition of auto-antibody production [Moake et al. 1985]. It is unclear whether prednisone played a role in maintaining the remission in the boy we report.

The boy we report had atypical HUS. Atypical HUS is a heterogenous disorder likely with multiple causes. Atypical HUS may be familial. Atypical HUS has been reported in association with renal transplant, pregnancy, snake venom, rhabdomyolysis, bromide poisoning, chemotherapy, malignant hypertension, malignancy, immunodeficiency, Addison's disease, systemic lupus erythematosus, immunization reactions, phenylbutazone, Kawasaki disease, and ingestion of fresh apple juice [Robson et al. 1988]. None of these associated problems were present by history, physical examination, or laboratory testing in the boy we report. In addition, there was no family history of HUS. This child, therefore, likely had an idiopathic atypical HUS. Since plasmapheresis was so successful in the treatment of this child, we recommend that plasmapheresis be considered in the treatment of children with idiopathic atypical HUS. In addition to the advantage of either adding or removing a factor important to the pathogenesis of HUS, plasmapheresis may be the only way of infusing sufficient fresh frozen plasma in those children with oligo-anuria.

Acknowledgment

The authors would like to thank Joan Willmott for her expert transcription services.

REFERENCES

Ansell CK, Beaser RS, Chet L 1978 Thrombotic thrombocytopenic purpura fails to respond to fresh frozen plasma infusion. Annals Intern Med *89:* 647–648

Bukowski RM, King JW, Hewlett JS 1977 Plasmapheresis in the treatment of thrombotic thrombocytopenic purpura. Blood *50:* 413–417

Cole BR 1988 Plasma infusion therapy in hemolytic uremic syndrom: is it warranted? Pediatr Nephrol *2:* 286–287

Eddy AA, Geary DF, Balfe JW, et al 1989 Prolongation of acute renal failure in two patients with hemolytic-uremic syndrome due to excessive plasma infusion therapy. Pediatr Nephrol *3:* 420–423

Levin M, Elkon KB, Nokes TJC et al, 1983 Inhibitor of prostacyclin production in sporadic haemolytic uraemic syndrome. Arch Dis Child *58:* 703–708

Loirat C, Sonsino E, Hinglais N, et al 1988 Treatment of the childhood haemolytic uraemic syndrome with plasma. Pediatr Nephrol *2:* 279–285

Misiani R, Appiani AC, Edefonti A, et al 1982 Hemolytic-uremic syndrome: therapeutic effect of plasma infusion. Br Med J *285:* 1304–1306

Moake JL, Rudy CK, Troll JH, et al 1985 Therapy of chronic relapsing thrombotic thrombocytopenic purpura with prednisone and azathioprine. Am J Hematol *20:* 73–79

Powell HR, McCredie DA, Taylor CM, et al 1984 Vitamin E treatment of haemolytic uraemic syndrome. Arch Dis Child *59:* 401–404

Remuzzi G, Misiani R, Marchesi D, et al 1978 Haemolytic-uraemic syndrome: deficiency of plasma factor(s) regulating prostacylin activity? Lancet *2:* 871–872

Remuzzi G, Misiani R, Marchesi D, et al 1979 Treatment of the hemolytic uremic syndrome with plasma. Clin Nephrol *12:* 279–284

Rizzoni G, Claris-Appiani A, Edefonti A, et al 1988 Plasma infusion for hemolytic-uremic syndrome in children: Results of a multicenter controlled trial. J Pediatr *112:* 284–290

Robson WLM, Fick GH, Wilson PCG 1988 Prognostic factors in typical postdiarrhea hemolytic-uremic syndrome. Child Nephrol Urol *89:* 203–207

Rossi EC, Redondo D, Borges WH 1974 Thrombotic thrombocytopenic purpura. JAMA *228:* 1141–1143

Sheth KJ, Gill JC, Hanna J, et al 1988 Failure of fresh frozen plasma infusions to alter the course of hemolytic uremic syndrome. Child Nephrol Urol *89:* 38–41

Siegler RL 1987 Hemolytic uremic syndrome: Clinical observations from the Southwest Pediatric Nephrology Study Group and laboratory findings from the University of Utah Health Sciences Center. In: *Murakami K, Kitagawa T, Yabuta K, Sakai T, (eds)* Recent Advances in Pediatric Nephrology. Elsevier Science, Amsterdam, pp 581–584

Vickers DW, Coulthard MG 1989 Letter to the editors. Pediatr Nephrol *3:* 225–226

Clinical Nephrology, Vol. 35 No. 3 – 1991 (123–129)

Efficacy of percutaneous renal biopsy in obese patients under computerized tomographic guidance

S.-M. K. Lee[1], J. King[2] and B. H. Spargo[3]

[1]*Division of Nephrology, Department of Medicine and* [2]*Department of Radiology, St. Elizabeth Hospital, Beaumont, Texas, USA*
[3]*Specialized Center of Research and Diagnosis in Renal Pathology, Department of Pathology, University of Chicago, Chicago, Illinois, USA*

Abstract. The performance of percutaneous renal biopsy under ultrasound guidance in markedly obese patients is associated with technical difficulties because of the production of poor image quality. Fluoroscopy can be potentially used as an alternative guidance method when the kidneys are not visualized sonographically. However, the presence of uremia in an obese patient imposes an additional risk when fluroscopy is used because of possible nephrotoxicity from the use of radiocontrast dye. Computerized tomography (CT) provides advantages over these two methods because of the production of excellent spatial resolution of images leading to accurate localization of the kidneys. We performed 59 consecutive percutaneous renal biopsies in 58 patients using CT as guidance. The body mass index (BMI) defined as weight in kilograms/(height in meter)^2 [Watson et al. 1979], was used to assess the severity of obesity. Twenty-nine patients had Grade 0 (BMI ≤24.9), 17 had Grade I (BMI 25–29.9), 7 had Grade II (BMI 30–39.9) and 5 had Grade III (BMI ≥40) obesity. Thirty-two patients had superimposed uremia of varying degrees. Image quality was maintained in all four groups, and tissues adequate for diagnosis were obtained in 98% of the attempts. Complications were minimal with no deaths, nephrectomies or surgical interventions attributable directly to the biopsy procedure itself. We recommend the use of CT guidance in the grossly obese patients (Grade II or III) when their kidneys are poorly visualized by sonography.

Key words: CT Scan – morbidity – obesity – percutaneous – renal biopsy success rate

Introduction

Over the past three decades percutaneous renal biopsy has been established as a valuable tool in the diagnosis and management of many renal parenchymal diseases. Various imaging methods have been developed to improve the accuracy of kidney localization and hence the success of the biopsy with minimal morbidity. Static ultrasound and image amplification fluoroscopy are used as guidance methods [Tisher 1989]. However, fluoroscopy with contrast infusion is rarely used for visualization today. Indeed, Farrington et al. [1989] stated that since 1981 they have used ultrasound instead of fluoroscopy as a guidance method in their center.

Received August 6, 1990; in revised form December 6, 1990.

Reprints requests to Dr S. M. K. Lee, 2955 Harrison Street, Suite 305, Beaumont, Texas 77702, USA

The performance of percutaneous renal biopsy in obese patients poses special problems under sonographic guidance. Thus Windler et al. [1985], using ultrasound, found a negative correlation between the severity of obesity and image quality. Whelan et al. [1985] found that marked obesity caused technical interference when the ultrasound method was used. Charboneau et al. [1990] stated that the amount of subcutaneous fat interferes with the visualization of the needle tip under sonographic guidance, supporting the observations of Windler et al. [1985].

The presence of uremia in an obese patient imposes an additional risk. Thus Whelan et al. [1985] described the case of an azotemic patient whose renal contours or collecting systems were not adequately delineated under sonographic guidance. This patient subsequently underwent percutaneous renal biopsy successfully under computerized tomography (CT) guidance. The use of fluoroscopy with contrast infusion in this situation would be prohibitive due to the potential nephrotoxicity of radiocontrast dye. Thus

Table 1 Clinical and demographic characteristics of patients under study.

Number of patients	58
Mean age ± SD	45.2 ± 18.6 years
Range	7 to 70 years
Number of pediatric patients (less than 16 years of age)	6
Number of adult patients (greater than 16 years of age)	52
Male : Female ratio	29:29
Race/Ethnic distributions	Number (%)
Black	32 (55%)
White	21 (36%)
Hispanic	4 (6.8%)
American Indian	1 (1.7%)

Gault et al. [1983] considered the presence of obesity and moderate or severe uremia as relative contraindications for percutaneous renal biopsy. Bolton et al. [1977] used open biopsy in these patients.

Computerized tomography (CT) provides excellent spatial resolution of the kidneys as well as the accurate image of the location of the needle tip [Rosenbaum et al. 1978]. Thus, it is a potentially useful guidance method for percutaneous biopsy in obese patients, regardless of the underlying renal status. The present study was therefore undertaken to evaluate the clinical utility of the CT method as applied to obese patients whose kidneys are poorly visualized by sonography.

We studied patients with different grades of obesity and varying degrees of uremia. Our data showed that the CT method is an accurate and safe imaging modality for the guidance of percutaneous renal biopsy and proper use of this technique may eliminate the use of open biopsy in these high-risk patients.

Patients and methods

From January, 1986, to June, 1989, we performed 59 consecutive percutaneous renal biopsies in 58 patients. Informed consent was obtained from every patient subjected to percutaneous renal biopsy. The study was approved by the Hospital Institutional Review Committee. Coagulation profile (hemoglobin and hematocrit levels, platelet counts, prothrombin and partial thromboplastin times) was assured to be normal 24 hours before each biopsy. Twenty-four hours before each biopsy serum creatinine, blood urea nitrogen levels, routine urinalysis, height and weight were determined. The clinical and demographic characteristics of these patients are summarized in Table 1.

The severity of obesity was classified according to a grading system based on body mass index (BMI) [Watson et al. 1979] where

$$\text{BMI} = \frac{\text{Weight in kilograms}}{(\text{height in meters})^2}$$

Patients were then assigned different grades of obesity [Pi-Sunyer et al. 1988] as follows:

Grade 0	≤24.9 BMI
Grade I	=25–29.9 BMI
Grade II	=30–39.9 BMI
Grade III	≥40 BMI

The biopsy procedure was carried out in three phases:

Localization phase

The patient was placed in a prone position on the cradle of the CT scanner (CT9800 Model, General Electric, Milwaukee, Wisconsin). The lower poles of both kidneys were scanned and multiple images were taken to select an appropriate site for biopsy. This site was determined with the help of a computer cursor. An imaginary "needle pathway" was designed for the biopsy needle to reach the target position with the computer cursor. This pathway was drawn so as to avoid major vascular structures, bowel loops, renal pelvis and other intra-abdominal organs. The imaginary angle of the needle from the spinous process of the vertebrae (predicted angle) and the depth of the kidney under the skin (predicted depth) were measured. These two parameters were used as reference markers for the accurate placement of the biopsy needle.

Biopsy phase

Using the laser coordinated system of the CT scanner as guidance, the corresponding point marked on the console screen was transposed on the skin surface. This specific needle entry point was marked. The skin surface was then prepared, draped and locally anesthetized. A vertical incision of approximately 2 mm was made with a number II Bard-Parker blade (Becton Dickinson, Lincoln Park, New Jersey). A Tru-Cut disposable needle (Travenol, Deerfield, Illinois) was used for the biopsy. The needle was inserted with the specimen notch fully exposed and the inner cannula fully extended. The needle was inserted to the predetermined depth using the two previously measured reference markers (predicted angle and depth) as guidance. The patient was then moved back to the gantry via the mobile cradle. Multiple images of the kidneys were taken to ensure the correct position of the needle tip. The kidney depth, defined as the distance between the needle entry point on the skin to the surface of the renal capsule, was then measured. The biopsy specimen was obtained by puncturing the kidney in the conventional fashion. In order to ensure the procurement of adequate tissues, a minimum of two attempts were made in each patient. No exploring needle was used. The tissue core obtained was immediately submitted to one of us (BHS) for immunofluorescent, electron and light microscopic studies.

Post biopsy phase

For 24 hours post biopsy the patients were observed in the medical unit with close monitoring of blood pressure and other signs of potential complications. All patients were examined for signs of bleeding around the biopsy site, infections, lacerations, or any clinical evidence of intra-abdominal bleeding in 24 hours. Complete blood count, urinalysis, and urine for culture and sensitivities were obtained 24 hours post biopsy. Evidence of gross hematuria or increased microscopic hematuria was noted. If clinically indicated, CT scan of the abdomen was performed in the first 47 patients. In the remaining 11 consecutive patients we routinely performed CT scan of the abdomen in the immediate post-biopsy period regardless of the presence of symptoms to evaluate the presence of hematomas or any other immediate complications.

The number of glomeruli seen on the histological sections was quantitated and evaluated by one of us (BHS) who had no knowledge of the localization method used.

The results were statistically analysed with student's t test according to standard methods [Matthews et al. 1988].

Table 2 Pathological diagnosis of biopsied specimens

Pathological diagnosis	Number
Acute glomerulonephritis	3
Acute tubular necrosis	3
Chronic focal glomerulonephritis	6
Chronic non-specific glomerulonephritis	2
Diabetic glomerulosclerosis	12
Epithelial cell disease	2
Focal segmental glomerulosclerosis	3
IgA nephropathy	4
Interstitial nephritis	4
Membranous nephropathy	6
Nephrosclerosis	12
Non-diagnostic tissues	1
Thin basement membrane nephropathy	1
Total	59

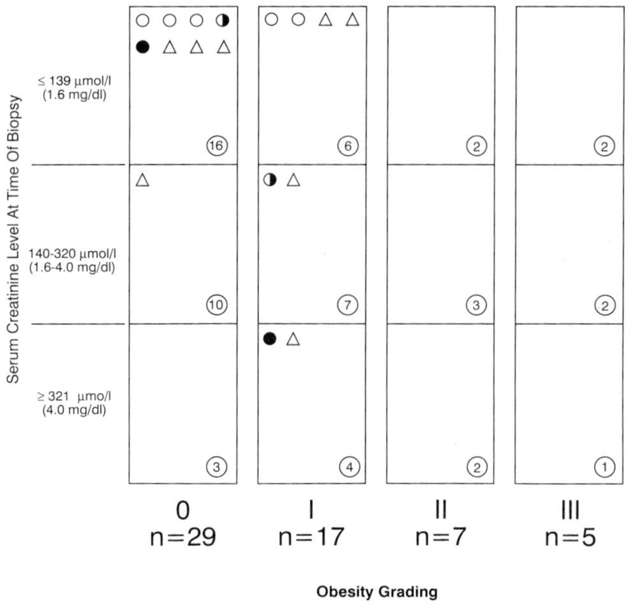

Fig. 1 shows the distribution of complications among the 4 different obesity groups. These patients were further stratified into different groups according to the degree of uremia at the time of biopsy. Open circles (○) represent patients with pain in the biopsy site. Half closed circles (◑) represent persistent pain in the biopsy site that led to the discovery of subcapsular hematomas. Closed circles (●) represent pain in the biopsy site with macroscopic hematuria and subcapsular hematoma. Triangles (△) represent asymptomatic perinephric hematomas. Each symbol represents one patient. The number with the circle on the right hand corner of each subgroup represents the number of patients in that subgroup.

Results

The lower poles of both kidneys were adequately visualized using the CT method in every patient. Image quality was maintained and the needle tip was visualized adequately in each one of the patients studied. Twenty-nine patients had normal body habitus, obesity Grade 0, 17 were in Grade I, 7 in Grade II and 5 in Grade III. In 52 adult patients the mean body weight was 79.5 kg (175 lb) with SD of 23.6 kg (52 lb). The range was 50.9 kg (112 lb) to 164 kg (361 lb) kg. The mean body weight in six pediatric patients was 52.7 kg (116 lb), the SD was

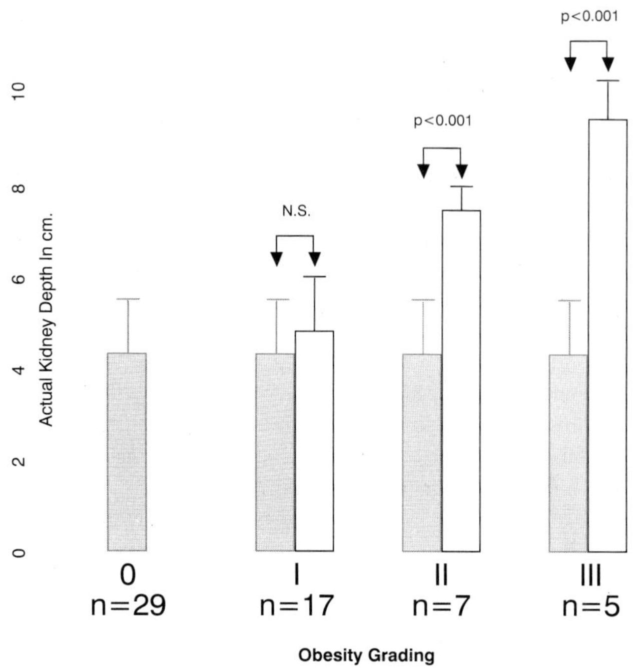

Fig. 2 shows the actual kidney depth measured with the insertion of a biopsy needle at the time of biopsy in the 4 different obesity groups. Patients in obesity Grade 0 were used as control and their kidney depths were compared with patients in Grades I, II and III. Statistical analysis showed no difference between Grade 0 and Grade I, but there was a statistically significant difference between Grade II vs Grade 0 ($p \leq 0.001$) and Grade III vs Grade 0 ($p \leq 0.001$).

19.5 kg (43 lb) and the range was 26.4 kg (58 lb) to 80.9 kg (178 lb). Thirty-two patients had renal failure with serum creatinine greater than 139 µmoles/l (1.6 mg/dl) and ten of these had advanced renal failure with serum creatinine greater than 320 µmoles/l (4 mg/dl).

Fifty-nine consecutive attempts were made in 58 patients. Tissues adequate for diagnosis were obtained in 58 attempts and the success rate was 98%. The pathological diagnosis of the biopsied specimen is summarized in Table 2. In one attempt, nondiagnostic tissues were obtained in one patient who had normal body habitus (Grade 0) but had advanced uremia. Forty-nine biopsies were performed on the right kidney and ten biopsies were done on the left side.

The distribution of complications among the 4 obesity groups is summarized in Figure 1. Two patients developed gross hematuria following biopsy. Both of them developed severe pain in the biopsy site. One of them had advanced uremia secondary to post-streptococcal glomerulonephritis and had Grade I obesity. The other patient had systemic lupus erythematosus but had normal body habitus and renal functions. Both of these patients required transfusion with 8 units and 2 units of packed red cells respectively. CT scan of both patients in 48 hours following biopsy showed subcapsular hematomas. Both patients were treated conservatively and recovered uneventfully without any surgical interventions. Including

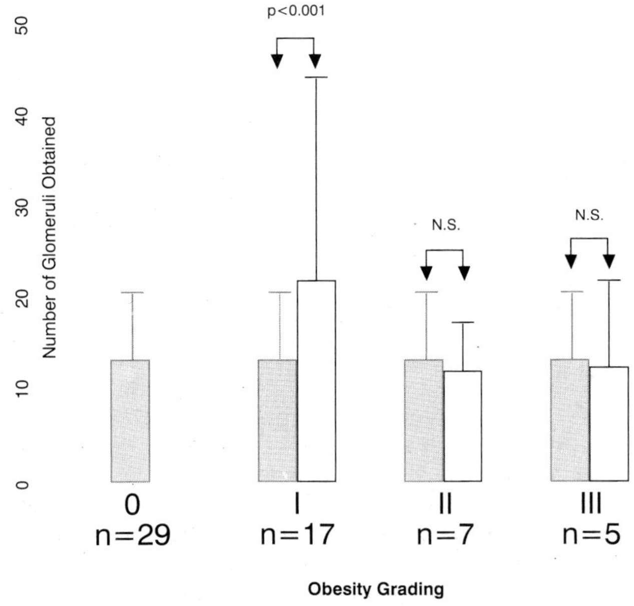

Fig. 3 shows the number of glomeruli obtained (sample size) in the 4 obesity groups. Grade 0 patients served as control. There were no statistical differences in Grade II vs Grade 0 and Grade III vs Grade 0. Grade I vs Grade 0 was statistically significant at $p \leq 0.001$.

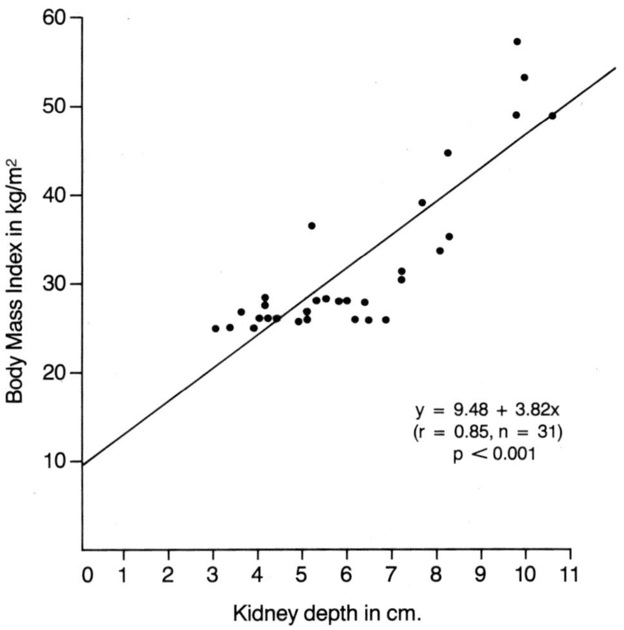

Fig. 4 shows the relationship between the body mass index and the actual kidney depth. Patients in Grade 0 showed no statistical correlation between BMI and actual kidney depth but patients in Grade I, II and III showed a strong correlation as shown in the graph.

these two patients a total of 10 patients developed pain in the biopsy site. Eight patients were treated with oral analgesics for pain which subsided in two to three days and the other two had persistent pain for one week. These two patients had CT scan of the abdomen because of persistence of pain in the biopsy site and showed subcapsular hematomas. Both patients were treated conservatively and recovered without any problems. Thus we had four patients who developed subcapsular hematomas and two of them required transfusions. The complication rate for symptomatic hemorrhage was therefore 6.9% (4/58). In the eleven patients who had routine CT scan of the abdomen regardless of symptoms in the immediate post-biopsy period, 73% (8/11) showed asymptomatic small perinephric hematomas. None of our remaining 56 patients showed any increase in microscopic hematuria following biopsy. No deaths, nephrectomies, or any other complications attributable directly to the biopsy procedure were recorded.

The actual kidney depth measured by insertion of the biopsy needle at the time of biopsy in the 4 obesity groups is shown in Figure 2. The number of glomeruli obtained as evaluated on the histological sections in the 4 obesity groups is shown in Figure 3. A strong correlation was found between the kidney depth and the BMI and this relationship is shown in Figure 4.

Discussion

The successful outcome of a percutaneous renal biopsy depends on the accurate localization of the kidney which in turn relies on the image quality obtained at the time of biopsy. The effect of obesity on kidney localization under ultrasound was summarized by Charboneau et al. [1990], who stated that the surrounding fat in an obese patient causes poor visualization of the needle tip and deeply located kidneys in obese patients are difficult to biopsy. In order to evaluate the effect of obesity on the kidney localization under CT guidance we used the body mass index (BMI) to assess the severity of obesity because it has the highest correlation with body fat [Bolton et al. 1977]. Indeed we found a strong correlation ($r = 0.85$) between the BMI and kidney depth as measured by insertion of biopsy needle at the time of biopsy (see Figure 4). Furthermore, as shown in Figure 2, we found that patients with Grade II or III obesity have statistically significant "deeper" kidneys when compared with the Grade 0 patients. Thus, the BMI and the assignment of different obesity grades based on the BMI is a reliable indicator of obesity and the amount of subcutaneous fat.

After the validity of this obesity grading system was confirmed, we evaluated the effects of obesity on the kidney localization, image quality and the outcome of the biopsy under CT guidance. In the present study, the image quality was subjectively evaluated in 53 patients and was judged to be well maintained with adequate visualization of the kidneys. In order to evaluate the image quality objectively, we assessed the outcome of the biopsy by measuring the number of glomeruli obtained (sample size) and complication rates in the four different obesity groups. The sample size was used as an indicator of outcome because Corwin et al. [1988] proved mathematically that this parameter is important in the interpretation of the renal biopsy and the diagnosis of glomerular diseases. Saitol [1984] shared the same view and further stressed that the ability to obtain sufficient glomeruli depends on selective placement of the needle to the cortex, which is highly dependent on the image quality and the accuracy of kidney localization. We hypothesized that if the image quality were compromised, the accuracy of kidney localization would be smaller due to "misplacement" of the needle to the medulla or adjacent organs, thus missing the cortex. In our study we found that the number of glomeruli obtained in patients with Grades II and III obesity were not statistically different from patients with Grade 0 obesity (see Figure 3). On the contrary, patients with obesity Grade I have statistically more glomeruli than patients with Grade 0. The complication rates in the obese patients (Grades I, II, III) were not different from Grade 0 patients (see Figure 1). Therefore, our data showed that obesity does not affect the image quality and the outcome of the biopsy under CT guidance.

It is speculated that in the American population about 26% of those aged between 20 to 75 years are overweight, totaling about 24 million adult Americans [Pi-Sunyer 1988]. Thus it is conceivable that a substantial percentage of patients undergoing percutaneous renal biopsy are obese. The cost of a percutaneous renal biopsy using CT is about US$ 550 in our institution. Rao [1984] quoted that the cost of the procedure in Minnesota in 1984 was US$ 315.00. However, the cost of an open biopsy would be three or four times higher than this price. Thus, the CT method also offers a substantial cost saving as well as avoiding the potential risks of anaesthetic or surgical complications of an open biopsy.

Twelve patients (20%) in our study had diabetic glomerulosclerosis. This is due to the fact that a large proportion of patients in our study populations were from the lower socio-economic groups and most had no periodic health examinations or adequate maintenance health care. Nine of these diabetic patients were biopsied because of an apparent simultaneous onset of nephrotic syndrome and renal failure. Duration of their diabetes was not known to us; in fact, some of these patients were not aware of their diabetes prior to the biopsy. Some claimed they had taken insulin or hypoglycemic agents in the past but had stopped when they felt well. Most nephrologists would not biopsy a patient with diabetes unless another disease was suspected. However, this view has recently been challenged. Mauer et al. [1990], in a recent article, argued that renal biopsy in diabetic patients may serve as a predictor of renal risk and would identify the patients who are developing significant lesions during the "silent phase" of the disease. Thus, these authors suggest that more diabetic patients should be biopsied.

Three of these diabetic patients in our study had persistent microscopic hematuria and proteinuria. Thorough medical and urological evaluations failed to establish an etiology for the urinary abnormalities. Hence, these patients were subjected to a percutaneous biopsy.

Twenty percent of our biopsied patients showed nephrosclerosis. However, 42 percent (5/12) of these had an underlying systemic disease such as Wegener's granulomatosis (1), systemic lupus (1), scleroderma (2) and vasculitis of unknown etiology (1). Nephrosclerosis was listed as the renal diagnosis, but the overall medical diagnosis followed that of the respective systemic diseases. The remaining seven patients were primarily from lower socio-economic groups with no adequate medical information or periodic health examinations prior to their referral to us. Thus, we elected to biopsy these patients after other causes of renal failure, collagen vascular disease or hypertension were carefully excluded. The main indications for biopsy in these patients classified as having nephrosclerosis were renal failure or proteinuria of unclear etiology.

The success rate of 98% in our study is higher than the current methods which varied from 85% to 95% [Almkuist et al. 1979]. Only in one attempt were nondiagnostic tissues obtained. This took place at the beginning of our study when the radiologists were not familiar with the procedure and two to three radiologists were assisting the biopsies. Hence the radiologists were not "experienced". Thus in all subsequent 53 biopsies only one radiologist was assigned to do all the biopsies, with one of us adopting a "clinician-radiologist"-team approach as recommended by the American College of Physicians [1988].

The complication rate of 6.9% for symptomatic hemorrhage in this study was low considering the high proportion (55%) of uremic patients biopsied. Thus, Patil et al. [1974] found 4% of his uremic patients died as a result of an open biopsy. Farrington et al. [1989] reported that 9 (8.3%) of his 109 uremic patients who had percutaneous renal biopsy using ultrasound or fluoroscopy as guidance developed symptomatic hemorrhage. Six of these patients required transfusions and one of them died as a direct result of the biopsy. In our study it appears that patients with obesity and uremia do not have a higher complication rate than patients with a normal body habitus (see Figure 1). The low complication rate in our study is probably because CT is an accurate method for kidney localization with maintained image quality and clear visualization of the needle tip. Finally, in eleven consecutive patients we found a 73% incidence of asymptomatic small perirenal hematomas in the immediate post-biopsy period. This agrees with an earlier observation by Rosenbaum et al. [1978] that 14 of his 20 patients developed asymptomatic perirenal hematomas diagnosed by using CT scanning. None of our 11 patients developed any further clinical problems and they all recovered uneventfully.

Charboneau et al. [1990] in a recent editorial commented: "Sonographic guidance is optimal for the biopsy of lesions located superficially or at moderate depth in the thin to average-sized individual. Deeply located masses or masses in obese patients can be hard to biopsy under sonographic guidance because of difficulty in lesion visualization due to sound attenuation in the soft tissues." Thus, the use of real-time ultrasound in obese patients was associated with difficulties as pointed out by Yoshimoto et al. [1988], Rao [1984] and Charboneau et al. [1990]. Based on these observations, it is conceivable that the ability to visualize the kidneys in obese patients follows a continuous spectrum. In the "less obese" patients, the kidneys may still be seen adequately by ultrasound. In our study we showed that patients with obesity Grades II and III have statistically "deeper" kidneys (Figure 2). We further demonstrated the direct correlation between BMI and actual kidney depth, which is a reflection of severity of obesity and the amount of subcutaneous fat in patients with Grade I, II or III obesity (Figure 4). The kidney depth of the patients with Grade I obesity were not statistically different from the control patients. Thus, in these "less obese" patients (Grade I), ultrasound may be used for biopsy. The choice of the biopsy method depends on the preference and experience of the clinician and radiologist performing the biopsy. We do not recommend the routine use of the CT method in percutaneous renal biopsy because of its high cost.

In our study we found no complications among the high-risk patients, whereas all the complications took place in the control group or in the mildly obese patients (Grade I). These observations are clearly demonstrated in Figure 1 where patients in the right-hand corner of the matrix had no complications. This group consisted of patients with Grade II or III obesity with varying degrees of azotemia. These patients' kidneys are statistically deeper than the control. Therefore, based on the hypothesis of Charboneau et al. [1990], these kidneys would be poorly visualized by sonography. However, our data showed that the biopsy of patients with Grade II and Grade III obesity is safe. We therefore recommend the use of CT in the grossly obese patients (Grade II or III) when their kidneys are poorly visualized by sonography. Application of this method may eliminate the use of a surgical approach in these high-risk patients [Bolton et al. 1977].

Acknowledgements

We thank Cheryl Dana for typing the manuscript and the Administrative Staff of St. Elizabeth Hospital, Beaumont, Texas, for their help in the preparation of this study. We also thank Dr. Paul Chu of the Department of Mathematics, Lamar University, Beaumont, for his helpful comments on the statistical analysis of our data.

REFERENCES

Almkuist RD, Buckalew VM 1979 Techniques of renal biopsy. Urol Clin North Am *6:* 503–517

Bolton WK, Vaughan ED 1977 A comparative study of open surgical and percutaneous renal biopsies. J Urol *117:* 696–698

Charboneau JW, Reading CC, Welch TJ 1990 CT and Sonographically guided needle biopsy – current techniques and new innovations. AJR *154:* 1–10

Corwin HL, Schwartz MM, Lewis FJ 1988 The importance of sample size in the interpretation of the renal biopsy. Am J Nephrol *8:* 85–89

Farrington K, Levison PA, Greenwood RN, Cattell WR, Baker LRI 1989 Renal biopsy in patients with unexplained renal impairment and normal kidney size. QJ Med *263:* 221–233

Gault MH, Muehrcke RC 1983 Renal biopsy: current views and controversies. Nephron *34:* 1–34

Health and public policy committee, American College of Physicians 1988 Clinical Competence in percutaneous renal biopsy. Ann Intern Med *108:* 301–303

Matthews DE, Farewell VT 1988 Using and understanding medical statistics. 2nd ed. Basel (Switzerland): Karger AG, 124–134

Mauer SM, Chavers BM, Steffes MW 1990 Should there be an expanded role for kidney biopsy in the management of patients with type I diabetes? Am J Kidney Dis *16:* 96–100

Patil J, Bailey GL, Mahoney EF 1974 Open renal biopsy in uremic patient. Urology *3:* 293

Pi-Sunyer FX 1988 Obesity. In: *Wyngaarden* and *Smith* (eds). Textbook of Medicine. 18th ed., Philadelphia: W. B. Saunders, 1219

Rao KV 1984 Percutaneous renal transplant biopsy under CAT Scanner guidance. Nephron *38:* 273–275

Rosenbaum R, Hoffsten PE, Stanley RJ, Klahr S 1978 Use of computerized tomography to diagnose complications of percutaneous renal biopsy. Kidney Int *14:* 87–92

Saitol M 1984 Selective renal biopsy under ultrasonic real-time guidance. Urol Radiol *6:* 30–37

Tisher CC 1989 Clinical Indications for Kidney Biopsy. In: *Tisher CC, Brenner BM* (ed). Renal pathology with clinical and functional correlations. Philadelphia: J. B. Lippincott, Vol I, 1st Ed., p3

Watson PE, Watson ID, Batt RD 1979 Obesity indices. Am J Clin Nutr *32:* 730–737

Whelan TV, Healy GF, Patel TG 1985 Renal biopsy: localization using computed tomography. Urol Radiol *7:* 94–96

Windler EE, Lempp FL 1985 US of the upper abdomen: factors influencing image quality. Radiology *157:* 513–515

Yoshimoto M, Gujisawa S, Sudo M 1988 Percutaneous renal biopsy well visualized by orthogonal ultrasound application using linear scanning. Clin Nephrol *30:* 106–110

Clinical Nephrology, Vol. 35 No. 3 – 1991 (130–133)

Correction of hypophosphatemia in patients on hemodialysis using a calcium-free dialyzate with added phosphate

M. Kaye, M. Vasilevsky and E. Barber

Division of Nephrology, Montreal General Hospital, Montreal, Quebec, Canada

Abstract. Three patients on long term hemodialysis were found to be hypophosphatemic. They were treated using a calcium-free dialysate to which phosphate was added to give a final concentration of 1 or 2 mmol/l. All corrected their low phosphates. Hypocalcemia developed in two patients when the calcium infusion rate was 15 ml/hour of 10% $CaCl_2$. It is recommended that this should be increased to 20 ml/hour. Under these circumstances, correction of hypophosphatemia is possible with the transfer of approximately 30–35 mmol phosphate over a four-hour dialysis.

Key words: dialysis – phosphate – deficiency

Introduction

Patients with renal failure are usually hyperphosphatemic. Occasionally, however, the reverse is found which may be accompanied by symptoms and signs of phosphate depletion [Gagnon et al. 1983, Kurtin and Kouba 1987]. In a patient undergoing regular hemodialysis, considerable loss of inorganic phosphorus (Pi) occurs with each dialysis. The total loss is directly related to the pre-dialysis Pi level, the dialyzer characteristics and the blood flow [Shinaberger et al. 1987]. Phosphate replacement under these circumstances requires intravenous phosphate administration. A suitable parenteral preparation may not always be available, Pi will continue to be lost by dialysis and the dose required can be difficult to estimate. Under any, or all of these circumstances, the addition of Pi to the dialysate would prevent further loss of Pi and, if high enough, would replenish body stores. Pi cannot be added to acetate concentrate because of the precipitation of calcium phosphate however, it can be added to the bicarbonate component of the concentrate used to make a bicarbonate dialyzate but a dual proportioning system is required [Ing et al. 1983, Ross and Nissenson 1988].

We have recently described the development and application of a bicarbonate concentrate for dialysis which is calcium free [Kaye et al. 1989]. Calcium is infused, usually at 10 mmol/hour (15 ml of 10% $CaCl_2$ per hour), into the venous drip chamber. This concentrate provides bicarbonate dialysis using single proportioning machines, it can be used for citrate anticoagulation and it provides a very flexible system for calcium replacement so that calcium balance can be precisely varied. One further application is in hypophosphatemia which is the subject of the present report.

Materials and methods

The first three patients treated for hypophosphatemia are included in this report. All were patients on long term hemodialysis and a brief historical background on each is given below. The only source for Pi repletion in each instance, other than the diet, was the dialyzate.

Case 1 A 69-year-old Chinese male with end stage renal disease (ESRD) due to nephrosclerosis dialyzed for four hours, was treated three times weekly with sulcralfate since January 1989 following gastric bleeding. In January 1990 he presented with severe fatigue, weakness and the inability to walk. Following Pi repletion and stopping sulcralfate he has been well.

Case 2 A 63-year-old woman with lymphoma and ESRD due to glomerulonephritis dialyzed for four hours, three times a week. Associated with chemotherapy, her food intake was poor and she was fatigued and found to be hypophosphatemic. Following correction of the low Pi, there were several subsequent recurrences associated with poor food intake.

Received July 16, 1990; in revised form September 18, 1990.

Reprint requests to Dr. M. Kaye, Director, Division of Nephrology, Montreal General Hospital, 1650 Cedar Avenue, Montreal, Quebec H3G 1A4, Canada

Table 1

		Case 1		Case 2		Case 3	
Duration of dialysis (h)		4		4		4	
Type of dialyzer		Gambro 120 M		Gambro 120 M		Filtral/2	
Blood flow (ml/min)		250		185		250	
Calcium infusion rate (ml/h)		15		20		15	
(mmol/h)		10		13.3		10	
Dialyzate calcium (mmol)		40.6		48.8		43.5	
Calcium balance (mmol)		−0.6		+4.2		−3.5	
Dialysate Pi (mmol/l)		1 for 0–2 h 2 for 2–4 h		2		2	
Pi balance (mmol)		+29.4		+36		+35.5	
	(normal)	Pre	Post	Pre	Post	Pre	Post
Weight (kg)		54.0	52.2	46.6	46.5	71.8	70.4
Blood pressure (mmHg)		150/80	170/80	210/112	224/120	160/80	120/80
Urea (mmol/l)	(3.0–8.9)	16.0	4.9	11.2	4.6	35.7	15.5
Creatinine (μmol/l)	(40–130)	843	298	528	223	911	389
Phosphate (mmol/l)	(0.8–1.45)	0.63	1.31	0.71	1.49	0.43	1.46
Ionized Ca (mmol/l)	(1.15–1.28)	1.16	0.93	1.08	1.42	1.03	0.58
Total Calcium (mmol/l)	(2.11–2.51)	2.17	1.89	2.05	2.46	2.35	1.48
Magnesium (mmol/l)	(0.75–1.05)	0.94	1.10	0.7	0.89	0.95	1.02
PTH (pg/ml)	(10–65)	13.9	86.3	48.6	12.8	3.0	2.3
Total Protein (g/l)	(60–80)	61	62	56	47	76	68
Bicarbonate (mmol/l)	(22–27)	18	25	26	25	20	23

Case 3 A 34-year-old male with ESRD due to glomerulonephritis dialyzed for four hours, three times a week. He had a total parathyroidectomy for severe hyperparathyroidism in January, 1988 and was stable on 3 g/day of calcium as $CaCO_3$. In January 1990 he was started on prednisone 30 mg daily for myopathy, identified as idiopathic inclusion body myositis. One month later he was asymptomatic but markedly hypophosphatemic. He was repleted and Pi was subsequently normal.

Calcium-free dialysis was carried out as described previously using a concentrate (Biopharm, Laval, Quebec) which, after 1:13.5 dilution, with a Hospal Monitral/S proportioning unit, gave a dialysate with a Na of 142 mmol/l, a Cl of 108 mmol/l, a bicarbonate of 34 mmol/l, a Mg of 0.8 mmol/l and a pH of 8.3. Potassium was added on an individual basis. This was usually 1.5 mmol/l final concentration. Calcium was infused into the venous drip chamber as 10% $CaCl_2$, injectable USP, at rates of 15 or 20 ml/hour (10 or 13.3 mmol/hour of elemental calcium) using an Abbott/Shaw Lifecare pump – Model 3. All spent dialyzate was collected, the volume determined by weighing and an aliquot taken for calcium and Pi analysis. The flow rate was 0.5 l/min.

Pi was initially added to the concentrate container (10 l) as a solid mixture of mono and dibasic sodium phosphate, Case 1. Because of the time and shaking required to solubilize, the addition of a liquid solution is preferable. This can be made but is available commercially as either Fleet Enema® or Fleet Phospho-Soda® buffered saline laxative as suggested previously [Ing et al. 1983]. 100 ml of the former, or 35 ml of the latter added to 10 l of concentrate will give 1 mmol/l Pi after dilution and was used for Cases 2 and 3.

Biochemistry was done in the Clinical Chemistry laboratory except for ionized calciums which were measured in the Research laboratory using a Nova II analyzer. Similarly, parathyroid hormone was determined using the Nichols Allegro IRMA Kit which employs a two-site antibody technique for measuring only intact hormone. All results in this paper were from a single assay.

Results

The findings for each patient are shown in Table 1. In each instance, hypophosphatemia was

® C. B. Fleet Co. Inc., Lynchburg, VA, 24506, USA.

corrected into the normal range by the end of the four hour dialysis. This occurred with a transfer of Pi from the dialysate into the body (29.4–35.5 mmol). Associated with the rise in serum Pi was a fall in calcium unless sufficient calcium was infused as in Case 2. The drop in calcium was particularly striking in Case 3. This patient was totally parathyroidectomized and was unable to mobilize calcium from bone by secreting PTH. Net calcium balance calculated from the calcium infused, minus that analyzed in the spent dialyzate, was close to equilibrium being −0.6, +4.2 and −3.5 for each of the three cases. In subsequent dialyses, using the same parameters but without added Pi, the calcium balance for Case 1 was +1.2 and +1.0 mmol, for Case 2 it was +9.5 and +9.5 mmol and for Case 3 it was +1.5 mmol. Each value is for a single dialysis.

Discussion

A simple technique for correcting or preventing Pi loss from patients on hemodialysis is desirable. The use of a calcium-free dialysate has multiple applications and is particularly useful in these circumstances. Although Pi can be added to regular bicarbonate concentrate, it requires a double proportioning system and careful removal of precipitated calcium phosphate from the equipment after use. This is not necessary with the present system as it is calcium-free until distal to the dialyzer and can be used with a single proportioning system.

The fall in total and ionized calcium when only 15 ml/hour of $CaCl_2$ is infused, is of interest. As calcium cannot be lost in the urine and the parathyroid glands are stimulated (if present), then the hypocalcemia could be due to calcium lost into dialyzate, metastatic calcification or a change in the flux of calcium into or out of bone. The dialyzate loss of −0.6 mmol for Case 1 is unlikely to have decreased the serum calcium. In Case 3, the loss of −3.5 mmol in a parathyroidectomized patient on steroids could be responsible for some of the fall in serum calcium. The larger negative balance in this patient was due to the use of a high flux dialyzer without compensatory increase in the calcium infusion rate. Precipitation can probably be excluded as the fall in calcium occurred with a normal or low (Case 3) calcium phosphorus product and the serum calcium is improved, rather than worsened, when the calcium infusion rate was increased (Case 2). Based on in vitro data, it was found that an increase of 1 mmol/l in inorganic phosphorus would produce a fall of 0.018 mmol in ionized calcium [Adler et al. 1985]. Using Case 3, where the compensatory effect of increased PTH secretion is absent, there was a drop in ionized calcium of 0.45 mmol/l which was more than twenty times the expected fall. Previous studies have shown that Pi can affect bone resorption [Thompson et al. 1975, Baylink et al. 1971] and that acute changes in Pi can alter calcium efflux from bone [Somerville and Kaye 1982]. This would seem the most likely explanation for these findings. Extra calcium would need to be infused to compensate for the temporary decrease entering the extracellular fluid from the bone compartment. 20 ml/hour of $CaCl_2$ will do this safely as shown by the result in Case 2. Subsequently, two further dialyses were carried out in this patient using 2 mmol/l Pi in the dialysate and a 20 ml/hour $CaCl_2$ infusion. There was a rise in post dialysis ionized calcium on each occasion (1.16 to 1.21 and 1.20 to 1.21). In a separate study, in a random group of dialysis patients, we have shown that 20 ml/hour of 10% $CaCl_2$ is equivalent to dialysis with 1.75 mmol/l calcium in standard bicarbonate and will consistently elevate the post dialysis ionized calcium and suppress PTH [Kaye and Fischer 1990]. It is recommended that this dose should be used for calcium free dialysis when Pi is added to the dialysate. The only exception might be a patient who is already hypercalcemic and post dialysis hypocalcemia is desired. In someone who is both hypophosphatemic and hypocalcemic, increasing the infusion rate to 25 ml/hour might be required. This could be assessed by following the calcium levels during the procedure. Finally, when using calcium free dialyzate with a large or high flux dialyzer, quantitation of calcium lost is necessary to achieve the correct replacement infusion rate.

Acknowledgements

We wish to thank Dr. P. Somerville for reviewing the manuscript, the nurses of the dialysis unit for their help and Baxter Corporation for financial support. Ms. J. Sears provided expert secretarial assistance.

REFERENCES

Adler AJ, Ferran N, Berlyne GM 1985 Effect of inorganic phosphate on serum ionized calcium concentration in vitro: a reassessment of the "trade-off hypothesis". Kidney Int *28:* 932–935

Baylink D, Wergedal J, Stauffer M 1971 Formation, mineralization and resorption of bone in hypophosphatemic rats. J Clin Invest *50:* 2519

Gagnon RF, Pajel P, Kaye M 1983 Hypophosphatemia-induced hypercalcemia during acute renal failure. Clin Exper Dialysis and Apheresis *7:* 207–218

Ing TS, Purandara VV, Daugirdas JT, Reid RW, Pierce JS, O'Neill CT 1983 Preparation of phosphate-containing dialysate for use in hemodialysis and peritoneal dialysis. Int J Artif Organs *6:* 321–322

Kaye M, Barber E, Vasilevsky M, Langer K 1989 Calcium-free dialyzate: development and applications. Clin Nephrol *31:* 133–138

Kaye M, Fischer D 1990 Changes in intact parathyroid hormone levels following exposure to either differing dialyzate calcium concentrations or calcium-free dialysis with varying calcium infusion rates. Clin Nephrol 34: 84–87

Kurtin P, Kouba J 1987 Profound hypophosphatemia in the course of acute renal failure. Amer J Kidney Dis *10:* 346–349

Ross EA, Nissenson AR 1988 Acid-Base and Electrolyte Disturbances. In: *Daugirdas JT, Ing TS* (eds) Handbook of Dialysis. Little, Brown and Co, Boston/Toronto, ch 22, p 313

Shinaberger JH, Miller JH, von Albertini B, Gardner PW, Coburn JW 1987 Phosphate (P) removal by conventional dialysis (CHD), high efficiency dialysis (HEHD) and high flux hemodiafiltration (HFHDF). Abstract. Kidney Int *31:* 245

Somerville PJ, Kaye M 1982 Action of phosphorus on calcium release in isolated perfused rat tails. Kidney Int *22:* 348–354

Thompson ER, Baylink DJ, Wergedal JE 1975 Increases in number and size of osteoclasts in response to calcium or phosphorus deficiency in the rat. Endocrinol *97:* 283–289

LETTERS TO THE EDITOR

IgA nephropathy: characterization of the light chains
(Smith SM 1990 Clin Nephrol *34:* 93–94)

Dear, Sir, – We read with interest the comments of Dr. Smith on our paper on immunohistochemical characterization of glomerular IgA deposits in IgA nephropathy (IgAN). He refers to his own study on the light chains, in which lambda light chain IgA is the predominant immunoglobulin in IgAN. This may explain the existence of monoclonality of glomerular IgA deposition. We cannot confirm this observation on the monoclonality, glomerular deposition of only IgA1 and lambda light chain, as we found the glomerular deposits of both kappa and lambda light chain in the all cases of both idiopathic and secondary IgAN. On the other hand, some Japanese researchers (1987 Jap. J. Nephrol. 26: 1395) reported that 3 out of 42 patients with IgAN had glomerular deposits of only kappa light chain. This may explain that the diversity of immunopathogenetic mechanisms relates to geographic differences as well as to methodology without ethnic differences.

Sincerely,
Satoru Suzuki, Hirokazu Sato, Masaaki Arakawa

Tubulointerstitial disorders in the kidney associated with primary biliary cirrhosis (PBC)

Sir, – Tubulointerstitial disorders in the kidney associated with primary biliary cirrhosis (PBC) have been described previously. Furthermore, the disorder has been reported to improve both clinically and histologically after undergoing glucocorticoid therapy [Macdougall et al. 1987 Clin Nephrol 27: 36–40]. We have recently seen a PBC patient associated with interstitial nephritis, Sjögren's syndrome and chronic thyroiditis. We therfore attempted to treat her with glucocorticoid.

A 58-year-old Japanese woman was admitted to our hospital because of an evaluation of hypokalemia and an increased serum creatinine level in March 1986. She had been in good health until 1975, when she initially complained of thirst, polydipsia and polyuria. In 1983, she presented at our hospital with liver dysfunction, an increased serum creatinine level and hypokalemia. Diffuse goiter had also gradually developed since 1985. Laboratory data on admission were as follows: SGOT 75 IU/l, SGPT 95 IU/l, alkaline phosphatase 422 IU/l (normal range 30–110), total bilirubin 1.0 mg/dl. The level of serum potassium was 2.9 mEq/l, sodium 142 mEq/l, chloride 101 mEq/l. Serum copper concentration was 209 μg/dl (normal 70–130). Creatinine clearance was 25 ml/minute with a serum creatinine level of 2.0 mg/dl. The values of an arterial blood gas study were within the normal range. Urinary pH after an oral ammonium chloride load was persistently greater than 6.0 (normal below 5.4). Schirmer's test was positive and the salivary flow was diminished. A sialography of the parotid glands showed diffuse sialectasia. The findings of a wedge liver biopsy and thyroid gland biopsy were compatible with stage II of PBC as classified by

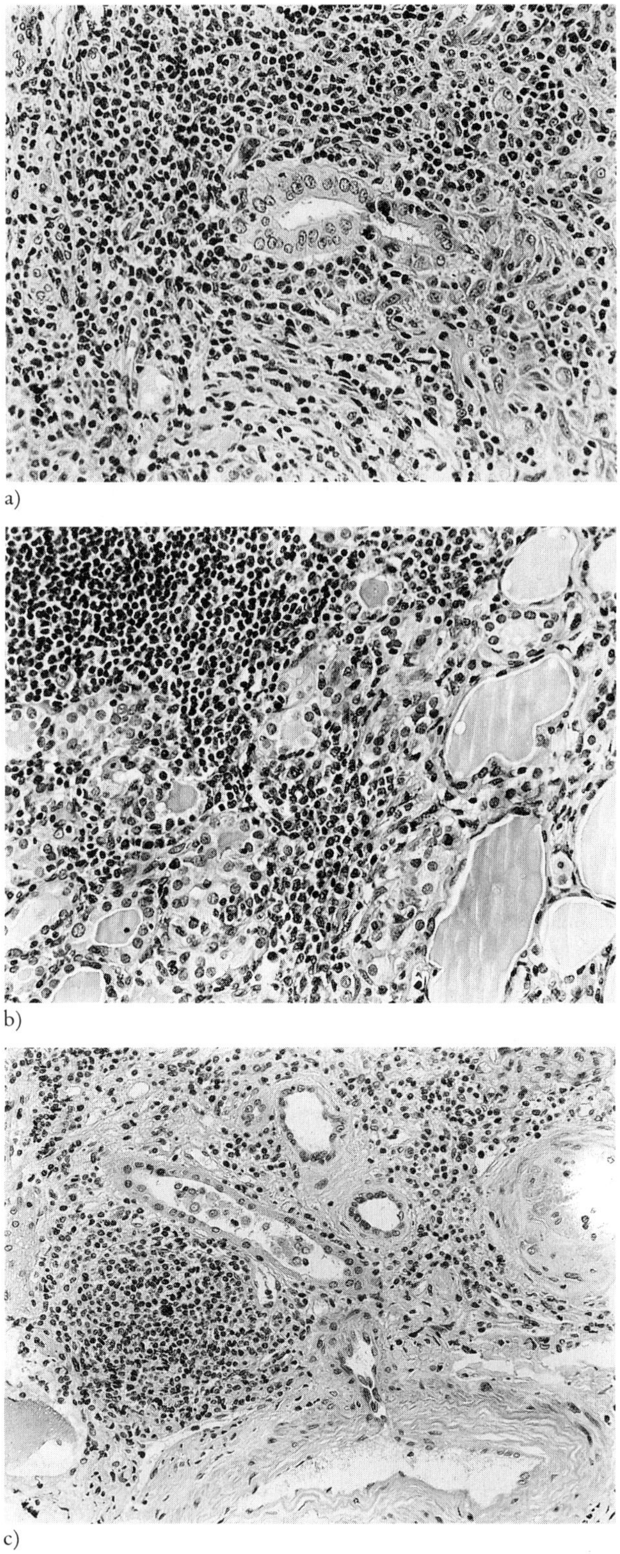

Fig. 1 Biopsy specimens of the liver (panel A, ×250), thyroid gland (panel B, ×200) and kidney (panel C, ×240) showing inflammatory cell infiltration composed predominantly of lymphocytes. This histological similarity suggests that multiple lesions in the liver, thyroid gland and kidney were possibly caused by an autoimmune mechanism characterized by lymphocytic infiltration.

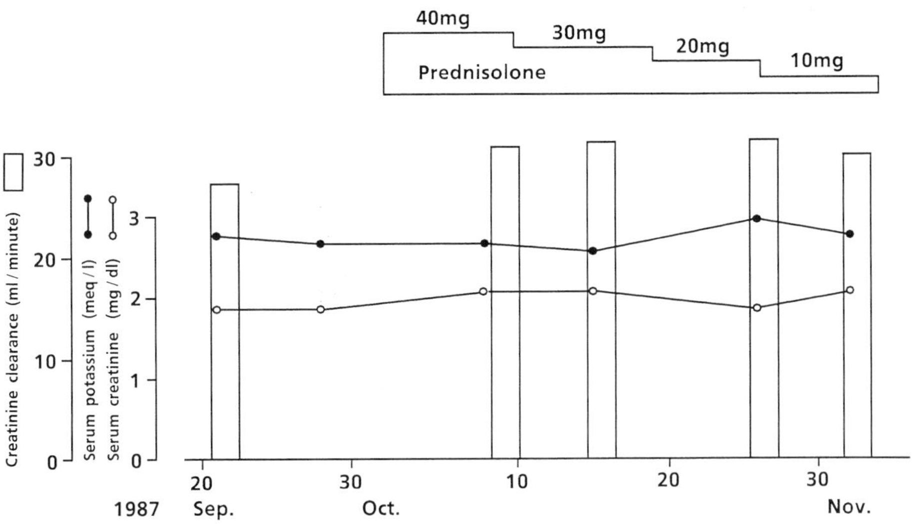

Fig. 2 Serum potassium, creatinine level and creatinine clearance during prednisolone therapy.

Sheuer and struma lymphomatosa. A kidney biopsy specimen contained eight glomeruli and three of them were sclerosed. Tubular epitheliums were partly atrophic and interstitial fibrosis with lymphocyte infiltration were scattered. Immunofluorescent staining showed no fluorescence with IgA, IgG or IgM antisera, or with antisera to C_3 or C_{1q}.

We treated her with a potassium supplement, 24 mEq daily, using potassium chloride. However, the decreased serum potassium level did not improve. Therefore, we initiated glucocorticoid therapy with her consent. She was treated with 40 mg prednisolone daily for nine days. However, the prednisolone also showed no effect on either the serum potassium level or creatinine level (Figure 2). In addition, no improvement in liver or thyroid function was obtained after the prednisolone therapy.

In PBC, extrahepatic lesions and autoimmune disorders have been reported to occur. To our knowledge, there has been no previous report on the co-occurrence of these four diseases including PBC, interstitial nephritis, chronic thyroiditis and Sjögren's syndrome.

An ammonium chlorid loading test revealed a defect in urinary acidification in our case. An association between renal tubular acidosis (RTA) and Sjögren's syndrome has been previously recorded [Shioji et al. 1970 Am J Med 48: 456–463]. RTA has also been known to occur in PBC. It has been postulated that either an inadequate peritubular circulation due to hyperglobulinemia [Pasternack et al. 1970 Acta Med Scand 187: 123–127], the deposition of copper in the distal renal tubules [Leeson and Fourman 1969 Am J Med 43: 620–635, Parés et al. 1981 Gastroenterology 80: 681–686] or a cell-mediated immune response [Golding 1975 Postgrad Med J 51: 550–556, Tsantoulas et al. 1974 Br Med J 4: 491–494] might be the mechanisms for RTA associated with PBC. In our case, a kidney biopsy revealed interstitial fibrosis with lymphocyte infiltration. These findings suggest that RTA is associated with the cell-mediated immune response.

We attempted a four-week course of glucocorticoid therapy (prednisolone 10–40 mg a day). El-Mallakh et al. [1985 Am J Med 79: 509–514] have reported that RTA and focal plasma-lymphocytic interstitial infiltrate in the kidney associated with Sjögren's syndrome improved with a low-dose glucocorticoid therapy (prednisolone 7.5–30 mg a day) over 5½ years. Macdougall et al. [1987 Clin Nephrol 27: 36–40] have also reported both clinical and histological improvements in interstitial nephritis associated with PBC after a seven-week course of high-dose glucocorticoid (prednisolone 40 mg a day). However, in our patient, glucocorticoid did not affect either the serum potassium level, serum creatinine level or the creatinine clearance. Since both glomerular sclerosis and interstitial fibrosis were apparent before glucocorticoid therapy was begun in our case, the desired effects might not have been obtainable by glucocorticoid, which is known to regress tissue mononuclear cell infiltration.

We, therefore, conclude that glucocorticoid should be used to improve renal function as long as glomerular sclerosis and interstitial fibrosis have not yet progressed. Since the optimum dose and period of administering glucocorticoid for improving clinical findings has yet to be elucidated, we should carefully consider both the benefits of glucocorticoid therapy and the increased risk of side reactions.

M. Kamouchi, H. Tsuji, H. Hirakata, K. Okamura, T. Ishitsuka, K. Murai, K. Onoyama, M. Fujishima
Second Department of Internal Medicine, Faculty of Medicine, Kyushu University, Maidashi 3-1-1, Higashi-ku, Fukuoka 812, Japan

Hypozincemia in nephrotic syndrome

Sir, – Zinc deficiency has been reported in patients with nephrotic syndrome [Lindeman et al., 1978, Reimold 1980, Mahajan et al. 1985]. The cause of hypozincemia in nephrotic syndrome is not clear. It may be related to increased urinary excretion of Zn, decreased dietary intake of Zn or decreased intestinal absorption of Zn, but studies on the latter have not been done.

In this study we used the increase in plasma Zn concentration following a test dose of 22.5 µg elemental Zn given as ZnSO4 to determine the intestinal absorption of Zn.

Patients and methods

Seventeen patients with "minimal changes" nephrotic syndrome were included in the study. Their ages ranged from 4 to 12 years (13 males and 4 females). All patients had nephrotic range proteinuria (>2 g/m 2/24 hours) and hypoalbuminemia (<3 g/ 100 ml). All patients had normal renal functions and blood pressure. None had any illness or gastrointestinal disorder. Seventeen healthy subjects served as controls.

Oral Zn tolerance test was performed in patients and controls by a previously described method [Solomons et al. 1981].

The increase in plasma Zn was estimated at the 2nd and 4th hours after the test dose of 22.5 µg elemental zinc given as ZnSO4. The results were demonstrated as mean increase (mean + SEM) in plasma zinc levels over fasting values plotted against time in hours and were analyzed statistically.

Blood samples for plasma Zn were drawn in the fasting state. Zinc concentration in plasma were measured by atomic absorption spectrophotometer (Perkin-Elmer Model 2380) as previously described (Perkin-Elmer 1971).

Statistical analyses were done on the basis of Student's t-test.

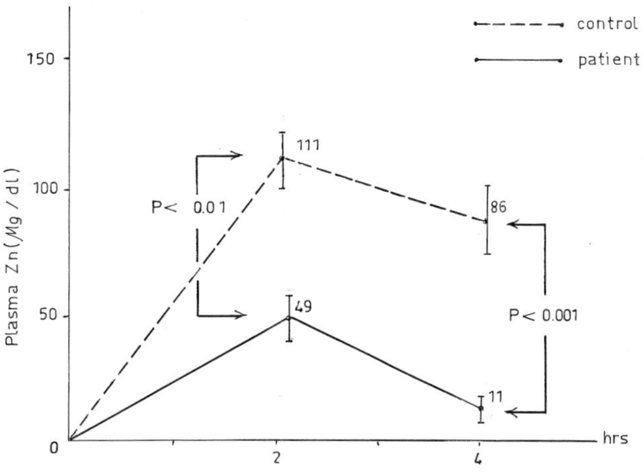

Patient n=17	49.41 ± 8.18	11.41 ± 4.66
Control n=17	111.7 ± 11.81	86.5 ± 13.48

Data are mean ± SEM

Fig. 1 The mean increase in plasma Zn levels in normal and nephrotic children.

Results

The results of oral zinc absorption tests measured on 17 patients and 17 controls are shown in Figure I. The mean increase in plasma Zn concentration over those of fasting values at the 2nd and 4th hours after the test dose of Zn in patients and controls were 49.41 ± 8.18 µg/100 ml vs. 111.7 ± 11.81 µg/100 ml ($p < 0.01$) and 11.41 ± 4.66 µg/100 ml vs. 86.5 ± 13.48 µg/100 ml ($p < 0.001$), respectively.

Discussion

Decreased plasma and serum Zn levels have been reported in patients with nephrotic syndrome. In addition decreased erythrocyte and hair Zn levels have also been demonstrated [Reimold 1980, Mahajan et al. 1985].

The cause of Zn deficiency in nephrotic syndrome is not clearly understood. It has been suggested that the low plasma Zn level may be due to increased urinary excretion of Zn (Mahajan et al. 1985). However, some investigators have not observed significant urinary Zn losses in these patients (Lindeman et al. 1978, Reimold 1980).

We have previously shown that patients with minimal change nephrotic syndrome have low plasma Zn levels. Hyperzincuria was not present in any of our patients. And the low plasma Zn level could not be explained by an increased rate of urinary Zn excretion [Tümer et al. 1989].

Besides hyperzincuria it has also been suggested that decreased dietary intake of zinc and decreased intestinal absorption of zinc may lead to zinc deficiency [Mahajan et al. 1985].

Therefore, Zn absorption was examined in 17 patients with minimal change nephrotic syndrome using the oral zinc tolerance test and comparing results to a healthy control group. Fasting plasma zinc levels (mean + SEM) in our patients before the oral test were significantly lower than those in normal controls (52.411 ± 4 µg/100 ml vs. 81.4 ± 4.2 µg/100 ml $p < 0.01$). After 22.5 µg elementary zinc was given, the increase in plasma zinc was significantly lower in the nephrotic patients than in the control group with $p < 0.01$ in the second hour and $p < 0.001$ in the fourth hour.

Serum protein binding zinc levels were not studied. And the test was not performed when the patients were in remission.

The results of our study suggest that the patients with nephrotic syndrome are Zn deficient and it also suggests that Zn deficiency in nephrotic syndrome may in part be due to decreased intestinal absorption of Zn.

We may conclude that intestinal edema observed in these patients or other unknown factors may cause changes in intestinal epithelial cells accounting for malabsorption of zinc.

N. Tumer, S. Baskan, A. Arcasoy, A. O. Cavdar, M. Ekin
Department of Pediatric Nephrology, Medical School of Ankara University, Ankara, TURKEY

REFERENCES

Lindeman RD, Baxter DJ, Yunice AA, Kreikitpanich S 1978 Serum concentration and urinary excretions of zinc in chirrosis, nephrotic syndrome and renal insufficiency. Am J Med Sci *275:* 17

Mahajan SK, Speck J, Varghese G, Abu-Hamdan D, Migdal S, Briggs W, Prasad A, McDonald F. 1985 Zinc metabolism in nephrotic syndrome. Nutr Res Suppl *I:* 360

Perkin-Elmer 1971 Clinical method's for atomic absorption spectroscopy, determination of zinc in serum. Perkin-Elmer Nowarlk, Connecticut

Reimold EW 1980 Changes in zinc metabolism during the course of the nephrotic syndrome. Am J Dis Child *134:* 46

Solomons NW, Pineda D, Viteri F 1981 Studies on the bioavailability of zinc in humans. Mechanism of the intestinal interaction of nonheme iron and zinc. J Nutr *13:* 31

Tumer N, Baskan S, Arcasoy A, O. Çavdar A, Ekim M 1989 Zinc Metabolism in nephrotic syndrome, Nephron *52:* 95

Infectious mononucleosis

Sir, – Renal complications of infectious mononucleosis are rare and usually benign. We present here a case of infectious mononucleosis in which the diagnosis was arrived at in an unusual fashion.

A 19-year-old male rugby player presented to his personal physician with an 8-day history of anorexia, vomiting and right upper quandrant pain followed by 3 days of diarrhea. He denied muscle pain and did not take any medications or use illicit drugs.

Laboratory evaluation showed a WBC of 10.10^9/l with 0.60 segmented neutrophils and 0.25 lymphocytes. Transaminases were elevated (50 IU/l), while total bilirubin was normal. Most noteworthy was a serum creatinine value of 900 μMol/l. A nephrology consult was obtained. He noted a 10-pound weight gain and dependent edema in the patient. Blood pressure was 165/85 mmHg. Normal urine output was preserved. The patient was hospitalized.

Admission laboratory values were noteworthy for: serum creatinine 2,330 μMol/l; BUN 63.3 mMol/l; serum bicarbonate 18 mMol/l; phosphorus 4.43 mMol/l; potassium 5 mMol/l; uric acid 400 μMol/l; ASLO titer <200 IU/l; and normal values for complement, calcium, and the hemogram. Stool culture and serologic testing for salmonella were negative. Microscopic hematuria was present, and the value for 24-hour urinary excretion of protein was 300 mg. Chest x-ray, plain film of the abdomen, and abdominal ultrasound were normal.

For the first two days, the patient's general condition remained unchanged with persistance of anorexia and profound fatigue.

Approximately 48 hours after admission, the patient developed an erythematous pharyngitis associated with a morbilliform rash. Skin biopsy revealed areas of spongiosis with a discrete exocytosis of mononuclear cells and perivascular inflammation. At this time, serologic investigation for EBV infection was undertaken. A monospot test was positive, and heterophil antibodies were present in a titer of 1:160. VCA titer was 1:32 and EA titer was 1:80. A diagnosis of infectious mononucleosis was made.

The patient's clinical course was favorable, with resolution of his rash within 48 hours after its appearance, as well as a steady decrease in his creatinine level. One month later, his creatinine level has normalized.

This type of presentation has not been reported often within the literature. When it has been, the initial clinical impression does not point to EBV infection, and a correct diagnosis is often made with incidental serologic testing.

Various renal complications have been described but they are usually transitory [Eknoyan and Dillman 1978 Med Clin North Am *52:* 979–1003]. Clinically, one finds renal insufficiency that is usually transient, hematuria, nephrotic syndrome, hemolytic-uremic syndrome, or rhabdomyolysis [Friedman and Libby 1986 Clin Ped *25:* 228–229]. Pathologically, one finds interstitial or tubulointerstitial nephritis with an infiltration of mononuclear cells or glomerulopathies with proliferation of mesangial cells and periglomerular fibrosis [Lowery et al. 1976 South Med J *69:* 1212–1215]. Immunofluorescence is positive for IgA and IgM. The pathogenesis has been attributed to a direct viral effect, hyperuricemia (frequent with infectious mononucleosis), hemolysis, and the cytotoxic effects of certain drugs; however, to this day, the exact cause is unknown.

E. Cassuto-Viguier, D. Barrillon, T. Tibi, P. Jambou, C. Roux, H. Duplay.
Clinique Néphrologique, Hôpital Pasteur, 06000 Nice, France.

ANNOUNCEMENTS

The **Arbeitsgemeinschaft für Klinische Nephrologie e. V.** would be pleased to receive submission of papers from candidates for the Nils-Alwall-Prize- This Prize is awarded to young scientists engaged in clinical research in German speaking regions in the field of nephrology, with particular emphasis on activities involving dialysis or similar methods of extracorporeal elimination or kidney transplants.

The award comprises the Nils-Alwall Medal, a certificate and prize money of DM 15000,–.

The prize may be awarded to up to three nominees.

Candidates up to 45 years of age are required to submit either non-published work, work published up to one year before submission or a summary of original extended research work (but not a habilitation thesis).

If this work involved patients it must explicitly confirm that all relevant ethical principles have been observed (Helsinki Agreement 1964, Tokyo Agreement 1975).

A total of six copies of the paper submitted are required. These are to be in anonymous form and accompanied by a short curriculum vitae and information regarding the candidates present professional activities. These documents are to reach the Chairman of the Prize Committee, Professor Dr. G. A. Jutzler, former Director of the Department of Nephrology *not later than April 15, 1991,* at the following address:

Am Brunnen 2
W-6650 Homburg/Saar, Germany

The **Fourth International Course on Peritoneal Dialysis** will be held in Vicenza, Italy, from May 21–24, 1991. English will be the official language but English-Italian simultaneous translations will be provided.

For further information please write to Dr. M. Feriani, Secretariat of the 4th International Course on Peritoneal Dialysis, Department of Nephrology, St. Bortolo Hospital, I-36100 Vicenza, Italy.

The **XXth Annual Conference of the European Dialysis and Transplant Nurses Association – European Renal Care Association** will take place in Brussels, from June 23–26, 1991. Conference secretariat: Mr. Hervé Bosquet, EDTNA/ERCA Conference, c/o ICSA, Rue Defacqz 1, bte 1, 1050 Brussels, Belgium. Tel.: 32–2–537 4608, Fax: 32–2–537 4800. Scientific secretariat: Mr. Tony Goovaerts, EDTNA/ERCA Conference, c/o UCL St-Luc, Home Dialysis, Avenue Hippocrate 10, 1200 Brussels, Belgium. Tel.: 32–2–764 1862 and Fax: 32–2–764 2836.

The **International Workshop on Alport Syndrome** will take place August 23–24, 1991 in Oulu, Finland. The objective of this workshop is to give a concise picture of the clinical aspects of Alport syndrome. The workshop will also cover the new available approaches for diagnosis. It will be of interest to nephrologists, pathologists, clinical geneticists and to molecular biologists specializing in kidney disease and basement membranes.

Deadline for application is July 1, 1991. Please contact Secretariat, International Workshop on Alport Syndrome, Biocenter and Department of Biochemistry, University of Oulu, SF-90570 Oulu, Finland, Tel: 358–81–352355, Fax: 358–81–352356.

The **VIth International Congress on Nutrition and Metabolism in Renal Disease** will be held August 26–30, 1991 in Harrogate, UK. Topics will include all aspects of nutrition and metabolism in relation to acute and chronic renal disease, with State of the Art lectures, free communications, posters and debates.

For further information, contact Dr. A. Meguid El Nahas (UK Organizing Secretary), Sheffield Kidney Institute, Northern General Hospital, Herries Road, Sheffield S5 7AU, UK. Tel.: 0742-434343 (ext 4017), Fax: 0742-560472.

The **XXVIIIth Congress of the European Dialysis and Transplant Association – European Renal Association** (EDTA/ERA) will be held in Belgrade, Yugoslavia from September 1 to 4, 1991.

For further information, contact the Organizing Secretariat: Yugotours, Congress, Incentive & Exhibition Department, Djure Djakovića 31, Y-11000 Belgrade, Yugoslavia. Tel.: 3811/763-028, 764-622; Telex: 11000, 12902; Fax: 3811/766-447.

The **Second Seminar on Renal Involvement in Systemic Vasculitis** will take place September 21, 1991 in Vimercate, a city near Milan in Italy. Contemporary issues relating to immunopathology of Systemic Lupus Erythematosus, with special regard to anti-endothelial and anti-cardiolipin antibodies, clinicopathological correlations and treatment will be discussed.

For further information please contact Dr. Adalberto Sessa, Unità Operativa di Nefrologia e Dialisi, Ospedale di Vimercate, 20059 Vimercate/Milan, Italy

A **Festakt in honor of Priscilla Kincaid-Smith** will be held on November 5–8th, 1991 in Melbourne, Australia. Events will include state of the art lectures and symposia.

For further information contact The Festschrift Organizing Committee, c/o Department of Nephrology, The Royal Melbourne Hospital, Victoria 3050, Australia.

The **IIIrd International Conference on SLE** will be held in the Queen Elizabeth II Conference Centre, Westminster, London, April 13–15, 1992.

For further details, please contact Dr. Graham Hughes or Mrs. Denzil Fletcher, Rheumatology Department, St. Thomas' Hospital, London SE1 7EH. Tel. and Fax: 016339422.

The **Third Symposium on Uroradiology** (Imaging and Intervention) will take place August 24–27, 1992 at Herlev Hospital, University of Copenhagen, Denmark.

For further information, please contact Dr. Henrik S. Thomsen, Department of Diagnostic Radiology 54E2, Herlev Hospital, Herlev Ringvej 75, DK-2730 Herlev, Denmark. Tel.: 4544/535300, Ext. 278; Fax: 4544/535332.

Clinical Nephrology, Vol. 35 No. 4–1991 (139–147)

Wegener's granulomatosis with renal involvement: patient survival and correlations between initial renal function, renal histology, therapy and renal outcome

K. Andrassy[1], A. Erb[1], J. Koderisch[1], R. Waldherr[2] and E. Ritz[1]

Medizinische Universitätsklinik[1] und Institut für Pathologie[2] der Universität, Heidelberg, Germany

Abstract. Patient survival and renal outcome were followed in 25 patients with biopsy confirmed Wegener's granulomatosis and renal involvement. Fourteen out of 25 patients required dialysis on admission, 11/25 patients did not. All patients were treated with a novel protocol comprising methylprednisolone and cyclophosphamide. The median follow-up observation was 36 months (12–113 months). With the exception of 1 patient (who died from causes not related to Wegener's granulomatosis) all patients are alive. Among the patients initially requiring dialysis (n = 14) 4 are in terminal renal failure after 0, 7, 21 and 38 months respectively. In the nondialysis group (n = 11) only 1 patient subsequently required chronic dialysis 30 months after clinical admission. Renal failure was due to non-compliance with immunosuppressive therapy in at least 2 patients. Percentage of obsolescent glomeruli and the degree of tubulointerstitial lesions, but not active glomerular lesions (crescents, necroses) predicted renal outcome. The major cause of renal functional impairment was relapse of Wegener's granulomatosis usually within 2 years after clinical remission. Therefore prolonged treatment with cyclophosphamide for at least 2 years after clinical remission is recommended. Two patients with initially negative immunohistology had a second renal biopsy which revealed de novo appearance of mesangial IgA deposits.

Key words: Wegener's granulomatosis – rapidly progressive glomerulonephritis – IgA glomerulonephritis – antineutrophil cytoplasmic antibodies

Introduction

Wegener's granulomatosis (WG) is a systemic vasculitis characterized by necrotizing granulomata involving the upper and lower respiratory tract and by crescentic glomerulonephritis. Histological evidence of renal involvement has been demonstrated in 80% of patients at initial evaluation and in 94% on follow-up [Appel et al. 1981]. In the past the most frequent causes of death in untreated patients had been renal and/or pulmonary failure (>80%). Death usually occured [Walton 1958] within 2 years after onset of generalized disease. Since the introduction of treatment with cytotoxic agents, it has been claimed that complete remission can be achieved in over 80% [Fauci et al. 1983]. This form of treatment, however, carries the risks of severe intercurrent infections and toxicity. Undoubtedly treatment of WG with cytotoxic agents has effectively changed survival, but renal prognosis remains still uncertain. According to Appel [Appel et al. 1981], chronic renal failure is less likely to occur in patients with serum creatinine of <1.2 mg/dl or proteinuria of <1 g/day at presentation. The predictive value of serum creatinine prior to treatment is also illustrated by the statement of Fauci [Fauci et al. 1983] that "the risk of ultimate progression to end-stage renal disease in WG was approximately 30% in those patients with glomerulonephritis and azotemia before immunosuppressive therapy was introduced". This has also been emphasized by Pinching et al. [1983] who reported that 10/18 patients with initially severe renal disease had died within 3 years, 7/10 patients during the first months of therapy. Weiss et al. [1985] and Croker et al. [1987] noted that global glomerular sclerosis rather than serum

Received May 30, 1990; in revised form January 2, 1990.

Reprint requests to Dr. K. Andrassy, Medizinische Universitätsklinik, Bergheimerstr. 56A, W-6900 Heidelberg, Germany.

creatinine on admission was the most useful predictor of renal prognosis, adverse renal outcome being certain when more than 65% of glomeruli were sclerosed.

The above conclusions are based on observations in cohorts of limited size. We observed a large series of patients with WG and renal involvement on admission. This prompted us to reexamine renal prognosis and to reassess predictors of adverse renal outcome in our series where patients received cytotoxic treatment which differed from previous studies by being initially more limited in intensity but more prolonged in duration.

Patients

From January 1980 to December 1989 we observed a total of 70 patients with Wegener's granulomatosis. The annual number of admission was 2 patients until 1985 and increased subsequently to 14 patients. This was mainly due to the availability of the ANCA test and the consequent referal of many patients from outside centers. Of these patients 22/70 had limited Wegener's granulomatosis (WG) without urinary abnormalities, 3/48 had abnormal urinary sediment without elevated serum creatinine and 45/48 had elevated serum creatinine, i. e. >1.4 mg/dl. Of

Table 1 Clinical presentation

Pat. No.	Age/ Sex*	History (months)	Organ-Involvement** kidney	lung	ear	nose	eye	nervous system	arthralgia	Duration of dialysis treatment (days)
Conservative treatment group										
1	48 M	8	+	–	+	+	+	+	+	–
2	64 F	6	+	–	–	+	+	–	–	–
3	39 F	2	+	+	+	–	–	–	–	–
4	50 M	2	+	+	+	+	+	–	+	–
5	49 M	1	+	+	+	+	–	+	+	–
6	47 M	6	+	+	–	+	–	–	+	–
7	28 F	4	+	+	–	+	–	–	–	–
8	52 F	3	+	–	+	–	–	–	+	–
9	65 F	12	+	+	–	+	+	–	+	–
10	52 M	6	+	–	–	+	+	–	–	–
11	67 F	1	+	+	+	+	–	–	–	–
										–
Dialysis group***										
12	56 F	8	+	+	+	+	+	–	+	#¹
13	49 M	3	+	+	+	+	+	–	+	16
14	50 F	2	+	+	+	+	+	+	+	39
15	70 M	6	+	+	–	+	–	–	–	17
16	63 M	2	+	+	–	+	–	–	–	60
17	50 F	3	+	+	–	–	+	–	+	14
18	61 M	1	+	+	–	+	–	–	+	5
19	49 F	5	+	+	+	+	–	–	–	17
20	62 F	2	+	+	+	+	–	–	+	7
21	58 M	11	+	+	+	–	–	+	–	3
22	54 M	9	+	+	–	+	+	–	+	#²
23	53 M	12	+	+	+	+	+	–	+	#³
24	17 F	1	+	+	+	–	+	–	+	21
25	58 M	2	+	–	+	+	–	–	–	14

* F = female, M = male,

** + = positive/present, – = negative/absent

*** dialysis required on admission

#¹ = on chronic hemodialysis 60 months after clinical admission.

#² = on chronic hemodialysis since admission.

#³ = on chronic hemodialysis 7 months after admission.

the 45 patients 25 (13 males, 12 females, median age 52 years, range 17–70 years) had been initially either treated by us or continuously followed in our outpatient clinic. Three patients (pat. No. 12, 13, 23) are included, who had been treated elsewhere and in whom our treatment protocol was not performed; they were later seen in our unit on a consultant basis. Median follow up was 36 months (range 12–113 months). Clinical features are summarized in Table 1. All patients had multiorgan involvement. Clinical diagnosis was based on the involvement of the respiratory tract and the presence of glomerulonephritis. Biopsies documenting a granulomatous process in the upper respiratory tract (nasal mucosa and/or paranasal sinuses) suggestive of WG were available in 20/25 patients, and biopsies of granulomatous inflammation in the lower respiratory tract in 5/25 patients. Patients were analyzed separately in two groups according to whether they initially required hemodialysis (serum urea concentration >200 mg/dl) or not. A relapse was diagnosed if one of the following occured: 1. new development of granuloma; 2. reappearance of hematuria (unrelated to cyclophosphamide induced bladder damage) or erythrocyte casts; 3. rise of ANCA titers by more than two dilutions upon repeated examinations but only in association with clinical signs [Andrassy et al. 1989].

Treatment of patients

Once the diagnosis of WG had been supposed usually before histological confirmation of the disease was available – treatment with immunosuppressive drugs was started. All patients were treated with steroids and cyclophosphamide although the mode of treatment was not uniform (Table 2). The type of treatment chosen depended primarily on clinical acuity and presence of contraindications (e.g. gastrointestinal ulcers, septicemia etc.). Patients with less severe involvement were usually treated with steroid boli, i.e. 250 mg methylprednisolone for 3 days and 100 mg methylprednisolone for further 3 days followed by methylprednisolone (1 mg/kg/day) per os for 8 weeks. Until 1986 patients with severe clinical presentation initially received also oral cyclophosphamide as originally proposed by Fauci [Fauci et al. 1983]; in the following years cyclophosphamide boli were administered i.e. 3 boli of 1 g each within 6–12 weeks depending on the severity of the disease with dose reduction to 750 mg of serum creatinine >5 mg/dl. In some cases with severe intensity of the disease which was initially not controlled, cyclophosphamide po was added in the initial 3–6 weeks. Mesna (Uromitexan®; ASTRA Co., Germany) (sodium 2-mercaptoethanesulphonate; 200 mg every 4 hours for 12 h) was coadministered with i.v. cyclophosphamide to reduce bladder toxicity and a fluid intake of three liters was subsequently maintained in all patients with frequent measurements of urine osmolality to check compliance. In oliguric patients, where the dose of cyclophosphamide was reduced by 25%, urine volume was "pushed" by furosemide and in dialysis dependent patients hemodialysis was performed 6 hours after i.v. cyclophosphamide. Oral cyclophos-

Table 2 Treatment

Pat. No.	Follow up (months)	Total duration of therapy (months)	Cyclophosphamide bolus-therapy (parenteral)#	Oral cyclophosphamide therapy (duration of respective treatment in months)	Relapse after onset of therapy (months)	Time off therapy (months)
Conservative treatment group						
1	36	36	C –	C (15) P (33) A (21)	17	0
2	18	18	C P	C (17) P (18)	–	0
3	13	13	C P	C (11) P (13)	–	0
4	14	14	C P	C (14) P (14)	–	0
5	12	12	– –	C (12) P (12)	–	0
6	36	17	– –	C (17) P (12)	–	19
7	37	31	– –	C (8) P (31) A (19)	–	6
8	104	47	C P	C (17) P (29) A (30)	71	57
9	36	36	C –	C (36) P (31)	–	0
10[1]	25	25	– –	C (25) P (25)	–	0
11	12	12	C P	C (12) P (12)	–	0

Table 2 (Continued)

Pat. No.	Follow up (months)	Total duration of therapy (months)	Cyclophosphamide bolus-therapy (parenteral)#	Oral cyclophosphamide therapy (duration of respective treatment in months)	Relapse after onset of therapy (months)	Time off therapy (months)
Dialysis group						
12[2]	100	36	– –	C (31) P (36)	24, 32, 47, 57	64
13[3]	28	28	– –	C (11) P (10) T (8) A (3)	11	0
14[4]	24	24	C P 7× PF**	– P (24)	12	0
15[5]	36	36	C P	C (15) P (31) A (23)	16	0
16[6]	38	33	C –	C (27) P (23) A (6)	30	5
17	36	36	C –	C (25) P (25) A (11)	–	0
18	101	73	– –	C (73) –	11	28
19	48	21	– P	C (21) P (19)	–	27
20	80	44	– P	C (44) P (38)	60	36
21	113	24	– P	C (23) P (2)	–	89
22[7]	31	31	C P	C (2) P (28) A (10)	–	0
23[8]	68	56	– –	C (?) P (?)	–	12
24	61	61	– – 10× PF**	C (10) P (11) A (51)	43	0
25	72	31	– –	C (25) P (9) A (6)	–	41

\# C = cyclophosphamide, P = methylprednisolone

* A = azathioprine, T-trimethoprim-sulfamethoxazole

** PF = plasmapheresis

[1] = chronic dialysis 21 months after clinical admission.

[2] = patient had 4 relapses when she stopped therapy after each episode of clinical improvement. She had to be put on chronic hemodialysis 60 months after clinical admission.

[3] = after 10 months patient was taken off cyclophosphamide and started on T in an outside center. This was followed by a severe relapse with deterioration of renal function. Clinical remission with residual renal dysfunction was achieved with cyclophosphamide-boli administered according to ANCA-serology.

[4] = treatment with oral cyclophosphamide was prevented by severe chronic Non-A-Non-B-hepatitis. Treatment of relapse possible only with cyclophosphamide-boli and small doses of steroids.

[5] = early switch from cyclophosphamide to azathioprine.

[6] = patient died 38 months after clinical admission because of respiratory failure due to asbestosis; no evidence of active WG-disease.

[7] = on chronic hemodialysis since clinical admission.

[8] = chronic hemodialysis 7 months after admission with admitted non-compliance. Renal transplantation after 4 years of chronic hemodialysis.

phamide was started after 6–12 weeks in combination with steroids. The oral dose of cyclophosphamide was chosen according to leukocyte counts initially twice per week (Table 3). Leukocyte counts below 4000/µl were avoided. Ten to 12 months after clinical remission steroids were discontinued. All patients were treated with cyclophosphamide for at least 2 years after clinical remission before an attempt was made to switch to azathioprine or to stop treatment. Relapses were given the induction therapy (Table 3) irrespective of whether the patients had renal or extrarenal involvement. All patients received H_2 blockers, antacids and a local antifungal treatment (nystatin) including vaginal ovula until methylprednisolone dosage was below 12 mg/day. Although the majority of patients had fever on admission (24/25) or later in the course, antibiotic treatment was only given if bacteria could be isolated from blood, urine, bronchial or nasal sinus aspirates, or if X-ray examination was strongly suggestive of bacterial infections. A third generation cephalosporin (Cefotaxime) was effective in most patients.

Table 3 Scheme of therapy

Induction therapy
- Methylprednisolone 250 mg i. v. for 3 days
- Methylprednisolone 1 mg/kg/day per os for 8 weeks
- Cyclophosphamide 1000 mg i. v. (dose reduction for s-creatinine >5 mg/dl) at 2–4 week intervals; Mesna 200 mg i. v. every 4 hours for 12 hours; in severe cases cyclophosphamide (1–2 mg/kg/day) per os in addition;

Maintenance therapy
- Methylprednisolone per os, <20 mg/day, depending on disease activity for at least 9 months after clinical remission
- Cyclophosphamide per os for at least 2 years after clinical remission. Dosage dependent on leucocyte counts:

Leucocytes	>7000/µl	150 mg/day
	>5000/µl	100 mg/day
	>4000/µl	50 mg/day
	<4000/µl	interruption

Methods

Renal biopsies

Percutaneous renal biopsies were performed in 17/25 patients after a median of 26 days (2–570 days) following admission and after treatment had been started. Immunofluorescence microscopy was carried out as described [Waldherr et al. 1983] using FITC conjugated monospecific antisera to IgA, IgG, IgM, Clq, C4, C3c, C3d, properdin, fibrinogen related antigen and albumin (Behring Werke, Marburg, Germany; Dako Co., Copenhagen, Denmark). For light microscopy standard stainings were applied [Waldherr et al. 1989] i.e. hematoxylin and eosin, trichrome light green, periodic acid-shiff and chromotrope 2 R silver methenamine.

Laboratory investigations

Routine analysis, urinary protein, urine sediment, HBV, HCV, ANA, ds-DNA ab, GBM ab, cryoglobulins, complement factors and ANCA were measured as described elsewhere [Andrassy et al. 1989].

Results

Patient survival

A 11 patients except one are still alive. Death in the one patient was unrelated to WG; hemodialysis had to be reinstituted 38 months after clinical admission; he succumbed to respiratory failure from asbestosis 5 months after concluding cytotoxic therapy with no signs of active WG. The median duration of clinical signs and symptoms for the diagnosis of WG was 3 months (range 1–12 months) in the dialysis group and four months (range 1.1–12 months) in the conservative treatment group (Table 1).

Results of renal biopsy

Results of renal histology are shown in Table 4. "Crescentic" glomerulonephritis (including focal-segmental proliferative glomerulonephritis with crescents <50% of glomeruli and typical crescentic glomerulonephritis with crescents >50% of glomeruli) without significant immunoglobulin deposits was found in 8/8 patients of the conservative treatment group who had a kidney biopsy. Tubulointerstitial lesions were usually focal and mild; the percentage of sclerotic glomeruli never exceeded more than 20% of all glomeruli examined. Similarly, in the dialysis group all patients suffered from crescentic glomerulonephritis without significant immunodeposits. However, tubulointerstitial lesions were more severe than in the conservative treatment group and the percentage of obsolescent glomeruli ranged from 20–90%. No significant difference regarding the number of glomeruli affected by crescents or necrosis or the extent of glomerular crescent formation was noted between both groups. One patient (#24) had diffuse granulomatons (crescentic) glomerulonephritis. In 3 patients (#15, #16 and #24) biopsy was repeated after 6, 9 and 24 months following clinical admission because of deteriorating renal function and/or reappearance of urinary abnormalities. In all cases the number of sclerotic glomeruli had markedly increased. Two patients (#15 and #16) with originally negative non-specific renal immunohistology revealed mild to moderate mesangial IgA deposits on rebiopsy. Vasculitis of renal arterioles (arteriolitis) was observed in four patients. Additional inflammation of small and/or medium sized arteries was not noted in any patient.

Evolution of renal function

Ten of 11 patients of the conservative treatment group had stable renal function with normal serum creatinine levels at follow up but one patient required maintenance dialysis after 36 months despite immunosuppressive therapy and despite no extrarenal WG disease activity. In patients initially requiring dialysis, one patient had never been taken off dialysis and three patients who had had remission initially went subsequently into terminal renal failure after 7, 21 and 38 months respectively. The cause of the progression into end-stage renal failure was non-compliance with treatment in at least two patients. The cause of one further patient (#13) is of interest since after 10 months of immunosuppressive therapy he was switched to monotherapy with trimethroprim/sulfamethoxazole [DeRemee et al. 1985] in another institution; he had rapid deterioation of renal function but stabilised at an elevated serum creatinine level after reinstitution of immunosuppressive therapy. Of the patients who initially required hemodialysis only 3/14 had normal serum creatinine one year after admission and median serum creatinine at this time was signifi-

Table 4 Renal histology – correlation to renal outcome

Pat. No.	Glomeruli with crescents/necrosis (percent)	Glomerular obsolescence (percent)	Tubulointerstitial lesions*	Serum-creatinine (mg/dl) at 0 months after clinical admission	6 months after clinical admission	last follow up (months after admission)
Conservative treatment group						
1	67	8	1+	2.0	0.9	1.0 (36)
2	100	–	1+	2.3	1.4	1.4 (24)
3	33	17	1+	5.2	1.6	1.2 (24)
4	73	–	1+	3.2	1.3	1.1 (24)
5	–	–	–	0.8	1.3	1.3 (24)
6	–	–	–	1.8	1.0	1.4 (36)
7	–	–	–	1.3	0.9	0.9 (36)
8	92	–	1+	3.9	1.2	1.2 (104)
9	34	11	1+	1.5	2.7	1.7 (36)
10	70	–	1+	1.7	4.0	D[a] (21)
11	80	–	1+	4.6	0.9	0.9 (24)
Dialysis group						
12	50	50	2+	3.8	–	D[b] (60)
13	17	83	3+	8.8	3.8	5.0 (24)
14	–	–	–	8.9	1.0	0.9 (24)
15[1]	50 (33)	– (25)	2+ (2+)	7.0	1.8	1.8 (36)
16[1]	58 (–)	8 (67)	2+ (2+)	8.1	2.1	D[c] (37)
17	80	20	2+	9.6	1.8	1.0 (36)
18	50	25	2+	12.4	1.7	2.4 (101)
19	–	–	–	9.6	1.0	0.8 (48)
20	–	–	–	6.2	1.2	0.8 (80)
21	50	50	2+	9.6	2.4	3.6 (113)
22	–	–	–	10.2	D[d]	
23	100	–	1+	2.3	13.5	D[e] (7)
24[1]	100 (5)	– (90)	– (3+)	9.1	1.4	2.0 (61)
25	–	–	–	16.8	1.5	1.4 (72)

* tubular atrophy and interstitial fibrosis: 1+ (mild focal), 2+ (moderate), 3+ (severe)

[1] rebiopsy of kidney, in brackets findings at rebiopsy

D[a] chronic hemodialysis 21 months after clinical admission.

D[b] chronic hemodialysis 60 months after clinical admission.

D[c] chronic hemodialysis 37 months after clinical admission.

D[d] chronic hemodialysis since clinical admission.

D[e] chronic hemodialysis 7 months after clinical admission.

cantly higher (1.5; range 0.9–4.0 mg/dl) in the dialysis group than in the conservative treatment group (median 1.1; range 0.7–5.2 mg/dl).

Predictors of renal outcome

Apart from initial requirement of maintenance hemodialysis (see above) renal biopsy findings were predictive of renal outcome. Crescentic glomerulonephritis was found with similar severity in patients with conservative treatment and patients initially requiring hemodialysis. However, the number of obsolescent glomeruli and the degree of tubulointerstitial lesions (tubular atrophy, interstitial fibrosis) were more severe in the hemodialysis group. Hematuria and/or erythrocyte casts were initially demonstrable in all patients. After 1 year on immunosuppressive therapy, hematuria had completely disappeared in all patients who initially did not require hemodialysis (with the exception of patients who had a relapse), but was consistently present in those patients initially requiring dialysis. Marked proteinuria above 2 g/d was paradoxically more frequent in patients not requiring dialysis (5/11 vs 3/14). But under immunosuppression a transient increase of proteinuria into the nephrotic range (>3 g/d) was more frequent in the group requiring dialysis (5/14 vs 1/11). Proteinuria after 1 year was more marked in patients requiring dialysis median 1.4 (0.1–4.7) g/d vs median 0.8 (0.1–2.1) g/d.

Extrarenal disease

ESR was elevated in all patients, a hemoglobin level <12 g/dl was found in 21/25 patients. Leucocytosis (>10000/µl) was detected in 14/25 patients, thrombocytosis (>400.000/µl) in 10/25 patients. The frequency of elevated ESR, anemia, leucocytosis and thrombocytosis was similar in non-dialysis and dialysis dependent patients. The classical staining ANCA pattern was noted in 21/22 patients (median titer 1:160, range 1:20–1:1280; one patient had atypical perinuclear staining). ANA and other serological tests were negative upon repeated examination.

Discussion

Patients survival

The present report deals with the largest series of patients suffering from WG and renal failure seen in one center and treated according to uniform protocol. The salient features are (1.) renal outcome is not uniformly good: some patients having achieved partial renal remission progressed to end stage renal failure without extrarenal disease activity; this opposed previous opinion [Fauci et al. 1983] but is in line with more recent observations [Pinching et al. 1983]. (2.) present treatment protocol with initial bolus treatment (methylprednisolone and/or cyclophosphamide) yields excellent patient survival in contrast to high case fatality rates previously reported for other treatment schedules [Ten Berge et al. 1985, Adu et al. 1987, Gans et al. 1990]. In the present series only 1 patient was lost for causes unrelated to treatment and disease activity. It is useful to view current patient survival in historical perspective. Prior to introduction of immunosuppressive treatment median patient survival was 5 months, less than 20% surviving after 1 year and less than 10% after 2 years [Walton 1958]. Since the introduction of immunosuppressive drugs survival has steadily increased and remission is achieved in more than 80% [Fauci et al. 1983]. The immunosuppressive regimens originally introduced were fraught with considerable mortality mainly from bacterial and/or viral infections. In the study of Pinching [Pinching et al. 1983] 4/18 patients with WG or the related microscopic polyarteritis who had renal involvement died from infection during the induction phase. Similar observations were reported by Gans [Gans et al. 1989]; they noted 40% overall mortality after 3 years of therapy, all deaths resulting from infectious complications. In the series of Ten Berge [Ten Berge et al. 1985] 3/12 patients with severe renal disease died from infections in the induction phase and another 2 during relapse. Adu [Adu et al. 1987] reported a 62% actuarial 1 year survival in 43 patients with microscopic polyarteritis/WG and renal involvement. The major cause of death was again sepsis from pulmonary infections.

These unsatisfactory results prompted efforts to find out the optimal dosage of immunosuppression i.e. treatment intensive enough to control disease activity but restraint enough to avoid fatal infections. In this context our observation of no mortality during treatment is of interest. There are good arguments that renal failure at presentation is, in part, related to superimposed acute renal failure. If this is so, serum creatinine and urea are not good criteria for immune injury to the kidney. A high case fatality in the first months of treatment [Pinching et al. 1983, Ten Berge et al. 1985, Gans et al. 1990] prompted our policy to avoid prolonged high dose cyclophosphamide treatment in the induction phase. Low infection rates were seen as in the recent communication of Keller [Keller et al. 1989] on patients with rapidly progressive glomerulonephritis (RPGN). Keller noted only 2 deaths from infections in 46 patients. His protocol, however, may not have been aggressive enough, since of 25 patients initially requiring dialysis 22 had to continue on dialysis. This contrasts with our observation: only 1/25 patients failed to have initial remission which permitted to stop dialysis. A similar outcome was also reported by Falk [Falk et al. 1990] in a recent prospective study on 70 patients with ANCA positive glomerulonephritis, comprising WG and microscopic polyarteritis. Six deaths were noted among 70 patients. Death occured exclusively within the first days after clinical admission and was due to disease activity. Patient and renal survival were 78% after 22 months. This combined experience illustrates that excessive immunosuppression [Adu et al. 1987] can be avoided without the risk of undertreatment. In contrast to previous recommendations [Fauci and Wolff 1973] an effort should be made to avoid leukocyte counts below 4000/µl. Since today WG and related disorders can be readily diagnosed using the ANCA test [van der Woude et al. 1985] delay of treatment is easily avoided and this may also help to reduce the risk of infectious complications. The decision to stop maintenance therapy should consider clinical evidence of disease activity, routine laboratory tests (ESR, CRP, hemoglobin) and results of the ANCA test.

Renal course

Renal outcome in our patients deserves comment. We confirm recent suggestions of Couser et al. [1988] that adverse renal outcome is more likely in patients initially requiring dialysis. Our observations further extend this issue by showing that active glomerular lesions (crescents, necroses) on initial renal biopsy do not predict ultimate renal outcome. The percentage of sclerotic glomeruli and the degree of tubulointerstitial lesions, however, tended to be more severe in patients with adverse renal outcome. It is of note that serum creatinine at last follow-up was higher in patients requiring initial dialysis; whether this implies a long-term risk of progression of chronic renal disease [Brenner et al. 1982] remains to be seen. Most relapses in our series were seen within 2 years after clinical presentation. This may provide a rationale for the optimal duration of immunosuppressive treatment. Currently we prefer immunosuppression for least 2 years after clinical remission and serological stability have been achieved. It is of interest to compare renal outcome in our patients with past experience. The argument, that ultimate renal prognosis depends on duration of treatment, finds some support in the study of Kuross [Kuross et al. 1981]; he also analysed outcome of patients with WG who were admitted in renal failure requiring dialysis. In 9 patients immunosupression achieved partial renal remission but patients were mostly treated with azathioprine and prednisone and only infrequently with the more effective cylophosphamide. In some patients immunosuppression was stopped when renal function had stabilized. This led to a relapse in 3/9 patients, reminiscent of our observations in cases #12, #13 and #15. Similar results were obtained by Appel [Appel et al. 1981] who had used cyclophosphamide in some patients but – with the exception of 2 patients – gave treatment for less than 1 year. In contrast to our findings he saw frequent progression to end stage renal failure in those patients who initially had high serum creatinine or required dialysis. He found that glomerular histology and extent of proteinuria did correlate with ultimate renal prognosis; this observation is not in line with our findings.

In order to achieve a favourable renal outcome it seems important (1.) to maintain immunosuppression for an adequate period of time, i. e. no less than 2 years after clinical remission and (2.) to aggressively monitor patients to prevent relapses, since relapses were the most common cause of progression of renal failure in our patients. Due to the recent availability of ANCA testing earlier treatment of relapses should prevent cumulative renal damage.

REFERENCES

Adu D, Howie AJ, Scott DGI et al. 1987 Polyarteritis and the kidney. Q J Med *62:* 221–237

Andrassy K, Koderisch J, Rufer M et al. 1989 Detection and clinical implication of antineutrophil cytoplasm antibodies in Wegener's granulomatosis and rapidly progressive glomerulonephritis. Clin Nephrol *32:* 159–167

Appel GB, Gee B, Kashgarian M et al. 1981 Wegener's granulomatosis-clinical-pathologic correlations and long-term course. Am J Kidney Dis *1:* 27–37

Brenner B, Meyer T, Hostetter T 1982 Dietary protein intake and the progressive nature of kidney disease. New Engl J Med *307:* 652–659

Couser WG 1988 Rapidly progressive glomerulonephritis: classification, pathogenetic mechanisms, and therapy. Am J Kidney Dis *11:* 449–464

Croker BP, Lee T, Gunnells JC 1987 Clinical and pathologic features of polyarteritis nodosa and its renal-limited variant: primary crescentic and necrotizing glomerulonephritis. Hum Pathol *18:* 38–44

Falk RJ, Hogan SL, Jennette JC 1990 A prospective cohort study of 70 patients with anti-neutrophil cytoplasmatic autoantibody (ANCA)-associated glomerulonephritis (GN). Abstracts Am Kidney Int *37:* 256

Fauci AS, Haynes BF, Katz P et al. 1983 Wegener's granulomatosis: prospective clinical and therapeutic experience with 85 patients for 21 years. Ann Intern Med *98:* 76–85

Fauci AS, Wolff SM 1973 Wegener's granulomatosis: studies in 18 patients and a review of the literature. Medicine *52:* 535–561

Gans ROB, Kuizinga NÇ, Goldschmeding R et al. 1990 Clinical features and outcome in patients with glomerulonephritis and anti-neutrophil cytoplasmatic autoantibodies (ANCA). Abstracts Kidney Int *37:* 275

Keller F, Oehlenberg B, Kunzendorf U et al. 1989 Long-term treatment of rapidly progressive glomerulonephritis. Clin Nephrol *31:* 190–197

Kuross S, Davin T, Kjellstrand CM 1981 Wegener's granulomatosis with severe renal failure: clinical course and results of dialysis and transplantation. Clin Nephrol *16:* 172–180

Pinching AJ, Lockwood CM, Pussell BA et al. 1983 Wegener's granulomatosis: observations on 18 patients with severe renal disease. Q J Med *52:* 435–460

DeRemee RA, McDonald TJ, Weiland LH 1985 Wegener's granulomatosis: observations on treatment with antimicrobial agents. Mayo Clin Proc *60:* 27–32

Ten Berge IJM, Wilmink JM, Meyer CJLM et al. 1985 Clinical and immunological follow-up of patients with severe renal disease in Wegener's granulomatosis. Am J Nephrol *5:* 21–29

Van der Woude FJ, Rasmussen N, Lobatto S et al. 1985 Autoantibodies against neutrophils and monocytes. Tool for diagnosis and marker of disease activity in Wegener's granulomatosis. Lancet *1:* 425–429

Waldherr R, Seelig HP, Rambausek M et al. 1983 Deposition of polymeric IgA in idiopathic mesangial IgA glomerulonephritis. Klin Wschr *61:* 911–915

Waldherr R, Rambausek M, Duncker WD et al. 1989 Frequency of mesangial IgA deposits in a non-selected autopsy series. Nephrol Dial Transpl *4:* 943–946

Walton EW 1958 Giant-cell granuloma of the respiratory tract (Wegener's granulomatosis). Br Med J *2:* 265–270

Weiss MA, Crissman JD 1984 Renal biopsy findings in Wegener's granulomatosis: segmental necrotizing glomerulonephritis with glomerular thrombosis. Hum Pathol *15:* 943–956

Clinical Nephrology, Vol. 35 No. 4–1991 (148–150)

Renal failure in adult onset hypophosphatemic osteomalacia with Fanconi syndrome: a family study and review of the literature

N. A. Harrison[1], J. M. Bateman[1], J. G. G. Ledingham[2] and R. Smith[3]

[1]*Department of Medicine, John Radcliffe Hospital, Oxford, England*
[2]*Nuffield Department of Medicine, John Radcliffe Hospital, Oxford, England*
[3]*Nuffield Departments of Medicine and Orthopaedic Surgery, Oxford, England*

Abstract. Follow-up of a previously reported family with dominantly inherited adult onset hypophosphatemic osteomalacia with Fanconi syndrome and diabetes mellitus has shown that both the proposita and her affected sister have developed renal glomerular failure. We describe the evolution of renal failure in this family and discuss the possible mechanisms involved. The development of renal tubular acidosis in this condition further impairs renal function and we suggest that correction of systemic acidosis might improve renal function and prevent further decline in these patients.

Key words: Fanconi syndrome – hypophosphatemic osteomalacia – renal glomerular failure

Introduction

The first adult with the Debre – de Toni – Fanconi syndrome (usually called the Fanconi syndrome) was reported in 1947 [Stowers and Deut]. In 1976, Smith et al. described a family in which hypophosphatemic osteomalacia with Fanconi syndrome occurred in 4 generations. The proposita (DC) and her sister (PR) have now developed renal glomerular impairment. Both now have children who may develop the syndrome and be at risk of eventual renal failure. We discuss the development of renal failure within the family, and suggest that the rate of decline of renal function and the associated osteomalacia might benefit from early correction of associated renal tubular acidosis.

Family study

DC's family tree is presented at Figure 1, with the additions to the VI generation of her two children. DC, the "proposita", born in 1950, presented at the age of 17 with renal glycosuria. At the age of 20, she developed a waddling gait, and pains in the ribs and left thigh. Proteinuria was first detected at the age of 22, but her continuing symptoms were considered functional despite profound hypophosphatemia. A year later she was unable to climb stairs, and osteomalacia, characterized by Looser's zones in the femora, pseudo-fractures of several ribs, gross hypophosphatemia (0.54 mmol/l) and raised alkaline phosphatase (13 KA units), was confirmed by bone biopsy. Renal glomerular function was normal, but there was generalized aminoaciduria. She improved rapidly on oral phosphate supplementation.

In 1983, an intravenous urogram performed during investigation of infertility was normal. In 1985 her first child was born. Late in 1986, she developed intermittent facial twitching and carpopedal spasms. The plasma calcium was 1.14 mmol/l, and phosphate 1.1 mmol/l. The symptoms were improved when the oral phosphate (Sandoz-Phosphate) was reduced from 5 tablets to 3 daily, although the calcium remained low at 1.55 mmol/l. Investigations performed elsewhere in 1987, showed (for the first time) a raised plasma creatinine 195–218 mcmol/l, and a reduced creatinine clearance of 20–24 mls/min. There was impaired urinary acidification, systemic acidosis and hypokalemia (plasma K 2.8–3.0 mmol/l). The serum calcium was 1.55 mmol/l, phosphate 0.69 mmol/l and parathormone levels were normal (170 and 200 pg/ml). She began treatment with cholecalciferol 40,000 Units/day which was increased to 60,000 units per day 2 weeks later, and the phosphate therapy was stopped. No further follow-up took place, and shortly afterwards she became pregnant again.

Two weeks postpartum, she had nausea, vomiting, severe pains in her shins, and hypersentivity of

Received August 31, 1989; in revised form February 19, 1991.

Reprint requests to: N. A. Harrison, Consultant Physician, Department of Medicine, Princess Mary's RAF Hospital, Halton, UK-Aylesbury, Bucks, HP22 5PS, England.

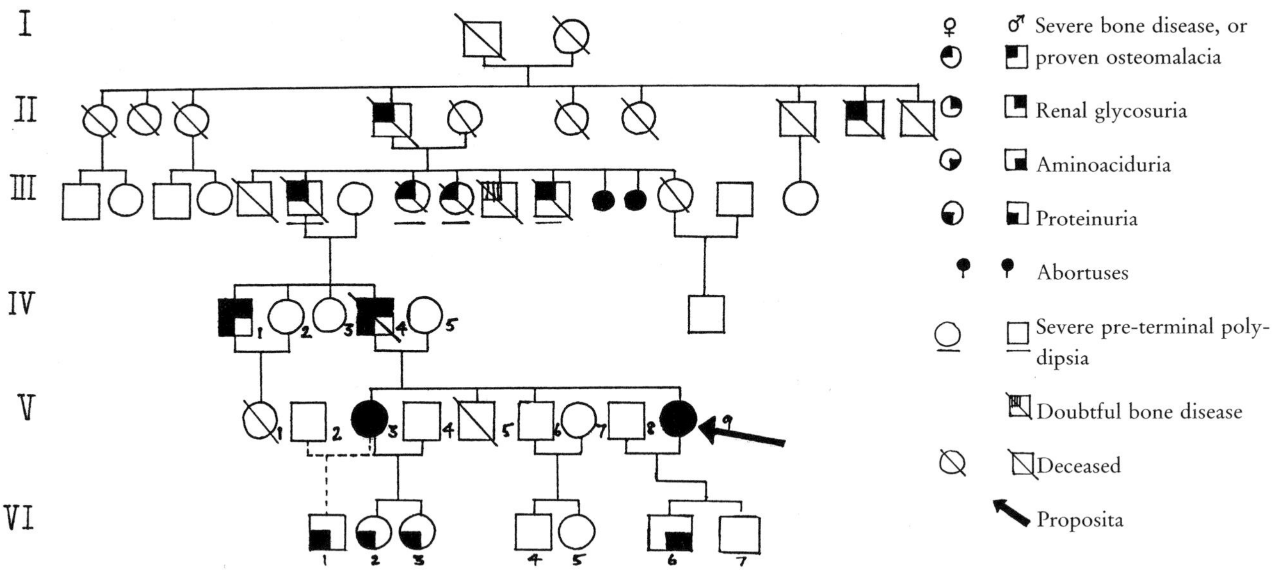

Fig. 1 Pedigree of family. Severe hypophosphatemia in: – IV (1) (4), V (3) (9). Renal failure in: – IV (4), V (3) (9). Diabetes mellitus in: – III (11), IV (4)

her teeth. Her plasma calcium was 3.43 mmol/l, phosphate 1.9 mmol/l, plasma creatinine 355 mcmol/l, and urea 21 mmol/l. A diagnosis of hypercalcemic nephropathy secondary to vitamin D intoxication was made, and the cholecalciferol was stopped. Intravenous saline, loop diuretics and oral prednisolone 20 mg daily were given. Because of a profound systemic acidosis (plasma bicarbonate 10.8 mmol/l, arterial blood pH 7.33 and pCO_2 20 mmHg), 45 mmol per day of sodium bicarbonate was commenced, orally.

Corticosteroids were given for 5 months before the plasma calcium fell to normal. This was associated with an improvement in glomerular function which is now stable with a plasma creatinine of 280–300 mcmol/l. The plasma calcium (2.29 mmol/l) and phosphate (0.9 mmol/l) are also normal without phosphate supplements, and she continues oral sodium bicarbonate 45 mmol/day.

DC's father – IV (4) was severely disabled by adult onset osteomalacia from age 40. At age 36, after 12 years of renal glycosuria he had developed diabetes mellitus, requiring on average 40 units of insulin per day. At age 46, his blood urea was 68 mg/100 ml (10.1 mmol/l), and he was acidotic with a total CO_2 14 mmol/l. An intravenous urogram showed shrunken kidneys. Shortly before his death aged 55, he had a blood urea of 200 mg/100 ml (33 mmol/l) and the 24-hour urinary protein excretion was 4 grams.

DC's elder sister (PR) – V (3) born in 1943, was found in 1974 to have intermittent hypophosphatemia (0.6–0.8 mmol/l), plasma bicarbonate 22 mmol/l, renal glycosuria, proteinuria (0.63 g/l) and generalized aminoaciduria. Bone biopsy and radiographs of her bones were normal. In 1988, she developed bone pains associated with a plasma calcium of 2.15 mmol/l, phosphate 0.6 mmol/l, and alkaline phosphatase 271 U/l (normal up to 300 U/l). At that time she was found to have +++ dipstick proteinuria and impairment of renal glomerular function, with a plasma creatinine concentration 195 mcmol/l. She is at present asymptomatic on oral phosphate replacement alone.

PR's children – VI (1), (2), (3) In 1974, PR's three children (ages 10, 7 and 2 years) all had trace dipstick proteinuria, and marginally low plasma bicarbonate levels (20–22 mmol/l). None has progressed yet within the syndrome. Their plasma phosphate levels are 0.94–1.3 mmol/l, and plasma creatinines 69–96 mcmol/l.

DC's children – VI (6), (7) DC's two children ages 6 and 2 years are well, and do not have aminoaciduria at present.

No other member of the family has evidence of renal disease, but DC's uncle – IV (1), had proteinuria in addition to osteomalacia and renal glycosuria and died aged 35 of undisclosed cause.

Discussion

Renal glomerular failure in the Fanconi syndrome may develop over 10 to 30 years, but its etiology remains obscure [Brodehl 1978]. Structurally the renal tubules are abnormal, with a very short thick proximal tubule joined to the glomerulus by a long thin "swan neck" [Brod 1973]. In the few reports of the histological appearances of biopsies taken from the kidneys of patients with the syndrome, glomerulosclerosis, marked tubular vacuolation and dilatation, and interstitial changes predominate. No glomerular lesion has been consistently observed [Neimann et al. 1968, Friedman et al. 1978, Hunt et al. 1966, Patrick et al. 1981]. The histological appearance of glomerulosclerosis without evidence of glomerular disease suggests that hyperfiltration damage may be instrumental in the glomerular loss [Hostetter 1984].

Functionally the tubules are also abnormal, with tubular leakage of substances normally reabsorbed by the proximal tubules, including glucose, aminoacids, phosphate, and bicarbonate. Losses of the latter two result in the osteomalacia or rickets and acidosis. Therapy in Fanconi syndrome has been based on the observations that replacement of phosphate and bicarbonate relieves symptoms and heals bone [Lanbert et al. 1951, Glorieux et al. 1972]. Phosphate replacement should be tailored to the degree of renal impairment. Impaired tubular function in Fanconi syndrome may affect the glomerulus in several ways. Sodium losses may be important resulting in a reduction of renal blood flow through activation of the renin-angiotensin glomerulo-tubular feedback mechanisms. Acidosis can profoundly reduce glomerular filtration rate (GFR), and also has effects on the pathogenesis of the osteomalacia as reported in both humans and animals. Sirota et al. [1954] reported that correction of acidosis reduced the hyperphosphaturia in an adult with Fanconi syndrome. Shvil et al. [1987] in a rat model of Fanconi syndrome found that in addition to improving GFR and consequently increasing phosphate delivery, correction of acidosis significantly reduced phosphaturia.

Correction of acidosis in DC's case, with the use of oral sodium bicarbonate has had marked benefits. The decline in her renal function, which was apparent before the hypercalcemic episode, has been arrested, and her plasma creatinine remains at 280–300 mcmol/l. Additionally, she no longer requires phosphate or vitamin D supplementation, and maintains normal plasma calcium and phosphate levels.

Of the family, three members have had proven renal failure (IV 4, V 3, and V 9). In addition to these, IV 1 had proteinuria. Unfortunately it is impossible to know how much of DC's father's renal failure was due to diabetic nephropathy.

PR's children, who are all in their early twenties now, are well except for trace dipstick proteinuria, and DC's children are normal. However, in a family pedigree exhibiting late adult-onset Fanconi syndrome, long-term follow-up is essential. Whether early correction of any detected acidosis will affect the progression to renal failure remains to be seen.

REFERENCES

Brod J 1973 "Hereditary and acquired metabolic disturbances of tubular function – Fanconi syndrome". In: The Kidney. Butterworth + Co. (Publishers) Ltd, p 579

Brodehl J 1978 The Fanconi Syndrome. In: Edelmann's "Peadiatric Kidney Diseases". Little Brown Comp, pp 955–987

Friedman AL, Trystad CW, Chesney RW 1978 Autosomal dominant Fanconi syndrome with early renal failure. Am J Med Genetics *2:* 225–232

Glorieux FH, Scriver CR, Reade TM, Goldman H, Roseborough A 1972 Use of phosphate and vitamin D to prevent dwarfism and rickets in X-linked hypophosphatemia. N Engl J Med *287:* 481

Hostetter TH 1984 "The Hyperfiltering Glomerulus" in Symposium on Renal Disease, Medical Clinics of North America *68:* 387–398

Hunt DD, Stearns G, McKinley JB, Froning E, Hicks P, Bonfiglio M 1966 Long-term study of family with Fanconi syndrome without cystinosis (De Toni – Debre – Fanconi Syndrome). Am J Med *40:* 492–510

Lambert PP, de Heinzelin de Braucourt C 1951 Syndrome de Fanconi; un cas chez l'adulte. Acta clin belg *6:* 13–41

Neimann N, Pierson M, Marchal C, Rauber G, Grignon G 1968 Nephropathie familiale glomerulo-tubulaire avec syndrome de Toni-Debre-Fanconi. Arch Fr Pediat *24:*43

Patrick A, Cameron JS, Ogg CS 1981 A family with a dominant form of idiopathic Fanconi syndrome leading to renal failure in adult life. Clin Nephrol *16:* 289–292

Shvil Y, Wald H, Popovtzer MM 1987 Effect of bicarbonate and phosphate on renal phosphate leak in experimental Fanconi syndrome. Am J Physiol *252F:* 310–316

Sirota JH, Hamerman D, Jaffe EE 1954 Renal function studies in an adult subject with the Fanconi syndrome. Am J Med *16:* 138–152

Smith R, Lindenbaum RH, Walton RJ 1976 Hypophosphataemic osteomalacia and Fanconi syndrome of adult onset with dominant inheritance. Quart J Med *179:* 387–400

Stowers JM, Dent CE 1947 Studies on the mechanisms of the Fanconi syndrome. Quart J Med *64:* 275–290

Clinical Nephrology, Vol. 35 No. 4 – 1991 (151–157)

The effect of prostacyclin on intracranial pressure in patients with acute hepatic and renal failure

A. Davenport, E. J. Will and A. M. Davison

Department of Renal Medicine, St. James's University Hospital, Beckett Street, Leeds LS9 7TF, England

Abstract. Prostacyclin was administered on 20 occasions to 12 patients with fulminant hepatic failure complicated by acute renal failure prior to commencing dialysis at a dose of 5 ng/kg·min. Intracranial pressure was noted to increase during the infusion from a median of 12 mmHg (95% confidence limits 9–14) to 17 mmHg (12–25), $p < 0.01$, at the same time the mean arterial blood pressure declined from 79 mmHg (65–82) to 64 (56–70), $p < 0.01$, and the cerebral perfusion pressure from 62 mmHg (53–67) to 44 mmHg (41–55), $p < 0.01$. The changes were greater for those patients who subsequently died from cerebral edema. Patients with fulminant hepatic and acute renal failure are at risk of dying from cerebral edema. The direct administration of prostacyclin, used for extracorporeal anticoagulation, may cause a further increase in intracranial pressure and reduce cerebral perfusion, thus resulting in patient morbidity and mortality.

Key words: intracerebral pressure – liver failure – prostacyclin

Introduction

Patients with fulminant hepatic failure [Bernuau et al. 1986] have a high mortality despite advances in the management of critically ill patients [O'Grady et al. 1988]. Although death usually occurs in the setting of multi-organ failure, cerebral edema remains the most common mode of death [Ware et al. 1971]. Those patients who develop acute renal failure in addition to hepatic failure have been reported to have an even higher mortality [Forbes et al. 1989], due to the increased incidence of cerebral edema and the difficulty in controlling intracranial pressure (ICP) [Forbes et al. 1989].

Patients with fulminant hepatic failure have abnormalities of blood clotting [O'Grady et al. 1986] and are at increased risk of gastrointestinal hemorrhage. This may be due to a maldistribution of blood flow to the gastric mucosa [Knight et al. 1985]. In addition patients with acute liver failure exhibit an abnormal hemodynamic state characterized by an increased cardiac output and reduced peripheral vascular resistance state [Bihari 1985]. This altered distribution of tissue blood flow also occurs in the brain [Ede et al. 1988] and may result in development of cerebral edema [Davenport 1990; Sherlock 1990].

Prostacyclin is produced from arachidonic acid by the vascular endothelium and it is the most potent endogenous inhibitor of platelet aggregation [Moncada and Vane 1979]. Studies have shown that the exogenous administration of prostacyclin can be successfully used as an extracorporeal anticoagulant, either alone [Turney et al. 1981] or in combination with heparin [Turney et al. 1980]. Further studies have shown the benefit of using prostacyclin in patients requiring hemodialysis who were at risk of hemorrhage [Keogh et al. 1984] and in whom conventional heparin extracorporeal anticoagulation was contraindicated.

We have successfully used prostacyclin as an extracorporeal anticoagulant in patients with fulminant hepatic and acute renal failure who had suffered recent hemorrhage and/or marked peripheral thrombocytopenia [Davenport et al. 1988]. However, it was noted that in one patient with grade IV hepatic coma and increased ICP the administration of prostacyclin prior to commencing extracorporeal therapy as directed by the manufacturer's data sheet was associated with a marked increase in ICP. To study this further we carefully evaluated the effect of the administration of prostacyclin when administered for 30 minutes directly into patients prior to commencing dialysis.

Received July 7, 1990; in revised form December 14, 1990.

Reprint requests to Dr. A. Davenport, Department of Renal Medicine, Southmead Hospital, Westbury on Trym, Bristol BS10 5NB, England.

Table 1 Patient details.

Patient no.	Age (years)	Sex	Etiology of FHF	Grade of coma	Serum creatinine (μmol/l)
1	44	M	paracetamol	4	760
2	29	F	fatty liver of pregnancy	4	990
3	26	M	paracetamol	4	650
4	34	F	paracetamol	4	490
5	25	F	paracetamol	4	585
6	26	F	paracetamol	4	760
7	46	M	paracetamol	4	550
8	22	M	paracetamol	4	490
9	22	M	paracetamol	4	660
10	35	M	paracetamol	4	890
11	35	M	paracetamol	4	630
12	25	M	paracetamol	4	760

paracetamol = paracetamol (acetaminophen) self-poisoning

Subjects and methods

Twelve patients with fulminant hepatic failure (FHF) who also developed oliguric acute renal failure, urine output <10 ml/h, were studied on 20 occasions. Patient details are set out in Table 1. At the time of study all patients were treated with elective hyperventilation, $PaCO_2$ <4.5 kPa (34 mmHg) in an attempt to reduce intracranial pressure (ICP) [Ede et al. 1988], sedated with propofol, median dose 100 mg/h (range 50–200 mg/h), paralyzed with atracurium, median dose 1 mg/h (range 0.5–2 mg/h) and given the analgesic alfentanyl, median dose 1 mg/h (range 0.5–2.0 mg/h). In addition all patients were inotrope dependent and all patients were in receipt of a dopamine infusion, median dose 10 μg/kg·min (range 5–50). Eight patients were also treated with dobutamine, median dose 15 μg/kg·min (range 10–50), and seven with noradrenaline, median dose 10 μg/min (range 5–100).

All patients had been referred for dialysis treatment, and prostacyclin was chosen instead of heparin as the extracorporeal anticoagulant on clinical grounds. Nine patients had had recent hemorrhage requiring blood transfusion (8 gastrointestinal and 1 scalp wound), and seven also had marked peripheral thrombocytopenia (platelet count less than 30×10^9/l).

Prostacyclin (Epoprostenol, Wellcome, Beckenham, Kent UK) was made up as per the manufacturer's instructions, and as suggested by the manufacturer's data sheet initially administered centrally at a dose of 5 ng/kg·min before switching the site of the infusion to the extracorporeal circuit. Prior to commencing prostacyclin the pulmonary artery wedge pressure was checked to make sure that the patient was not hypovolemic, then prostacyclin was commenced at 2 ng/kg·min which was increased by 1 ng/kg·min every 5 minutes and then run at 5 ng/kg·min for 30 minutes before starting dialysis.

Measurements were made prior to commencing prostacyclin and then after 30 minutes at 5 ng/kg·min. During this period no additional fluids were given or alteration in inotropic support made unless a life-threatening increase in ICP or reduction in cerebral perfusion pressure occurred.

Measurements

All patients were monitored with indwelling radial arterial catheters and pulmonary artery wedge catheters (American Edwards Laboratories, AHS del Caribe inc, Anasco, Puerto Rico). In addition ICP was monitored using a subdural catheter which had been aseptically inserted in an adjacent operating theatre. All pressures were transduced (Gould P10, Ez, Spectromed, Illinois, USA) and displayed on a single monitor (Mennen Horizon, Mennen Medical, Buffalo, New York, USA). ICP was measured with respect to the frontal burr hole and the cerebral perfusion pressure taken as the difference between the mean arterial blood pressure measured at the level of the carotid bifurcation and the ICP [Davenport et al. 1990].

Arterial blood gas tensions were also measured using a hemoximeter (ABL3, Radiometer, Copenhagen, Denmark). Anticoagulation with prostacyclin was assessed using a thromboelastograph (Hellige, Freiburg, Germany).

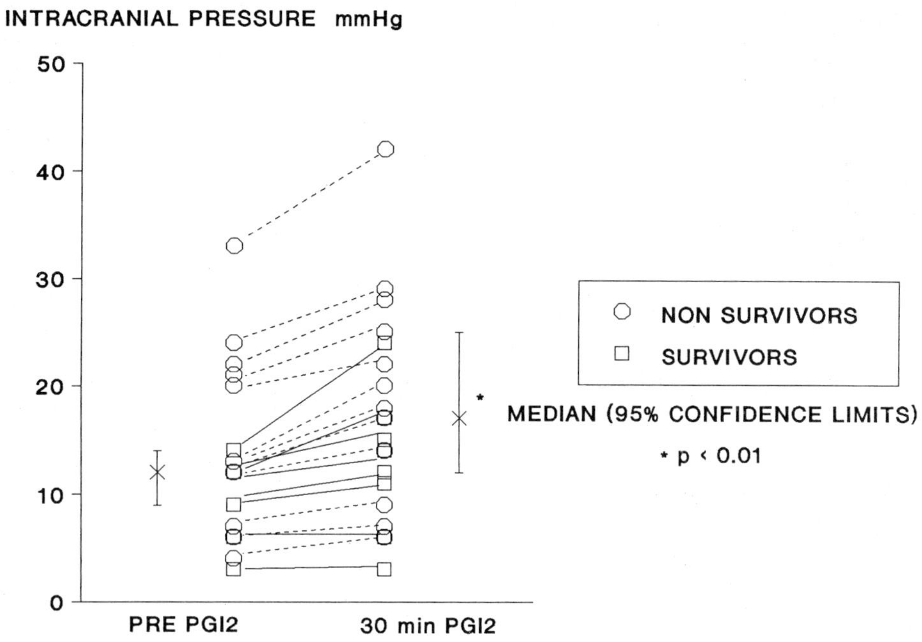

Fig. 1 The effect of prostacyclin infused at 5 ng/kg·min for 30 minutes on intracranial pressure (ICP)

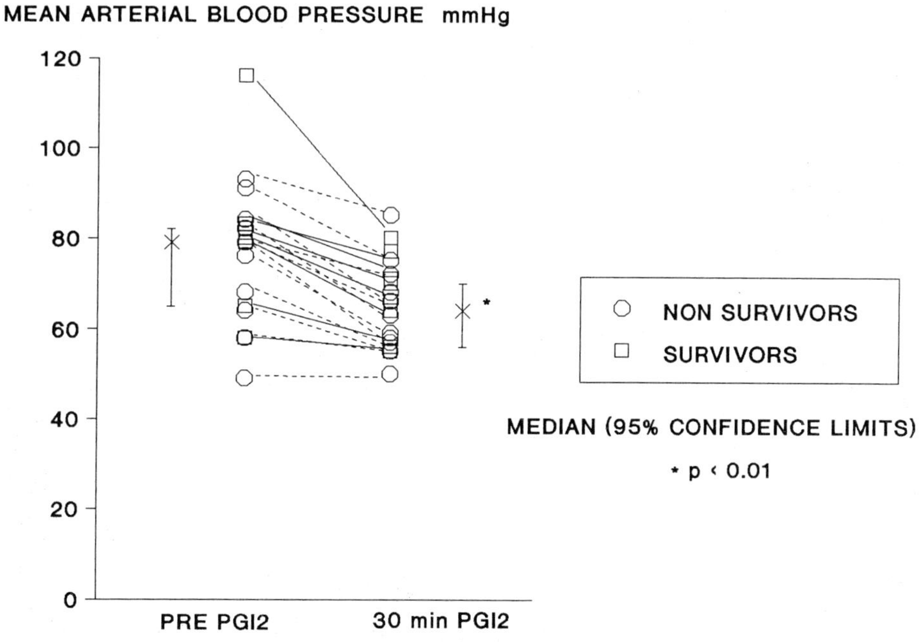

Fig. 2 The effect of prostacyclin infused at 5 ng/kg·min for 30 minutes on mean arterial blood pressure (MAP)

Statistical analysis

Wilcoxon rank sum pair test and analysis of variance were used to analyze the data, and statistical significance was taken at or below the 5% level.

Results

Intracranial pressure increased from a median of 12 mmHg (95% confidence limits 9–14) to 17 mmHg (12–25) following the administration of prostacyclin (Figure 1). At the same time there was a reduction in mean arterial blood pressure from 79 mmHg (65–82) to 64 mmHg (56–70) (Figure 2). Thus the cerebral perfusion pressure was also reduced from 62 mmHg (53–67) to 44 mmHg (41–55) (Figure 3).

Five patients subsequently died from cerebral edema, which was confirmed at autopsy, and 2 others died from endotoxic shock. Five patients survived. The ICP was greater prior to prostacyclin administration in those who died from cerebral edema, median

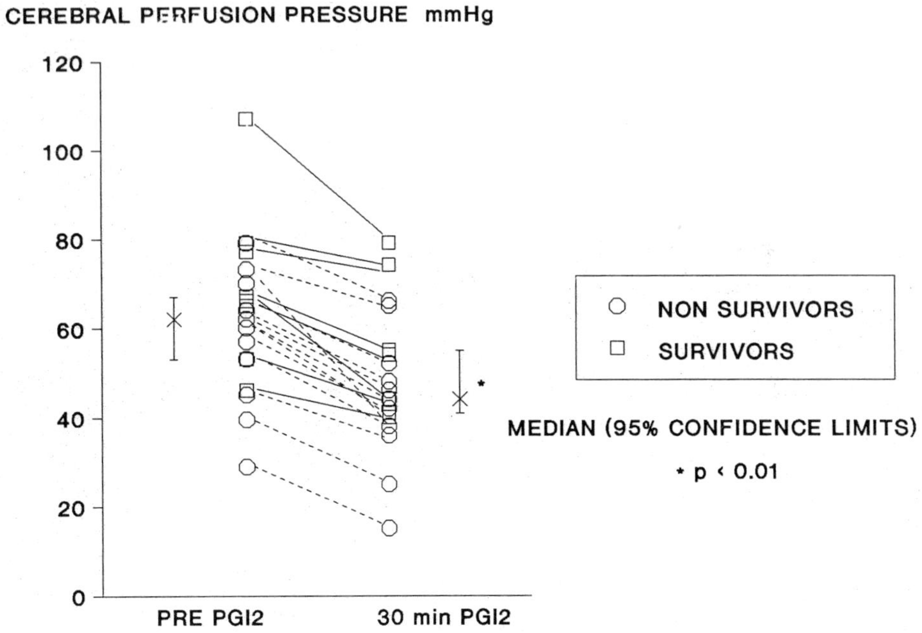

Fig. 3 The effect of prostacyclin infused at 5 ng/kg·min for 30 minutes on the cerebral perfusion pressure (CPP)

22 mmHg (range 6–33) compared to the 7 others, median 12.5 mmHg (range 3–24), $p < 0.05$. Similarly the mean increase in ICP caused by prostacyclin was greater in the group who subsequently died from cerebral edema, 5 ± 2 mmHg (SEM) compared to 1 ± 1 mmHg in the other group. All those who subsequently died from cerebral edema required noradrenaline to sustain the arterial blood pressure compared to only one of the survivors. Similarly the group who died from cerebral edema had a lower cerebral perfusion pressure prior to the administration of prostacyclin than the others, mean 59 mmHg (range 27–79) compared to 70 mmHg (46–107), $p < 0.05$, and prostacyclin produced a greater fall in the former group to 41 mmHg (15–66) compared to the others 55 mmHg (36–74), $p < 0.05$. Prior to prostacyclin the cerebral perfusion pressure was less than 50 mmHg in 20% of cases and following prostacyclin was below 50 mmHg in 65% of cases.

Prostacyclin also caused a reduction in the median pulmonary artery pressure from 12 mmHg (9–14) to 10 mmHg (8–13), $p < 0.05$; and a reduction in the right atrial pressure from 10 mmHg (7–12) to 7 mmHg (5–9). Despited elective hyperventilation, prostacyclin also caused a reduction in arterial oxygen tensions from a median of 17.3 kPa (11.6–17.3) to 14.6 (10.7–18.0), $p < 0.05$. There were no changes in arterial carbon dioxide tensions [pre 3.93 kPa (3.5–4.5) vs 4.1 kPa (3.6–4.4)]. There was a minor, but statistically significant increase in arterial hydrogen ion concentration following the administration of prostacyclin from a median of 30 nmol/l (22–47) prior to prostacyclin, to 31 nmol/l (23–51) following 30 minutes of prostacyclin, $p < 0.05$.

The administration of prostacyclin resulted in an increase in both the reaction time from a median of 7.5 min (4–10) to 11 min (8–22), $p < 0.05$; and clot formation time from 7 min (4–37) to 17 min (11–37), $p < 0.05$; and a reduction in the maximum amplitude recorded by the thromboelastograph [Hartert 1971] from 78 mm (43–150) to 53 mm (20–75), $p < 0.05$, a function of both platelet and fibrinogen activity [Marchal et al. 1962].

Discussion

Despite strenuous efforts to control ICP prior to commencing dialysis using elective hyperventilation [Ede et al. 1988], sedation with propofol [Davenport et al. 1989], and optimal positioning all but one patient had an increased ICP prior to commencing prostacyclin. As expected the ICP was greater in those patients who subsequently died from cerebral edema, and cerebral edema accounted for the majority of deaths in this study, confirming the work of others [Ware et al. 1971]. Similarly the cerebral perfusion pressure was also lower prior to the commencement of prostacyclin in those who subsequently died from cerebral edema. Currently there is no recommended cerebral perfusion pressure for patients with FHF complicated by acute renal failure. Previous work based on animal experiments using a mechanical model has suggested a critical perfusion pressure of

40 mmHg, although others have pointed out that in hepatic encephalopathy the blood-brain barrier is abnormal [Ede et al. 1989], and under these circumstances a greater cerebral perfusion pressure is required [Lassen and Christensen 1976], the majority of authors have suggested that a minimal perfusion pressure of 50 mmHg is required to ensure survival [Davenport et al. 1989, Price 1980]. In this study a suboptimal perfusion pressure was present in 20% of cases prior to the administration of prostacyclin, and only one patient with a perfusion pressure of less than 50 mmHg survived, and no patient survived with a perfusion pressure of less than 40 mmHg. The cerebral perfusion pressure dropped to less than 50 mmHg either prior to or during prostacyclin treatment in all seven patients who subsequently died. Although the normal brain has an autoregulated blood flow [Bryan-Brown 1988], at cerebral perfusion pressures of 50 mmHg or less in patients with a metabolic encephalopathy cerebral autoregulation can fail [Price 1980] and the brain becomes a supply dependent organ [Bryan-Brown 1988]. In this study there was a small but statistically significant increase in arterial hydrogen ion concentration, which may suggest that prostacyclin had an adverse effect on the distribution of oxygenated blood within tissues, including the brain.

Patients with FHF have an abnormal cardiovascular state characterized by an increased cardiac output and reduced vascular resistance [Sherlock 1990], with evidence of shunting of blood at the tissue level [Bihari et al. 1985], including intracerebral shunting [Ede et al. 1988]. Some studies have suggested that the excess vasodilatation observed is due to the activity of increased circulating levels of endogenous prostacyclin and other prostaglandins [Sherlock 1990]. In this study the administration of prostacyclin produced an increase in ICP, a reduction in mean arterial blood pressure with a consequent reduction in cerebral perfusion pressure. Other workers have shown that prostacyclin can cause a dose related increase in ICP [Seifert and Stolke 1985]. Under normal circumstances prostacyclin, by reducing vascular resistance, would be expected to decrease ICP by causing pooling of blood in the spinal venous sinuses, so reducing the intracranial blood volume. However in patients with cerebral edema these compensatory mechanisms may have already been maximally utilized [Davenport et al. 1990], and further cerebral vasodilatation produces a paradoxical increase in intracerebral blood volume with a corresponding increase in ICP. Prostacyclin could also have produced an increase in ICP secondary to a reduction in cerebral perfusion pressure and by aggravating the shunting of blood at the neuronal level, as neuronal hypoxia results in the local production and release of vasodilator substances which result in arteriolar vasodilatation and an increase in ICP [Kontos and Wei 1985].

Anticoagulation with prostacyclin was effective as shown by the thromboelastograph recordings [Scott-Blair and Matchett 1972], and it would have been unlikely that these observations were due to cerebral arteriolar thrombosis or hemorrhage.

In this study prostacyclin produced a reduction in both left and right ventricular filling pressures due to its vasodilator properties [Moncada and Vane 1979], this was despite attempts to correct hypovolemia using 4.5% human albumin solution prior to the administration of prostacyclin. Prostacyclin has been reported in other studies to increase [Bihari et al. 1987] or have no effect on cardiac output [Chelly et al. 1982]. As the cardiac filling pressures were reduced in this study then any increase in output must be due to an increase in heart rate. Some investigators have shown that prostacyclin may cause a reduction in heart rate due to the activation of cardiac vagal receptors [Triuzli et al. 1983]. In addition patients with FHF who die from cerebral edema have been reported to have macroscopic evidence of myocardial damage [Weston et al. 1976], and the increased blood endotoxin levels observed in these patients [Wilkinson et al. 1974] would also be expected to impair cardiac output [Suffredini et al. 1990]. In addition prostacyclin would have produced a fall in the coronary artery perfusion pressure [Cunnion et al. 1986] and other workers have shown that prostacyclin can produce coronary artery vasoconstriction in a dose dependent manner [Darius et al. 1987], these factors would be expected to further impair cardiac performance.

Even if prostacyclin had caused an increase in cardiac output, other workers have shown that prostacyclin can cause both a reduction in total cerebral blood flow [Pickles et al. 1984] and alter the distribution of blood flow to the brain, unfortunately causing a redistribution away from actively respiring neurones [Feddersen et al. 1986]. In addition in this study, despite elective hyperventilation, prostacyclin caused a reduction in arterial oxygen tension, presumably by altering the normal physiological response of pulmonary hypoxic vasoconstriction [Pierpont et al. 1980]. Thus, in this study prostacyclin caused an increase in pulmonary shunting and could have reduced oxygen delivery to the brain by both reducing oxygen delivery and exacerbating intracerebral shunting [Sherlock 1990]. This effect of reducing oxygen delivery would be expected to cause an increase in ICP [Kontos and Wei 1985].

As hepatic transplantation increases then so will the nephrologists's role in supporting patients with acute liver failure both pre- and perioperatively

[Delaney and Nasir 1990]. More patients at risk of dying from increased ICP will require renal support while waiting for urgent liver transplantation.

The nephrologist will have to consider dialysis treatments designed to provoke least change in ICP and cardiac output [Davenport et al. 1987]. In certain clinical circumstances prostacyclin will be the preferred anticoagulant. In this study the direct administration of prostacyclin to a critically ill group of patients with increased ICP caused a further increase in ICP, a reduction in arterial blood pressure and a reduction in cerebral perfusion pressure, to critical values in the majority of cases. These adverse effects were greater in those patients who subsequently died from cerebral edema. Although all but one of the patients studied had developed fulminant hepatic failure following paracetamol (acetaminophen) self-poisoning, these observations would be expected in other patients who had developed fulminant hepatic failure due to other etiologies and who had also progressed to acute oligo-anuric renal failure.

To prevent these adverse effects three management steps could be considered. Firstly, not only should the intravascular volume be checked with a pulmonary artery flotation catheter, but a fluid challenge with colloid given, as static measurements of pulmonary artery wedge pressures may not give an accurate assessment of the intravascular volume in critically ill patients [Shippy et al. 1984]. Patients with FHF are at risk of an adult respiratory-like syndrome, hence some workers have suggested an optimal wedge pressure of 8 mmHg [Bihari et al. 1986], although more recently it has been suggested that higher pressures should be used [Bihari et al. 1987]. In this study the median wedge pressure prior to prostacyclin was 12 mmHg (9–14), and this may have resulted in some patients being given prostacyclin who had not had their effective circulating volume maximized.

Secondly, the majority of these critically ill patients were inotrope dependent and in receipt of sedative agents which may also have vasodilatory properties. The administration of a further potent vasodilator, prostacyclin, would be expected to produce further cardiovascular instability. To prevent this effect vasoconstrictor support should either be temporarily increased to cover the start of the prostacyclin infusion, or be close at hand to prevent precipitate reductions in arterial blood pressure and cerebral perfusion pressure. In view of the underlying pathophysiological state of FHF [Sherlock 1990], noradrenalin would appear the most suitable vasoconstrictor.

Thirdly, prostacyclin is lost during its passage through the extracorporeal circuit, due to losses in the filtrate/dialysate and protein binding [Zobel et al. 1988], thus the effective dose reaching the patient is much reduced. As some of the adverse effects of prostacyclin including increased ICP, coronary artery vasoconstriction, reported in other studies have been shown to be dose dependent, it would appear logical not to directly infuse prostacyclin into the patient prior to commencing extracorporeal treatment, but only to administer prostacyclin into the extracorporeal circuit.

By utilizing these measures the advantages of prostacyclin as an extracorporeal anticoagulant may be gained [Davenport et al. 1988] without the adverse effects demonstrated in this study. Subsequent to this study we have implemented these proposals and have been able to reduce the incidence of precipitous increases in ICP and reductions in cerebral perfusion pressure. This has allowed to continue to successfully utilize prostacyclin as an effective extracorporeal anticoagulant in this group of critically ill patients.

Acknowledgements

We wish to thank Professor M. S. Losowsky for referring his patients for treatment, our neurosurgical colleagues for inserting the subdural catheters and Dr. A. T. Cohen and his intensive care staff for their co-operation.

We wish to acknowledge the generous and continued support of the Yorkshire Kidney Research Fund.

REFERENCES

Bernuau J, Rueff R, Benhamou J 1986 Fulminant and subfulminant hepatic failure: definitions and causes. Semin Liv Dis *6:* 97–106

Bihari D 1985 Acute liver failure. Clinics in Anaesthes *3:* 973–997

Bihari DJ, Gimson AES, Williams R 1986 Cardiovascular, pulmonary and renal complications of fulminant hepatic failure. Semin Liv Dis *2:* 119–128

Bihari D, Smithies M, Gimson A, Tinker J 1987 The effects of vasodilatation with prostacyclin on oxygen delivery and uptake in critically ill patients. N Engl J Med *317:* 397–403

Bryan-Brown CW 1988 Blood flow to organs: parameters for function and survival in critical illness. Crit care Med *16:* 170–178

Chelly J, Fabiani JN, Chahine R, Tricot AM, Carpentier A, Passelecq J, Dubost C 1982 Hemodynamic and metabolic effects of prostacyclin after coronary artery bypass surgery. Circulation *66:* (suppl 1) 145–149

Cunion RE, Schoer GL, Parker MM 1986 The coronary circulation in human septic shock. Circulation *73:* 637–644

Darius H, Thomsen T, Schror K 1987 Cardiovascular actions in vitro and cardioprotective effects in vivo of nileprost a mixed type prostacyclin/prostaglandin E2 agonist. J Cardiovasc Pharmacol *10:* 144–152

Davenport A 1990 Studies in hepatic and renal failure. MD thesis. University of Cambridge 1990

Davenport A, Will EJ, Losowosky MS, Swindells S 1987 Continuous arteriovenous hemofiltration in patients with hepatic encephalopathy and renal failure. Br Med J *295:* 1028

Davenport A, Davison AM, Will EJ 1988 Anticoagulation with prostacyclin in patients treated by continuous hemofiltration. Nephrol Dial Transplant *3:* 547

Davenport A, Will EJ, Davison AM, Swindells S, Cohen AT, Miloszewski KJA, Losowosky MS 1989 Changes in intracranial pressure during hemofiltration in oliguric patients with grade IV hepatic encephalopathy. Nephron *53:* 142–146

Davenport A, Will EJ, Davison AM 1990 The effect of posture on intracranial pressure in patients with fulminant hepatic failure and oliguric renal failure following paracetamol (acetaminophen) self-poisoning. Crit Care Med *18:* 286–289

Delaney V, Nasir M 1990 Liver transplantation: a challenge to the nephrologist. Nephron *55:* 353–360

Ede RJ, Gove CD, Williams R 1988 Increased cerebral blood flow in fulminant hepatic failure due to paracetamol overdose. In: *Soeters PB, Wilson JHP, Meijer AJ, Holm E* (eds), Advances in ammonia metabolism and hepatic encephalopathy. Elsevier science publishers, Amsterdam, pp 567–570

Ede RJ, Keays R, Williams R 1989 Intracranial pressure monitoring and management of encephalopathy. Crit Care Ill *5:* 46–48

Feddersen K, Aren C, Nilsson NJ, Radegran K 1986 Cerebral blood flow and metabolism during cardiopulmonary bypass with special reference to effects of hypotension induced by prostacyclin. Ann Thorac Surg *41:* 395–400

Forbes A, Alexander GJM, O'Grady J, Keays R, Gullen R, Dawling S, Williams R 1989 Thiopental infusion in the treatment of intracranial pressure complicating fulminant hepatic failure. Hepatol *3:* 306–310

Hartert H 1971 Thromboelastography. In: *Bang NO, Beller FK, Deutsch E, Mammen EF* (eds), Thrombosis and bleeding disorders. Theory and methods, Georg Thieme, Verlag, Stuttgart, Germany, pp 70–76

Keogh AM, Rylance PB, Weston MJ, Parsons V 1984 Prostacyclin (epoprostenol) hemodialysis in patients at risk of hemorrhage. Proc Eur Dial Transplant Nurses Assoc *13:* 51–54

Knight A, Bihari D, Tinker J 1985 Stress ulceration in the critically ill patient. Brit J Hosp Med *33:* 216–219

Kontos HA, Wei EP 1985 Oxygen dependent mechanisms in cerebral autoregulation. Ann Biomed Engin *13:* 329–334

Lassen NA, Christensen MS 1976 Physiology of cerebral blood flow. Br J Anaesthes *48:* 719–734

Marchal G, Leroux ME, Samma M 1979 Atlas de thrombodynamographie. Service de propagande edition information, Paris, France

Moncada S, Vane JR 1979 Pharmacology and endogenous roles of prostaglandin endoperoxides, thromboxane A2 and prostacyclin. Pharmacol Rev *30:* 293–331

O'Grady JG, Langley PG, Isola LM, Williams R 1986 Coagulopathy of fulminant hepatic failure. Semin Liv Dis *6:* 159–163

O'Grady JG, Gimson AES, O'Brien CJ, Pucknell A, Hughes RD, Williams R 1988 Controlled trials of charcoal hemoperfusion and prognostic factors in fulminant hepatic failure. Gastroenterol *94:* 1186–1192

Pickles H, Brown MM, Thomas M, Hewazy AH, Redmond S, Zilkha E, Marshall J 1984 Effect of indomethacin on cerebral blood flow, carbon dioxide sensitivity and the response to epoprostenol infusion in man. J Neurol Neurosurg Psych *47:* 51–55

Pierpoint G, Hale KA, Franciosa JA, Cohn JN 1980 Effects of vasodilators on pulmonary hemodynamics and gas exchange in left ventricular failure. Am Heart J *99:* 208–216

Price DJ 1980 Intracranial pressure monitoring. Br J Clin Equip *5:* 92–98

Scott-Blair GW, Matchett RH 1972 On the interpretation of thromboelastograms. Hemostasis *1:* 93–100

Seifert V, Stolke D 1985 Experimental investigations on the behaviour of intracranial pressure under prostacyclin application. Neurochir *28:* 40–45

Sherlock S 1990 Vasodilatation associated with hepatocellular disease: relation to functional organ failure. Gut *31:* 365–366

Shippy LR, Appel PL, Shoemaker WC 1984 Reliability of clinical monitoring to assess blood volume in critically ill patients. Crit Care Med *12:* 107–112

Suffrendini AF, Fromm RE, Parker M, Brenner M, Kovacs JA, Wesley RA, Parillo JE 1989 The cardiovascular response of normal humans to the administration of endotoxin. N Engl J Med *321:* 180–187

Triuzli MD, Sansonetti G, Signovini G, Mattioli R, Maggi BC, Aguggini G 1983 Prostacyclin effect on heart rate in the pig. Prost Leukot Med *10:* 269–278

Turney JH, Williams LC, Fewell MR, Parsons V, Weston MJ 1980 Platelet protection and heparin sparing with prostacyclin during regular dialysis therapy. Lancet *2:* 219–222

Turney JH, Dodd NJ, Weston MJ 1981 Prostacyclin in extracorporeal circulations. Lancet *1:* 1101

Ware AJ, D'Agostino A, Coombes B 1971 Cerebral oedema: a major complication of massive hepatic necrosis. Gastroenterol *61:* 877–884

Weston MJ, Talbot IC, Howarth PJN, Mant AK, Cupiledo R, Williams R 1976 Frequency of arrhythmias and other cardiac abnormalities in fulminant hepatic failure. Br Heart J *38:* 1179–1188

Wilkinson SP, Arroyo V, Gazzard BG, Moodie H, Williams R 1974 Relation of renal impairment and hemorrhagic diathesis to endotoxaemia in fulminant hepatic failure. Lancet *1:* 521–524

Zobel G, Trop M, Muntean W, Ring E, Gleispach TA 1988 Anticoagulation for continuous arteriovenous hemofiltration in children. Blood Purif *6:* 90–95

Clinical Nephrology, Vol. 35 No. 4 – 1991 (158–164)

Effect of osmolar changes on plasma arginine vasopressin (PAVP) in dialysis patients

S. J. Rosansky[1], R. Rhinehart[2] and R. Shade[3]

[1]*Medical Service, WJB Dorn Veterans Hospital and* [2]*Department of Medicine, University of South Carolina School of Medicine, Columbia, South Carolina and the* [3]*Southwest Foundation for Biomedical Research, San Antonio, Texas, USA*

Abstract. The effect of changes in plasma osmolality and changes in plasma arginine vasopressin (PAVP) were analyzed in 10 stable chronic hemodialysis patients utilizing four protocols. During regular hemodialysis opposing influences on PAVP (decrease in blood pressure and intravascular volume and increase in serum calcium) resulted in no significant change in PAVP (by analysis of variance). In the second protocol low dialysate calcium (2.5 meq/l) isovolemic hemodialysis was used. PAVP and serum osmolality levels declined from 2.0 ± 0.4 to 1.4 ± 0.2 μU/ml ($p < 0.05$), and 285 ± 2.5 mOsm/l to 275 ± 3.2 mOsm/l respectively. Removal of PAVP by hemodialysis did not occur as evidenced by no difference in arterial-venous PAVP levels and no "rebound" of PAVP for three hours after completion of dialysis (second protocol). Isovolemic low calcium high dialysate sodium (145 meq/l) hemodialysis was utilized in the third protocol. Serum osmolality and PAVP did not change. Addition of a very high dialysate sodium (155 meq/l) to isovolemic low calcium hemodialysis resulted in an increase in plasma sodium, osmolality and AVP (139.7 ± 0.62 to 144 ± 0.67 meq/l, 294 ± 2.79 to 304.3 ± 2.4 mOsm/l and 1.8 ± 0.3 to 2.7 ± 0.5 μU/ml ($p < 0.05$ for each) respectively. In conclusion, PAVP responds to changes in plasma osmolality in chronic hemodialysis patients.

Key words: vasopressin – osmolality – hemodialysis – volume

Introduction

The relationship of plasma arginine vasopressin (PAVP) to plasma osmolality has been well described in normals. In patients who regularly receive dialysis, plasma osmolality and plasma volume, the two main stimuli to (PAVP), can be altered in a controlled manner. Previous studies which investigated changes in vasopressin secretion in response to osmolar changes during hemodialysis have produced conflicting results. These discrepancies may be due to failure to adequately account for all the factors that influence vasopressin secretion.

The current paper describes methodology used to account for factors that alter PAVP levels including plasma calcium, plasma osmolality, plasma volume, mean arterial blood pressure, and dialytic removal of PAVP. After controlling for these factors, we have shown that PAVP responds to changes in plasma osmolality in chronic dialysis patients.

Received August 24, 1990; in revised form December 20, 1990.

Reprint requests to Dr. S. J. Rosansky (111F), Chief, Renal Section, VA Hospital, Columbia, SC 29201

Methods

Ten stable chronic dialysis patients were studied. The mean age of the patients was 58. Patients were treated with hemodialysis for a mean of 2.4 years. All patients gave informed consent and the study was approved by the Columbia SC VA Hospital Human Studies Committee. In order to standardize results, patients were only studied if their weight gain was less than or equal to 2.5 kg above their estimated dry body weight. Dry body weight was defined as a weight below which a patient consistently developed hypotension during dialysis or a post dialysis weight where the patient exhibited orthostatic hypotension. All studies were done in recumbency except where indicated. Patients withheld their medications for at least 12 hours prior to being studied, and were not studied if they were taking any medication that could affect PAVP levels. Futhermore, subjects were not studied if they were overtly anxious. If subjects experienced nausea or vomiting, or hypotension, the protocol was terminated and data were excluded from analysis. All patients were anemic (hematocrit 19 to 30 percent). None had symptoms of overt cardiac or hepatic failure.

Protocols

Conditions common to all protocols

Prior to hemodialysis treatment, baseline data were obtained in all subjects 30 minutes after needle insertion. This data included systolic, diastolic and mean arterial blood pressure; heart rate; (all of which were measured at baseline and every 15 minutes during the study). Body weight was measured hourly during each study. Blood was sampled hourly for determination of PAVP, osmolality, calcium, potassium, urea nitrogen, glucose, and hematocrit. All studies utilized: a Gambro 1.0 m^2 dialyzer; Sentry 2 Rx dialysis machine; dialysate dextrose of 200 mg%; magnesium of 1.5 mEq/l; and potassium of 2 mEq/L. Changes in corrected osmolality (measured osmolality corrected to a BUN of 10 mg/dl) rather than measured osmolality were reported since urea is not considered an effective osmole with respect to PAVP stimulation (Trasher et al. 1980). Four different protocols were carried out.

1. The first protocol utilized standard dialysis with combined ultrafiltration and diffusion dialysis. In this protocol, a dialysate sodium of 134 mEq/l and ionized calcium of 3.25 mEq/l was used for a four-hour treatment. A relatively low dialysate sodium was utilized to exacerbate the drop in plasma osmolality.
2. To control the changes in plasma volume which could effect changes in PAVP the second protocol utilized isovolemic hemodialysis. Isovolemic hemodialysis was achieved by continuous infusion of 0.9% saline at a rate equal to a subject's obligatory ultrafiltration rate (dependent upon the venous resistance). Ultrafiltration rates were checked and and justed every 15 minutes by putting the Sentry 2 dialysis machine in a bypass ultrafiltration mode. To stabilize calcium levels (which also may affect PAVP levels), a dialysate ionized calcium of 2.5 mEq/l was used. In order to emphasize the drop in osmolality during this protocol, a dialysate sodium of 130 mEq/l was chosen. To evaluate PAVP removal during dialysis, simultaneous arterial and venous samples of PAVP were obtained during the second hour of this protocol for each subject. In addition, PAVP levels were measured for three hours after completion of a four-hour dialysis treatment. If significant amounts of PAVP were removed by diffusion dialysis or ultrafiltration, one would expect a "rebound" of PAVP post dialysis.
3. The third protocol utilized isovolemic low calcium (2.5 meq/l) hemodialysis as used in protocol 2. A high dialysate sodium of 145 mEq/l was used in this protocol, to prevent the drop in osmolality and PAVP seen in protocol 2. The variable sodium device on the Sentry 2 hemodialysis machine was set to a dialysate of sodium of 145 mEq/l. In order to check the accuracy of the variable sodium device, two dialysate samples during the second hour of the study were obtained for each subject. The protocol was carried out for three hours. During the fourth hour of the patients' dialysis treatment, ultrafiltration was carried out in order to bring the patients' weight close to their "dry body weight". Blood sampling during this final hour was not carried out.
4. The fourth protocol utilized isovolemic low dialysate calcium hemodialysis with a very high dialysate sodium of 155 mEq/l. In this protocol, an attempt was made to increase plasma corrected osmolality and PAVP by increasing plasma sodium concentration. Dialysate sodium was adjusted and monitored in the same way as in protocol 3. Isovolemic hemodialysis was carried out during the first three hours of the protocol. During hour four subjects were ultrafiltrated to their dry body weight. In addition, during this final hour dialysate sodium was decreased to 150 mEq/l to prevent post dialysis hypernatremia.

Analytical methods

Blood samples for measurement of plasma osmolality, sodium, urea, and glucose were drawn into a vacuated tube containing a small amount of heparin. After mixing, duplicate capillary tubes were filled from the specimen for determination of hematocrit. Next the tubes were centrifuged and the plasma was removed. Osmolality was measured by freezing piont depression (Osmette microosmometer-Precision Systems). Plasma sodium and potassium concentration were measured by ion specific electrodes (Orion Research 1026). Total and ionized calcium was determined by ion specific electrode (AVL Model 984 Electrolyte Analyzer). Total calcium was determined colorimetrically by the o-cresolpthalein complexone method (Sigma Diagnostic, Procedure No. 586). Plasma urea nitrogen was measured colorimetrically (Sigma Diagnostics Procedure No. 640). Plasma glu-

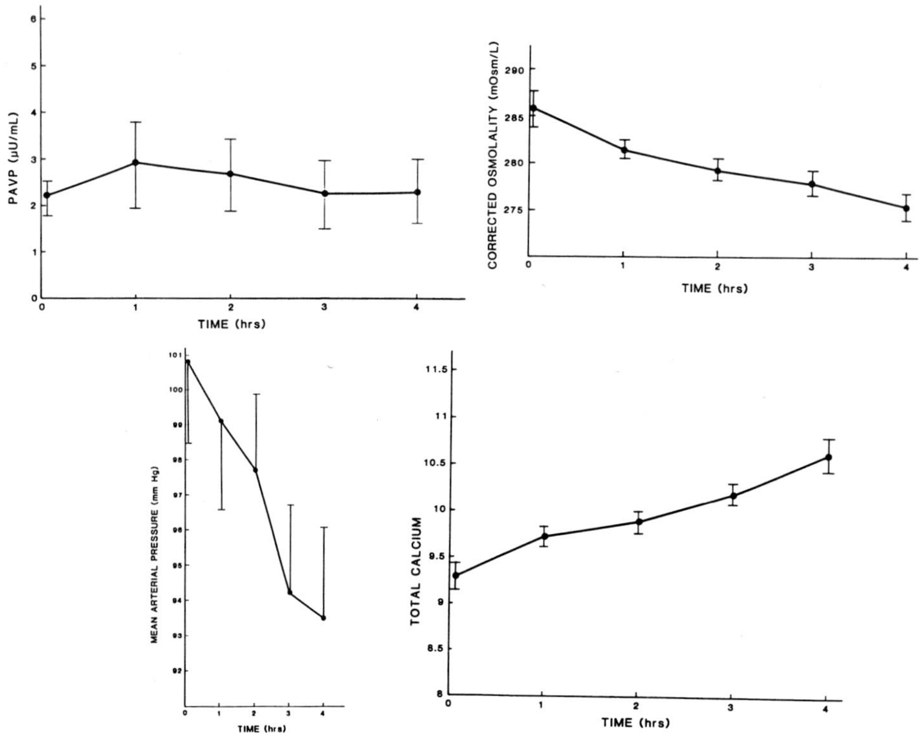

Fig. 1 Changes in plasma arginine vasopressin (PAVP) during four-hour regular hemodialysis. PAVP levels remain unchanged (by analysis of variance, ANOVA). Factors that stimulate PAVP include decline in mean arterial pressure and weight (intravascular volume) and an increase in serum calcium. Decline in corrected osmolality and possible clearance of PAVP (not shown in Figure), could decrease PAVP levels.

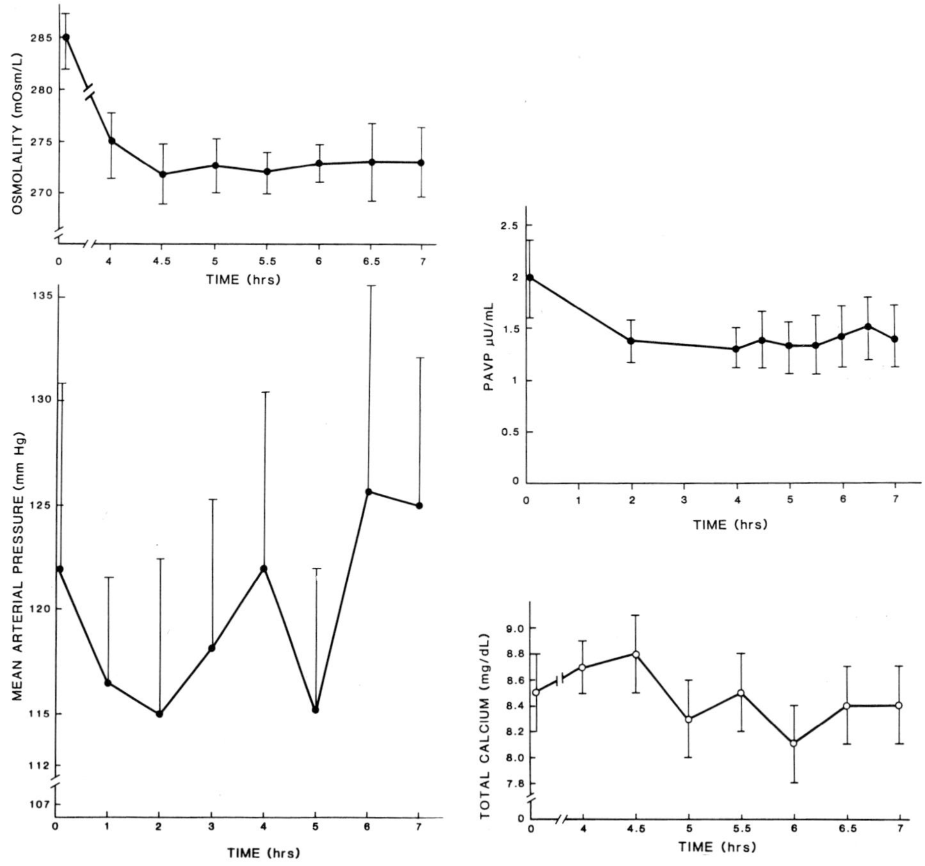

Fig. 2 Low calcium (2.5 meq/l), isovolemic hemodialysis and post dialysis (hours 4–7) evaluation for "rebound" of PAVP. PAVP declines by hour 2 ($p < 0.05$ by ANOVA), in conjunction with a decline in corrected osmolality. Other factors that increase PAVP – decline in mean arterial pressure, decrease in weight, increase in calcium, are all prevented by isovolemic high calcium dialysis. PAVP levels do not increase post dialysis (by ANOVA) providing evidence against PAVP removal (clearance) during dialysis.

cose was measured by the Hexokinase Method (Sigma Diagnostics Procedure No. 115).

Blood samples for PAVP were drawn into chilled evacuated tubes containing small amounts of dipotassium EDTA and centrifuged at 3000 rpm for 15 minutes at 4 degrees C. PAVP was measured on extracted plasma samples utilizing a radioimmunoassay previously described (Hinojosa et al. 1986). PAVP values from 11 normal subjects using this assay ranged from 0.4–1.5 μU/ml with a mean ± S. E. of 0.73 ± 0.10 μU/ml.

Calculations and statistical analysis

All values were expressed as the mean ± SEM. Data were analyzed by two-way analysis of variance, (ANOVA, patients, periods) or Student's t-test for paired values.

Results

1. Utilizing standard dialysis (Figure 1) several factors that could stimulate PAVP were uncovered. These included an increase in total calcium from 9.3 ± 0.31 to 10.6 ± 0.3 mg/dl; a decrease in mean arterial blood pressure from 100.8 ± 2.3 to 93.5 ± 27 mmHg; decreased intravascular volume as reflected by a decrease in weight from 72 ± 2.5 to 69 ± 2.6 kg and an increase in hematocrit from 27.8 ± 0.9 to 29.7 ± 1.7%. Factors that could lower PAVP during standard dialysis included a decline in corrected osmolality from 286 ± 1.7 mOsm/l to 275.8 ± 1.2 mOsm/l and removal of PAVP by dialysis (diffusion and or ultrafiltration). As a result of these opposing effects, PAVP levels remained unchanged during the four-hour regular dialysis treatment.
2. Utilizing the isovolemic low dialysate calcium dialysis protocol, there were no significant changes in total calcium, mean arterial pressure, or weight during the four hours of hemodialysis (Figure 2). On the other hand, corrected osmolality declined significantly from 285 ± 2.5 mOsm/l to 275 ± 3.2 mOsm/l respectively. A decline in PAVP from 2.0 ± 0.4 to 1.4 ± 0.2 μU/ml ($p < 0.05$ by ANOVA) occurred by hour 2 and then remained stable until the end of the dialysis procedure. (A two-hour osmolality

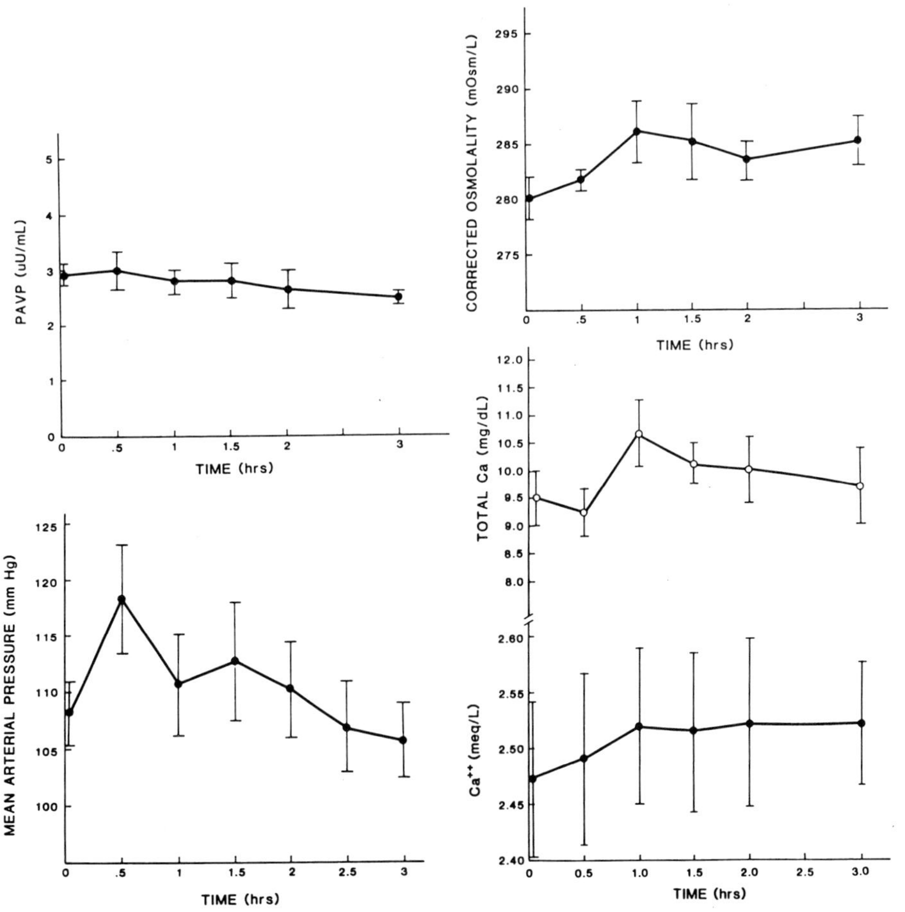

Fig. 3 Low calcium, high sodium, isovolemic hemodialysis. By utilizing a high dialysate sodium (145 meq/l) corrected osmolality does not decline and PAVP levels remain unchanged (by ANOVA). Both ionized and total calcium also remain unchanged (by ANOVA).

sample was not obtained). As seen in Figure 2, for three hours postdialysis PAVP levels and other parameters that could affect PAVP (osmolality, calcium, and mean aterial pressure) remained stable. Simultaneous arterial venous samples for PAVP obtained during the second hour of this protocol revealed no significant differences between arterial (1.50 ± 0.17 μU/ml) and venous (1.51 ± 0.20 μU/ml) PAVP values. The mean arterial venous difference was −0.05 ± 0.11 μU/ml.

3. During the isovolemic low calcium hemodialysis with a high dialysate sodium (145 mEq/l) protocol a measured dialysis sodium of 143 ± 0.9 mEq/l was produced. Although the variable sodium device alters the dialysate to water ratio, there was no significant change in total or ionized calcium (Figure 3). In addition, there was no significant change in plasma osmolality or mean arterial blood pressure (by analysis of variance). Prevention of a significant decline in corrected osmolality, may have led to no significant change in PAVP (2.9 ± 0.2 μU/ml to 2.5 ± 0.1 μU/ml, no significant change by ANOVA).

4. In the final protocol, a dialysate sodium of 158 ± 1.2 meg/l was produced. As seen in Figure 4, there was a significant increase in PAVP ($p < 0.05$ by ANOVA) from a baseline value of 1.8 ± 0.3 μU/ml to 2.7 ± 0.5 μU/ml at 1 hour. PAVP remained stable during hours 2 and 3. Plasma sodium paralleled the increase in PAVP from 139.7 ± 0.62 mEq/l at baseline to 144.0 ± 0.67 mEq/l at hour 1 and no change after hour 2. Corrected osmolality increased from 249 ± 2.79 mOsm/l at baseline to 304.3 ± 2.4 mOsm/l at hour 1 and 311.6 ± 3.1 mOsm/l at hour 2. Corrected osmolality stabilized at hours 3 and 4.
During the final hour of this protocol patients were ultrafiltrated to their dry body weight and the dialysate sodium was reduced to 150 mEq/l. During this hour a significant rise in PAVP was noted, presumably related to the decrease in weight (75.5 ± 2.8 kg to 73.8 ± 2.9 kg) and intravascular volume.

Discussion

There are several parameters that are altered during hemodialysis that could affect PAVP levels. Changes in blood constituents including plasma sodium, calcium, and osmolality, may affect PAVP. Changes in plasma sodium may affect PAVP through changes in plasma osmolality. The effect on PAVP of a decrease in plasma osmolality during hemodialysis is controversial. Seven studies demonstrated a parallel change between PAVP and plasma osmolality during hemodialysis (Horky et al. 1979, Nord and Danovitch et al. 1979, Iitake et al. 1985, Fasanella d'Amore et al. 1985, Papadoliopoulou-Diamandopoulou et al. 1987, Quillen et al 1984, Pastoria-Munoz et al. 1976). On the other hand four studies failed to show a relationship between plasma osmolality and PAVP changes during hemodialysis (Vaziri et al. 1980, Shimamoto et al. 1977, Elias et al. 1989). Two studies attempted to isolate PAVP changes due to osmolar changes during dialysis from those due to ultrafiltration (Fasanella d'Amore et al. 1985, Ardaillou et al. 1986). Neither of these studies recorded intradialytic body weight changes. In addition isovolemic dialysis was not produced since obligatory ultrafiltrate was not replaced with a constant infusion of saline.

In addition to changes in osmolality, changes in intravascular volume and blood pressure may effect PAVP levels during dialysis. The effect of ultrafiltration, with accompanying decrease in intravascular volume and blood pressure, on PAVP levels is also controversial. One study demonstrated a strong correlation between the amount of volume removed by ultrafiltration and the increase in PAVP (Ardaillou et al. 1984, Sorensen et al. 1986). Five other studies reported little or no change in PAVP with changes in weight or posture (Fasanella d'Amore et al. 1985, Quillen et al. 1984, Ardaillou et al. 1986, Zabetakis et al. 1987, Hammer et al. 1980).

In addition to plasma osmolality, plasma volume and blood pressure changes, total and/or ionized calcium may effect PAVP changes in chronic dialysis patients (Varizi et al. 1980a, Varizi et al. 1980b).

Our study attempted to control changes in intravascular volume, blood pressure and plasma calcium while we examined the effect of changes in plasma sodium and plasma osmolality on PAVP levels in chronic dialysis patients. As found in all previous studies, PAVP levels were elevated in our chronic dialysis patients. Although elevated, the baseline PAVP levels varied from 1.8 μU/ml to 2.9 μU/l in the four protocols. These variations might have been due to differences in interdialytic dietary salt and fluid control.

Protocol 1 (Figure 1) utilized a standard high calcium dialysate with combined ultrafiltration and diffusion dialysis. PAVP levels did not change. Several opposing factors may have effected PAVP. A decrease in intravascular volume and blood pressure secondary to ultrafiltration and an increase in serum calcium all could have raised PAVP. The decrease in plasma corrected osmolality could have lowered PAVP. The net effect was no significant change in PAVP during the protocol.

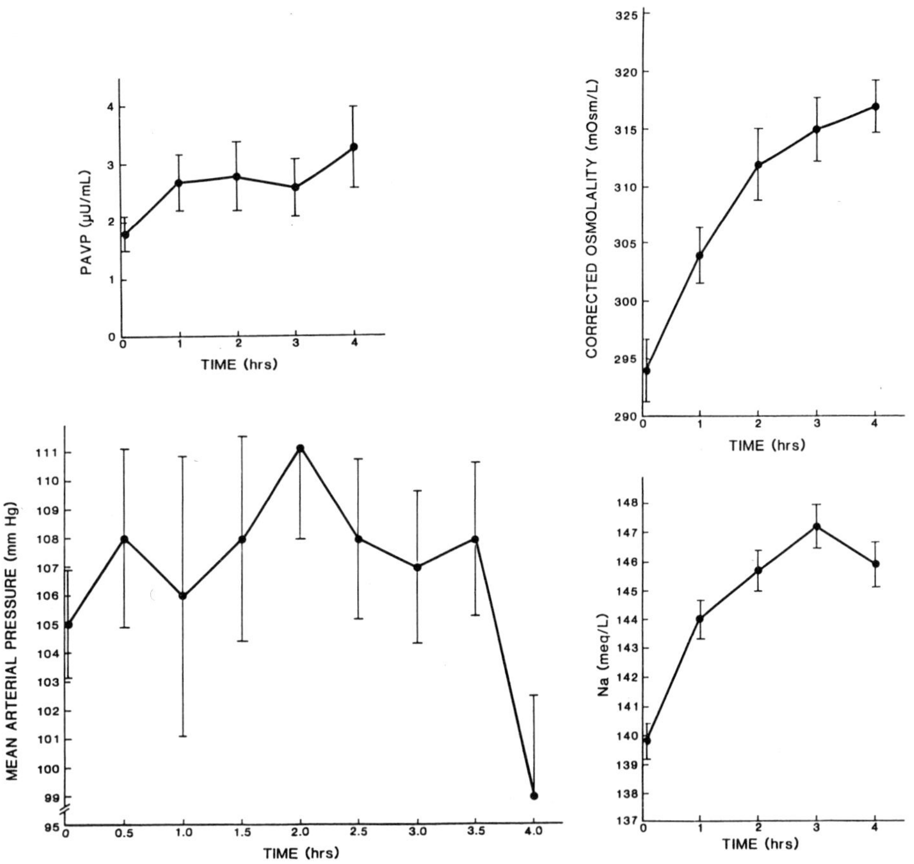

Fig. 4 Very high sodium, low calcium, isovolemic hemodialysis. By utilizing a dialysate sodium of 155 meq/l a significant increase in serum sodium and corrected osmolality occurs between hours 0 and 1 and 1 and 2 ($p < 0.05$ for both). This leads to a significant increase in PAVP which occurs by the end of hour 1 ($p < 0.05$). A significant increase in PAVP during hour four ($p < 0.05$ by ANOVA) may be due to ultrafiltration (weight declined from 74.5 ± 2.8 kg to 73.8 ± 2.9 kg).

Isovolemic high calcium hemodialysis prevented the change in calcium, weight (intravascular volume) and blood pressure seen in protcol 1. Thus, the drop in osmolality that occurred with dialysis may have caused a decline in PAVP. Another factor which could have explained this decline in PAVP is dialytic (by diffusion dialysis or ultrafiltration) removal of PAVP.

In protocol 2, we found, as did Jawadi et al. 1986, that PAVP was not removed by diffusion dialysis. It is unlikely that significant amounts of PAVP were removed by either diffusion or ultrafiltration since PAVP levels failed to rebound during three hours of observation, post dialysis.

Further evidence for a definitive effect of changes in plasma osmolality on PAVP levels during dialysis is seen in protocols 3 and 4. The drop in PAVP and plasma osmolality found during isovolemic high calcium hemodialysis in protocol 2 was prevented in protocol 3 by the utilization of a high sodium dialysate. As predicted, PAVP levels remained unchanged. Further evidence that PAVP levels are effected by plasma corrected osmolality was found in protocol 4. Utilizing the very high sodium dialysate PAVP levels increased significantly. PAVP levels seemed to parallel the change in serum sodium more than the change in plasma corrected osmolality (Figure 4). One could hypothesize that serum sodium is the main determinant of PAVP changes in dialysis patients.

Alternatively, urea may be a partly effective osmole with respect to PAVP stimulation. Zerbe and Robertson [1983] reported that for the same increase in plasma osmolality, hypertonic urea infusion produced a smaller increase in PAVP than did intravenous hypertonic saline. This partial response to urea may be the reason why baseline PAVP levels are elevated in chronic hemodialysis patients. As well, it may explain the lack of full inhibition of PAVP in protocol 2 when corrected plasma osmolality was reduced to 275 mOsm/l while PAVP levels remained rather high (1.4 ± 0.2 μU/ml).

The standard method for evaluating PAVP responses to changes in plasma osmolality involves infusion of hypertonic saline. This results in an increase in plasma volume. In protocol 4, by utilizing a very high sodium dialysate in isovolemic hemodialysis, we were able to raise plasma osmolality without simultaneously increasing plasma volume. Thus, the hemodialysis patient may serve as a good model to study osmolality-PAVP relationships without the confounding effect of changes in plasma volume.

REFERENCES

Ardaillou R, Benmansour M, Rondeau E, Caillens H 1984 Metabolism and secretion of antidiuretic hormone in patients with renal failure, cardiac insufficiency and liver insufficiency. Adv Nephrol *13:* 35–49.

Ardaillou R, Pruszcynski W, Benmansour M 1986 Secretion and catabolism of antidiuretic hormone in renal failure. Contrib Nephrol *50:* 46–53.

Elias AN, Vaziri ND, Pandian MR, Daupke J 1989 Plasma concentrations of artrial natriuretic peptide, arginine vasopressin and hormones of the renin-angiotensin system in patients with end-stage renal disease. Int J Artif Organs *12:* 153–158.

Fasanella d'Amore T, Wauters JP, Waeber B, Nussberger J, Brunner HR 1985 Response of plasma vasopressin to changes in extracellular volume and/or plasma osmolality in patients on maintenance hemodialysis. Clin Nephrol *23:* 299–302.

Hammer M, Ladefoged J, Madsen S, Olgaard K, Tvedegaard E 1980 Calcium-stimulated vasopressin secretion in uremic patients; an effect mediated via parathyroid hormone? J Clin Endocrinol Metab *51:* 1078–1084.

Hinojosa C, Shade RE, Haywood JR 1986 Plasma vasopressin concentration in high sodium renal hypertension. J Hypertens *4:* 529–534.

Horky K, Sramkova J, Lachmanova J, Tomasek R, Dvorakova J 1979 Plasma concentration of antidiuretic hormone in patients with chronic renal insufficiency on maintenance dialysis. Horm Metab Res *11:* 241–246.

Iitake K, Kimura T, Matsui K, Ota K, Shoji M, Inoue M, Yoshinaga K 1985 Effect of hemodialysis on plasma ADH levels, plasma renin activity and plasma aldosterone levels in patients with end-stage disease. Acta Endocrinol (Copenh) *110:* 207–213.

Jawadi MH, Ho LS, Dipette D, Ross DL 1986 Regulation of plasma arginine vasopressin in patients with chronic renal failure maintained on hemodialysis. Am J Nephrol *6:* 175–181.

Nord E, Danovitch GM 1979 Vasopressin response in hemodialysis patients. Proc Eur Dial Transplant Assoc *16:* 238–243.

Papdoliopoulou-Diamandopoulou N, Papagalanis N, Gavras I, Gavras H 1987 Vasopressin in end-stage renal disease: relationship to salt, catecholamines and renin activity. Clin Exp Hypertens [A] *9:* 1197–1208.

Pastoriza-Munoz E, Easterling RE, Malvin RL 1976 The effect of plasma calcium on plasma ADA levels in anephric patients. Nephron *16:* 449–461.

Quillen EW Jr, Skeleton MM, Rubin J, Cowley AW Jr 1984 Osmotic control of vasopressin with chronically altered volume states in nephric dogs. Am J Physiol *247 (3 Pt 1):* E355–361.

Shimamoto K, Watarai I, Miyahara M 1977 A study of plasma vasopressin in patients undergoing chronic hemodialysis. J Clin Endocrinol Metab *45:* 714–720.

Sorensen SS, Danielsen H, Jespersen B, Pedersen EB 1986 Hypotension in end-stage renal disease: effect of postural change, exercise and angiotensin 11, aldosterone and arginine vasopressin in hypotensive patients with chronic renal failure treated by dialysis. Clin Nephrol *26:* 288–296.

Thrasher TN, Brown CJ, Keil LC, Ramsay DJ 1980 Thirst and vasopressin release in the dog: an osmoreceptor or sodium receptor mechanism? Am J Physiol *238:* R333–339.

Vaziri ND, Skowsky R, Saiki J 1980a Antidiuretic hormone in end-stage renal disease. J Dial *4:* 73–81.

Vaziri ND, Skowsky R, Saiki J, Warner A 1980b Hemodialysis studies of antidiuretic hormone. J Dial *4:* 185–190.

Zabetakis PM, Kumar DN, Gleim GW, Gardenswartz MH, Agrawal M, Robinson AG, Michelis MF 1987 Increased levels of plasma renin, aldosterone, catecholamines and vasopressin in chronic ambulatory peritoneal dialysis (CAPD) patients. Clin Nephrol *28:* 147–151.

Zerbe R, Robertson GL 1983 Osmoregulation of thirst and vasopressin secretion in human subjects: Effect of various solutes. Am J Physiol *244* (endocrinol metab 7): E 607–E 614.

Clinical Nephrology, Vol. 35 No. 4 – 1991 (165–170)

Influence of erythropoietin treatment on urea kinetic parameters in hemodialysis patients

J. A. van Geelen, M. J. Nubé, P. A. Zuurbier

Dialysis Department, Medical Center Alkmaar, Alkmaar, The Netherlands

Abstract. Urea kinetic parameters were studied by means of dialysate collection in 8 stable hemodialysis patients before and after treatment with recombinant human erythropoietin (r-HuEPO), in order to investigate the impact of a rising hematocrit (Ht) on dialyzer performance and nutritional status. After 6 months, the average in vivo dialyzer urea clearance had fallen from 152 to 132 ml/min and consequently Kt/V values had become undesirably low in most of the patients in whom the relatively short dialysis regimens had been kept unchanged. There was also a significant decrease of protein intake. As a result of both changes there was only a moderate increase of predialysis mean blood urea concentration. These findings indicate that after correction of anemia by r-HuEPO dialyzer performance decreased. The concomitant decrease of protein intake seems to contrast to the improved general physical condition and appetite as indicated in the questionnaires. Although body weight remained the same, there might have been a tendency to avoid protein consumption with maintained total calory intake as a result of slight underdialysis. Therefore, in individual cases dialysis prescriptions may need reconsideration when Ht levels rise after r-HuEPO administration, especially in short dialysis regimens.

Key words: hemodialysis – recombinant human erythropoietin – urea kinetics

Introduction

One of the major breakthroughs in hemodialysis in the last decade is the introduction of recombinant human erythropoietin (r-HuEPO) for the treatment of uremic anemia. In hemodialysis patients r-HuEPO usually causes an increase in hematocrit, improvement of general condition, increased exercise tolerance and better appetite [Eschbach et al. 1987, Bommer et al. 1987]. As a result of improved calorie and protein intake, an increase of body mass and total body potassium content were reported. Also r-HuEPO may have direct anabolic effects [Zehnter et al. 1988]. However, after a sufficiently long period of administration a new steady state will probably ensue in which anabolism and catabolism are balanced again.

On the other hand, from urea kinetic studies it is known that hemodialysis patients sometimes have a poor nutritional status. From these studies it has also become apparent that uremic morbidity is partly associated with poor nutritional status and that short dialysis regimens may contribute to this condition [Harter et al. 1983, Gotch and Sargent 1985].

At high hematocrit (Ht) levels dialysis efficiency may decrease because of a reduction of blood water content [Zehnder 1989, Shinaberger et al. 1989, Zehnder et al. 1988]. Bosch reported solute clearances to be inversely related to plasma flow in high flux hemodiafiltration. The reduction of plasma flow that occurs at high Ht has only a small impact on urea clearances, because there is a rapid exchange of urea between red cells and plasma during the passage of blood through the dialyzer. Thus, in contrast to other solutes, the decrease of urea clearance is less than the reduction of plasma flow would predict [Bosch et al. 1989].

Nevertheless, if after r-HuEPO therapy a rising Ht as well as an increase of protein intake exist together, one would expect to find rather high predialysis urea concentrations. This however does not reflect the general experience after r-HuEPO therapy. In order to clarify this issue we have gathered urea kinetic data in stable hemodialysis patients by mass balances calculated from spent dialysate. This was done before and after prolonged r-HuEPO administration.

Received May 11, 1990; in revised form October 13, 1990.

Reprints requests to Dr. J. A. van Geelen, Dept. Internal Medicine, Medical Center Alkmaar, Wilhelminalaan 12, 1815 JD Alkmaar, The Netherlands.

Methods

Patients

Hemodialysis patients with Ht levels <28% were considered for treatment with r-HuEPO. Eleven patients without residual diuresis were selected for urea kinetic studies at the beginning of r-HuEPO administration and after 6 months. Three of them were withdrawn because of intercurrent changes in dialysis prescription or r-HuEPO administration. (In one patient hyperkalemia necessitated a permanent increase in duration of the dialysis session, another patient had fistula problems interfering with stability of blood flow, and the third patient interrupted r-HuEPO administration because of headache.) The remaining 8 patients (7 female) had a mean age of 54 years (range 31–73) and had been on dialysis therapy for an average period of 92 months (range 12–240). Six patients were dialyzed twice weekly, and 2 patients underwent 3 sessions per week (patients number 2 and 3 in Tables 1 and 2). The dialysis time was calculated uniformly by a standard procedure according to Babb [Babb et al. 1971] from in vitro dialyzer data, body mass and residual kidney function, resulting in an average treatment time of 9.5 hours/week (range 7–10.5). The patients were on different types of dialyzers (capillary cuprophane, Gambro; capillary polysulphone normal and high flux, Fresenius; polyacrilonitrile plate, Hospal; and capillary cellulose acetate, Cordis Dow), but each patient used the same type of dialyzer throughout the study period. The patients were on the same volumetric ultrafiltration control machine (Fresenius A2008C) throughout the study period. The patients were not allowed to handle the machine themselves and the nursing staff fixed the blood pump speed throughout the dialysis session at 200 ml/min. Blood flow was measured automatically by counting pump revolutions. Heparin was administered as an initial bolus of

Table 1 Kinetic parameters before (left column) and after (right column) r-HuEPO

Pt	Age	BW (kg)	V (l) pre post	Kd (ml/min) pre post	N. Kt/V pre post	PCR (g/d) pre post	TAC (mmol/l) pre post
1	67	53.5	25.2–26.3	112–125	2.40–2.60	42–36	19.5–18.6
2	54	56.0	29.7–30.5	140–129	3.30–2.90	71–62	20.7–22.4
3	31	63.0	39.2–40.1	180–134	2.90–2.10	59–65	17.3–22.1
4	43	56.5	39.1–36.2	165–125	2.00–1.90	63–55	22.6–23.6
5	69	71.0	30.4–29.3	125–120	2.70–2.70	46–44	17.8–17.8
6	58	51.5	33.8–29.1	152–144	2.80–2.80	49–34	17.1–15.7
7	37	55.8	32.5–29.2	173–144	3.20–3.00	55–48	16.9–17.4
8	73	71.3	31.7–29.6	168–137	2.70–2.50	39–34	14.1–16.7
mean	54	60	32.7–31.2	152–132*	2.75–2.55	53–47*	18.3–19.3
SEM	5.8	2.7	1.56– 1.5	8.6–3.2	0.14–0.13	3.9–4.4	0.93–1.05

* $p < 0.05$; Pre vs post. (Pts 2 and 3: 3 sessions/week.)

Table 2 Predialysis laboratory values before (left column) and after (right column) r-HuEPO

Pt	Ht	Urea mmol/l	Creatinine µmol/l	Potassium mmol/l	Phosphate mmol/l	Bicarbonate mmol/l
1	0.20–0.27	33.6–26.7	1225–1008	5.9–5.5	0.97–1.49	21.3–23.3
2	0.16–0.33	33.6–35.3	1165–1300	6.2–6.8	1.50–2.35	20.4–17.8
3	0.15–0.26	32.4–33.4	1235–1430	7.4–6.4	2.69–2.17	17.6–17.2
4	0.19–0.26	34.6–32.8	1386–1536	6.0–6.8	1.52–1.67	19.3–20.2
5	0.23–0.27	25.1–27.1	1200–1288	5.3–6.1	1.53–1.67	22.3–21.8
6	0.19–0.25	28.3–26.5	1305–1364	5.6–5.5	1.30–1.43	19.8–18.8
7	0.18–0.31	30.9–33.5	1700–1711	5.7–5.9	1.90–2.05	20.5–17.9
8	0.20–0.31	24.8–30.4	0873–0949	4.7–6.5	1.79–2.49	17.6–19.8
mean	0.19–0.28	30.4–30.7*	1261–1323*	5.9–6.2*	1.65–1.92*	19.9–19.6*
SEM	0.01–0.01	1.38–1.25	0082–0054	0.3–0.2	0.18–0.14	0.59–0.75

* = N. S. pre vs post.

40 IU/kg, followed by continuous infusion of 10 IU/kg/hour. In case of visible clotting in the extracorporeal circuit, the heparin dose was increased during the course of the study. All other dialysis prescriptions were carefully kept constant troughout the 6 months study period. All patients received phosphate binding drugs, vitamins and iron preparations if ferritine levels were below 150 µg/l. One patient was on antihypertensive drugs. None of the patients was suffering from aluminum overload (mean serum concentration 54.5 µg/l; upper limit 100), hyperparathyroidism (mean 1–84 PTH concentration 5.5 pmol/l; upper limit 15), pericarditis or infectious diseases.

r-HuEPO (Boehringer Mannheim, Almere, The Netherlands) was administered intravenously at the end of each dialysis session at a dose of 40 U/kg three times per week or 60 U/kg twice weekly. This low dose regimen was chosen in order to obtain a gradual increase of Ht to 30–35% in the course of 12–18 weeks, avoiding undue risks of thrombosis or development of hypertension. All patients completed monthly questionnaires about their general condition, appetite, and social activities.

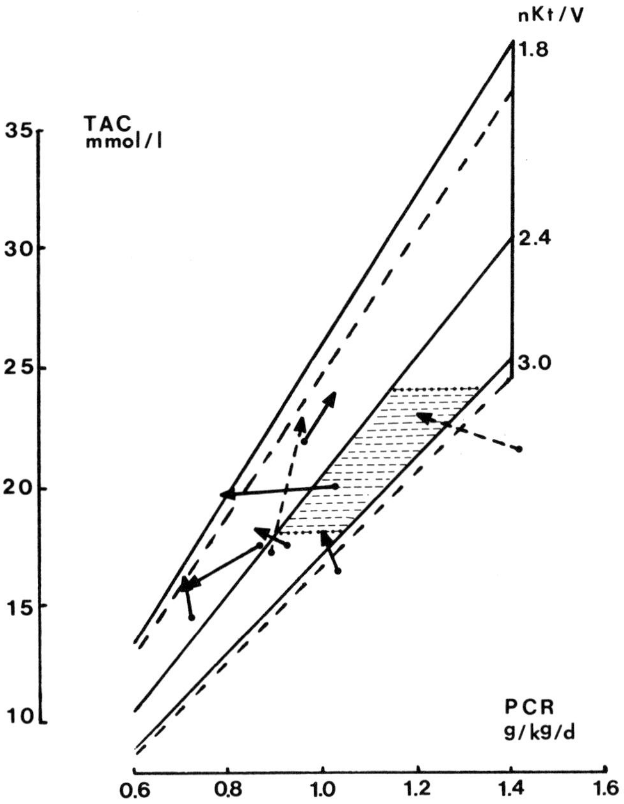

Fig. 1 Change of urea kinetic parameters in 8 patients after 6 months treatment with r-HuEPO. Solid lines: total week Kt/V values for 2 dialysis sessions per week (6 patients); broken lines: 3 sessions per week (2 patients). Shaded area: target domain. See also appendix B for calculations: equations 14 and 15

Urea kinetic studies

Mass balance studies with collection of spent dialysate were performed at the beginning of treatment and after 6 months. The traditional approach as proposed by F. Gotch et al. [1985] using a fixed value of V corresponding to 60% of BW and an estimate of dialyzer clearance derived from in vitro data of the manufacturer, were not considered appropriate for this study. The direct dialysis quantification method of Malchesky, based upon dialysate collection was preferred [Malchesky et al. 1982, Sargent and Gotch 1978, Lowrie and Teehan 1983]. This approach provides reliable values for average in vivo dialyzer clearance (K) and urea distribution volume in the body (V), which are calculated as described previously [Van Geelen and Flendrig 1985]. All dialysate and ultrafiltrate are collected and after stirring a representative sample is drawn in duplicate for determination of urea. Dialysate collection can be facilitated by means of a sampling device that measures total dialysate flow and deviates 1% into a measuring glass (Organon Teknica, Turnhout, Belgium). Urea values were measured in blood from the arterial (predialyzer) line at the beginning (pre-C1) and end (post-C2) of the test dialysis (neglecting rebound phenomena), and immediately prior to the next dialysis (C3). Dialyzer clearance was calculated using equation 2, which takes into account the exponential decline of urea during dialysis. In the absence of residual diuresis the simplified calculation of V according to equation 1 was considered justified. In this equation Vd can be predicted a priori from the time and dialysate flow of the machine, which provides a control of accurate sampling. This equation will yield reproducible values for V in the same patient although it may not reflect actual total body water because it depends on the value of C2, which is not considered to be totally accurate as hemoconcentration at the end of dialysis and rebound phenomena are not taken into account. Protein catabolic rates (PCR) were calculated from the interdialytic interval, which was always planned in the middle of the week, and also expressed per kg of lean body weight (pcr) (appendix A). Time averaged concentration of urea (TAC) is given in mmol/l and is expressed as a function of pcr and Kt/V for 2 and 3 sessions per week to construct the plot in Figure 1 (appendix B). As patients with variable degrees of residual renal function, as well as dialysis schedules with 2 and 3 sessions per week with variable length of time are sometimes compared, we felt that it might be appropriate to formulate a week value of Kt/V in which K is the sum of total dialyzer and renal clearance per week (appendix formula 7). Traditionally Kt/V is given for a midweek dialysis session of 4 hours duration and its target value is equal to 1 [Gotch et al. 1985]. Considering the fact that our in vivo dialyzer clearances (K) are on the average 15% lower than the in vitro estimations in the traditional approach, and that the average value for V is 5% lower, the target index for a 7 day period can be calculated to be 2.7 ± 0.3. However, the validity of this target week index needs to be confirmed by more clinical experience. At the beginning and at the end of the study as well as every month, all other relevant hematological and chemical parameters were determined in duplicate by standard laboratory methods. Results are expressed as the mean and standard error of the mean, and for statistical comparison the student's paired t test was used. P <0.05 was selected as the level of statistical significance.

Results

After 6 months of r-HuEPO treatment, Ht had increased from 18% to 28%, which was still slightly below the target value of 30% (p <0.01). This rise was associated with iron consumption: mean ferritine decreased from 303 to 83 µg/l at the end of the study. Body weight did not increase: 59.9 vs 59.6 kg. The average fluid intake between dialysis sessions did not show significant changes: 2400 vs 2100 ml. Protein catabolic rate (PCR), however, decreased significantly (p <0.05) from 53 to 47 gram/day (Table 1, Figure 1). The average pcr decreased from 0.95 to 0.88 g/kg/d and urea generation rate decreased from 0.165 to 0.146 mmol/min. There was a significant (p <0.05) decrease of average dialyzer clearance from 152 to 132 ml/min, associated with a decrease of weekly values for Kt/V from 2.75 to 2.55. The increase of TAC was relatively small: 18.3 to 19.3 mmol/l (N.S.). Patients number 2 and 3 (Table 1) underwent 3 dialysis sessions per week. Their Kt/V values were slightly higher but the decrease of Kd and Kt/V after 6 months was comparable to that of the other patients. In contrast to the others the PCR values in patient number 3, who was the only male patient, showed a small increase. Decreased efficiency of dialysis was also reflected in the predialysis laboratory data (Table 2), although these changes were not significant, probably due to the small number of patients. As expected (see discussion), predialysis mean urea concentration increased only 1%, whereas creatinine increased 5%, potassium 6% and phosphate 16%. Predialysis pH decreased significantly from 7.37 to 7.34. Reproducibility of the sampling procedures was satisfying as the variation of measured volume of distribution (V) was on the average only 5% (Table 1).

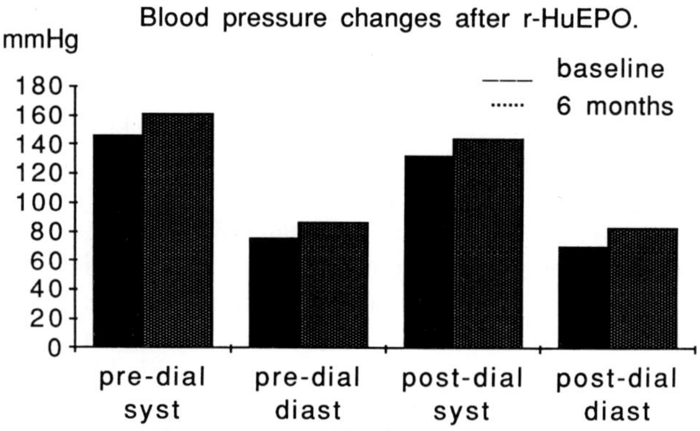

Fig. 2 Pre- and post-treatment blood pressures in 8 patients before (left columns) and after (right columns) 6 months treatment with low dose r-HuEPO

There was a significant (p <0.05) increase of systolic (SBP) and diastolic blood pressure (DBP) before as well as after dialysis in all patients (Figure 2). The mean (SEM) pre-treatment SBP increased from 147 (6.1) to 160 (3.5) mmHg, and DBP from 76 (5.2) to 86 (4.1) mmHg. The mean (SEM) post-treatment SBP increased from 133 (7.5) to 144 (9.1) mmHg and DBP from 71 (3.8) to 84 (3.3) mmHg. In one patient anti-hypertensive drugs were started and in another patient, who already received anti-hypertensive drugs, the dose was increased. Although we did not find significant changes in clotting parameters (bleeding time, clotting time, APTT, PTT, platelet count), in 5 out of 8 patients the heparin dose was increased because of visible fiber clotting in the dialyzers. During the 6 months period we did not observe changes in parathyroid status, aluminum load or vitamin profiles.

All patients completed the questionnaires, which indicated improvement of general condition and expansion of social activities in most of them. Anorexia was not reported.

Discussion

The patients in this study were stable dialysis patients without specific complaints but with relatively short dialysis prescriptions. None of them complained of anorexia. Their dietary compliance was adequate. As there have been no intercurrent diseases, we have assumed that after 6 months of r-HuEPO therapy a new steady state would exist in which protein intake balanced protein catabolic rate. From the fact that body weight remained constant but protein intake decreased we tend to conclude that some avoidance of protein foods may have occurred. Inspection of the individual data in Figure 1 indicates that most patients obtained a steep relationship between TAC and PCR. Thus, small increases in protein intake would have caused large increases of urea with concomitant uremic symptoms. Although body weight remained constant, there was a small decrease in V. This can, however, be explained in different ways. Because V was calculated from an equation that contained C2 as post dialysis urea concentration, there is some methodological inaccuracy involved, caused by the fact that rebound phenomena and hemoconcentration were neglected in C2. On the other hand there might have been a real decrease of distribution volume if, as suggested by Keshaviah, at high Ht there is some restauration of membrane integrity, opposing rapid shifts of urea from one compartment to another. We have no indication that better ultrafiltration was achieved after 6 months r-HuEPO therapy. These explanations however remain speculative. After 6 months of r-HuEPO therapy Ht had gradually increased by 50%. The only change in dialysis prescription was an increase of the heparin dose if indicated by visible clotting in the extracorporeal circuit. Otherwise there had been no alterations in the dialysis schedules. Mean dialyzer urea clearance fell 13% although predialysis values of other uremic markers after 6 months would suggest a less dramatic effect. The corresponding fall of Kt/V was smaller (7%) due to a concomitant decrease of V (55% of body weight before versus 52% after r-HuEPO). As the patients served as their own controls in this study our data indicate that dialyzer function is adversely affected at high Ht levels after r-HuEPO therapy. Casati et al. [1989] found similar changes only at Ht levels over 40%. The small decrease of blood water content at higher Ht, however, does not sufficiently explain these data, especially since the high permeability of the erythrocyte membrane to urea does not restrict transport. Some other influences such as deteriorating rheologic conditions or clotting phenomena might play an additional role, but this cannot be deduced from our data. Clotting parameters did not change significantly during the study and were not useful for the estimation of the increased need for heparin in 5 out of 8 patients. Our findings correspond to those of Paganini et al. [1988] except for the decrease in PCR. This difference may be related to the higher dialysis dose in Paganini's population, with consequently less steep relationships between TAC and PCR. The existence of a decrease of both PCR and dialyzer clearance in our study has opposite effects on predialysis urea concentrations and explains the relatively small increase of urea concentration as compared to predialysis values of other solutes.

Surprisingly, the "low and slow" dosage regimen of r-HuEPO administration which necessitated a dose adaptation in 5 out of 8 patients (average weekly dose from 120 IU/kg to 195 IU/kg) in order to reach the target Ht after 18 weeks, did not prevent the occurrence of hypertension in these patients. This happened in spite of a more moderate fluid intake towards the end of the study.

From this study we are tempted to conclude that the rise of Ht after r-HuEPO leads to decreased dialyzer efficiency, which in short dialysis regimens may lead to underdialysis. The mechanism of decreased dialyzer efficiency remains to be elucidated. As a consequence, in susceptible patients, protein intake may deteriorate, although this study does not suggest real catabolism to occur. Questionnaires did not reveal anorexia and were dominated by responses indicating improvement of general well-being. Obtaining urea kinetic data by means of dialysate sampling, facilitated by a small sampling device, may be considered a feasible and reliable approach when compared to the standard method according to Gotch et al. [1985], which is based upon in vitro clearances and a fixed assumed value for distribution volume.

Acknowledgements

The authors wish to thank Boehringer Mannheim b. v. Almere, The Netherlands, for their collaboration and supply of r-HuEPO.

Appendix A

Definition of kinetic parameters.

Abbreviations:

C1 = urea concentration before dialysis (mmol/l).
C2 = urea concentration after dialysis.
C3 = urea concentration before next dialysis.
Cd = urea concentration in dialysate.
Vd = total volume of spent dialysate (liters).
Kd = dialyzer clearance (ml/min).
Kr = residual renal clearance (ml/min).
Td = dialysis time (min).
Tid = interval between dialysis sessions (min).
V = urea distribution volume in the body (liters).
ΔV = volume of ultrafiltrate.
G = urea appearance rate (mmol/min).
TAC = time averaged concentration of urea in blood (mmol/l).
PCR = protein catabolic rate (g/d).
pcr = normalized protein catabolic rate (g/l/d).

Calculations:

In case of anuria the following mass balance is assumed:

$$Vd * Cd = (V + 0.5\ \Delta V)C1 - (V - 0.5\ \Delta V)C2 \quad (1)$$

Considering the exponential decrease of blood urea concentration during the dialysis session, the average clearance is calculated as described before (10):

$$Kd = \frac{Vd * Cd * \ln C1/C2}{(C1 - C2) * Td} \quad (2)$$

From the interval between the dialysis sessions the urea appearance rate is calculated:

$$G = \frac{V * (C3 - C2)}{Tid} + \frac{Kr\ (C3 + C2)}{2000} \quad (3)$$

The second term is neglected when residual renal clearance (Kr) is less than 0.5 ml/min. (In the present study all patients had neglectable residual functions.) TAC is calculated from the total observation period (Td + Tid):

$$TAC = \frac{(C1 + C2) * Td + (C2 + C3) * Tid}{2\,(Td + Tid)} \quad (4)$$

PCR is calculated according to Sargent et al. (12), with conversion of urea (mmol/l) to protein (g/d):

$$PCR = 262\ G + 0.294\ V \quad (5)$$

pcr is normalised to theoretical lean body weight, assuming a body water content of 58%:

$$pcr = PCR/1.72\ V \quad (6)$$

In the table Kt/V is expressed as the weekly combined renal and dialyzer clearance if residual renal clearance is more than 0.5 ml/min; n = the number of dialysis sessions per week.

$$Kt/V = \frac{Kd * Td * n + 10080\ Kr}{1000\ V} \quad (7)$$

Appendix B

Expression of TAC as a function of pcr and Kt/V for 2 and 3 dialysis sessions per week.

In Figure 1 the following simplifications were applied: TAC = 0.5 (C1 + C2) and Kt/V relates to only one dialysis session. Furthermore we assume: C3 = C1.

Defining $\Delta C = C1 - C2$,
and $C2 = C1\ \exp\text{-}Kt/V$, (8)

then: $\Delta C = C1\,(1 - \exp\text{-}Kt/V)$ and $TAC = 0.5\ C1\,(1 + \exp\text{-}Kt/V)$ (9)

$$TAC = \frac{0.5\ \Delta C\ (1 + \exp\text{-}Kt/V)}{(1 - \exp\text{-}Kt/V)} \quad (10)$$

As C3 = C1, expression (3) can be written as:
$G = V * \Delta C/Tid$, and substituted in (10):

$$TAC = \frac{0.5\ (G * Tid/V) * (1 + \exp\text{-}Kt/V)}{(1 + \exp\text{-}Kt/V)} \quad (11)$$

Rearranging (5): $G = (PCR - 0.294\ V)/262$,
or $G = 0.00382\ PCR - 0.00112\ V$ and substitution in (11) gives:

$$TAC = \frac{[0.5\ Tid\ (0.00382\ PCR - 0.00112\ V)/V] * [1 + \exp\text{-}Kt/V]}{[1 - \exp\text{-}Kt/V]} \quad (12)$$

Rearrangement of (6) and substitution to solve for V yields:

$$TAC = \frac{0.5\ Tid\ (0.00658\ pcr - 0.00112) * (1 + \exp\text{-}Kt/V)}{(1 - \exp\text{-}Kt/V)} \quad (13)$$

Then, for a 2 sessions/week schedule the average value for Tid is approximately 4000 minutes and for a 3 sessions/week schedule 2650 minutes, which, substituted in (13) gives:

$$TAC = \frac{(13.2\ pcr - 2.24) * (1 + \exp\text{-}Kt/V)}{(1 - \exp\text{-}Kt/V)} \quad (n = 2) \quad (14)$$

and

$$TAC = \frac{(8.72\ pcr - 1.48) * (1 + \exp\text{-}Kt/V)}{(1 - \exp\text{-}Kt/V)} \quad (n = 3) \quad (15)$$

REFERENCES

Babb AL, Popovich RP, Christopher TG, Scribner BH 1971 The genesis of the square meter-hour hypothesis. Trans Am Soc Artif Internal Organs *17:* 81–92

Bommer J, Alexiou C, Müller-Bühl U 1987 Recombinant human erythropoietin therapy in hemodialysis patients. Dose determination and clinical experience. Nephrol Dial Transplant *2:* 238–242

Bosch JP, Barlee V, Von Albertini B 1989 Impact of hematocrit (Hct) on solute transport in hemodialysis. Kidney Int *35:* 241 (abstr)

Casati S, Campise M, Crepaldi M, Lobo J, Graziani G, Ponticelli C 1989 Haemodialysis efficiency after long-term treatment with recombinant human erythropoietin. Nephrol Dial Transplant *4:* 718–720

Eschbach JW, Egrie JC, Downing MR, Browie JK, Adamson JW 1987 Correction of anemia of end stage renal disease with recombinant human erythropoietin: result of a phase I and II clinical trial. N Engl J Med *310:* 73–78

Van Geelen J, Flendrig J 1985 Evaluation of in vivo solute clearances during hemodialysis and hemodiafiltration. Dialysis Transplant *14:* 85–88

Gotch FA, Sargent JA 1985 A mechanistic analysis of the National Cooperative Dialysis Study (NCDS). Kidney Int *28:* 526–534

Harter HR et al 1983 Review of significant findings from the National Cooperative Dialysis Study and recommendations. Kidney Int *23:* S107–S112

Lowrie EG, Teehan BP 1983 Principles of prescribing dialysis therapy: Implementing recommendations from the National Cooperative Dialysis Study. Kidney Int *23 (Suppl 13):* 113–122

Malchesky PS, Ellis P, Nosse S, Magnusson M, Lankhorst B, Nakamoto S 1982 Direct quantification of Dialysis. Dial Transplant *11:* 42

Paganini E, Garcia J, Ellis E, Bodnar D, Magnusson M 1988 Clinical sequellae of correction of anemia with recombinant human erythropoietin (r-HuEPO): urea kinetics, dialyzer function and reuse. Am J Kidney Dis *11:* A16 (abstr)

Sargent J, Gotch F 1978 Urea kinetics: a guide to nutritional management of renal failure. Am J Clin Nutr *31:* 1696–1702

Shinaberger JH, Miller JH, Gardner PW, West LA 1989 Disadvantages and risks of normal hematocrit (Hct) hemodialysis (HD). Kidney Int *35:* 264 (abstr)

Zehnder C 1989 Erythropoietin treatment: influence of hemoglobin concentration on dialyzer creatinine clearance in hemodialysed patients. Nephron *51:* 424–425

Zehnder C, Glück Z, Decoeudres C, Uehlinger DE, Blumberg A 1988 Human recombinant erythropoietin in anaemic patients on maintenance hemodialysis, secondary effects of the increase of hemoglobin. Nephrol Dial Transplant *3:* 657–660

Zehnter E, Pollok M, Ziegenhagen D et al 1988 Urea kinetics in patients on regular dialysis treatment before and after treatment with recombinant human erythropoietin. Contr Nephrol *66:* 149–155

Clinical Nephrology, Vol. 35 No. 4 – 1991 (171–175)

Acute encephalopathy due to thiamine deficiency (Wernicke's encephalopathy) in a chronic hemodialyzed patient: a case report

E. Descombes[1], C.-A. Dessibourg[2] and G. Fellay[1]

[1] *Dialysis Unit, Hopital Cantonal, CH-1700 Fribourg, Switzerland*
[2] *Neurology Consultant, Medicine Departement, Hopital Cantonal, CH-1700 Fribourg, Switzerland*

Abstract. We report the case of a patient with terminal renal disease on chronic hemodialysis who developed acute thiamine deficiency as confirmed by erythrocyte transketolase determinations. The patient presented with a confusional state and severe memory disturbances, but other classical features of Wernicke's encephalopathy were absent. Almost all central nervous system symptoms rapidly disappeared after thiamine therapy. Therefore the possibility of thiamine deficiency must be considered in patients on chronic dialysis who present with central nervous system disturbances, even if all of the classical features of Wernicke's encephalopathy are not present.

Key words: thiamine deficiency – erythrocyte transketolase activity – hemodialysis – Wernicke's encephalopathy – electroencephalogram

Introduction

Central nervous system dysfunction due to thiamine deficiency is one known complication of dialysis [Raskin and Fishman 1976, Dreyfus 1979, Mahoney and Arieff 1982, Arieff 1986]. However only a few cases of Wernicke's encephalopathy in dialyzed patients are reported in literature, and all concern diagnosis made postmortem [Lopez and Collins 1968, Faris 1972, Ebels 1974, Jagadha et al. 1987]. We recently observed a patient on chronic hemodialysis who developed severe neurological disturbances due to acute thiamine deficiency and in whom thiamine therapy almost completely reversed symptoms.

As appropriate therapy can be life-saving or prevent irreversible neurological damage, thiamine deficiency must be considered in differential diagnosis of diffuse neurological abnormalities occurring in dialyzed patients. However thiamine deficiency seems to occur more frequently than Wernicke's encephalopathy and this point is briefly commented.

Case report

A 77-year-old man had a 10-year history of renal disease. In 1936, after an appendectomy, agenesia of the left kidney was diagnosed; gout was diagnosed in 1957. Since 1979 his renal function had become progressively impaired and hemodialysis had to be started in February 1987. As a residual diuresis of more than 1000 ml/day was still present, the patient was dialysed for 4 hours twice a week using a cellulose acetate filter (CA 210) with a bicarbonate dialysate and a Fresenius monitor. Although the patient was relatively thin we considered him to be satisfactorily nourished. He was on a free diet with only recommendations for a salt consumption of 3–4 g/day. There was no history of alcohol abuse. Current therapy consisted of Lasix 125 mg/day, aluminum hydroxide 2,4 g/day, calcium carbonate 3 g/day, Rocaltrol 0,25 microg/day and Laroxyl 25 mg/day.

In November 1988, a vitamin screening performed on all patients attending our center, showed a normal red blood cells transketolase activity (alpha-ETK ratio = 1.07; N <1.13)$^{\text{Note}}_{\text{p. 5}}$. At that time no thiamine supplementation was given to patients attending our center.

On January 13 1989, the patient had an operation for cataract of the left eye which was performed in our hospital under general anesthesia. Postoperative progress was favorable and the patient returned home on January 23, after a dialysis session. During this session the nurses noticed slight character disturbances and slight disorientation. At home, the patient complained of abdominal pain which was associated with inappetence, nausea and diarrhea. Due to these symptoms he ate very poorly for 3 days.

Received April 17, 1990; in revised form September 27, 1990.

Table 1 Laboratory Data

Date	BUN mmol/l	Glucose mmol/l	Na mmol/l	K mmol/l	Ca mmol/l	P mmol/l	Mg mmol/l	Al µmol/L	Hb g/L
12.1	32/18	5.8/–	139/136	5.8/4.8	2.75/2.70	1.2/1.3	1.05/0.95	–	107
26.1	–/25	–/5.1	–/142	–/6.0	–/2.80	–	–	–	88
27.1	26/13	5.9/4.8	139/139	5.7/4.0	2.25/2.60	–	–	–	103
28.1	16/–	5.8/–	142/–	4.0/–	–	–	–	–	–
2.2	14/6	–	142/143	–	2.30/2.50	0.8/0.9	0.90/0.80	–	107
20.2	13/8	–	143/140	4.2/3.8	2.55/–	–	–	1.6	90
Normal	3.8–7.0	3.9–6.1	136–150	3.7–5.0	2.20–2.80	0.8–1.6	0.89–1.00	<0.4	>120

/: values before and after dialysis

On January 26 (day 1), when arriving at the dialysis center, the patient showed marked character changes. After 2 hours of dialysis he became agitated, confused, disoriented and pulled away the dialysis needles. On clinical examination he was disoriented in time and space, showed symmetrical myoclonic jerks of the extremities and talked as if in quasi-delirium. His axillary temperature was 36.5° C, his pulse rate was 100/min and his blood pressure was 120/80 mmHg; abdominal examination showed diffuse tenderness, particularly in the right upper quadrant, with peritoneal symptoms; neurological assessment showed no meningeal symptoms, no gross sensory or motor losses and no ocular abnormalities; reflexes were symmetrical but knee-jerks were diminished and ankle-jerks were absent; cutaneous plantar was in flexion bilaterally. Some laboratory data are reported in Table 1. Other relevant data revealed white blood cells 20,300 cells/mm^3, platelets 252,000/mm^3, SGOT 91 UI/L (N <40), SGPT 162 UI/L (N <40), alkaline phosphatase 958 UI/L (N <246), gamma-GT 497 UI/L (N <50), total bilirubin 22 U/L (N <18.8), direct bilirubin 15 UI/L (N <3.4), serum amylase 65 UI/L (N <100), total protein 69 g/L, bicarbonate 17.6 mmol/L (N 23–27). The electroencephalogram (EEG) showed a bilateral theta and even delta diffuse but predominantly frontal bradyarrhythmia, without triphasic waves or spikes, which accords with a non-specific metabolic encephalopathy (Figure 1). A laparotomy was performed in the afternoon and, as acute cholecystitis was found, cholecystectomy was performed. During the operation the patient was perfused with a normal saline solution and transfused twice; after the operation a 5–10% glucose solution was perfused.

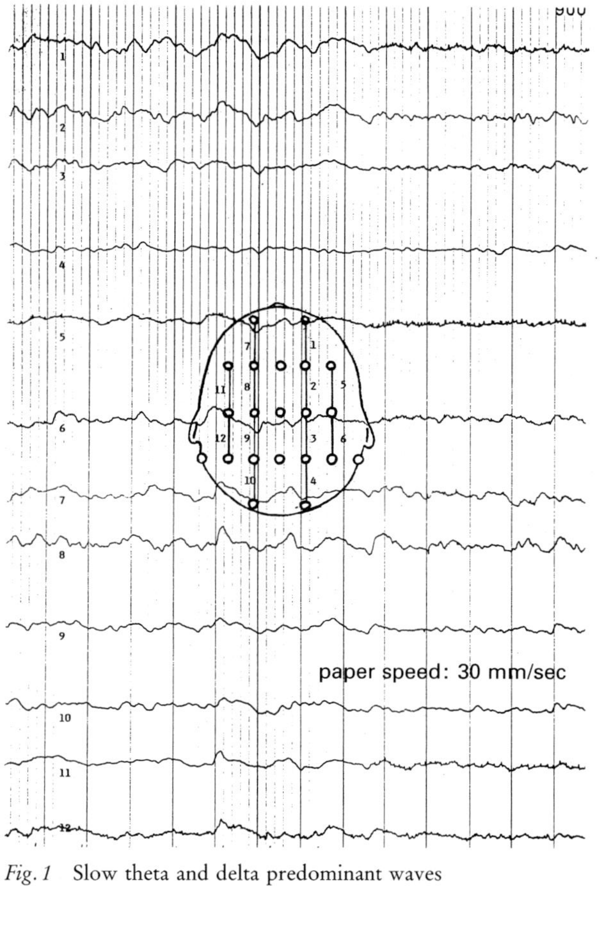

Fig. 1 Slow theta and delta predominant waves

On the second day, the patient was still intubated and presented some bilateral myoclonic jerks. A pericardial rub consistent with an uremic pericarditis was present. Considering this finding and neuro-psychological abnormalities compatible with an uremic encephalopathy, it was decided to intensify dialysis; so the patient was dialyzed six times in the following seven days.

On the third day, the patient was disoriented with intermittent periods of restlessness and showed considerable memory disturbances: he didn't know his name and birthday, didn't recognize his wife or the physician or dialysis nurses he had known for a long time; when meeting the physician many times a day he didn't remember previous visits. When asked about those previous points the patient looked perplex but, on the other hand, when asked about a concrete item, i.e. pain or thirst, he answered adequately. On neurological examination there were no lateralized signs, no oculomotor palsies, no speech disturbances nor dyspraxia; on the fourth and the fifth days the patient could stand up and walked slowly but was not frankly atactic.

With daily dialysis we obtained good laboratory results (Table 1), the pericardial rub rapidly disappeared but no changes were produced in the mental state of the patient. As no neuropsychiatric improvement was observed, thiamine deficiency was considered on the sixth day. Blood samples were taken for measurement and thiamine was given orally at a dose of 900 mg/day (3 × 300 mg, Benerva®). The blood taken on the sixth day was highly deficient in RBC transketolase activity (alpha-ETK ratio = 1.30, N <1.13).

Some hours after the first dose of thiamine the patient already showed improvement of central nervous system functions and in the next 48 hours he became progressively more oriented and memory disturbances almost completely disappeared. Owing to dysfunction the arterio-venous fistula had to be repeated on the eighth day and the operation was well tolerated. On day 13 the patient was able to go back home in a good physical and psychic state; he was well oriented, had no more memory problems and the character changes noticed prior to admission had disappeared. Thus no Korsakoff syndrome was to be observed at that time. To rule out a concomitant aluminum intoxication, serum aluminum was determined on February 20 and was 1.6 micromol/L (40 microg/L). A control EEG performed some weeks later after a dialysis session was nearly normal with a well-distributed and reactive alpha rhythm of 8 c/s (Figure 2).

Discussion

Since its original description by Carl Wernicke in 1881, Wernicke's encephalopathy (WE) has been considered to be a syndrome occurring mostly in chronic malnourished alcoholics, and taking either an acute, subacute or chronic course [Harper 1979, Adams and Victor 1981]. However, since then, some reports have pointed out that WE can occur in other clinical circumstances, mostly associated with insufficient nutrition [Reuler et al. 1985, Victor and Martin 1987]. Dialysis is generally considered as a predisposing factor to thiamine deficiency and WE, but, to our knowledge, only 8 cases of WE have been reported in literature, and in all cases diagnosis was made retrospectively at autopsy [Lopez and Collins 1968, Faris 1972, Ebels 1974, Jagadha et al. 1987].

Some recent clinical and anatomo-clinical reports have pointed out that clinical presentation of WE may be quite variable and that the classical triad of confusional state, ataxia and ophthalmoplegia is present in only a minority of cases (16–44%) [Brew 1986, Harper et al. 1986, Naidoo 1988]. According to those results some authors consider that WE is underdiagnosed in clinical practice. In autopsy series prevalence of WE varied between 0.8% and 2.8%, with no more than 25% of the cases being diagnosed before death [Cravioto et al. 1961, Ebels 1974, Torvik et al. 1982, Harper et al. 1986]. Mental changes, particularly confusional state and memory problems, are the most frequent clinical features reported (50–100%). Ocular abnormalities, generally considered a striking feature of WE, are reported with quite different frequencies in clinical (53% to 95%) [Brew 1986, Wood et al. 1986, Naidoo 1988] or anatomopathological studies (29% to 32%) [Cravioto et al. 1961, Harper et al. 1986]. This difference is partly due to the fact that in clinical studies the presence of these clinical signs is one of the criteria by which the patients are selected. It is clear that if diagnosis of WE is considered only in patients with all of the clinical signs, many cases of limited

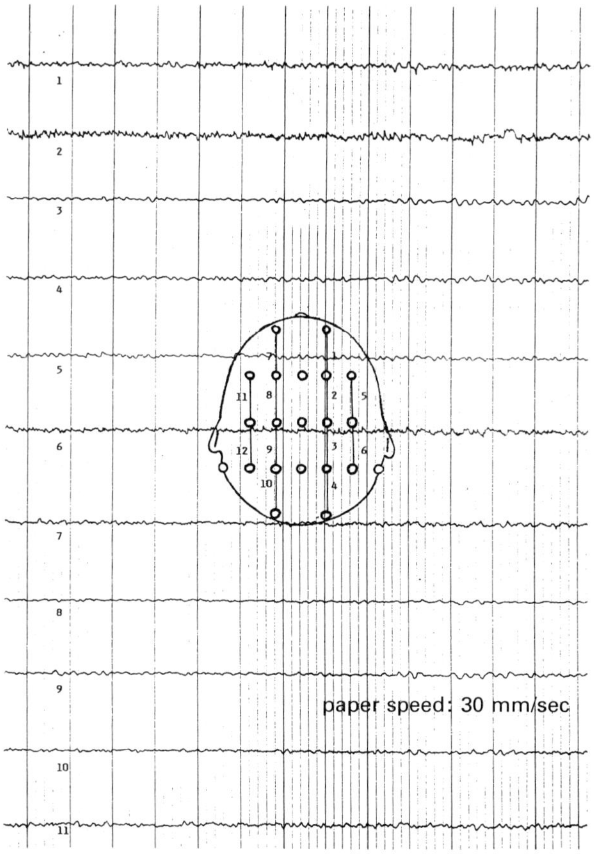

Fig. 2 Alpha dominant nearly normal EEG

forms of WE will not be recognized, and therefore not treated. RBC transketolase activity is a good indicator of thiamine deficiency, although it may be normal in some patients with clinical features of WE [Leigh et al. 1981, Wood et al. 1986].

For our patient positive diagnosis of WE was made on the basis of: 1) central nervous system disturbances with considerable loss of memory; 2) rapid clinical improvement after thiamine supplementation; 3) deficient RBC transketolase activity (which had been normal two months before). Clinically there was no ophthalmoplegia or frank ataxia. When compared to the clinical data of the five cases reported by Jagadha et al. [1987] quite similar features were present in our patient such as personality changes, confusion, loss of memory and myoclonic jerks. Some of these clinical features are also commonly observed in aluminum intoxication; however aluminum encephalopathy has a quite different clinical course and occurs in patients who have been on HD much longer and who have serum aluminum concentrations much higher than our patient [Mc Kinney et al. 1982, Winney et al. 1985, Alfrey 1986, Rovelli et al. 1988]. Furthermore most patients with aluminum encephalopathy have typical EEG features, characterized by bursts of slow activity with rather normal background activity between bursts, which are almost pathognomic of dialysis encephalopathy [Hughes and Schreeder 1980, Alfrey 1986]. On the other hand EEG is nonspecific in WE and shows a general slowing of the background activity with an excess of theta and delta waves which are bilaterally synchronous and, as a rule, symmetrical [Adams and Victor 1981, Kiloh et al. 1981]; similar nonspecific features may be found in other encephalopathies associated with uremia and/or dialysis [Raskin and Fishman 1976, Mahoney et Arieff 1982]. Lastly, we have to note that myoclonic jerks did not find any expression on our EEG recording, which can be the case in many metabolic encephalopathies.

Some general considerations can be outlined from these clinical observations:

a) occurrence of neurological disturbances is not rare in dialysis patients and the differential diagnosis must consider a wide range of etiologies, related or unrelated to the dialytic therapy itself [Raskin and Fishman 1976, Mahoney and Arieff 1982, Arieff 1986, Victor and Martin 1987]. A positive clinical diagnosis is sometimes quite difficult, particularly in elderly patients who may present several concomitant uremic and/or degenerative problems, which may further confuse the clinical picture. Concerning WE it is interesting to note that the mean age of the 8 autopsy-diagnosed cases reported in the literature was 44 years (range 12 to 66 years) and that the clinical diagnoses were as follows: uremic encephalopathy (3), dysequilibrium syndrome (1), dialysis dementia (1), brainstem hemorrhage (1), sepsis with associated drug toxicity (1) and not reported (1). Three of these cases had ocular abnormalities which may have suggested WE, but WE was not considered as there was no history of alcohol abuse. Uremic encephalopathy was also the initial diagnosis in our patient, and it was only as no improvement was obtained with daily HD that the alternative diagnosis of WE was considered. Due to the small number of cases reported in literature WE seems to be a rare complication of dialysis. However we question if, due to the nonspecific clinical picture in most patients, the diagnosis of WE is not overlooked in some dialysis patients. As WE is readily treatable we consider therefore that thiamine deficiency must be considered in the differential diagnosis of dialysis patients presenting with unexplained diffuse disturbances of the central nervous system, even if all the classical clinical signs of WE are not present.

b) biochemical thiamine deficiency is not so rare in dialyzed patients [Kuriyama et al. 1980, Marumo et al. 1986, Ramirez et al. 1986]; a general screening performed in Nov 1988 in patients attending our center showed that 18% out of 46 had a deficient RBC transketolase activity (alpha-ETK ratio ranging from 1.17 to 1.24 unpublished data). A similar incidence of biochemical thiamine deficiency has also been reported in asymptomatic patients with alcoholic liver disease [Camilo et al. 1981]. So it is of interest that only a few patients develop clinical manifestations of WE. This is attributed by some authors to individual predisposition due to a genetic defect in transketolase activity [Blass and Gibson 1977, Leigh et al. 1981, Reuler et al. 1985]; in an experimental study Goto et al. [1986] showed that, in rats, the more serious lesions of CNS occur when thiamine deficiency is associated with insufficient magnesium intake; previously also Traviesa [1974] suggested a possible role of hypomagnesemia in clinical resistance to thiamine therapy in a patient with WE. However, as already pointed out by Jaghada et al. [1987], we have to note that WE generally occurs in dialysis patients who are severely ill with subsequent poor vitamin intake (febrile illness, infection, operation, poor eating and/or vomiting, intravenous alimentation without adequate vitamin supplement, etc.) and that often the clinical course is aggravated by intravenous glucose loading, which increases thiamine requirement, as was probably the case in our patient.

c) many centers give systematic vitamin supplement to dialysis patients, but data concerning water-soluble vitamins needs in patients on maintenance hemodialysis are controversial [Kurijama et al. 1980, DeBari et al. 1984, Stein et al. 1985, Marumo et al. 1986, Ramirez et al. 1986, Allman et al. 1989]. For this reason a prospective study concerning needs for systematic supplementation is presently being conducted at our center. Anyway considering thiamine, since the amount of thiamine stored in the body is in any case limited [Schaeffer et al. 1977], it would probably be a wise policy to provide a preventive supplement of this vitamin in high doses at time of particular stress, such as acute illness or operation.

Note: vitamin activity determinations were performed by Hoffman-La Roche Research Laboratories (Basel, Switzerland), using the transketolase test (ETK) according to the method described by Schouten and colleagues (Transketolase in blood. Clinica Chim Acta 10, 474, 1964).

REFERENCES

Adams RD, Victor M 1981 The Wernicke-Korsakoff syndrome. In Principles of Neurology (2nd ed). New York, McGraw-Hill Book Company

Alfrey AC 1986 Dialysis encephalopathy. Kid Int Suppl *18:* 53–57

Allman MA, Truswll AS, Tiller DJ, Stewart PM et al 1989 Vitamin supplementation of patients receiving haemodialysis. Med J Aust *150:* 130–133

Arieff AI 1986 Neurological complications of uremia. In: *Brenner BM, Rector FC (eds)* The kidney (3rd ed). Philadelphia, WB Saunders

Blass JP, Gibson GE 1977 Abnormality of a thiamine-requiring enzyme in patients with Wernicke-Korsakoff syndrome. N Engl J Med *297:* 1367–1370

Brew BJ 1986 Diagnosis of Wernicke's encephalopathy. Aust N Z J Med *16:* 676–678

Camilo ME, Morgan MY, Sherlock S 1981 Erythrocyte transketolase activity in alcoholic liver disease. Scand J Gastroent *16:* 273–279

Cravioto H, Korein J, Silberman J 1961 Wernicke's encephalopathy. A clinical and pathological study of 28 autopsied cases. Arch Neurol *4:* 510–519

DeBari VA, Franck O, Baker H, Needle MA 1984 Water-soluble vitamins in granulocytes, erythrocytes, and plasma obtained from chronic hemodialysis patients. Am J Clin Nutr *39:* 410–415

Dreyfus PM 1979 Nutritional disorders of de nervous system. In: *Beeson PB, McDermott W, Wyngaarden JB (eds)* Textbook of medicine (15th ed.). Philadelphia, Saunders

Ebels EJ 1974 Underlying illness in Wernicke's encephalopathy. Analysis of possible causes of under-diagnosis. Europ Neurol *12:* 226–228

Faris AA 1972 Wernicke's encephalopathy in uremia. Neurology *22:* 1293–1297

Goto I, Nagara H, Tateishi J, Kuroiwa Y 1986 Thiamine-deficient encephalopathy in rats: effects of deficiencies of thiamine and magnesium. Brain Res *372:* 31–36

Harper CG 1979 Wernicke's encephalopathy: a more common disease than realized. A neuropathological study of 51 cases. J Neurol Neurosurg Psychiat *42:* 226–231

Harper CG, Giles M, Finlay-Jones R 1986 Clinical signs in the Wernicke-Korsakoff complex: a retrospective analysis of 131 cases diagnosed at necropsy. J Neurol Neurosurg Psychiat *49:* 341–345

Hughes JR, Schreeder MT 1980 EEG in dialysis encephalopathy. Neurology *30:* 1148–1154

Kiloh LG, McComas AJ, Osselton JW, Upton ARM 1981 Acute thiamine deficiency. In: Clinical Electroencephalography (fourth ed). London. Butterworths

Kuriyama M, Mizuma A, Yokomine R, Igata A, Otuji Y 1980 Erythrocyte transketolase activity in uremia. Clinica Chim Acta *108:* 169–177

Jagadha V, Deck JH, Halliday WC, Smyth HS 1987 Wernicke's encephalopathy in patients on peritoneal dialysis or hemodialysis. Ann Neurol *2:* 78–84

Leigh D, McBurney A, Ilwain H 1981 Wernicke-Korsakoff syndrome in monozygotic twins: a biochemical peculiarity. Brit J Psychit *139:* 156–159

Leigh D, McBurney A, McIlwain H 1981 Erythrocyte transketolase activity in the Wernicke-Korsakoff syndrome. Brit J Psychiat *139:* 153–155

Lopez RI, Collins GH 1968 Wernicke's encephalopathy. A complication of chronic hemodialysis. Arch Neurol *18:* 248–259

Mahoney CA, Arieff AI 1982 Uremic encephalopathies: clinical, biochemical and experimental features. Am J Kidney Dis *2 (3):* 324–336

Marumo F, Kamata K, Okubo M 1986 Deranged concentrations of water-soluble vitamins in the blood of undialyzed and dialyzed patients with chronic renal failure. Int J Artif Org *9:* 17–24

McKinney TD, Basinger M, Dawson E, Jones MM 1982 Serum aluminum levels in dialysis dementia. Nephron *32:* 53–56

Naidoo DP 1988 Wernicke's encephalopathy in Durban. A retrospective analysis. S Afr Med J *74:* 293–294

Ramirez G, Chen M, Boyce HW et al 1986 Longitudinal follow-up chronic hemodialysis patients without vitamin supplementation. Kidney Int *30:* 99–106

Raskin NH, Fishman RA 1976 Neurologic disorders in renal failure. N Engl J Med *294 (3 and 4):* 143–148 (first part) and 204–210 (second part)

Reuler JB, Girard DE, Cooney TG 1985 Wernicke's encephalopathy; current concepts. N Engl J Med *312 (16):* 1035–39

Rovelli E, Luciani L, Pagani C, Albonico C, Colleoni N, D'Amico G 1988 Correlation between serum aluminum concentration and signs of encephalopathy in a large population of patients dialyzed with aluminum-free fluids. Clin Nephrol *29 (6):* 294–298

Schaeffer G, Quirin H, Kern U, Mix A, Nakayama T 1977 Zur Frage der Vitaminzufuhr bei dialysen Patienten. Akt Ernährung 1–4: Georg Thieme Verlag, Stuttgart

Stein G, Sperschneider H, Koppe S 1985 Vitamin levels in chronic renal failure and need for supplementation. Blood Purification *3:* 52–62

Torvik A, Lindboe CF, Rogde S 1982 Brain lesions in alcoholics: a neuropathological study with clinical correlations. J Neurol Sci *56:* 233–248

Traviesa DC 1974 Magnesium deficiency: a possible cause of thiamine refractoriness in Wernicke-Korsakoff encephalopathy. J Neurol Neurosurg Psychiat *37:* 959–962

Victor M, Martin JB 1987 Nutritional and metabolic diseases of nervous system. In: Harrison's principles of internal medicine (11th ed). New York, McGraw-Hill Book Company

Winney RJ, Cowie JF, Robson JS 1985 What is the value of plasma/serum aluminum in patients with chronic renal failure? Clin Nephrol *24 (Suppl 1):* 2–8

Wood B, Currie J, Breen K 1986 Wernicke's encephalopathy in a metropolitan hospital. Med J Aust *144:* 12–16

Uremic polyneuropathy: a clinical and electrophysiological study in 135 short- and long-term hemodialyzed patients

C. Bazzi[1], C. Pagani[2], G. Sorgato[1], G. Albonico[2], G. Fellin[1] and G. D'Amico[1]

[1]*Division of Nephrology and Dialysis, San Carlo Borromeo Hospital, and*
[2]*Division of Neurology, San Carlo Borromeo Hospital, Milano, Italy*

Abstract. Twenty neurophysiological parameters were employed to evaluate the presence and the degree of peripheral neuropathy (PNP) in a cohort of 135 patients (pts) on regular dialysis treatment (RDT) for 2 to 184 months. The 135 pts were divided into 3 groups according to the duration of RDT (group I: 52 pts with less than 5 yrs; group II: 46 pts 5 to 10 yrs; group III: 37 pts 10 to 15 yrs). Each group was then divided into two subgroups according to age (less or more than 47 yrs) to evaluate the influence of age on PNP. Correlations of electrophysiological parameters with some biochemical parameters (urea, creatinine, PTH) were looked for. The presence of clinical PNP was evaluated according to the Bolton classification: in group I, 50% of pts have mild PNP; in group II, 45.7% of pts have mild PNP; in group III, 81.1% have mild, 10.8% have moderate and 2.7% of pts have severe PNP. In as many as 84.4% of the 135 pts at least one of the 20 parameters studied had abnormal values and in 63% two or more parameters were abnormal. Of 20 parameters evaluated separately in the 3 groups only three showed abnormal mean values: sural nerve latency in all 3 groups; sural nerve Sensory Conduction Velocity (SCV) and peroneal nerve Max. Motor Conduction Velocity (MCV) in group III. Five parameters referring to ulnar nerves and two referring to the sural nerve were significantly more impaired in the group of pts with the longest duration of RDT and in this group the impairment was more severe in older patients. Ulnar nerve MCV was significantly more impaired in pts with higher levels of PTH. In summary, long-term dialysis treatment does not prevent persistence of mild signs of PNP, which is worse in pts with more than 10 yrs of RDT and older than 47 yrs.

Key words: uremic polyneuropathy – electrophysiology – hemodialysis

Introduction

While earlier studies suggested that the polyneuropathy (PNP) present in the severe stages of uremia progressively regressed during regular dialysis treatment (RDT) [Konotey-Ahulu et al. 1965, Jebsen et al. 1967], more recent studies [Mariani et al. 1971, Nielsen 1974, Bolton et al. 1975, Mc Comas et al. 1975, Caccia et al. 1977, Albertazzi et al. 1981, Di Paolo et al. 1988] have documented that on long-term RDT there may be disappearance of overt clinical signs of PNP, but not complete regression of electrophysiological abnormalities, which tend to improve and eventually to stabilize. However, no study conducted on a large population of RDT patients has analyzed the effect of a protracted hemodialytic treatment (over 10 years) on the electrophysiological derangement. The world-wide diffusion of "short-dialysis" strategies, which do not ensure sustained depuration of "middle molecular size" toxins, thought to be some of the major neurotoxic substances [Babb et al. 1973, Savazzi et al. 1982], could in the long run lead to a slowly progressive course of PNP.

Electrophysiological parameters of peripheral nerve function are not a very sensitive short-term index of insufficient dialysis [Teschan et al. 1983]; comparison of these parameters in large enough groups of patients with widely differing durations of regular hemodialysis treatment is necessary to establish whether such treatment, even when protracted over more than 10 years, still guaranties sufficient control of peripheral nerve alterations [Savazzi 1981]. Moreover, the most commonly used motor conduc-

Received April 4, 1990; in revised form January 1, 1991.

Reprint requests to Dr. Claudio Bazzi, Division of Nephrology, San Carlo Borromeo Hospital, Via Pio II, 3, 20153 Milano, Italy.

tion tests (median, ulnar, peroneal and tibial nerves), especially when only a few of them are performed, as is very often the case [for example, Wesely et al. 1989], are not sufficient to exhaustively demonstrate PNP. In fact, they might be still normal in subjects who have PNP that could be proved by a study of the sensory electrophysiological parameters (median, ulnar and sural nerves), probably more sensitive but not widely used by nephrologists [Nielsen 1973, Nielsen 1974, Fraser 1988].

We report the results of an analysis of a wide spectrum of clinical and electrophysiological signs of PNP in 135 patients who had been on RDT for periods ranging from a few months to 15 years. Because we have shifted to short-dialysis treatment since 1973, all the patients with less than 10 years of treatment at the time of the study had been treated from the beginning with the schedule proposed by Cambi [Cambi et al. 1975] and reported by us at the VIth International Congress of Nephrology in 1975 [D'Amico et al. 1976].

Table 1 Regular dialysis treatment modalities

Membrane	Cuprophan
Surface area	1 mq
Hours of dialysis/Day	11–12 until 1972 4–5 from 1973
Number of hemodialysis/Week	2/week until 1972 3/week from 1973
Dialysis fluid composition	Na 132 mEq/l until 1972 K 1.5 mEq/l until 1972 Ca 2.5 mEq/l until 1972 Na 138–142 mEq/l from 1973 K 1.5–3.5 mEq/l from 1973 Ca 4.0 mEq/l from 1973 Mg 1.5 mEq/l Acetate 37 mEq/l Glucose 0 g/l Q. D. 500 ml/min
Blood flow	325 ml/min from 1973

Patients

All the patients on regular dialysis treatment (RDT) at the Renal Unit of our hospital, with the exception of those with diabetes mellitus, chronic alcoholism, exposure to neurotoxic agents, collagen-vascular diseases, amyloidosis and sarcoidosis, were analyzed during the course of a few months. All patients were treated only with hemodialysis. A total of 135 patients on RDT for 2 to 184 months (mean: 72.6 ± 52) were evaluated. The mean age was 47.3 years ± 11.2 (range 21–72 years); 86 were men (63.8%) and 49 women (36.2%). Table 1 shows how hemodialysis was carried out before and after 1973. The 135 patients were divided into 3 groups according to the different durations of RDT. Then, each group was divided into 2 subgroups of different age (cutoff: 47 years), to see how in the 6 subgroups so formed (Table 2) this variable affected the electrophysiological parameters that in the literature are shown to be correlated with age [Buchthal et al. 1966, Ludin 1980]. The mean ages of the various groups and subgroups were not significantly different, with the one exception indicated in Table 2. Serum urea, creatinine and PTH, expressed as means of the values in the 6 months before the examination, were recorded in order to look for possible correlations with the degree of PNP.

Methods

For the neurologic examination, we followed Bolton's classification [Bolton et al. 1971, Bolton 1976], which divides uremic PNP into mild, moderate and severe on the grounds of specific subjective and objective criteria.

Table 2 Number and mean age of all patients, and of the 3 groups with different duration of RDT

	Patients subdivided according to the duration of hemodialysis treatment			
	Group I (<5 yrs RDT)	Group II (5 to 10 yrs RDT)	Group III (10 to 15 yrs RDT)	All patients
Total no. of patients	52	46	37	135
No. of patients <47 yrs	21	26	20	67
No. of patients ≥47 yrs	31	20	17	68
Mean age of total population (yrs)	48.2 ± 12.2	45.0 ± 11.0	49.1 ± 10.1	47.3 ± 11.2
Mean age of patients <47 yrs	36.2 ± 7.4 *	37.3 ± 7.0	42.0 ± 4.9 *	
Mean age of patients ≥47 yrs	56.4 ± 6.8	55.0 ± 5.2	57.5 ± 6.2	

* $p < 0.05$ (Scheffe's Multiple Range Test)

For neurophysiological evaluation, we measured the Maximum Motor Conduction Velocities (Max. MCVs) of the median, ulnar and peroneal nerves, the distal motor latency and the amplitude (negative phase) of the Muscle Action Potential (MAP) evoked by stimulation of these nerves, recorded with surface electrodes. We determined the latency (at the negative peak) and the amplitude (from peak to peak) of the orthodromic Sensory Action Potentials (SAPs) of the median and ulnar nerves bilaterally. These were recorded at the wrist with surface electrodes following stimulation with ring electrodes of the digital nerves of the index and fifth fingers. Sural nerve SAP was studied by the antidromic method (recording behind and below the lateral malleolus and stimulation 7, 14 and 21 cm from the recording point, along the course of the sural nerve on the posterior surface of the leg); latency (to the negative peak) and amplitude (from peak to peak) were measured at 14 cm; finally, the sensory conduction velocity (SCV) of the sural nerve along a tract of 14 cm (between the points 7 and 21 cm from the recording electrode) was calculated. We employed a Medelec MS 6 Electromyograph with DAV 62 Averager. Cutaneous temperature was monitored and maintained at 34–36° C. Standardized normal values proposed by Schoenhuber et al. [1978] and Lambert et al. [1979] have been used for comparison in Table 5: they refer to normal subjects with mean ages and range of age that are comparable with those of our total population of hemodialyzed patients and of the 3 groups with different duration of RDT. Pathological thresholds were fixed at 2.5 S. D. from mean normal values.

Plasma urea and creatinine were determined by standard methods; parathyroid hormone by C-terminal radioimmunoassay.

The data were analyzed statistically by the SPSS-PC package [Norusis 1984]; the groups with different lengths of treatment were compared by one-way ANOVA and by the Scheffé test.

Results

Serological parameters

Mean serum urea and creatinine levels did not differ significantly in the various groups and subgroups, but PTH differed significantly in groups I and III (Table 3).

Clinical signs of PNP

Only 1 (0.7%) of the 135 patients showed signs of severe polyneuropathy according to the criteria described by Bolton, and only 4 (3.0%) showed signs of moderate PNP, while 77 (57%) patients had mild signs. There were no clinical signs in the remaining 53 (39.3%) patients (Table 4). When analyzed separately according to the duration of RDT treatment and to age, it appeared that all 5 patients with moderate or severe clinical signs had been on RDT for more than 10 years and that 3 of the 4 subjects with moderate PNP and the patient with severe PNP were older than 47 years. In the group with the most prolonged duration of RDT, only 5.4% showed no signs of PNP, versus more than 50% of those on RDT for less than 10 years (Table 4).

Electrophysiological signs of PNP

Mean values for the neurophysiological parameters, evaluated separately for the 3 groups of patients with different durations of RDT, are reported in

Table 3 Mean predialysis values of some serum parameters in the 3 groups of patients with different durations of RDT

	Blood urea (mg/dl)	Serum Creatinine (mg/dl)	PTH ng/ml
Group I (5 yrs RDT)	190.0 ± 37.8	13.3 ± 2.7	3.31 ± 2.4
Group II (5 to 10 yrs RDT)	206.4 ± 34.7	14.6 ± 2.4	4.39 ± 2.4*
Group III (10 to 15 yrs RDT)	199.8 ± 44.3	13.7 ± 1.9	5.87 ± 3.9

* $p < 0.05$ (Scheffe's Multiple Range Test)
PTH: normal values: ≤1.0 ng/ml

Table 4 Incidence of signs of clinical peripheral neuropathy in the total population of 135 patients and in the 3 groups of patients with a different duration of RDT (% of patients)

	Total Population	Group I (<5 yrs RDT)	Group II (5 to 10 yrs RDT)	Group III (10 to 15 yrs RDT)
Absent	39.3%	50%	54.3%	5.4%
Mild	57.0%	50%	45.7%	81.1%
Moderate	3.0%	0%	0%	10.8%
Severe	0.7%	0%	0%	2.7%

Table 5. (Parameters referring to median and ulnar nerves for the 11 subjects with carpal tunnel syndrome and the 2 patients with overt ulnar neuropathy were not considered). Although almost all mean results were still within normal values, with the exception of sural nerve latency in all 3 groups and of sural SCV and peroneal nerve Max MCV in the group with the most prolonged duration of RDT (Table 5), in as many as 84.4% of the 135 patients, at least one of the 20 parameters was abnormal and two or more parameters were abnormal in 63%. When the values in the groups with different durations of RDT, were compared by Scheffé's multiple range test, it was found that 5 parameters referring to ulnar nerves and two parameters referring to sural nerve were significantly more impaired in the group of patients with the longest duration of RDT than in the two other groups, which did not differ significantly from each other.

The effect of the duration of RDT on each of the various electrophysiological parameters was investigated separately after stratification of the patients of each of the 3 groups into two subgroups according to age (<47 years; ≥47 years). None of the parameters was significantly different in the 3 subgroups with different durations of RDT when only patients younger than 47 years were considered. As Table 6 shows, when patients older than 47 years with different durations of RDT were compared in the 3 groups, some of the ulnar parameters considered in the previous analysis of the total cohorts (SAP amplitude and latency) plus two additional parameters (median nerve Muscle Action Potential and peroneal nerve Max. MCV) were significantly more impaired in patients with more than 10 years of RDT than in the two other subgroups which did not significantly differ from each other.

Table 5 Mean values of neurophysiological parameters for the median, ulnar, peroneal and sural nerves in the 3 groups of patients with different durations of RDT

				Group I (<5 yrs RDT)	Group II (5 to 10 yrs RDT)	Group III (10 to 15 yrs RDT)	Normal Values	
R. Median	N. SAP°	Ampl.	(μV)	10.7 ± 4.5	10.5 ± 5.1	9.37 ± 4.7	7	
		Lat.	(mS)	3.2 ± 0.37	3.19 ± 0.37	3.3 ± 0.34	3.6	
L. Median	N. SAP	Ampl.	(μV)	11.8 ± 5.5	12.7 ± 6.7	9.7 ± 4.2	7	
		Lat.	(mS)	3.1 ± 0.44	3.01 ± 0.32	3.26 ± 0.34	3.6	
R. Ulnar	N. SAP	Ampl.	(μV)	7.7 ± 4.1	8.5 ± 5.3	6.18 ± 3.8	5	* (II vs III)
		Lat.	(mS)	2.87 ± 0.36	2.76 ± 0.35	3.01 ± 0.39	3.3	* (II vs III)
L. Ulnar	N. SAP	Ampl.	(μV)	8.2 ± 4.6	7.11 ± 4.2	5.6 ± 3.6	5	* (I vs III)
		Lat.	(mS)	2.77 ± 0.34	2.83 ± 0.31	3.02 ± 0.49	3.3	* (I vs III)
Median	N. Max.	MCV°°	(m/s)	50.4 ± 4.7	51.1 ± 3.9	48.6 ± 4.5	59.1 ± 5.2 (49–79)	
		MAP°°°	(mV)	7.06 ± 2.7	7.6 ± 2.5	6.5 ± 2.5	10.7 ± 3.7 (4.1–21.4)	
		DL°°°°	(mS)	3.6 ± 0.47	3.58 ± 0.59	3.6 ± 0.47	3.4 ± 0.5 (2.5–4.6)	
Ulnar	N. Max.	MCV°°	(m/s)	52.9 ± 4.7	52.0 ± 4.4	49.6 ± 4.7	59.0 ± 5.5 (47–75)	* (I vs III)
		MAP°°°	(mV)	7.5 ± 2.3	7.5 ± 2.3	6.4 ± 1.7	11.1 ± 2.6 (5.6–20)	
		DL°°°°	(mS)	2.7 ± 0.39	2.7 ± 0.34	2.88 ± 0.39	2.7 ± 0.4 (1.6–4.0)	
Peroneal	N. Max.	MCV	(m/s)	41.5 ± 4.9	41.6 ± 4.7	40.2 ± 5.5	50.7 ± 3.7 (41–59)	
		MAP	(mV)	5.4 ± 1.9	6.25 ± 2.05	4.99 ± 1.7	7.3 ± 2.6 (2.2–14.6)	
		DL	(mS)	3.99 ± 0.87	4.04 ± 0.82	4.18 ± 0.9	3.9 ± 0.6 (2.3–5.7)	
Sural	N. SAP	Ampl.	(μV)	8.4 ± 4.8	7.8 ± 3.97	5.5 ± 3.5	4	* (I vs III)
		Lat.	(mS)	4.43 ± 0.44	4.47 ± 0.42	4.6 ± 0.46	4.4	
Sural	N. SCV §§		(m/s)	43.3 ± 4.8	41.8 ± 5.1	39.9 ± 4.9	49.0 ± 3.3 (42–56)	* (I vs III)

* p <0.05 (Scheffe's Multiple Range Test); ° SAP: Sensory Action Potential; °° MCV: Motor Conduction Velocity; °°° MAP: Muscle Action Potential; °°°° DL: Distal Latency; §§ SCV: Sensory Conduction Velocity; ___: Pathological Mean values underlined

Correlation between electrophysiological and serological parameters in single patients

The only significant correlations between any of the 20 electrophysiological parameters and the blood urea, serum creatinine or PTH levels, was the MCV of the ulnar nerve, which was significantly more impaired ($p < 0.03$) in patients with higher levels of PTH.

Discussion

Although reduced in frequency and severity when RDT is started early, PNP is still one of most frequent neurological manifestations of untreated or unadequately controlled uremic syndrome. While earlier studies suggested the possibility of consistent improvement of PNP during hemodialytic treatment, more recent studies have shown that PNP was unchanged or even slightly worsened during RDT. Nevertheless, the majority of studies of PNP were of groups of patients with short-term dialytic treatment, and there are very few clinical and electrophysiological observations on long-term RDT patients.

Our study of PNP using a large number of electrophysiological motor and sensory parameters in a large population of patients with variable durations of RDT (from 2 to 184 months) shows that as many as 60% of the patients have clinical signs of PNP, usually very mild according to Bolton's criteria, and 84.4% have pathological values of at least one of the 20 electrophysiological parameters. These results confirm that long-term dialysis treatment even when performed correctly (actuarial survival of our total unselected population of RDT patients is 62% at 15 years; the age at the beginning of RDT was 36.5 ± 10.8 years) does not prevent the persistence of mild, usually clinically inapparent signs of PNP. A more selective analysis of the incidence of the pathological signs according to the duration of RDT and to age demonstrated that up to 10 years of treatment the impairment of nervous system is very mild and requires the contemporary study of many sensitive electrophysiological parameters to be detected, while patients older or those with more prolonged treatment

Table 6 Mean values of neurophysiological parameters for median, ulnar, peroneal and sural nerves in the 3 groups of patients with different durations of RDT, subdivided according to age

				Group I (<5 yrs RDT)		Group II (5 to 10 yrs RDT)		Group III (10 to 15 yrs RDT)	
				47 yrs	≥47 yrs	47 yrs	≥47 yrs	47 yrs	≥47 yrs
R. Median	N. SAP	Ampl.	(μV)	13.02 ± 3.7	9.2 ± 4.6	11.2 ± 4.9	9.6 ± 5.1	11.9 ± 4.3	6.4 ± 3.1
		Lat.	(mS)	3.16 ± 0.35	3.26 ± 0.39	3.17 ± 0.32	3.22 ± 0.43	3.2 ± 0.31	3.4 ± 0.34
L. Median	N. SAP	Ampl.	(μV)	12.9 ± 4.6	11.1 ± 5.80	14.4 ± 6.40	10.4 ± 6.5	11.1 ± 4.5	8.1 ± 3.3
		Lat.	(mS)	3.05 ± 0.48	3.12 ± 0.42	3.0 ± 0.31	3.03 ± 0.34	3.19 ± 0.39	3.34 ± 0.28
R. Ulnar	N. SAP	Ampl.	(μV)	9.7 ± 4.4	6.47 ± 3.3	8.9 ± 4.5	8.0 ± 6.30	8.8 ± 3.4	3.1 ± 2.0
		Lat.	(mS)	2.85 ± 0.3	2.89 ± 0.4	2.76 ± 0.28	2.77 ± 0.43	2.8 ± 0.38	3.25 ± 0.3
L. Ulnar	N. SAP	Ampl.	(μV)	10.0 ± 5.4	7.0 ± 3.6	8.2 ± 4.5	5.7 ± 3.2	6.8 ± 4.1	4.2 ± 2.4
		Lat.	(mS)	2.74 ± 0.26	2.8 ± 0.39	2.8 ± 0.29	2.88 ± 0.34	2.84 ± 0.63	3.24 ± 0.27
Median	N. Max.	MCV	(m/s)	51.8 ± 4.9	49.4 ± 4.5	51.6 ± 4.1	50.6 ± 3.6	50.1 ± 4	46.8 ± 4.6
		MAP	(mV)	7.5 ± 2.8	6.76 ± 2.6	8.4 ± 2.6	6.6 ± 1.8	8.1 ± 2.1	4.6 ± 1.4
		D. L.	(mS)	3.6 ± 0.59	3.53 ± 0.39	3.5 ± 0.51	3.68 ± 0.68	3.4 ± 0.48	3.87 ± 0.3
Ulnar	N. Max.	MCV	(m/s)	53.1 ± 4.4	52.7 ± 5.1	51.9 ± 4.9	52.2 ± 3.4	50.5 ± 5.21	48.6 ± 4.5
		MAP	(mV)	7.76 ± 2.4	7.39 ± 2.3	7.76 ± 2.4	7.14 ± 2.1	6.7 ± 1.7	6.12 ± 1.9
		D. L.	(mS)	2.73 ± 0.47	2.67 ± 0.31	2.73 ± 0.27	2.66 ± 0.42	2.96 ± 0.44	2.79 ± 0.34
Peroneal	N. Max.	MCV	(m/s)	41.7 ± 5.1	41.4 ± 5	42.2 ± 4.7	40.8 ± 4.6	42.1 ± 4.2	38 ± 5.9
		MAP	(mV)	5.97 ± 1.9	5 ± 1.8	6.4 ± 1.8	6.05 ± 2.4	5.4 ± 1.2	4.5 ± 2.4
		D.L.	(mS)	4.01 ± 0.87	3.97 ± 0.88	4.09 ± 0.77	3.97 ± 0.89	4 ± 0.65	4.4 ± 1.1
Sural	N. SAP	Ampl.	(μV)	10.3 ± 4.6	7.14 ± 4.8	9.05 ± 4.2	6.26 ± 3.1	6.79 ± 3.6	4.1 ± 2.7
		Lat.	(mS)	4.34 ± 0.49	4.5 ± 0.39	4.45 ± 0.44	4.49 ± 0.41	4.46 ± 0.39	4.7 ± 0.45
Sural	N.	SCV	(m/s)	44.4 ± 4.8	42.3 ± 4.6	42.4 ± 5.4	40.8 ± 4.5	41 ± 5	38.8 ± 4.5

* $p < 0.05$ (Scheffe's Multiple Range Test)

have more significant and clinically apparent signs of such impairment. All our patients with less than 10 years of RDT have been dialyzed with short-dialysis strategies since the beginning of treatment, while patients with more than 10 years of treatment were dialyzed at the beginning with the less efficient modalities based on the Kiil dialyzers and a twice-weekly schedule. Therefore, our data appear to confirm that short-dialysis treatment for as long as 10 years does not impair the peripheral nerve system in any worrisome way (none of the patients had severe or even moderate clinical signs of neuropathy) in spite of the incomplete depuration of middle molecular size toxins. It is possible that more evident abnormality of all the parameters we found in patients with more than 10 years of RDT is due to the persisting irreversible toxic effects of the less efficient treatment that was offered to all dialyzed patients until the early 70's. The analysis of the data for patients older than 47 years with different durations of RDT confirms that the values of the electrophysiological parameters are correlated to age and deteriorate with age [Buchthal et al. 1966, Ludin 1980].

The most sensitive electrophysiological parameters that appear also the most useful to point out neurophysiological derangement are sural nerve SCV, sural and ulnar SAP amplitude and latency and peroneal nerve Max MCV: therefore these six parameters should be used in a shortened electrophysiological evaluation of uremic PNP.

REFERENCES

Albertazzi A, Di Paolo B, Gambi D, Rossini P 1981 Electrophysiological assessment in encephalopathy and peripheral neuropathy in chronic uremia. In: Giordano C, Friedman EA (eds). Uremia, Pathobiology of patients treated for 10 years or more. Wichtig Ed., Milano, p 130

Baab AL, Johansen PJ, Strand MJ, Tenckhoffeh H, Scribner BH 1973 Bidirectional permeability of the human peritoneum to middle molecules. Eur Dial Transp Ass *10:* 247

Bolton CF, Baltzan HA, Balban RB 1971 Effects of renal transplantation on uremic neuropathy. New Engl J Med *284:* 1170

Bolton CF, Kaibara 1975 Electrophysiological signs of peripheral neuropathy during chronic hemodialysis. Communication at the fifth International Congress of Electromyography-Rochester, Minnesota

Buchthal F, Rosenfalck A 1966 Evoked action potentials and conduction velocity in human sensory nerves. Brain Res *3:* 1

Caccia MR, Mangili A, Mecca G, Ubiali E, Zanoni P 1977 Effects of hemodialytic treatment on uremic polyneuropathy. J Neurol *217:* 123

Cambi V, Bignardi L, Garini G, Rossi E, Savazzi G, Migone L 1975 Short dialysis after three years; progress report. Proc Garda Meeting, Opuscula Med Tech Lundensia

D'Amico G, Petrella E, Orlandini G, Cambi V, Savazzi G, Migone L 1976 Long term multicentric experience with short dialysis treatment. In: Giovannetti S, Bonomini V, D'Amico G (eds). Advances in Nephrology, Sixth Int Congr of Nephrol. Karger Ed, Basel, p 629

Di Paolo B, Di Marco T, Cappelli P, Spisni C, Del Rosso G, Palmiere PF, Evangelista M, Albertazzi A 1988 Electrophysiological aspects of nervous conduction in uremia. Clin Nephrol *29:* 253

Fraser C, Arieff AI 1988 Nervous system complications in uremia. Ann Int Med *109:* 143

Jebsen RM, Tenckoff H, Honet JE 1967 Natural history of uremic polyneuropathy and effects of dialysis. New Engl J Med *277:* 327

Konotey-Ahulu FID, Baillod R, Comty CM, Heron JR, Shaldon S, Thomas PK 1965 Effect of periodic dialysis on the peripheral neuropathy of end-stage renal failure. Brit Med J *2:* 1212

Lambert EH, Daube JR 1979 Special course 16: Clinical Electromyography. American Academy of Neurology Meeting, Chicago

Ludin HP 1980 Electromyography in practice. Georg Thieme Verlag (ed), Stuttgart

Mariani G, Cosi V, Faggi L, Zelaschi F 1971 La polineuropatia uremica precoce: studio clinico-elettro-miografico in soggetti trattati (e non) con dialisi extracorporea. Riv Neurobiol *17:* 67

Mc Comas AJ, Upton ARM, Brandstanter ME, Shimizu A, Toyonaga K 1975 Serial neurophysiological studies in renal failure. Communication at the fifth International Congress of Electromyography – Rochester, Minnesota

Nielsen VK 1973 The peripheral nerve function in chronic renal failure. VI The relationship between sensory and motor function and kidney function, azotemia, age, sex and clinical neuropathy. Acta Med Scandin *194:* 455

Nielsen VK 1974 The peripheral nerve function in chronic renal failure. VII Longitudinal course during terminal renal failure and regular dialysis. Acta Med Scandin *195:* 155

Nielsen VK 1974 The peripheral nerve function in chronic renal failure. A survey. Acta Med Scandin *196: 7*

Norusis M 1984 SPSS/PC for the IBM PC. SPSS inc., Chicago

Savazzi GM 1981 Nerve conduction times in uremia. Int Artif Org *4:* 211

Savazzi GM, Buzio C, Migone L 1982 Lights and shadows on the pathogenesis of uremic polyneuropathy. Clin Nephrol *18:* 219

Schoenhuber R, Pagani C, Prattichizzo F 1978 Relationship between arm paresthesias and entrapment syndromes in 397 patients: EMG findings. In: *Canal N, Pozza G* (eds). Peripheral Neuropathies. Elsevier – North Holland, Biomedical Presse, p 345

Teschan PE, Bourne JR, Reed RB, Ward JW 1983 Electrophysiological and neurobehavioral response to therapy: the national cooperative dialysis study. Kidney Int *23* (13): 58

Weseley SA, Liebowitz B, Katims JJ 1989 Neuropathy of uremia: evaluation by nerve conduction velocity versus neurospecific current perception threshold. Nephron *52:* 317

LETTERS TO THE EDITOR

Comment on "Use of aminohydroxypropylidene bisphosphonate (AHPrBP, "APD") for the treatment of hypercalcemia in patients with renal impairment" by Yap et al., Clin Nephrol, *34:* 225–229

Sir, – We read with interest the paper by Yap et al [1990] on their reported use of APD in the treatment of hypercalcemia due to immobilisation and hyperparathyroidism in a patient undergoing hemodialysis. We have previously reported [Kwan and Cunningham 1990] the use of APD in chronic dialysis patients with severe hyperparathyroidism and parathyroid dependent hypercalcemia (PDH). We used intravenous APD in 4 stable dialysis patients (3 hemodialysis and 1 CAPD) with PDH. All had persistently raised corrected serum calcium (sCa) (>2.8 mmol/l) and ionised calcium (iCA) (>1.2 mmol/l), greatly elevated parathyroid hormone (>80 ng/ml, NR <1.5 ng/ml, mid-molecule assay), raised alkaline phosphatase (ALP) (NR <100 iu/l), radiological evidence of hyperparathyroid bone disease and enlarged parathyroids on radionuclide imaging. All the patients were awaiting elective parathyroidectomy.

APD was given as weekly intravenous injections of 10 mg APD in 250 ml of saline infused over 4 hours post-dialysis for 6 weeks. Biochemical values (mean [SD]) pre-treatment, at the end of the sixth week of treatment and 3 week post-treatment were:

		Pre-treatment	End of treatment	3 week post-treatment
sCa	mmol/l	3.01 (0.21)	2.91 (0.12)	3.05 (0.08)
iCa	mmol/l	1.31 (0.14)	1.27 (0.07)	1.35 (0.08)
Pi	mmol/l	1.93 (0.61)	2.01 (0.37)	1.83 (0.46)
ALP	iu/l	176 (40)	200 (59)	208 (84)

Although 1 patient showed a transient resolution of hypercalcemia following APD, the other 3 did not, and in the group as a whole there was no significant response to APD given according to the above schedule. All 4 patients tolerated the treatment well.

Contrary to Yap et al.'s single case report, we have found that intravenous APD was ineffective in the treatment of PDH in 4 stable dialysis patients, even when given at doses effective in treating some cases of malignant hypercalcemia. It is possible that a larger dose of APD is required in dialysis related PDH.

Nephrologists have understandably been cautious when giving APD to dialysis patients. Although very safe, effective and well tolerated in patients with malignant hypercalcemia of Paget's disease [Sawyer et al. 1990], APD does persist in the skeleton for many months and its long term safety in patients with abnormal renal function has not been established. Further study is required to demonstrate whether APD can be given safely to these patients either as a bridging manoeuvre pending parathyroidectomy, or possibly in combination with intravenous calcitriol in an attempt to regain control of parathyroid dependent hypercalcemia without recourse to surgery.

JTC Kwan, J Cunningham
Department of Nephrology, The Royal London Hospital, Whitechapel, London E1 1BB, England.

REFERENCES

Yap AS, Hockings GI, Fleming SJ, Khafagi FA 1990 Use of aminohydroxypropylidene bisphosphonate (AHPrBP, "APD") for the treatment of hypercalcemia in patients with renal impairment. Clin Nephrol *34:* 225–229

Kwan JTC, Cunningham J 1990 Intravenous (IV) pamidronate disodium (APD) does not lower serum calcium (sCa) in dialysis patients with parathyroid dependent hypercalcemia (PDH). XIth Int Cong Neph Abstracts 409A

Sawyer N, Newstead C, Drummond A, Cunningham J 1990 Fast (4-H) or slow (24-H) infusions of Pamidronate disodium (Aminohydroxypropylidene diphosphonate [APD]) as single shot treatment of hypercalcemia. Bone and Mineral *9:* 122–128

Prevalence of HLA-B27 antigens in patients with dialysis-related β_2-M amyloidosis

Sir, – A major complication in patients undergoing long-term hemodialysis is destructive arthropathy which has been observed in association with the carpal tunnel syndrome and characterized by chronic joint pain, subchondral bone cysts and histological evidence of synovial β_2-microglobulin (β_2-M) amyloid deposits [Bardin et al. 1987].

Since β_2-M is part of the HLA class I molecule, we determined the HLA phenotypes in 36 patients (21 males, 15 females) treated by intermittent hemodialysis for more than 6 years. Twenty-one patients had β_2-M destructive amyloid arthropathy (mean age 52.1 ± 2.7 years, duration of hemodialysis therapy 113.9 ± 6.5 months). Fifteen patients had no β_2-M amyloid-related syndrome (mean age 45.2 ± 2.7 years, duration of hemodialysis therapy 134.9 ± 7.7 months). A comparison of the HLA antigens frequency was established with a control population of 322 healthy donors. The HLA typing performed by employing two-stage NIH microlymphocytotoxicity testing revealed the presence of HLA-B27 and HLA-A9 antigens with a higher frequency in patients with β_2-M amyloidosis (statistical evaluation of deviations observed was done using χ^2-test) (Table 1).

It has been demonstrated that β_2-M amyloid deposition tends to occur mainly in joints [Zingraff et al. 1990]. We also know that the HLA-B27 antigen has been found more frequently in rheumatological disorders such as ankylosing spondylitis than in the general population. The pathogenesis of β_2-M amyloid arthropathy is still debated but HLA seems to play a role with other factors previously described such as long-term dialysis, plasma concentration of β_2-M, dialysis membranes, dialysate, patients age or aluminium overload.

J. P. Charmes[1], M. Drouet[1], C. Leroux-Robert[1], H. Ton That[2] and G. Bouteiller[2]
Service de Néphrologie[1], CHU Dupuytren, 87042 Limoges and Service de Néphrologie[2], CHU Rangueil, 31054 Toulouse, France.

REFERENCES

Bardin T, Zingraff J, Shirahama T, Noël LH, Droz D, Voisin MC, Drüeke T, Dryll A, Skinner M, Cohen AS, Kuntz D 1987 Hemodialysis-associated amyloidosis and β_2-microglobulin: Clinical and immuno-histochemical study. Am J Med *83:* 419–24.

Zingraff J, Noël LH, Bardin T, Kuntz D, Dubost C, Drüeke T 1990 β_2-microglobulin amyloidosis: a sternoclavicular joint biopsy study in hemodialysis patients. Clin Nephrol *33:* 94–97.

Table 1 Frequency of HLA-B27 and HLA-49 antigens in long-term hemodialysis patients, with and without β_2-M amyloid arthropathy compared to a control of healthy donors. ( ) antigen frequency.

	n	HLA-B27	HLA-A9
Healthy donors	322	29 (9%)	78 (24.2%)
Dialysis patients with β_2-M amyloidosis	21	5 (23%)	9 (42.8%)
Dialysis patients without β_2-M amyloidosis	15	1 (6.6%)	4 (26.6%)
RR		4.37 $p < 0.001$	2.01 $p < 0.01$

Comment on "Portions of basement membrane with decreased negative charge in various glomerulonephritis" [Clin Nephrol 1990; *34:* 9–16]

To support the proposition that the anionic charge layer is important in the development of proteinuria Wada et al. [1990] investigated the anionic charge layer in glomeruli in biopsies from subjects with different types of renal pathology. They found that in material from focal segmental glomerulosclerosis and membrano-proliferative glomerulonephritis there were fewer intramembranous particles of a cationic probe than in equivalent tissue from subjects with IgA nephropathy, Henoch-Schoenlein purpura nephritis and controls. It was claimed that the observed differences in basement membrane charge layers suggested "...different developmental mechanisms."

The relevance of this suggestion needs to be assessed in terms of the literature which describes proteinuria occurring with normal renal function as in exercise-induced proteinuria. We showed [Simpson and Shand 1983] that in temporary, albumin-overload-induced proteinuria high molecular weight urinary proteins appeared by 16 hours after the albumin injection. These large proteins persisted in the urine for as long as the albumin overload continued but 24 hours after the last albumin injection large molecular weight proteins were no longer present in the urine. That and numerous other studies have confirmed beyond doubt that damage to the glomerular basement membrane is not a necessary prerequisite for proteinuria.

It has been proposed that glomerular permeability is due to the thixotropic nature of the basement membrane [Simpson 1981]; the relevance of basement membrane research to its functional role has been discussed [Simpson 1986] and the excretion of negatively charged molecules such as albumin has been considered in detail [Simpson et al. 1987]. As increased blood viscosity will have an adverse influence on postglomerular blood flow, proteinuria can be a consequence of increased blood viscosity [Simpson 1984]. It has been suggested that IgA nephropathy could be due to altered blood rheology [Simpson et al. 1987a] and subsequently this has been found to be so [Shand et al. 1988]. Gordge et al. [1988] and Solerte and Fioravanti [1987] reported direct correlations between blood viscosity and proteinuria. Furthermore, when blood viscosity was reduced therapeutically there was "...a marked reduction in proteinuria and albumin excretion rate" [Solerte and Ferrari 1985].

The only way in which blood viscosity can influence renal function is by the effect on intraglomerular pressure because of the increased resistance to flow in postglomerular vessels. As glomerular filtration increases postglomerular blood viscosity the problems of flow in the peritubular plexus will be exacerbated when preglomerular blood viscosity is increased.

In the face of this information, which has been available for some time, it is difficult to accept the conclusion that the status of an anionic charge layer at a single point in time represents "...different development mechanisms of various glomerular diseases."

L. O. Simpson
University of Otago, Department of General Practice, Medical School, P.O. Box 913, Dunedin, New Zealand

REFERENCES

Gordge MP, Faint RW, Rylance PB, Nield GH 1988 Abnormal blood rheology in progressive renal failure: a factor in non-immune glomerular disease. Nephrol Dial Transplant *3:* 257–262

Shand BI, Bailey RR, Simpson LO 1988 Blood rheology in IgA nephropathy. Clin Nephrol *29:* 288–293

Simpson LO 1983 Glomerular permeability: an alternative to the pore theory. Lancet *2:* 251–252

Simpson LO 1984 Blood viscosity induced proteinuria. Nephron *36:* 280–281

Simpson LO 1986 Is current research into basement membrane chemistry and ultrastructure providing any new insights into the way the glomerular basement membrane functions? Nephron *43:* 1–4

Simpson LO, Shand BI 1983 The implications of the changes in the nature of the urinary proteins which occur in albumin

overload-induced proteinuria in normal mice. Br J Exp Path *64:* 6–14
Simpson LO, Shand BI, Olds RJ 1987 A reappraisal of the influence of blood rheology on glomerular filtration and its role in the pathogenesis of diabetic nephropathy. J Diabetic Complications *1:* 137–144
Simpson LO, Shand BI, Olds RJ 1987a IgA nephropathy. Nephron *45:* 253–254
Solerte SB, Ferrari E 1985 Diabetic retinal complications and erythrocyte filtrability: results of a 2-year follow-up study with pentoxifylline. Pharmatherapeutica *4:* 341–350
Solerte SB, Fioravanti M 1987 Hemodynamic alterations in long-term insulin-dependent diabetic patients with overt nephropathy: role of blood hyperviscosity and plasma protein changes. Clin Nephrol *28:* 138–143
Wada N, Ueda Y, Iidaka K, Inaga A, Kikkawa Y, Kitagawa T 1990 Portions of basement membrane with decreased negative charge in various glomerulonephritis. Clin Nephrol *34:* 9–16

The treatment of mesangial IgA nephropathy with cyclophosphamide, dipyridamole and warfarin

Sir, – We read with great interest the paper by Walker et al. [1990 Clin Nephrol 34: 103–107] which reported a prospective two-year controlled therapeutic trial in patients with IgA nephritis using cyclophosphamide, dipyridamole and "anti-coagulant" doses of warfarin which showed that even though there was a significant decrease in the proteinuria in the treatment group compared with the control group, there were no significant differences in the pre and post-trial serum creatinine values in both groups.

Reference was made to our earlier therapeutic trial [Woo et al. 1987 Clin Nephrol 27: 56–64] on IgA nephritis also using the triple regimen consisting of cyclophosphamide, dipyridamole and low dose or "anti-thrombotic" dose of warfarin for 3 years. (Thrombotest was maintained between 30%–50%.) Our study showed that patients in the treatment group had a significant decrease in proteinuria and more stable renal function compared with those in the control group. Furthermore, repeat biopsies at the end of the trial showed less histological progression among patients in the treatment group compared with those in the control group [Woo et al. 1987 Clin Nephrol 28: 304–305].

We would like to emphasize some significant differences between our trial and that of Walker et al.

Firstly, we treated our patients with the triple regimen for three years compared to Walker et al. whose trial lasted for 2 years.

When we initially analyzed the results of our original trial at 2 years, we found no significant differences in the pre and post-trial serum creatinine in both the treatment and control groups, though proteinuria had improved in the treatment group. However, at the end of the 3-year trial, we were able to demonstrate a small but significant deterioration in renal function among patients in the control group compared with those in the treatment group who had more stable renal function. In this respect, we hope that the Walker trial is still on-going as two years may be too short a period for patients with a slowly progressive disease like IgA nephritis to develop renal impairment. We have been following up our patients who entered the original trial for 10 years now and the results of our follow-up studies are enlightening (in press).

Secondly, we used "anti-thrombotic" doses of warfarin versus the "anti-coagulant" doses of warfarin used by Walker et al. We note that in the Walker trial, the urinary erythrocyte count of both groups at the start of the trial were not different but at the end of the trial, the treatment group had a significantly higher urinary erythrocyte count than the control group (5.49 ± 0.19 versus 5.21 ± 0.14 log rbc/ml, $p < 0.01$).

This may suggest that anti-coagulant doses of warfarin promote intraglomerular bleeding and hematuria and we suspect that this may account for the deterioration of renal function (serum creatinine 0.1 ± 0.01 mmol/l to 0.12 ± 0.01 mmol/l, $p < 0.05$) in the treatment group in the Walker trial in contrast to ours.

Lastly, we have post-trial biopsies which supported the clinical data of our trial and showed less histological progression among patients in the treatment group compared with those in the control group [Woo et al. 1987 Clin Nephrol 28: 304–305].

In a subsequent on-going study in patients with IgA nephritis with renal impairment using only dipyridamole and "anti-thrombotic" doses of warfarin, we have demonstrated [Lee et al. 1989 Clin Nephrol 31: 276] that patients in the treatment group have an improvement in proteinuria and more stable renal function compared with those in the control group and we believe that the use of cyclophosphamide is no longer justified in view of its side effects as in Walker's study, where one female patient developed amenorrhea and a male patient developed oligospermia.

Finally, we take this opportunity to acknowledge the help and advice of Professor Priscilla Kincaid-Smith in our early therapeutic trial on IgA nephritis.

K. T. Woo and G. S. L. Lee
Department of Renal Medicine, Singapore General Hospital, Outram Road, Singapore 0316

Comment on "Idiopathic acute interstitial nephritis associated with anterior uveitis in adults" by P. Cacoub et al.

Sir, – We appreciated the paper by Cacoub et al. [Clin Nephrol 1989; *31:* 307–310]. We agree that the actual incidence of tubulointerstitial nephritis with uveitis (TIN-U) may be underestimated, and that the evaluation of renal function is warranted in patients with uveitis. However, we differ on two things. Firstly, Cacoub et al. recommend the determination of plasma creatinine and routine urine examination for the evaluation of renal function. We would like to emphasize the measurement of urinary β_2-microglobulin, which reflects the severity of renal tubular damage [Portman et al. 1986], because our patients with TIN-U showed over 10,000 g/l in the spot urine [Itami et al.] and it is a good marker of TIN-U activity. Although urinalysis may provide the first hint of the diagnosis, in TIN-U, urinalysis usually reveals mild proteinuria, microhematuria and a few cells and casts which may cause a delay of the diagnosis and renal biopsy on the assumption that the process is mostly likely to be benign. Secondly, we also agree that systemic steroid therapy may reduce interstitial inflammation and subsequent fibrosis although no prospective, randomized, well-controlled trial has been reported. Like Cacoub et al. we reviewed the cases of TIN-U in adults. The patients in whom prednisone therapy was effective were diagnosed within three months after the onset of relatively uncharacteristic symptoms like weight loss, fever, and asthenia. On the other hand, the patients who developed chronic renal failure were diagnosed as having TIN-U seven or eight months or more after symptoms began. The likelihood of irreversible fibrotic changes occurring in these patients is great although there are rare reports of improvement in renal function after prolonged renal failure secondary to acute TIN [Frommer et al. 1979]. Even in children with TIN-U who showed spontaneous remission [Burghard et al. 1984, Koskimie et al. 1985], renal function began to improve within three months after the onset of disease. We consider early diagnosis to be more important for the prognosis of TIN-U than steroid therapy, and we believe a time frame exists for the potential use of steroids in TIN-U because the presence of chronic TIN-U mitigates against the use of high dose steroids due to their relative ineffectiveness in this situation and their potential for untoward side effects. Further study however is necessary.

In most reported cases of TIN-U, tubulointerstitial nephritis precedes uveitis. When uveitis is noted, it is possible that a long time has passed since the tubulointerstitial damage occurred and there may be little time left to prevent the progression of renal failure. These points aside, we still appreciate Cacoub's suggestions.

N. Itami, Y. Akutsu, K. Yasoshima, Y. Kusunoki
Hokkaido University, School of Medicine, Department of Pediatrics, Sapporo, Japan

REFERENCES

Burghard R, Brandis M, Hoyer PF, Ehrich JHH, Galaske RG, Brodehl J 1984 Acute interstitial nephritis in childhood. Eur J Pediatr *142:* 103

Frommer P, Uldall R, Fay WP, Deveber GA 1979 A case of acute interstitial nephritis successfully treated after delayed diagnosis. CMAJ *121:* 585

Itami N, Akutsu Y, Yasoshima K, Tochimaru H, Takekoshi Y Tubulointerstitial nephritis with uveitis. Arch Inter Med (in press)

Koskimies O, Holmberg C 1985 Interstitial nephritis of acute onset. Arch Dis Child *60:* 752

Protman RJ, Kissane JM, Robson AM 1986 Use of β_2-microglobulin to diagnose tubulointerstitial renal lesions in children. Kidney Int *30:* 91

ANNOUNCEMENTS

The **Fourth International Course on Peritoneal Dialysis** will be held in Vicenza, Italy, from May 21–24, 1991. English will be the official language but English-Italian simultaneous translations will be provided.

For further information please write to Dr. M. Feriani, Secretariat of the 4th International Course on Peritoneal Dialysis, Department of Nephrology, St. Bortolo Hospital, I-36100 Vicenza, Italy.

The **XXth Annual Conference of the European Dialysis and Transplant Nurses Association – European Renal Care Association** will take place in Brussels, from June 23–26, 1991. Conference secretariat: Mr. Hervé Bosquet, EDTNA/ERCA Conference, c/o ICSA, Rue Defacqz 1, bte 1, 1050 Brussels, Belgium. Tel.: 32–2–537 4608, Fax: 32–2–537 4800. Scientific secretariat: Mr. Tony Goovaerts, EDTNA/ERCA Conference, c/o UCL St-Luc, Home Dialysis, Avenue Hippocrate 10, 1200 Brussels, Belgium. Tel.: 32–2–764 1862 and Fax: 32–2–764 2836.

The **International Workshop on Alport Syndrome** will take place August 23–24, 1991 in Oulu, Finland. The objective of this workshop is to give a concise picture of the clinical aspects of Alport syndrome. The workshop will also cover the new available approaches for diagnosis. It will be of interest to nephrologists, pathologists, clinical geneticists and to molecular biologists specializing in kidney disease and basement membranes.

Deadline for application is July 1, 1991. Please contact Secretariat, International Workshop on Alport Syndrome, Biocenter and Department of Biochemistry, University of Oulu, SF-90570 Oulu, Finland, Tel: 358–81–352355, Fax: 358–81–352356.

The **VIth International Congress on Nutrition and Metabolism in Renal Disease** will be held August 26–30, 1991 in Harrogate, UK. Topics will include all aspects of nutrition and metabolism in relation to acute and chronic renal disease, with State of the Art lectures, free communications, posters and debates.

For further information, contact Dr. A. Meguid El Nahas (UK Organizing Secretary), Sheffield Kidney Institute, Northern General Hospital, Herries Road, Sheffield S5 7AU, UK. Tel.: 0742-434343 (ext 4017), Fax: 0742-560472.

The **XXVIIIth Congress of the European Dialysis and Transplant Association – European Renal Association** (EDTA/ERA) will be held in Belgrade, Yugoslavia from September 1 to 4, 1991.

For further information, contact the Organizing Secretariat: Yugotours, Congress, Incentive & Exhibition Department, Djure Djakovića 31, Y-11000 Belgrade, Yugoslavia. Tel.: 3811/763-028, 764-622; Telex: 11000, 12902; Fax: 3811/766-447.

The **Second Seminar on Renal Involvement in Systemic Vasculitis** will take place September 21, 1991 in Vimercate, a city near Milan in Italy. Contemporary issues relating to immunopathology of Systemic Lupus Erythematosus, with special regard to anti-endothelial and anti-cardiolipin antibodies, clinicopathological correlations and treatment will be discussed.

For further information please contact Dr. Adalberto Sessa, Unità Operativa di Nefrologia e Dialisi, Ospedale di Vimercate, 20059 Vimercate/Milan, Italy

A **Festakt in honor of Priscilla Kincaid-Smith** will be held on November 5–8th, 1991 in Melbourne, Australia. Events will include state of the art lectures and symposia.

For further information contact The Festschrift Organizing Committee, c/o Department of Nephrology, The Royal Melbourne Hospital, Victoria 3050, Australia.

The **IIIrd International Conference on SLE** will be held in the Queen Elizabeth II Conference Centre, Westminster, London, April 13–15, 1992.

For further details, please contact Dr. Graham Hughes or Mrs. Denzil Fletcher, Rheumatology Department, St. Thomas' Hospital, London SE1 7EH. Tel. and Fax: 0163394 22.

The **XXIXth Congress of the European Dialysis and Transplant Association** – European Renal Association (EDTA – ERA) will be held at the Palais des Congrès in Paris, France on June 28 – July 1, 1992. For further information contact Prof. C. Jacobs, Congress President, Service de Néphrologie, Hôpital de la Pitié, 83 bd de l'Hôpital, 75013 Paris, France (Fax: 33144 239984) or the organizing Secretariat: Convergences – EDTA 1992, 120 av. Gambetta, 75020 Paris, France (Fax: 3314030 0165).

The **Third Symposium on Uroradiology** (Imaging and Intervention) will take place August 24–27, 1992 at Herlev Hospital, University of Copenhagen, Denmark.

For further information, please contact Dr. Henrik S. Thomsen, Department of Diagnostic Radiology 54E2, Herlev Hospital, Herlev Ringvej 75, DK-2730 Herlev, Denmark. Tel.: 4544/535300, Ext. 278; Fax: 4544/535332.

The **VIth Congress of the International Society for Peritoneal Dialysis** will take place October 1–4, 1992 in Thessaloniki, Greece.

For additional information write to the First Department of Internal Medicine, AHEPA University Hospital, 54636 Thessaloniki, Greece. Tel. and Fax: (3031) 214606.

Clinical Nephrology, Vol. 35 No. 5 – 1991 (187–189)

Progression of a naproxen and amoxicillin induced acute interstitial nephritis with nephrotic syndrome: case report

J. Nortier[1], M. Depierreux[1], V. Bourgeois[2], J. Ducobu[2] and P. Dupont[2]

[1] *Service de Néphrologie et Département d'anatomie pathologique, Hôpital Erasme, Bruxelles, Belgium*
[2] *Service de Médecine interne, Département de Néphrologie et d'Hypertension, Hôpital de Tivoli, La Louvière, Belgium*

Abstract. This article reports an unusual case of acute interstitial nephritis associated with nephrotic syndrome which appeared after oral intake of naproxen and amoxicillin and led to end-stage renal failure. In the light of recent literature on this clinical entity, the authors formulate hypotheses accounting for this outcome.

Key words: acute interstitial nephritis – nephrotic syndrome – amoxicillin – naproxen.

Introduction

Acute interstitial nephritis associated with nephrotic syndrome has been frequently reported with the use of different drugs such as Non-Steroidal Anti-Inflammatory drugs (NSAID), antibiotics, lithium, interferon.... This clinical syndrome is, however, very rare (55 cases were reported in world literature in 1988). Moreover, a total or at least partial recovery usually follows the withdrawal of the incriminated drug.

In the present paper we would like to report and discuss an unusual case of acute interstitial nephritis with nephrotic syndrome after simultaneous intake of naproxen and amoxicillin. Progressive deterioration of renal function led the patient to chronic hemodialysis within a few months.

Case history

A 44-year-old male patient, usual blood donor without any pathological antecedent, ingested naproxen for 4 days (4 g) and amoxicillin for 10 days (24 g) with N-acetylcystein because he was suffering from acute pneumonia with thoracic pain.

During the following weeks, edema progressively increased, accompanied by a 12 kg-weight gain and hypertension at 180/120 mmHg. Clinical examination upon admission did not detect other significant signs, except papillar exsudates and retinal hemorrhages at the fundus of the eye. Biological tests showed alteration of renal function (urea 105 mg/dl, creatinine 4 mg/100 ml, C_{cr} 10 ml/min) and typical parameters of nephrotic syndrome (Table 1, first column). Eosinophilia ranging 2% – 6% of the total white blood cell count was noted. Complementemia was normal and the auto-immune panel was negative. A percutaneous renal biopsy was performed. Light microscopy revealed normal glomeruli, interstitial infiltration by inflammatory mononuclear cells and acute tubular necrosis.

Hydric restriction and diuretics led to a weight loss of 10 kg. Blood pressure values were then normalized as well as the funduscopic aspects. Considering the rather good prognosis of this non-oliguric acute renal failure, the patient was discharged from the hospital with the same therapeutic recommendations and an ambulatory clinical follow-up was set up. C_{cr} was back up to around 20 ml/min at that time. Other biological parameters are mentioned in Table 1, second column.

Three months later, the patient had to be admitted again with major edema and a serum creatinine of 7.7 mg/100 ml. Despite a creatinine clearance of 5 ml/min, the average daily proteinuria was 15 g (Table 1, last column). A second renal biopsy demonstrated a deterioration of the initial lesions with tubulo-interstitial and glomerular sclerosis.

The patient then commenced on chronic hemodialysis with a residual diuresis of 300–1200 ml/day. A daily proteinuria of 2–20 g without any monoclonal component was noted. Early failure of his first renal transplantation due to a Listeria monocytogenes cerebral abscess during the second post-operative month induced the discontinuation of immunosuppressive drugs. The patient is now waiting for a second transplantation.

Received September 14, 1990; revised January 21, 1991.

Reprint requests to Dr. J. Nortier, Service de Néphrologie, Hôpital Erasme, route de Lennik, 808, B-1070 Bruxelles, Belgium.

Table 1 Evolution of the most important laboratory findings

Biological parameters	First hospitalization		Second hospitalization
	Initial values	A week later	Three months later
Urea (mg/100 ml)	105	108	140
Creatinine (mg/100 ml)	4.2	3.9	7.7
White blood cells (cells/mm^3)	6680	11 530	11 630
Eosinophilia (%)	6.6	14.3	15.9
Protein (g/100 ml)	4.9	5.1	5.4
Albumin (%)	32.6	37.8	31.3
Triglycerides (mg/100 ml)	373	–	479
Cholesterol (mg/100 mg)	469	–	746
C_{cr} (ml/min)	9.7	17.8	4.3
Proteinuria (g/24 h)	11	4.8	16.7

Histological findings

The first renal biopsy contained twenty glomeruli without any significant abnormalities that would suggest primary glomerular disease (Figure 1). Interstitial areas were slightly enlarged by edema and infiltrated by scattered lymphocytes. These cells provoked some degree of tubular destruction. Foci of tubular epithelial damage were also apparent with cylinders and/or red blood cells in the luminae. The diagnosis of acute interstitial nephritis associated with NSAID was then proposed by the pathologists.

The second biopsy evidenced a worsening of the acute interstitial nephritis (Figure 2). The specimen was composed of fifteen glomeruli irregular in shape. One was sclerosed. Two others presented focal and segmental hyalinosis as well as sclerosis associated with mesangial and endocapillary proliferation mixed with foam cells. It was also possible to observe

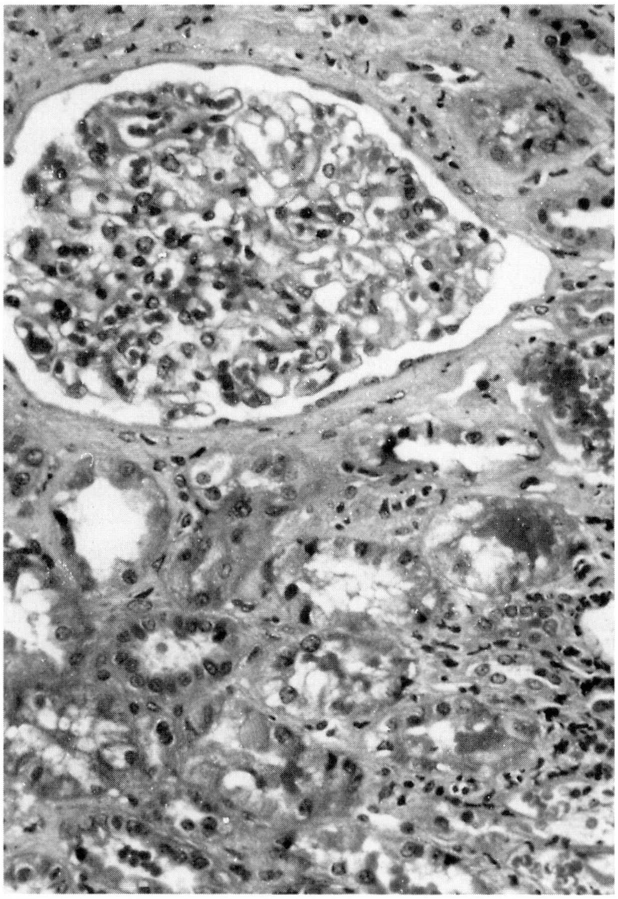

Fig. 1 Acute degeneration of tubes (loss of the brush border, dedifferentiation and mitosis) surrounded by edematous interstitium. Interstitial infiltration by inflammatory cells, mostly lymphocytes. No glomerular alteration is detectable. H. E. × 100.

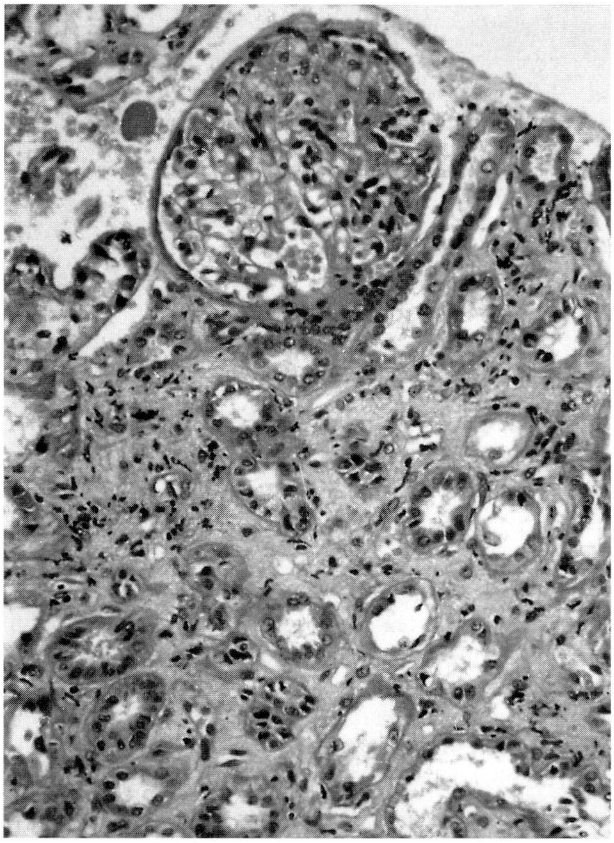

Fig. 2 Scarce lymphocytic infiltration of the interstitium associated with edema and fibrosis. Tubular damages are prominent. Segmental mesangial and endocapillary proliferation can be observed in the glomerular tuft. H. E. × 80.

pronounced fibrosis of the interstitium which was diffusely infiltrated by inflammatory cells with a majority of lymphocytes. In those areas, persisting tubular epithelial damages were encountered.

Direct immunofluorescence was performed on both biopsies. Glomeruli, tubular basement membrane and vessels were negative for IgG, IgM, IgA, C1q and fibrinogen. Spotty C3 deposits on the peripheral capillaries were noted in the first specimen but not in the second one.

Discussion

This clinical presentation of acute interstitial nephritis with nephrotic syndrome is interesting for several reasons. Indeed, the youth of the patient and the very short period of drug intake are quite unusual as well as the severely progressive course of renal dysfunction.

Recent compilations of reported cases of acute interstitial nephritis with nephrotic syndrome reveal an average age of 58 or 60 years among the affected patients [Deray et al. 1988, Maniglia et al. 1988]. Naproxen is one of the most frequently incriminated drugs. Studies report administration periods ranging from 4 weeks to one year [Maniglia et al. 1988, Brezin et al. 1979, Laxer et al. 1987]. Concerning antibiotics involved in such a syndrome, only two cases have been published on ampicillin, a β-lactam antibiotic close to amoxicillin [Linton et al. 1980; Reunke et al. 1980]. The medication period lasted for 5 to 11 days. In all these clinical reports, a total or partial recovery of renal function was observed after withdrawal of the drug. Neither the requirement to a transitory dialysis treatment nor the duration of the hemodialysis period seemed to interfere with the functional prognosis.

With regard to the intensity of renal lesions, our histological findings are not quite different from those observed in fenoprofen nephropathy, the most studied type of NSAID-induced acute interstitial nephritis with nephrotic syndrome [Brezin et al. 1979, Curt et al. 1980, Wendland et al. 1980, Finkelstein et al. 1982, Stachura et al. 1983, Bender et al. 1984, Maniglia et al. 1988]. Moderate to marked interstitial and/or glomerular fibrosis, even glomerular sclerosis are frequently observed in renal biopsy specimens as in ours [Wendland et al. 1980, Stachura et al. 1983, Maniglia et al. 1988]. Concomitant underlying pathology like systemic arterial hypertension is mentioned in several observations by these authors. Accordingly, the moderate degree of fibrosis, even though precocious for the age of our patient, could not by itself account for the pejorative evolution of renal function.

The combination of two drugs is perhaps a most important factor of bad prognosis. To our knowledge, this is the first clinical report in which deterioration followed oral intake of an NSAID and an antibiotic. In the literature, two cases have involved the successive oral intake of two NSAID, respectively ibuprofen and indomethacin in the first [Bender et al. 1984] and tolmetin and naproxen in the second [Laxer et al. 1987].

In both cases, deterioration of renal function was noted, leading to end-stage renal failure in the second case.

Pathogenic implication of T and B lymphocytes in acute interstitial nephritis with nephrotic syndrome has been suspected for several years. In fenoprofen nephropathy, the characterization of interstitial infiltrates using monoclonal antibodies and polyvalent antisera demonstrated the central role of T lymphocytes [Finkelstein et al. 1982] as well as a possible modulation by humoral immunity [Stachura et al. 1983]. Similar findings were extended to other NSAID such as ibuprofen, tolmetin and zomepirac [Bender et al. 1984]. No data are available about naproxen induced nephropathy. Despite the fact that the present immunological hypotheses concern only the NSAID mode of action, a cumulative effect of two drugs may be proposed to explain the impairment of our patient's renal function. Thus, if the combination of naproxen and amoxicillin may be incriminated, the specific role played by each drug in the deterioration process remains to be assessed. Furthermore, the slight interstitial fibrosis noted at the first renal biopsy may have constituted an additional precipitating factor.

REFERENCES

Bender WL, Whelton A, Beschorner WE, Darwish MO, Hall-Craggs M, Solez K 1984 Interstitial nephritis, proteinuria, and renal failure caused by nonsteroidal anti-inflammatory drugs. Am J Med *76:* 1006

Brezin JH, Katz SM, Schmartz AB, Chinitz JL 1979 Reversible renal failure and nephrotic syndrome associated with non-steroidal anti-inflammatory drugs. N Engl J Med *301 (23):* 1271

Clive D, Stoff JF 1984 Renal syndromes associated with non-steroidal anti-inflammatory drugs. N Engl J Med *310 (9):* 563

Curt GA, Kaldany A, Whitley LG, Crosson AW, Rolla A, Merino MJ, D'Elia JA 1980 Reversible rapidly progressive renal failure with nephrotic syndrome due to fenoprofen calcium. Ann Intern Med *92 (1):* 72

Deray G, Baumelou A, Cacoub P, Beaufils J, Anouar M, Jacobs C 1988 Néphropathies interstitielles d'origine médicamenteuse avec syndrome néphrotique. In: Séminaires d'uronéphrologie de la Pitié Salpétrière, p. 90

Finkelstein A, Fraley DS, Stachura I, Feldman HA, Gandy DR, Bourke E 1982 Fenoprofen nephropathy: lipoid nephrosis and interstitial nephritis. A possible T-lymphocyte disorder. Am J Med *72:* 81

Laxer RM, Silverman ED, Balfe JW, Poucell S, Baumal R 1987 Naproxen associated renal failure in a child with arthritis and inflammatory bowel disease. Pediatrics *80 (6):* 904

Linton AL, Clark WF, Driedger AA, Turnbull DI, Lindsay RM 1980 Acute interstitial nephritis due to drugs. Review of the literature with a report of nine cases. Ann Intern Med *93:* 735

Maniglia R, Schwartz AB, Moriber-Katz S 1988 Non-steroidal anti-inflammatory nephrotoxicity. Ann Clin Sci *18 (3):* 240

Rennke HG, Ross P, Wall SG 1980 Drug-induced interstitial nephritis with heavy glomerular proteinuria. N Engl J Med *302 (12):* 691 C

Stachura I, Jayakumar S, Bourke E 1983 T and B lymphocyte subsets in fenoprofen nephropathy. Ann J Med *75:* 9

Wendland ML, Wagoner RD, Holley KE 1980 Renal failure associated with fenoprofen. Mayo Clin Proc *55:* 103

Clinical Nephrology, Vol. 35 No. 5 – 1991 (190–197)

Immunohistochemical detection of renal carbonic anhydrase of patients with recurrent urolithiasis

L. Jonas[1], B. Klein[2], L. Hoffmann[3] and T. Kumpulainen[4]

[1] *Department of Pathological Anatomy and*
[2] *Urological Department of the University of Rostock, O-2500 Rostock, Germany*
[3] *Urological Department, Miners' Hospital Gera, O-6500 Gera, Germany*
[4] *Departments of Anatomy and Neurosurgery, University of Oulu, Oulu 90220, Finland*

Abstract. In renal exploratory excisions the isoenzyme C of the carbonic anhydrase was detected in 51 operative treated patients with recurrent urolithiasis and in 6 patients with ren mobilis or stenosis of the ureteral pelvic junction by using the immunohistochemical PAP-method. In the distal tubules and collecting ducts there is an alternating occurrence of cells with small and those with strong reactivity. This correlates with the distribution of mean or principal (P-, small reaction) and intercalated (I-, strong reaction) cells. The number of carbonic anhydrase rich cells and the degree of their cytoplasmic reaction to this enzyme seem to correlate with the ability of the urine to acidify. The patients were divided into four groups according to the mean urine pH estimated for a period of two weeks. The third group with predominantly acid urine (pH <5.8) showed a significantly increased number of carbonic anhydrase rich cells ($\bar{x}$ = 63% ± 6, n = 18) as compared to the first group (controls) without urolithiasis and normal urine (pH 5.8–6.8, $\bar{x}$ = 46% ± 8, n = 6) or the second group with urolithiasis and normal urine (pH 5.8–6.8, $\bar{x}$ = 46% ± 8, n = 28). The fourth group with predominant alkaline urine (pH >6.8) showed a significantly decreased number of intercalated cells ($\bar{x}$ = 42% ± 16, n = 5) in comparison to the third group. Indeed, the difference with the control group is not significant but the cytoplasmic reaction of I-cells decreases distinctly in comparison to all other groups.

Key words: carbonic anhydrase – kidney – exploratory excisions – recurrent urolithiasis – immunohistochemistry – urine pH

Introduction

There is increasing evidence of urinary acidification along the entire mammalian collecting duct [Giebisch 1986]. The enzyme carbonic anhydrase (E.C. 4.2.1.1.) plays a central role in this process [Pitss 1974, Warnock and Rector 1981]. Histochemical [Lönnerholm 1973, Lönnerholm and Ridderstrale 1980], immunohistochemical [Spicer et al. 1979], as well as biochemical studies [Eveloff et al. 1979, Wistrand 1979, Wistrand and Kinne 1977] on the rat kidney have shown the wide distribution of this enzyme in different nephron segments mainly in the intercalated cells (I-cells) of the distal tubules and collecting ducts. Similar results were obtained on the kidney of man and other primates [Jonas et al. 1983, Kumpulainen 1979, 1981, 1984, Lönnerholm 1971, 1983, Spicer et al. 1982]. Recent studies provided morphological evidence that the intercalated cells are involved in hydrogen ion secretion in the cortical and outer medullary collecting ducts [Dörup 1985, Clapp et al. 1987, Madsen and Tischer 1985, Zuvarov and Gonthmakher 1976].

In this paper we studied the distribution of carbonic anhydrase in the human kidney under pathological conditions by using an immunohistochemical method. The enzyme was detected in exploratory excisions of patients with recurrent urolithiasis to determine a possible correlation between the quantity of intercalated cells, their enzyme content and the urine pH of the patients, for a further characterization of the function of I-cells in the process of urinary acidification.

Received February 2, 1990; in revised form July 23, 1990.

Reprint requests to Dr. L. Jonas, Department of Pathological Anatomy, Electron Microscopic Centre, University of Rostock, Strempelstraße 14, O-2500 Rostock 1, Germany.

Patients and Methods

Patients

51 patients of both sexes (26 females, 25 males) with a mean age of 47 years representing 16 to

Table 1 Group 1 of patients (control group) without urolithiasis, normal urine pH (5.8–6.8)

No.	Name	Sex	Age (years)	Diagnosis	Degree of immuno-histochemical reaction	Percentage of CA-rich cells
1.	L. M.	m	46	Stenosis of ureteral pelvic junction	n	47.0
2.	R. L.	f	43	Ren mobilis	n	55.8
3.	Z. G.	f	53	Ren mobilis	n	47.2
4.	Z. W.	m	36	Stenosis of ureteral pelvic junction	n	53.8
5.	K. B.	f	39	Ren mobilis	n	38.4
6.	W. U.	f	22	Ren mobilis	n	35.4

n = normal degree of immunohistochemical reaction, degree of controls, m = male patient, f = female patient.

76 years were operated on recurrent urolithiasis (Tables 2–4). Six patients (4 females and 2 males; 22–53 years) without renal calculi and an average age of 40 years had an operation for ren mobilis or stenosis of ureteral pelvic junction and served as controls (Table 1). Patients with impaired renal function (increased serum creatinine concentration) were excluded from these studies. Furthermore, we did not investigate patients with abnormal impairments of acid-base equilibrium, as measured by blood analysis. The urine pH of all patients was established three times per day (in the morning, at noon, in the evening) by a test paper (Nitrazingelbpapier, Feinchemie Sebnitz, FRG) over a period of two weeks. In patients with significant bacteriuria a treatment with adequate antibiotics was carried out before the estimation of pH values. Preoperatively the antibiotic treatment was stopped for 7 days. Before we started the operation the sterility of urine was controlled. The patients were divided into four groups according to their diagnoses and the profile of urine pH (Tables 1–4). From all patients we determined the levels of creatinine, K^+, Na^+, Ca^{++}, Cl^-, pH, HCO_3^-, p CO_2, pO_2, and base excess in the serum. Patients with permanent urine pH above 6.0 were submitted to a tolerance test with ammonium chloride according to Wrong and Davis

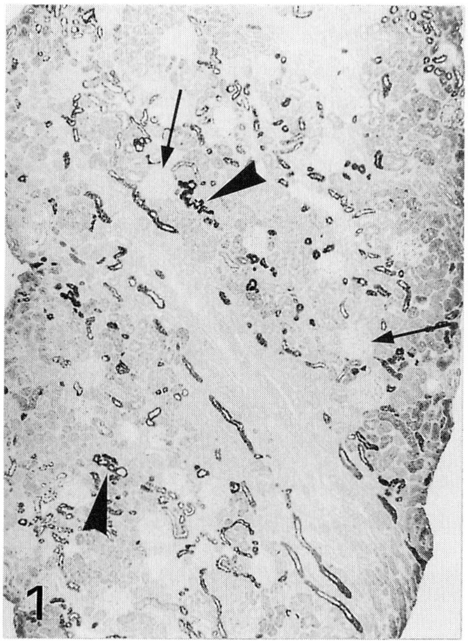

Fig. 1 Patient Z. G., 53 years, male, out of the group 1 (controls, Table 1, case No. 3); normal degree of immunohistochemical reaction, distal tubules and cortical collecting ducts (➤); glomeruli without reaction (↗) (×37)

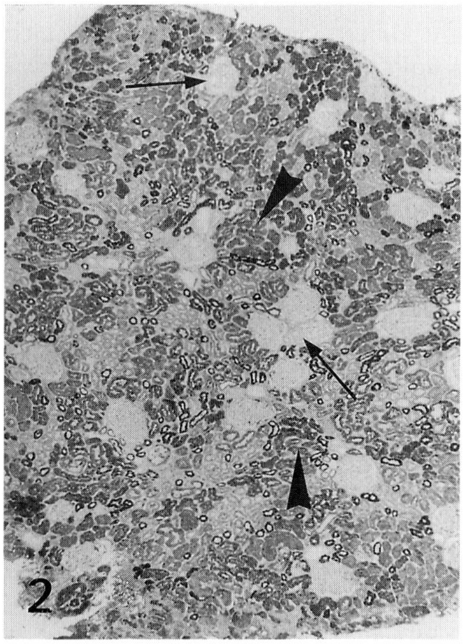

Fig. 2 Patient S. B., 62 years, female, out of the group 3 (patient with urolithiasis, urine pH 5.8, Table 3, case No. 6); strongly increased degree of immunohistochemical reaction for carbonic anhydrase; additional to the distal tubules and collecting ducts reaction in the proximal tubules (➤); glomeruli without reaction (↗) (×37)

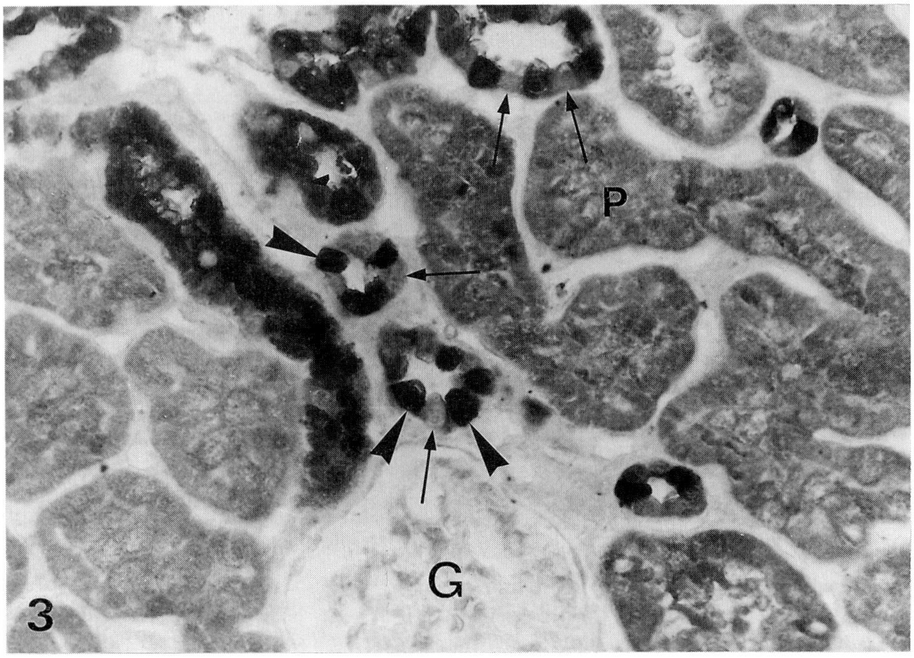

Fig. 3 Patient Z. W., 36 years, male, group 1 (control, Table 1, case No. 4, stenosis of ureteral pelvic junction); glomerulum (G) without reaction, proximal tubules (P) with diffuse reaction, cortical collecting ducts with an alternating pattern of P-(light, ↗) and I-(dark, ➘) cells (×200)

[1959]. All renal stones were analysed by x-ray diffraction.

Immunohistochemical methods

Exploratory excisions about 10–50 mm^3 were obtained from the kidney cortex with a special punch and fixed in Carnoys' mixture for 4 h. The tissue was dehydrated in alcohol, embedded in paraffin and sectioned. 5 µm thick sections were mounted on slides, deparaffinized in xylene, rehydratized and rinsed in PBS-buffer. For the detection of carbonic anhydrase we used the PAP-technique [Sternberger 1979]. The sections were incubated for 48 h with a polyclonal anti-serum against human carbonic anhydrase isoenzyme C, produced from human erythrocytes in rabbits [Kumpulainen 1979] in dilutions of 1:80 to 1:640. The sections were washed for several times and incubated with goat antirabbitserum (SIFIN Berlin, FRG) diluted 1:20 for 1 h. The slides were washed again and incubated for 1 hour with PAP-complex (E-Y Laboratories Inc. USA) diluted 1:40. To visualize the peroxidase activity the sections were incubated for 10 min in 100 ml of 0.05 mol/l TRIS-buffer pH = 7.6 containing 25 mg DAB and 50 µl 30% H_2O_2. The slides were washed, dehydrated in alcohol and embedded in Canada balsam. All incubation times and washing periods were timed by a stopwatch to allow the semiquantitative estimation of the immunohistochemical reaction. To control the specifity of immunohistochemical reaction, we incubated sections with non-immune rabbit sera or with antisera, preabsorbed through carbonic anhydrase powder [Kumpulainen 1979]. Furthermore, we used dilution controls, omitted single steps of the immunohistochemical procedure, or replaced it by PBS.

To quantify the results we semiquantitatively estimated the degree of immunohistochemical reactions in the light microscope. We used a magnification of 1:400. The degree of cytoplasmic reactions of intercalated cells was estimated (a scale from -- to ++). To estimate the quantity of principal and intercalated cells we counted the numbers of both cell types in all distal convoluted tubules and cortical collecting ducts of the sections as often as possible, finding at least 200 cells per section, and estimated the percentage of both. To minimize the subjective factor all results were estimated independently by two authors. The reactivity of intercalated cells of the control group (patients without urolithiasis and normal urine pH) served as a standard of comparison.

Results

Qualitative findings

Figure 1 shows a picture of a kidney biopsy of a patient from the control group. The enzyme carbonic anhydrase isoenzyme C is demonstrable in the proximal and distal tubules of the nephron as well as in the collecting ducts. The glomeruli with the Bowman's capsule are unreactive with the exception of the erythrocytes in the capillaries. The proximal tubules are slightly coloured and homogeneous in all cells in contrast to the distal tubules and collecting ducts, where there is an alternating occurrence of strongly and slightly reacting cells. It is possible to distinguish between strongly reacting intercalated cells (I-cells) and slightly reacting principal cells (P-cells) (Figure 3). There are qualitatively no distinctions between patients without urolithiasis (control group) and those with renal calculi and different urine pH (Figure 2).

Quantitative findings

Tables 1–4 show the clinical data and immunohistochemical findings (estimated degree of the reaction, percentage of I-cells) of all individual patients divided into four groups. The immunohistochemical reaction in the distal tubules and cortical collecting ducts seems to correlate with the urine pH. Group 3 (Table 3) with predominantly acid urine (pH <5.8) shows only one out of 18 cases with a normal degree of immunohistochemical reactivity (Table 1). The other 17 patients had elevated or strongly increased reactions. In contrast to this, we found only diminished or strongly decreased reactions in the group 4 (Table 4) (5 cases with predominantly alcaline urine, pH >6.8). In the second group (Table 2) (28 cases with urine pH 5.8–6.8) there was a big variation of cytoplasmic reactions.

In some cases with strongly elevated immunohistochemical reactions we found, apart from the typical alternating pattern in the distal tubules and collecting ducts, distal tubules with only very strongly reacting cells and a strongly increased diffuse reaction in the proximal tubules.

Table 5 shows the estimated mean values and standard deviations from the mean in the percentage

Table 2 Group 2 of patients, patients with urolithiasis and normal urine pH (5.8–6.8)

No.	Name	Sex	Age (years)	Analysis of urinary stones	Degree of immuno-histochemical reaction	Percentage of CA-rich cells
1.	T. R.	f	45	Apatite/Potass. apatite	–	49.5
2.	W. J.	m	42	Oxalate	+	49.8
3.	K. O.	m	49	Apatite/Oxal./Uric acid	n	45.3
4.	H. K.	f	16	Oxalate	++	64.4
5.	M. U.	f	59	Oxal./Apatite/Struv./Potass. apatite	–	54.95
6.	A. E.	m	56	Oxalate	++	56.6
7.	H. A.	f	21	Cystine	––	35.5
8.	K. H.	f	52	Oxalate	++	51.9
9.	H. W.	m	33	Struv./Potass. apatite	–	49.8
10.	P. E.	f	41	Oxalate	n	43.8
11.	B. E.	f	49	Oxalate	n	46.8
12.	K. M.	f	37	Oxalate/Potass. apatite	++	56.5
13.	K. I.	f	62	Struv./Potass. apatite	–	46.1
14.	C. A.	f	56	Struv./Potass. apatite	–	41.7
15.	M. D.	m	63	Oxalate	–	47.4
16.	B. M.	m	32	Struv./Potass. apatite	–	45.1
17.	S. C.	f	41	Oxalate	n	47.4
18.	P. H. G.	m	52	Oxalate	n	46.4
19.	H. R.	f	52	Oxalate	n	48.0
20.	G. E.	f	65	Oxal./Uric acid	+	47.8
21.	S. H.	f	39	Oxal./Uric acid	–	22.2
22.	S. E.	m	63	Oxalate	n	45.4
23.	P. R.	m	29	Oxalate/Uric acid	–	43.9
24.	H. H. C.	m	39	Oxalate	+	45.9
25.	S. K. P.	m	31	Cystine	––	27.4
26.	T. C.	m	26	Oxal./Uric acid	––	36.1
27.	F. R.	m	57	Oxalate	++	46.8
28.	W. L.	f	59	Oxalate	+	51.8

Degree of immunohistochemical reactions, (––) strongly diminished, (–) diminished (n) normal, the same as of controls, (+) increased, (++) strongly increased

Table 3 Group 3 of patients, patients with urolithiasis and predominantly acid urines (pH <5.8)

No.	Name	Sex	Age (years)	Analysis of urinary stones	Degree of immuno-histochemical reaction	Percentage of CA-rich cells
1.	T. D.	m	41	Oxalate	+	64.3
2.	S. W.	m	67	Oxalate/Uric acid	+	63.3
3.	M. P.	m	37	Oxalate/Uric acid	++	60.4
4.	L. R.	m	21	Oxalate	+	49.7
5.	B. E.	f	39	Oxalate	+	64.8
6.	S. B.	f	62	Oxalate	++	71.1
7.	P. K. H.	m	57	Oxalate	++	67.9
8.	W. M.	m	69	Oxalate/Uric acid	++	66.5
9.	B. R.	f	41	Oxalate/Uric acid	++	62.7
10.	K. S.	m	42	Oxalate/Uric acid	n	57.0
11.	M. G.	m	60	Oxalate/Uric acid	+	60.1
12.	H. I.	f	70	Oxalate/Uric acid	++	63.0
13.	K. M.	m	53	Oxalate	++	60.1
14.	G. G.	f	43	Oxalate/Uric acid	+	78.8
15.	S. G.	m	46	Oxalate/Uric acid	+	65.4
16.	H. M.	f	62	Oxalate	++	64.7
17.	Z. G.	f	51	Oxalate/Uric acid	++	62.8
18.	H. B.	m	29	Oxalate	+	55.4

Estimated degree of immunohistochemical reaction, n = degree of controls, normal degree; + = increased; ++ = strongly increased degree of reaction; m = male; f = female.

Table 4 Group 4 of patients, patients with urolithiasis and predominantly alkaline urines (pH >6.8)

No.	Name	Sex	Age (years)	Analysis of urinary stones	Degree of immuno-histochemical reaction	Percentage of CA-rich cells
1.	M. C.	f	47	Struv./Potass. apatite	–	42.2
2.	K. L.	f	57	Potass. apatite	––	46.2
3.	K. H.	f	25	Oxal./Potass. apatite/Brush.	–	52.0
4.	P. I.	f	29	Oxal./Uric acid	––	15.4
5.	H. H.	f	44	Potass. apatite	–	53.0

f = female patients, estimated degree of immunohistochemical reaction, – = decreased, –– = strongly decreased degree of reaction

Table 5 Summary of the data of the 4 groups of patients. Percentage of CA-rich cells

Groups of patients	1	2	3	4
n	6	28	18	5
means	46.3%	46.2%	63.2%	41.9%
±SD	8.1	8.4	6.2	15.5

of I-cells in the four groups. There is a significant difference between group 3 with predominantly acid urine ($\bar{x}$ = 63% ± 6) and group 1 ($\bar{x}$ = 46% ± 8) or group 2 ($\bar{x}$ = 46% ± 8) with normal urine pH. Furthermore we found a significantly decreased number of I-cells in the group 4 of patients with predominantly alcaline urine ($\bar{x}$ = 42% ± 16) in comparison to group 3 ($\bar{x}$ = 63% ± 6), whereas the difference to the control group is, indeed, not significant.

Discussion

The distribution of the enzyme carbonic anhydrase in the kidney biopsies of patients with recurrent urolithiasis does not differ qualitatively from that of the normal healthy kidney. In accordance with other studies on human kidneys [Lönnerholm 1973, 1984, Lönnerholm and Wistrand 1984, Kumpulainen 1981, 1984, Spicer et al. 1982, Jonas et al. 1983] we found the main quantity of the enzyme in the distal tubules and collecting ducts. Similar results were obtained from studies on rat and other vertebrate kidneys [Lönnerholm 1971, 1974, 1983, Lönnerholm and Ridderstrale 1974, 1984, Ridderstrale 1976, Rosen 1972, Spicer et al. 1979, Jonas 1982, Brown et al. 1982, 1983, Holthöfer et al. 1987].

The occurrence of cells with alternatingly weak and strong reactivity for carbonic anhydrase correlates with the distribution of principal (P-) and intercalated (I-)cells [Dobyan and Bulger 1982, Holthöfer et al. 1987]. The carbonic anhydrase rich I-cells are considered to be involved in regulating the acid-base equilibrium and in the exchange of potassium and hydrogen ions [Giebisch 1986, Hansen et al. 1980, Kaissling et al. 1981, Kaissling 1985a, b, Madsen and Tisher 1984, 1985, Rastegar et al. 1980, Stetson et al. 1980, Zufarov et al. 1976].

The number of investigated human kidneys in all preceding studies was small. In addition, the kidneys were obtained by autopsy. Quantitative data, e. g. on the number of I- and P-cells were not obtained. As far as we know there have not been any studies on the human kidney for carbonic anhydrase in a great number of cases until now.

In a preliminary study we used 22 exploratory excisions of patients with urolithiasis, ren mobilis or stenosis of ureteral pelvic junction, for obtaining qualitative results [Jonas et al. 1983]. In this quantitative study we used 57 new cases.

The immunohistochemical techniques are not quantitative, but we consider it possible to analyse the preparations semiquantitatively, if all preparation steps are reproducible. Therefore, we consider the degree of immunohistochemical reaction as indicative of the enzyme quantity. We found a great variability in the degree of immunohistochemical intensity. This seems to correlate with urine acidification or the mean urine pH.

Furthermore, the number of carbonic anhydrase-rich I-cells in the distal tubulus and collecting ducts of the cortical exploratory excisions differs in the four patient groups. It seems to be correlated to a definite quantity of acid excretion. But we are not able to distinguish between the primary and secondary effect. It is not clear whether the capacity of I-cells and of carbonic anhydrase is a constitutionally genetic (primary) question or a sign of adaptation to a special necessity to excrete protons or to regulate a certain acid-base equilibrium. An adaptation of the enzyme quantity and/or activity of carbonic anhydrase in the I-cells and in other nephron parts such as proximal tubules was suggested [Lönnerholm et al. 1986]. Indeed, the adaptability of the number of I-cells in the kidney is not confirmed. Whereas Oliver et al. [1957], Holliday et al. [1959], Hagege et al. 1968, 1969, 1974] and Richet et al. [1970, 1975] found an increased number of I-cells after metabolic alcalose by administration of bicarbonate or after respiratoric acidosis, Hansen et al. [1980] were not able to reproduce these results.

In addition to the acid-base-regulation, the I-cells play a role in the maintenance of potassium homeostasis [Hansen et al. 1980, Rastegar et al. 1980, Stetson et al. 1981, Madsen and Tisher 1985, Kaissling 1985]. Ordonez and Spargo [1976] and Kaissling [1985a, b] found an increased number of I-cells by chronic potassium depletion. Furthermore Stetson et al. [1980] described an increased number of I-cells with special so-called rodshaped particles in their apical plasma membranes by freeze fracture studies after potassium depletion on rats, whereas the total number of I-cells in ultrathin sections appeared to be unchanged. Indeed, other investigators found no changes in the percentage of I-cells in the renal cortex after experimental loading or depletion of potassium [Richet and Hagege 1975, Toback et al. 1976, Hansen et al. 1980, Stanon et al. 1981]. Methodological differences in detection of I- and P-cells, as shown by Stetson et al. [1980] are a possible explanation for the different results.

We investigated our tissue samples immunohistochemically only with regard to carbonic anhydrase. It is not evident, whether the number of ultrastructural detectable I-cells would be significantly changed in our material. Furthermore, it is doubtful whether the detections of I-cells by the scanning electron microscope, or by light microscopical immunohistochemistry would give the same results. This would require further experimentation.

We were not able to correlate individual risk factors for urolithiasis such as urinary tract infections, hypercalciuria, hyperuricosuria, hypomagnesuria, and hyperphosphaturia, with the quantity of carbonic anhydrase. Only in the case of two patients with cystinuria did we detect a remarkably low level of this enzyme and a small number of I-cells. But two cases are insufficient from which to reach a valid conclusion.

REFERENCES

Brown D, Roth J, Kumpulainen T, Orci L 1982 Ultrastructural immunocytochemical localization of carbonic anhydrase. Histochem *75:* 209

Brown D, Roth J, Kumpulainen T, Orci L 1983 Immunohistochemical localization of carbonic anhydrase in postnatal and adult rat kidney. Am J Physiol *245:* F 110

Clapp WL, Madsen KM, Verlander JW, Tisher CC 1987 Intercalated cells of the rat inner medullary collecting duct. Kidney Int *31:* 1080

Dobyan DC, Bulger RE 1982 Renal carbonic anhydrase. Am J Physiol *243:* F 311

Dörup J 1985 Structural adaptation of intercalated cells in rat renal cortex to acute metabolic acidosis and alkalosis. J Ultrastr Res *92:* 119

Eveloff J, Swenson ER, Maren TH 1979 Carbonic anhydrase activity of brush border and plasma membranes prepared from rat kidney cortex. Biochem Pharmacol *28:* 1434

Giebisch G 1986 Mechanism of renal tubular acidification. Klin Wochenschr *64:* 853

Hagege J, Gabe M, Richet G 1968 Augmentation du nombre des cellules intercalaires rénales du rat soumis a une surcharge en bicarbonate alcaline. C R Acad Sci *267:* 1611

Hagege J, Richet G, Gabe M 1969 Effect de l'acidose grazeuse sur les parties distales du néphron de rat albinos. C R Acid Sci *269:* 1539

Hagege J, Gabe M, Richet G 1974 Scanning of the apical pole of distal tubular cells under different acid-base conditions. Kidney Int *5:* 137

Hansen GP, Tisher CC, Robinson RR 1980 Response of the collecting duct to disturbances of acid-base and potassium balance. Kidney Int *17:* 326

Holliday MA, Winter RW, Welt LG, MacDowell M, Oliver J 1959 The renal lesions of electrolyte imbalance: II. The combined effect of renal architecture of phosphate loading and potassium depletion. J Exp Med *110:* 161

Holthöfer H, Schulte BA, Spicer SS 1987 Expression of binding sites for Dolichos biflorus agglutinin at the apical aspect of collecting duct cells in rat kidney. Cell Tissue Res *249:* 481

Jonas L 1982 Immunfluoreszenzhistochemischer Nachweis von Carboanhydrase in der Magenmukosa und Niere des Rindes. Acta histochem *70:* 43

Jonas L, Hoffmann L, Serfling D 1983 Der Nachweis von Carboanhydrase in der menschlichen Niere unter dem Aspekt der Säure-Basen-Regulation. Z Urol Nephrol *76:* 311

Kaissling B 1985a Structural adaptation to altered electrolyte metabolism by cortical distal segments. Federation Proc *44:* 2710

Kaissling B 1985b Cellular heterogenity of the distal nephron and its relation to function. Klin Wochenschr *63:* 868

Kaissling B, Koeppen BM, Wade JB, LeHir M 1981 Effect of mineralocorticoids on the structure of intercalated cells. Acta Anat *111:* 72A

Kumpulainen T 1979 Immunohistochemical localization of human carbonic anhydrase isoenzyme C. Histochemistry *62:* 271

Kumpulainen T 1981 Human carbonic anhydrase isoenzyme C. Histochemistry *72:* 425

Kumpulainen T 1984 Immunohistochemical localization of human carbonic anhydrase isoenzymes. Ann NY Acad Sci *429:* 359

Lönnerholm G 1971 Histochemical demonstration of carbonic anhydrase activity in the rat kidney. Acta Physiol Scand *81:* 433

Lönnerholm G 1973 Histochemical demonstration of carbonic anhydrase activity in the human kidney. Acta Physiol Scand *88:* 455

Lönnerholm G 1974 Carbonic anhydrase histochemistry. A critical study of Hanssons cobalt-phosphate method. Acta Physiol Scand *418 (Suppl):* 1

Lönnerholm G 1983 Carbonic anhydrase in the monkey kidney. Histochemistry *78:* 195

Lönnerholm G 1984 Carbonic anhydrase in the human kidney. A histochemical and immunocytochemical study. Kidney Int *25:* 866

Lönnerholm G, Ridderstrale Y 1980 Intracellular distribution of carbonic anhydrase in the rat kidney. Kidney Int *17:* 162

Lönnerholm G, Ridderstrale Y 1974 Distribution of carbonic anhydrase in the frog nephron. Acta Physiol Scand *90:* 764

Lönnerholm G, Wistrand PJ 1984 Carbonic anhydrase in the human kidney. A histochemical and immunocytochemical study. Kidney Int *25:* 886

Lönnerholm G, Wistrand PJ, Barany E 1986 Carbonic anhydrase isoenzymes in the rat kidney. Effects of chronic acetazolamide treatment. Acta Physiol Scand *126:* 51

Madsen KM, Tisher CC 1984 Response of intercalated cells of rat outer medullary collecting duct to chronic metabolic acidosis. Lab Invest *51:* 268

Madsen KM, Tisher CC 1985 Structure-function relationships in H^+-secreting epithelia. Federation Proc *44:* 2704

Oliver J, MacDowell M, Welt MA, Holliday MA, Hollander W, Winter RW, William FF, Segar WE 1957 The renal lesions of electrolyte imbalace: I. The structural alterations in potassium depleted rats. J Exp Med *106:* 563

Ordonez NG, Spargo BH 1976 The morphologic relationship of light and dark cells of the collecting tubule in potassium-depleted rats. Am J Pathol *84:* 317

Pitts RF 1974 Physiology of kidney and body fluids. Year Book Med Publ Inc, Chicago

Rastegar A, Biemersderfer D, Kashgaria M, Hayslett JP 1980 Changes in membrane surfaces of collecting duct cells in potassium adaptation. Kidney Int *18:* 293

Richet G, Hagege J 1975 Dark cells of the distal convuluted tubules and collecting ducts. II. Physiological significance. Fortschr Zool *23:* 299

Richet G, Hagege J, Gabe M 1970 Correlations entre les transferts de bicarbonate et la morphologie du segment terminal du néphron chez le rat. Nephron *7:* 413

Ridderstrale Y 1976 Intercellular localization of carbonic anhydrase in the frog nephron. Acta Physiol Scand *98:* 465

Rosen S 1972 Localization of carbonic anhydrase activity in the vertebrate nephron. Histochem J *4:* 35

Spicer SS, Stoward PJ, Tashian RE 1979 The immunohistolocalization of carbonic anhydrase in rodent tissue. J Histochem Cytochem *27:* 820

Spicer SS, Sens MA, Tashian RE 1982 Immunocytochemical demonstration of carbonic anhydrase in human epithelial cells. J Histochem Cytochem *30:* 864

Stanton BA, Biemesderfer D, Wade JB, Giebisch G 1981 Structural and functional study of the rat distal nephron: Effects of potassium adaptation and depletion. Kidney Int *19:* 36

Sternberger LA 1979 Immunocytochemistry. Wiley, New York, Chishester – Brisbane – Toronto – Singapore

Stetson DL, Wade JB, Giebisch G 1980 Morphologic alterations in the rat medullary collecting duct following potassium depletion. Kidney Int *17:* 45

Toback FG, Ordonez NG, Bortz SL, Spargo BH 1976 Zonal changes in renal structure and phospholipid metabolism in potassium-deficient rats. Lab Invest *34:* 115

Warnock DG, Rector FC 1981 Renal acidification mechanism. In: *Brenner BM, Rector FC* (eds). The Kidney, Vol. I, chapter 10. WB Saunders, Philadelphia, p 440

Wistrand PJ 1979 Renal membrane-bound carbonic anhydrase: Purifications and properties. Upsala J Med Sci *26 (Suppl): 75*

Wistrand PJ, Kinne R 1977 Carbonic anhydrase activity of isolated brush border and basal-lateral membranes of renal tubular cells. Pfluegers Arch *370:* 121

Wrong O, Davies HEF 1959 The excretion of acid in renal disease. Quart J Med *28:* 259

Zuvarov KA, Gontmakher VM 1976 On cells secreting hydrogen ions in renal tubules. Arch Pathol (Moscow) *38:* 13

Clinical Nephrology, Vol. 35, No. 5 – 1991 (198–206)

Vaccination for prevention of CAPD associated staphylococcal infection: Results of a prospective multicentre clinical trial

L. A. Poole-Warren, M. D. Hallett, P. W. Hone, S. H. Burden and P. C. Farrell

University of New South Wales

Center participants

R. Atkins[1], D. Berry[2], J. Burgess[3], T. Cahill[4], S. Campbell[5], B. Cocksedge[6], P. Collett[7], J. Collins[8], T. Garland[9], J. Hayes[9], R. Hernadez[4], D. Hunt[6], L. Ibels[6], M. Ku[4], F. Lynn[1], J. Mahony[6], J. Moran[10], J. Neale[3], C. Pollock[6], L. Potts[3], J. Ridder[11], S. Riordan[11], H. Scott[8], G. Stewart[7], J. Stewart[5], L. H. Tan[2], L. Walker[11], M. Wallace[11], C. Wood[1]

[1]Prince Henry's Hospital, Melbourne; [2]Prince of Wales Hospital, Sydney;
[3]Wellington Hospital, New Zealand; [4]Lidcombe Hospital, Sydney;
[5]Westmead Hospital, Sydney; [6]Royal North Shore Hospital, Sydney;
[7]Concord Hospital, Sydney; [8]Auckland Hospital, New Zealand;
[9]St. Vincent's Hospital, Sydney; [10]St. Vincent's Hospital, Melbourne;
[11]Waikato Hospital, New Zealand

Abstract. 124 stable CAPD patients from 8 Australian and 3 New Zealand centers were randomly assigned in a blinded fashion to one of two groups to study the effect of vaccination using commercial preparations consisting of a combined staphylococcus toxoid and whole killed staphylococci (SB) or normal saline solution (SS) on the incidence of peritonitis and exit site infection and *S. aureus* nasal carriage over a 12-month prospective period. In addition, levels of IgG, IgA, IgM, C3 and C4 were monitored during the trial period in serum and dialysate; serum levels of anti-α hemolysin and dialysate levels of fibronectin and specific anti-staphylococcal antibodies were also measured. Over the period, treatment with SB or SS did not affect the incidence of peritonitis, catheter-related infection or *S. aureus* nasal carriage. However, vaccination with SB elicited a significant increase in the level of serum anti-α hemolysin throughout the 12 month duration of the study, although the level of increase was unrelated to the subsequent rate of peritonitis. Vaccination with SB but not SS elicited a significant increase in the dialysate level of specific antibodies against *S. aureus*. Serum levels of IgG, IgA, IgM, complement C3 and C4 were within the normal range in the CAPD patients studied and remained unaffected by vaccination with SB. In addition, dialysate levels of IgG, IgA, IgM, complement C3 and C4 were 50–100 times lower than corresponding serum levels and remained unaffected by vaccination. In summary, immunisation with an anti-staphylococcal agent was not successful in reducing peritonitis or exit site infection in CAPD patients.

Key words: staphylococcal vaccination – CAPD – immunoglobulins – complement – peritonitis – exit site infection – nasal carriage – dialysate

Introduction

Peritonitis and catheter-associated infections are significant contributors to morbidity and, to a lesser extent, mortality in patients treated with continuous ambulatory peritoneal dialysis (CAPD). In the USA, for example, peritonitis occurs at an average rate of 1.4 episodes per patient year [National CAPD Registry 1988]. Attempts at prevention of infection in patients established on CAPD have been based on either barrier methods, aimed at preventing microbial entry [Maiorca et al. 1983], or on prophylaxis using antibiotics [Low et al. 1980, Churchill et al. 1988] or immunization [Scatizzi and Strippoli 1986, Lamperi et

Received June 6, 1990; in revised form January 21, 1991.

Reprint requests to: Prof. P. C. Farrell, University of New South Wales, PO Box 1, Kensington, NSW 2113, Australia.

al. 1986]. Although some barrier methods have proved highly successful, such as the disconnect systems pioneered by Maiorca [Maiorca et al. 1983], they are solely aimed at reducing the level of peritonitis.

Antibiotic prophylaxis has generally been unsuccessful for prevention of infection in CAPD patients [Low et al. 1980, Churchill et al. 1988]. This lack of success, combined with the likelihood of developing resistant strains, discourages further investigation of antibiotic prophylaxis. Immunological prophylaxis, on the other hand, has the potential to reduce the risk of both peritonitis and catheter-related infections, thereby improving patient quality of life. Prevention of peritonitis by enhancing the immune response has been examined in the past [Scatizzi and Strippoli 1986, Lamperi et al. 1986, Lamperi and Carozzi 1986, Chan 1988]. This may be achieved by either passive immunization, using immunoglobulins, or by active immunization with vaccines.

In vitro examination of phagocytic cell function in dialysate has suggested functional impairment due to deficient opsonic levels [Keane et al. 1984]. Addition of IgG to these *in vitro* systems restored phagocytic function of cells in opsonin-poor CAPD effluents. Additionally, confirmatory *in vivo* results were believed to demonstrate a significant correlation between IgG levels in spent peritoneal dialysate and patient's peritonitis rate [Lamperi and Carozzi 1986]. Putative prophylactic and therapeutic efficacy of intraperitoneal administration of human immunoglobulin in the treatment of bacterial peritonitis has also been reported [Lamperi and Carozzi 1986, Chan 1988]. These results would suggest that passive immunization may be successful in reducing the peritonitis rate in the CAPD population.

Passive immunization, however, merely supplements host defense mechanisms by providing an exogenous defence against antigens and, therefore, there is a continual requirement for administration of immunoglobulin to maintain passive immunity. Active immunization is based on presenting an appropriate antigenic stimulus to the host immune system. While passive immunization provides immediate protection, active immunization requires at least 7 to 10 days for development of antibodies by the host, depending on the antigenicity of presented epitopes. In the latter case, subsequent exposure to administered immunogens potentially results in a rapid secondary immune response.

Since staphylococcal species are responsible for up to 80% of CAPD peritonitis episodes [Everett and Bodem 1984, West et al. 1986], vaccines against staphylococci have been proposed as potentially useful in conferring immunity to a large proportion of infections in these patients. A staphylococcal vaccine for prevention of *S. aureus* CAPD peritonitis was reported to have been applied successfully [Scatizzi and Strippoli 1986], reducing peritonitis rate and eliminating peritonitis caused by *S. aureus*. Protective mechanisms of the vaccine were found to include production of an anti-staphylococcal effect in dialysate, thereby preventing proliferation of the organism.

The precedent established by these favourable preliminary results, and the potential impact such prophylaxis would have on the quality of life offered CAPD patients, encouraged further investigation of the efficacy of staphylococcal vaccine. The aim of this multi-centre trial was to compare, prospectively, the efficacy of a commercially available staphylococcal toxoid and whole killed bacterial suspension for reduction of peritonitis and catheter-associated infection rates in CAPD patients. The vaccine, Staphypan Berna, was identical in composition to that used by Scatizzi and Strippoli [1986]. This study reports the results of the comparative performance of Staphypan Berna (Swiss Serum and Vaccine Institute, Berne) versus a saline placebo.

Materials and methods

A double-blind, placebo-controlled design was undertaken. The vaccine studied was a combined toxoid/whole killed bacterial formulation, Staphypan Berna (SB). Patients were randomly assigned by an independent third party to either the vaccinated group or the saline solution (SS) placebo (0.9% NaCl solution, John Bull Laboratories, Melbourne) administered group. Peritonitis and catheter related infection incidence was prospectively monitored over a 12 month period and the rates compared with up to 1 year pre-study incidence. The protocol and details of both vaccines were submitted to and approved by all participating hospital's ethics committees prior to patient enrolment.

Patients

All patients included were currently undergoing chronic CAPD and were stabilized on the therapy. Exclusion criteria included current peritoneal infection, receipt of an antibiotic course within the 2 week period prior to study enrolment or use of assist devices or disconnect systems. Eligible patients were randomly assigned to either the SB or SS groups. The assigned injection group was not known to either patient or staff immediately connected with the patient's care at any time during the study. Patient particulars and data were assembled by the study direction team at the coordinating center.

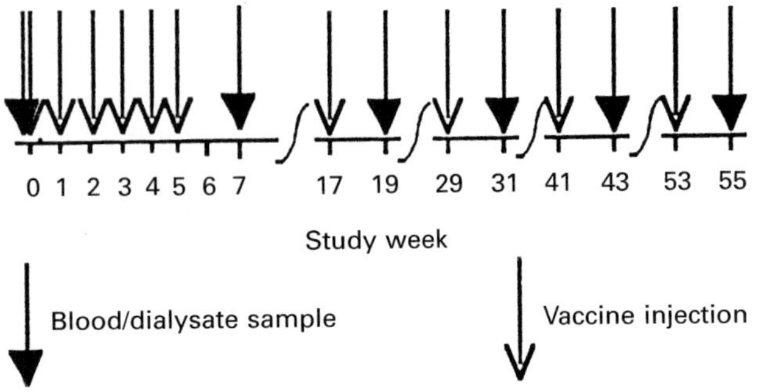

Fig. 1 Injection and sampling schedule versus study week

Patient data collection, both pre-enrolment and intra-study, included: patient name, identification no., date of birth, center name, primary renal lesion, injection group and scheduling, date of CAPD commencement; bag connection system, pre-study infection record (up to 1 year); peritonitis and catheter infections and antibiotic usage during study, interruptions to CAPD; use of antibiotics other than for peritonitis and catheter infections.

Patients were withdrawn from the study, prior to the completion of the 12-month injection schedule and follow up, for any one of the following reasons: 1) renal transplantation, 2) transfer from CAPD to other dialysis modes, 3) recommendation by the patient physician that it was in the patients' interest to withdraw, and, 4) withdrawal of patient consent. The sample size required was determined by biostatisticians at Siromath Pty Ltd (Sydney, Australia) using a method based on calculation of the differences between two Poisson expectations. The mean peritonitis rate in the general CAPD population was assumed to be 1.5 episodes per patient year based upon mean USA rate (9). The total years of experience required in each treatment group to obtain a 95% probability of detecting a 50% reduction in peritonitis rate, in a test conducted with a 5% significance level, was 43 patient years.

Injection schedules

Injection schedules for the vaccine were based on manufacturers' recommendations. All injections were given intramuscularly (IM). Six IM injections of SB were given in increasing concentrations (1%, 5%, 10%, 20%, 50% and undiluted) over six weeks (week 0 to week 5). Four booster injections of 1 ml of undiluted SB were given every 12 weeks thereafter (on weeks 17, 29, 41 and 53). Normal saline placebo was given at the same intervals as for the vaccine in 1 ml volumes injected IM. Injections were administered by qualified medical personnel.

Sample collection

Immediately prior to commencing an injection schedule, each patient had pre-study blood and overnight dwell dialysate samples taken and a nasal swab performed. The timing of this sample was deemed equivalent to week 0 in the schedule. Blood and dialysate samples and nasal swabs were subsequently taken at week 7, 2 weeks after completion of the first course of 6 injections and approximately 2 weeks following each booster injection at weeks 19, 31, 43 and 55. Each blood sample was separated into two serum samples. All serum and dialysate samples were either analyzed following collection or frozen at −70° C prior to analysis. (Injection and sampling protocols are summarized in Figure 1.)

Clinical diagnosis of infection

Peritonitis was diagnosed as the presence of any 2 of the following 3 criteria: cloudy dialysate, culturable microorganisms present in dialysate and abdominal pain [Vas 1985]. Dialysate specimens were cultured using at least one enrichment or concentration step at the patient's hospital laboratory.

Clinical diagnosis of exit-site infection was defined by either erythema alone or in combination with purulent exudate. Swabs of exit-sites and tunnels with suspected infection were cultured on enriched plates, such as blood agar. All isolates were identified using standard microbiological techniques and reported.

Recurrent infection was defined as one which occurred within 14 days of antibiotic cessation for the treatment of a previous infection. Reinfections were counted only once together with the first occurrence. Cumulative time at risk of infection was calculated by taking the total time of all patient experience during the study period and subtracting both days on antibiotics and those off CAPD.

Statistical analysis of infection rates

Infection rates were statistically compared using a chi-squared test, where infections were assumed to follow a Poisson distribution. The null hypothesis tested at the 5% significance level was that the Poisson rates of infection were equal in all treatment groups (2 groups in Australia, 2 groups in New Zealand). Overall analysis was conducted initially and, if a significant difference was found, individual 2 × 2 analyses, using a significance level of 0.05/no. comparisons [Armitage and Berry 1987], were used to identify groups representing a different population mean.

Prospective peritonitis data obtained during the study period were also analyzed using the Cox proportional hazards model [Cox 1972] in which the risk of peritonitis in the vaccinated group was assessed relative to the placebo group. Analysis was conducted using BMDP statistical software (Program P2L: University of California, Los Angeles).

Results were expressed as relative risk (RR), and the 95% confidence intervals for RR.

Serum assays

Australian serum samples were assayed by the Prince of Wales Hospital Department of Clinical Chemistry, Sydney, for immunoglobulins IgG, IgA and IgM and complement components C3 and C4. Serum immunoglobulins were assayed by nephelometry on a Kallestead QM-300 nephelometer using Kallestead standards and antibodies (Kallestead, USA). The detection limit for immunoglobulins and complement components was 0.07 g/l.

Serum anti-staphylolysin (AStaL) was assayed by the Prince Henry's Hospital, Melbourne, Department of Biochemistry and Wellington Hospital, Department of Microbiology using a kit based on hemolysis of rabbit erythrocytes (Calbiochem Behring, Marburg, Germany). Serum complement was inactivated by treating for 30 min at 56° C prior to assay. The upper limit of normal levels given by the manufacturer is 2 IU/ml. In this study AStaL levels above this were considered to indicate positive response to the vaccine or possible staphylococcal infection.

Statistical analysis of between group differences in serum proteins over time was conducted by two-way analysis of variance according to Armitage and Berry [1]. The significance level was set at 5%.

Dialysate assays

Dialysate samples were assayed by Prince Henry's Hospital Department of Chemical Pathology, Melbourne. IgG, IgA, IgM, complement C3, C4 and fibronectin (Fn) were assayed by nephelometry using a Behring nephelometer and Behring standard antibodies (Behring, Marburg, Germany). Atlantic Antibodies calibrator CA1 (Maine, USA) was used for calibration of IgG, IgA, IgM, C3 and C4 assays and N Protein Standard Plasma (Behring, Germany) was used for calibrating the Fn assays. The detection limits (mg/l) for the above assays were: IgG 6.5; IgA 5.4; IgM 4.8; C3 1.8; C4 0.8; Fn 1.8. Statistical analyses were conducted as for serum proteins.

Dialysate samples taken at baseline (week 0) and at week 7 were randomly selected from the SB (n = 21) and SS (n = 9) treatment groups and qualitatively assayed for specific antibodies against *S. epidermidis* (ATCC 12228) and *S. aureus.* (ATCC 10832) by ELISA. Analyses were performed at the Baxter Life Sciences Center, Round Lake, Ill. Samples were tested either undiluted or with four-fold dilution.

Antibody activity was quantitated by comparing the optical density (OD) values in test well with OD values of a serially diluted standard sample. Standards were assigned an antibody activity unit (AAU) which allowed a relative value for each test sample based on the slope of the dilution to be assigned. Baseline AAU's were statistically compared with week-7 levels for each study group and each bacteria using a Wilcoxon sign-rank test [Armitage and Berry 1987].

Table 1 Population statistics

	SB	SS
Age at commencement (yr)	54 ± 11	52 ± 14
Sex (ratio m:f)	1.5	0.7
Time on CAPD (yr)	1.5 ± 1.3	1.7 ± 1.9
Connector system*		
System I	40	36
System II	25	23
Primary disease		
Glomeruloneph.	16	18
Analgesic neph.	7	9
Diabetic neph.	12	9
Renal vascular dis.	11	5
Reflux neph.	5	2
Others/unknown	8	6
Total	65	59

Figures quoted mean ± SD where appropriate
* System 1 – spike connect system; System 2 – luer lock connect system

Table 2A Peritonitis infection rates (episodes/year)[1]

	SB	SS
Pre-study		
New Zealand	1.13 (19.5)	0.99 (17.2)
Australia	1.83[2] (24.1)	1.05 (22.9)
Total	1.51 (43.6)	1.03 (40.1)
During study		
New Zealand	1.28 (21.0)	0.96 (22.8)
Australia	1.20 (25.0)	1.27 (22.8)
Total	1.24 (46.0)	1.12 (45.6)

[1] Patient years at risk given in brackets
[2] $0.01 < p < 0.05$ cf other placebo pre study groups.

Nasal swabs

Patient anterior nares were swabbed using a moist, sterile swab. Swabs were screened for *S. aureus* by plate culture. For the purposes of subsequent analyses, patients were defined as carriers if more than half of the swabs taken from an individual during the study were positive for *S. aureus*.

Microbial growth

Growth of *S. aureus* in drained overnight dialysate was assessed in a randomly selected sample (n = 5) of patients from each treatment group. Dialysate for this study was filtered prior to examination through a 0.45 µm filter. Growth was measured over 12 hours at 37° C. A standard inoculum of the test bacteria was prepared by harvesting bacteria from an 18-hour culture (37° C) in tryptone soya broth (Oxoid, Basingstoke, UK).

Quantitative culture at 0, 3, 6 and 12 hours was conducted by spread plating 0.1 ml samples of undiluted sample and diluted sample, to 10^{-6} in 10-fold steps, on tryptone soya agar [Oxoid, UK]. Plates were incubated for 24 hrs at 37° C and colonies counted on plates with densities within the range of 30–300 colonies. Results were expressed as colony forming units (CFU)/ml. Pre-study counts in each group were statistically compared with mid-study counts at 12 hours using two-way analysis of variance with replication and a significance level of 5% [Armitage and Berry 1987].

Table 2B Tunnel and exit site infection rates (episodes/year)[1]

	SB	SS
Pre-study		
New Zealand	1.09 (19.4)	1.09 (16.4)
Australia	0.65 (24.8)	0.34 (23.3)
Total	0.84 (44.2)	0.65 (39.7)
During study		
New Zealand	1.53 (21.0)	1.50 (22.0)
Australia	0.42 (26.1)	0.39 (23.2)
Total	0.91 (47.1)	0.93 (45.2)

[1] Patient years at risk given in brackets

Table 3 Microorganisms isolated in dialysate during peritonitis pre- and during study in vaccinated and placebo patients

Microorganism	Pre-study		Study	
	SB	SS[1]	SB	SS[1]
Gram positive (GP)				
S. aureus	9	9	8	8
CNS[4]	16	13	20[2]	14
Other GP	8	3	16	9
Gram negative (GN)				
E. coli	3	3	2	2
Pseudomonas sp.	3	0	1	2
Enteric GN	3	1	1	2
Other GN	5	3	3	6
Fungi	1	0	4[3]	2
No Growth	18	9	5	6
Total	66	41	60	51

[1] placebo

[2] 1 episode mixed CNS/*Acinetobacter*

[3] 2 episode mixed yeast/*E. coli*

[4] Coagulase negative Staphylococci

Results

A total of 124 patients from 11 centres in Australia and New Zealand participated in the study. The distribution of patients according to age, primary renal lesion, time on CAPD and connection system were similar in the 2 groups as shown in Table 1.

Infection incidence

Peritonitis rate data gathered both retrospectively prior to study commencement and prospectively during the study are summarized in Table 2A; peritonitis rates were not significantly different between vaccine groups. More stringent analyses by Cox's proportional hazards model corroborated these findings, showing the relative risk of peritonitis was similar in saline placebo and vaccinated groups. More specifically it was found that the relative risk of staphylococcal peritonitis was also similar in vaccinated and placebo groups. These results were also reflected by the overall rate of catheter-related infection in the 2 groups as summarized in Table 2B. In contrast to peritonitis data, however, it was found that catheter-related infection overall was significantly higher in New Zealand patients compared to their Australian counterparts, possibly due to differing catheter insertion methods and exit site management.

Microorganisms isolated from dialysate sampled during peritonitis and swabs taken from exit sites during catheter-related infection pre- and post-immunization in the two treatment groups, are summarized in Tables 3 and 4, respectively. The proportion of Gram positive microorganisms isolated during peritonitis increased during the study in the vaccinated group. No-growth peritonitis decreased in both groups during the study compared with retrospectively gathered pre-study data. Gram positive microorganisms, particularly *S. aureus*,, were the most common etiologic agent in catheter infection in both pre-study and during study periods.

Serum and dialysate immunochemistry

Mean serum levels of the immunoproteins IgG, IgA, IgM, complement C3 and C4, were within normal ranges in both groups at all monitoring points during the study. Mean dialysate immunoprotein levels of IgG, IgA, IgM, complement C3, C4 and fibronectin (Fn) were, with the possible exception of IgM which was below the detectable limit in dialysate, 50–100 times lower than equivalent serum concentrations; no significant variation was evident between the groups or with time.

The mean serum anti-α hemolysin (AStaL) levels in the SB group were significantly higher after completion of the initial injection course compared with pre-study ($p < 0.01$ ANOVA) at all time points. Pre-study levels in the SB group were 0.9 ± 0.2 IU/ml (n = 65). Mean levels peaked at week 7 (11.6 ± 1.9 IU/ml) and dropped gradually to 4.6 ± 0.8 IU/ml (n = 34) at week 55. There appeared to be no relation between the level of individual initial response and the subsequent incidence of peritonitis in this group. Although the levels in the SB exhibited a downward trend from the initially elevated levels, values were not significantly different from one another during the study. In addition, the levels at all monitoring points in the SB group during the study after the initial injection course were significantly higher than those in the SS group ($p < 0.01$) which were consistently under the normal level of 2 IU/ml throughout the study.

Results of ELISA for specific anti-staphylococcal antibodies in dialysate showed that the pre-study antibody levels against *S. epidermidis* were not significantly different from mid-study levels in either the SS or SB groups. Specific antibodies against *S. aureus* were significantly higher, compared with pre-study levels, in the SB group (Wilcoxon sign rank test; $p < 0.002$).

S. aureus nasal carriage

Table 5 gives the number of *S. aureus* positive nasal swabs relative to the total swabs taken at each time point, in the 2 groups. Chi squared analysis indicated no significant difference in *S. aureus* nasal carriage, at any time point, between the groups. Table 6 shows the incidence of *S. aureus* and total infections divided according to carrier status (carriers were defined as patients with greater than 50% positive *S. aureus* nasal swabs). In the carrier group, 80% of 210 swabs were positive, whereas in the non-carrier group, 11% of 490 swabs were positive. Statistical analysis demonstrated no relationship between nasal carriage and *S. aureus* peritonitis or catheter infection.

Microbial innocula growth

S. aureus multiplied equally as well in dialysate samples taken pre- and post-immunization (week 7) from SB and SS administered patients. Growth curves representing the mean bacterial levels in dialysate from vaccinated and placebo patients, over 12 hours, are given in Figure 2 (a and b). There was no significant difference in the bacterial concentration in the dialysate at 12 hrs, either between patients or between groups.

Table 4 Microorganisms isolated from infected exit-site/tunnel pre-study and during study in vaccinated and placebo patients

Microorganism	Pre-study		Study	
	SB	SS[1]	SB	SS[1]
Gram positive (GP)				
S. aureus	22	21	29	25
CNS	9	3	4[2]	6
Other GP	2	0	0	3
Gram negative (GN)				
E. coli	1	0	1	0
Pseudomonas sp.	0	1	0	1
Other GN	0	1	3	3
No growth	3	0	6	4
Total	37	26	44	42

[1] placebo
[2] 1 episode CNS/*S. aureus*

Table 5 *S. aureus* nasal carriage vs weeks following injection 1 expressed as number of carriers/group total

	SB	SS
Pre study	13/40	11/36
7 Weeks	19/50	14/44
19 Weeks	11/51	14/46
32 Weeks	9/29	5/20
44 Weeks	2/22	6/25
57 Weeks	10/20	6/22

$\chi^2 = 13.9$, df = 22

Table 6 Incidence of infection vs. *S. aureus* nasal carriage

Peritonitis Inj. type	Nasal carriage	Years at risk	*S. aureus* peritonitis	Total peritonitis
SB	+	18.4	3	27
SB	–	27.7	1	31
SS	+	13.3	3	11
SS	–	32.6	5	36

Exit-site Infection Inj. type	Nasal carriage	Years at risk	*S. aureus* ESIs	Total ESIs
SB	+	18.2	9	13
SB	–	27.0	11	21
SS	+	13.0	9	14
SS	–	32.0	11	19

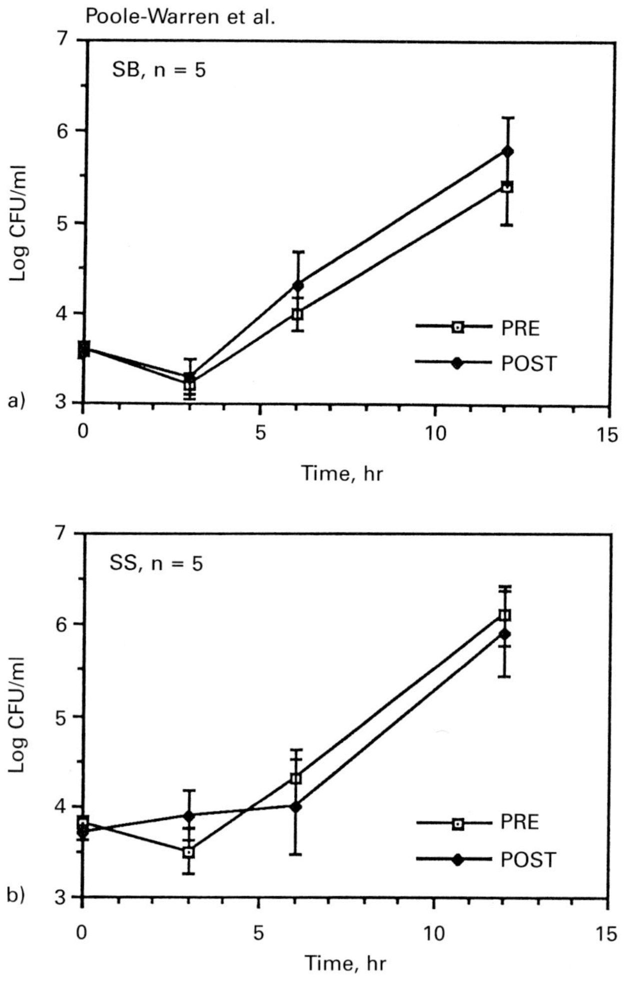

Fig. 2 *S. aureus* innocula growth rates in overnight dialysate drained from patients in groups SB (fig. a) and SS (fig. b) did not differ significantly pre-post immunization

Discussion

In this study, vaccination using Staphypan Berna had no effect on the rate of peritonitis or catheter infection in CAPD patients. Microbial growth was similar in dialysate from SB and SS patients and nasal swab culture indicated no difference in the carriage rate of *S. aureus* between vaccinated and placebo groups. In direct contrast, the work by Scatizzi and Strippoli [1986], suggested SB vaccination to be effective in preventing Staphylococcal peritonitis, in reducing morbidity associated with *S. aureus* tunnel infections, and in reversing *S. aureus* carriage. The findings reflected by this study are based upon results which are more representative than those reported by Scatizzi and Strippoli. Their preliminary data were not subject to the full range of controls required of a well designed prospective double-blind study involving appropriately sized cohorts. The lack of efficacy of vaccination with SB observed in this study may be due to either the inability of patients to mount a response to the vaccine as a result of local (peritoneal) or systemic immune deficiencies, a failure of the vaccine to stimulate the appropriate protective immune response or a combination of these two factors.

Serum immunoglobulin and complement levels were within the normal range in both groups and serum AStaL levels rose significantly in response to SB vaccination as did specific anti-*S. aureus* antibody levels. These observations suggest intact humoral immune responses to antigenic stimuli. Other studies have also suggested that both humoral and cell-mediated immunity in CAPD patients remain unimpaired [Chan et al. 1983, Rubin et al. 1983]. Since infection rates were not influenced by vaccination, regardless of the level of response invoked, as evidenced by the absence of any relation between serum AStaL levels in the SB group and the peritoneal infection rate, deficient systemic immunological factors are unlikely to have been responsible for the unaltered rate of infection seen in this study.

The dilution of peritoneal opsonins, compared to corresponding levels in serum, particularly those considered critical for uptake of staphylococci, such as IgG and Fn [Keane et al. 1984, Duwe et al. 1981, Khan et al. 1987] would appear an important factor in local diminution of immunological protective mechanisms. However, while immunoglobulin levels in this study were similar to those reported elsewhere [Khan et al. 1987, Lamperi and Carozzi 1989, Verbrugh et al. 1983] and appeared to be uninfluenced by vaccination, optimal dialysate levels are not well defined. Scatizzi and Strippoli [1986] suggested the appearance of a factor or factors in dialysate, following SB immunization, which prevented microbial growth thereby reducing *S. aureus* peritonitis. The results of this study showed that *S. aureus* was able to multiply equally as well in spent overnight dialysate from both placebo patients and patients immunised with SB. Although only one strain of *S. aureus* was tested, the efficacy of a vaccine for prevention of peritonitis would be strongly dependent on the vaccine conferring protection against a broad spectrum of staphylococcal strains. These observations are consistent with peritoneal dilution of protective immunological mechanism.

The hypothesis that staphylococcal vaccines are unable to elicit a sufficiently appropriate immunological response is also a likely contributing factor to the lack of efficacy seen in this study. The virulence factors of *S. aureus* are numerous and their pathogenic mechanisms are not fully understood [Mathews 1970]. The organisms possess hemolysins (α-hemolysin being the best characterised), coagulase, lipase, leukocidin, enterotoxin, exfoliatin and protein A [Mathews 1970]. In addition, encapsulated strains have been shown experimentally to be most susceptible to immunization stimulated capsular antibody-initiated phagocytosis [Cohen 1984]. This has also been suggested in studies using capsular Staphylococcal vaccines for prevention of mastitis in cows [Yoshida et al. 1984, Opdenbeeck and Norcross 1985]. Induction of protective antibodies against strains without capsules would appear, therefore, to be less successful. The many virulence factors of staphylococci are likely to influence the ability to produce a vaccine which will mimic the functional immunogens. Historically, vaccines against bacteria with few virulence factors or a small number of different serotypes have been shown to be most successful [Mathews 1970].

Prevention of staphylococcal infection is unlikely to be achieved using vaccination with toxoids or whole killed bacteria. Even in the event of production of a successful vaccine based on capsular antigens, unencapsulated staphylococcal strains could still cause infection. Strategies which rely on prevention of microbial invasion, as opposed to augmenting the immune system, would appear to be the approach preferred for prevention of infection in CAPD patients.

Conclusions

Vaccination with SB did not reduce the incidence of peritonitis, catheter related infection or *S. aureus* nasal carriage. These observations are most likely a result of an inappropriate response to the vaccine and/or deficient immune mechanisms. Vaccination with SB elicited a significant increase in the level of serum anti-α hemolysin throughout the 12 month duration of the study. However, the level of increase in serum anti-α hemolysin elicited by SB was unrelated to the subsequent rate of peritonitis. Vaccination with SB also elicited a significant increase in the dialysate level of specific antibodies against *S. aureus* but not *S. epidermidis*. The serum levels of IgG, IgA, complement C3 and C4 were within the normal range in all CAPD patients and remained unaffected by vaccination. In addition, dialysate levels of IgG, IgA, IgM, complement C3 and C4 were 50–100 times lower than corresponding serum levels and remained unaffected by vaccination. In short, vaccination with a whole killed staphylococci preparation to prevent staphylococcal related peritonitis and catheter related infection in CAPD was found to be ineffective in a prospective multi-centre clinical trial conducted over 2 years.

Acknowledgement

Funding for this project was provided by the Baxter Healthcare Corporation, Deerfield Ill.

REFERENCES

Armitage P, Berry G 1987 Statistical methods in medical research. 2nd Ed. Blackwell Scientific Publications, Oxford

Chan MK 1988 Intraperitoneal gammaglobulin as an adjunct in the treatment of high risk patients with peritonitis. Perit Dial Int *8:* 287

Chan MK, Baillod RA, Varghese Z, Sweeny P, Moorhead JF 1983 Immunoglobulins and complement components (C3, C4) in CAPD and haemodialysis patients. Dial Transplant *12:* 777–778

Churchill DN, Taylor DW, Vas SI, Singer J, Beecroft ML, Wu G, Manuel A, Paton T, Walker S, Smith EKM, Oreopoulos DG 1988 Peritonitis in continuous ambulatory peritoneal dialysate (CAPD) patients: A randomised prospective clinical trial of Cotrimoxazole prophylaxis. Perit Dial Int *8:* 125–128

Cohen SN 1984. Immunization. In: Basic and Clinical Immunology. 5th Ed. *Stites DP, Stobo JD, Fudenberg HH, Wells JV* (eds). Lange Medical Publications, Los Altos. pp 728–743

Cox DR 1972 Regression models and life tables. J R Stat Soc B *34:* 187

Duwe AK, Vas SI, Weatherhead JW 1981 Effects of composition of peritoneal dialysis fluid on chemiluminescence, phagocytosis and bactericidal activity *in vitro*. Infect Immun *33:* 130–135

Everett ED, Bodem CR 1984 Catheter and shunt infections in dialysis patients. In: Infections associated with prosthetic devices. *Sugarmen B, Young EJ* (eds.) CRC Pres Inc Boca Raton, Florida. p 165

Keane WF, Compty CM, Verbrugh HA, Peterson PK 1984 Opsonic deficiency of peritoneal dialysis effluent in continuous ambulatory peritoneal dialysis. Kidney Int *25:* 539–543

Khan RH, Klein M, Vas SI 1987 Fibronectin in the normal peritoneal fluids of patients on chronic ambulatory peritoneal dialysis (CAPD) and during peritonitis. Perit Dial Int *7:* 69–73

Lamperi S, Carozzi S 1986 Defective opsonic activity of peritoneal effluent during continuous ambulatory peritoneal dialysis (CAPD): importance and prevention. Perit Dial Bull *6:* 87–92

Lamperi S, Carozzi S 1989 Immunological defenses in CAPD. Current concepts of CAPD. Blood Purif. *7:* 126–143.

Lamperi S, Carozzi S, Grazia Nasini M 1986 Peritoneal membrane defense machanism in CAPD. In: Immune and Metabolic Aspects of Therapeutic Blood Purification Systems. *Smeby LC, Jorstad S, Wideroe TE* (eds). Karger, Basel. pp 112–116

Low DE, Vas SI, Oreopoulos DG 1980 Prophylactic cephalexin ineffective in chronic ambulatory peritoneal dialysis. Lancet *II:* 753–754

Maiorca R, Cantaluppi A, Cancorini GC, Scalamogna A, Broccoli R, Grazianig, Brasa S, Poticelli C 1983 Prospective controlled trial of a Y-connector and disinfectant to prevent peritonitis in continuous ambulatory peritoneal dialysis. Lancet *ii:* 642–644

Mathews JD 1970 New aspects of immunology. In: Modern Medicine of Australia. The journal of diagnosis and treatment. Modern Medicine Publications, Australia. pp 6–15

National CAPD Registry of the National Institutes of Health: Patient characteristics, selected outcome measures and special topics for the period January 1, 1981 through January 31, 1988. Clinical Coordinating Centre: University of Missouri, Columbia and Data Coordinating Centre: The Emmes Corporation, 1988

Opdenbeeck JP, Norcross NL 1985 Antibodies in bovine serum and lacteal secretions to capsular antigens in *Staphylococcus aureus.* Am J Vet Res *46:* 1561–1564

Rubin J, Lin LM, Lewis R, Cruse J, Bower JD 1983 Host defense mechanisms in continuous ambulatory peritoneal dialysis. Clin Nephrol *20:* 140–144

Scatizzi A, Strippoli P 1986 Prevention of *Staphylococcus aureus* peritonitis in continuous ambulatory peritoneal dialysis. In: Immune and Metabolic Aspects of Therapeutic Blood Purification Systems. *Smeby LC, Jorstad S, Wideroe TE* (eds). Karger, Basel. pp 191–196

Vas SI 1985 Peritonitis. In *Nolph KD* (ed) Peritoneal Dialysis, 2nd ed. Martinus Nijhoff Publishers, Boston, pp 403–439

Verbrugh HA, Keane WF, Hoidal RJ, Freiberg MR, Eliott GR, Peterson PK 1983 Peritoneal macrophages and opsonins: antibacterial defense in patients undergoing peritoneal dialysis. J Infect Dis *147:* 1018–1029

West TE, Walshe JJ, Krol CP, Amsterdam D 1986 Staphylococcal peritonitis in patients on continuous ambulatory peritoneal dialysis. J Clin Micro *23 (5):* 809–812

Yoshida K, Ichiman Y, Narikawa S, Evans B 1984 Staphylococcal capsular vaccine for preventing bovine mastitis in two herds in Georgia. J Dairy Sci *67:* 620–627

Clinical Nephrology, Vol. 35 No. 5 – 1991 (207–212)

Correction of anemia in patients on continuous ambulatory peritoneal dialysis with subcutaneous recombinant erythropoietin twice a week: a long-term study

I. K. P. Cheng[1, 3], C. Cy[3], M. K. Chan[1, 3], L. Yu[1], G. X. Fang[1] and D. Wei[2]

Department of Medicine[1] and Pathology[2], University of Hong Kong, Queen Mary Hospital and Renal Unit[3], Tung Wah Hospital, Hong Kong

Abstract. Subcutaneous recombinant human erythropoietin (rHuEPO) was given for 12 months twice weekly to 10 patients on continuous ambulatory peritoneal dialysis (CAPD) with anemia (hemoglobin <9.0 mg/dl). All patients responded to a median weekly dose of between 37.5 to 100 (mean 55 to 105) units/kg and reached a target hemoglobin of 10–12 mg/dl in a mean of 11.7 weeks (range 5–24). Serum iron, iron saturation and ferritin were significantly lower and serum potassium was significantly higher than the pre-treatment level from 1 month onwards. Five patients without pre-treatment iron overload required oral iron supplement and 3 required oral potassium-binding resin. No significant change in other serum biochemical parameters was observed. Blood pressure remained stable during the treatment period but additional or increased dosage of antihypertensive drugs was required in 5 patients. Peritoneal small solute clearance and ultrafiltration and residual renal clearance did not change significantly after correction of anemia. The incidence of peritonitis and exit site infection was similarly unaffected. One patient developed a severe headache which was not associated with hypertension and responded to withdrawal of rHuEPO treatment. Most of the remaining patients showed improvement in subjective well-being. It was concluded that the subcutaneous route twice a week is a safe, convenient and cost-effective way to administer rHuEPO to patients on CAPD.

Key words: recombinant erythropoietin – continuous ambulatory peritoneal dialysis – anemia

Introduction

Intravenous recombinant human erythropoietin (rHuEPO) has been used successfully in the treatment of anemia in patients with advanced renal failure [Eschbach et al. 1989, Lim et al. 1989a] and in those on chronic hemodialysis [Winearls et al. 1986, Eschbach et al. 1987, Casati et al. 1987]. Pharmacokinetic studies have shown that the bioavailability of rHuEPO given by the subcutaneous route is superior to the intraperitoneal route and is about 20% of the intravenous route [MacDougal et al. 1989a, Boelaert et al. 1989]. Compared to the latter, the subcutaneous route produces a more sustained plasma level. Short-term studies have shown that subcutaneous rHuEPO is effective in correcting anemia in patients on hemodialysis and peritoneal dialysis [Bommer et al. 1989, Sinai-Trieman, Salusky and Fine 1989, Liu et al. 1990, Hughes et al. 1990, Zehnder and Blumberg 1990]. Therefore the subcutaneous route of administration should be a cost-effective means of treating anemia in patients with end-stage renal failure on continuous ambulatory peritoneal dialysis (CAPD) and this will be more convenient than the intravenous route because it will allow them to administer rHuEPO at home and alleviate the need for repeated venepunctures. Herein we report our twelve months experience of the use of subcutaneous rHuEPO in the treatment of anemia in 10 patients on CAPD.

Patients and methods

Patients between 15 to 75 years of age whose hemoglobins were less than 9 mg/dl and who were on CAPD for not less than 6 months were eligible for the

---

Received May 23, 1990; in revised form January 2, 1991.

Reprint requests to Dr. Ignatius K. P. Cheng, Department of Medicine, University of Hong Kong, Queen Mary Hospital, Pokfulam, Hong Kong.

Table 1 Demographic and clinical parameters in CAPD patients treated with rHuEPO

	Mean ± SD	Range
Age (yrs)	27 ± 11.6	16–57
Male : female ratio	4 : 6	
Duration on CAPD (months)	36.3 ± 19.0	10–69
Previous transfusion (units/year)	4.9 ± 3.3	1–12
Underlying renal diseases		
Chronic glomerulonephritis	7	
Obstructive uropathy	1	
Polycystic kidney disease	1	
Unknown	1	

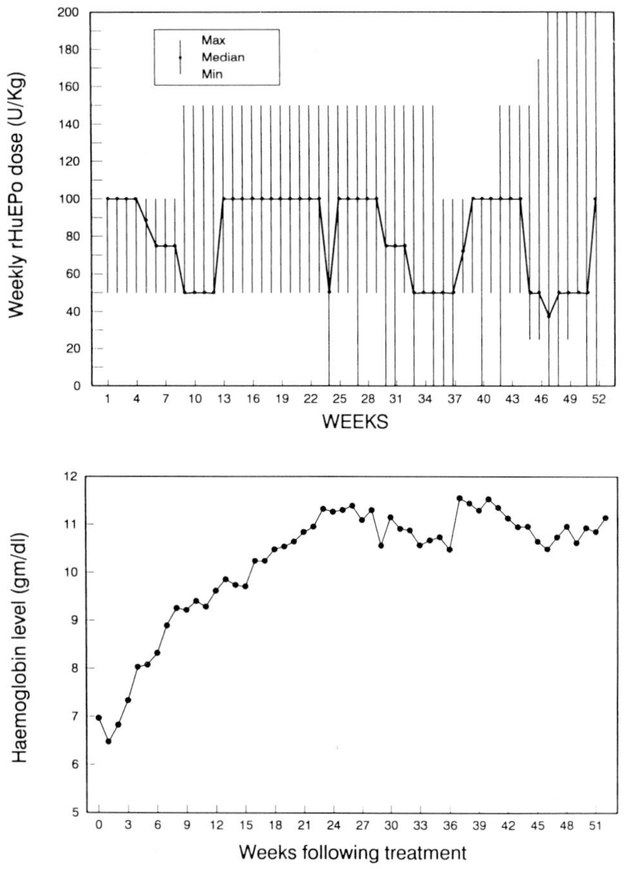

Fig. 1 Serial median rHuEPO dosage (upper panel) and mean hemoglobin level (lower panel) in patients receiving rHuEPO

study. All patients who were entered into the study gave informed consent. Exclusion criteria included the following:

1. Anemia from causes other than chronic renal failure
2. Serum ferritin <100 ng/ml
3. B_{12} and folic acid deficiency
4. Uncontrolled hypertension (diastolic blood pressure >90 mmHg)
5. Drug and alcohol abuse
6. Abnormal liver function test
7. Previous rHuEPO or androgen therapy

After establishing that the patients had a stable hemoglobin over a 3-week period, rHuEPO was given subcutaneously twice a week in the forearm. Injections were given in the hospital by the nursing staff. The starting dose was 25 U/kg if the baseline hemoglobin was equal to or exceeded 8.0 mg/dl and 50 U/kg if it was lower. Dose adjustment was made by a stepwise increase or decrease of 25 U/kg every 4 weeks in the initial 8 weeks of treatment to achieve a target hemoglobin level of between 10–12 mg/dl.

Hemoglobin (Hb) and hematocrit (Hct) were measured weekly after treatment. Red blood cell count, mean corpuscular hemoglobin concentration (MCHC) and mean corpuscular volume (MCV), reticulocyte count, white blood cell and differential count and platelet count were measured just prior to treatment and weekly thereafter. Serum sodium, potassium, calcium, phosphate, albumin, creatinine, bilirubin, aspartate and alanine transaminases, alkaline phosphatase, iron, total iron binding capacity and ferritin were measured at baseline for 4 weeks using routine laboratory techniques. The reticulocyte index was calculated using the following formula:

Reticulocyte count (%) × (patient's Hct/normal Hct).

All patients performed CAPD using standard spike technique and had 3 daily exchanges of 2-liter 1.5% to 4.25% Dianeal solution (Baxter). Residual renal function was measured using endogenous creatinine clearance at baseline and every 3 months. Peritoneal ultrafiltration rate and clearance of urea and creatinine were measured after a period of 4 hours of 1.5% and 4.25% Dianeal solution at baseline and at 9 months. Routine medications were continued and the dose of antihypertensive drugs were adjusted to maintain the diastolic blood pressure <90 mmHg. Oral iron supplement was given if the serum ferritin fell below 200 ng/ml or was showing a rapid downward trend.

Statistical analysis was done using the Statistical Package for Social Sciences. Difference between post-treatment value and baseline and between groups was analyzed respectively by the paired and pooled Student's t-test. Correlation analysis was performed by the least square method. P <0.05 was considered as significant.

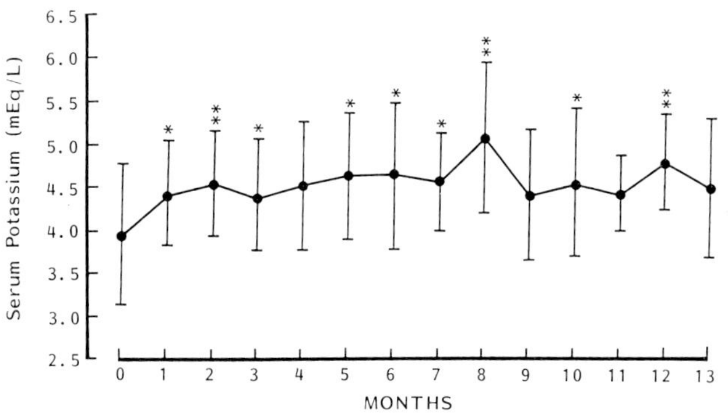

Fig. 2 Serial serum potassium level in patients receiving rHuEPO. *p <0.05, **p <0.001 versus level at 0 time

Results

The demographic and baseline clinical parameters of the study patients were shown in Table 1. No patient had a previous renal transplant. None had previous nephrectomy. All were free of hepatitis B antigenemia.

All patients responded to subcutaneous rHuEPO injections (Figure 1). Hemoglobin level and hematocrit were significantly higher than baseline 4, 3 weeks respectively following treatment. However, the time required to achieve a target hemoglobin level of 10 mg/dl ranged from 5 to 24 weeks (mean 11.7). This weakly correlated inversely with the pre-treatment serum iron ($r = -0.368$, $p = 0.296$) and iron saturation ($r = -0.393$, $p = 0.261$) but not with serum ferritin level. A significantly elevated reticulocyte index was observed from the first month onwards (data not shown). No significant change in the white cell counts was observed but platelet count increased slightly, but transiently during the first 2 months of treatment (273 ± 51 and 280 ± 68 versus 229 ± 36 × 10^9/l at baseline, $p <0.05$). The serial median weekly rHuEPO dosages were shown at the top of Figure 1 and ranged from 37.5 to 100 (mean 55 to 105) units/kg. The highest dosage used was 200 units/kg and was required in only 1 patient for 6 weeks.

No significant change in body weight, serum urea, creatinine, calcium, phosphate, albumin and liver enzymes was observed following treatment. Serum potassium increased significantly from 1 month onwards (Figure 2). Three patients required oral resonium C for 2–4 days for control of severe hyperkalemia (5.9–6.4 mmol/l). None of them received such treatment prior to rHuEPO therapy. Potassium restricted diet was prescribed to all 3 patients with normalization of serum potassium level in 2, but in the remaining patient a further course of resonium was needed for treating a recurrent episode of hyperkalemia. Serum iron, iron saturation and ferritin decreased significantly from 1, 1 and 2 months onwards and in the case of serum ferritin, there was a progressive downward trend due mainly to the progressive reduction in patients with initially high levels (Figure 3). Five patients required oral iron supplement because their serum ferritin level fell below 200 ng/ml and the level was restored to >200 ng/ml in all over a mean period of 1.8 (range 1–4) months. Systolic and diastolic blood pressure did not change significantly following treatment (129 ± 34 and 79 ± 20 mmHg at baseline versus 112 ± 11 and 71 ± 11 mmHg at the end of the study). Increase in the dosage or the addition of antihypertensive drugs were required in 2 and 3 patients respectively between 12–16 weeks after rHuEPO treatment when the

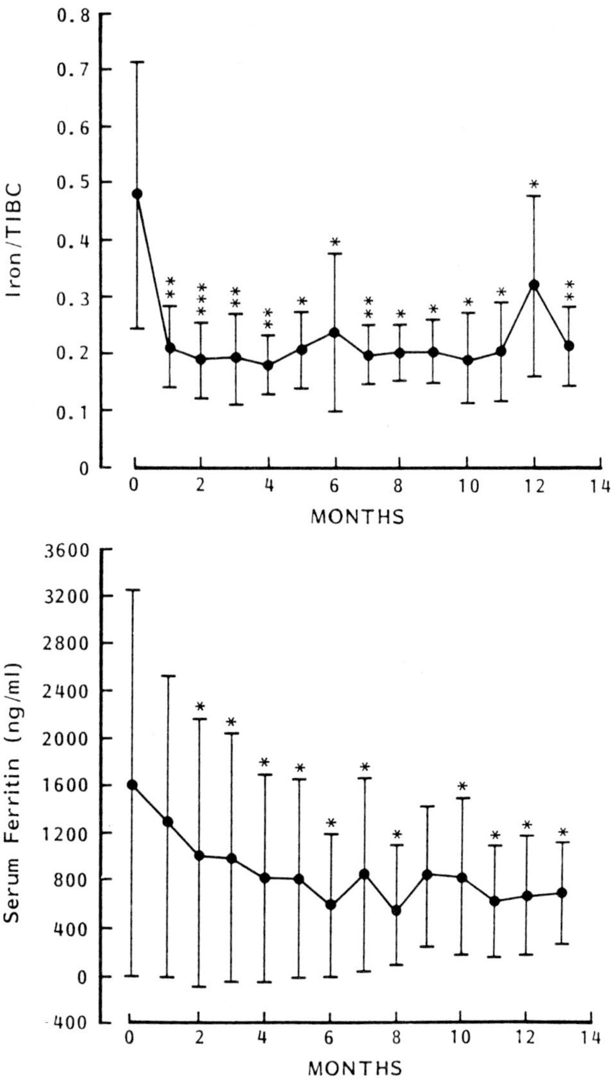

Fig. 3 Serial serum iron status in patients receiving rHuEPO. *p <0.05, **p <0.005, ***p <0.0001 versus level at 0 time

Table 2 Peritoneal clearance of urea and creatinine and ultrafiltration rate before and 9 months after rHuEPO therapy

		Before	After
Peritoneal clearance (ml/min)			
Urea	1.5%	7.7 ± 1.5	8.8 ± 0.8
	4.25%	10.7 ± 1.9	11.5 ± 1.5
Creatinine	1.5%	7.2 ± 2.1	6.9 ± 0.9
	4.25%	8.6 ± 1.9	9.0 ± 1.5
Ultrafiltration rate (ml/min)			
	1.5%	0.46 ± 0.62	0.54 ± 0.52
	4.25%	3.5 ± 0.7	3.8 ± 0.5

hemoglobin level reached the target range. The additional antihypertensive drugs required for control of blood pressure included nifedipine and nadolol in 2 patients and captopril and prazocin in the remaining patient. Reduction of dosage or cessation of antihypertensive drugs was possible in 2 patients generally from 20 weeks onwards when the hemoglobin level had already plateaued. The dosage of antihypertensive drugs was unchanged in one patient. There was no difference in the age, sex ratio, pre-treatment number of antihypertensive drugs and time to achieve target hemoglobin between those who required more antihypertensives and those who did not.

Only 3 patients have urine output and in these, there was slight reduction in residual renal clearance at the end of 12 months which was not significantly different from baseline levels (0.88 + 0.36 versus 1.53 + 1.45 ml/min). There was no significant change in the ultrafiltration rate and in the peritoneal clearance of urea and creatinine following treatment (Table 2). Peritonitis rate during the 12-month treatment period was 1/15 patient-months compared to 1/20 in the 12-month pre-treatment period. The overall peritonitis rate in our CAPD population in the same period was 1/17.2 patient-months. Four patients developed 3 exit site and 2 tunnel infections during the treatment period. In the 12-month pre-treatment period, 5 exit site infections were observed in 4 patients. One patient with severe tunnel infection required catheter removal and re-insertion. Two patients had a reduction in hemoglobin level and an increase in the requirement of rHuEPO during an episode of tunnel infection or peritonitis and they had a lower pre-treatment serum ferritin level than the 5 patients who did not have such experience (152, 547 versus 486–4410 ng/ml). When measurement coincided with an episode of peritonitis, a transient decrease in serum iron and a marked increase in serum ferritin level was observed.

One patient developed persistent headaches 10 months after treatment. At the time his hemoglobin overshot the upper limit of the target range of 12 mg/dl. Temporary stoppage of rHuEPO for 2 weeks with the hemoglobin level dropping back to 10 mg/dl did not result in improvement. Extensive investigations including CT scan of brain and lumbar puncture failed to reveal any abnormal findings. Blood pressure remained well-controlled during the treatment period. rHuEPO was stopped at 12 months. His headache slowly improved over the next 4 weeks. No other side effects attributable to rHuEPO were observed. Subjective improvement in appetite, physical energy, feeling of warmth and general well-being were reported by 20%, 50%, 60% and 80% of patients with only 1 patient reporting a worsening of appetite and physical energy after rHuEPO treatment. Nine patients elected to continue treatment but only 7 could afford to pay for the injections.

Discussion

The present study shows that rHuEPO given subcutaneously twice a week is effective in correcting anemia in patients with end-stage renal failure on CAPD. The mean weekly dose required to achieve and maintain a hemoglobin of between 10–12 mg/dl was around 105 units per week which was substantially lower than that reported using the intravenous route [Casati et al. 1987]. This confirms the preliminary data of Bommer et al. [1988] and the data from recently published short-term studies [Sinai-Trieman, Salusky and Fine 1989, Liu et al. 1990, Hughes et al. 1990, Zehnder and Blumberg 1990] and suggests that lower and more sustained blood level achieved by the subcutaneous route is not only more physiological and provides a more convenient way to administer rHuEPO especially in patients on CAPD or not yet on dialysis but is also more economical. Our study also shows that prior priming of the erythroid precursors with a high intravenous dose of rHuEPO is not required for a low maintenance subcutaneous dose as suggested previously [Lim et al. 1989b] because the mean weekly subcutaneous dose needed to achieve and to maintain a target hemoglobin in our patients was similar.

No treatment failure was observed among our patients but the time to achieve a target hemoglobin level may take up to 24 weeks. The delay in response is most likely secondary to suboptimal delivery of iron to the erythroid precursors because the time to achieve a target hemoglobin tended to correlate inversely with the pre-treatment serum iron and iron saturation. This occurs despite all the pre-treatment serum iron parameters falling within the normal range. Recently, MacDougall et al. [1989b] reported 5 patients with normal serum ferritin level and iron saturation of <20% who initially had a poor response to intravenous rHuEPO but responded well after the iron saturation was increased to >20% by intravenous iron therapy. It is therefore quite likely that an approach using serum iron saturation instead of serum ferritin as an index of adequate functional iron store would further improve the response to subcutaneous rHuEPO in our patients.

Hypertension and hypertensive encephalopathy has been reported in patients on hemodialysis receiving intravenous rHuEPO [Winearls et al. 1986, Eschbach et al. 1987]. This was not observed in our patients but increased dosage and the addition of antihypertensive drugs were required in 50% of patients to maintain the blood pressure under control. The severity of pre-existing hypertension and the rapidity of hemoglobin response did not predict those patients who would develop more severe hypertension requiring an increase in antihypertensive drugs following treatment, a finding also confirmed in hemodialysis patients receiving the equivalent dose of intravenous rHuEPO [Levin 1989].

Severe hyperkalemia has been observed in hemodialysis patients receiving rHuEPO and has been attributed to increase in appetite and enhanced release of potassium into the plasma from a greater number of red cells hemolyzed daily [Eschbach et al. 1987, Casati et al. 1987]. Although the control of serum potassium is usually better in patients on CAPD than on hemodialysis, we have observed a significant rise in serum potassium level after rHuEPO treatment.

Recent studies have shown that correction of anemia may affect solute clearances and require adjustment of dialysis prescription in patients on hemodialysis [Paganni et al. 1989]. A preliminary short-term study in CAPD patients has shown that ultrafiltration rate increased while solute clearance remained unchanged after correction of anemia with rHuEPO [Steinhauer et al. 1989]. As we did not measure these parameters serially, we could not exclude the possibility that similar changes may have occurred in our patients during the first few months of treatment. However, the absence of significant alteration of these parameters at 9 months post-treatment suggests that if increased ultrafiltration does occur, it is not sustained. In 3 patients with residual urine output, the residual renal clearance did not change significantly after correction of anemia. This finding is similar to that in pre-dialysis patients [Eschbach et al. 1989, Lim et al. 1989b] but at variance with the observation in rats with 5/6 nephrectomy [Garcia et al. 1989]. These preliminary data therefore suggests that the relative advantage of preservation of residual renal clearance in patients on CAPD versus hemodialysis [Rottenbourg et al. 1982] is likely to be retained following correction of anemia with rHuEPO.

The rate of peritonitis among our study patients was not different from that before treatment was started and was comparable to that of our overall population. Similarly, there was no increase in the incidence of exit site or tunnel infection following treatment with rHuEPO. Peritonitis and tunnel infection were shown to reduce the erythrocyte response to rHuEPO mainly in patients with lower pre-treatment body iron stores. Therefore, early adequate iron supplement e.g. in the form of parental iron may ensure adequate erythrocytic response even during an episode of systemic infection. Since peritonitis was associated with a transient decrease in serum iron and a marked increase in serum ferritin level, caution must be exercized in the interpretation of this serum parameter during an episode of peritonitis or tunnel infection.

Subcutaneous rHuEPO is well tolerated in our patients. "Flu" like symptoms which have previously been described during intravenous therapy [Winearls et al. 1986, Casati et al. 1987] were not reported in our patients and local reaction to the subcutaneous injection was minimal. The development of a severe headache in one patient was intriguing but appeared to be related to rHuEPO therapy as no medical cause of his headache could be found after extensive investigations and it resolved after cessation of treatment.

In summary, the subcutaneous route twice a week is a convenient, economical, safe and effective way to administer rHuEPO to patients on CAPD. Although alteration of dialysis prescription is not necessary, as in hemodialysis patients, careful monitoring of blood pressure, serum potassium and iron status and attention to dietary restriction is still needed.

Acknowledgement

The authors wish to thank Mrs. Jenny Watt for secretarial help and the nurses in the Renal Unit, Tung Wah Hospital for caring for the patients involved in this study. This study was supported by a grant from Cilag Research who also provided the recombinant erythropoietin.

REFERENCES

Boelaert JR, Schurgers ML, Matthys EF et al 1989 Comparative pharmacokinetics of recombinant erythropoietin administered by the intravenous, subcutaneous, and intraperitoneal routes in continuous ambulatory peritoneal dialysis (CAPD) patients. Perit Dial Int *9:* 95–98

Bommer J, Ritz E, Weinreich TH et al 1988 Subcutaneous erythropoietin (letter). Lancet *ii:* 406

Casati S, Passerini P, Campise MR et al 1987 Benefits and risks of protracted treatment with human recombinant erythropoietin in patients having hemodialysis. Brit Med J *295:* 1017–1020

Eschbach JW, Michael RK, Haley NR et al 1989 Treatment of the anemia of progressive renal failure with recombinant human erythropoietin. N Eng J Med Vol *321:* 158–163

Eschbach JW, Egrie JC, Downing R et al 1987 Correction of the anemia of end-stage renal disease with recombinant human erythropoietin. N Eng J Med *316:* 73–78

Garcia DL, Anderson S, Rennke HG et al 1988 Anemia lessens and its prevention with recombinant human erythropoietin worsens glomerular injury and hypertension in rats with reduced renal mass. Proc Natl Acad Sci *85:* 6142–6146

Hughes RT, Cotes PM, Pippard MJ et al 1990 Subcutaneous administration of recombinant human erythropoietin to subjects on continuous ambulatory peritoneal dialysis: an erythrokinetic assessment. Brit J Hematol *75:* 268–273

Levin N 1989 Management of blood pressure changes during recombinant human erythropoietin therapy. Semin Nephrol *9 (Suppl 2):* 16–20

Lim VS, DeGowin RL, Zavala D et al 1989a Recombinant human erythropoietin treatment in pre-dialysis patients. Ann Int Med *110:* 108–114

Lim VS, Kirchner PT, Fangman J et al 1989b The safety and the efficacy of maintenance therapy of recombinant human erythropoietin in patients with renal insufficiency. Am J Kid Dis *14:* 496–506

Liu SF, Chung WWM, Leung CB et al 1990 Pharmacokinetics and pharmacodynamics of subcutaneous and intraperitoneal administration of recombinant human erythropoietin in patients on continuous ambulatory peritoneal dialysis. Clin Nephrol *33:* 47–51

MacDougall IC, Roberts DE, Neubert P et al 1989a Pharmacokinetics of recombinant human erythropoietin in patients on continuous ambulatory peritoneal dialysis. Lancet *I:* 425–427

MacDougall IC, Hutton RD, Cavill I et al 1989b Poor response to treatment of renal anemia with erythropoietin corrected by iron given intravenously. Brit Med J *299:* 157–158

Paganini EP, Latham D, Abdulhadi M 1989 Practical considerations of recombinant human erythropoietin therapy. Am J Kid Dis *14 (Suppl 1):* 19–25

Rottenbourg J, Issad B, Degoulet P et al 1982 Evolution of residual renal function in patients undergoing maintenance hemodialysis or continuous ambulatory peritoneal dialysis. Proc EDTA *19:* 397–403

Sinai-Trieman L, Salusky IB, Fine RN 1990 Use of subcutaneous recombinant human erythropoietin in children undergoing continuous cycling peritoneal dialysis. J Pediatr *114:* 550–554

Steinhauer HB, Lubrich-Birkner I, Dreyling KW, Schollmeyer P 1989 Increased ultrafiltration after erythropoietin-induced correction of renal anemia in patients on continuous ambulatory peritoneal dialysis. Nephron *53:* 91–92

Winearls CG, Oliver DO, Pippard MJ et al 1986 Effect of human erythropoietin derived from recombinant DNA on the anemia of patients maintained by chronic hemodialysis. Lancet *II:* 1175–1178

Zehnder C, Blumberg A 1990 Behandlung der Anämie von Hämodialysepatienten mit rekombinantem humanem Erythropoietin: Vergleich zwischen intravenöser und subkutaner Verabreichung. Schweiz Med Wochenschr *120:* 217–220

Clinical Nephrology, Vol. 35 No. 5 – 1991 (213–217)

Removal of trace metals by continuous ambulatory peritoneal dialysis after desferrioxamine B chelation therapy

J. A. Navarro[1], V. A. Granadillo[1], B. Rodríguez-Iturbe[2], R. García[2], O. Salgado[2] and R. A. Romero[1]

[1]Analytical Instrumentation Laboratory, Faculty of Sciences, Universidad del Zulia and [2]Renal Service and Laboratory, Hospital Universitario, Maracaibo, Venezuela

Abstract. We studied the removal of aluminum (Al), iron (Fe), copper (Cu), lead (Pb) and zinc (Zn) with continuous ambulatory peritoneal dialysis, before and after desferrioxamine B (DFO) administration (2 g intravenously) in two patients with chronic renal failure and Al-related osteopathy. Both patients had 4 peritoneal dialysis exchanges (2 liters each) per day. Blood concentrations of Al increased 413% (patient A) and 190% (patient B) after DFO. Patient B had a 15% increase in Fe; other metals remained unchanged. Dialysate efflux Al concentrations had peak post-DFO increments of 761% and 840% in patients 1 and 2, respectively. Peak post-DFO increments in Fe dialysate concentration were 342% and 89.5% in the respective patients. Dialysate/plasma (D/P) concentration ratios of Al increased from pre-DFO levels (mean ± SEM) of 0.370 ± 0.048 to 0.523 ± 0.061 after DFO; similarly, Fe D/P ratios increased from 0.259 ± 0.053 to 0.446 ± 0.075 with DFO therapy. These results indicate an increase in the ultrafiltrable proportion of Al and Fe in plasma after DFO administration. During 3 days after DFO, patient 1 had a total removal of Al and Fe of 2.9 mg and 4.9 mg, respectively. Metal removal in patient 2 was 7.6 mg of Al and 2.7 mg of Fe. Peritoneal extraction of other trace metals was minor.

Key words: aluminum – copper – iron – lead – zinc – metal removal – desferrioxamine B – CAPD

Introduction

Trace metal levels in blood and tissues of uremic patients have been extensively studied in the last few years. The chelating agent desferrioxamine B (DFO) was initially intended for the management of iron overload; however, since the report of Ackrill et al. [1980], it has been widely used to treat Al-induced dialysis encephalopathy [Winterberg et al. 1984, Navarro et al. 1988a], osteodystrophy [Milliner et al. 1984, Malluche et al. 1984, Ott et al. 1986], and microcytic anemia [Altmann et al. 1988] in patients with chronic renal failure.

The removal of the Al-DFO complex via hemodialysis requires a favorable plasma/dialysis bath concentration gradient and reverse osmosis treatment of dialysis water is necessary to assure its low metal content; unfortunately, water treatment systems are expensive and not universally available in dialysis units in third world countries. Continuous ambulatory peritoneal dialysis (CAPD) is a reasonable alternative because of the low content of trace metals in the CAPD dialysate but relatively few reports [Andreoli et al. 1985, Hercz et al. 1986, Molitoris et al. 1987, Passlick et al. 1989] have studied DFO-mobilized Al removal by this route, and little information exists on the concomitant removal of other trace metals.

In this work we evaluate the effectiveness of CAPD in the removal of aluminum (Al), copper (Cu), zinc (Zn), lead (Pb) and iron (Fe) in two patients with chronic renal failure that received intravenous DFO.

Patients and methods

Patients

Patient 1: A 36-year-old female patient with chronic renal failure (CRF) had been undergoing periodical hemodialysis treatment for 2 years. During that time, she was dialyzed with untreated tap water containing (mean ± SEM) 847 ± 89 µg Al/l [Navarro et al. 1988c] and urine output was less than 100 ml/day. Whole blood Al concentration varied consider-

Received February 27, 1990; in revised form November 23, 1990.

Reprint requests to Prof. Dr. R. A. Romero, Apartado postal 1430, Maracaibo 4001-A, Venezuela.

Table 1 Blood metal concentrations before and after DFO chelation therapy

	Pre-DFO	Post-DFO* 24 h	48 h	72 h	Mean post-DFO increment (%)
Patient 1					
Al (µg/l)	46 ± 4	224	312	172	413
Fe (mg/l)	225 ± 2	239	198	198	–6
Pb (µg/l)	105 ± 1	155	187	178	65
Cu (µg/l)	866 ± 4	883	840	840	–1
Zn (mg/l)	4.87 ± 0.05	4.83	4.07	4.00	–12
Patient 2					
Al (µg/l)	152 ± 4	486	440	398	190
Fe (mg/l)	286 ± 1	342	325	322	15
Pb (µg/l)	213 ± 1	235	224	231	8
Cu (µg/l)	750 ± 2	800	800	967	14
Zn (mg/l)	6.87 ± 0.04	7.60	8.47	5.80	6

* After 2 g of desferrioxamine B (Desferal®, Ciba-Geigy) given intravenously.

ably but reached as high as 166 µg/l. After a test dose of DFO of 2 g intravenously [Milliner et al. 1984], whole blood Al had an increment of 379 µg Al/l. Bone biopsy showed histological findings of Al accumulation: heavy Al staining in a mixed osteopathy with an osteomalacic predominance. Bone Al content was 272 mg/kg.

Patient 2: A 30-year-old female patient had been on periodical hemodialysis treatment for 8 years. Tap water used in the bath preparation was untreated and contained 800 µg/l of Al. During the year prior to the studies, the patient had no urine output. The patient maintained whole blood Al concentrations above 280 µg/l, and increased after the infusion of 2 g of DFO, with a peak of 487 µg Al/l. The bone biopsy revealed Al content of 257 mg/kg and a histomorphometric finding of a mixed osteopathy with predominant osteomalacia.

Because reverse osmosis treatment for the tap water was not available, the patients were switched from hemodialysis to CAPD and received this treatment modality for 6 months (patient 1) and 12 months (patient 2) prior to the DFO studies. Just before the start of this investigation, they had mean hemoglobin and hematocrit values of 6.5 g/dl and 22% for patient 1, and 9.8 g/dl and 33% for patient 2.

Metal removal studies

Mobilization of trace metals during CAPD was evaluated as follows: each patient received intravenously 2 g of DFO (Desferal®, Ciba-Geigy), equivalent to 40 mg/kg of body weight, diluted in 200 ml of 5% dextrose solution, over a period of 2 h. Blood samples were collected before the DFO infusion and 24 hours, 48 hours, and 72 hours afterwards. CAPD dialysate (4 bags of 2 liters each, daily in each patient) used during this 3-day period were measured and analyzed before use and at the end of the peritoneal exchange period. Metal content of the unused peritoneal dialysis solution was as follows: Al <1 µg/l, Fe <0.8 µg/l, Pb <0.1 µg/l, Zn <0.2 µg/l, Cu <0.2 µg/l. Peritoneal exchanges were of a duration of 4 hours during the day (3 exchanges) and 8 hours in the night (1 exchange). The amount of metal removed attributable to DFO chelation in the CAPD exchange was calculated subtracting the pre-DFO values from those found afterwards. Since patients had virtually no urine output, urinary losses of metals were not considered.

Table 2 Dialysate metal concentrations before and after DFO chelation therapy

	Dialysate Metal Concentrations Al (µg/l)	Fe (µg/l)	Pb (µg/l)	Cu (µg/l)	Zn (µg/l)
Patient 1					
Pre-DFO	15.2 ± 13.1	59.6 ± 15.7	6.60 ± 1.91	26.8 ± 6.5	19.4 ± 1.57
24 h	107.0 ± 26.9*	263.8 ± 45.8*	7.75 ± 1.32	24.3 ± 3.9	17.3 ± 1.70
48 h	143.0 ± 21.8*	212.8 ± 36.7*	6.33 ± 2.85	24.0 ± 4.2	21.3 ± 2.29
72 h	106.0 ± 14.8*	110.8 ± 12.1*	8.75 ± 1.84	20.0 ± 4.0	17.0 ± 0.58
Patient 2					
Pre-DFO	41.0 ± 7.8	69.3 ± 2.8	9.00 ± 4.04	26.3 ± 3.3	27.3 ± 2.60
24 h	268.0 ± 68.4*	131.3 ± 31.7*	3.50 ± 0.29	27.0 ± 4.1	23.5 ± 1.19
48 h	353.0 ± 7.2*	124.0 ± 11.1*	8.00 ± 1.73	33.0 ± 5.4	21.5 ± 2.10
72 h	314.0 ± 14.9*	67.5 ± 8.9	6.00 ± 1.58	23.0 ± 2.1	16.5 ± 2.06

Values represent mean ± SEM of 4 determinations. * $p < 0.01$ vs pre-DFO levels.

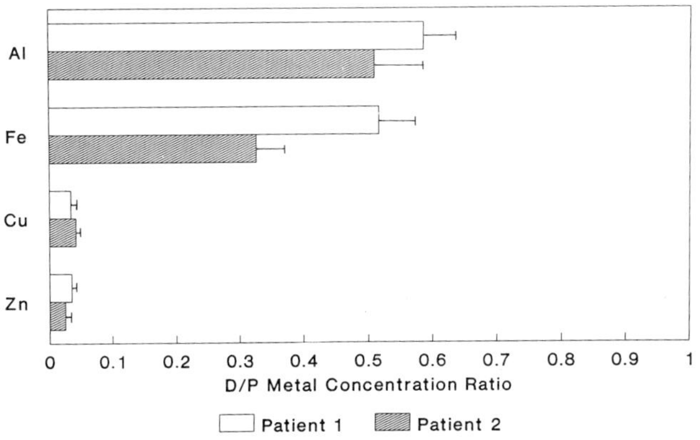

Fig. 1 Mean dialysate/plasma (D/P) metal concentration ratios after desferrioxamine B (DFO) administration. Values represent mean ± SEM of 12 peritoneal exchanges (4 exchanges per day × 3 days) in each patient.

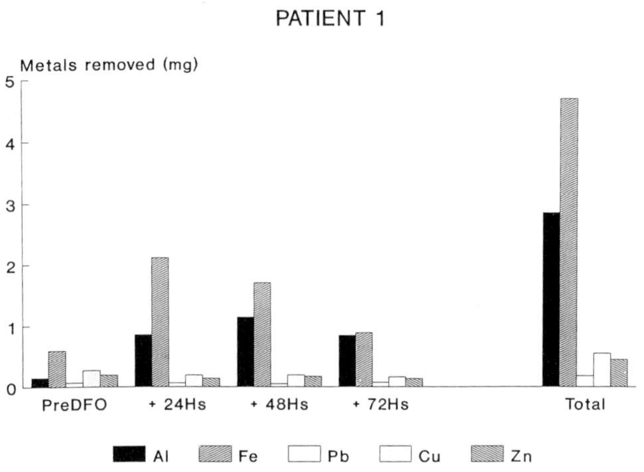

Fig. 3A

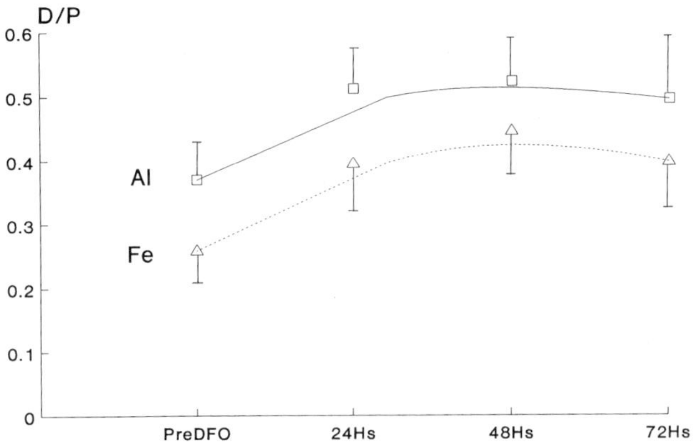

Fig. 2 Aluminum (Al) and iron (Fe) dialysate/plasma (D/P) concentration ratios before (pre-DFO) and 24, 48 and 72 hours after desferrioxamine B (DFO) administration. Each value represents mean ± SEM of 4 determinations in each patient (4 peritoneal exchanges at each time).

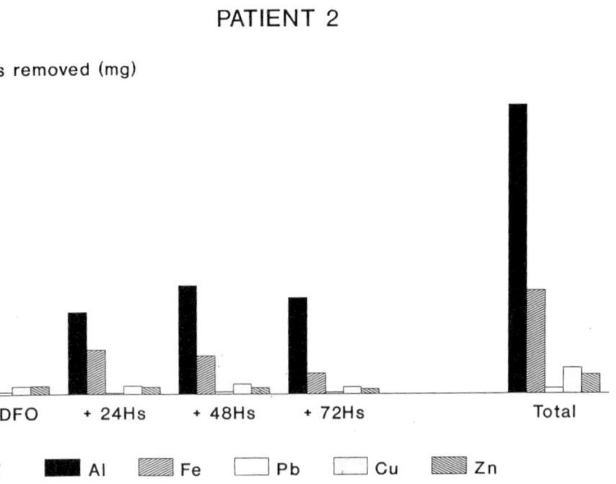

Fig. 3B

Fig. 3 Removal of aluminum (Al), iron (Fe), lead (Pb), copper (Cu) and zinc (Zn), before (pre-DFO) and 24, 48 and 72 hours after desferrioxamine B (DFO) therapy. The values shown as Total correspond to the cumulative removal obtained after DFO administration. Patients 1 (3A) and 2 (3B) are described in the text.

Aluminum, Cu, Fe, Zn and Pb in blood, plasma and CAPD solutions were determined by graphite furnace atomic absorption spectrometry following methodologies reported previously [Navarro et al. 1988b and 1989, Parra et al. 1988, Navarro and Romero 1988].

Dialysate to plasma (D/P) metal concentration ratios were calculated for all metals except for Pb which had undetectable plasma concentrations.

Statistical comparisons of data obtained sequentially after DFO chelation were done by repeated measurement analysis of variance ([Wallenstein et al. 1980]; significant F values were tested with Tukey's test with the help of a statistical commercial package (Statgraphics, STSC Inc., Rockville, Md); p values <0.05 were considered significant.

Results

As shown in Table 1, DFO administration induced in both patients increments in blood Al concentration representing 6.8 and 3.2 times the baseline pre-DFO levels; in addition, Fe levels increased in Patient 2. Other metals tested did not change significantly after DFO (Table 1).

Table 2 shows the dialysate metal concentrations before and after DFO chelation therapy in both patients. The pre-DFO values in Table 2 are those found in the outflow dialysate, representing the removal accomplished with CAPD before the DFO chelation. As shown, Al and Fe concentrations increased significantly after intravenous DFO administration while dialysate concentrations of Pb, Cu and Zn remained at pre-DFO levels.

Figure 1 shows the mean post-DFO D/P metal concentration ratios and Figure 2 shows that Al and Fe D/P ratios tend to increase gradually after intravenous DFO administration. The combined data in both patients indicated mean increases of 38% and 58% in the D/P ratios of Al and Fe, respectively, 1 to 3 days after DFO administration. Figure 3 shows the metal removal accomplished by 4 daily changes of 2 liters of peritoneal dialysate in the 72 hours following DFO treatment.

As shown, 2.9 mg and 7.6 mg of Al were removed in patients 1 and 2, respectively. Extraction of Fe with the peritoneal dialysis totaled 4.9 mg and 2.7 mg, in patients 1 and 2, respectively. Minor cumulative removal of Pb (circa 200 µg), Cu (circa 600–700 µg) and Zn (circa 400–500 µg) was observed during the study (Figure 3).

Discussion

The use of DFO to chelate Al for its extraction via hemodialysis or peritoneal dialysis is an accepted therapy of Al intoxication in renal failure. Yet little attention has been devoted to CAPD as a method of metal extraction and to the effects of DFO treatment on trace metal removal other than Al and Fe [Falk et al. 1983, Andreoli et al. 1985, Hercz et al. 1986, Taber et al. 1986, Molitoris et al. 1987].

Both patients kept very high blood Al while on hemodialysis (166 µg/l and >280 µg/l in patients 1 and 2, respectively) and after switching to CAPD, the blood Al decreased considerably: 46 µg/l and 152 µg/l (Table 1, pre-DFO data). This is expected when dialysate with low Al concentration is used [Ackrill et al. 1986].

Blood and plasma levels of Al increase after intravenous or intraperitoneal DFO administration [Hercz et al. 1986, Molitoris et al. 1987, Navarro et al. 1988a]. In Table 1, we use whole blood metal concentrations since they may be more representative of the total Al burden [Navarro 1989, Navarro et al. 1988b, Romero et al. 1990] and increments of 413% and 190% were observed in patients 1 and 2, respectively. These results are expected in patients with toxic Al tissue levels [Milliner et al. 1984], in agreement with the results of bone biopsy studies. Interestingly, patient 1 showed a 65% increase in blood Pb after DFO but no significant increment in dialysate Pb concentration was observed (Table 2); the lack of significant dialysis removal of Pb is not surprising since practically all the Pb found in the content of the blood is located in red blood cells and, therefore, unavailable for dialysis exchange.

Patient 2 had a 20% increase in blood Fe concentration in the first 24 hours after DFO (Table 1), and the dialysate Fe concentration increased 84% over the pre-DFO levels (Table 2). It is likely that the proportion of ultrafiltrable Fe available for transperitoneal transfer had increased with DFO. This possibility is strengthened by the results in patient 1 who did not show significant changes in total blood Fe concentration (Table 1) but presented a 343% increment in the efflux peritoneal dialysate Fe 24 hours after DFO administration (Table 2).

Dialysate/plasma concentration ratios of both Al and Fe showed a tendency to increase after DFO therapy (Figure 2) which is indicative of a rise in the ultrafiltrable fraction of these metals after DFO. Similar findings with respect to Al D/P ratios were also observed by Hercz et al. [1986].

Blood and peritoneal dialysis concentration of Pb, Cu and Zn was unchanged after DFO administration.

Total Al removal in the period of study was 2.85 mg and 7.5 mg in patients 1 and 2, respectively. This is a significant amount that is higher than the efficiency of 4–6 hours of hemodialysis [Hercz et al. 1986, Navarro et al. 1988a]. The D/P ratios observed for Al (Figures 1 and 2) are somewhat higher than the values found by Hercz et al. [1986] who reported mean D/P Al concentration ratios of about 0.15 and 0.32, before and after intravenous DFO, respectively. It is possible that our higher values are due to longer intraperitoneal dialysate dwelling time, which was 4 hours for the day exchanges and 8 hours for the night exchange; Hercz et al. [1986] used 2-hour nocturnal cycles and a single half-volume daytime dwell. Peritoneal removal of Fe was 4.7 mg in patient 1 and 2.7 mg in patient 2 (Figure 3); this is in contrast with the lack of significant Fe losses in hemodialysis during intravenous DFO treatment [Navarro 1989]. In circumstances of severe iron overload, CAPD has been used in association with the administration of DFO to remove large amounts of this metal [Falk et al. 1983, Andreoli and Cohen 1989].

The removal of Cu, Zn and Pb is small in CAPD (less than 200 µg/day) and remains unchanged after chelation therapy. The low removal of these metals is expected because the stability constants of Zn-DFO, Cu-DFO and Pb-DFO complexes are $10^{11.07}$, $10^{14.12}$ and 10^{10} [Anderegg et al. 1963] which are much smaller than the stability constants of Al-DFO (circa $10^{22.08}$) and Fe-DFO (circa $10^{30.50}$) [Romero 1982]. The low effectiveness of DFO chelation for Pb contrasts with the results obtained by Mehbod [1967] with EDTA chelation (Pb-EDTA stability constant ca. 10^{18}; [Skoog and West 1976]). Improvement of Al-induced osteomalacia, myopathy and anemia have been found after 4 months of DFO therapy in association with CAPD [Passlick et al. 1989]; therefore, the efficiency and safety of long-term DFO chelation therapy in patients undergoing CAPD should be investigated.

Acknowledgements

This research was partially supported by Grant S1-1994 from the Consejo Nacional de Investigaciones Científicas y Tecnológicas (CONICIT), Inbiomed (FUNDACITE) and Asociación de Amigos del Riñón, Maracaibo, Venezuela. Authors gratefully acknowledge the supply of Desferal by Ciba-Geigy, S. A. (División Farmacéutica, Venezuela) and the bibliographic grant given by the Deutsche Forschungsgemeinschaft (DFG) of the Federal Republic of Germany.

REFERENCES

Ackrill P, Ralston AJ, Day JP, Hodge KC 1980 Successful removal of aluminum from patient with dialysis encephalopathy. Lancet *2:* 692–693

Ackrill P, Ralston AJ, Day JP 1986 Role of desferrioxamine in the treatment of dialysis encephalopathy. Kidney Int *29:* 104–107

Anderegg G, Leplanttenier F, Schwartzenbach G 1963 Hydroxamatkomplexe II. Die Anwendung der pH-Methode. Helvetica Chim Acta *46:* 1400–1408

Andreoli SP, Dunn D, DeMyer W, Sherrard DJ, Bergstein JM 1985 Intraperitoneal desferrioxamine therapy for aluminum intoxication in a child undergoing continuous peritoneal dialysis. J Pediatr *107:* 760–763

Andreoli SP, Cohen M 1989 Intraperitoneal desferrioxamine therapy for iron overload in children undergoing CAPD. Kidney Int *35:* 1330–1335

Altmann P, Marsh F, Plowman D, Cunningham J 1988 Aluminium chelation therapy in dialysis patients: evidence for inhibition of haemoglobin synthesis by low levels of aluminium. Lancet *1:* 1405–1406

Falk RJ, Mattern WD, Lamanna RW, Gitelman HJ, Parker NC, Cross RE, Rastall JR 1983 Iron removal during continuous ambulatory peritoneal dialysis using desferrioxamine. Kidney Int *24:* 110–112

Hercz G, Salusky IB, Norris KC, Fine RN, Coburn JW 1986 Aluminum removal by peritoneal dialysis: Intravenous vs intraperitoneal desferrioxamine. Kidney Int *30:* 944–948

Malluche HH, Smith AJ, Abreo K, Faugere M 1984 The use of desferrioxamine in the management of aluminum accumulation in bone in patients with renal failure. N Engl J Med *311:* 140–144

Mehbod H 1967 Treatment of lead intoxication. Combined use of peritoneal dialysis and Edetate Calcium Disodium. J Amer Med Ass *201:* 972–974

Milliner DS, Nebeker HG, Ott SM, Andress DL, Sherrard DJ, Alfrey AC, Slatopolsky EA, Coburn JW 1984 Use of the desferrioxamine infusion test in the diagnosis of aluminum-related osteodystrophy. Ann Intern Med *101:* 775–780

Molitoris BA, Alfrey PS, Miller NL, Hasbargen JA, Kaehney WD, Alfrey AC, Smith BJ 1987 Efficacy of intramuscular and intraperitoneal desferrioxamine for aluminum chelation. Kidney Int *31:* 986–991

Navarro JA, Romero RA 1988 Determination of whole blood and serum iron by graphite furnace atomic absorption spectrometry. XV FACSS Meeting, Boston, MA, USA. Paper No. B93

Navarro JA, García R, Rubio PD, Rodríguez-Iturbe B, Virla J, Méndez G, Romero RA 1988a Aluminum transfer and desferrioxamine treatment in dialysis units in Maracaibo, Venezuela. Trace Elem Med *5:* 104–108

Navarro JA, Parra OE, Romero RA 1988b Aluminum determination in whole blood, dialysis solution, and tap water samples from Maracaibo dialysis units (Venezuela) by graphite furnace atomic absorption spectrometry. J Trace Elem Electrolytes Health Dis *2:* 3–8

Navarro JA, Parra OE, García R, Rodríguez-Iturbe B, Rubio D, Romero RA 1988c Niveles de aluminio en el agua de consumo de la ciudad de Maracaibo y Costa Oriental del Lago, Estado Zulia, Venezuela. Invest Clin *29:* 37–45

Navarro JA, Granadillo VA, Parra OE, Romero RA 1989 Determination of lead in whole blood by graphite furnace atomic absorption spectrometry with matrix modification. J Anal At Spectrom *4:* 401–406

Navarro JA 1989 Estudio sobre la transferencia de hierro y aluminio en procesos de hemodiálisis y durante la quelación con desferrioxamina B (chemistry Thesis). Faculty of Sciences, University of Zulia. Maracaibo, Venezuela

Ott SM, Andress DL, Nebeker HG 1986 Changes in bone histology after treatment with desferrioxamine. Kidney Int *29:* 108–113

Parra OE, Navarro JA, Granadillo VA, Romero RA 1988 Graphite furnace determination of trace metals in whole blood and dialysis solution samples of chronic renal failure patients. 1st Symposium on furnace atomic absorption spectrometry. Rio de Janeiro, Brazil. Paper No. 30

Passlick J, Whilhelm H, Busch T, Grabensee B, Ohnesorge FK 1989 Chronische Aluminium-Intoxikation bei kontinuierlicher ambulanter Peritonealdialyse. Therapie mit Desferrioxamin. Dtsch Med Wochenschr *114:* 253–257

Romero RA 1982 The application of electrochemical methods of analysis to problems in clinical chemistry. PhD Thesis. University of Manchester, UK

Romero RA, Navarro JA, Rodríguez-Iturbe B, García R, Parra OE, Granadillo VA 1990 Distribution of trace metals in blood compartments of patients with chronic renal failure undergoing periodical hemodialysis treatment. Trace Elem Med *7:* 176–181

Skoog DA, West DM 1976 Fundamentals of analytical chemistry. Holt-Saunders International Editions. Third Edition. New York, p 274

Taber T, Hegeman T, York S, Miller R 1986 Removal of aluminum with intraperitoneal desferrioxamine. Perit Dial Bull *6:* 213–215

Wallenstein S, Zucher CL, Fleiss JL 1980 Some statistical methods useful in circulation research. Circ Res *47:* 1–9

Winterberg B, Lison AE, Bertram HP, Spieker C, Kellinghaus H, Zumkley H 1984 Aluminum intoxication: Treatment with desferrioxamine. Trace Elem Med *1:* 111–114

Clinical Nephrology, Vol. 35 No. 5 – 1991 (218–223)

Vasoactive hormones in uremic patients on continuous ambulatory peritoneal dialysis

K. N. Lai[1], P. K. T. Li[1], K. S. Woo[1], S. F. Lui[1], J. C. K. Leung[1], E. Law[2] and M. G. Nicholls[1]

Departments of Medicine[1] and Chemical Pathology[2], Prince of Wales Hospital, The Chinese University of Hong Kong

Abstract. Plasma levels of atrial natriuretic peptide (ANP), renin activity (PRA), and endothelin (ET) are often elevated in uremic patients on hemodialysis treatment. The profile of these vasoactive hormones and their relationships with hemodynamic indices in patients on continuous ambulatory peritoneal dialysis (CAPD), however, are not clear. We therefore measured plasma concentrations of ANP, PRA, ET, together with parathyroid hormone (PTH) in 17 patients (mean age 38.5 years) on maintenance CAPD over a period of 12 weeks. Baseline ANP, PRA, and ET levels were significantly higher than those of healthy subjects, and no significant changes in these indices were observed over the 12 week period. There was a significant positive correlation between levels of plasma ANP and PRA [rank correlation coefficient, R(s) = 0.496, p <0.05] as has been reported in cardiac failure. Despite the absence of clinically overt heart failure, a significant proportion (approximately 50%) of our patients demonstrated evidence of myocardial dysfunction on echocardiography. Furthermore, a significant positive correlation was demonstrated between plasma ANP and left atrial size [R(s) = 0.61, p <0.01] and an inverse correlation existed between plasma ANP and the left ventricular ejection fraction [R(s) = 0.51, p <0.05]. Twelve patients (71%) had biochemical evidence of hyperparathyroidism with raised levels of serum PTH. Our study demonstrates increased levels of plasma ANP, PRA, and ET in uremic patients on long-term CAPD. A positive correlation exists between plasma ANP and PRA suggesting their myocardial function may be compromized and this was confirmed on echocardiography. The possibility that high circulating PTH concentrations contribute to impaired cardiac function in such patients, deserves further study.

Key words: continuous ambulatory peritoneal dialysis – chronic renal failure – atrial natriuretic peptide – endothelin – renin activity – uremic cardiomyopathy

Introduction

Continuous ambulatory peritoneal dialysis (CAPD) has emerged as an effective replacement therapy for end stage renal failure [Popovich et al. 1978]. There have been a number of studies comparing the control of blood pressure in hypertensive patients on hemodialysis and on CAPD [Wu, 1983, Young et al. 1984, Youmbissi et al. 1986]. Hemodialysis appears to be more effective than CAPD in controlling blood pressure, despite similar levels of exchangeable sodium, renin, and aldosterone [Youmbissi et al. 1986]. Nonetheless, 30–68% of medicated hypertensive patients were normotensive after one year of CAPD [Wu, 1983, Stablein et al. 1988]. Plasma levels of atrial natriuretic peptide (ANP), renin activity (PRA), and endothelin (ET) are often elevated in uremic patients on hemodialysis treatment [Schalekamp et al. 1973, Ando et al. 1988, Koyama et al. 1989]. There is now evidence that volume expansion in azotemia is associated with increased levels of ANP [Rascher, Tulassay, and Lang 1985, Walker et al. 1987] which may serve to offset excessive vasoconstrictor factors. Furthermore, plasma ANP levels is sensitive to volume status even in chronic hemodialysis patients [Ando et al. 1988].

Continuous ambulatory peritoneal dialysis differs from hemodialysis as continuous rather than intermittent removal of fluid by ultrafiltration is carried out. Hence, plasma concentrations of vasoactive hormones in CAPD patients should reflect a steady-state measurement rather than a single point in a fluctuating cycle. The profile of these vasoactive hormones has not previously been studied in CAPD. In the present study, we examined the profile of vasoactive hormones including ANP, PRA, and ET in a group of hemodynamically stable patients on

Received April 17, 1990; in revised form November 23, 1990.

Reprint requests to Dr. K. N. Lai, Department of Medicine, The Chinese University of Hong Kong, Shatin, Hong Kong.

Table 1 Reasons governing the choice of CAPD therapy

	Number of patients
Cardiac	
History of heart failure	1
Rheumatic valve disease	1 (mild mitral insufficiency)
Inadequate hemodialysis facilities	2
Age	
Young patient	2
Elderly patient	1
Patient preference	2
Lack of vascular access	4
Hepatitis B virus carrier	2
Diabetes mellitus	1

Table 2 Plasma levels of ANP, PRA, and ET, and mean arterial pressure in 17 CAPD patients over a 12-week period

	0 week	6 week	12 week
MAP (mmHg)	97.3 ± 3.7	100.6 ± 3.5	99.9 ± 1.5
ANP (pg/ml)	201.7 ± 32.4	202.6 ± 31.8	214.8 ± 34.9
PRA (ng/ml/hr)	3.79 ± 1.00	3.89 ± 1.06	3.76 ± 1.00
ET (pg/ml)	2.91 ± 0.20	3.28 ± 0.19	3.06 ± 0.23

Results are expressed as mean ± SEM.
MAP = mean arterial pressure.

maintenance CAPD and related these indices to blood pressure and to simple hemodynamic measurements.

Patients and methods

Patient selection

Seventeen patients, 5 males and 12 females with end stage renal failure were studied. All except one were older than 18 years (aged 13–62 years, mean age 38.5). The causes of renal failure included chronic glomerulonephritis 14, lupus nephritis 1, polycystic disease 1, and diabetic nephropathy 1. Their daily fluid intake was limited to 1–1.5 liters and the urine output ranged from 0.15 to 0.6 litre/day. Their residual glomerular filtration rate (measured by endogenous creatinine clearance ranged from 3.5 to 8.5 ml/min/1.73 m^2 (mean 5.1). They had been on CAPD for at least 12 months and were hemodynamically stable. The reasons governing the choice of CAPD over hemodialysis are depicted in Table 1. Two of these patients received CAPD treatment for their underlying heart disease. One had mild rheumatic mitral insufficiency and the other had symptoms of heart failure which disappeared with the commencement of maintenance dialysis. None of these patients had an arterio-venous fistula. Patients with a hemoglobin less than 6.5 gm/dl, clinically evident fluid retention, or uncontrolled hypertension were excluded from the study. Medications (including antihypertensive drugs), the dialysis regime and dialysate requirements had not altered for two months prior to and during the study. The patients received no blood transfusion, and their dry weight (body weight measured without intraperitoneal installation of dialyzate) remained unchanged throughout this period.

Vasoactive hormones were measured three times over a period of 12 weeks. Blood was collected (the plasma separated at 4° C and stored at –20° C) at baseline, then at 6 and 12 weeks for measurement of plasma ANP, ET, and PRA. The venous blood samples were collected in the morning after patients had been resting in the supine position for one hour and two hours after change of peritoneal dialyzate. Chest X-ray for cardio-thoracic ratio (CTR) and M-mode echocardiography were performed at the end of the study period. Echocardiographic measurements (left atrial size, left ventricular end-diastolic diameter, and ejection fraction) were determined by standard techniques as previously described [Pombo et al. 1971, Lai et al. 1985]. The echocardiographic measurements were highly reproducible provided the patients' dry weight remained unchanged and consistent pattern was observed in serial measurements from patients on stable maintenance dialysis [Lai et al. 1985].

Assays

All samples from an individual patient were measured in the same assay. Atrial natriuretic peptide was measured by radioimmunoassay after extraction using Sep-pak C18 cartridge (Waters Associates, Milford, MA) as described previously [Yandle et al. 1986]. The sensitivity of the assay was 2 pg/tube and the within-assay coefficient of variation was 8%. The plasma ANP concentration in normal healthy controls was 42 ± 3 pg/ml (mean ± sd).

Plasma endothelin concentrations were measured by radioimmunoassay using a commercially available kit (Amersham, UK) after extraction using Sep-pak C18 cartridges. The assay measures endothelin-1 and endothelin-2 but not endothelin-3. The lowest detectable level was 1.25 pg/tube. The intra-assay coefficient of variation was 5%. The plasma ET concentration in 10 healthy non-uremic controls was less than 1 pg/ml.

Plasma renin activity was measured by radioimmunoassay of generated angiotensin I using a commercially available kit (Pharmacia Diagnostics, Uppsala, Sweden). This assay could detect less than

0.2 ng/ml/h of angiotensin I and the intra-assay coefficient of variation was 10%. The mean supine plasma renin activity in 479 healthy controls was 0.96 ng/ml/h (range 0.4–4.1) [Data from Pharmacia AB].

Serum parathyroid hormone (PTH) was measured by a two-site chemiluminometric immunoassay [Magic-Lite Intact PTH immunoassay, Ciba Corning Diagnostic, USA] which employed a constant amount of two sequence specific anti-PTH antibodies. The patient's serum was initially incubated with an acridinium-ester labelled sheep anti-human amino-terminal (1–34) PTH antibody. Subsequently, a mouse monoclonal anti-human (44–68)-region-PTH antibody covalently coupled to paramagnetic particles was added. The minimum detectable concentration was 1.4 pg/ml and the serum PTH levels in healthy controls was 11–54 pg/ml.

Statistical analysis

The data (mean ± SEM) were analyzed using the Wilcoxon signed-rank test, Rank-Sum test, and Spear-

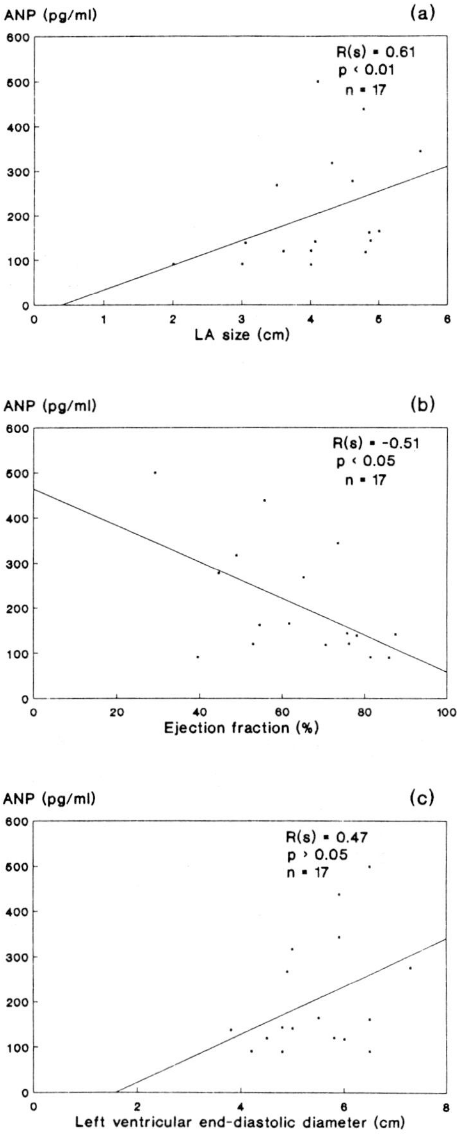

Fig. 1 The plasma ANP, PRA, and ET levels in 17 patients on CAPD. A significant correlation was demonstrated between ANP and PRA (Figure 1a), but not between endothelin and PRA (Figure 1b) or ANP (Figure 1c).

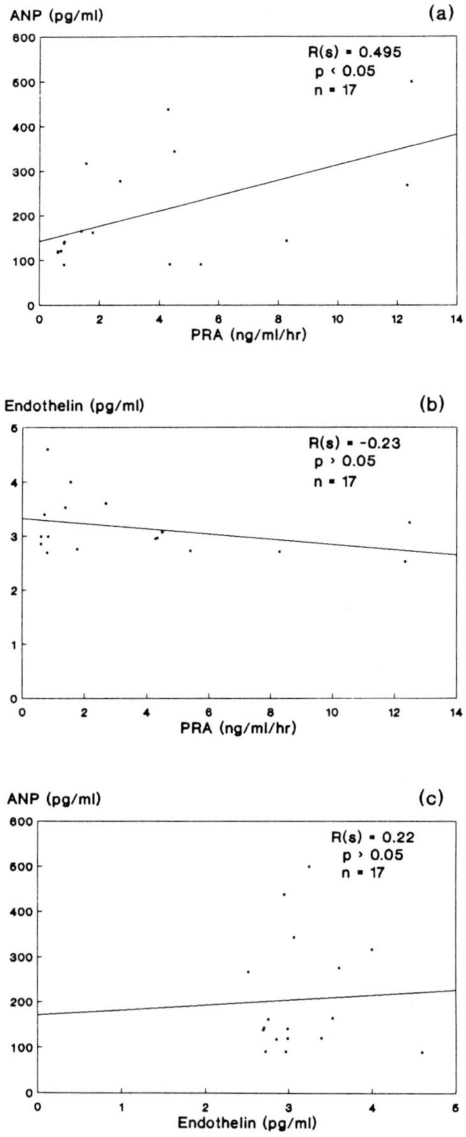

Fig. 2 The correlation between plasma ANP levels and echocardiographic measurements. A significant correlation was demonstrated between ANP and left atrial size (Figure 2a) or ejection fraction (Figure 2b), but not with left ventricular end-diastolic diameter (Figure 2c).

man's rank correlation when appropriated. All p values quoted are two-tailed.

Results

Clinical features

Five of the 17 patients had symptoms of fluid overload prior to the onset of CAPD treatment. Their symptoms improved after the commencement of CAPD. The average hemoglobin level was 7.1 gm/dl. Eight patients practised three 2-liter exchanges daily and nine patients required four 2-liter exchanges daily. Most used 1.5% dextrose peritoneal dialyzate and 8 required supplementary 2.5% dextrose peritoneal dialyzate: hypertonic 4.25% dialyzate was not required. Their mean plasma creatinine were 958 umol/l (range 770–1230). Nine patients were receiving antihypertensive treatment (nadolol, metoprolol, or prazosin) for optimal control of blood pressure throughout the study. The mean arterial pressure remained stable (Table 2). None of the patients received diuretic therapy.

Echocardiography

Despite the absence of clincally overt heart failure, the cardio-thoracic ratio exceeded 0.5 in 12 patients (70%). Echocardiography revealed an increase in left atrial size (normal 1.9–4.0 cm) in 8 patients (47%), a reduction in left ventricular ejection fraction (normal >65%) in 8 patients (47%), and an increased left ventricular end-diastolic diameter (normal 3.7–5.6 cm) in 8 patients (47%). No patients had significant pericardial effusion.

Vasoactive hormones

The baseline ANP, PRA, and ET levels were 201.7 ± 32.4 pg/ml (range 87.3–516.8), 3.79 ± 1.00 ng/ml/h (range 0.3–13.5), and 2.91 ± 0.20 pg/ml (range 1.30–4.59) respectively (Table 2). These values were all significantly higher than those of healthy subjects. No significant fluctuation in these measurements was observed over the twelve weeks (Table 2). Correlations between vasoactive hormones were determined using mean values at zero, six, and twelve weeks. There was a significant positive association between levels of plasma ANP and PRA [rank correlation coefficient, R(s) = 0.495, $p < 0.05$] but there was no significant relationship of plasma ET with ANP or PRA (Figure 1). Furthermore, mean arterial pressure did not correlate significantly with the plasma ANP, PRA, or ET levels.

Table 3 Rank correlation coefficient [R(s)] between various vasoactive hormones and hemodynamic indices

	ANP	PRA	ET
Mean arterial pressure	0.34	–0.025	–0.20
Cardio-thoracic ratio	0.47	0.61*	0.21
Parathyroid hormone	–0.09	–0.36	0.475
Left atrial size	0.61*	0.069	0.23
Ejection fraction	–0.51**	–0.33	–0.093
Left ventricular end-diastolic diameter	0.47	0.27	0.19

* $p < 0.01$
** $p < 0.05$

Relationships between vasoactive hormones and echocardiographic indices

A significant positive correlation was demonstrated between plasma ANP and left atrial size (LA) [R(s) = 0.61, $p < 0.01$] (Figure 2a). Similary, an inverse correlation existed between the plasma ANP and left ventricular ejection fraction [R(s) = –0.51, $p < 0.05$] (Figure 2b). No statistically significant correlation was demonstrated between endothelin or PRA and other hemodynamic indices although there was a positive relationship between plasma renin activity and cardio-thoracic ratio on chest X-ray, which achieved statistical significance [R(s) = 0.61, $p < 0.01$].

PTH measurement

Twelve patients (71%) had a raised level of serum PTH (mean ± sd, 242.9 ± 103.9 pg/ml; range 11–1757 pg/ml). However, no statistically significant correlation was demonstrated between serum PTH levels and the vasoactive hormones (Table 3). Nor was there any significant relationship between serum PTH and left atrial size, left ventricular end-diastolic diameter, ejection fraction, or mean arterial pressure [R(s) = 0.125, –0.002, 0.20, and –0.08 respectively].

Discussion

In view of the possibility that changes in circulating levels of vasoactive hormones could contribute to hypervolemia and hypertension associated with uremia, we studied the plasma levels of ANP, PRA, and ET in patients who were well maintained on CAPD treatment. Elevated plasma ANP has been reported in end-stage renal failure [Crozier et al. 1988, Weidmann et al. 1988], which probably relates to the volume-overload state of chronic renal failure [Weidmann et al. 1988]. Plasma ANP correlated positively with volume status in uremic patients and fell with fluid removal during ultrafiltration or hemodialysis [Rascher et al. 1985, Wilkins et al. 1986]. Levels of renin are extremely variable in end-stage renal failure, and are not infrequently elevated [Schalekamp et al. 1973, Iitake et al. 1985]. Nonetheless, a fall in PRA is observed with fluid removal by hemodialysis [Rascher et al. 1985]. Plasma ET levels, normally at or below the level of detection in healthy subjects are reportedly elevated in patients with uremia [Koyama et al. 1989, Webb & Cockcroft 1989]. Plasma endothelin levels are reported to be higher in patients on hemodialysis than in non-dialysis uremic patients, and the levels fell with hemodialysis [Koyama et al. 1989]. The physiological significance of elevated ET in uremia remains speculative. Animal studies suggest that ET is cardiotoxic and may induce sudden death due to arrhythmia and hypertension [Terashita et al. 1989, Cao and Banks 1990]. Furthermore, a marked reduction of glomerular filtration rate is observed with intravenous infusion of ET [Cao and Banks 1990].

Continuous ambulatory peritoneal dialysis is distinctly different from hemodialysis, as continuous rather than intermittent removal of fluid by ultrafiltration is carried out. Hence, plasma concentrations of vasoactive hormones in CAPD patients should reflect a steady-state measurement rather than a single point in a fluctuating cycle. The profile of these vasoactive hormones has not previously been studied in CAPD. Our present study shows that the levels of plasma ANP, PRA, and ET are elevated in patients on CAPD treatment, as has been reported in pre-dialysis uremia and in patients on maintenance hemodialysis. The pathophysiological mechanisms leading to elevation of these vasoactive hormones in CAPD patients, remains speculative. The increased ANP most likely relates to volume and sodium overload in renal failure, but our data suggest that impaired cardiac function may also contribute (see below). The increased renin levels are somewhat surprising in view of the fluid-replete state, hypervolemia of the central circulation, and treatment in some patients with beta blockers. Nevertheless, poor cardiac function leads, both experimentally and in man to increased renin levels perhaps due to a continuation of reduced blood flow to the afferent renal arteriole, a slow rate of delivery of chloride and sodium to the macula densa, and increased sympathetic activity to the juxtaglomerular apparatus [Davis and Freeman 1984]. The elevated PRA in our patients could be secondary to the combined effect of hypertension related to uremia and impaired cardiac function [Weidman et al. 1971]. Elevation of endothelin may be due either to increased synthesis and release or to reduced degradation removal because of impaired renal function [Koyama et al. 1989].

Of interest in our patients was the positive relationship between ANP and PRA which is in contrast to an inverse correlation seen in healthy subjects [Crozier et al. 1988]. In that a positive relationship has previously been reported in patients with heart failure [Crozier et al. 1988], these data suggested the possibility that myocardial function was compromized in our patients despite the absence of overt heart failure. The significant positive correlation between plasma ANP and left atrial size, and inverse relationship with left ventricular ejection suggests that the raised plasma ANP may reflect not only the hypervolemic state of uremia, but also myocardial dysfunction [Lai et al. 1985].

Myocardial function was further investigated by echocardiography. Despite the absence of clinically overt heart failure cardiomegaly on chest X-ray, decreased myocardial contractility (reduced ejection fraction), and a dilated left atrium and left ventricle were frequently observed. Several factors, including anemia [Neff et al. 1971], acetate in dialysate [Aizawa et al. 1977], arterio-venous fistula [Daniel et al. 1972], coronary artery disease [Ikram et al. 1983], and hyperparathyroidism [Drueke et al. 1977, Drueke et al. 1980, Lai et al. 1985], have been implicated in the pathogenesis of myocardial dysfunction in hemodialysis patients. The prevalence of myocardial dysfunction has rarely been studied in CAPD patients since older patients or those with cardiovascular diseases tend to have been preferentially treated with CAPD [Wu 1983]. Our CAPD patients were young compared with patients from other centers [Wu 1983, Gokal et al. 1986], but a significant proportion (approximately 50%) nevertheless demonstrated clear evidence of myocardial dysfunction. Although our study does not elucidate the pathophysiological mechanism, anemia is likely to be an important contributory factor, whereas other factors such as acetate dialysate, fistula, and coronary artery disease did not contribute or are likely to be less important. Treatment with beta-blockers may have exacerbated the poor cardiac function. Previous work has suggested that myocardial function may be impaired by high levels of parathyroid hormone [Drueke et al. 1977]. We documented raised concentrations of PTH in most of our patients which, through a negative inotropic action, may have contributed to cardiac dysfunction. Further studies are needed to elucidate this possibility.

In conclusion, we have demonstrated increased levels of plasma ANP, PRA, and ET in uremic patients on long-term CAPD. Despite the absence of clinically overt heart failure, a positive correlation existed between plasma ANP and PRA suggesting their myocardial function may be compromized, and this was confirmed by echocardiographic studies. The underlying mechanism of cardiac dysfunction remain to be clarified, but anemia and high parathyroid hormone levels may contribute, and the use of beta-blockers to control arterial pressure might be questioned.

Acknowledgement

The research was supported by the Mr. and Mrs. L. C. Liu Research Fund. We thank Pharmacia Diagnostics AB for providing Phadabas Angiotensin I test.

REFERENCES

Ando R, Matsuda O, Miyake S, Yoshiyama N 1988 Plasma levels of human atrial natriuretic factor in patients treated by hemodialysis and continuous ambulatory peritoneal dialysis. Nephron *50:* 225–228

Cao L, Banks RO 1990 Cardiovascular and renal actions of endothelin: effects of calcium-channel blockers. Am J Physiol *258:* F254–F258

Crozier IG, Richards AM, Nicholls MG, Espiner EA, Ikram H, Yandle TG 1988 Atrial natriuretic factor in human pathophysiology. Clin Exp Pharmacol Physiol *15:* 173–183

Daniel J, Ahearn MD, Maher JF 1972 Heart failure as a complication of hemodialysis arteriovenous fistula. Arch Intern Med *77:* 201–205

Davis JO, Freeman RH 1984 Renin release mechanism in congestive heart failure. J Hypertension 2 (suppl 1): 89–94

Drueke T, Le Pailleur C, Meilhac B, Koutoudis C, Zingraff J, DiMatteo J, Crosnier J 1977 Congestive cardiomyopathy in uremic patients on long-term hemodialysis. Br Med J *1:* 350–353

Drueke T, Fauchet M, Fleury J, Toure Y, Le Pailleur C, De Vernejoul P, Crosnier J 1980 Effect of parathyroidectomy on left ventricular function in hemodialysis patients. Lancet *1:* 112–114

Gokal R, Lloyd C, Baillod R, Marsh F, Ogg C, Oliver O, Ward M, Wilkinson R 1986 Multi-center study on the outcome of patients on CAPD and hemodialysis. In: Frontiers in peritoneal dialysis. *Maher JF, Winchester JF* (eds) Field, Rich & Assoc, New York, pp 293–296

Iitake K, Kimura T, Matsui K, Ota K, Shoji M, Inoue M, Yoshinaga K 1985 Effect of hemodialysis on plasma ADH levels, plasma renin activity and plasma aldosterone levels in patients with end-stage renal failure. Acta Endocrinol *110:* 207–213

Ikram H, Lynn KL, Bailey RR, Little PS 1983 Cardiovascular changes in chronic hemodialysis patients. Kidney Int *24:* 371–376

Koyama H, Tabata T, Nishzawa Y, Inoue T, Morii H, Yamaji T 1989 Plasma endothelin levels in patients with uraemia. Lancet *1:* 991–992

Lai KN, Ng J, Whitford J, Buttfield I, Fassett RG, Mathew TH 1985 Left ventricular function in uremia: echocardiographic and radionuclide assessment in patients on maintenance hemodialysis. Clin Nephrol *23:* 125–133

Neff MS, Kim KE, Persoff M, Onesti G, Swartz G 1971 Hemodynamics of uremic anemia. Circulation *43:* 876–883

Pombo J, Troy BL, Russell R 1971 Left ventricular volumes and ejection fraction by echocardiography. Circulation *43:* 480–490

Popovich RP, Moncrief JW, Nolph KD, Ghods AJ, Twardowski ZJ, Pyle WK 1978 Continuous ambulatory peritoneal dialysis. Ann Intern Med *88:* 449–456

Rascher W, Tulassay T, Lang RE 1985 Atrial natriuretic peptide in plasma of volume-overloaded children with chronic renal failure. Lancet *ii:* 303–305

Schalekamp MA, Beevers DG, Briggs JD, Brown JJ, Davies DL, Fraser R, Lebel M, Lever AF, Medina A, Morton JJ, Robertson JI, Tree M 1973 Hypertension in chronic renal failure. Am J Med *55:* 379–390

Stablein DM, Hamburger RJ, Lindblad AS, Nolph KD, Novak JW 1988 The effect of CAPD on hypertension control: a report of the National CAPD Registry. Perit Dial Int *8:* 141–144

Terashita Z, Shibouta Y, Imura Y, Iwasaki K, Nishikawa K 1989 Endothelin-induced sudden death and the possible involvement of platelet activating factor. Life Sciencs *45:* 1911–1918

Walker RG, Swainson CP, Yandle TG, Nicholls MG, Espiner EA 1987 Exaggerated responsiveness of immunoreactive atrial natriuretic peptide to saline infusion in chronic renal failure. Clin Sci *72:* 19–24

Webb DJ, Cockcroft JR 1989 Plasma immunoreactive endothelin in uraemia. Lancet *1:* 1211 (letter)

Weidman P, Maxwell MH, Lupu AN, Lewin AJ, Massry SG 1971 Plasma renin activity and blood pressure in terminal renal failure. N Engl J Med *285:* 957–962

Weidmann P, Saxenhofer H, Ferrier C, Shaw SG 1988 Atrial natriuretic peptide in man. Am J Nephrol *8:* 1–14

Wu G 1983 Cardiovascular deaths among CAPD patients. Perit Dial Bull *3, (suppl 3):* S23–S26

Yandle TG, Espiner EA, Nicholls MG, Duff H 1986 Radioimmunoassay and characterization of atrial natriuretic peptide in human plasma. J Clin Endocrinol Metabol *63:* 72–79

Youmbissi J, Sellars L, Shore AC, Poon T, Wilkinson R 1986 Blood pressure on CAPD: relationship to sodium status, renin, and aldosterone, compared with hemodialysis. In: Frontiers in peritoneal dialysis. *Maher JF, Winchester JF* (eds) Field, Rich & Assoc, New York pp 450–456

Young MA, Nolph KD, Dutton S, Prowant B 1984 Antihypertensive drug requirements in continuous ambulatory peritoneal dialysis. Perit Dial Bull *4:* 85–88

Clinical Nephrology, Vol. 35 No. 5 – 1991 (224–226)

Hypersensitivity reactions during hemodialysis related to the use of acetate dialysate. A case report

J. T. Papadakis[1], A. Patrikarea[1], S. Saradi[2], K. Papakostas[1], A. Leondi[2], A. Kravaritis[1] and S. Vafiadis[1]

[1] *Renal Unit of NIMTS Hospital, 10 M. Petraki Str., Athens 115 21, Greece*
[2] *Nuclear Medicine Department "Alexandra" Hospital, V. Sofias and Lourou Str., Athens 115 28, Greece*

Abstract. A patient developed a hypersensitivity reaction two weeks after being put on hemodialysis with acetate dialysate. The reactions appeared exclusively during hemodialysis and were relieved immediately after its termination. These allergic manifestations disappeared with substitution of bicarbonate for acetate dialysate and reappeared upon rechallenge with acetate dialysate. The rest of the dialysis materials were excluded as possible causes of allergy by scheduled dialysis sessions with varying materials. Acetate dialysate is implicated as the cause of allergy reaction in this case.

Key words: hemodialysis – acetate – hypersensitivity reactions

Introduction

Hypersensitivity reactions during hemodialysis, although relatively uncommon, are of great concern because they can be life-threatening. The most frequently recognized causes of these reactions include: ethylene oxide (ETO) and its breakdown products [Rockel et al. 1988], other toxic or undesirable materials [Kjellstrand et al. 1978], dialyzer membranes [Hakim et al. 1984, Daugirdas et al. 1985], contaminated dialysate [Man et al. 1987] and Interleukin-1 production [Giacchino et al. 1985]. In addition the use of acetate dialysate has been implicated in a small number of cases of anaphylactoid hypersensitivity reactions [Ei et al. 1979, Caravaca et al. 1987]. A case is presented in which acetate dialysate is implicated as a cause of hypersensitivity reactions expressed with anaphylactic signs and symptoms during hemodialysis.

Case report

The patient was a 23-year old female with end-stage renal failure due to focal segmental glomerulosclerosis. Her past medical history was negative for any other illness or allergic problems. In March 1989, she was put on regular hemodialysis thrice weekly with a cuprophan hollow fiber dialyzer Sorin spiraflo NT 1108 1.1 m^2 sterilized with ETO. The dialysis machine was Gambro AK-10. The dialysate had the following composition: Na 137.24 mEq/l, K 1.64 mEq/l, Cl 104.73 mEq/l, Ca 3.34 mEq/l, Mg 0.98 mEq/l and acetate 38.46 mEq/l. It was prepared proportionally from concentrate dialysate, commercially available and water pretreated with softener, granural carbon filter and reverse osmosis. No medication was given. She tolerated dialysis without any problem for the first six sessions, but in the first 30 minutes of the seventh session she experienced generalized pruritus associated with a feeling of burning, mild dyspnea, urticaria and lacrimation that subsided soon after discontinuation of the dialysis. The same symptoms reappeared in the next dialyses in spite of the substitution of gamma ray sterilizer, using a dialyzer Secon S-122 Gamma 1.2 m^2, for ETO and of cellulose acetate (FB Nipro 110-T and FB Nipro 110 T-GA 1.1 m^2) for cuprophan dialyzer. Accidentally, she was put on bicarbonate dialysate that has had the following composition: Na 137 mEq/l, K 1.5 mEq/l, Cl 104 mEq/l, Ca 3.5 mEq/l, Mg 1.0 mEq/l, HCO_3 39 mEq/l and acetate 5 mEq/l and no reactions appeared.

In an effort to elucidate if acetate dialysate was the cause of the hypersensitivity reactions in this patient and after obtaining her informed consent, we

Received September 12, 1989; in revised form October 17, 1990.

Reprint requests to Dr. John Papadakis, Renal Unit, NIMTS Hospital, 10 M. Petraki Str., 115 21 Athens, Greece.

Table 1 Dialysis materials and hypersensitivity reactions in the dialysis sessions with alternate use of bicarbonate and acetate dialysate

Dialyzer	Cuprophan	Cuprophan	Cuprophan	Cellulose acetate	Cellulose acetate	Cellulose acetate
Sterilizer	ETO	ETO	γ-ray	ETO	γ-ray	ETO
Blood tubing	PVC sterilized with ETO	PVC sterilized with ETO	PVC sterilized with ETO	PVC sterilized with ETO	PVC sterilized with ETO	PVC sterilized with ETO
Dialysate buffer	Bicarbonate	Acetate	Acetate	Acetate	Acetate	Bicarbonate
Heparin	Porcine	Porcine	Porcine	Porcine	Porcine	Porcine
Dialysis sessions	2	2	2	2	2	2
Hypersensitivity reactions	Negative	Positive	Positive	Positive	Positive	Negative

The dialyzers were rinsed with 2 liters of 0.9% normal saline.
ETO: ethylene oxide; PVC: polyvinylchloride

scheduled a number of dialyses with varying combination of the dialysis materials (Table 1) and we observed that hypersensitivity reactions, such as described above, appeared only when acetate buffer was used. At the commencement and the termination of one dialysis using acetate and one with bicarbonate buffer the arterial blood gases were measured and no particular differences were found in pH, pO_2, pCO_2 and HCO_3 between the corresponding values. At the end of each of these scheduled dialysis sessions and the next three weeks, while the patient was constantly on bicarbonate dialysate, the level of total serum IgE and blood eosinophils were determinated. Both increased during the use of acetate dialysate and returned to normal values when bicarbonate dialysate was used again (Figure 1). The ETO-radio-allergy sorbent test (RAST) as well as the RAST for inhalant and food allergens which included (Greer labs inc. Holister-stier labs), Dermatophagoides pteronyssinus, Dermatophagoides farinae, egg white, milk, fish-cod, honey bee venom, yellow jacket wasp, paper wasp venom, cat epithelium, dog dander, pine tree, olive tree, Cynodon dactylon, Parietaria officinalis, Altenaria tenuis, Aspergillus fumigatus, goose feathers, chicken feathers, duck feathers were negative. Since the studies were completed the permanent use of bicarbonate dialysate has provided the patient with hemodialysis free of allergic reactions independently of the type of any dialysis material used other than the dialysate buffer.

Discussion

The use of acetate as a dialysate buffer has been linked to hypotension, myocardial depression, hypoxemia and abnormal lipid metabolism [Diamond and Henrich 1987]. Its association with hypersensitivity reactions during hemodialysis has been reported in a very limited number of cases. Ei et al. [1979] described a case of hemodialysis-induced asthmatic attacks which subsided soon after an acetate-free dialysate was used. More recently, Caravaca et al. [1987] reported another case of hypersensitivity reactions, quite similar to those observed in our patient, which were attributed either to the use of acetate dialysate or to celluse acetate membrane.

A relation between hypersensitivity reactions and the acetate dialysate is strongly suggested in our case by the appearance of clinical manifestations when acetate was used initially and when the patient was retreated with acetate dialysate. In particular the

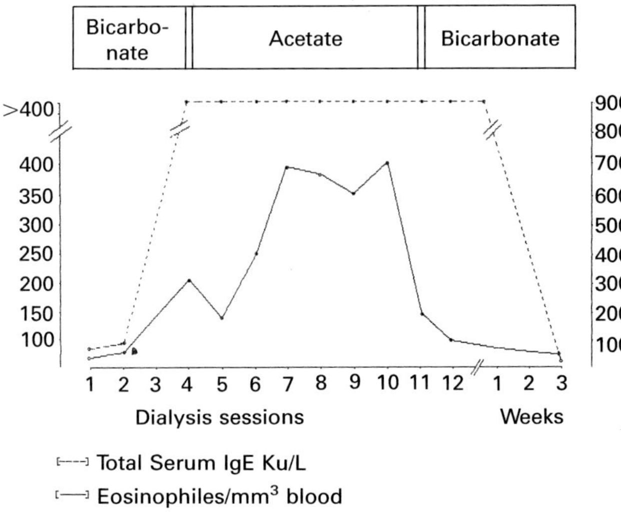

Fig. 1 Total serum IgE and blood eosinophils in the dialysis sessions with alternate use of bicarbonate and acetate dialysate

dialyzer membranes and the materials of sterilization cannot be implicated in the generation of the hypersensitivity reactions in our patient, since they appeared, independently of their composition, in the same frequency and severity always and only on acetate and never on bicarbonate dialysate (Table 1). It is also noteworthy that the ETO-RAST, that is usually positive in the ETO-dependent hypersensitivity reactions, was negative in our patient.

It remains unexplained how acetate dialysate induces hypersensitivity reactions. It seems to be dose dependent since the small quantity of acetate in the bicarbonate dialysate did not trigger hypersensitivity reactions. In addition the above mentioned reactions subsided soon after the discontinuation of acetate dialysate supply and the obvious reduction of acetate burden in the blood via its metabolism.

Although the implications of complement activation or Interleukin-1 production cannot be proved or excluded, the appearance of the hypersensitivity reactions two weeks after institution of dialysis and the increase in the serum IgE levels, along with eosinophilia, during the acetate dialysis sessions (Figure 1) suggest that either acetate itself may act as an antigen or as a hapten, or the physiochemical differences between acetate and bicarbonate dialysate may cause, during the use of acetate, leaching of another antigen or hapten from the blood circuit, which in conjunction with substance present or produced during dialysis, lead to Type-I hypersensitivity reactions.

REFERENCES

Daugirdas JT, Ing TS, Roxe DM, Ivanovich PT, Krumlovsky F, Popli S, Mc Laughlin MM 1985 Severe anaphylactoid reactions to cuprammonium cellulose hemodialyzers. Arch Intern Med *145:* 489–494

Diamond SM, Henrich WL 1987 Acetate Dialysate versus Bicarbonate Dialysate: A Continuing Controversy. Am J Kidney Dis *IX:* 3–11

Ei K, Hanai I, Horiuchi T, Hanai J, Gotoh H, Hirasawa Y, Gejyo F, Aizawa Y 1979 Hemodialysis-associated asthma in a renal failure patient. Nephron *25:* 247–248

Garavaca F, Pizarro JI, Arrobas M, Cubero JJ, Antona JM, Sanchez E 1987 Hypersensitivity Reactions Related to Acetate Dialyzate and Cellulose Acetate Membrane. Nephron *45:* 158–159

Giacchino F, Pozzato M, Landolfo SS, Quarello F, Garetto A, Gangemi C, Girando G, Piccoli G 1985 Interleukin-1 in hypersensitivity reactions during hemodialysis. Proc EDTA-ERA *22:* 192–195

Hakim RM, Breillatt J, Lazarus JM, Port FK 1984 Complement activation and hypersensitivity reactions to dialysis membranes. N Engl J Med *311:* 878–882

Kjellstrand CM, Alfrey AC, Eaton JW, Friedman EA, Ginn HE, Hull AR, Ogden D 1978 Toxicity of materials and medications used in dialysis. Trans Am Soc Artif Intern Organs *24:* 764–769

Man NK, Ciancioni CH, Guyomard S, Blais D, Delons S, Funck-Brentano JL 1987 Risk and hazards of contaminated dialysate associated with high flux membranes. In: *Buccianti G* (ed): Prevention in Nephrology, Milano, Masson Italia Editore, pp 227–234

Rockel A, Hertel J, Wahn U, Perschel WT, Thiel C, Abdelhamid S, Fiegel P, Walb D 1988 Ethylene oxide and hypersensitivity reactions in patients on hemodialysis. Kidney Int *33* (suppl 24): 62–67

Clinical Nephrology, Vol. 35 No. 5 – 1991 (227–232)

Shoulder ultrasound in dialysis related amyloidosis

L. P. McMahon[1], J. Radford[2] and J. K. Dawborn[1]

Renal Unit, Department of Medicine[1] and Department of Radiology[2], Austin Hospital, Heidelberg, Victoria 3084, Australia

Abstract. Ultrasonographic changes around the shoulder joint were compared in ten symptomatic patients with dialysis related amyloid (DRA) and seventeen patients without symptoms. All patients had been on long-term (>7 years) hemodialysis (HD). Three control groups were used: 8 predialysis patients, 10 continuous ambulatory peritoneal dialysis (CAPD) and 9 HD patients who had been on dialysis for less than two years. Dry bodyweight, sex, handedness, length of hemodialysis and fistula side were not significantly different between the study groups. Proven amyloid patients were significantly older than other groups ($p < 0.001$). Parameters assessed included cross-sectional area of long head of biceps tendon (LHB), diameter of supraspinatus tendon (SS), and general features (bursae, deposits) around the joint. Results demonstrated significant differences in all parameters in patients with symptomatic amyloid compared with other long-term patients: [SS: 7.4 mm ± 0.7, mean ± SEM, vs 5.1 ± 0.2 (right, R), p = 0.001; 6.7 ± 0.7 vs 4.9 ± 0.2 (left, L), p = 0.01. LHB : 140.0 mm^2 ± 11.1 vs 79.6 ± 5.1 (R), $p < 0.001$; 114.5 ± 10.5 vs 80.8 ± 5.4 (L), p = 0.004. Bursae: 5 vs 1 (patients), p = 0.006]. Compared with controls changes in the amyloid group were less marked though in most cases still significant. There was no significant difference between control groups nor between controls and asymptomatic long-term HD patients in any parameter. We conclude that shoulder ultrasound may have a role in identifying patients with dialysis related amyloid. Serial measurements may also help to elucidate the pathogenesis of the tendon changes.

Key words: dialysis related amyloidosis – shoulder ultrasound – symptomatic – asymptomatic

Introduction

Dialysis related amyloid is an insidious disease with an increasing incidence in the long-term dialysis community. Diagnosis currently rests on histological confirmation, usually obtained at the time of carpal tunnel release, although other means such as joint aspiration are also described [Kleinmann and Coburn 1989]. In order to facilitate earlier diagnosis of DRA as well as obtain insight into its pathogenesis other non-invasive techniques have been investigated, however most are still of limited value [Hawkins et al. 1988, Sethi et al. 1990]. We describe the results of detailed ultrasonography of the shoulder joint as an aid to diagnosis and, potentially, to following the progression of this disease.

Received May 21, 1990; in revised form December 27, 1990.

Reprint requests to Dr. L. P. McMahon, Renal unit, Churchill Hospital, Oxford Ox3 7 LJ, England, UK.

Patients and methods

Patients

Study group: all patients from the Renal Unit at the Austin Hospital on HD (conventional cuprophane membrane) for more than seven years (range seven to fifteen) were included in the study (n = 27) and were tested over a period of three months. All those (n = 10) who had symptoms of persistent shoulder pain (more than six weeks) and/or carpal tunnel syndrome (uni or bilateral symptoms, confirmed by nerve conduction test) were proven to have amyloid through routine histological (congo red) staining of synovial tissue obtained either at the time of carpal tunnel release (n = 4), or shoulder (n = 4) or other joint aspiration (n = 2). Amyloid was found at multiple sites in two patients (shoulder joint and carpal tunnel synovium and carpal tunnel and hip joint synovium). Eight of seventeen patients who were symptom free also consented to joint aspiration, however in none of these was synovial tissue able to be obtained.

Table 1 Clinical data in patients and controls

	Age (years)	Bodyweight* (kg)	Length of HD (years)	Sex M : F	Hours of HD (per week)	Handedness L	Handedness R	Fistula side L	Fistula side R
Amyloid	63.6 ± 2.8	62.2 ± 5.9	9.6 ± 1.0	6 : 4	13.2 ± 0.54	0	10	6	4
Asymptomatic	43.1 ± 3.2	60.8 ± 3.0	9.5 ± 0.6	11 : 6	13.9 ± 0.44	1	16	10	7
HD <2	53.2 ± 4.2	63.0 ± 4.9	1.0 ± 0.0	5 : 4	12.2 ± 0.39	not assessed		not assessed	
CAPD <2	60.0 ± 4.5	62.8 ± 3.2	0.8 ± 0.2	3 : 7	–	not assessed		–	
Predialysis	50.5 ± 5.3	65.6 ± 4.3	–	4 : 4	–	not assessed		–	

*Weight post dialysis where applicable

Table 2 Correlation matrix of tendon size, age, weight and length of HD of each tendon estimate in long-term HD patients (asymptomatic and amyloid-proven) and tendon size, age and weight in controls (grouped, n = 27). Statistical significance as shown

	Symptomatic Age (years)	Symptomatic Weight (kg)	Symptomatic Length of HD (years)	Asymptomatic Age (years)	Asymptomatic Weight (kg)	Asymptomatic Length of HD (years)	Controls Age (years)	Controls Weight (kg)
LHB (R)	–0.37	0.02	–0.16	–0.05	0.51*	–0.03	0.20	0.31
LHB (L)	0.23	–0.13	–0.03	0.15	0.53*	–0.29	0.21	0.51**
SS (R)	–0.21	–0.29	–0.26	–0.23	0.41	0.31	0.09	0.23
SS (L)	–0.37	0.13	–0.22	–0.11	0.30	–0.17	0.14	0.39*

*p <0.05, **p <0.01

Table 3 Results of ultrasound examination of the shoulder joints in all patients

	Long-term HD Proven amyloid (n = 10)	Asymptomatic (n = 17)	p[1]	Controls HD <2 (n = 9)	CAPD <2 (n = 10)	Predialysis (n = 8)	p[1]
SS (R)	7.4 ± 0.7	5.1 ± 0.2	0.001	5.0 ± 0.6	5.4 ± 0.3	5.4 ± 0.4	0.03, 0.02, 0.06
SS (L)	6.7 ± 0.7	4.9 ± 0.2	0.01	5.1 ± 0.4	5.0 ± 0.2	5.1 ± 0.3	0.07, 0.03, 0.08
LHB (R)	140.0 ± 11.1	79.6 ± 5.1	<0.001	76.9 ± 8.4	76.8 ± 6.4	95.4 ± 14.1	<0.001, <0.001, 0.02
LHB (L)	114.7 ± 10.5	80.8 ± 5.4	0.004	72.4 ± 5.6	90.9 ± 6.4	99.7 ± 13.1	0.003, 0.07, 0.39
Bursae (patients per group)	5	1	0.006	1	1	0	0.15, 0.05, <0.02

SS: supraspinatus tendon (diameter, mm), LHB: long head of biceps tendon (area, mm^2), (R) (L): right and left side, [1]: p values represent comparison of group results with "proven amyloid" group in each case.

Control groups: Three control groups were used: HD <2 years (n = 9), CAPD <2 years (n = 10), predialysis (n = 8).

No patient had amyloid as their primary illness, nor any other disease known to be associated with other types of amyloid deposition.

Ultrasound: A conventional ultrasound scanner (Toshiba SSA-90A 7.5 mega-hertz) was used. All measurements were performed on the same machine by one operator who was unaware of patient details. Joint parameters were recorded only after three consistent values for each tendon had been obtained.

Specifications: Linear array, 64-element, 57 mm field of view. Maximum depth required: 3 cm, with no standoff. Dynamic near-field focusing technique with two-fold magnification used.

Long head of biceps and supraspinatus tendons were chosen within the rotator cuff group. These two tendons had previously been found to be the most accessible thereby allowing reproducible measurements.

Long head of biceps: Position: shoulder in adduction, elbow flexion, wrist clenched.

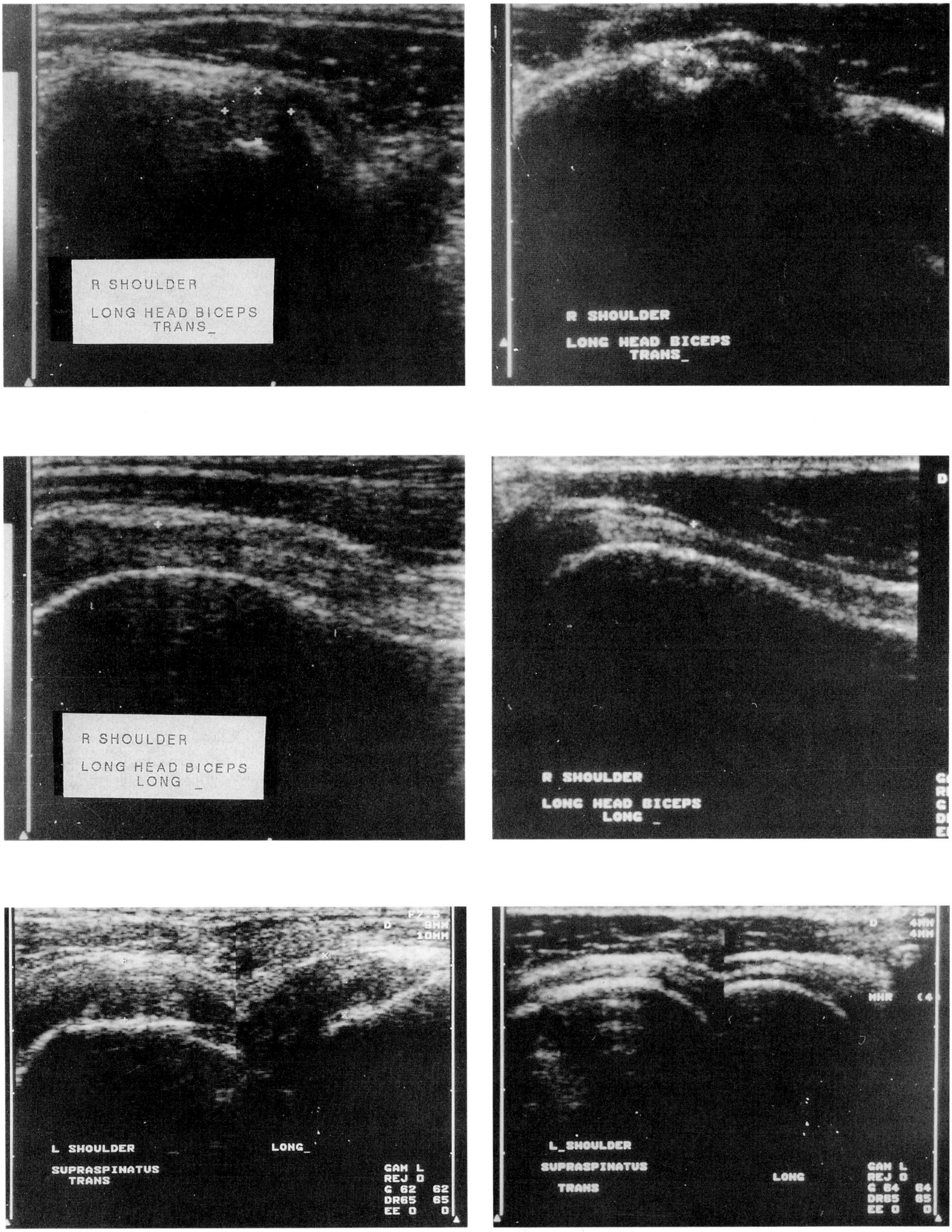

Fig. 1 Ultrasonographic images of LHB (upper photographs, transverse view; middle, longitudinal view) and SS (lower photographs) tendons in long-term HD patients. Patients with proven amyloid are on the left, asymptomatic patients on the right. Long head of biceps tendon is delineated at bicipital notch in upper photographs. (Calibration points at the sides are at 1 cm intervals.)

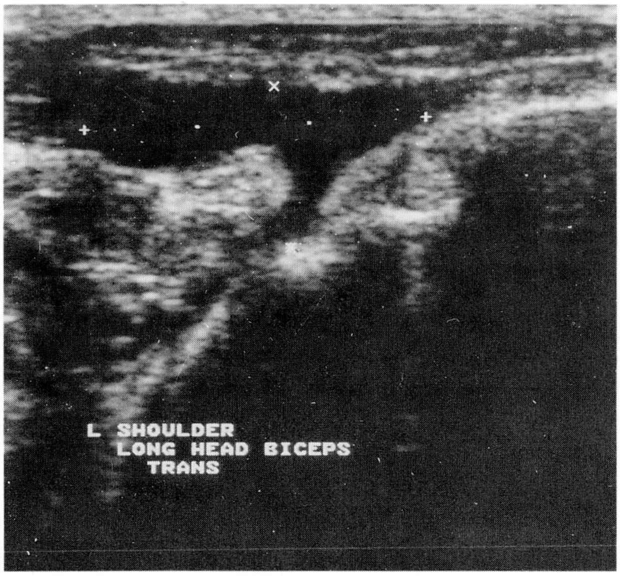

Fig. 2 Deltoid bursa (LHB, transverse view) in patient with symptomatic amyloid, with dimensions as indicated.

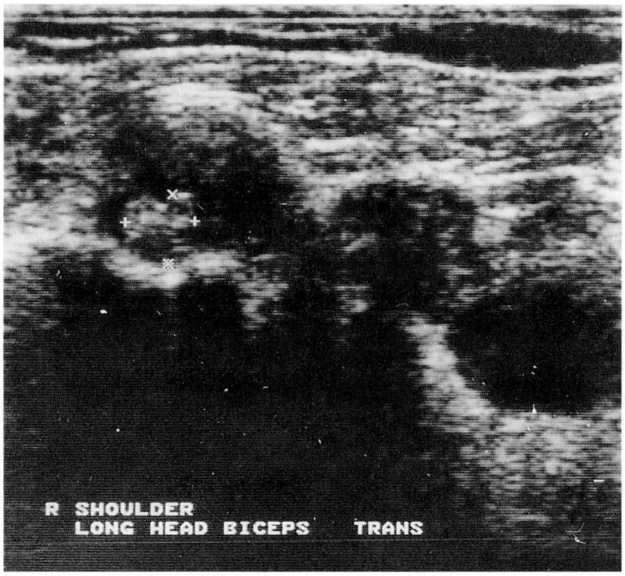

Fig. 3 View of LHB (transverse view) in patient with symptomatic amyloid, indicating large tissue deposits in relation to head of humerus.

View: (a) transverse: level of bicipital groove. 30–40° downtilt anterior approach. Transverse (tdt) and vertical (vdt) diameters were measured. View sufficiently wide to show peritendinous tissue and bursae.

View: (b) longitudinal: at right angles to (a), same arm position. Vertical diameter (vdl) measured.

Supraspinatus. Position: shoulder in abduction to 45° with elbow bent and hand behind back to expose tendon beneath acromion.

View: (a) transverse: probe moved posteriorly and superiorly to head of humerus immediately behind posterior ridge of bicipital groove. Approached at an angle of 45–60°. Measurements of tendon diameter (dt) taken at mid-point of parallel region between symmetrical lateral narrowing of tendon.

View: (b) sagittal: view taken and diameter (ds) measured at point where tendon emerges beneath acromial shadow.

Computations: Long head of biceps: vertical diameters in transverse (vdt) and longitudinal (vdl) views were averaged (vdt + vdl/2). Cross sectional area of biceps tendon was approximated to an ellipse and calculated according to the standard formula: $\pi[(vdt + vdl/2) \times dt]$.

Supraspinatus: measurements of tendon diameters were averaged (dt + ds/2).

Statistics: All results are expressed as mean ± SEM except where otherwise indicated. Statistical comparisons were made using the Student's unpaired *t* test and by Pearson Correlation. Significant differences were defined by a p value <0.05.

Results

There was no significant difference between the study groups for bodyweight (post dialysis), sex, length of time of HD, number of hours HD per week, fistula side or handedness. Control groups also did not differ significantly from the asymptomatic study group for age, weight and sex, nor from the amyloid group for weight and sex (Table 1).

Patients with proven amyloid were significantly older than asymptomatic patients (64 ± 3 vs 42 ± 3, $p < 0.001$), however no correlation was found between age and tendon size for either group (Table 2). No correlation was observed either between tendon size and length of hemodialysis. Tendon size did show some relationship however to bodyweight in the asymptomatic group, and when controls were treated as a single group (n = 27) a similar correlation was also observed (Table 2).

Long-term HD patients showed no clear relationship between the presence of symptomatic amyloid and length of HD, although four of nine patients who had dialysed eleven years or more had symptoms compared with six of eighteen patients on dialysis for less than eleven years.

Diameter of supraspinatus tendon, estimated area of long head of biceps tendon and prevalence of bursae within the shoulder joint were all significantly greater in the proven amyloid group than in the asymptomatic long-term HD group (Table 3, Figures 1 and 2). For those with proven amyloid, most parameters were also significantly greater than control groups. There was no appreciable difference in any measurement between control groups and asymptomatic long-term HD patients. Tendon abnormalities were not observed within the latter group for any tendon, measurements in all patients being within two standard deviations of the calculated mean (data not shown).

In addition to tendon changes, large tissue deposits were seen in two patients. In each case these were adjacent to the LHB tendon, and were best demonstrated on transverse views (Figure 3). In contrast to the relatively high incidence of bursae (50%) within the amyloid group only three of forty-seven patients (6%) otherwise displayed bursae, and two of these had previously suffered trauma to the shoulder joint. Bursae were also best seen on transverse view of LHB (Figure 2).

Within the control groups the following mean (± SD) tendon sizes were found. SS: 5.0 ± 0.8 mm (L); 5.2 ± 1.4 (R). LHB: 27.6 ± 8.6 mm^2 (L), 26.2 ± 8.5 (R). Defining an abnormal test as at least 2 tendons greater than the mean ± 2 SD or at least one tendon plus a bursal sac, 7 of the 10 proven amyloid patients displayed positive tests, indicating a sensitivity of about 70%.

Discussion

The study demonstrates significant differences in ultrasonographic findings between symptomatic patients with proven DRA and similar asymptomatic patients. There were no obvious differences between study groups except that those with proven amyloid were older. No correlation between age and tendon size was observed within either study group nor in controls. In addition, a recent report [Van Ypersele de Strihou et al. 1990] has demonstrated a relationship between age and DRA irrespective of the length of dialysis or type of membrane used. It seems unlikely therefore that the observed increase in tendon size was simply a result of aging although this cannot be excluded.

Some relationship was found between LHB tendon size and bodyweight in both long-term asymptomatic HD patients and controls. This was not observed, perhaps because of amyloid deposition, in the symptomatic group.

It has been convincingly demonstrated [Laurent et al. 1988] that the onset of symptoms due to DRA is directly related to the duration of HD. In our study, tendon size did not show a correlation with length of HD. This might be because, in contrast to other studies, the current analysis is restricted to patients on HD for between seven and fifteen years. Although there was some trend towards longer duration of dialysis in symptomatic patients it was not statistically significant. This is in contrast to recent similar work [Jadoul et al. 1990], and might be partly explained by the limited numbers (n = 10) in our study.

It is possible that ultrasonographic assessment of increased tendon size, particularly in symptomatic patients, is related to factors other than just amyloid deposition. Depierreux et al. [1988] and others [Ogawa et al. 1990], for instance, have demonstrated an inflammatory process in histological sections of amyloid deposits, indicating there might be an inflammatory component to DRA in some cases. Tendon diameters in patients with symptoms could be related to varying degrees of inflammation as well as amyloid infiltration.

Large tissue deposits were seen in two of the three patients who had been previously diagnosed with amyloid (Figure 3), one of whom demonstrated positive staining for amyloid after shoulder joint aspiration. We believe these deposits are likely to be composed of amyloid. The presence of bursae was also more pronounced in the symptomatic group and could allow confirmation of DRA where required by needle aspiration.

It is unclear why asymptomatic long-term HD patients did not show some increase in tendon diameter when compared with controls. It is possible, though not proven, that the asymptomatic patients involved in the study were free from significant amyloid deposition, as marked individual differences in the rate of symptomatic amyloid deposition have been described [Laurent et al. 1988]. Although ultrasonic scanning does not allow specific identificaton of tissues, sequential studies of the same patients over several years may contribute to understanding the pathogenesis of symptomatic amyloid deposition.

The place of joint aspiration as a routine means of detecting amyloid tissue is uncertain. Patients with symptoms were readily identified as having DRA by this technique, however in the eight of the seventeen asymptomatic patients who had consented to joint aspiration no tissue was able to be obtained, despite multiple attempts in most patients. As alluded to above, it is not known if this group were free from amyloid or whether the technique is unsatisfactory for detecting asymptomatic aymloid infiltration of a focal nature similar to that reported in patients with longstanding symptoms [Flöege et al. 1989], although Flöege's three patients were all symptomatic and had radiological abnormalities. More invasive diagnostic tissue sampling was precluded in our patients because of ethical considerations.

Although sensitivity was calculated at around 70%, this is an approximation because of the limited numbers (n = 10). Because it is unknown whether some asymptomatic patients had DRA, an estimate of specificity could not be determined.

At present there is only scant reference to shoulder ultrasound of DRA in the literature [Van Ypersele de Strihou et al. 1988, Jadoul et al. 1990]. This study suggests it might be of use in monitoring long-term dialysis patients to predict the development of DRA without invasive tissue sampling and to assess response to modalities of treatment.

REFERENCES

Depierreux M, Goldman M, Fayt I, Richard C, Quintin J, Dhaene M, Van Herweghem J-L 1988 Osteoarticular amyloidosis associated with haemodialysis: an immunoultrastructural study. J Clin Pathol *41:* 158–162

Flöege J, Nonnast-Daniel B, Gielow P, Brandis A, Spindler E, Hundeshagen H, Koch KM, Shaldon S 1989 Specific imaging of dialysis-related amyloid deposits using ^{131}I-beta-2-microglobulin. Nephron *51:* 444–447

Hawkins PN, Lavender JP, Myers MJ, Pepys MB 1988 Diagnostic Radionuclide Imaging of Amyloid: Biological targeting by circulating human serum amyloid P component. Lancet *i:* 1413–1418

Jadoul M, Malghem J, Van de Berg B, Van Ypersele C 1990 Ultrasonographic detection of thickened joint capsules and tendons: an early marker of dialysis related amyloidosis (DRA)? XIth International Congress of Nephrology. Abstracts. p 18 A

Kleinmann KS, Coburn JW 1989 Amyloid syndromes associated with hemodialysis (Editorial). Kidney Int *35:* 567–575

Laurent G, Calemard E, Charra B 1988 Dialysis related amyloidosis. Kidney Int *33 (Suppl. 24):* S 32 – S 34

Ogawa H, Ono M, Saito A 1990 X-ray and histological analysis of cystic radiolucent lesions of bones in patients with dialysis related amyloidosis. XIth International Congress of Nephrology Abstracts, p 206

Sethi D, Naunton Morgan TC, Brown EA, Jewkes RF, Gower PE 1990 Technetium-99-Labelled Methylene diphosphanate uptake scans in patients with dialysis arthropathy. Nephron *54:* 202–207

Van Ypersele de Strihou C, Honhon B, Vandenbrouke JM, Huaux JP, Noel H, Maldague B 1988 Dialysis amyloidosis. In: *Grundfeld J-P, Bach JF, Crosnier J, Funck-Brentano J-L, Maxwell MH* (eds). Advances in Nephrology® from the Necker Hospital. Volume 17 Year Book Medical Publishers, Inc.

Van Ypersele de Strihou C, Jadoul M, Jamart F, Noel H and the Working Party on Dialysis Amyloidosis 1990 Age is an important determinant of dialysis related amyloidosis (DRA). XIth International Congress of Nephrology Abstracts, p 205 A

LETTERS TO THE EDITOR

Nephropathia epidemica in a patient with renal transplant

Sir, – recently we read with interest a case report on acute interstitial nephritis caused by herpes simplex virus in a renal allograft [Silbert et al. 1990]. Last year we treated a patient with renal transplant who had nephropathia epidemica, the Scandinavian type of hemorrhagic fever with renal syndrome caused by Puumala virus. As we found no document in the literature on this kind of clinical experience, we want to report on our patient.

The patient was a 38-year-old Finnish male who had terminal uremia due to congenital bladder atony and hydronephrosis. In 1978 chronic hemodialysis treatment was begun, and a successful renal transplantation was performed in the same year. From then on his serum creatinine was in the range of 100–120 μmol/l and urinalysis was continuously normal. He was normotensive without medication. Immunosuppression included azathioprine 150 mg per day and methylprednisolone 6 mg every other day.

In July 1989 the patient was admitted to hospital with temperature up to 39.3° C for five days. Other symptoms were headache, arthralgia, myalgia and transiently blurred vision. The patient had also noticed slightly reduced urine volume.

In hospital fever subsided after four days. One week after admission he had polyuria up to 6520 ml/24 hours and during polyuria the weight loss was 4.6 kg. Blood pressure was continuously normal.

Serum creatinine rose to 248 μmol/l and urinalysis revealed transient proteinuria (1.04 g/24 hours) and microscopic hematuria. The patient had transient anemia (hemoglobin 110 g/l), leukocytosis (12,900/mm^3) and thrombocytopenia (70/mm^3). The ESR rose to 52 mm/hour and C-reactive protein to 77 mg/l. Urine and blood cultures for bacteria were repeatedly negative.

Chest X ray and ultrasound examination of renal allograft yielded normal findings. Fine-needle aspiration biopsy [Pasternack 1968] did not show acute rejection; some solitary activated lymphocytes and plasma cells probably associated with the acute infection were seen in the aspirate.

By using immunofluorescence assay a clear seroconversion in Puumala virus antibody titer was observed. There was a fourfold rise (80–320) in antibody titer in samples taken on the 7th and 17th days after onset of clinical symptoms.

The patient recovered completely. Antibiotics were not administered and previous immunosuppressive medication was continued. At a control visit three weeks later the patient was in good condition. Serum creatinine was 117 μmol/l and urinalysis was normal.

The symptoms of our patient, fever, headache and blurred vision as well as transient thrombocytopenia, are very typical of nephropathia epidemica [Lähdevirta et al. 1984, Settergren et al. 1988]. The clinical course of the renal disease was also strongly suggestive of acute interstitial nephritis caused by Puumala virus. The diagnosis was serologically confirmed. Acute nephritis caused only transient deterioration of renal function. Transplant rejection was not observed. We thus believe that our patient had acute nephropathia epidemica infection, also affecting his renal allograft.

To our knowledge nephropathia epidemica in a patient with renal transplant has not previously been described. Previous reports on virus-caused nephritis in a renal allograft include cytomegalovirus [Cameron et al. 1982], Epstein-Barr virus [Griffiths et al. 1980], varicella zoster virus [Bourbigot et al. 1986], and herpes simplex virus [Silbert et al. 1990]. According to the experience of the present case Puumala virus should also be added to this list. In transplanted patients with acute nephritic syndrome viral diseases should be taken into account in the differential diagnosis of acute rejection. Some viruses such as cytomegalovirus can even induce acute rejection.

J. Mustonen[1], *H. Saha*[1], *A. Pasternack*[1], *M. Brummer-Korvenkontio*[2]
[1] Department of Clinical Sciences, University of Tampere, Teiskontie 35, SF-33520 Tampere, Finland
[2] Department of Virology, University of Helsinki, Haartmaninkatu 3, SF-00290 Helsinki, Finland

REFERENCES

Bourbigot B, Quillen MC, Airiau J, Hardy E, Quiserix J, Leroy JP, Cledes J, Chastel C 1986 Renal failure in the course of reactivation of varicella-zoster virus infection in a renal transplant recipient. J Infection *13:* 159–162

Cameron J, Rigby RJ, van Deth AG, Petrie JJB 1982 Severe tubulo-interstitial disease in a renal allograft due to cytomegalovirus infection. Clin Nephrol *18:* 321–325

Griffiths PD, Lechler RI, Edwards JBM 1980 Primary Epstein-Barr virus infection associated with a rejection episode in a human renal allograft recipient. Clin Nephrol *13:* 296–297

Lähdevirta J, Savola J, Brummer-Korvenkontio M, Berndt R, Illikainen R, Vaheri A 1984 Clinical and serological diagnosis of Nephropathia epidemica, the mild type of haemorrhagic fever with renal syndrome. J Infection *9:* 230–238

Pasternack A 1968 Fine-needle aspiration biopsy of human renal homografts. Lancet *2:* 82–84

Settergren B, Juto P, Trollfors B, Wadell G, Norrby SR 1988 Hemorrhagic complications and other clinical findings in Nephropathia Epidemica in Sweden: a study of 355 serologically verified cases. J Infect Dis *157:* 380–382

Silbert PL, Matz LR, Christiansen K, Saker BM, Richardson M 1990 Herpes simplex virus interstitial nephritis in a renal allograft. Clin Nephrol *33:* 264–268

Comment on Huttunen K, Grönhagen-Riska C and Fyhrquist F, 1989 Enalapril treatment of a nursing mother with slightly impaired renal function. Clin Nephrol *31:* 278.

Dear Sir, – Huttunen et al. described the measurement of enalaprilat levels (active moiety of enalapril) in serum and breast milk of three hypertensive women [1989], one of whom had impaired renal function. Using a competitive inhibitor binding assay, enalaprilat concentrations were determined in these women both before and four hours after 5 and 10 mg doses of enalapril. There was no detectable enalaprilat in the breast milk. However, these investigators did not measure unchanged enalapril which would presumably be better absorbed by the infant than would enalaprilat. Although it is possible that infants, in contrast to adults, may absorb enalaprilat, it is likely that enalapril is the analyte of greater interest. We would like to report a case in which we assayed serum, urine and breast milk for enalapril and enalaprilat.

A 31-year old caucasian woman had been receiving 10 mg enalapril once daily for essential hypertension for 11 months. At the time of study she was 12 months postpartum. After ingesting 10 mg of enalapril (24 hours after the previous dose), timed serum samples were obtained as well as a 24-hour collection of both breast milk and urine. Samples were analyzed by radioimmunoassay [Hichens et al.] (lower limit for detection of serum enalaprilat is 0.4 ng/ml). Enalapril is routinely analyzed as enalaprilat following hydrolysis but the usual enzymatic method of hydrolysis (normal rat serum or rat liver homogenate) was not satisfactory in the presence of breast milk. Hydrolysis of enalapril in breast milk was achieved by incubating the samples overnight at room temperatur with a one third volume of 1 N NaOH. In breast milk, the detection limit for unchanged enalaprilat plus the increment due to hydrolysis of enalapril was 1.2 ng/ml. Standards and quality control samples were assayed in normal breast milk to maintain a constant matrix.

Serum

Time after dosing (hr)	Enalaprilat ng/ml	Enalapril ng/ml
0	4.9	0.0
1	5.0	5.8
2	8.4	30.0
3	18.1	22.7
4	24.8	14.3
6	32.1	2.1
8	30.6	0
12	23.8	0
24	6.3	0

Breast milk

Time after dosing (hr)	Vol. (ml)	Enalaprilat Concentration (ng/ml)	Enalaprilat Quantity (ng)	Enalapril Concentration (ng/ml)	Enalapril Quantity (ng)
Prestudy	13	0.57	7.4	0.63*	8.2*
4	18	0.55	9.9	2.05	36.9
8.75	15	0.75	11.3	1.85	27.8
24	11	0.68	7.5	0.82	9.0
Total	57		36.1		81.9

*Marginal accuracy due to the 1.2 mg/ml detection limit for enalaprilat plus enalapril.

Results for the patient's serum and breast milk are given in the table below. Urinary clearance of enalaprilat in this patient was as expected.

Fifty-seven milliliters of breast milk were collected in the study period containing at most 82 ng of enalapril and 36 ng of enalaprilat; the dosage to the infant is probably clinically insignificant [Biollaz et al. 1982]. Even younger infants consuming larger volumes of breast milk would receive an exceedingly small dose. Our data in this single patient suggest, however, that enalapril may be more efficiently secreted in breast milk than enalaprilat and that studies to address this issue should include measurement of both enalapril and enalaprilat levels.

An additional case has recently been published by Redman et al., confirming the low enalaprilat levels measured by Dr. Fyhrquist and the enalaprilat and enalapril levels detected by our laboratory [Redman et al. 1990]. Similar conclusions have been reported with respect to benazepril, a new ACE inhibitor [Kaiser et al. 1989].

Janet E. Rush, M. D.; Dianne L. Snyder, B. A.
Andrea Barrish, B. S.; Martin Hichens, D. Phil.

REFERENCES

Huttunen K, Grönhagen-Riska C, Fyhrquist FF 1989 Enalapril treatment of nursing mother with slightly impaired renal function. Clin Nephrol *31:* 278

Hichens M, Hand EL, Mulcahy WS Radioimmunoassay for angiotensin converting enzyme inhibitors. Ligand Quarterly, *4:* 43

Biollaz J, Schelling JL, Jacot des Combes B et al. 1982 Enalapril maleate and a lysine analogue (MK 521) in normal volunteers; relationship between plasma drug levels and the renin angiotensin system. Br J Clin Pharmacol *14:* 363–368

Redman CWG, Kelly JG, Cooper WD 1990 The excretion of enalapril and enalaprilat in breast milk. Eur J Clin Pharmacol *38:* 99

Kaiser G, Ackermann R, Dieterle W, Fleiss PM 1989 Benazepril and benazeprilat in human plasma and breast milk. Eur J Clin Pharmacol *36:* Suppl A303J

Evaluating the recirculation in hemodialysis without peripheral venipuncture

Sir, – Pederson [Pederson et al. 1990 Clin Nephrol *33:* 203–206] recently described a "two needle calculation" of recirculation in hemodialysis. The method required however a short (15 minutes) prolongation of the dialysis session and does not seem to be adequate for repeated measurement. We evaluated another method, also eliminating the necessity of puncturing a peripheral vein, and suitable for multiple determinations in the same patient. In 50 instances, recirculation (R1) was calculated either according to the classical formula using urea concentrations in arterial (Ua), venous blood lines (Uv), and in a peripheral vein (Up), or (R2) using (Up') instead of (Up): (Up') is the urea concentration in the blood drawn from the arterial line after the blood pump has been switched off for one minute, then turned on at a 50 ml/min flow rate for another minute [Gibson et al. 1990 Reproducible measurement of recirculation without peripheral venipuncture Kidney Int *37 (1):* 297 a].

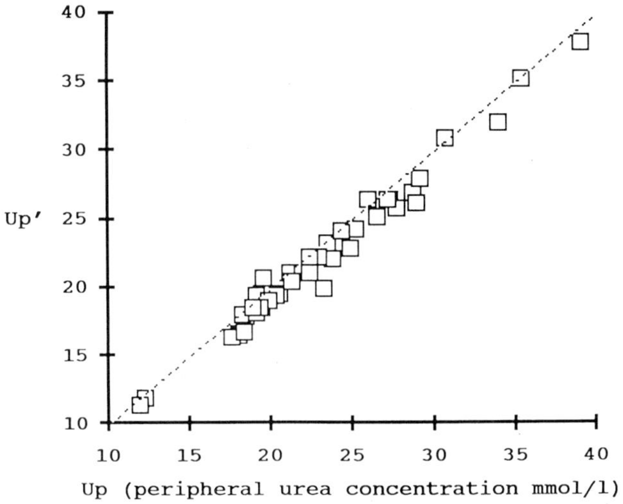

Fig. 1

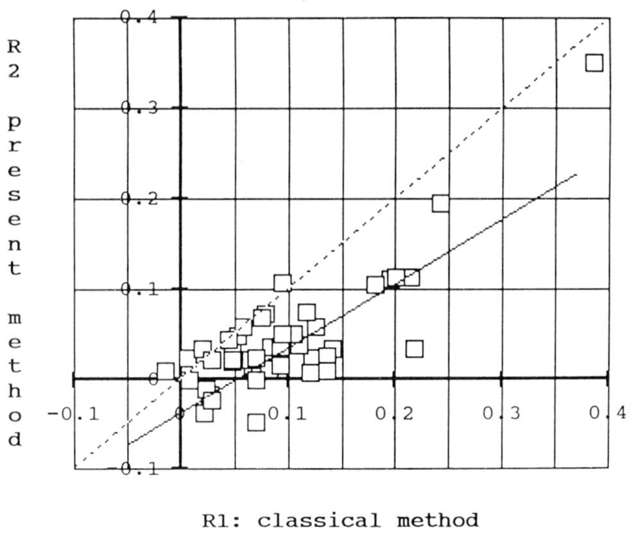

Fig. 2

An excellent correlation was evident between both measurements of peripheral urea (Up' = 0.035 + 0.966 · Up, r = 0.988, $p < 0.001$, Figure 1) and both values of fractional recirculation: R2 = – 0.025 + 0.734 · R1, r = 0.812, $p < 0.001$ (Figure 2). The value of recirculation was underestimated by R2 (mean difference R2–R1 = 0.052 ± 0.044). However, assuming that a 15% level of recirculation is unacceptable, a value of R2 = 10% correctly classified 97.7% of cases with R1 <15% and 83.3% of cases with R1 >15% (Figure 2).

The method proposed by Pederson appears to reflect R1 more precisely than the present one. However intraindividual variation of recirculation is quite high [Gibson et al. 1990]. Besides obvious factors such as different puncture sites and various flow rates, emphasis should be made on the precision of measuring urea concentration; using common values of Ua = 20, Uv = 8, Up = 21 mmoles/l, it can be easily calculated that, given the usual 5% precision on Up or Ua, the calculated recirculation rate ranges from 0 to 15%. Therefore, the accuracy of the method calculating the rate of recirculation appears less crucial than initially thought.

In practice, measuring recirculation can be used for several purposes: 1) to evaluate hemodialyzed patients with unsatisfactory results in term of clearances of small molecules; 2) to yield realistic values of blood flow rate in prescribing dialysis on the basis of urea kinetics; 3) to regularly evaluate the blood access. While in the first case, permanently and markedly elevated levels of recirculation are suspected and would be evidenced by a single measurement, in the others, the clinician might better rely on multiple determinations. In this regard, the method described here appears convenient and in any case well accepted by the patient.

N. Hosni, A. Caillette, S. Baretto, E. Gimenez, M. Labeeuw
Service de Nephrologie, Hôpital E. Herriot, Place d' Arsonval, Lyon Cedex 3, France

ANNOUNCEMENTS

The **International Workshop on Alport Syndrome** will take place August 23–24, 1991 in Oulu, Finland. The objective of this workshop is to give a concise picture of the clinical aspects of Alport syndrome. The workshop will also cover the new available approaches for diagnosis. It will be of interest to nephrologists, pathologists, clinical geneticists and to molecular biologists specializing in kidney disease and basement membranes.

Deadline for application is July 1, 1991. Please contact Secretariat, International Workshop on Alport Syndrome, Biocenter and Department of Biochemistry, University of Oulu, SF-90570 Oulu, Finland, Tel: 358–81–352355, Fax: 358–81–352356.

The **VIth International Congress on Nutrition and Metabolism in Renal Disease** will be held August 26–30, 1991 in Harrogate, UK. Topics will include all aspects of nutrition and metabolism in relation to acute and chronic renal disease, with State of the Art lectures, free communications, posters and debates.

For further information, contact Dr. A. Meguid El Nahas (UK Organizing Secretary), Sheffield Kidney Institute, Northern General Hospital, Herries Road, Sheffield S5 7AU, UK. Tel.: 0742-434343 (ext 4017), Fax: 0742-560472.

The **XXVIIIth Congress of the European Dialysis and Transplant Association – European Renal Association** (EDTA/ERA) will be held in Belgrade, Yugoslavia from September 1 to 4, 1991.

For further information, contact the Organizing Secretariat: Yugotours, Congress, Incentive & Exhibition Department, Djure Djakovića 31, Y-11000 Belgrade, Yugoslavia. Tel.: 3811/763-028, 764-622; Telex: 11000, 12902; Fax: 3811/766-447.

The **22nd Annual Congress of the Nephrology Society** will take place from September 15–18, 1991 in Heidelberg, Germany.

The Nephrology Society will be awarding a prize for the best doctoral thesis dealing with a nephrological theme. Eligible theses and further inquiries should be sent to the following address: Dr. M. Walla, c/o Prof. Ritz, Med. Univ. Clinic/Section of Nephrology, Bergheimerstr. 56a, W-6900 Heidelberg.

The **Second Seminar on Renal Involvement in Systemic Vasculitis** will take place September 21, 1991 in Vimercate, a city near Milan in Italy. Contemporary issues relating to immunopathology of Systemic Lupus Erythematosus, with special regard to anti-endothelial and anti-cardiolipin antibodies, clinicopathological correlations and treatment will be discussed.

For further information please contact Dr. Adalberto Sessa, Unità Operativa di Nefrologia e Dialisi, Ospedale di Vimercate, 20059 Vimercate/Milan, Italy

The **Seventh International Symposium of Nephrology at Montecatini,** October 14–16, 1991. The title of the symposium is "Kidney, Proteins and Drugs". Advances in protein hormones research, proteinuria, proteins and progression of kidney disease and nephrotoxicity of drugs will be discussed.

For further information please contact Dr. Claudio Bianchi, Unita di Nefrologia, Clinica Medica 2, University of Pisa, I-56100 Pisa, Italy. Tel.: 050–592573.

A **Festakt in honor of Priscilla Kincaid-Smith** will be held on November 5–8th, 1991 in Melbourne, Australia. Events will include state of the art lectures and symposia.

For further information contact The Festschrift Organizing Committee, c/o Department of Nephrology, The Royal Melbourne Hospital, Victoria 3050, Australia.

The **IIIrd International Conference on SLE** will be held in the Queen Elizabeth II Conference Centre, Westminster, London, April 13–15, 1992.

For further details, please contact Dr. Graham Hughes or Mrs. Denzil Fletcher, Rheumatology Department, St. Thomas' Hospital, London SE1 7EH. Tel. and Fax: 0163394 22.

The **XXIXth Congress of the European Dialysis and Transplant Association** – European Renal Association (EDTA – ERA) will be held at the Palais des Congrès in Paris, France on June 28 – July 1, 1992. For further information contact Prof. C. Jacobs, Congress President, Service de Néphrologie, Hôpital de la Pitié, 83 bd de l'Hôpital, 75013 Paris, France (Fax: 33144 239984) or the organizing Secretariat: Convergences – EDTA 1992, 120 av. Gambetta, 75020 Paris, France (Fax: 3314030 0165).

The **Third Symposium on Uroradiology** (Imaging and Intervention) will take place August 24–27, 1992 at Herlev Hospital, University of Copenhagen, Denmark.

For further information, please contact Dr. Henrik S. Thomsen, Department of Diagnostic Radiology 54E2, Herlev Hospital, Herlev Ringvej 75, DK-2730 Herlev, Denmark. Tel.: 4544/535300, Ext. 278; Fax: 4544/535332.

The **VIth Congress of the International Society for Peritoneal Dialysis** will take place October 1–4, 1992 in Thessaloniki, Greece.

For additional information write to the First Department of Internal Medicine, AHEPA University Hospital, 54636 Thessaloniki, Greece. Tel. and Fax: (3031) 214606.

Clinical Nephrology, Vol. 35 No. 6 – 1991 (237–242)

Effect of dietary proteins and lipids in patients with membranous nephropathy and nephrotic syndrome

G. D'Amico[1], G. Remuzzi[2], G. Maschio[3], M. G. Gentile[1], E. Gotti[2], L. Oldrizzi[3], G. Manna[1], G. Mecca[2], C. Rugiu[3] and G. Fellin[1]

[1] *Division of Nephrology, S. Carlo Hospital, Milano, Italy*
[2] *Division of Nephrology, Ospedali Riuniti and Mario Negri Institute, Bergamo, Italy*
[3] *Department of Nephrology, University of Verona, Italy*

Abstract. Twenty-four patients with idiopathic membranous nephropathy, long-lasting nephrotic syndrome and serum creatinine <2 mg/dl ate sequentially, in a randomized cross-over design, a normal protein diet containing 1.1 ± 0.3 g/kg/day of proteins and a low protein diet containing 0.7 ± 0.1 g/kg/day of protein, each diet for a period of 3 months. Both diets were low in fat (<30% of total calories) and cholesterol (<200 mg/day) content and rich in polyunsaturated fatty acids and in linoleic acid (10% of energy). Random assignment to one of the two 3 month diet periods was done after a RUN-IN period of at least one month on the hypolipidic normal protein diet. Glomerular filtration rate (inulin clearance), 24 hour urinary protein loss and serum albumin concentration did not significantly differ at the end of the two diet periods, indicating that long-term restriction of protein intake does not modify GFR or urinary protein loss in nephrotic patients. Serum total and LDL-cholesterol and daily proteinuria were significantly lower at the end of both diet periods than at the beginning and at the end of the RUN-IN period. We suggest that these changes were a consequence of the manipulation of dietary fat intake.

Key words: nephrotic syndrome – hyperlipidemia – dietary manipulation

Introduction

For many years, high protein diets were used for management of nephrotic patients in the hope that albumin synthesis and serum albumin concentration could be increased [Blainey et al. 1954, Coggins 1982]. However, it has been well known since the first observation reported by Farr [1938] that when nephrotic patients are fed a diet rich in protein, urinary protein excretion increases but serum protein concentration does not. More recently, since it has become apparent that progression of some renal diseases may be slowed down by a low protein diet, the effect of dietary protein intake on albumin homeostasis in nephrotic animals and humans has been investigated more carefully. Kaysen et al. [1986, 1989] have demonstrated that in nephrotic patients and in experimental nephrosis reduction of dietary proteins reduces the rate of albumin synthesis, but plasma albumin concentration increases significantly because of a concomitant reduction in urinary albumin loss that occurs on the low protein diet, offsetting the reduced rate of albumin synthesis. The reduction of urinary albumin loss in nephrotic patients without concomitant decrease in serum albumin by feeding low protein diets has been confirmed in short-term experiments [Kaysen et al. 1986, Rosenberg et al. 1987, Olmer et al. 1989]. No studies are available so far about the long-term effects of reducing dietary proteins in patients with nephrotic syndrome. In particular, we do not know whether a reduction in dietary protein from a normal content to the lowest limit that can be prescribed without risk as a chronic regimen would reproduce the beneficial effects observed in animals or in humans treated for a few days. In the present study in nephrotic patients with idiopathic membranous nephropathy we wanted to investigate: 1) whether a long-term regimen of low protein intake, from normal to 0.6 g/kg/day, reduces proteinuria; 2) whether such a regimen has any influence on parameters of renal function; 3) whether dietary intervention will influence the lipid abnormalities that usually accompany nephrotic syndrome and might expose patients to major cardiovascular complications.

Received July 9, 1990; in revised form January 2, 1991.

Reprint requests to Prof. G. D'Amico, Division of Nephrology, S. Carlo Hospital, via Pio II, 3-20153 Milano, Italy

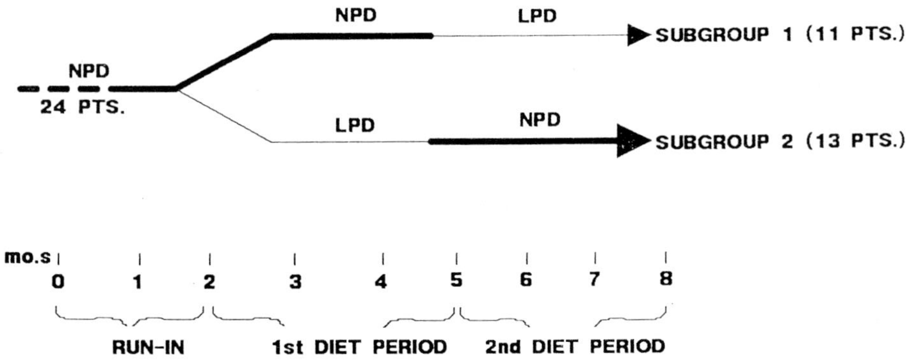

Fig. 1 Schematic representation of the study protocol.
—— Normal protein diet (NPD) = 1.3 g/kg/day of proteins.
—— Low protein diet (LPD) = 0.6 g/kg/day of proteins.

Methods

Patient population

Twenty-four patients, 14 men and 10 women, with biopsy proven primary membranous glomerulopathy were studied. Mean age was 52.8 ± 14.9 years. Admission criteria were proteinuria in the nephrotic range (>3 g/24 hrs) for at least three months before entry into the study and normal or slightly reduced renal function (serum creatinine <2 mg/dl; creatinine clearance >50 ml/min). Patients who had been treated with steroids, immunosuppressive drugs, non-steroidal anti-inflammatory drugs or ACE-inhibitors in the last three months were excluded. For hypertensive patients, the only drug regimen used included diuretics and/or calcium antagonists. Informed consent was obtained prior to entry into the study.

Study protocol

Three sequential study periods were scheduled (Figure 1). The initial period of observation, ranging from 30 to 60 days (RUN-IN PERIOD), was established to assess the patient's renal function, nutritional status and compliance, to correct fluid retention, if any, and to control blood pressure when necessary. The patients were given intensive dietary education during this period, changing their protein, calorie and fat intake to the standards corresponding to the normal protein diet (NPD) used in one of the subsequent diet periods (diet compositions are described in detail in the next section).

Baseline evaluations included a complete history, physical examination, blood chemistry (plasma creatinine, urea, glucose, sodium, potassium, chloride, uric acid, calcium, phosphorus, alkaline phosphatase, serum electrophoresis, complete and differential blood count, creatinine clearance, serum lipids, liver function tests), urinalysis, 24 hour urinary protein (standard biuret technique), urea, sodium, potassium, calcium and phosphorus excretion.

As Figure 1 shows, at the end of the RUN-IN PERIOD, patients were randomly allocated either to a three months period on the same diet as in the observation period (NPD PERIOD) or to a low protein diet (LPD PERIOD). Eleven patients (Subgroup 1) were started on NPD and thirteen on LPD (Subgroup 2). At the end of this first period, all patients were crossed over to the alternative diet for three additional months. Therefore, the sequence of the 3 study periods was NPD → LPD → NPD or NPD → NPD → LPD, according to whether they had been first allocated to the low or to the normal protein diet after the RUN-IN period (the diet of the RUN-IN period being actually the same normal protein diet for all patients).

During each of the three experimental periods patients were seen every two weeks by one of us, body weight and blood pressure were recorded and 24 hour proteins excretion, urinary sodium, potassium, calcium, phosphorus and urea excretion were measured and blood chemistry done. At the end of the RUN-IN period and of each diet period renal inulin clearance was determined after an overnight fasting with 3 exactly timed urine collections of about 30 minutes, as previously described [Remuzzi et al. 1989]. The last oral administration of aminoacid-ketoanalogue supplement had been given at meal time the evening preceding the test.

Lipid analysis

Total serum cholesterol and total serum triglyceride concentrations were determined by enzymatic reagents in an autoanalyzer. HDL-cholesterol was determined enzymatically, following precipitation of serum with phosphotungstic acid 0.55 mmol/l and magnesium chloride 25 mmol/l. LDL-cholesterol was calculated as described by Friedwald et al. [1972].

Diet composition

Two isocaloric (30 kcal/kg of ideal body weight (IBW) dietary regimens were employed, differing in amount and quality of proteins: 1) a low proteins diet (LPD) containing 0.6 g/kg/IBW of protein, all of vegetable origin, supplemented by a mixture of essential aminoacids and their ketoanalogues prepared in the proportions proposed by Zimmermann et al. [1979]; 2) a diet containing 1.3 g/kg/IBW day of mixed proteins (0.9 g/kg of animal origin), which is the equivalent of a normal Italian protein diet (NPD) moderately adjusted to compensate for urinary loss of proteins. The nutritional requirements were referred to the patient's ideal body weight according to the Metropolitan Insurance Company diagrams. Both diets were hypolipidic (fat intake less than 30% of total calories), with a high polyunsaturated/saturated (P/S) fatty acid ratio, high linoleic acid (10% of energy) and low cholesterol (<200 mg/day) content. However, the vegetarian diet (LPD) had higher P/S ratio (2.1 vs 1.1) and a lower cholesterol content (nearly zero).

Sodium content was controlled at about 90 mEq/day. Carbohydrate calories were substituted for protein calories in the low protein diet. Patients on the protein restricted diet were given a B vitamin complex tablet and calcium and iron supplementation every day, to provide an adequate intake. Each diet was composed of natural food products and care was taken to give intensive dietary education to the patients. Compliance with the diet was assessed, every 15 days, by means of dietary interviews performed by an expert dietician and by control of urinary phosphate and urea excretions according to the methodology already described [Gentile et al. 1987]. Dietary protein intake was calculated from urinary urea nitrogen by the standard formula of Maroni et al. [1985].

Statistics

Statistical analysis was performed with SPSS/PC package. The results were expressed as means ± standard error (S. E.). The groups' means were compared by the Student t-test for paired samples.

Results

For valid comparison of data, the clinical and laboratory parameters reported in Table 1 were calculated as the mean for the last two weeks determinations at the end of the initial observation period (RUN-IN period) and for the two 3 month-periods of dietetic control, on the low protein diet (LPD period) or the normal protein diet (NPD period). The first determination, performed at the beginning of the observation period, referred to as To, was also recorded for comparison.

Table 1 Values at first observation (To) and at the end of the three study periods for the whole population (24 PTS), with one of both diets (mean ± SE)

	To	End of RUN-IN (a) period	End of LPD (a) period	End of NPD (a) period
Serum creatinine mg/dl	1.16 ± 0.7	1.19 ± 0.1	1.12 ± 0.1	1.27 ± 0.1
Inulin clearance[b]		51.2 ± 4.5	48.2 ± 3.8	46.4 ± 4
Creatinine clearance ml/min		88.5 ± 7.2	88 ± 9.7	85.1 ± 9.1
Total Cholesterol mg/dl	380 ± 26	360 ± 25	284 ± 17***	304 ± 19*
LDL-Cholesterol mg/dl	319 ± 27	306 ± 24	229 ± 15***	251 ± 16*
HDL-Cholesterol mg/dl	47.7 ± 4	49 ± 3	47 ± 3#	56 ± 3*#
Triglycerides mg/dl	237 ± 26	219 ± 24	226 ± 29	209 ± 30
Serum albumin g/dl	2.7 ± 0.1	2.8 ± 0.1	3.0 ± 0.2*	3.1 ± 0.1*
Proteinuria g/day	8.9 ± 1.1	7.9 ± 1.1	5.6 ± 0.8*	5.6 ± 0.8*
Phosphorus excretion mg/day	849 ± 90	812 ± 83	439 ± 50**##	729 ± 50##
Urea excretion g/day	27 ± 2	23 ± 1.5	13.1 ± 0.7***##	22 ± 1.1##
Estimated protein intake g/kg/day	1.4 ± 0.9	1.2 ± 0.2	0.68 ± 0.1	1.1 ± 0.3
Body weight kg	67.7 ± 2	66.5 ± 2	64.7 ± 2**	65.1 ± 2**

* $p \leq 0.01$, ** $p \leq 0.001$, *** $p \leq 0.0001$ in comparison with the end of the RUN-IN

$p \leq 0.01$, ## $p \leq 0.0001$ in comparing LPD vs NPD

[a] The values of the last two determinations of the period were used for each patient (only data for urinary urea excretion refer to the whole observation period)

[b] Data refer only to 18 patients

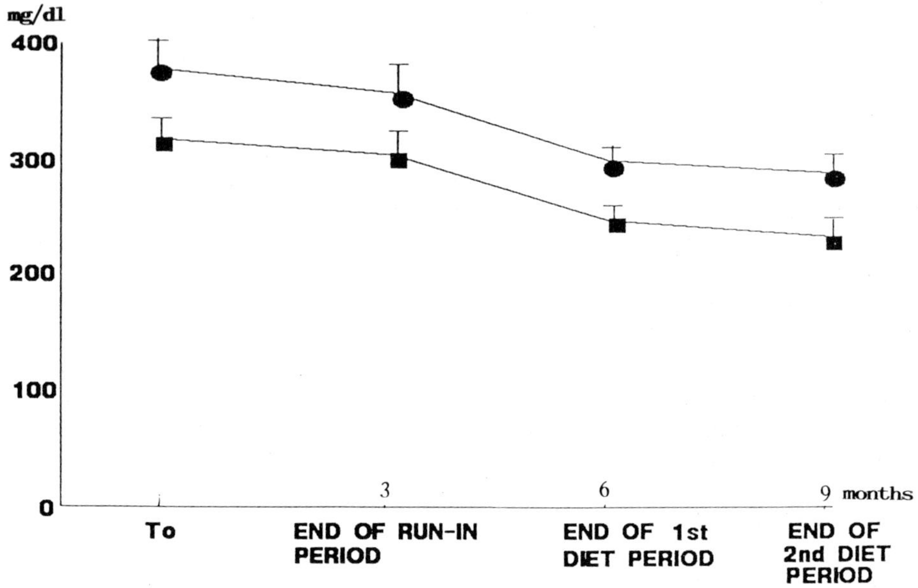

Fig. 2 Serum total cholesterol (●) and LDL-cholesterol (■) (means ± S. E.) in the 24 patients, in chronological sequence from the time of enrollment (To) to the end of the second diet period.

The average protein intake, calculated from urinary urea excretion, was 1.4 ± 0.9 g/kg/day at the time of enrollment in the study, 1.2 ± 0.2 at the end of the RUN-IN period, 0.68 ± 0.1 at the end of the LPD period and 1.1 ± 0.3 at the end of the NPD period, showing that protein intake was comparable at the end of the RUN-IN and of the NPD diet periods, but was significantly lower at the end of the LPD period. Dietary interviews indicated that patients generally had higher fat and cholesterol intake at To than in all three study periods.

Mean serum creatinine level and inulin clearance did not change from baseline values during the two diet periods. Body weight at the end was the same on both diets, but significantly lower than at time To or at the end of the RUN-IN period. No significant differences in blood pressure levels between the RUN-IN period and the two diet periods were observed: Systolic blood pressure was 141.4 ± 6.6 at the end of the RUN-IN period, 137.5 ± 4.9 at the end of the LPD period and 139.5 ± 5.1 at the end of the NPD period; diastolic blood pressure was 85.8 ± 2.7 at the end of the RUN-IN period, 82.7 ± 2.6 at the end of the LPD period and 85.6 ± 2.2 at the end of the NPD period. Such stability of arterial pressure was achieved by giving during the two diet periods a slightly lower dosage of anti-hypertensive and diuretic drugs than at the beginning of the observation period.

Serum concentrations of albumin were comparable in the two diet periods, although for both periods they were slightly but significantly higher than at To and at the end of the RUN-IN period. Similarly, urinary protein excretion was not significantly different at the end of the LPD period and of the NPD period (whichever the sequence of the two diet periods), although for both diet periods the mean 24 hour proteinuria was significantly lower than at the end of the RUN-IN period, and even more than at To, i. e., the time of enrollment of patients.

Serum concentrations of total and LDL-cholesterol were significantly lower at the end of both diet periods than at the start and at the end of the RUN-IN period, while serum concentration of HDL-cholesterol was higher only at the end of the NPD period and triglyceride levels were unchanged. Serum total and LDL cholesterol and triglycerides concentrations were not significantly different at the end of the two 3 month diet periods, although the average concentrations of total and LDL-cholesterol tended to be higher on the NPD. On the contrary, HDL-cholesterol was significantly higher ($P = .002$) at the end of the NPD diet than at the end of the LPD diet. When the mean values of the serum total and LDL-cholesterol concentration in the total population of our patients were plotted according to a chronological sequence (Figure 2), considering consecutively the time of the enrollment, the end of the observation period, the end of first diet period, and the end of the second diet period (whichever the sequence of the protein intake for a single patient) we found a total progressive decrease from 380 ± 26 mg/dl to 289 ± 19 mg/dl for serum total cholesterol and from 319 ± 19 mg/dl to 233 ± 17 for LDL-cholesterol, i. e. a 25% reduction at the end of the 7–8 months total duration of the study.

Discussion

Measurements of urea excretion during the three study periods documented that the patients tended to eat more proteins than prescribed during the LPD period and less than prescribed during NPD. However, protein intake was still effectively reduced during LPD, compared to NPD, by about 35–40% on the average.

The results of the present study did not confirm previous short-term studies that document for both experimental nephrosis [Kaysen et al. 1989, Feehally et al. 1988, Diamond and Karnovsky 1987, Beukers et al. 1988, Motomura et al. 1988] and in nephrotic patients [Kaysen et al. 1986, Rosenberg et al. 1987, Olmer et al. 1989] that reducing the protein content of the diet reduces urinary protein loss. In our 24 patients with nephrotic syndrome and moderately impaired renal function, urinary protein excretion and serum albumin concentration at the end of a 3 month period on a low protein diet were not significantly different from the corresponding values observed at the end of a 3 month period on a normal protein diet, the sequence of the two diet periods being randomly assigned. In the present study, the difference in the protein content of the two diets tested was lower than in the previous quoted studies, and each diet was given for a definitely longer period of time. Moreover, our low protein diet was supplemented with a mixture of essential aminoacids and their ketoanalogues, and we cannot exclude that the administration of these mixtures may have contributed to blunt the anti-proteinuric effect of the low protein diet. No significant changes in glomerular filtration rate were seen on either normal or low protein intake, confirming recent data on the effects of chronic dietary protein intake on renal function in healthy male subjects [Wiegmann et al. 1990].

There were considerable reductions in serum total and LDL-cholesterol during both diet periods, more evident when the protein intake was low (LPD period). There was a significant increase in HDL-cholesterol concentration only at the end of the 3 month period of normal protein intake. It is conceivable that these favourable decreases were due to the manipulation of fat intake of our diets starting at To, a manipulation which was both quantitative (fat intake <30% of caloric intake) and qualitative (high P/S fatty acid ratio, high linoleic acid intake, low cholesterol intake). If this hypothesis is correct, our study offers the first evidence, to our knowledge, that protracted dietary manipulation of lipid intake can be effective in reducing hyper-cholesterolemia, which is considered an important risk factor for cardiovascular complications in patients with long-lasting nephrotic syndrome [Alexander et al. 1974, Curry and Roberts 1977, Mallick and Short 1981]. However, we cannot exclude that the reduction of serum cholesterol found in our study was a consequence of the concomitant reduction of urinary protein loss and increase of serum albumin during both diet periods. Even though correlation of changes in urinary protein loss and serum cholesterol has already been demonstrated in both experimental nephrosis and nephrotic patients [Appel et al. 1985, Kaysen et al. 1987, Wheeler et al. 1989], this alternative hypothesis seems to us less probable, since the increase in serum albumin was very small (0.2–0.3 g/dl) and the decrease in urinary protein excretion was moderate.

This reduction in proteinuria during both diet periods, in comparison with the RUN-IN period, may reflect a spontaneous favourable evolution of the disease, favoured by persistent accurate control of such influencing factors as blood pressure and fluid retention. However, these complicating factors had been corrected at the end of the RUN-IN period, and it is unlikely that the subsequent further decrease in proteinuria during the two diet periods was due to the slight non-significant reduction in the average systolic and diastolic blood pressure from the beginning of the observation period to the end of the study (systolic blood pressure decreased from 143.3 ± 6.3 to 140.9 ± 5.6 and diastolic blood pressure from 86.8 ± 2.6 to 84.3 ± 2.8).

An alternative explanation for the changes in albumin homeostasis seen at the end of both diet periods is that the lipid manipulation of our diets, from the beginning of the observation period to the end of the study, may have contributed to the improvement in the urinary albumin loss through an effect on the permselectivity of the glomerular capillary wall or on the tubular handling of albumin. There are no data in the literature, to our knowledge, on the effect of changes in dietary lipid composition on urinary protein loss in humans. However, three groups of investigators have recently reported that a diet rich in polyunsaturated fatty acids (fish oil or safflower oil) reduced urinary protein loss in rats with subtotal renal ablation [Barcelli et al. 1982, Heifets et al. 1987, Clark et al. 1990]. Fish oil feeding was more effective than severe protein restriction in lessening both the gammaglobulinuria and albuminuria in this remnant nephron model [Clark et al. 1990]. An enhanced renal production of arachidonic acid metabolites via the cyclooxygenase pathway, with a consequent increase in the ratio of vasodilator to vasoconstrictor prostaglandins, has been suggested as one of the potential mechanisms for these effects [Clark et al. 1990].

Our data suggest that quantitative and qualitative modification of fat intake is able to reduce hyper-cholesterolemia even when it is not associated with a drastic reduction in protein intake. In fact, the concomitant increase in serum HDL-cholesterol we achieved by a hypolipidic diet with a normal protein content could be beneficial "per se" to reduce the risk of atherosclerosis, as demonstrated in non-nephrotic patients [Crouse 1989]. Thus, a hypolipidic diet with a moderate reduction in protein intake deserves the future controlled trials necessary to confirm the efficacy of the present approach, at least for correcting the lipid abnormalities of nephrotic syndrome.

Acknowledgements

We thank Farma-Biagini (Pisa, Italy), who kindly provided the capsules of aminoacid and ketoanalogue mixture; S. Cristina Zanoni and Enrica Raschioni for their valuable help with the dietary interviews; S. Mascia Marchesini and Viviana Baretto for their secretarial assistance.

REFERENCES

Alexander JH, Schapel GJ, Edwards KDG 1974 Increased incidence of coronary heart disease associated with combined elevation of serum triglycerides and cholesterol concentrations in the nephrotic syndrome in man. Med J Austr *2:* 119

Appel GB, Blum CB, Chien S, Cumis CL, Appel AS 1985 The hyperlipidemia of the nephrotic syndrome. Relation to plasma albumin concentration, oncotic pressure, and viscosity. N Engl J Med *312:* 1544

Barcelli UO, Weiss M, Pollack VE 1982 Effects of a dietary prostaglandin precursor on the progression of experimentally induced chronic renal failure. J Lab Clin Med *100:* 786

Beukers JJB, Hoedemaeker PJ, Weening JJ 1988 Pharmacological and dietary intervention in experimental models of chronic renal disease. Contrib Nephrol *60:* 101

Blainey JD 1954 High protein diets in the treatment of the nephrotic syndrome. Clin Sci *13:* 567

Clark WF, Parbtani A, Philbrick D, et al. 1990 Comparative efficacy of dietary treatments on renal function in rats with sub-total nephrectomy: renal polyunsaturated fatty acid incorporation and prostaglandin excretion. Clin Nephrol *33:* 25

Coggins CH Management of nephrotic syndrome 1982. In: *Brenner BN, Stein JH* (eds). Contemporary issues in Nephrology. New York: Churchill Livingstone, Vol IX, p 283

Crouse JR 1989 Gender, lipoproteins, diet, and cardiovascular risk. Lancet *i:* 318

Curry R, Roberts W 1977 Status fo the coronary arteries in the nephrotic syndrome. Am J Med *63:* 183

Diamond JR, Karnovsky MJ 1987 Ameliorative effects of dietary protein restriction in chronic aminonucleoside nephrosis. J Lab Clin Med *109:* 538

Farr LE 1938 The assimilation of protein by young children with the nephrotic syndrome. Am J Med *195:* 70

Feehally J, Baker F, Walls J 1988 Dietary protein manipulation in experimental nephrotic syndrome. Nephron *50:* 247

Friedwald WT, Levy RI, Fredrickson DS 1972 Estimation of the concentration of low density lipoprotein cholesterol in plasma without the use of the preparation ultracentrifuge. Clin Chem *18:* 499

Gentile MG, Fellin G, Manna G, et al. 1987 Dietetic education and assessment of compliance in patients with chronic renal insufficiency. Contrib Nephrol *55:* 36

Heifets M, Morrissey JJ, Purkenson ML, Morrison AR, Klahr S 1987 Effect of dietary lipids on renal function in rats subtotal nephrectomy. Kidney Int *32:* 335

Kaysen GA, Gambertoglio J, Jimenez I, Jones H, Hutchison FN 1986 Effect of dietary protein intake on albumin homeostasis in nephrotic patients. Kidney Int *29:* 572

Kaysen GA, Gambertoglio J, Felts J, Hutchison FN 1987 Albumin synthesis, albuminuria and hyperlipemia in nephrotic patients. Kidney Int *31:* 1368

Kaysen GA, Jones H, Martin V, Hutchison FN 1989 A low-protein diet restricts albumin synthesis in nephrotic rats. J Clin Invest *183:* 1623

Mallick N, Short C 1981 The nephrotic syndrome and ischemic heart disease. Nephron *27:* 54

Maroni BJ, Steinman TI, Mitch WE 1985 A method for estimating nitrogen intake of patients with chronic renal failure. Kidney Int *27:* 58

Motomura K, Okuda S, Sanai T, et al. 1988 Importance of early initiation of dietary protein restriction for the prevention of experimental progressive renal disease. Nephron *49:* 144

Olmer M, Pain C, Dussol B, Berland Y 1989 Protein diet and nephrotic syndrome. Kidney Int *36 (Suppl 27):* 152

Remuzzi A, Schieppati A, Battaglia C, Remuzzi G 1989 Angiotensin-converting enzyme inhibition ameliorates the defect in glomerular size selectivity in hyponatremic hypertensive syndrome. Am J Kidney Dis *14:* 170

Rosenberg ME, Swanson JE, Thomas BL, Hostetter TH 1987 Glomerular and hormonal responses to dietary protein intake in human renal disease. Am J Physiol *253:* F 1083

Wheeler DC, Varghese Z, Moorhead JF 1989 Hyperlipidemia in nephrotic syndrome. Am J Nephrol *9 (Suppl 1):* 78

Wiegmann TB, Zlomke AM, Mac Dougall ML, Kipp DE 1990 Controlled changes in chronic dietary protein intake do not change glomerular filtration rate. Am J Kidney Dis *15:* 147

Zimmermann EW, Meisunger E, Weinel B, Strauch M 1979 Essential aminoacid/ketoanalogue supplementation: an alternative to unrestricted protein intake in uremia. Clin Nephrol *11:* 71

Clinical Nephrology, Vol. 35 No. 6 – 1991 (243–251)

Crescentic glomerulonephritis in Wegener's granulomatosis: morphology, therapy, outcome

W. Grotz[1], C. Wanner[1], E. Keller[1], J. Böhler[1], H. H. Peter[2], R. Rohrbach[3] and P. Schollmeyer[1]

Department of Medicine, Division of Nephrology[1], Division of Rheumatology and Clinical Immunology[2], and Department of Pathology[3], University of Freiburg, Hugstetterstr. 55, W-7800 Freiburg, Germany

Abstract. Fourteen patients with Wegener's granulomatosis (WG) and severe renal and extrarenal involvement were studied (serum creatinine on admission 5.8 ± 3.4 mg/dl). Renal histology showed a necrotizing, crescentic glomerulonephritis in all patients. Despite advanced renal disease on admission cyclophosphamide, steroids (in 13 patients) and plasma exchange (in 9 patients) caused a rapid and sustained improvement of renal function. Four patients required intermittent hemodialysis over a period of one week. After 2 weeks of treatment serum creatinine values below 2 mg/dl (n = 4) indicated a nearly complete recovery of renal function in the long-term follow up (mean serum creatinine achieved after 12 months therapy: 1.1 ± 0.1 mg/dl (n = 4). Therefore serum creatinine values observed after 2 weeks of therapy, appear to be of prognostic value with regard to renal outcome. No relapse of active WG or progressive renal deterioration was observed during follow-up (22 ± 13 months) except in one patient with persisting renal impairment. Three patients died (staphylococcus sepsis, intracerebral hemorrhage during hypertensive crisis, pulmonary embolism) during the first two months of therapy. The decline of serum creatinine seemed to be a better indicator of successful therapy than the decrease of anticytoplasmatic antibody (ANCA), erythrocyte sedimentation rate (ESR) and hematuria. On admission ANCA titer neither correlated with serum creatinine, the degree of renal involvement, nor was it of prognostic value. ANCA, serum creatinine and hematuria normalized within 2 to 8 months, whereas ESR and proteinuria remained elevated. Our data indicate a good prognosis of WG even with advanced renal involvement and generalized vasculitis provided aggressive treatment is performed early.

Key words: Wegener's granulomatosis – crescentic glomerulonephritis – rapidly progressive glomerulonephritis

Introduction

Wegener's granulomatosis (WG) is a disease of unknown origin, histopathologically characterized by a necrotizing granulomatous inflammation of the upper and lower respiratory tract often associated with glomerulonephritis. A generalized vasculitis may involve small vessels in a variety of tissues. Before cytotoxic drugs were introduced for therapy, most patients died of renal failure. The average survival time from the onset of clinically evident renal disease was 5 months, and death occurred with the first year in 79% of the patients [Walton 1958].

Cyclophosphamide and corticosteroids have been found to induce complete remissions in 93% of the patients [Fauci et al. 1983]. The one year survival rate under therapy ranged from 72 to 100% [Wolff et al. 1974, Reza et al. 1975, Fauci et al. 1983, Martens and Verberckmoes 1983]. In advanced renal disease the three year survival rate was 44% [Pinching et al. 1983]. In the individual patient long term survival may be up to ten years [Brandwein et al. 1983, Koretz et al. 1983, Bohn et al. 1985]. If remission can be induced, only a small subgroup of patients will suffer a relapse within 4 years [Fauci et al. 1983].

Despite markedly improved patients survival, the course of renal disease is questionable. Since today no histological, laboratory or clinical parameter is given to estimate or to predict the outcome of renal disease in severe WG. Therefore, we retrospectively investi-

Received July 16, 1990; in revised form December 27, 1990.

Reprint requests to Dr. W. Grotz, Medizinische Universitätsklinik, Hugstetterstr. 55, W-7800 Freiburg, Germany.

gated fourteen patients with severe WG and acute deterioration of renal function.

Patients and methods

Fourteen patients (7 male, 7 female, mean age 56 ± 10 years) with WG and severe renal involvement were investigated retrospectively. The patients were admitted to our unit within a period of 4 years (1985–1988) due to acute deterioration of renal function.

Diagnosis of WG was established histopathologically by evidence of necrotizing granulomatous inflammation in various organs (upper respiratory tract, lung, prostate, nerve, spleen, skin) and clinically by the presence of a pulmo-renal syndrome. Renal biopsies were performed in 11 patients. Immunofluorescence studies were done by direct immunofluorescence on native tissue immediately after biopsy. Additionally indirect immunofluorescence was performed (Biotin-Avidin method, monoclonal anti-C3 APAAP) to compare the various slices. In 4 patients electron microscopy was performed.

The ANCA test was performed by indirect immunofluorescence according to Van der Woude et al. 1985. Cytoplasmatic (c-ANCA) and perinuclear (p-ANCA) staining patterns were distinguished [Falk and Jennette 1988]. In 4 patients ANCA testing was performed retrospectively with frozen sera of the time of acute disease. ESR was performed by Westergreen method and serum creatinine was measured by the method of Jaffe.

Initially 13 out of 14 patients received prednisone and cyclophosphamide. Prednisone was given orally in a dose of 1 mg/kg body weight daily, six cases started with a 0.5–1.0 g bolus injection intravenously. Cyclophosphamide was administered orally in a dose of 2–3 mg/kg body weight daily. In 4 cases this therapy was started with a 0.5–1.0 g initial bolus injection intravenously. In one patient cyclophosphamide was administered in 3 boluses to 1 g every 2 weeks (patient AM, Table 1). Cyclophosphamide therapy was guided by serial measurements of leukocyte counts. Dose reduction was performed when peripheral leukocyte count or total neutrophil count fell below 4,000/µl and 1,500/µl, respectively.

Membrane plasma exchange (Plasmaflux P II® Fresenius, Oberursel, Germany) was performed in 9 out of 14 patients 3 to 9 times using fresh frozen plasma (30 ml/kg) and 500 ml 5% human albumin for substitution. Four patients required 3 to 5 consecutive intermittent hemodialysis treatments (Table 1).

For long term treatment prednisone was used in a maintenance dose of 7.5–25 mg/day. Corticosteroide were tapered off gradually and were stopped in 6 out of 11 patients after a period of 0.5 years (n = 3) and 1.5 years (n = 3). Cyclophosphamide was given over a period of one year after induction of remission. In three patients (HI, BE, MB; Table 1) cyclophosphamide was switched to azathioprin due to leukopenia (n = 2) or cyclophosphamide induced exanthema (n = 1). In a fourth patient (KH) therapy was stopped after 5 months because of noncompliance. In a fifth patient (SF) cyclosporine therapy was instituted after severe cyclophosphamide associated bone marrow depression. Cyclosporine was given in a dose of 80 mg twice daily resulting in whole blood through levels of 200–300 ng/ml (Radioimmunoassay, nonspecific polyclonal antibody, Sandoz®, Basel, Switzerland).

Mean values are given as standard deviation (± SD), and in the figures as standard error of the mean (± SEM). For statistically evaluation Wilcoxon test was used for paired and unpaired samples. Patients who died shortly after initiation of therapy (JM, ME, WR) were not considered for the longterm statistical evaluation. ANCA titers which were not estimated prior to the initiation of therapy were not considered for statistical evaluation (Table 1, ANCA titer in brackets).

Results

History and clinical signs on admission

Table 1 shows the various involved organs of the 14 patients at the time of hospital admission. History findings revealed that first clinical symptoms were noted 1 to 6 months before a rapid rise of serum creatinine was detected and admission to the hospital occurred. The diagnosis of WG was made by a biopsy supported pulmo-renal syndrome. Necrotizing granulomatous vasculitis was found in 11 out of 14 patients (Table 1): the upper respiratory tract (4 out of 11 biopsies), lung (3 out of 3 biopsies), as well as prostate, middle ear, trachea, spleen (respectively 1 out of 1 biopsy). Renal biopsies often showed a periglomerular granuloma-like infiltration located preferentially at the vascular pole (6 out of 12). Bronchial biopsy (n = 9) and biopsies of the digestive tract (n = 5) showed only nonspecific inflammation without evidence of granuloma or vasculitis. Immunosuppressive treatment was immediately instituted (13 out of 14). In one patient (JM) WG was diagnosed one year after initiation of chronic hemodialysis treatment when respiratory lesions became evident. After one month on immunosuppressive treatment the patient died of pneumonia.

Table 1 Initial presentation, treatment and outcome of 14 patients with WG

		Initial presentation				Treatment			Outcome					
patient	age	months from onset of symptoms to ARF	organs involved	ANCA	serum creatinine	initial treatment	maintenance treatment	months on treatment	ANCA	serum creatinine	proteinuria	hematuria	months of follow up	months after withdrawal of treatment
SF	58	3	nose, lung, spleen, kidney, joint	(c-100)	7.2	150 C. 100 P.	CyA	5 C. →30 CyA 18 P.	0	2.0	1.3	–	52	17
NG	50	1	eye, trachea, kidney	c-80	11.7	220 C. 100 P. + 1 × 0.5 g 7 PP 4 HD	50 C. 20 P.	36 C. 6 P.	c-10	CAPD	1.0	(+)	36	c. t.
BE	35	1	ear, nose, lung, kidney, skin	c-50	6.3	150 C. 75 P. 3 PP	100 C. 10 P.	11 C. 11 P.	0	1.2	0.5	–	29	18
KR	72	6	nose, kidney, joint, skin	(c-100)	4.0	150 C. 100 P. 6 PP	100 C. 12.5 P.	20 C. 15 P.	0	1.3	0.3	–	38	18
KH	55	2	ear, nose, lung, kidney	0	2.8	100 C. 40 P.	50 C. 10 P.	5 C. 5 P.	p-10	1.1	0.6	–	30	24
MB	48	8	nose, paranasal sinus, kidney, joint	p-80	8.1	200 C. 150 P. + 3 × 0.5 g 3 PP 3 HD	100 C. 7.5 P.	25 C. 20 P.	c-40	1.2	0.7	–	25	c. t.
SW	49	3	ear, nose, cheek, tongue, lung, kidney, joint	c-80	3.5	200 C. 300 P. + 1 × 0.5 g 3 PP	150 C. 10 P.	18 C. 18 P.	0	1.1	1.2	–	18	c. t.
HE	51	2	nose, lung, kidney, skin	c-20	5.2	150 C. + 1 × 1 g 100 P. + 3 × 0.5 g 9 PP	100 C. 25 P.	18 C. 8 P.	c-10	1.0	1.5	+++	18	c. t.

Age in year, ARF = acute renal failure, organs biopsied with granuloma, organs biopsied without granuloma, c-ANCA = cytoplasmatic ANCA titer, p-ANCA = perinuclear ANCA titer, titer in brackets = titer measured after starting immunosuppressive therapy, serum creatinine in mg/100 ml, C. = mg/day cyclophosphamide, P. = mg/day prednisone, Aza. = mg/day azathioprine, CyA = cyclosporine A, proteinuria in g/day, c. t. = currently on treatment.

Laboratory values on admission

On admission all patients exhibited hematuria, proteinuria (1.5 ± 1.4 g/day) and renal failure (mean serum creatinine 5.8 ± 3.4 mg/dl). ANCA-titers were positive in all but one patient (KH). In this case a positive p-ANCA staining pattern was observed 30 months later. However, diagnosis of WG was supported by clinical symptoms and histology. In another patient (MB) p-ANCA initially observed changed into a c-ANCA pattern under therapy. The initial ANCA-titers were not correlated to the serum creatinine levels on admission. In a control group of 4 patients with other forms of crescentic glomerulonephritis (1987–1988), routinely assayed ANCA-titers were negative.

Table 2 summarizes inflammatory parameters of the patients. Beside elevated ESR and serum

Table 1 Continued

		Initial presentation				Treatment			Outcome					
patient	age	months from onset of symptoms to ARF	organs involved	ANCA	serum creatinine	initial treatment	maintenance treatment	months on treatment	ANCA	serum creatinine	proteinuria	hematuria	months of follow up	months after withdrawal of treatment
AM	50	3	nose, lung, kidney, joint, nerves	c-80	3.3	3 × 1 g C. 200 P. 9 PP	75 C. 20 P.	17 C. 17 P.	0	1.4	5.6	–	17	c. t.
PE	60	1	nose, paranasal sinus, lung, kidney	c-80	6.7	150 C. + 1 × 1 g 100 P. + 1 × 1 g 3 PP 4 HD	75 Aza. 25 P.	11 C. 11 P.	0	1.5	0.5	–	11	c. t.
HI	65	6	lung, kidney, lymph nodes	c-80	3.3	150 C. + 1 × 0.5 g 150 P.	150 Aza. 7.5 P.	15 Aza. 15 P.	c-20	1.3	0.2	++	15	c. t.
ME	64	5	nose, kidney, nerves	c-40	2.2	100 C. + 1 × 0.5 g 100 P. 3 PP	100 C. 40 P.	2 C. 2 P.	0	1.5	0.4	(+)	2	died
WR	52	2	eye, ear, nose, lung, kidney, prostate	c-30	5.1	200 C. 200 P. + 3 × 0.5 g 3 HD	200 C. 100 P.	1 C. 1 P.	c-30	2.6	1.4	+++	1	died
JM	68	6	kidney, retroperitoneal hematoma	(c-100)	13.8	100 C. 50 P.	100 C. 50 P.	1 C. 1 P.	c-50	chron. HD	anuria	anuria	13	died

Age in year, ARF = acute renal failure, organs biopsied with granuloma, organs biopsied without granuloma, c-ANCA = cytoplasmatic ANCA titer, p-ANCA = perinuclear ANCA titer, titer in brackets = titer measured after starting immunosuppressive therapy, serum creatinine in mg/100 ml, C. = mg/day cyclophosphamide, P. = mg/day prednisone, Aza. = mg/day azathioprine, CyA = cyclosporine A, proteinuria in g/day, c. t. = currently on treatment.

creatinine, anemia, leukocytosis and thrombocytosis were the most prominent features.

Renal histology

Percutaneous renal biopsies were performed in 11 patients. The obtained tissue showed 7 or more glomeruli (mean 16 ± 9) in all cases. A nearly uniform picture of a focal segmental necrotizing glomerulonephritis with extracapillary proliferation was found (Table 3). These extracapillary cellular crescents were focal and involved 30 to 100% of the glomeruli. Extensive glomerular mesangial and/or endocapillary hypercellularity was absent. In some specimen extracapillary cell proliferation extended beyond Bowman's capsule, which was partially destroyed. In 6 patients Bowman's capsule was penetrated by a periglomerular lymphohistiocytic infiltrate with epitheloid cells and mononuclear and polymorphonuclear leukocytes. However, multinucleated giant cells were not present. In 5 patients thrombosis of glomerular capillaries were observed. In only 3 out of 11 renal biopsies signs of a preglomerular arteriolitis were observed ranging from intimal fibrinoid insudation to fibrinoid necrosis comprising more than the inner half of the vessel wall. In the adjoining glomerular capillaries fibrin thrombosis was observed regularly. Eight specimens showed a focal or diffuse interstitial edema and lymphohistiocytic infiltration. In all biopsies proximal tubuli were irregularly dilated and showed swollen epithelial cells. The tubular lumen was filled with protein casts. Tubular basement membranes were sometimes interrupted.

The immunofluorescence studies were performed directly on native tissue immediately after biopsy. Ten out of 11 biopsies showed a coarse granular type of immunofluorescence in all glomeruli. This was consistent with a segmental deposition of immune complexes containing C3, IgM, and/or IgG or IgA deposits in the mesangium and preferentially attached basement membrane. Controls with albumin staining were negative throughout. In comparable slides made from paraffine embedded biopsy material indirect immunofluorescence studies against C3 showed immune deposits in necrotic but not in undamaged glomerular tissue. In electron microscopy (n = 4) dense deposits could not be demonstrated. Fibrin antigen was present in 9 specimen in the glomerular tuft and urinary space crescents mostly in a focal manner. Fibrin exudation into the urinary space was usually associated with crescents.

In one patient (KH), a second biopsy exhibited a decrease of cellular proliferation within the mesangium two months after starting immunosuppressive therapy. Few glomeruli were still affected and extracapillary cell proliferation had progressed to sclerosing crescents; whilst in the former biopsy 100% cell-rich crescents were observed. Acute signs of necrosis or thrombosis were no longer detectable.

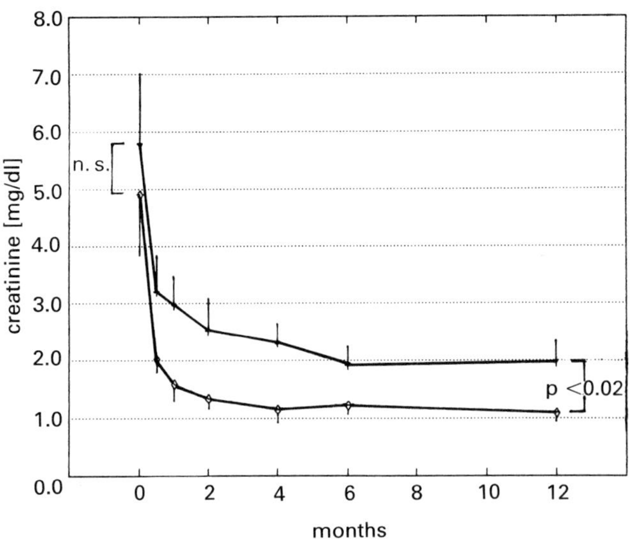

Fig. 1: Serum creatinine as a prognostic factor of renal outcome. Group 1 (◇) with serum creatinine ≤2 mg/dl (mean 2.0 ± 0.1 mg/dl) after 2 weeks of therapy. Group 2 (+) with serum creatinine >2 mg/dl (mean 3.2 ± 1.4 mg/dl) after 2 weeks of therapy. Mean values ± SEM.

Table 2 Laboratory values on admission in 14 patients with WG.

Parameter	Number of patients	Mean ± SD
anemia (Hb <12 g/dl)	14/14	9.5 ± 1.6 g/dl
thrombocytosis (>300,000/μl)	14/14	542,000 ± 195,000/μl
leukocytosis (>10,000/μl)	11/14	13,692 ± 4,598/μl
(>15,000/μl)	5/14	
ANCA-titer	13/14	1:82 ± 17
rheumatic factor (latex fixation > 1:8)	6/11	
elevation of ESR	14/14	106 ± 32/141 ± 34 mm
elevation of CRP (>0.5 mg/dl)	10/11	11.2 ± 8.0 mg/dl
elevation of complement (CH50 >50/ml)	3/8	49 ± 19/ml
elevation of creatinine (>1.5 mg/dl)	14/14	5.8 ± 3.4 mg/dl
elevation of urea (>40 mg/dl)	14/14	173 ± 66 mg/dl
proteinuria (>0.5 g/day)	13/14	1.5 ± 1.4 g/day
microhematuria (>10/hpf)	14/14	54 ± 28 cells/hpf

Abbreviations: CRP = C-reactive protein, CH50 = half maximal total hemolytic complement activity, hpf = high power field 1:40.

Outcome

Under therapy the extrarenal B-symptoms disappeared in all patients within days. In one patient mouth and tongue ulcers disappeared within one week. On chest x-ray pulmonary infiltrations regressed within 21 ± 6 days. Necrotizing granulomas, seen in pulmonary biopsy of one patient prior to immunosuppressive therapy, were scarred on autopsy 28 days after institution of therapy. While in one patient acute hearing loss was irreversible, renal improvement measured by serum creatinine was seen in all patients between 1 to 10 days after starting treatment. On the average serum creatinine decreased during the first month from 5.8 ± 3.4 mg/dl to 2.4 ± 1.3 mg/dl. A further regression to 1.7 ± 1.0 mg/dl could be observed within 6 months of follow up. All early treated patients (n = 13) recovered from acute renal failure.

All patients with serum creatinine below 2 mg/dl (n = 4) after 2 weeks of therapy recovered almost completely within 12 months regarding serum creatinine values (1.1 ± 0.1 mg/dl). Creatinine clearance was 86 ± 26 ml/min, proteinuria 1.0 ± 0.4 g/day and 1 out of 4 patients had hematuria. Those patients

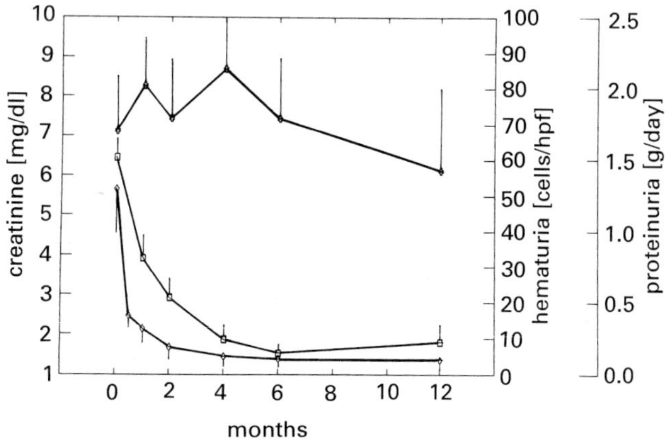

Fig. 2: Serum creatinine (◇), hematuria (□) and proteinuria (+) during 12 months of therapy in 11 patients with WG. Mean values ± SEM.

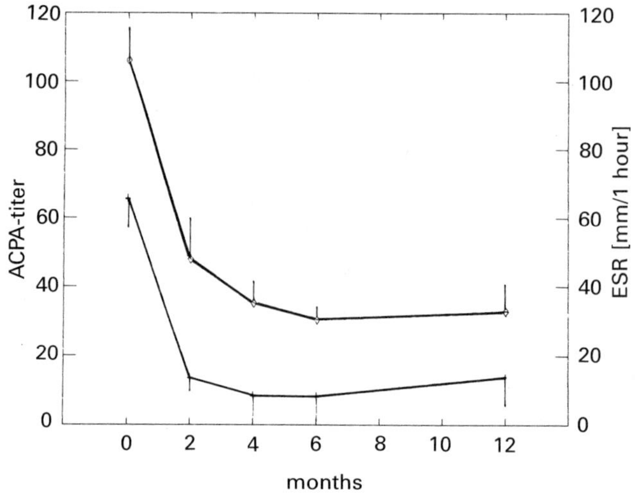

Fig. 3: ACPA/ANCA (+) and ESR (◇) during 12 months of therapy in 11 patients with WG. Mean values ± SEM.

(n = 7) with a serum creatinine above 2 mg/dl after two weeks on therapy did not demonstrate a full recovery (follow up at 12 months: serum creatinine 2.1 ± 1.1 mg/dl, $p < 0.02$; proteinuria 1.34 ± 1.9 g/day, one patient with persisting hematuria). Only one patient (NG) has had progressive impairment of renal function over 34 months and is now on continuous ambulatory peritoneal dialysis. Her lowest serum creatinine was 3.7 mg/dl after 4 months of therapy.

Serum creatinine of patients treated with plasmapheresis (n = 9) decreased from 5.7 ± 3.3 mg/dl to 2.3 ± 1.6 mg/dl within one month. In the same time serum creatinine of patients treated only with cyclophosphamide and prednisone (n = 5) decreased from 4.4 ± 1.8 mg/dl to 2.6 ± 0.7 mg/dl. No differences between these two groups were observed initially and during the follow up.

In the early phase of the disease serum creatinine, ANCA, ESR and hematuria dropped rapidly. Normalizing of ANCA, serum creatinine and hematuria was usually achieved within 2, 6 and 8 months of therapy, respectively (Fig. 2 + Fig. 3).

Despite a rapid decrease of ESR from 106 ± 32 mm (1st hour) to 48 ± 36 mm achieved after 2 months on therapy, ESR was still elevated after 1 year of treatment (33 ± 26 mm) and continued to be elevated after 2 years of follow up (25 ± 13 mm; n = 4). In 7 patients proteinuria (>0.5 g/day) persisted even after 22 ± 13 months (1.6 ± 1.4 g/day). Despite improvement of renal function (serum creatinine <1.5 mg/dl in 9 out of 11 patients) and despite of antihypertensive therapy (6 out of 11 patients) blood pressure tended to rise from 132 ± 18/78 ± 10 mmHg to 154 ± 28/91 ± 10 mmHg ($p < 0.05$) within one year.

ANCA-titers determined before therapy were not significantly correlated to the response of treatment. In 6 out of 14 patients ANCA-titer decreased from 1:80 to 0 within 2 months. In another four patients a lower titer persisted. Two of these patients had persisting hematuria but stable renal function.

Table 3 Renal histology in 14 patients with WG

Patient	Diagnosis	Glom. with cresc.	Extra-glomerular vasculitis	Thrombosis of glom. capillaries	Granuloma-like infiltrations
SF	cresc. GN + necr.	50%	+		(+)
NG	cresc. GN + necr.	<50%		+	
BE	cresc. GN + necr.	100%	+		(+)
KR	cresc. GN + necr.	50%			
KH	cresc. GN + necr.	100%			
MB	cresc. GN + necr.	50%			(+)
SW	cresc. GN + necr.	<50%		+	(+)
HE	cresc. GN + necr.	>50%	(+)	+	
AM	cresc. GN + necr.	100%		+	
PE	cresc. GN + necr.	75%			
HI	n. p.				
ME	cresc. GN + necr.	50%		+	(+)
WR	n. p. (in autopsy 1 month after start of therapy: cresc. GN + necr.	<50%	+ aneurysm)		
JM	n. p. (in autopsy complete shrinkage 1 year after acute renal deterioration)				

Abbreviations: cresc. GN + necr. = crescentic glomerulonephritis with necrosis, n. p. = not performed.

One of these four patients (NG) had progressive deterioration of renal function, another had stable renal function, both in the absence of hematuria. Another three patients died, so outcome of their ANCA-titers could not be observed (Table 1).

The patient (SF, Table 1), switched to cyclosporine, has been in remission with negative ANCA-titers for a total of 52 months (30 months with cyclosporine). After 30 months of treatment a carcinoma of the sigmoid colon was surgically removed. So far there is no evidence for metastases or local recurrence. Cyclosporine treatment was stopped shortly before operation and the patient is now 17 months without treatment.

In three other patients immunosuppressive therapy has also been discontinued: The patients (KH) who was treated for only 5 months is still in remission after 24 months without treatment. In patients KR and BE treatment was stopped 12 months after onset of remission. By now, both patients are without therapy for 18 months and are still in remission. Three out of 14 patients died, 60, 28 and 20 days after institution of therapy, respectively. One patient (JM) died from staphyloccocal pneumonia, one (WR) from an acute cerebral hemorrhage during hypertensive crisis, and one (ME) from pulmonary embolism. Eleven patients are surviving between 12 to 52 months after institution of treatment and 10 have resumed normal activities.

Discussion

Fourteen patients with WG and predominant renal involvement were studied retrospectively. In all cases rapid deterioration of renal function was the cause of admission. Clinical symptoms consisting of progressive renal failure, either upper respiratory tract and/or pulmonary symptoms, arthralgia, malaise, fever, and weight loss were similar in frequency to those described by Fauci and Wolff [1973].

Uniformly, renal histology of all the cases showed a focal necrotizing glomerulonephritis with crescents. This differs from the data of Fauci et al. [1983], who showed a broad scope from mild focal, segmental glomerulonephritis to diffuse necrotizing glomerulonephritis with proliferative and crescentic changes. However, we emphasize the severity of the disease in our selected group of patients. Previous reports also showed that with deterioration of renal function focal necrotizing glomerulonephritis with crescents is apparent [Pinching et al. 1983, Dahlberg et al. 1984, Weiss and Crissmann 1984, Ten Berge et al. 1985]. In cases in which renal involvement was not dominant, focal glomerulitis seems to be the most common lesion [Fauci and Wolff 1973, Wolff et al. 1974]. Furthermore, in 10 out of 11 biopsies a positive immunofluorescence characterized by a coarse granular type was seen. In controls there was evidence of stained necrotic or damaged tissue, although all albumin controls were negative. In electronmicroscopy accumulation of dense deposits could not be observed. Although, immunofluorescent deposits revealed a focal segmental distribution pattern as seen in necrosis and sclerosis, a secondary insudation of complement and immunoglobulins could not be excluded. This would be an explanation for the discrepancies described in the literature [Horn et al. 1974, Wolff et al. 1974, Juncos et al. 1979, Novac et al. 1982, Martens and Verberckmoes 1983, Pinching et al. 1983, Weiss and Crissmann 1984, Ten Berge et al. 1985, Bhathena et al. 1987, Furlong et al. 1987].

Appel et al. [1981] found that early kidney biopsies were useful with regard to prognosis. They mentioned that the initial severity of renal involvement, as determined by serum creatinine, proteinuria, and light microscopic morphology correlated well with prognosis. In our patients, the severity of histological alterations, even in patients with 100% crescents which is believed to have a negative outcome, did not allow any prediction of outcome. Conversely, both patients with poor renal outcome had 50 or less percent crescents.

Early treatment with prednisone and cyclophosphamide lead to a rapid disappearance of most extrarenal symptoms within days and to a rapid improvement of renal function within weeks independently from initial findings. Additional plasmapheresis (9 out of 14 patients) did not yield greater or faster amelioration of serum creatinine in the first month of treatment. Plasmapheresis was without influence on long-term prognosis. Despite advanced disease and severe renal involvement (serum creatinine >4 mg/dl in 8 out of 14 patients on admission) improvement of renal function was impressive especially in view of the histological alterations.

According to some reports endstage renal failure developed over a period of several years despite initial improvement of renal function [Koretz et al. 1980, Kuross et al. 1981, Brandwein et al. 1983, Dahlberg et al. 1984, Littlejohn et al. 1985, Weiss and Crissmann 1985, Andrassy et al. 1986]. So far only one of our patients treated (observation time 22 ± 13 months), proceeded to endstage renal failure. Long-term results seemed to depend on serum creatinine achieved after 2 weeks of treatment. A serum creatinine below 2 mg/dl indicated nearly complete recovery of renal function in the follow-up period. Kuross et al. [1981] described 9 patients, who did progress to endstage renal failure. Their serum creatinine remained at least above 2 mg/dl. According to Brenner et al. [1982] progressive glomerulosclerosis can develop despite adequate control of vasculitis. Ten Berge et al. [1985] observed no isolated deterioration of renal function without nonrenal manifestations over a follow up of 15 years. Therefore, serum creatinine, achieved after 2 weeks of aggressive treatment, might be a prognostic parameter for renal outcome.

Although, no arterial hypertension was observed on admission in 13 out of 14 patients, an increase in blood pressure was observed later on. Proteinuria did not seem to correlate with serum creatinine and might be a symptom of defective healing after initial therapy. Heinicke [1986] observed a proteinuria of 40–200 mg/day during remission when follow-up biopsies showed no focal sclerosis. Higher urinary protein (1,8–2,5 g/day) was present when follow-up biopsies revealed sclerosis.

Since 1985, when ANCA-antibody was discovered as a marker for WG [Van der Woude 1985], a highly specific and sensitive parameter is available in WG with a close correlation to the activity of the disease [Nölle et al. 1989]. Moreover, it allows the distinction between superinfection and recurrence of vasculitis [Lüdemann et al. 1988]. Serial ANCA measurements indicated a response to initial therapy earlier than the change in hematuria or erythrocyte sedimentation rate. However, in contrast to Andrassy et al. [1989], initial ANCA titer correlated neither with the number of organs involved nor with serum creatinine on admission nor was it predictive for the initial response to therapy.

In summary, our data show severe necrotizing crescentic glomerulonephritis accompanied with poor renal function in WG and substantial renal recovery under immunosuppressive treatment. Plasmapheresis therapy did not induce a faster decrease of serum creatinine. Outcome was independent from initial clinical, pathological or laboratory findings. Long-term results and progressive renal failure seemed to depend on serum creatinine achieved after initial treatment. Our data indicate a good prognosis of WG even in advanced renal involvement and generalized vasculitis if an aggressive treatment is performed.

REFERENCES

Andrassy K, Koderisch J, Ritz E 1986 Therapie und Verlauf der Glomerulonephritis (GN) bei M. Wegener. Nieren/Hochdruckkrankheit *15:* 390 (abstract)

Andrassy K, Koderisch J, Rufer M et al 1989 Detection and clinical implication of antineutrophil cytoplasm antibodies in Wegener's granulomatosis and rapidly progressive glomerulonephritis. Clin Nephrol *32:* 159–167

Appel GB, Gee B, Kashgarian M, Hayslett JP 1981 Wegener's granulomatosis – Clinical-pathologic correlations and long-term course. Am J Kidney Dis *1:* 27–37

Bhathena DB, Migdal SD, Julian et al 1987 Morphologic and immunohistochemical observations in granulomatous glomerulonephritis. Am J Pathol *126:* 581–591

Bohn Th, Hunstein W, Ho AD 1985 Langzeitbeobachtungen bei Morbus Wegener. Erfolge der Rezidivtherapie. Dtsch Med Wschr *110:* 642–644

Brandwein S, Esdaile J, Danoff D, Tannenbaum H 1983 Wegener's granulomatosis. Clinical features and outcome in 13 patients. Arch Intern Med *143:* 476–479

Brenner BM, Meyer TW, Hostetter TH 1982 Dietary protein intake and the progressive nature of kidney disease: the role of hemodynamically mediated glomerular injury in the pathogenesis of progressive glomerular sclerosis in aging, renal ablation, and intrinsic renal disease. N Engl J Med *307:* 652–659

Dahlberg PJ, Newcomer KL, Yutuc WR, Kalfayan B 1984 Renal failure in Wegener's granulomatosis: recovering following dialysis and cyclophosphamide-prednisone therapy. Am J Med Sci *287:* 47–50

Falk RJ, Jennette JC 1988 Anti-neutrophil cytoplasmatic autoantibodies with specificity for myeloperoxidase in patients with systemic vasculitis and idiopathic necrotizing and crescentic glomerulonephritis. N Engl J Med *318:* 1651–1657

Fauci AS, Wolff SM 1973 Wegener's granulomatosis. Studies in eighteen patients and a review of the literature. Medicine *52:* 535–561

Fauci AS, Haynes BF, Katz P, Wolff SM 1983 Wegener's granulomatosis: Prospective clinical and therapeutic experience with 85 patients for 21 years. Ann Intern Med *98:* 76–85

Furlong TJ, Ibels LS, Eckstein RP 1987 The clinical spectrum of necrotizing glomerulonephritis. Medicine *66:* 192–201

Heinicke HJ 1986 Verlaufsbeobachtungen bei Wegenerscher Granulomatose mit Nierenbeteiligung. Z Urol Nephrol *79:* 163–169

Horn RG, Fauci AS, Rosenthal AS, Wolff SM 1974 Renal biopsy pathology in Wegener's granulomatosis. Am J Path *74:* 423–440

Juncos LI, Alexander RW, Marbury TC 1979 Intravascular clotting preceding crescent formation in a patient with Wegener's granulomatosis and rapidly progressive glomerulonephritis. Nephron *24:* 17–20

Koretz SH, Feigenbaum PA, Raitt JW 1980 Long-term follow up of Wegener's granulomatosis patients treated with cytotoxic agents plus steroids. Arthritis Rheum *23:* 706–707

Kuross S, Davin T, Kjellstrand CM 1981 Wegener's granulomatosis with severe renal failure: clinical course and results of dialysis and transplantation. Clin Nephrol *16:* 172–180

Littlejohn GO, Ryan PJ, Holdsworth SR 1985 Wegener's granulomatosis: Clinical features and outcome in seventeen patients. Aust NZ J Med *15:* 241–245

Lüdemann G, Nölle B, Rautmann A et al 1988 Antizytoplasmatische Antikörper als Seromarker und Aktivitätsparameter der Wegenerschen Granulomatose. Dtsch Med Wschr *113:* 413–417

Martens J, Verberckmoes R 1983 Wegener's granulomatosis: Retrospective analysis of eleven patients. Acta Clinica Belgica *83:* 148–157

Novak RF, Christiansen RG, Sorensen ET 1982 The acute vasculitis of Wegener's granulomatosis in renal biopsies. Am J Clin Path *78:* 367–371

Nölle B, Specks U, Lüdemann G et al 1989 Anticytoplasmatic autoantibodies: their immunodiagnostic value in Wegener granulomatosis. Ann Intern Med *111:* 28–40

Pinching AJ, Lockwood CM, Pussell BA et al 1983 Wegener's granulomatosis: Observations on 18 patients with severe renal disease. Quart J Med *208:* 435–460

Reza MJ, Dornfeld L, Goldberg LS et al 1975 Wegener's granulomatosis: Long-term follow-up of patients treated with cyclophosphamide. Arthritis Rheum *18:* 501–506

Ten Berge IJM, Wilmink JM, Meyer C et al 1985 Clinical and immunological follow-up of patients with severe renal disease in Wegener's granulomatosis. Am J Nephrol *5:* 21–29

Van der Woude FJ, Rasmussen N, Lobatto et al 1985 Autoantibodies against neutrophils and monocytes. Tool for diagnosis and marker of disease activity in Wegener's granulomatosis. Lancet *1:* 425–429

Walton EW 1958 Giant-cell granuloma of the respiratory tract. (Wegener's granulomatosis). Br Med J *2:* 265–270

Weiss MA, Crissmann JD 1984 Renal biopsy findings in Wegener's granulomatosis: Segmental necrotizing glomerulonephritis with glomerular thrombosis. Hum Pathol *15:* 943–956

Weiss MA, Crissmann JD 1985 Segmental necrotizing glomerulonephritis: Diagnostic, prognostic, and therapeutic significance. Am J Kidney Dis *4:* 199–211

Wolff SM, Fauci AS, Horn RG et al 1974 Wegener's granulomatosis. Ann Intern Med *81:* 513–525

Clinical Nephrology, Vol. 35 No. 6 – 1991 (252–254)

Very late recurrence of renal vasculitis

A. Innes[1], R. E. Cotton[2], P. A. Rowe[1] and R. P. Burden[1]

Renal Unit[1] and Department of Histopathology[2], City Hospital, Nottingham, England

Abstract. We report a case of renal vasculitis with a relapse occurring 9 and a half years after the original presentation. The plasma creatinine six months before relapse was only 118 µmol/l. During the initial illness there was histological evidence of glomerular damage but at the time of relapse renal biopsy showed the remaining glomeruli to be normal with the destructive process causing fibrinoid necrosis of arteries.

Key words: late relapse – renal vasculitis

Introduction

Both microscopic polyarteritis and Wegener's granulomatosis produce a necrotizing crescentic glomerulonephritis and necrotizing vasculitis of arteries and arterioles [Balow and Fauci, 1988]. These conditions can be difficult to differentiate histologically in the absence of granulomata [Fauci et al., 1983]. Relapses can occur in both but the time course and nature of these has been poorly documented. We report a case presenting with a very late relapse of renal vasculitis, in which the plasma creatinine six months previously was only 118 µmol/l. The histological target of the destructive process appears to have been different sizes of vessels in the original presentation and at the time of relapse.

Case report

A 62-year-old male initially presented in March 1979 with a two-week history of cough productive of blood stained sputum, arthropathy and malaise. He also complained of sinusitis and epistaxis. Examination revealed pallor, fluid overload, oliguria, conjunctivitis of the right eye and a swollen, inflamed right wrist. Blood and protein were present in the urine. On admission plasma creatinine was 1100 µmol/l, urea 46.6 mmol/l and hemoglobin 6.2 g/dl. Serum complement and autoantibodies were normal. Chest X-ray revealed small bilateral pleural effusions and opacities in the apical and anterior segments of the right upper lobe and central parts of the middle lobe. Percutaneous renal biopsy was performed and 21 glomeruli were obtained; five were normal and 16 showed cellular crescent formation with the presence of abundant fibrin in the capsular space and segmental necrosis. Vessels greater than capillaries in size (both arteries and arterioles) were normal. The histological appearances were therefore those of crescentic glomerulonephritis of recent onset with focal segmental necrosis (Figure 1). Immunocytochemistry was negative except for the presence of fibrinogen.

The patient was initially treated with peritoneal dialysis and thereafter with hemodialysis by means of an A-V shunt. As the prognosis for recovery of renal function was initially in some doubt, an A-V fistula was created in the left forearm. He received 1G IV methylprednisolone on four successive days followed by oral prednisolone and cyclophosphamide. On this regime, the lung opacities gradually resolved over three weeks and renal function improved such that hemodialysis was discontinued after six weeks. His convalescence was complicated by a perforated duodenal ulcer for which a vagotomy and pyloroplasty was performed in May 1979. Cyclophosphamide was discontinued in June 1979 and oral steroids were eventually stopped in January 1980.

The patient was followed up on a regular basis and serum creatinine measurements never exceeded 120 µmol/l. ESR never exceeded 10 mm/hr during follow-up and only a trace of proteinuria was observed. Hypertension was noted in 1985 and this responded to treatment with atenolol.

He was readmitted in December 1988 with a six-week history of arthralgia, eye discomfort and hemoptysis. He had been oliguric for two days. He was again pale and fluid overloaded and had bilateral conjunctivitis. Urinalysis demonstrated hematuria and proteinuria. Serum creatinine was 690 µmol/l, urea was 40 mmol/l and hemoglobin 7.8 g/dl. At the clinic visit six months previously these values were 118 µmol/l, 8.2 mmol/l and 14.2 g/dl respectively and

Received September 21, 1990; in revised form December 30, 1990.

Reprint requests to Dr. Andrew Innes, Renal Unit, City Hospital, Nottingham NG5 1PB, England

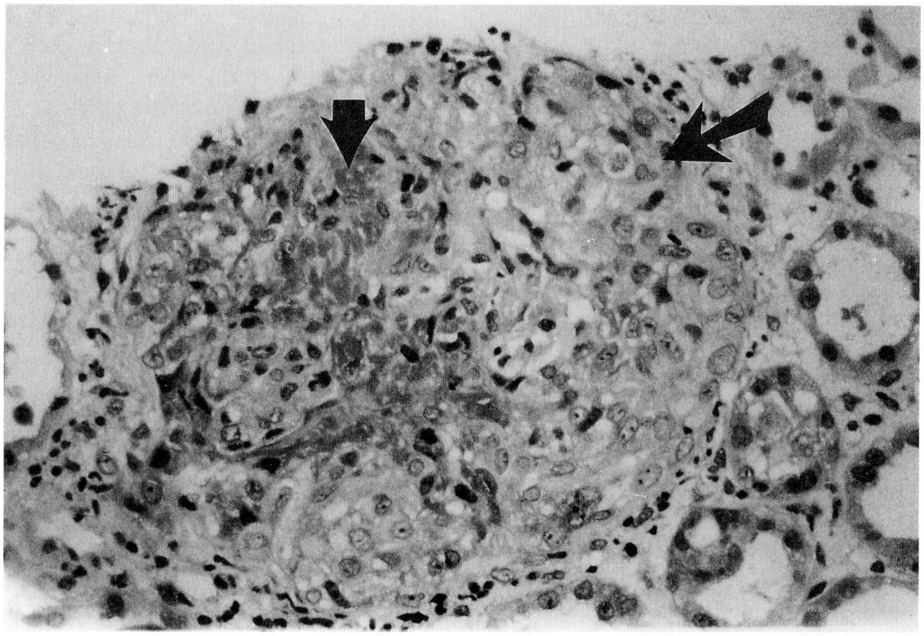

Fig. 1 First (1979) renal biopsy showing a glomerulus with obliterated capsular space associated with a cellular crescent (large arrow). The glomerular tuft is much distorted and contains foci of dark staining fibrin. Hematoxylin and eosin ×400.

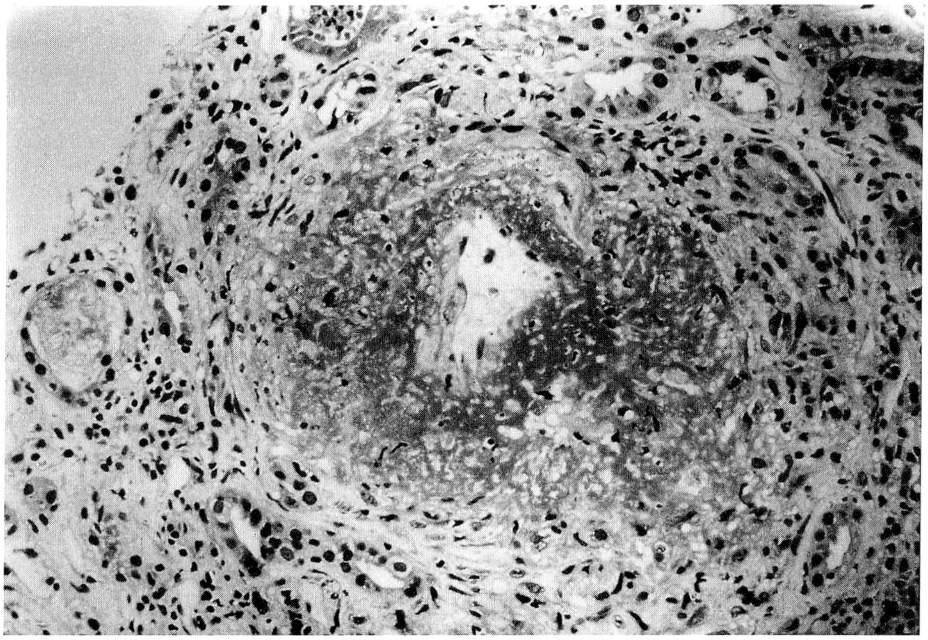

Fig. 2 Second (1988) renal biopsy in which there were no fresh glomerular abnormalities but several blood vessels showed necrosis of the wall with the associated presence of dark staining fibrinoid material. Hematoxylin and eosin ×260.

the blood pressure was 150/85. Chest X-ray demonstrated widespread rounded opacities. Immunological tests were again normal with the exception of the presence of anti-neutrophil cytoplasmic antibody (ANCA) with a cytoplasmic staining pattern in a titre of 1/64. A second renal biopsy contained 16 glomeruli, 10 of which were completely sclerosed. Of the remainder, one glomerulus showed a segment of fresh fibrinoid necrosis. The major abnormality lay in the arteries three of which showed fibrinoid necrosis of their walls without significant inflammatory cell infiltrate. There was marked tubular atrophy and nephron loss (Figure 2).

Clinically and histologically this was necrotizing vasculitis affecting small arteries in a patient who had sustained considerable nephron loss due to the previous crescentic glomerulonephritis in 1979.

Early hemodialysis was again required (using the A-V fistula fashioned in 1979). Despite the use of high dose steroids and intravenous cyclophosphamide the patient remains dialysis-dependent.

Discussion

The initial episode (in 1979) of crescentic glomerulonephritis with lung involvement suggested three possible diagnoses – Wegener's granulomatosis, microscopic polyarteritis or Goodpasture's syndrome. Goodpasture's syndrome was excluded by the absence of characteristic staining on immunocytochemistry. Differentiation between the other two conditions is more difficult and we were unable to demonstrate the presence of granulomatous lesions although it is well known that these are rarely found in renal biopsies where the appearances are by no means pathognomic [Fauci et al., 1983]. The radiological and clinical evidence of pulmonary lesions in both episodes and the clinical involvement of the upper respiratory tract would favor a diagnosis of Wegener's granulomatosis but pulmonary involvement is also observed in over 50% of cases of microscopic polyarteritis [Serra et al., 1984]. These features emphasize the problems of classifying renal vasculitides [Serra et al., 1984; Balow, 1985] and in this case the absence of granulomata make a definitive diagnosis of Wegener's granulomatosis difficult. The most accurate pathological description is microscopic polyarteritis.

An interesting feature of the present case was the difference in histological appearances on the two biopsies over nine years apart. On the first biopsy 16 glomeruli showed crescent formation with the presence of segmental tuft necrosis. Arteries and arterioles in this biopsy were entirely normal. In the second biopsy there was evidence of old damage (sclerosis) to many glomeruli but with the exception of one glomerulus showing fibrinoid necrosis, there was no fresh damage to the remaining glomeruli. On this occasion, however, the arteries showed severe abnormalities with massive destruction and fibrinoid necrosis. It would appear that a different size of blood vessel has been the target of immune damage – the capillaries of the glomerulus during the first episode and the arteries during the recurrence. Although the disease may be focal and therefore prone to sampling error, it is unusual that, in the first biopsy, the arteries were completely spared and the glomeruli affected, whereas in the second biopsy exactly the opposite occurred. The pathogenesis of microscopic polyarteritis remains poorly understood [Balow, 1985] and the reason that the destructive immunological process affected a different vessel size during relapse is unknown.

Other authors have demonstrated that relapse is a frequent feature of microscopic polyarteritis [Savage et al., 1985]. Relapses have been documented by these authors up to five years after the first presentation. In our case, relapse occurred nine and a half years after first presentation in a gentleman whose serum creatinine had been under 120 µmol/l for eight years. Furthermore, he had been off immunosuppressive agents for almost nine years.

This case illustrates that very late acute recurrences of renal vasculitis can occur, many years after immunosuppressive agents have been discontinued, even in the face of seemingly "normal" creatinine levels, ESR and urinary sediment. These patients need to be kept under careful review and presumably cannot be deemed "cured" but it is questionable whether such review would have detected an acute relapse earlier. This patient's original presentation preceded the introduction of ANCA testing. In Wegener's granulomatosis, however, regular measurements of ANCA titres can be used to monitor disease activity and, indeed, treatment to prevent relapse has been based on rising ANCA titres [Cohen Tervaert et al., 1990]. The case also suggests that the vasculitic process may affect a different size of vascular target during a relapse.

REFERENCES

Balow JE 1985 Renal vasculitis. Kidney Int *27:* 954

Balow JE, Fauci AS 1988 Vasculitic diseases of the kidney: polyarteritis nodosa, Wegener's granulomatosis, allergic angiitis and granulomatosis and other disorders. In: *Schrier RW, Gooschalk CW* eds. Diseases of the kidney. Boston/Toronto. Little Brown, p 2335.

Cohen Tervaert JW, Huitema MG, Hené RJ, Sluiter WJ, The TH, Van der Hem GK, Kallenbert CGM 1990 Prevention of relapses in Wegener's granulomatosis by treatment based on antineutrophil cytoplasmic antibody titre. Lancet *336:* 709.

Fauci AS, Haynes BF, Katz P, Wolff SM 1983 Wegener's granulomatosis: prospective clinical and therapeutic experience with 85 patients for 21 years. Ann Intern Med *98:* 76

Savage COS, Winearls CG, Evans DJ, Rees AJ, Lockwood CM 1985 Microscopic polyarteritis: presentation, pathology and prognosis. Q J Med *56:* 467

Serra A, Cameron JS, Turner DR, Hartley B, Ogg CS, Neild GH, Williams DG, Taube D, Brown CB, Hicks JA 1984 Vasculitis affecting the kidney: presentation, histopathology and long-term outcome. Q J Med *53:* 181

Clinical Nephrology, Vol. 35 No. 6 – 1991 (255–262)

Glomerular proteinuria as an early sign of renal-transplant rejection

J. Steinhoff, A. Feddersen, W. G. Wood, J. Hoyer and K. Sack

Klinik für Innere Medizin, Medizinische Universität Lübeck, Ratzeburger Allee 160, W-2400 Lübeck 1

Abstract. The introduction of cyclosporin gave rise to an additional problem in the surveillance of renal transplant patients, namely the differentiation between cyclosporin toxicity and acute transplant rejection. The development of assays for specific proteins in urine has produced a non-invasive solution to this problem. In 55 renal transplant patients the following proteins were determined daily in 24 h-urine samples: IgG, transferrin (TF), albumin, β_2-microglobulin (β_2-MG), retinol binding protein (RBP), α_1-microglobulin (α_1-MG) and α_1-antitrypsin (α_1-AT). All proteins were determined quantitatively using immunoluminometric assays and 10 µl urine in dilutions from 1:1 – 1:100. The urinary protein excretion was related to the actual creatinine clearance as this index gave the best differentiation between normal and abnormal status. In 24 h-urine, intraindividual peaks of IgG, TF and albumin were seen regularly in acute rejection episodes. However, a peak in the "tubular" proteins (RBP, β_2-MG, α_1-MG) could not be detected. After effective treatment of the rejection episode, the renal function improved and the protein excretion returned to pre-rejection episode levels. In bacterial infection of the urogenital tract, urinary α_1-AT levels rose. They returned to normal after successful antibiotic treatment.
In two cases of cyclosporin toxicity neither glomerular nor tubular proteins were excreted in abnormal amounts when compared with transplant patients without complications, the only changes being an increase in serum creatinine as a result of reduced renal function.

Key words: renal transplantation – transplant rejection – proteinuria – cyclosporin – immunometric assays

Introduction

An early warning of a rejection episode in patients who have undergone renal transplantation is important in assessing the future function of the transplanted kidney. The diagnostic procedures used at present often have a low specificity due to their unspecific nature. Sonographic techniques and the measurement of serum creatinine are good examples of such methods. The other alternatives are invasive techniques such as biopsy, which are not without hazard, at least in the early post transplant phase.

The study of proteinuria as a rejection parameter has been published by several groups [Burghard et al. 1986, Frey et al. 1977, Krishua et al. 1987, Lapia et al. 1986, Lison et al. 1985]. The use of sodium dodecyl sulphate – polyacrylamide gel electrophoresis (SDS-PAGE) allows the definition of "tubular" and "glomerular" proteinuria, although the disadvantage of these methods is their qualitative nature. Urine concentration procedures often recommended in SDS-PAGE lead to misinterpretation of results as well as to a non-standardisation of the method [Frey et al. 1977, Lapia et al. 1986, Lison et al. 1985].

The quantitative determination of specific proteins in urine is seen by many groups to be an important contribution to the routine diagnosis and follow-up procedure [Burghard et al. 1986, Dati and Lammers 1988, Frey et al. 1977, Petersen et al. 1989, Schmitt and Schneider 1988]. At the time of writing, nephelometric methods are the most popular as they are rapid and commercially available [Dati and Lammers 1988, Guder 1988, Schmitt and Schneider 1988, Weber et al. 1985]. A disadvantage is the often insufficient lower detection limit as well as the possi-

Received May 21 1990; in revised form March 6 1991.

Requests for reprints to Dr. J. Steinhoff.

Abbreviations: MP = methyl prednisolone; ATG = anti-human T-lymphocyte globulin; ALG = anti-lymphocyte globulin; PS = plasmapheresis; IgG = Immunoglobulin G; TF = Transferrin; Alb = Albumin; d = day; Cl-Crea = creatinine clearance (ml/min); α_1-AT = α_1-anti proteinase inhibitor; α_1-MG = α_1-microglobulin; β_2-MG = β_2-microglobulin; RBP = retinol-binding protein.

Table 1 Flow scheme of the immunoluminometric assay for urine proteins

10 µl sample/standard
200 µl assay buffer*
1 antibody coated ball
Incubate – 120 minutes at room temperature
Wash with 2 × 5 ml aqua demin.
200 µl ABEN – labelled antibody**
Incubate – 60 minutes at room temperature
Wash with 2 × 5 ml aqua demin.
Transfer ball to measuring cuvette, add catalyst, initiate light reaction and integrate signal over 2 seconds.

* 0.05 mol/l phosphate, 0.15 mol/l NaCl, 0.25 ml/l Tween 20 pH 7,5.
** ABEN = 9-[N-(4-aminobutyl)-N-ethyl] aminobenzo(f) phthalazine-1,4(2H, 3H)-dione.

Table 2 Lower detection limit of urinary proteins measured by ILMA. Zero plus 3 standard deviations – data from 20 assays

Protein	Mr(kD)	Detection limit (mg/l)
Immunoglobulin G	150.0	<0.2
Transferrin	76.5	<0.05
Albumin	66.0	<0.23
Alpha-1-antitrypsin	54.0	<0.1
Alpha-1-microglublin	33.0	<0.03
Retinol-bind.-protein	21.0	<0.04
Beta-2-microglobulin	11.8	<0.04

α_1-antitrypsin = α_1-proteinase inhibitor.

Table 3 Reference ranges for healthy volunteers (n = 44); nd = non-detectable; urine values = mg/l; values = 2.5 – median – 97.5 percentiles

Parameter	urine values
Immunoglobulin G	nd – 0.83 – 5.4
Transferrin	nd – 0.30 – 2.54
Albumin	nd – 2.49 – 22.7
Alpha-1-proteinase inhibitor	nd – 0.16 – 1.45
Retinol-binding-protein	nd – 0.52 – 0.90
Alpha-1-microglobulin	nd – 3.66 – 23.4
Beta-2-microglobulin	nd – 0.16 – 0.90

bility that the accuracy of the present methods is questionable.

In order to monitor transplant patients during the first 14–28 days post-operatively, methods are needed which are precise, economical, rapid and have an acceptable lower detection limit.

This article describes the practical application of immunoluminometric assays (ILMA) developed in this laboratory in the daily surveillance of renal transplant patients using seven selected proteins. The results form part of an ongoing study which has been in progress since July 1989, and which encompasses 55 renally transplanted patients with observation times between 20 and 300 days post-operatively. In cases of acute tubular necrosis (ATN) after renal transplantation, the assays could not be performed during the anuric phase.

Materials and methods

All 55 patients who received an allogenic renal transplant in the Medical University of Lübeck during the period July 1989 to August 1990 have been included in the study. The median ages of the 29 men and 26 women was 45.9. The 24 h-urines were collected daily during the hospitalization period and were analyzed within 24 h of receipt, except on Saturdays where the samples were stored at 4° C for maximally 48 h.

Prior to analysis, the urine was centrifuged for 10 min at 3000 min^{-1}. Urines were only stored deep-frozen at −37° C as part of a stability study published elsewhere [Wood 1989, Wood et al. 1990, Wood et al. 1990].

The following proteins were analyzed quantitatively: immunoglobulin-G (IgG), transferrin (Tf), albumin (Alb), α_1-proteinase inhibitor (α_1-AT), retinol binding protein (RBP), α_1-microglobulin (α_1-MG) and β_2-microglobulin (β_2-MG).

Table 1 shows the assay flow scheme used for all proteins. Further details of the ILMA have been published in detail elsewhere [Braun et al. 1986, Wood 1989, Wood et al. 1990, Wood et al. 1990]. The lower detection limits of the assays used here is shown in Table 2. The reference values for excretion of proteins in healthy individuals are shown in Table 3.

All measurements were made in duplicate on a semi automatic 250-sample luminometer (Berthold LB 952/16T, EG & G – Berthold, Wildbad, D). The labelling of antibodies was performed using an active ester method as already described [Braun et al. 1986, Wood et al. 1990, Wood et al. 1990]. Serum and urine standards were either produced in the laboratory or were purchased from Behringwerke, Marburg a. d. L., D. All standards were calibrated, where possible, against the international reference preparation of the NBSB/WHO (for IgG – 1. IRP 1970 [67/86] for albumin and transferrin-1. B. S. 1975 [74/520]).

The antibodies used were obtained from the following sources: DAKO-Hamburg D, Atlantic Antibodies (Baxter) Munich D, Cappel (Organon

Table 4 Protein excretion per day/creatinine clearance at the time of diagnosis

Patient	IgG	Tf	Alb	α_1AT	β_2MG	RBP	α_1MG	Diagnosis
Pat. Ze.	++	++	++	+	=	−−	−−	* interstitial Rejection
Pat. He	++	++	++	+	=	+	=	interstitial Rejection
Pat. Ba.	++	+++	++	+	=	=	=	* interstitial Rejection
Pat. Ja.	+++	+++	+++	++	−−	−−	−−	* interstitial Rejection
Pat. Wi.	+++	+++	+++	+++	=	=	−−	interstitial Rejection
Pat. Jo.	+++	+++	+++	=	−	−−	−−	* interstitial Rejection
Pat. Fr.	++	+++	+++	++	=	−−	−−	* interstitial Rejection
Pat. Öt.	+++	+++	+++	+++	=	=	=	* interstitial Rejection
Pat. Hö.	++	++	++	+	=	−−	−	* interstitial Rejection
Pat. Bl.	+++	+++	+++	++	=	+	+	* interstitial Rejection
Pat. Gr.	++	++	++	++	−	−	−	interstitial Rejection
Pat. Be.	++	++	+++	++	=	=	+	interstitial Rejection
Pat. St.	+++	++	++	++	=	=	−	interstitial Rejection
Pat. Lub.	+++	++	++	++	=	=	=	* interstitial Rejection
Pat. Sei	++	++	++	++	−	−	−−	* interstitial Rejection
Pat. Fed.	+++	+++	++	++	=	=	=	interstitial Rejection
Pat. Lew.	++	++	++	+	=	=	+	* interstitial Rejection
Pat. Len.	+++	+++	+++	+++	=	−	−	interstitial Rejection
Pat. Ris.	+++	+++	+++	++	=	−	−−	* interstitial Rejection
Pat. Un.	++	++	++	+	=	+	+	* vascular Rejection
Pat. Jo.	++	++	++	+	=	=	=	* vascular Rejection
Pat. Sch.	++	++	++	+	+	+	−	* vascular Rejection
Pat. Gür.	+++	+++	+++	+++	+	+	+	* vascular Rejection
Pat. Baa.	+++	+++	+++	+++	+	+	+	* vascular Rejection
Pat. Zap.	+++	+++	+++	+++	+	+	+	* vascular Rejection
Pat. Wa.	=	=	=	=	=	=	=	uncomplicated course
Pat. Mü.	=	=	=	=	=	=	=	uncomplicated course
Pat. Ku.	=	=	=	=	=	=	=	uncomplicated course
Pat. Ja.	=	=	=	=	=	=	=	uncomplicated course
Pat. Fe.	=	=	=	=	=	=	=	uncomplicated course
Pat. Eh.	=	=	=	=	=	=	=	uncomplicated course
Pat. Kö.	=	=	=	=	=	=	=	uncomplicated course
Pat. Bac.	=	=	=	=	=	=	=	uncomplicated course
Pat. Tim.	=	=	=	=	=	=	=	uncomplicated course
Pat. Dür.	=	=	=	=	=	=	=	uncomplicated course
Pat. Kra.	=	=	=	=	=	=	=	uncomplicated course
Pat. Schl.	=	=	=	=	=	=	=	uncomplicated course
Pat. Sev.	=	=	=	=	=	=	=	uncomplicated course
Pat. Bad.	=	=	=	=	=	=	=	uncomplicated course
Pat. Wal.	=	=	=	=	=	=	=	uncomplicated course
Pat. Wul.	=	=	=	=	=	=	=	uncomplicated course
Pat. Schm.	=	=	=	=	=	=	=	uncomplicated course
Pat. Gla.	=	=	=	=	=	=	=	uncomplicated course
Pat. Lie.	=	=	=	=	=	=	=	uncomplicated course
Pat. Kru.	=	=	=	=	=	=	=	uncomplicated course
Pat. La.	=	=	=	=	=	=	=	acute Ciclosporin-Tox.
Pat. Ro.	=	=	=	=	+	=	=	acute Ciclosporin-Tox.
Pat. Bal.	=	=	=	+++	+++	=	+	Urosepsis after Ntx
Pat. Ehl.	=	=	=	=	=	=	=	Anal abscess
Pat. He.	=	=	=	=	=	=	=	bact. gastro enteritis
Pat. Bä.	=	=	=	=	++	=	=	CMV-infection

Table 4 Continued

Patient	IgG	Tf	Alb	α_1AT	β_2MG	RBP	α_1MG	Diagnosis
Pat. Frö.	=	=	=	++	++	=	=	CMV-infection
Pat. Lin.	=	=	=	=	++	=	=	CMV-infection
Pat. Lub.	=	=	=	=	++	=	=	CMV-infection
Pat. Kru.	=	=	=	=	+++	=	=	CMV-infection

+ = Rise in quotient value up to 2× compared with previous day; ++ = Rise in quotient from 2–5× compared with previous day; +++ = Rise in quotient from greater than 5× compared with previous day; – = Drop in quotient by up to ⅓ compared with previous day; –– = Drop in quotient by up to ½ compared with previous day; = = No change when compared with previous day; * = Result confirmed histologically; # = CMV – Cytomegalovirus.

Teknica) Turnhout NL, Paesel-Lorei Frankfurt a. M., D and Biogenesis (Quartett) Berlin, D.

The treatment of the data was made in terms of the quotient between daily protein excretion (mg/d) and the creatinine clearance measured on the same day (ml/min) for each patient. The quotients were given without dimensions as only a numerical increase or decrease was of importance diagnostically. The intraindividual change in the quotient value was evaluated as shown in Table 4. Day 0 was defined as the onset of diuresis after renal transplantation. This is to be taken into account when interpreting Figures 1–5.

All patients received the same immunosuppressive therapy, after an initial dose of 250 mg methyl prednisolone, comprising prednisolone (2.5–7.5 mg/d), azathioprine (2 mg/kg/d) and cyclosporin (3–5 mg/kg/d). Therapeutic cyclosporin whole blood levels were normally between 80–120 ng/ml measured with a specific RIA (Sandoz). The diagnostic sensitivity and specificity were estimated according to accepted methods [Immich 1979].

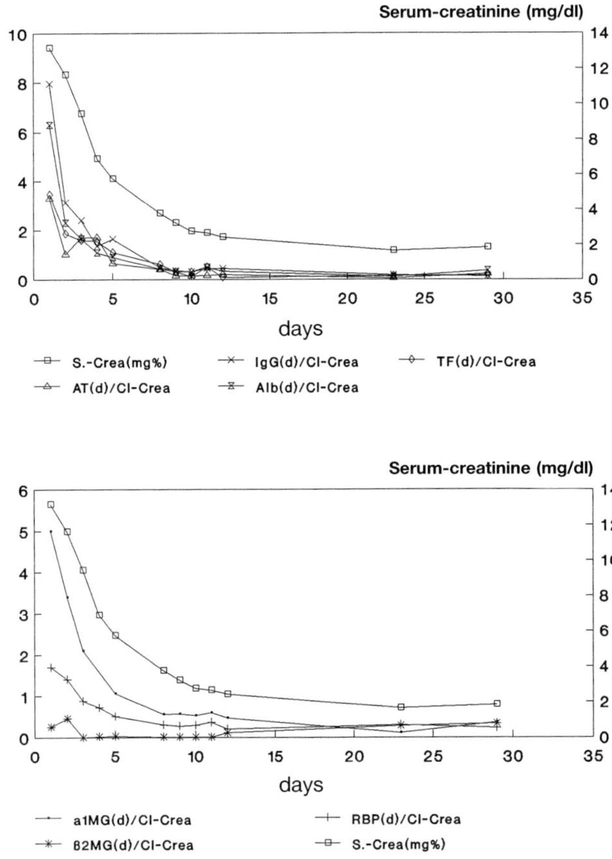

Fig. 1 Uncomplicated case (43-year-old female – Pat. Pen.) after renal transplantation with initial low proteinuria.

Results

1. Uncomplicated course

Figure 1 indicates the course of protein excretion in one patient without a rejection episode. This shows a progressive fall in the quotient value parallel to the fall in serum creatinine concentrations. This pattern is seen in all patients who do not present with post-operative complications.

2. Rejection episodes

Figure 2 represents one patient with histologically confirmed interstitial rejection and shows the urinary protein pattern which is typical for a rejection episode.

There is a rise in serum creatinine, which is accompanied by an increase in IgG, albumin and transferrin. There is also a smaller but significant increase in the α_1-proteinase inhibitor concentration. The "tubular" proteins, especially α_1-microglobulin, either show a decrease in concentration, or remain unchanged. After successful treatment, these proteins rise significantly and are accompanied by a concomitant fall in the levels of the "glomerular" proteins.

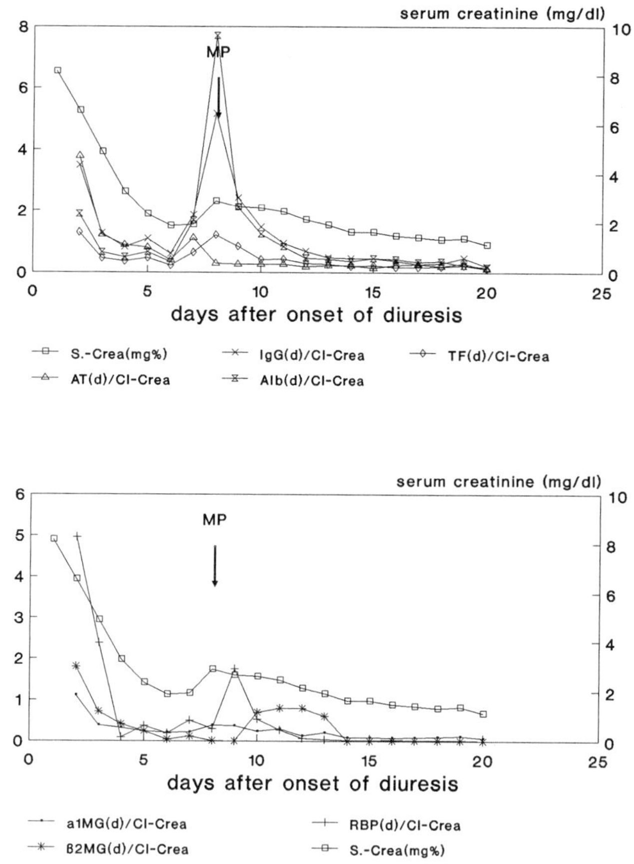

Fig. 2 28-year-old man (Pat. Ris.) after renal transplantation with initially good renal function. On day 7 histologically confirmed interstitial rejection with increase in excretion of the glomerular proteins IgG, TF, Alb. together with an increase of α_1-AT. After successful treatment with methyl prednisolone (MP) an increase of the tubular proteins α_1-MG, RBP and β_2-MG is seen.

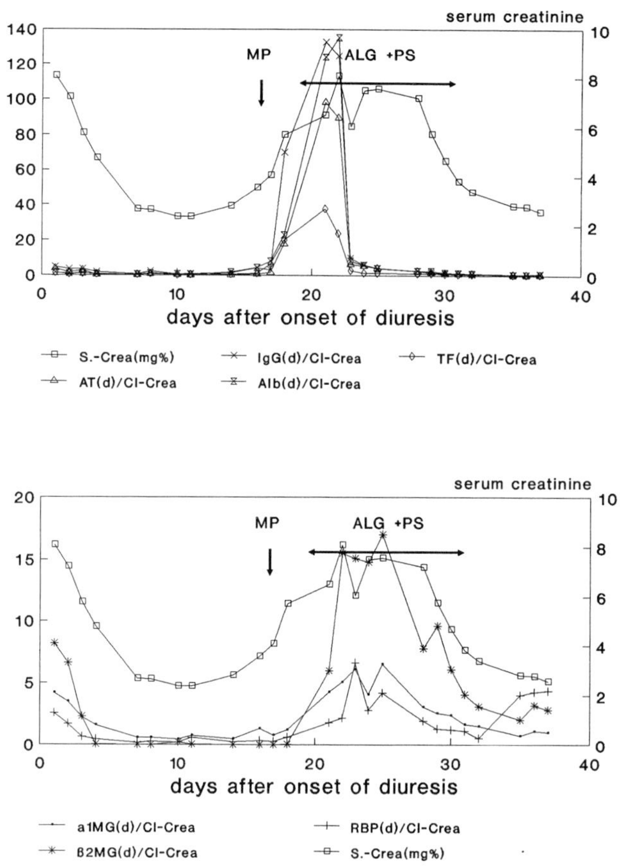

Fig. 3 48-year-old woman (Pat. Gür.) after renal transplantation with initially good renal function. On day 17 histologically confirmed vascular rejection with extreme increase in proteinuria due to glomerular proteins IgG, TF and Alb. Therapy with methyl prednisolone (MP) was ineffective, but the therapy with anti-lymphocyte globulin (ALG) and plasmapheresis (PS) was successful, with subsequent increase in tubular proteinuria seen by increased α_1-MG, RBP and β_2-MG values. The glomerular protein concentration (IgG, TF, Alb.) is reduced during this time.

Although a clear-cut differentation between interstitial and vascular rejection is not possible at the present time, it appears that the rise in the "glomerular" proteins is more marked in the cases of vascular rejection (see Figure 3).

The "glomerular" lesion is only seen in rejection episodes but in all cases and therefore has a diagnostic specificity of 100% and a sensitivity of 100%. A peak of "glomerular" proteins was detected in all of the 25 rejection cases (Table 4). The criterium which was used for the specificity/sensitivity was an increase in total glomerular protein excretion of more than 100% over that in previous 24-hour period. Using the Poisson distribution, the probability of the occurrence of "glomerular" proteinuria as a rejection criterium is at least 86.3% in the 25 confirmed cases of rejection in this study [Immich 1979].

3. Cyclosporin toxicity

Figure 4 presents data from one patient with acute cyclosporin renal toxicity. The diagnosis was made when, after reduction of the dosage of cyclosporin, the serum creatinine concentration decreased. The case in Figure 4 shows that under these circumstances the treatment with methyl prednisolone resulted in no change in serum creatinine. In the only two cases of cyclosporin toxicity without additional complications, no changes in the excretion of urinary proteins were seen.

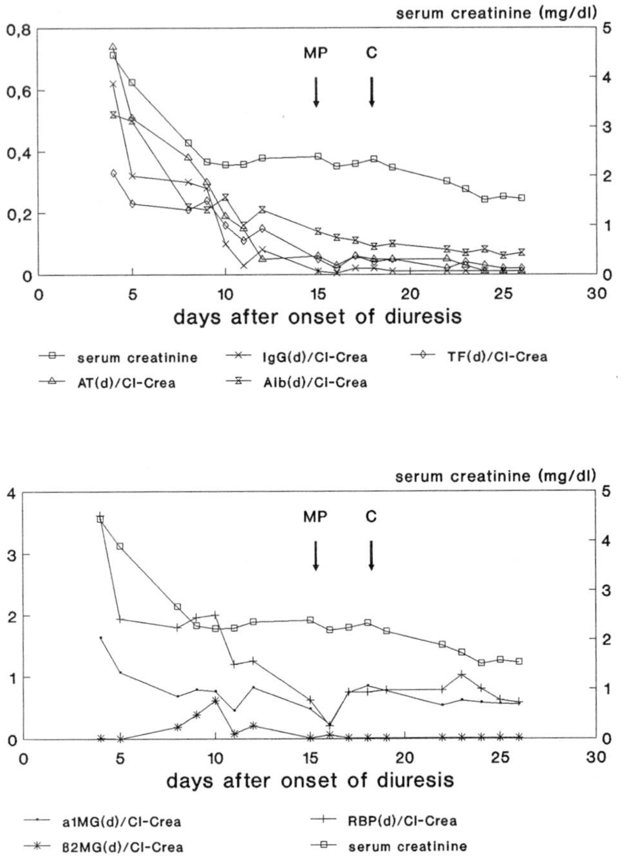

Fig. 4 44-year-old woman (Pat. La.) after renal transplantation with accompanying cyclosporin-nephrotoxicity. Initially good renal function but with continuing high serum creatinine from day 10. An exjuvantibus therapy with methyl prednisolone (MP) was ineffective, but after reduction of cyclosporin (C) serum creatinine decreased. The cyclosporin blood level was 380 ng/ml. No changes were seen in the proteins excreted.

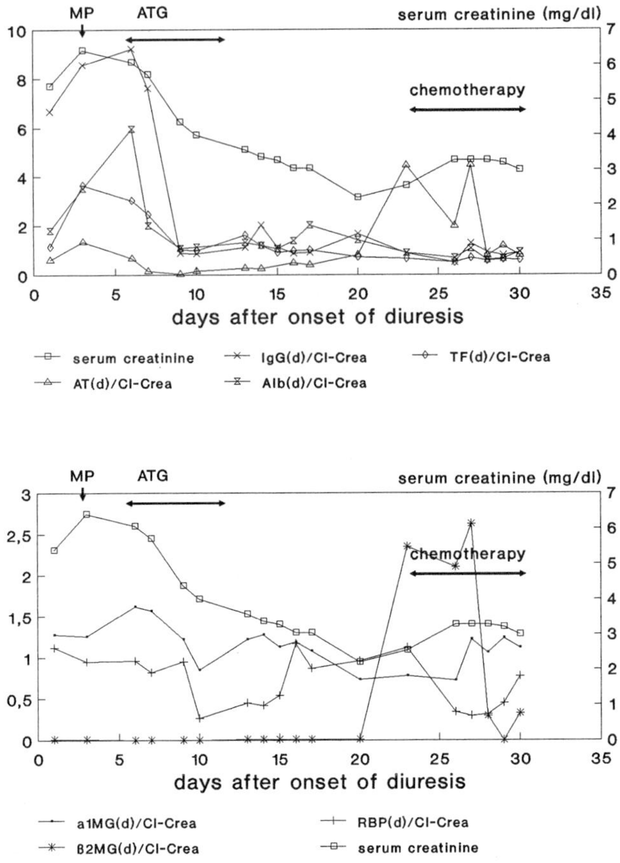

Fig. 5 52-year-old woman (Pat. Bal.) after renal transplantation showing rejection on day 3. After therapy with methyl prednisolone (MP) and anti-human T-lymphocyte globulin (ATG) the serum creatinine and glomerular protein levels both fell (IgG, TF, Alb.). On day 20 the excretion of α_1-AT and β_2-MG increased, this being concomitant with the diagnosis due to urosepsis with streptococcus fecalis. After antibiotic therapy proteinuria due to α_2-AT and β_2-MG fell to pre-infection levels.

4. General points

A point of interest is that all transplanted patients showed a marked excretion of "tubular" proteins which was independent of any complications. In view of these findings, the excretion of β_2-microglobulin, retinol binding protein and α_1-microglobulin were always in the pathological range, when compared with healthy controls. As an example, the concentration of α_1-microglobulin in healthy control urine lay between 3–8 mg/l whereas 25–180 mg/l are found in post renal transplant patients (20).

The levels of IgG fell to within the reference range for healthy non-transplanted persons (<25 mg/d) within 2 weeks post operatively (18). In rejection episodes, the IgG levels reach 450 mg/d in extreme cases. The excretion of albumin can rise to 2000 mg/d and transferrin to 200 mg/d in the same set of patients.

Figure 5 shows the case of a patient who first presented with an interstitial rejection, which was successfully treated with methylprednisolone and anti-human T-lymphocyte globulin. This patient contracted an urosepsis from streptococcus fecalis which was then treated with antibiotics. Whereas during the rejection episode, the usual "glomerular" pattern was seen, the pattern at the time of urosepsis was an increase in α_1-proteinase inhibitor (an acute-phase protein) and β_2-microglobulin – i.e. a "tubular" protein. The "glomerular" proteins, (IgG, albumin and transferrin) showed no changes at this time. The successful treatment of the streptococcus infection was accompanied by a normalisation of the protein pattern.

Discussion

The occurrence of proteinuria in renal transplant rejection episodes has been known for many years [Bear et al. 1988, Frey et al. 1977, Krishua et al. 1987, Lapia et al. 1986] and is well documented [Burghard et al. 1986, Lapia et al. 1986, Lison et al. 1985]. In contrast to results from other groups a "glomerular" pattern of excreted proteins was always seen at the time of rejection, whereas the "tubular" proteins either remained constant or sank. An increase in the "tubular" proteins at the time of rejection was seldom seen (Table 4). In 12 out of 19 cases of interstitial rejection, the typical "glomerular" proteinuria pattern was confirmed by renal biopsy and histological examination, i.e. using the "golden standard" as the reference method.

The remaining 7 cases were not subjected to biopsy, but success in therapy with methyl prednisolone (MP) is most probably due to correct clinical diagnosis (Table 4). All the vascular rejections were proved histologically (Table 4). The urinary protein/creatinine ratio was sufficient in diagnosis of rejection in most cases, however the correct diagnosis of rejection was made more certain when the protein/creatinine clearance ratio was used as far as "background oscillations" were eliminated.

From the results, it can be postulated that a vascular lesion occurs together with the rejection, thus resulting in a "glomerular" protein pattern.

The reduction in "tubular" proteins is probably associated with the reduction in the glomerular filtration rate, and that at this time the tubulus is still capable of clearing the small proteins from the primary urine.

This is supported by the rise in tubular proteins excreted following successful medication and resulting in a normalisation of the glomerular filtration rate. The tubulus in the transplanted kidney does not appear to be able to reabsorb all small proteins completely and this has been confirmed by others [Frey et al. 1977, Lison et al. 1985, Onitsuka et al. 1989].

Although a "glomerular" protein pattern has been documented by other groups [Burghard et al. 1986, Lapia et al. 1986, Manaligod et al. 1986, Onitskuka et al. 1989] this was inconstant. The constancy shown in this article is due in part to the lower detection limits of the assays used. This explains that the IgG urine-peaks seen in rejection may only be 5–15 mg/l whereas for tubular proteins – for example α_1-microglobulin more than 100 mg/l may be found.

The advantage of the methods described here, is that a daily surveillance is possible as the results can be returned to the ward within 4 hours. It has been shown that the rise in "glomerular" urine proteins occurs suddenly. Although the diagnosis of renal transplant rejection may sometimes not be quicker than by observing the rise in serum creatinine, it is possible to differentiate between rejection and cyclosporin neprhotoxicity and other causes of reduced renal function, important facts for determining the course of medication.

We believe that IgG, TF and α_1-MG are the 3 proteins which are necessary for proven diagnosis of rejection.

The much favoured β_2-microglobulin as rejection parameter [Ametor et al. 1985, Odlind et al. 1988, Prischl et al. 1989] receives no support in this publication, as β_2-microglobulin increases are seen in cytomegalovirus infections as well as in urosepsis. Furthermore the stability of β_2-microglobulin in acid urine has been questioned [Ametor et al. 1985, Prischl et al. 1989, Weber et al. 1985]. Some authors report elevated β_2-microglobulin by cyclosporin toxicity [Odlind et al. 1988, Prischl et al. 1989]. β_2-microglobulin increases are also seen after the successful treatment of rejection crises, as a result of the treatment. This is in agreement with the observation that "β_2-microglobulin increases occur too late to monitor rejection crisis" [5].

Whether the rise in IgG is purely due to glomerular "leakage" is questionable, and it may be due in part to secretory processes. Several authors have found [Autignac et al. 1988, Solling 1985, Zevin et al. 1985] massive deposits of IgG during the rejection episode not only along the glomerular, but also the tubular basal membranes. This problem is being investigated in terms of the IgA- and IgM-excretion during early and late rejection episodes, as well as specific proteins and immune complexes.

To conclude, the results published here have been made possible by using sensitive, specific and robust immunoluminometric assays and have served to throw more light on the course of renal rejection as monitored by proteins excreted in the urine of transplanted patients. In addition the differentiation between drug overdose and rejection or urosepsis allows a rapid and accurate choice of medication.

Acknowledgements

The authors wish to thank Frau Hildegard Jaensch and Frau Christine Wolanin for excellent technical assistance in performing the immunoluminometric assays as well as Frau Bettina Polke for the layout and typing of the manuscript.

REFERENCES

Ametov AS, Toritsina LK, Gurera IV 1985 β_2-microglobulin in clinical practice. Med Radiol Mosk *30:* 83

Autignac C, Hinglais N, Gubler MC, Gaguadoux MF, Broyer M, Habib R 1988 Novo membranous glomerulo-nephritis in renal allografts in children. Clin Nephrol *30:* 1

Bear RA, Aprile M, Sweet J, Cole PH 1988 Proteinuria in renal transplant recipients: incidence, cause, prognostic importance. Transplant Proc *20:* 1235

Braun J, Schultek Th, Tegtmeier KF, Florenz A, Rohde C, Wood WG 1986 Luminometric assays of seven acute-phase proteins in minimal volumes of serum, plasma, sputum and bronchioalveolar lavage. Clin Chem *31:* 743

Burghard R, Galaske RG, Offner G, Ehrich JH, Leititis JU, Brodehl J 1986 Urinary protein analysis in the early detection of acute rejection episodes after renal transplantation in children. Clin Nephrol *26:* 1

Dati F, Lammers M 1988 Nierenschädigungen: Früherkennung durch neue Methoden zum Nachweis einer Proteinurie. Diagnose + Labor *38:* 24

Frey BM, Frey FJ, Wegmüller E, Holder G 1977 Proteinurie nach Nierentransplantation. Schweiz Med Wschr *107:* 1181

Guder WG 1988 Die Proteinurie: Ursachen, Formen, Bestimmungsmethoden. Diagnose + Labor *38:* 2

Immich H 1979 Medizinische Statistik, Schattauer Verlag, Stuttgart – New York, S 259

Krishua KS, Pandey AP, Kirnbakaran MG, Kanagasabapathy AS 1987 Urinary protein/creatinine ratio as an indicator of allograft function following live related donor renal transplantation. Clin Chim Acta *163:* 51

Lapia A, Zyman H, Gabl F, Kopsa H, Zazgornik J 1986 Monitoring of urinary proteins by SDS electrophoresis in kidney transplant patients. J Clin Chem Clin Biochem *24:* 221

Lison AE, Brandt U, Weisshaar Ch, Meyer E, Buchholz B, Zastrow F 1985 Frühzeitige Diagnose der Abstoßungsreaktion nach Nierentransplantation mit Hilfe der SDS-Disk-Elektrophorese? Nieren- und Hochdruckkrankheiten *14:* 537

Manaligod JR, Jao W, Mozes MF, Jonasson O 1986 Glomerular changes in renal allografts. Am J Kidney Dis *7:* 29

Odlind B, Backman U, Forbes MA, Cooper EH 1988 Proteinuria after renal transplantation. Contrib Nephrol *68:* 149

Onitsuka S, Yamaguchi Y, Toma H, Yagisawa T, Takahashi K, Teraoka S, Ota K 1989 Glomerular rejection in kidney allografts under cyclosporin. Transplant Proc *21:* 1680

Petersen KG, Schultheiss M, Rosak C, Schuler G, Khalaf N, Schmidt P, Hecker W, Haug H, Kerp L 1989 Diabetische Proteinurie, was sagen Markerproteine? Akt. Endokr. Stoffw. *10:* 58

Prischl F, Gremmel F, Schwabe M, Schindler J, Balcke P, Kopsa H, Pinter G, Schwarzmeier J, Zagornik J 1989 Beta-2-microglobulin between ciclosporin A nephrotoxicity and graft rejections in renal transplant recipients. Nephron *51:* 330

Schmitt Y, Schneider H 1988 Die Ausscheidung der Plasmaproteine Albumin, Transferrin, Immunglobulin G (IgG) und retinolbindendes Protein (RbP) im Urin gesunder Testpersonen zur Ermittlung von Referenzwerten. Nieren- und Hochdruckkrankheiten *17:* 512

Solling J 1985 Circulating immune complexes in patients with glomerulonephritis and in renal transplant patients. Scand J Urol Nephrol Suppl *97:* 1

Weber MH, Scholz P, Stibbe W, Scheler F 1985 Alpha-1-Mikroglobulin in Urin und Serum bei Proteinurie und Niereninsuffizienz. Klin Wschr *63:* 711

Wood WG 1989 Radioimmunoassay versus nicht-radioisotopischer Immunoassay 1989. Pro und contra. Lab Med *13:* 345

Wood WG, Herhahn D, Steinhoff J, Schulz E, Sack K 1990 Zur diagnostischen Relevanz von Harnproteinanalysen nach Nierentransplantation. Focus MHL *7:* 33

Wood WG, Herhahn D, Steinhoff J, Feddersen A, Schulz E, Sack K 1990 The diagnostic relevance of specific urinary Proteins after renal transplantation. Ärztl Lab *36:* 260

Zevin D, Ben-Bassat M, Weinstein T, Shapira Z, Levi J 1985 Rejection-related nephrotic syndrome associated with massive antiglomerular and antitubular basement membrane deposits. Isr J Med Sci *21:* 915

Clinical Nephrology, Vol. 35 No. 6 – 1991 (263–269)

Familial juvenile gouty nephropathy with renal urate hypoexcretion preceding renal disease

F. Moro[1], C. S. Ogg[2], H. A. Simmonds[1], J. S. Cameron[2], C. Chantler[3], M. B. McBride[1], J. A. Duley[1] and P. M. Davies[1]

[1] *Purine Research Laboratory,* [2] *Renal Unit, and Department of Paediatrics*[3], *Guy's Campus UMDS, London, England*

Abstract. This paper reports investigations in a young woman with renal disease and six other seemingly healthy young members of a new kindred (four male: two female) with familial juvenile gouty nephropathy (McKusick 16200). The family had previously been known to have a "familial" renal disease, but came to attention through an isolated episode of gout in the propositus when renal function was already impaired. A reduced GFR was found in three of the other six subjects. Hyperuricemia associated with a grossly reduced fractional uric acid clearance ($C_{ur}/C_{cr} \times 100$) was present in the propositus and five kindred members, three of whom were children. The finding of this abnormality in two subjects with normal GFR suggests that this apparent hallmark of the disease precedes the onset of renal damage. The results confirm the dominant nature of the disorder, and highlight the need to investigate all kindred members of patients with juvenile gout and renal failure. Early recognition is important, since allopurinol therapy in doses adjusted to the reduced renal function may ameliorate the progression of the renal lesion.

Key words: familial gout – precocious gout – hyperuricemia – renal failure – gouty nephropathy – allopurinol – fractional urate clearance

Introduction

Gout is unusual in the young, particularly in young women [Lally et al. 1986, Wyngaarden et al. 1983, Simmonds 1987]. Two inherited X-linked disorders have been described presenting as gout in young adolescent males: hypoxanthine guanine phosphoribosyltransferase (HGPRT) deficiency and phosphoribosylpyrophosphate synthetase (PRPS) superactivity [Wyngaarden et al. 1983, Simmonds 1987]. In PRPS superactivity carrier females may also present with gout, but both are very rare disorders accounting for less than 1% of the gouty population [Wyngaarden et al. 1983], and although acute urate nephropathy can occur in HGPRT deficiency [Simmonds 1987], these genetic defects are not generally associated with chronic renal disease.

Familial juvenile gouty nephropathy (FJGN: McKusick 16200), was first described by Duncan and Dixon [1960], and has been documented since in many countries, although much of the evidence is anecdotal [Simmonds et al. 1980, Simmonds et al. 1980, Rosenbloom et al. 1967, Treadwell 1971, Van Goor et al. 1971, Westberg et al. 1979, Massari et al. 1980, Richmond et al. 1981, Leumann et al. 1983]. The condition has several distinctive features: it affects young men and women equally and, in the few kindreds studied in detail, renal disease has been rapidly progressive, usually leading to end stage renal disease between 30 and 40 years of age [Wyngaarden et al. 1983, Simmonds 1987, Duncan et al. 1960, Simmonds et al. 1980, Simmonds et al. 1980, Hollingworth et al. 1983]. Two groups have reported medullary cystic disease in juvenile gouty nephropathy [Thompson et al. 1978, Burke et al. 1982], one of which questioned whether these were not all manifestations of underlying medullary cystic disease [Burke et al. 1982], reflecting a continuing debate as to whether the hyperuricemia preceded the renal disease or vice versa. However, no cause and effect relationship between hyperuricemia and renal failure has been demonstrated unequivocally. Recently we reported studies in 21 young men and women with precocious onset of gout or hyperuricemia which first drew attention to the underlying renal disease [Calabrese et al. 1990]. The consistent finding in the majority was a

Received July 29, 1990; November 28, 1990.

Reprint requests to Dr. F. Moro, Purine Research Laboratory, Clinical Science Laboratories, 18th Floor Tower Block, Guy's Hospital, London Bridge, SE1 9RT, England.

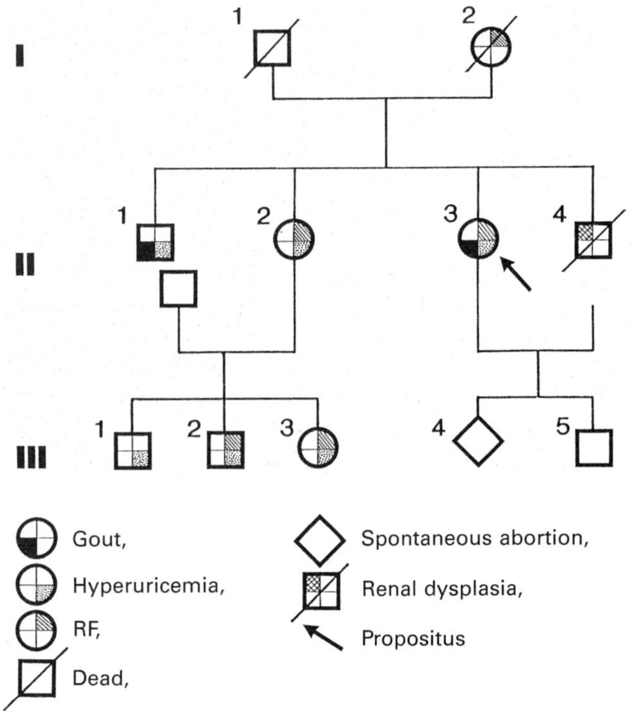

Fig. 1 The dominant inheritance in this new kindred with FJGN is shown, and the presence of gout and/or hyperuricemia and renal disease, as indicated by the key given on the right hand side, in young seemingly healthy kindred members. The strong penetrance affecting young males and females equally over three successive generations (1–111), and the absence of renal disease in two males (II 1, III 1) with hyperuricemia only, is evident.

grossly reduced fractional urate clearance (FE_{ur}: uric acid clearance factored by creatinine clearance × 100) for age, sex or renal function (4.4 ± 1.4%).

In this study we describe a new kindred, which came to attention through an isolated episode of gout in a young woman previously designated as having a familial renal disease. Family investigations revealed early manifestations of the disorder in young apparently healthy subjects, both male and female: hyperuricemia associated with a reduced fractional urate clearance in the majority and a less severe renal impairment in some. These studies demonstrate that renal hypoexcretion of urate may precede the onset of renal disease in this dominantly inherited defect, and that this reduced fractional excretion of urate is probably the central event in the disorder.

Patients and methods

Patients

The propositus LJ (born 19.9.61) (II 3, Figure 1) was originally diagnosed as having "familial renal disease". Proteinuria was discovered during pregnancy which led to a normal delivery (III 5) in 1979. At the age of 16, she had suffered an antepartum hemorrhage with intrauterine death (III 4, Figure 1). She was symptomless when first investigated for renal impairment in 1981. Her weight was 44 kg, BP 120/85, urine deposit and culture were normal, and 24 hr protein excretion was 1.9 G. Plasma creatinine was found to be 145 μmol/l, urea 8.1 mmol/l, urate 460 μmol/l, GFR (single injection of ^{51}Cr edetate) 35 ml/min/1.73 m^2. On IVU both kidneys were small with smooth outlines. She did not return to our clinic until 1985, when she was still symptomless, BP was 100/70, plasma creatinine 189 μmol/l, urea 9.9 mmol/l and she was started on a low protein diet. Two years later she suffered a single episode of gout which was attributed to her renal impairment, until the surviving brother (II 1, Figure 1) also developed gout, suggesting a familial gouty disorder. Detailed purine metabolic studies were carried out in 1988, by which time her plasma creatinine and urate had risen (Table 1), and the FE_{ur} was found to be low for the degree of renal dysfunction [Calabrese et al. 1990]. Her renal function deteriorated steadily to end stage renal failure in 1989, when plasma creatinine was 808 μmol/l, requiring hemodialysis and CAPD. Cadaveric renal transplantation was unsuccessful with rejection leading to infarction of the kidney, and transplant nephrectomy. She is currently maintained on CAPD.

MB, the mother of LJ (I 2, Figure 1), died of chronic renal failure at age 43 whilst on hemodialysis in our Renal Unit; an aunt was reported to have died of "blood disease". In addition to LJ there were two other reputedly healthy surviving offspring: JB and SR (see below). A fourth pregnancy had resulted in the normal delivery of a male infant who died at age 10 weeks with a diagnosis of "bilateral total renal dysplasia" made at postmortem (II 4, Figure 1). MB was first studied in 1969 following referral for investigation of low back pain and renal failure. She was small and had a normal BP; her plasma creatinine was 550 μmol/l, urea 25 mmol/l, and she had a trace of protein in urine. IVU showed that both kidneys were grossly contracted. Bone X-ray showed renal osteodystrophy, and treatment was begun with dihydrotachysterol. In 1972, her plasma creatinine had risen to 900 μmol/l, urate 660 μmol/l. Hemodialysis was commenced in 1973, and in 1974 splenectomy was performed for hypersplenism and anemia. Death occurred in 1976 from pneumonia, with fluid overload and access problems.

The isolated episodes of gout in LJ and JB, coupled with the family history of renal disease and the results of the detailed metabolic studies in LJ, prompted the present studies in JB and SR, the two siblings of LJ, and in LuJ the son of LJ, and subsequently the three children of SR: DR, StR and CR (Figure 1).

JB (born 31.3.55), a seemingly healthy brother of LJ, was studied at the age of 33 (II 1, Figure 1) because of the family history of renal failure and a recent attack of clinical gout. Values for plasma creatinine, plasma urate, GFR and FE_{ur} are shown in Table 1. Although the GFR was normal, the plasma urate level was high by the specific enzymic method used, associated with a grossly reduced FE_{ur}. Allopurinol was commenced at 100 mg per day.

SR (born 2.4.57), the seemingly healthy sister, (II 2, Figure 1) was first seen aged 32. There was a history of recurrent urinary tract infections and occasional bilateral loin pain. For two years she had had frequent headaches, for which up to 3 Sulphadeine® tablets per day (paracetamol, caffeine and codeine) had been taken. On investigation there were no apparent abnormalities: BP 120/80, and plasma creatinine was normal. Urine deposit and culture were also normal. However, both GFR, and FE_{ur} were reduced and the plasma urate was raised (Table 1). Renal ultrasonography showed both kidneys to be slightly reduced in size, but no calculi or obstruction were present. She was started on allopurinol at 100 mg/day.

Results in the three healthy children of SR, investigated subsequently because of the abnormal findings in the mother (Table 1), were as follows: DR, the eldest son (III 1, Figure 1) aged 14 (born 8.1.75) appeared normal on clinical examination, with BP 120/75 and normal urine test. Plasma creatinine, and GFR were normal (Table 1). Plasma urate, however, was greatly elevated associated with a grossly reduced FE_{ur}. He was commenced on allopurinol at 50 mg per day and progress will be assessed at regular intervals.

StR, the second son (III 2, Figure 1), aged 12, (born 25.3.77) was reported to have always been thirsty, to pass large quantities of urine, and to have been enuretic till the age of 7. Height appeared normal in the third centile, BP was 110/70. Plasma urea, creatinine, and urate were all elevated for age and GFR was reduced (Table 1); FE_{ur} was also low for age and reduced renal function. X-Ray of the hands showed incipient changes of renal osteodystrophy. He was started on a hypercaloric diet low in purines and phosphate. Treatment was commenced with allopurinol 50 mg, and alphacalcidol 0.25 μg daily.

CR, the daughter (III 3, Figure 1), aged 9 (born 26.3.80), had a history of dysuria and vulval soreness and sometimes complained of central abdominal pain. Repeated urine cultures had been normal, as was an IVU and ultrasonography of the urinary tract. BP was normal (98/55). Investigations revealed a normal plasma creatinine, but increased plasma urate associated with a grossly reduced FE_{ur} for age (Table 1).

Table 1 Plasma uric acid and creatinine concentrations in the propositus and six seemingly healthy members of the same kindred with FJGN and the husband of one member. The normal range for plasma uric acid by the specific enzymic method used is listed in parenthesis; the control range for creatinine is 50–130 μmol/l for adults. The urinary UA/Cr excretion ratio (mmol/mmol), FE_{ur}%, GFR (ml/min corrected to 1.73 m^2) and activity of the purine enzymes APRT and PNP in lysed erythrocytes (RBC) are also listed (normal range in the UK population for APRT is 16–32 nmol/mgHb/h and 3000–7000 for PNP).

Subject	Plasma UA (μmol/l)	Cr	UA/Cr	Urine FE_{ur} %	GFR ml/min 1.73 m^2	RBC enzymes APRT (nmol/mgHb/h)	PNP
LJ (f, 28)	490	449	0.08	8.2	–	28	4120
SR (f, 31)	430	105	0.24	5.8	59	19	2500
control (f)	(140–280)		<0.30	12.2 ± 1.9			
JB (m, 34)	440	91	0.20	4.0	107*	28	3250
PR (m, 32)**	320	88	–	–	–	6	4340
control (m)	(180–340)		<0.25	8.2 ± 1.2			
LuJ (m, 9)	170	61	0.36	12.9	114	24	4160
CR (f, 9)	370	79	0.24	5.2	57	4	4040
StR (m, 12)	340	212	0.19	11.1	19	8	3140
DR (m, 14)	390	76	0.19	3.8	134	22	3000
control (c)	(130–250)		+	18.5 ± 3.2			

* creatinine clearance, – not investigated, ** husband of SR, + varies with age, UA uric acid, Cr creatinine

GFR was also reduced. Allopurinol was commenced at 50 mg daily.

LuJ (III 5, Figure 1), the only surviving and apparently healthy child of LJ, aged 9 (born 20. 12. 79), was found to have a normal plasma creatinine urate, FE_{ur} and GFR (Table 1).

Methods

Detailed biochemical studies were performed in all the above subjects on a low purine caffeine-free diet and no medication. Venous blood was taken into lithium heparin at the end of a 24 hour urine collection (toluene preservative) and centrifuged and separated immediately. Creatinine was measured by standard rate-dependent Jaffe based methods. GFR was evaluated using a single injection of ^{51}Cr labelled edetate. Uric acid and other endogenous purines were investigated using sensitive methods described previously [Simmonds et al. 1980, Fairbanks et al. 1987, Morris et al. 1986]. The normal range for plasma urate by the specific enzymic method used in UK subjects on a normal diet (generally low in purine) is 140–280 μmol/l for females, 180–340 μmol/l for males aged 10 to 40 years, and 130–250 μmol/l for children from 1–10 years. Purine production was evaluated from the ratio of the urine uric acid excretion in mmol/24 h relative to creatinine excretion in mmol/24 h (UA/Cr). Fractional uric acid clearance (uric acid clearance factored by creatinine clearance ×100 : FE_{ur}) was calculated in all subjects. Values for FE_{ur} in a healthy UK population differ between adult males (8.2 ± 1.2%), pre-menopausal females (12.2 ± 1.9%), and children of either sex (18.5 ± 3.2%). FE_{ur} is reduced (5.4 ± 1.7%) in the majority of middle-aged male gouty patients compared with age matched UK controls [Calabrese et al. 1990, Cameron et al. 1981]. Purine enzyme activities (HGPRT and PRPS, adenine phosphoribosyltransferase [APRT] and purine nucleoside phosphorylase [PNP] were also investigated in intact and lysed erythrocytes by methods adapted to high performance liquid chromatography (HPLC) as described [Fairbanks et al. 1987, Morris et al. 1986].

Results

The family tree shown in Figure 1 summarizes the results in individual family members (see key for explanation) and confirms the high penetrance and dominant nature of the disorder.

Table 1 compares the results of the biochemical investigations in the propositus LJ and the six apparently healthy members of the kindred, together with the renal function studies. Studies from PR, the healthy husband of SR, are listed for comparison. In addition to the propositus, hyperuricemia was found in two other adults and three of the children studied (Table 1). Purine production, as estimated from uric acid excretion on a creatinine basis, was normal or low in all instances. Concentrations of the other minor purine bases in plasma and urine were all within the normal range (data not shown). The activities of the two enzymes associated with X-linked gout (HGPRT and PRPS) were also within the normal range in all subjects (Table 1). The combined findings would exclude uric acid overproduction as the basis of the gout and hyperuricemia in this kindred. The clearance studies demonstrate that the metabolic basis for this lies rather in a grossly reduced FE_{ur}. The absence of detectable renal disease in two kindred members with a reduced FE_{ur} is noteworthy. SR was found coincidentally to be heterozygous for PNP deficiency (Table 1), and two of her children, StR and CR were heterozygotes for APRT deficiency. The latter defect was shown to be inherited from the father, PR.

Discussion

This new kindred with FJGN is remarkable for several reasons. Firstly, until an isolated episode of gout in a young woman being treated for renal failure prompted study of other seemingly healthy members, the kindred was considered to suffer from an undefined familial renal disease, the mother having died previously of renal failure, and an infant brother of bilateral renal dysplasia. The second important feature is the presence of hyperuricemia in such young subjects and the ability to define the cause of this at the level of the renal handling of uric acid by the kidney. The third is the finding of this extreme renal tubular retention of urate in two individuals who still had normal renal function. The fourth is the occurrence of the disorder in young normotensive subjects of such slight build, in contrast to "typical" or "primary" gout in which hypertension and obesity are frequent accompaniments [Wyngaarden et al. 1983], exacerbating the already reduced FE_{ur}. The confirmation that plasma creatinine alone is a poor guide to early renal impairment in such subjects is equally noteworthy, as is the need for early recognition of the familial disorder which allows treatment of the associated hyperuricemia.

Gout in this kindred, and others like it, is obviously an important symptom of an underlying disease associated with a grossly reduced FE_{ur}. The number of seemingly healthy yet affected members in the present kindred underlines the need for detailed investigation of all such kindred members. Had the mother presented with gout, attention would have been drawn to the kindred, and the need for purine metabolic studies highlighted. Consequently, the propositus would have been investigated annually, as have children of earlier kindreds [Simmonds et al. 1980, Simmonds et al. 1980, Calabrese et al. 1990, Cameron et al. 1981]. The familial disease could thus have been diagnosed and treated much earlier, and the rapid progression to renal failure might have been avoided [Wyngaarden et al. 1983, Simmonds 1987]. The decline in renal function over eight years in the propositus treated only for familial renal disease, contrasts with the apparent amelioration of the renal lesion in three other subjects with FJGN studied by us and treated with allopurinol over similar or even longer periods (Figure 2). The latter kindreds were fortunate in that the index case presented initially with gout, which made early instigation of allopurinol therapy possible in all hyperuricemic kindred members, but at a dose commensurate with the degree of renal disease in those with a reduced GFR [Simmonds 1987, Simmonds et al. 1980, Cameron et al. 1987].

FJGN is clearly an unusual disorder within the spectrum of gout [Precocious familial gout 1990, Cameron et al. 1990]. Although the majority of gouty patients (over 90%) have a reduced FE_{ur} (5.4 ± 1.7%), the reduction is not as great as in FJGN [Wyngaarden et al. 1983, Calabrese et al. 1990]. Moreover, they are usually middle-aged and male with normal renal function for age [Wyngaarden et al. 1983] and hypertension, a frequent accompaniment of this so-called "primary" gout [Wyngaarden et al. 1983], and of renal disease per se, is not a feature of FJGN [Calabrese et al. 1990, Cameron et al. 1981]. It is worth reiterating that today gout is equally rare in renal failure [Simmonds et al. 1980, Cameron et al. 1981] and the FE_{ur} generally increases with progressive reduction in GFR [Calabrese et al. 1990, Cameron et al. 1981]. The other two genetic disorders presenting as gout in the young are both X-linked and again renal function and FE_{ur} are generally normal. The present studies have confirmed the dominant nature of FJGN and its early onset and demonstrate that both purine production and purine enzymes associated with uric acid overproduction are normal in this disorder. Although two carriers for APRT deficiency were found, this was inherited from the father, thereby supporting earlier contentions that the association of heterozygosity for APRT deficiency with juvenile gout as reported in several kindreds [Simmonds et al. 1989], was coincidental. The finding of heterozygosity for PNP deficiency in one affected kindred member was equally unusual, but again seemingly unrelated to the disease.

There are several possible genetic mechanisms for FJGN. First, an as yet unidentified metabolite might be produced which alters tubular urate handling, probably by competing with one of the transporters recently identified on the brush-border or baso-lateral membranes of the proximal tubule [Werner et al. 1986]. Second, there could be a genetic defect in the transporter of uric acid itself. Animal studies have shown that the pig, a net secretor of uric acid, lacks the brush-border anion-exchange transporter [Werner et al. 1986]. Conversely a breed of gouty chickens apparently possess a genetic defect in the urate secretory mechanism on the baso-lateral membrane [Zmuda et al. 1975]. Although a grossly reduced FE_{ur} of even greater magnitude than that found in FJGN has been reported in the Maori and other Polynesians [Prior et al. 1966, Gibson et al. 1984], the Maori do not suffer progressive renal disease [Gibson et al. 1984]. This raises the possibility that the renal damage may not relate directly to the hyperuricemia, and there may be two separate defects closely linked on the same gene,

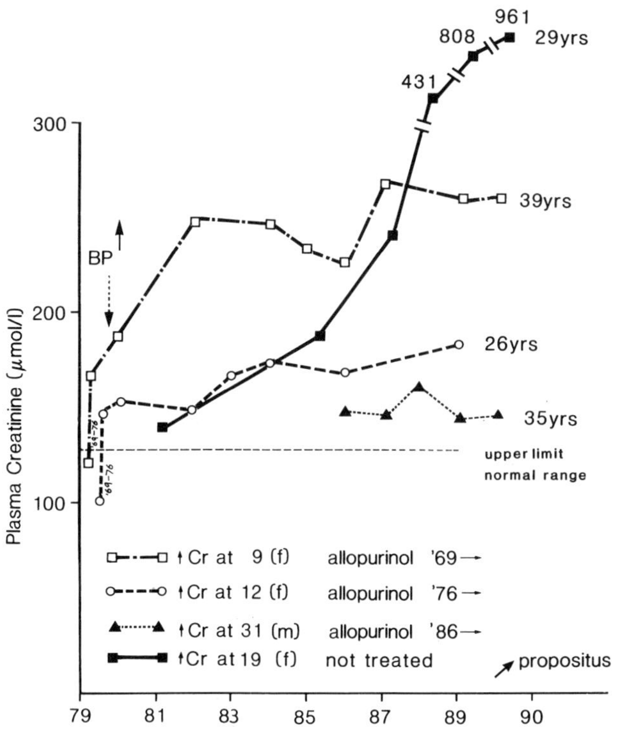

Fig. 2 Plasma creatinine values from 1981 to the present time in the propositus (LJ, solid line) compared with data from two adult females from a previously reported kindred with FJGN [Simmonds et al. 1980] from 1980, and a male from another kindred, identified in 1986 [Calabrese et al. 1990]. The relative stabilization of creatinine levels in these patients following introduction of allopurinol contrasts with the relentless progression in the propositus LJ, treated only for renal impairment over a similar period. (The sharp increase in creatinine in the young woman now aged 39 coincided with the onset of a raised BP following commencement of contraceptive therapy which was subsequently discontinued.)

one affecting renal urate handling, the other associated with progressive renal disease [Calabrese et al. 1990]. The findings in the present kindred would be consistent with any of the above possibilities, but it would not be ethical to withold allopurinol from the few members with a normal GFR as yet and only a reduced FE_{ur} as evidence of the familial disorder, in order to test the latter hypothesis. The presence of hyperuricemia and a low FE_{ur} in these kindreds is an indication for allopurinol therapy. According to our observations [Simmonds et al. 1980, Moro et al. 1991] allopurinol appears to ameliorte the progression of the renal damage. The degree of renal function at the time of commencing treatment is an important factor determining therapeutic effect.

The other interesting observation is the considerable heterogeneity in expression of FJGN, also evident in previous kindreds [Simmonds et al. 1980, Simmonds et al. 1980]. Although presentation is generally around or soon after puberty, in the few kindreds investigated in detail by us there is a similar history of death in utero or in the neonatal period [Simmonds et al. 1980]. This suggests that severe forms of the defect may be lethal, and underlines the need to identify the defective gene(s). Only the index case has been studied to date in many families in which there is an equally strong family history [Calabrese et al. 1990]. In several kindreds there are young children for whom the parents wish to determine prognosis; development of DNA based tests would enable presymptomatic determination of genetic status. Members of earlier kindreds have reached marriagable age, and it would be advantageous to be able to offer prenatal diagnosis for a disorder of this severity. Although the genetic basis is unknown, our combined experience leads us to speculate that FJGN may not be such a rare disorder as has been thought. We have studied patients with all the known inherited purine and pyrimidine disorders [Simmonds 1987, Fairbanks et al. 1987], and the largest number of cases diagnosed in the UK with any one such defect [Morgan et al. 1987] amounts to less than half the number of subjects identified by us with FJGN.

The results in this new kindred highlight the fact that the recognition of FJGN is easily (and possibly frequently) missed by nephrologists. The data underline the importance of early identification [Cameron et al. 1990], since allopurinol treatment in appropriately reduced dosage may ameliorate the progression of the renal lesion [Cameron et al. 1987, Moro et al. 1991]. Finally, they provide the first clear evidence that the hyperuricemia is associated with extreme renal hypoexcretion of uric acid, and that this hallmark of the disease by preceed renal disease. However, they do not enable us to suggest which of the genetic mechanisms discussed above may be operative.

Acknowledgement

This study was supported by the Arthritis and Rheumatism Council for Research.

REFERENCES

Burke JR, Inglis JA, Craswell PW, et al. 1982 Juvenile nephronophthisis and medullary cystic disease. Clin Nephrol *18:* 1

Calabrese G, Simmonds HA, Cameron JS 1990 Precocious familial gout with reduced fractional urate clearance and normal purine enzymes. Q Jl Med *75:* 441

Cameron JS, Ogg CS, Moro F, Chantler C, Simmonds HA 1990 Precocious familial gout. Lancet (letter) *ii:* 745

Cameron JS, Simmonds HA 1981 Uric acid, gout and the kidney. J Clin Pathol *34:* 1245

Cameron JS, Simmonds HA 1987 Use and abuse of allopurinol. BMJ (editorial) *294:* 1504

Duncan H, Dixon AStJ 1960 Gout, familial hyperuricemia and renal disease. Q Jl Med *29:* 127

Fairbanks LD, Simmonds HA, Webster DR 1987 Use of intact erythrocytes in the diagnosis of inherited purine and pyrimidine disorders. J Inher Metab Dis *10:* 174

Gibson T, Waterworth R, Hatfield P, et al. 1984 Hyperuricemia in young New Zealand Mori men. Adv Exp Med Biol *165A:* 123

Hollingworth P, Scott JT 1983 Familial gout, hyperuricemia and renal impairment. Ann Rheum Dis *42 (Suppl 1):* 87

Lally EW, Ho G, Kaplan SR 1986 The clinical spectrum of gouty arthritis in women. Arch Intern Med *146:* 2221

Leumann EP, Wegmann W 1983 Familial nephropathy with hyperuricemia and gout. Nephron *34:* 51

Massari PU, Hsu CH, Barnes RV, et al. 1980 Familial hyperuricemia and renal disease. Arch Intern Med *140:* 680

Morgan G, Levinsky RJ, Hugh-Jones K, Fairbanks LD, Morris GS, Simmonds HA 1987 Heterogeneity of biochemical, clinical and immunological parameters in severe combined immunodeficiency due to adenosine deaminase deficiency. Clin Exp Immunol *70:* 491

Moro F, Simmonds HA, Cameron JS, Ogg CS, Williams DG 1991 Does allopurinol affect the clinical progression in FJGN? Abstract 7th International/3rd European Joint Symposium on Purine and Pyrimidine metabolism in man, Bournemouth GB

Morris GS, Simmonds HA, Davies PM 1986 Use of biological fluids for the rapid diagnosis of potentially lethal inherited disorders of human purine and pyrimidine metabolism. Biomed Chromatog *1:* 109

Precocious familial gout 1990 Lancet (editorial) *ii:* 412

Prior IA, Rose BS, Harvey HP, Davidson F 1966 Hyperuricemia, gout and diabetic abnormality in Polynesian people. Lancet *i:* 333

Richmond JM, Kincaid Smith P, Whitworth JA, Becker GJ 1981 Familial urate nephropathy. Clin Nephrol *16:* 163

Rosenbloom FM, Kelley WN, Carr AA, Seegmiller JE 1967 Familial nephropathy and gout in a kindred (abstract). Clin Res *15:* 270

Simmonds HA 1987 Purine and pyrimidine disorders. Chapter 6. In: *Holton JB* (ed). The inherited metabolic diseases. Churchill Livingstone, Edinburgh, p 215

Simmonds HA, Cameron JS, Potter CF, Farebrother DA 1980 Familial gout and renal failure in young women. Clin Nephrol *14:* 176

Simmonds HA, Cameron JS, Potter CF, et al. 1980 Renal failure in young subjects with familial gout. Adv Exp Med Biol *122A:* 15

Simmonds HA, Van Acker KJ, Sahota A 1989 Adenine phosphoribosyltransferase deficiency: 2,8-dihydroxyadenine lithiasis. In: *Scriver CR, Beaudet AL, Sly WS, Valle D* (eds). The metabolic basis of inherited disease. McGraw-Hill, New York, 6th edition, Chapter *39:* p 1029

Simmonds HA, Webster DR, Becroft DMO, Potter CF 1980 Purine and pyrimidine metabolism in hereditary oroticaciduria. Eur J Clin Invest *10:* 333

Thompson GR, Weiss JJ, Goldman RT, Rigg GA 1978 Familial occurrence of hyperuricemia, gout, and medullary cystic disease. Arch Int Med *138:* 1614

Treadwell BLJ 1971 Juvenile gout. Ann Rheum Dis *30:* 279

Van Goor W, Kooiker CJ, Doorhout Mees EJ 1971 An unusual form of renal disease associated with gout and hypertension. J Clin Pathol *24:* 354

Werner D, Martinez F, Roch Ramel F 1986 Urate and PAH transport in the brush border membrane of the pig kidney. J Pharm Exp Therapeut *237:* 636

Westberg NG, Rosen E, Waldenstrom J 1979 Recessive X-linked hyperuricemia with gout and renal damage, normal activity of hypoxanthine-guanine phosphoribosyltransferase and resistance to azaguanine. Acta Med Scand *205:* 163

Wyngaarden JB, Kelley WN 1983 Gout. In: *Stanbury JB, Wyngaarden JB, Fredericksen DA, Goldstein JL, Brown MS* (eds). The metabolic basis of inherited disease. McGraw Hill, New York, 5th Edition, Chapter 50, p 1043

Zmuda MJ, Quebbmann AJ 1975 Localisation of the renal tubular uric acid defect in gouty chickens. Am J Physiol *229:* 820

Clinical Nephrology, Vol. 35 No. 6 – 1991 (270–279)

Nutritional assessment in anemic hemodialysis patients treated with recombinant human erythropoietin

P. BÁRÁNY[1], E. PETTERSSON[1], M. AHLBERG[1], E. HULTMAN[2] and J. BERGSTRÖM[1]

Departments of Renal Medicine[1] and Clinical Chemistry[2], Huddinge University Hospital, Karolinska Institute, Stockholm, Sweden

Abstract. Nutritional status was assessed in 25 anemic hemodialysis patients before and during erythropoietin treatment. Nutritional assessment included regular blood chemistry determinations, anthropometric measurements, analysis of protein content in skeletal muscle, and estimation of daily protein intake from protein catabolic rate determinations (using urea kinetic modelling) and dialysis efficiency for urea. These measurements were done immediately prior to erythropoietin treatment, after anemia correction and after one year of maintenance erythropoietin treatment. Both relative body weights and subcutaneous fat stores were low at the start, but increased significantly ($p < 0.05$) during the study. Sixteen of the 25 patients gained weight and eight patients lost weight. The patients with weight gain had at the start of the study low weight indices (body weight 89.9 ± 7.6% of ideal body weight, body mass index 20.6 ± 1.6), significantly ($p < 0.005$) lower than the patients with weight loss. Although protein malnutrition was not obvious from arm anthropometrics, alkali soluble protein/DNA ratio or from serum albumin determinations, ASP/DNA ratio, increased in three of five patients investigated after one year on erythropoietin treatment. Neither protein catabolic rate nor dialysis efficiency changed significantly during the study. We conclude that anemia correction with erythropoietin has a positive effect on malnutrition in hemodialysis patients. In patients with underweight, an adjustment of fat stores was initially observed, followed possibly by an improvement in muscle protein content.

Key words: anemia – erythropoietin – hemodialysis – nutrition – uremia

Introduction

Malnutrition is a frequent problem in patients with chronic renal failure [Acchiardo et al., Schoenfeld et al. 1983, Thunberg et al. 1981, Guarnieri et al. 1983]. Many patients experience nausea or a spontaneous loss of appetite. Inadequate control of uremia, altered sense of taste, medication, mental depression and physical inactivity may also contribute to anorexia. Metabolic and endocrine disturbances affect protein and energy metabolism. Catabolic stimuli are provided by hemodialysis itself [Bergström et al. 1986], metabolic acidosis [Papadoyannakis et al. 1984], and intercurrent illnesses, such as infections. Consequently, wasting may occur. Malnutrition increases the risk of further complications and a vicious circle with gradual deterioration may develop.

Although there is considerable adaptation to low hemoglobin values in uremia, anemia nevertheless leads to decreased work capacity, with physical inactivity as a consequence. Treatment with human recombinant erythropoietin has been a major advance in the control of anemia in hemodialysis patients [Winearls et al. 1986, Eschbach et al. 1987, Casati et al. 1987]. The treatment is successful in almost all cases and the hitherto noted adverse effects are usually well controlled. Most patients spontaneously report an improvement in appetite and well-being after correction of the anemia. Anemica correction with erythropoietin in hemodialysis patients has been suggested to improve amino acid and protein metabolism [Riedel et al. 1989, Fischer et al. 1989] and to have an anabolic effect [Zehnter et al. 1988].

Received November 19, 1990; in revised form February 2, 1991.

Reprint requests to Dr. P. Bárány, Dept. of Renal Medicine, Huddinge Univ. Hospital, S-141 86 Huddinge, Sweden

Abbreviations: AMC = arm muscle circumference, ASP/DNA = alkali soluble protein/deoxyribonucleic acid, BMI = body mass index, BW = body weight, EPO = recombinant human erythropoietin, MAC = mid-arm circumference, PCR = protein catabolic rate, TSF = triceps skinfold.

The present study was undertaken to elucidate the impact of anemia correction with erythropoietin upon the nutritional status of patients undergoing maintenance hemodialysis treatment. The nutritional assessment included regular blood chemistry determinations, anthropometric measurements, analysis of protein content in skeletal muscle, as well as estimates of daily protein intake from protein catabolic rate determinations (using urea kinetic modelling) and dialysis efficiency. These measurements were done immediately prior to erythropoietin treatment, after anemia correction and after one year of maintenance erythropoietin treatment.

Material and methods

Patients

Twenty-five hemodialysis patients (12 female, 13 male, aged 42 ± 13 years) participated in the study, which was approved by the hospital's Ethics Committee. Patient characteristics are given in Table 1. Patients with diabetes mellitus, severe malnutrition, severe hyperparathyroidism or severe heart diseases were excluded. The patients received intravenous recombinant human erythropoietin treatment (50–200 unit/kg BW) after each hemodialysis three times a week until a target hemoglobin of 10 g/dl was reached. The patients were then switched to maintenance therapy with reduced doses two or three times a week. Routine medication included B and C vitamins, phosphate binders and sodium bicarbonate. Dialysis was carried out three times a week, using standard dialysers (cellulose or cuprophane membranes – in one case polyacrylonitrile). Dietary recommendations were given routinely to maintain a daily protein intake exceeding 1.0 g/kg BW.

Nutritional evaluation

Anthropometric measurements and percutaneous needle biopsy of the quadriceps femoris muscle were

Table 1 Clinical data of 25 hemodialysis patients treated with human recombinant erythropoietin (EPO)

Patient No.	Age (y)	Sex	Diagnosis	Time on HD (months)	Transfusions (before EPO) (units)	Hemoglobin (g/dl) Start	Maintenance	Correction time (weeks)
1	24	F	CPN + MALF	76	64	6.0	10.3	5
2	24	F	CPN + MALF	75	69	5.9	10.2	10
3	38	F	CGN	72	62	6.7	9.9	24
4	33	F	CGN	5	17	8.7	10.5	5
5	53	F	CGN	6	13	7.8	10.2	6
6	44	M	CGN	48	0	7.8	10.4	4
7	45	M	CPN	280	90	8.6	10.2	7
8	24	F	JNE – NO	120	90	7.2	10.7	6
9	67	M	CGN	21	18	6.8	10.5	12
10	33	F	SLE	29	22	8.3	10.5	8
11	64	F	RENAL TB	76	75	8.5	10.6	4
12	35	F	CIN	8	4	7.2	10.0	17
13	51	F	SLE	1	9	8.5	10.0	12
14	30	M	CGN	12	2	5.7	10.2	21
15	34	M	CGN	105	10	6.4	10.5	13
16	36	M	CPN	12	2	8.2	10.5	15
17	41	F	CGN	48	20	6.3	10.0	22
18	45	M	CGN	7	2	7.0	9.7	33
19	53	M	PCKD	24	2	5.9	9.9	16
20	50	M	NS?	26	52	7.3	10.0	22
21	55	F	PCKD + NE	6	18	7.0	10.1	21
22	57	M	CGN	6	4	5.6	10.1	22
23	58	M	BL CA + HN	69	80	7.8	10.3	6
24	42	M	CGN	36	14	7.1	10.2	38
25	24	M	JNE – NO + NE	54	30	9.2	11.5	5
Mean ± SD	42 ± 13			49 ± 59	31 ± 31	7.3 ± 1.0	10.3 ± 0.4	14 ± 9

Table 1 Continued

Patient No.	Age (y)	Sex	Diagnosis	EPO dose (units/kg/week) Start	Maintenance	Hospitalisations (days/year) Before EPO (1 y)	During EPO	Remarks
1	24	F	CPN+MALF	300	200	9	1	Tx 12 m
2	24	F	CPN+MALF	300	200	2	0	Tx 17 m
3	38	F	CGN	300	300	0	0	
4	33	F	CGN	300	250	29	0	CAPD 15
5	53	F	CGN	300	250	66	4	
6	44	M	CGN	150	100	0	1	
7	45	M	CPN	150	100	0	0	
8	24	F	JNE-NO	240	90	8	2	
9	67	M	CGN	240	90	4	0	
10	33	F	SLE	240	180	0	0	Tx 18 m
11	64	F	RENAL TB	240	90	38	32	
12	35	F	CIN	150	100	4	0	
13	51	F	SLE	150	100	20	0	
14	30	M	CGN	150	400	37	5	
15	34	M	CGN	150	150	0	6	
16	36	M	CPN	150	225	0	0	Tx 9 m
17	41	F	CGN	240	180	0	0	Severe iron deficiency
18	45	M	CGN	150	150	24	11	PTX 10 m
19	53	M	PCKD	150	210	54	47	Fistula thrombosis 9 m, Tx 10 m (failed)
20	50	M	NS?	150	375	23	0	Tx 7 m
21	55	F	PCKD+NE	150	375	87	46	Tx 6 m
22	57	M	CGN	150	525	97	4	Deceased 11 m
23	58	M	BLCA+HN	240	90	5	62	Tx 7 m
24	42	M	CGN	150	130	0	17	Bowel dysfunction
25	24	M	JNE-NO+NE	150	150	14	16	Fistula thrombosis, EPO withdrawn 10 m
Mean ± SD	42 ± 13			202 ± 63	200 ± 116	21 ± 28	10 ± 18*	

Abbreviations are: Diagnosis: CGN (chronic glomerulonephritis), CPN (chronic pyelonephritis), MALF (urogenital malformations), J NE-NO (juvenile nephronophthisis), TB (tuberculosis), CIN (chronic interstitial nephritis), NE (bilateral nephrectomy), NS (nephrosclerosis), PCKD (polycystic kidney disease), BL CA (bladder cancer), HN (hydronephrosis). Remarks: Tx (kidney transplantation), PTX (parathyroidectomy).
* $p < 0.05$, Wilcoxon's signed-rank test.

performed on a day between dialyses. Investigations were carried out before the start of erythropoietin treatment and repeated when the target hemoglobin concentration (10 g/dl) was reached (mean 14 ± 9 weeks) and after one year on maintenance therapy.

Current body weight (BW, kg), assessed post-dialysis, (Mettler Multi-Range scale, accuracy between 0.02–0.05 kg, Mettler Instruments AG, Greifensee, Switzerland), was used for the calculation of the desired body weight (DBW = BW × 100/Ideal BW; normal: 100% of ideal BW) using actuarial tables from the Metropolitan Life Insurance Company as reference [Wright and Heymsfield 1984], for the determination of Broca's index (BW/height in cm − 100) and body mass index (BMI = BW/[height in m]^2).

Anthropometric evaluation included measurements of the triceps skinfold (TSF) and midarm circumference (MAC) [Heymsfield et al. 1984] from which the arm muscle circumference (AMC = MAC − 0.1 [$\pi \times$ TSF]) was calculated. Skinfold thickness was measured with a Harpenden skinfold caliper (British Indicators Ltd, St Albans, Herts, England). Hand-grip strength was measured with a Harpenden handgrip dynamometer (British Indicators Ltd, St Albans, Herts, England). All measurements were done by the same person, in order to minimize possible interpersonal variations. Age- and sexspecific American norms for upper arm anthropometry [Bishop et al. 1981] were used for comparison. A comparison with Swedish norms for an age- and sex-matched population [Eriksson et al. 1987] gave identical results.

Skeletal muscle biopsy and biochemistry

After local anesthesia of the skin only, muscle tissue samples were obtained from the lateral portion of the quadriceps femoris muscle by percutaneous needle biopsy [Bergström 1962]. After careful and rapid removal of visible fat and connective tissue, the specimen was weighed and immediately frozen in liquid nitrogen. The frozen material was freeze-dried and the fat extracted with petroleum ether. The dried muscle sample was carefully dissected under a magnifying glass to remove remaining flakes of connective tissue. The dried fat-free and connective tissue-free solids were powdered and intracellular alkali-soluble protein (ASP- i.e., non-collagen protein) and DNA were determined in 3–4 mg of the powder after precipitation of the protein. The powder was washed twice with perchloric acid (0.2 mol/l) and the supernatant discarded. The precipitate was incubated for one hour in KOH (0.3 mol/l) and ASP determined in an aliquot by the Lowry method [Bergström 1962, Lowry et al.1951]. DNA anaylsis was based on the Schmidt-Thunhauser method [Munro and Fleck 1966]. DNA was extracted by Schneider and Greco's method [Schneider and Greco 1971] and determined by a micromodification of the diphenylamine method [Giles and Myers 1965, Burton 1956].

Specimens earlier obtained from 45 healthy control persons (21 male, 24 female, median age 33, range 19–70 years) were similarly processed and analyzed.

Table 2 Nutritional characteristics and changes in body weight and anthropometrics during treatment with erythropoietin

Patient	Height	Body weight Δ BW kg					Desirable BW (10) % ideal BW	Broca's index	Body mass index Δ BMI kg/m²			
No.	cm	−6 m	At start	3 m	6 m	12 m	At start	At start	At start	3 m	6 m	12 m
1	177	59.5	59.0	3.9	4.3	2.5	85.5	0.77	18.8	1.2	1.4	0.8
2	*	47.8	48.4	0.3	0.3	2.7	–	–	–	–	–	–
3	162	49.0	49.0	0.4	1.4	1.9	81.0	0.79	18.7	0.2	0.5	0.7
4	178	68.0	66.2	1.8	1.8	1.8	95.8	0.85	20.9	0.6	0.6	0.6
5	150	–	48.5	2.5	2.5	4.0	89.3	0.97	21.6	1.1	1.1	1.8
6	187	75.5	77.9	0.1	0.1	1.1	98.6	0.90	22.3	0.0	0.0	0.3
7	184	70.5	68.0	0.0	2.0	3.0	88.9	0.81	20.1	0.0	0.6	0.9
8	160	42.5	43.7	−0.9	0.9	1.0	73.4	0.73	17.1	−0.4	0.4	0.4
9	181	70.0	69.0	0.5	2.0	2.0	92.0	0.85	21.1	0.2	0.6	0.6
10	174	60.0	59.0	2.0	2.5	0.5	88.1	0.80	19.5	0.7	0.8	0.2
11	160	55.5	52.0	−0.9	0.9	0.5	87.4	0.87	20.3	−0.4	0.4	0.2
12	174	66.0	71.5	0.9	1.0	1.0	106.7	0.97	23.6	0.3	0.3	0.3
13	172	61.4	62.0	2.0	3.0	6.9	93.9	0.86	21.0	0.7	1.0	2.3
14	169	61.5	60.0	3.0	8.0	8.0	88.2	0.88	21.1	1.1	2.8	2.8
15	181	69.0	69.5	0.0	0.5	0.5	92.7	0.86	21.2	0.0	0.2	0.2
16	159	55.0	54.5	1.0	0.5	–	86.5	0.92	21.6	0.4	0.2	–
17	171	59.5	60.5	−0.5	1.5	0.0	92.4	0.85	20.7	−0.2	0.5	0.0
18	178	87.0	79.0	0.0	1.6	−1.5	108.7	1.01	24.9	0.0	0.5	−0.5
19	192	81.0	84.0	0.7	2.0	−1.4	102.4	0.91	22.8	0.2	0.5	−0.4
20	183	86.0	86.0	−1.0	−1.0	–	113.2	1.04	25.7	−0.3	−0.3	–
21	164	–	70.3	−3.0	−3.0	–	114.3	1.10	26.1	−1.1	−1.0	–
22	176	60.4	64.7	−1.7	−1.7	–	90.5	0.85	20.9	−0.5	−0.5	–
23	175	83.0	84.0	−0.3	−4.0	–	117.8	1.12	27.4	−0.1	−1.3	–
24	174	57.0	60.5	−1.7	−2.5	−3.0	85.6	0.82	20.0	−0.6	−0.8	−1.0
25	150	51.5	55.7	−0.2	−1.3	–	96.9	1.11	24.8	−0.1	−0.6	–
Mean	172	64.2	64.1	0.4	0.9	1.7[a]	94.6	0.90	21.8	0.1	0.3	0.6[a]
SD	11	12.3	11.9	1.6	2.5	2.6	11.0	0.11	2.5	0.6	0.9	0.9
n	24	23	25	25	25	19	24	24	24	24	24	18

Table 2 Continued

Patient	Height	Triceps skinfold				Arm muscle circumference			
	cm	mm				cm			
No.		ref. [12]	0	2–6 m	12–18 m	ref. [12]	0	2–6 m	12–18 m
1	177	19.4	15.0	21.0	–	20.9	22.3	21.4	–
2	*	19.4	14.0	15.4	18.4	20.9	23.6	23.4	23.2
3	162	24.0	12.0	13.8	13.0	22.5	23.7	24.2	23.4
4	178	21.9	14.2	16.0	21.6	21.7	25.5	25.0	25.2
5	150	25.4	12.0	15.4	20.2	22.7	22.7	22.2	21.7
6	187	12.4	13.8	14.6	16.2	28.2	28.7	27.9	27.4
7	184	12.4	13.4	17.5	20.2	28.8	23.8	23.5	24.2
8	160	19.4	6.8	–	8.4	20.9	21.9	–	21.9
9	181	11.6	6.8	11.2	10.0	27.8	26.4	26.5	26.9
10	174	21.9	16.0	–	17.2	21.7	23.0	–	22.1
11	160	24.9	27.4	20.6	27.0	22.8	25.9	25.5	23.0
12	174	24.0	30.2	27.0	–	22.5	20.7	23.5	–
13	172	25.4	13.6	19.8	–	22.7	24.7	25.3	–
14	169	12.6	11.8	15.2	–	28.3	25.8	27.2	–
15	181	12.5	7.4	8.8	9.0	28.8	26.7	26.7	26.7
16	159	12.4	3.8	3.8	–	28.8	26.8	27.3	–
17	171	24.0	8.8	10.8	–	22.5	23.2	25.1	–
18	178	12.4	8.4	7.8	8.2	28.2	27.9	28.6	27.9
19	192	11.6	9.8	10.4	–	27.8	26.9	27.7	–
20	183	12.4	10.4	–	–	28.2	30.3	–	–
21	164	–	–	–	–	–	–	–	–
22	176	11.6	9.4	8.6	–	27.8	26.0	26.3	–
23	175	12.4	16.4		–	28.2	29.4		–
24	174	12.4	5.2	4.6	–	28.8	25.9	25.6	–
25	150	11.2	23.8	19.8	–	27.4	27.5	27.3	–
Mean	172	17.0	12.9	14.1	15.8[b]	25.4	25.4	25.5	24.4
SD	11		6.5	5.9	6.1		2.5	2.0	2.2
n	24		24	20	12		24	20	12

* Patient with prosthesis of both legs.
[a] $p < 0.05$; [b] $p < 0.01$

Blood chemistry

Blood samples were drawn pre-dialysis for determinations of hemoglobin, potassium, phosphate, urea and creatinine. Using routine methods, these analyses were performed regularly throughout the study.

Protein catabolic rate and adequacy of dialysis

Protein catabolic rate was calculated by urea kinetic modelling (variable-volume model) according to the method of Farrell and Gotch [Farrell and Gotch 1977]. KT/V (K × T/V) based on dialyser urea clearance K, dialysis time T (min), and the calculated urea distribution volume V [Farrell and Gotch 1977] was calculated to determine the adequacy of dialysis for urea. In the three patients with urine production, residual renal urea clearance was determined. These calculations were performed regularly every third month.

Hospitalization

The number of days spent in hospital per patient year at risk for the year before and during erythropoietin treatment were analyzed. Complete hospitalisation data were obtained from the hospital's computer files.

Statistical analysis

Analysis of variance [Snedecor and Cochran 1976] followed by Student's t test with the Bonferroni procedure, were used for calculation of statistical significance of paired data. Correlations between measured parameters were obtained using simple linear regression analysis. Values are expressed as means ± SD if not stated otherwise.

Results

Body weight

In 17 of the patients a retrospective analysis of the changes in body weight during the year preceding the study period showed no significant changes (Figure 1). In the whole group of patients body weight (Table 2) increased significantly ($p < 0.05$) 12 months after starting erythropoietin treatment. At the outset of the study mean body weight (BW), desired body weight (DBW), body mass index (BMI) and Broca's index were significantly lower ($p < 0.005$) in the 16 patients with weight gain compared to the eight patients with weight loss (for details see Table 2). An analysis of individual patients demonstrated that 10 of 25 patients had DBW <90%, five of 25 had BMI ≤20 and 14 of 25 had Broca's index <0.9 when the study started (Table 2). Five of eight patients with weight loss had Broca's index >1.0.

Anthropometry (Table 2)

Measures of triceps skinfold (TSF) were definitely lower in the patients than the reference values for healthy age- and sex-matched controls (mean TSF 76% of American healthy controls, 82% of Swedish norms). TSF increased significantly ($p < 0.01$) to normal values after one year on maintenance erythropoietin therapy. Arm muscle circumference

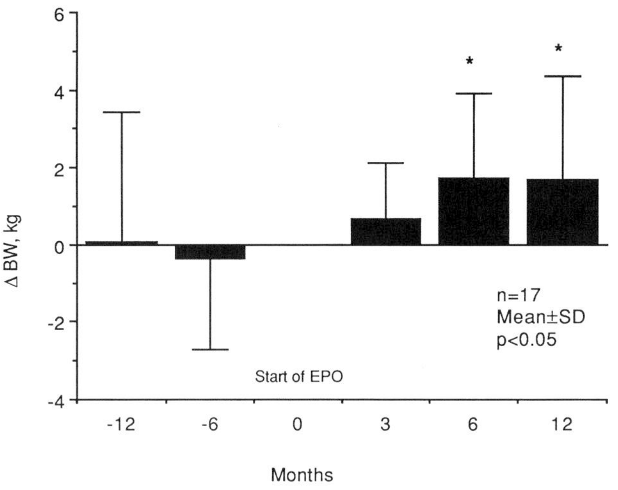

Fig. 1 Mean change in body weight (Δ BW) one year before and during erythropoietin treatment in 17 hemodialysis patients.

(AMC) was normal when compared with healthy age- and sex-matched controls (hemodialysis patients 101% of American norms, 106% of Swedish norms), but significantly less ($p < 0.005$) in patients with weight gain when compared to patients with weight loss. Hand-grip strength was unchanged 33 ± 8 kg (n = 24) at the start, 31 ± 9 kg (n = 19) after anemia correction, 28 ± 12 kg (n = 9) after one year of maintenance treatment.

Biochemical analysis of muscle

At the outset of the study the mean protein content in skeletal muscle, expressed as the ASP/DNA ratio, was 387 ± 71 (n = 18) and did not differ significantly from normal values (402 ± 63). One

Table 3 Results of predialysis blood chemistry analyses, protein catabolic rate calculations and index of dialysis adequacy (KT/V)

Month	0	3	6	12
n	25	25	25	20
Hemoglobin (g/dl)	7.0 ± 1.0	9.8 ± 1.0[c]	10.1 ± 0.7[c]	10.3 ± 1.0[c]
Albumin (g/l)	36 ± 4	36 ± 3	36 ± 4	37 ± 5
Phosphate (mmol/l)	1.8 ± 0.4	2.0 ± 0.5	2.1 ± 0.4	2.0 ± 0.6
Potassium (mmol/l	5.3 ± 0.7	5.7 ± 0.7[b]	5.8 ± 0.6[b]	5.5 ± 0.8
Urea (mmol/l)	31.1 ± 5.0	31.8 ± 5.8	33.6 ± 5.8	31.1 ± 5.0
Creatinine (μmol/l)	1123 ± 163	1203 ± 182[a]	1209 ± 215	1164 ± 179
n	20	20	19	16
PCR g/kg/day	1.3 ± 0.3	1.3 ± 0.3	1.3 ± 0.3	1.2 ± 0.2
KT/V	1.3 ± 0.3	1.3 ± 0.3	1.3 ± 0.3	1.3 ± 0.3

[a] $p < 0.05$ (3 vs. 0 months), [b] $p < 0.01$ (3 and 6 vs. 0 months), [c] $p < 0.001$ (3, 6 and 12 vs. 0 months)
Abbreviations are: PCR = Protein catabolic rate (Equations in ref. 21)

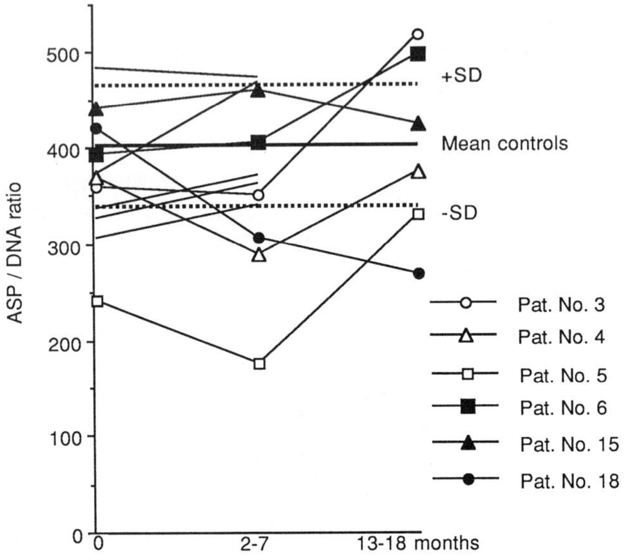

Fig. 2 ASP/DNA content in skeletal muscle in 11 hemodialysis patients before and during erythropoietin treatment. One of them (filled circles) developed secondary hyperparathyroidism during the study and parathyroidectomy was performed after 10 months.

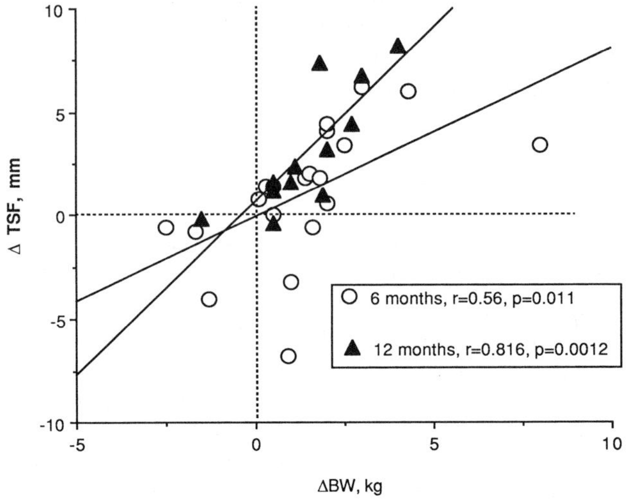

Fig. 3 Change in the triceps skinfold (Δ TSF) in relation (simple regression) to the change in body weight (Δ BW) during the correction period (n = 20) and after 12 months (n = 12) in the erythropoietin-treated hemodialysis patients.

patient (no. 18) was excluded from statistical analysis. He developed symptomatic secondary hyperparathyroidism and parathyroidectomy was performed after 10 months on erythropoietin treatment. The patient had muscle wasting and the ASP/DNA ratio decreased. Of the remaining patients, ten were investigated at the time of anemia correction. In these patients there was no significant change of the ASP/DNA ratio (363 ± 68 at the start and 370 ± 91 when hemoglobin was 10.0 g/dl). Five patients were followed for one year on maintenance erythropoietin treatment (Figure 2). Three of them had increased ASP/DNA ratios during the study period. The differences between the means were not significant (361 ± 74 at the start, 336 ± 110 after anemia correction, 428 ±79 at one year).

Blood chemistry (Table 3)

Significantly increased serum potassium and creatinine concentrations were found after the first 3–6 months of the study. During the study period no changes were seen in the pre-dialysis serum concentrations of phosphate, urea or albumin. Serum albumin concentrations, which were within the normal range, were significantly ($p < 0.01$) higher in patients who gained weight (38 ± 4 g/l) than in those who lost weight (34 ± 2 g/l) after 6 months of erythropoietin treatment.

Urea kinetics and dialysis efficiency

Details of the results of urea kinetic modelling and dialysis efficiency calculations are given in Table 3. Measures of protein catabolic rate (PCR) showed no notable changes during the study period. The target for dialysis prescriptions was KT/V equal to or above 1.0. Patients who lost weight had significantly ($p < 0.05$) lower KT/V (1.1 ± 0.1) after 6 months than patients with weight gain (KT/V 1.4 ± 0.3).

Correlations

AMC at the start of the study was significantly correlated to BW ($r = 0.63$, $p = 0.001$), weight indices ($p < 0.005$, relative BW, $r = 0.58$, Broca's I, $r = 0.59$, BMI, $r = 0.67$). AMC was also correlated to predialysis serum concentrations of creatinine at the start. The change in body weight (ΔBW) during the first 6 months after the start of erythropoietin treatment was significantly correlated to the change in TSF (ΔTSF 6 months, $r = 0.56$, $p = 0.011$, Figure 2) and serum albumin (Δ albumin, $r = 0.41$, $p = 0.043$). ΔBW and ΔTSF were also significantly correlated 12 months after the start of erythropoietin treatment. ΔBW at 6 months was inversely related to AMC values ($r = -0.42$, $p = 0.04$) and weight indices ($p < 0.05$, relative BW, $r = -0.45$, Broca's I, r =

−0.49, BMI, r = −0.5) at the outset of the study. ΔBW and the change in ASP/DNA after 12 months also showed a tendency to correlate (r = 0.75, p = 0.083). ΔBW was not correlated to the time on hemodialysis treatment.

Adverse events

The number of days spent in the hospital was lower during the study period than in the preceding year (10 ± 18 vs. 21 ± 28 days/year, p <0.05 Wilcoxon's signed-rank test, Table 1). The number of days spent in the hospital were higher in the patients with weight loss than in the patients with weight gain. Adverse events were seen in 18 of the 25 patients. Iron deficiency was observed in seven of the eight patients with correction time more than 20 weeks (Table 1). Fever reactions of 3–6 hours duration were reported by seven patients. Nine patients experienced hypertensive reactions, which were adequately controlled with anti-hypertensive drugs. In three of the patients (nos. 19, 23 and 25) thrombosis of the vascular access occurred with hospitalizations and operations as a consequence. This may have induced catabolism and subsequent weight loss in two of the patients. The third patient had already lost three kg in body weight when the fistula thrombosis occurred. Since recurrent thrombosis of the vascular access developed despite oral anticoagulant therapy, erythropoietin treatment was discontinued in one case (no. 25). Wasting in one patient (no. 22), who was underweight at the start, was probably related to a simultaneous deterioration in his cardiac function. A significant mitral valve insufficiency and later pericardial effusion was demonstrated by ultrasonography when he had already entered the study. He died at home 11 months after commencing erythropoietin treatment. The autopsy showed myocardial infarction. One patient (no. 18) was operated on for secondary hyperparathyroidism after 10 months on erythropoietin treatment. Patient no. 24 had bowel dysfunction with alternating diarrhea and constipation.

Discussion

The results of this study indicate that correction of anemia in hemodialysis patients with erythropoietin, influences amongst other parameters nutritional status. However, the effects are modest and seem to depend on other factors such as the nutritional status of the patients at the onset of therapy and/or ensuring intercurrent diseases and hospitalizations. Significantly increased body weight and triceps skinfold thickness were found after one year on maintenance erythropoietin treatment. A long-term positive effect on muscle content of protein was observed in three of five patients, who did not suffer from complications of chronic renal failure during the study period.

Most of the 25 patients included in the study had renal insufficiency due to primary renal disease. Patients with diabetes mellitus, severe malnutrition, or other diseases that might influence nutritional status had been excluded. The mean age (42 ± 13 years) of the patients was lower than for the general hemodialysis population in our region (57 ± 15 years). Consequently the patients selected for this study may have been better nourished than those usually requiring maintenance hemodialysis treatment and not fully representative of an elderly and more vulnerable hemodialysis population at large. Despite the selection, a positive effect on nutritional status was observed.

The low TSF (Table 2) values at the start of the study indicate mild energy malnutrition in the patient group. Protein malnutrition, which has been shown to be common in patients undergoing maintenance hemodialysis treatment [Acchiardo et al. 1983, Schoenfeld et al. 1983, Thunberg et al. 1981, Guarnieri et al. 1983], was not immediately obvious among the patients. The daily protein intake exceeded 1.1 g/kg BW, according to estimations from urea appearance rate. Serum albumin concentrations, the ASP/DNA ratio in skeletal muscle and the arm muscle circumference were not reduced when compared to the reference values (Tables 2, 3). Compared with previous studies [Acchiardo et al. 1983, Schoenfeld et al. 1983, Thunberg et al. 1981, Guarnieri et al. 1983] in non-selected hemodalysis patients our erythropoietin-treated patients seem to represent a less protein-malnourished selection.

The unchanged AMC during the study and the fact that we found no significant correlations between arm anthropometry and ASP/DNA may reflect the relative inaccuracy of antropometrics and the measurement of the skeletal muscle ASP/DNA ratio is probably a more sensitive indicator of borderline protein malnutrition than the conventional methods. According to the calculations of protein catabolic rate, dietary protein intake was unchanged. However, to detect a small increase in ingested protein is not possible with this method, because of the inexactness of the protein catabolic rate calculations. Data from dietary records were obtained during the study, but were insufficient for analysis of dietary intakes. The increase in subcutaneous fat stores suggests enhanced energy intake and perhaps also a better utilization of ingested protein. That decreased fat stores have a protein-wasting effect has been demonstrated in animal experiments [Li and Wassner 1986] and a high energy intake (>35 kcal/kg BW) improves nitrogen balance in hemodialysis patients [Slomowitz et al. 1989].

The correction of anemia in hemodialysis patients improves exercise capacity [Mayer et al. 1988] enabling increase in physical activity, which could have positive effects on the nutritional status per se. A reduction of proteolysis in muscle has been demonstrated after exercise training in chronically uremic rats [Davis et al. 1983] and in rat skeletal muscle incubated under slight tension protein balance was improved compared with muscles that were unrestrained [Baracos and Goldberg 1986]. Erythropoietin treatment of hemodialysis patients has been reported to correct the plasma amino acid pattern towards normal [Riedel et al. 1989]. The effect is in part the result of better food intake and a higher protein supply. However, an effect on amino acid metabolism of the improved oxygen transport after anemia correction has been proposed by Riedel et al. [1989].

Various factors may have contributed to the weight loss in eight of the participating patients (nos. 18–25). Five of the eight patients with weight loss during the study period had Broca's index >1.0 at start, indicating overweight. Two patients had increased subcutaneous fat stores (triceps skin folds thickness >120%) when compared with healthy matched subjects. The increase in daily physical activity and fitness reported by most patients, probably contributed to a desirable weight loss. However, some of these patients suffered from complicating illness and operations, which makes it more difficult to evaluate the effect of anemia correction, and as shown in Table 1 hospitalizations due to intercurrent diseases were higher in these patients than in the patients with weight gain.

An increased incidence of both hyperphosphatemia and hyperkalemia during erythropoietin treatment has been observed in previous studies [Winearls et al. 1986, Eschbach et al. 1987, Casati et al. 1987]. The cause of this is obscure, but it has been thought to be due to an increase in food intake, or a reduced dialysis efficiency [Winearls et al. 1986, Eschbach et al. 1987, Casati et al. 1987, Paganini et al. 1989]. In the present study there was a general tendency towards higher pre-dialysis serum concentrations of potassium, phosphate and creatinine. On the basis of urea kinetic modelling no reduction in dialysis efficiency was observed. However, a reduction in dialyser clearance of phosphate and creatinine cannot be excluded, and it has been demonstrated in other studies [Paganini et al. 1989].

The causes of malnutrition in hemodialysis patients are complex, involving many factors such as metabolic abnormalities and uremic toxins [Bergström and Fürst 1983, Delaprote et al. 1980]. However, one of the main causes may simply be an impaired nutritional intake. We have analyzed the physical, emotional and social well-being of our patients before and after anemia correction [Bárány et al. 1990]. The results indicated an improvement in all dimensions, particularly in physical well-being. It seems reasonable to assume that an increase in physical activities and a general improvement in emotional and social well-being will alleviate anorexia. The process of correcting that state of undernourishment is slow, and subcutaneous fat stores, as judged by triceps skinfold thickness, remained reduced despite anemia correction in our patients. Not until one year after anemia correction did TSF increase significantly and normalized in most patients. An effect on the muscle content of alkali soluble protein was observed in three of five patients after one year on maintenance erythropoietin therapy.

Acknowledgements

This work was supported by grants from the Swedish Medical Research Council (projects Nos. 1002 and 2647), Boehringer Mannheim GmbH, CILAG, the Swedish Society of Nephrology and the National Association of Kidney Patients in Sweden.

We thank Dr. Anand Saggar-Malik for collecting part of the data, Dr. Abdul Rashid Qureshi for assistance with the anthropometric measurements, Mrs Ann-Marie Forsberg and Mrs Eva Nilsson for analyzing the muscle specimens and Mrs Elsy Digréus and Mrs Ulla Pettersson for expert technical assistance.

REFERENCES

Acchiardo SR, Moore LW, Latour PA 1983 Malnutrition as the main factor in morbidity and mortality of hemodialysis patients. Kidney Int 24 (Suppl): S 199–203

Baracos VE, Goldberg AL 1986 Maintenance of normal length improves protein balance and energy status in isolated rat skeletal muscles. Am J Physiol (Cell Physiol). *251:* C 588–C 596.

Bárány P, Pettersson E, Bergström J 1990 Erythropoietin treatment improves quality of life in hemodialysis patients. Scand J Urol Nephrol (Suppl 131): 55–60

Bergström J 1962 Muscle electrolytes in man. Scand J Clin Lab Invest 14 (Suppl 68): 1–110

Bergström J, Alvestrand A, Gutierrez A 1986 Acute and chronic effects of dialysis. In: Immune and metabolic aspects of therapeutic blood purification systems. Karger, Basel, p 254–273

Bergström J, Fürst P 1983 Uremic toxins. In: *Drukker W, Parsons FM, Maher JF* (eds) Replacement of renal function by dialysis. Martinus Nijhoff Publishers, Boston, 354–390.

Bishop CW, Bown PE, Ritchey SJ 1981 Norms for nutritional assessment of American adults by upper arm anthropometry. Am J Clin Nutr *34:* 2530–2539.

Burton K 1956 A study of the conditions and mechanism of the diphenylamine method for the colorimetric estimation of deoxyribonucleic acid. Biochem J *62:* 315–323.

Casati S, Passerini P, Campise MR, Graziani G, Cesana B, Perisic M, Ponticelli C 1987 Benefits and risks of protracted treatment with human recombinant erythropoietin in patients having hemodialysis. Br Med J *295:* 1017–1020.

Davis TA, Karl IE, Goldberg AP, Harter HR 1983 Effects of exercise training on muscle protein catabolism in uremia. Kidney Int *24:* (Suppl 16) S 52–57.

Delaprote C, Gros F, Anagnostopoulos T 1980 Inhibitory effect of plasma dialysate on protein synthesis in vitro: Influence of dialysis and transplantation. Am J Clin Nutr *33:* 1407–1410.

Eriksson LS, Mossberg T, Wahren J 1987 Klinisk Nutrition. Norstedts Förlag, Stockholm.

Eschbach JW, Egrie JC, Downing MR, Browne JK, Adamson JW 1987 Correction of the anemia of end-stage renal disease with recombinant human erythropoietin, results of a combined phase I and II clinical trial. New Engl J Med *316:* 73–78.

Farrell PC, Gotch FA 1977 Dialysis therapy guided by kinetic modelling: Applications of a variable-volume single-pool model of urea kinetics. Proceedings of Second Australasian Conference on Heat and Mass Transfer. The University of Sydney, 29–37.

Fischer C, Scigalla P, Park W, Becker H, Schiller R, Paust H, Broesicke H, Kessel M 1989 Influence of rhEPO therapy on the protein metabolism of hemodialysis patients with terminal renal insufficiency. Contrib Nephrol. *76:* 250–256.

Giles KW, Myers A 1965 An improved diphenylamine method for the estimation of deoxyribonucleic acid. Nature *206:* 93.

Guarnieri G, Toigo G, Situlin R, Faccini L, Coli U, Landini S, Bazzato G, Dardi F, Campanacci L 1983 Muscle biopsy studies in chronically uremic patients: Evidence for malnutrition. Kidney Int 24 (Suppl): S 187–193.

Heymsfield SB, McManus III CB, Seitz SB, Nixon DW, Andrews JS. Anthropometric assessment of adult protein-energy malnutrition. In: *Wright RA, Heymsfield SB* (eds) 1984 Nutritional assessment. Blackwell scientific publications, Boston, p 27–82.

Li JB, Wassner SJ 1986 Protein synthesis and degradation in skeletal muscle of chronically uremic rats. Kidney Int. *29:* 1136–1143.

Lowry OH, Rosebrough NJ, Farr AL, Randall RJ 1951 Protein measurement with the Folin phenol reagent. J Biol Chem *193:* 265–275.

Mayer G, Thum J, Cada EM, Stummvoll HK, Graf H 1988 Working capacity is increased following recombinant human erythropoietin treatment. Kidney Int. *34:* 525–528.

Munro HN, Fleck A 1966 Recent development in the measurement of nucleic acids in biological materials. Analyst. *91:* 78–87.

Paganini EP, Abdoulhadi MH, Garcia J, Magnusson MO 1989 Recombinant human erythropoietin correction of anemia. Dialysis efficiency, waste retention, and chronic dose variables. ASAIO Transactions. *35:* 513–515.

Papadoyannakis NJ, Stefandis CJ, McGeown M 1984 The effect of the correction of metabolic acidosis on nitrogen and potassium balance of patients with chronic renal failure. Am J Clin Nutr *40:* 623–627.

Riedel E, Hampl H, Scigalla P, Nündel M, Kessel M 1989 Correction of amino acid metabolism by recombinant human erythropoietin therapy in hemodialysis patients. Kidney Int *36:* S 216–221.

Schneider WC, Greco AE 1971 Incorporation of pyrimidine deoxyribonucleosides into liver lipids and other components. Biochim Biophys Acta *228:* 610–626.

Schoenfeld PY, Henry RR, Laird NM, Roxe DM 1983 Assessment of nutritional status of the national cooperative dialysis study population. Kidney Int 23 (Suppl): S 80–88.

Slomowitz IA, Monteon FJ, Grosvenor M, Laidlaw SA, Kopple JD 1989 Effect of energy intake on nutritional status in hemodialysis patients. Kidney Int *35:* 704–711.

Snedecor GW, Cochran WG 1976 Statistical methods. Iowa State Univ Press, Iowa, USA.

Thunberg BJ, Swamy AP, Cestero RVM 1981 Cross-sectional and longitudinal nutritional measurements in maintenance hemodialysis patients. Am J Clin Nutr *34:* 2005–2012.

Winearls CG, Oliver DO, Pippard MJ, Reid C, Downing MR, Cotes PM 1986 Effect of human erythropoietin derived from recombinant DNA on the anemia of patients maintained by chronic hemodialysis. Lancet *2:* 1175–1177.

Wright RA, Heymsfield SB 1984 Nutritional assessment. Blackwell scientific publications, Boston, Appendix.

Zehnter E, Pollok M, Ziegenhagen D, Bramsiepe P, Longere F, Baldamus CA, Wellner U, Waters W 1988 Urea kinetics in patients on regular dialysis treatment before and after treatment with recombinant human erythropoietin. Contrib Nephrol *66:* 149–155.

Regression of left ventricular hypertrophy after partial correction of anemia with erythropoietin in patients on hemodialysis: a prospective study

J. Pascual[1], J. L. Teruel[1], J. L. Moya[2], F. Liaño[1], M. Jiménez-Mena[2] and J. Ortuño[1]

[1]*Department of Nephrology and* [2]*Department of Cardiology, Hospital Ramón y Cajal, Carr. Colmenar, Madrid, Spain*

Abstract. Myocardial effects of recombinant human erythropoietin (rhEPO) treatment were prospectively investigated in 15 hemodialysis (HD) patients with severe anemia (hematocrit [Ht] 19.7 ± 2.5%). Echocardiographic studies were performed after a midweek HD session just before and after a year of rhEPO. At the end of the study period, Ht had improved to 32.2 ± 3.5% and cardiac index significantly decreased (5.48 ± 1.54 vs 3.97 ± 0.94 l/min/m^2, p <0.001). Left ventricular mass index (LVMi) decreased with rhEPO (210.7 ± 48.3 vs 139 ± 50 g/m^2, p <0.05). This decrease was concomitant with a decrease of LV end-diastolic diameter (4.89 ± 0.44 vs 4.57 ± 0.64 cm, p <0.05), interventricular septum thickness (IVST, 1.42 ± 0.33 vs 1.07 ± 0.13 cm, p <0.01) and LV posterior wall thickness (LVPWT, 1.28 ± 0.21 vs 1.01 ± 0.11 cm, p <0.01). Eight patients were hypertensive well controlled with hypotensive drugs (group I) and 7 normotensive (group II). LVMi was higher in group I than in group II before rhEPO (235.2 ± 40 vs 182.7 ± 43.1 g/m^2, p <0.05) and significantly decreased after rhEPO in both groups (28.5% and 41.4% respectively). LVMi remained higher in group I than in group II at the end of the study (168.5 ± 0.9 vs 106.7 ± 24 g/m^2, p <0.025). A moderately elevated IVST/LVPWT was reduced with a year of rhEPO (1.14 ± 0.40 vs 1.05 ± 0.15, p <0.05), disclosing correction of asymmetric septal hypertrophy. We conclude that left ventricular hypertrophy (LVH) regression is obtained after partial correction of anemia with rhEPO. Previous hypertension with current need of antihypertensive treatment has also a significant effect in the development of LVH. Whether this regression would improve outcome in HD patients remains to be established.

Key words: recombinant human erythropoietin – chronic hemodialysis patients – chronic anemia – ventricular hypertrophy

Introduction

Cardiovascular complications still are the major cause of high morbidity and mortality in end-stage renal disease (ESRD) patients [Degoulet et al. 1982, Rostand et al. 1982]. Among cardiac alterations, left ventricular hypertrophy (LVH) is the most predominant finding in these patients [Harnett et al. 1988, Bullock et al. 1982]. It has been clearly demonstrated that LVH has an important and independent prognostic significance and is a determinant of survival in ESRD patients treated with all modalities of dialysis and transplantation [Silberberg et al. 1989, Parfrey et al. 1990] and in the general population [Levy et al. 1990]. Therefore, amelioration of LVH may contribute to improved cardiovascular survival in ESRD patients. Moreover, the regression of LVH after renal transplantation shown by our group and others [Teruel et al. 1987, Himelman et al. 1988] could contribute to the lower reported cardiovascular mortality for transplant patients than for patients on long-term hemodialysis (HD).

Evolution of LVH in HD patients has been observed in 3 recent studies [Deligliannis et al. 1984, Huting et al. 1988, Parfrey et al. 1990]. All of them concluded that LVH progressively increases with time. Progressive enlargement of LV wall usually affects the septum more importantly and results in an asymmetric septal hypertrophy (ASH) [Deligiannis et al. 1984, Huting et al. 1988]. It has not been possible to identify predisposing factors for LVH progression in these works, assuming therefore that LVH is produced by chronic increment of cardiac work and could be associated with HD treatment itself. In fact,

Received July 25, 1990; in revised form January 15, 1991.

Requests for reprints to Dr. J. Pascual, Department of Nephrology, Hospital Ramón y Cajal, Carr. Colmenar, km 9,100, ES-28034 Madrid, Spain.

in one study LVH and time on HD appears to be positively correlated [London et al. 1987]. Other factors such as age or hypertension have been associated with LVH in ESRD [Bernardi et al. 1985, Harnett et al. 1988, Deligliannis et al. 1984, Kramer et al. 1986]. Only one recent study correlates anemia and development of LVH [London et al. 1989] while others do not [Blake et al. 1989, Harnett et al. 1988, Huting et al. 1988, Huting et al. 1989, Kramer et al. 1986]. Thus, reviewing these conflicting results the question as to whether or not anemia is independently related to the development of LVH in ESRD remains unsolved.

Recombinant human erythropoietin (rhEPO) clearly is capable of improving anemia in almost all the patients treated with little change in other variables [Eschbach 1987, Winearls 1986], providing a good model for evaluation of the effect of anemia on LVH. The purpose of the present study was to assess prospectively the relationship between anemia and LVH and to quantitate the evolution of LVH by echocardiography after partial correction of anemia with rhEPO and further stabilization of hematocrit values.

Table 1 Clinical and biochemical characteristics and effects of erythropoietin treatment during one year

	Before rhEPO	One year	p value
Weight (kg)	60 ± 10	61.5 ± 10.7	NS
BSA (m^2)	1.61 ± 0.16	1.62 ± 0.17	NS
Hemoglobin (g/dl)	6.4 ± 0.9	10.5 ± 0.9	<0.001
Hematocrit (%)	19.7 ± 2.5	32.3 ± 3.5	<0.001
Calcium (mg/dl)	9 ± 0.9	9.2 ± 1	NS
Phosphorus (mg/dl)	5.8 ± 1.8	6 ± 1.8	NS
Potassium (mEq/l)	5.1 ± 0.7	5.2 ± 0.8	NS
iPTH (pg/ml)	194 ± 203	283 ± 300	NS
Patients with >55 (n = 8)	326 ± 198	496 ± 263	NS
Patients with <55 (n = 7)	43 ± 19	40 ± 21	NS
SAP (mmHg)			
Group I (n = 8)	159 ± 7	145 ± 12	<0.01
Group II (n = 7)	133 ± 10	122 ± 11	<0.01
DAP (mmHg)			
Group I (n = 8)	96 ± 8	87 ± 9	<0.01
Group II (n = 7)	82 ± 10	75 ± 9	<0.01

Values are mean ± SD. iPTH: intact parathyroid hormone. SAP: systolic arterial pressure. DAP: diastolic arterial pressure. Group I: patients under hypertensive therapy. Group II: normotensive without medication.

Methods

Patients

The study was performed in 15 nondiabetic patients (8 men and 7 women), aged 17 to 58 years (mean 38) with chronic renal failure undergoing chronic intermittent HD treatment for 10.5 to 12 hours weekly for 6 to 135 months (mean 54). Etiology of renal failure was: glomerulonephritis (6 patients), unknown (4 patients), interstitial nephritis, bilateral nephrectomy after urothelial tumors, tuberculosis, cortical necrosis and uropathy (one patient each). For the HD procedure, standard dialyzers with a cuprophan membrane and acetate as a buffer were used. Vascular access was achieved through arteriovenous shunts in the upper arm (n = 2) or forearm (n = 11), Thomas' shunt (n = 1) or permanent jugular catheter (n = 1). HD schedule was invariable during the study period. The selection criterion for entering the study was the need for regular transfusions of packed red blood cells during the last four months and the absence of angina pectoris, myocardial infarction, congestive heart failure or uncontrolled hypertension.

Predialysis blood pressure was determined in each patient by averaging supine blood pressure during the month before each echocardiographic study. All patients had normal blood pressure at the beginning of the study: 7 were treated with antihypertensive drugs before starting rhEPO (3 received propranolol plus hydralacine, 2 celiprolol plus captopril, 2 alpha-methyl-dopa) and one required low-dose captopril after several weeks. These 8 patients constituted the hypertensive group (group I). After a year of rhEPO treatment, antihypertensive treatment was largely uniformized and patients on celiprolol plus captopril and both on alpha-methyl-dopa were changed to propranolol plus hydralazine and low-dose enalapril. The other 7 patients remained normotensive without the need of drugs during the study period (group II). Only two patients had evidence of iron overload before rhEPO treatment but none had causes of anemia other than that related to renal failure or long-term HD. Only one patient had aluminum excess before rhEPO (579 µg/ml). Plasma parathyroid hormone concentrations were determined by radioimmunoassay using a specific antiserum against intact hormone (iPTH). Eight patients had normal values (10–55 pg/ml), five of them were hypertensive. Seven patients had values >55 pg/ml, 3 of them were hypertensive. None of the patients had severe secondary hyperparathyroidism or took vitamin D. Only one patient was anephric. During the year of the study period, survival was 100%.

Study protocol

The patients received 50 IU/kg body weight of rhEPO i.v. at the end of each HD. The dose was adjusted according to hematocrit response on a monthly basis, with a target level of 30–35%. Echocardiographic studies were performed immediately before the first dose of rhEPO and repeated after a year. All studies were accomplished 30 minutes after the midweek HD session, when the patient is on theoretical dry weight and circulatory volume overload factors are avoided.

Echocardiographic study

Echocardiography was performed with an automatic device (Ultramark 6) with 3.5 MHz transducer for M-mode, two-dimensional and Doppler echocardiography. Registration, measurements of cavities, cardiac walls and analysis were undertaken according to the recommendations of the American Society of Echocardiography [Sahn et al. 1978] using average values of five consecutive cardiac cycles. The studies were obtained with the patient in the left lateral recumbent position with 30 degree of head inclination from an echocardiographic window located in the 3rd or 4th intercostal space at the left sternal border. The LV stroke volume was calculated by multiplying the Doppler aortic flow velocity integral by the aortic area in systole at the level of the aortic valve. It is a well established technique whose effectiveness for measuring flow has been validated and correlated with the results obtained using invasive procedures [Lewis et al. 1984]. Cardiac output (CO) was computed as the product of LV stroke volume and heart rate; cardiac index (CI) was considered as the CO corrected for the body surface area of each patient, expressed in l/min/m^2. Control group for CI, constituted by 25 healthy volunteers, 14 males and 11 females, with an age of 35 ± 12 years, had a CI of 3.28 ± 0.26 l/min/m^2. Other echocardiographic measurements used in this report include left ventricular end-diastolic diameter (LVEDD) and end-systolic diameter (LVESD), interventricular septum thickness (IVST) and left ventricular posterior wall thickness (LVPWT). Left ventricu-

Table 2 Hemodynamic and myocardial effects of rhEPO treatment during one year

Group I	LVEDD (cm)		LVESD (cm)		IVST (cm)		LVPWT (cm)		IVST/LVPWT	
(n = 8)	A	B	A	B	A	B	A	B	A	B
M. P.	5.2	4.9	3.3	2.7	1.2	1.2	1.6	1.2	0.75	1
F. M.	4.6	4	2.8	2.2	1.3	1.2	1.6	1.2	0.81	1
J. M.	4.9	4.7	2.7	2.7	1.4	1.1	1.3	1.1	1.07	1
V. L.	5.5	5.3	3.1	3	1.1	1.1	1.2	1.1	0.91	1.1
P. M.	5.5	5.4	4	3.6	1.3	1.2	1.2	1.1	1.08	1.09
E. U.	4.9	4.9	2.7	3.2	1.7	1.2	1.6	0.9	1.06	1.33
N. M.	4.9	3.7	2.9	2	1.1	0.9	1.4	0.9	0.71	1
C. C.	4.3	4.9	2.7	3.3	2.2	1.2	1.3	1.1	1.69	1.09
Mean	4.97	4.72	3.02	2.83	1.41	1.13	1.40	1.06	1.01	1.07
+SD	± 0.41	± 0.59	± 0.44	± 0.54	± 0.37	± 0.10	± 0.17	± 0.11	± 0.3	± 0.11

Group I	LVMi (g/m^2)		SV (ml)		HR (bpm)		CO (l/min)		CI (l/min/m^2)	
(n = 8)	A	B	A	B	A	B	A	B	A	B
M. P.	278.5	200.7	66.2	72.2	86	72	7.98	5.20	5.70	3.66
F. M.	212.5	128.5	66.3	72.3	67	65	7.12	4.70	4.45	2.91
J. M.	195.9	134.8	73.9	81	76	79	5.62	6.40	3.26	3.65
V. L.	179.4	146.9	115.3	67.8	82	109	9.46	7.40	5.25	4.04
P. M.	245.2	212.9	165.7	130.8	69	68	11.40	8.90	7.70	6.05
E. U.	260	235.2	117.5	77.4	85	71	9.90	5.50	5.70	3.12
N. M.	218.8	87	52.2	60.4	100	81	5.22	4.90	3.76	3.52
C. C.	291.5	198.5	120	83.8	108	118	12.96	9.90	9.08	5.77
Mean	235.2	168	97.1	80.7	84.1	82.8	8.71	6.61	5.61	4.09
± SD	± 40	± 50.9*	± 38.6	± 21.5	± 14.2	± 19.7	± 2.73	± 1.94	± 1.95	± 1.17

Table 2 (continued)

Group II	LVEDD (cm)		LVESD (cm)		IVST (cm)		LVPWT (cm)		IVST/LVPWT	
(n = 7)	A	B	A	B	A	B	A	B	A	B
I. Z.	4.6	3.5	2.4	1.6	1.5	1.1	1.1	1.1	1.36	1
J. V.	4.5	5	2.2	3.1	1.2	0.8	1.2	1	1	0.8
C. L.	5.6	4.3	4.3	3	2.1	1	0.9	0.9	2.3	1.1
J. S.	4.7	4.2	3.1	2.2	1.3	1.1	1.4	0.9	0.92	1.22
A. D.	4.2	3.6	2.3	2	1.3	0.9	1	1	1.3	0.81
J. M.	4.7	4.8	3.2	3.6	1.3	0.9	1.3	0.9	1	1
L. V.	5.3	5.4	3.9	3.4	1.3	1.2	1.1	0.9	1.18	1.33
Mean	4.80	4.40	3.0	2.7	1.42	1.0	1.14	0.95	1.29	1.03
± SD	± 0.48	± 0.70	± 0.80	± 0.76	± 0.30	± 0.14	± 0.57	± 0.07	± 0.47	± 0.19
All (n = 15)										
Mean	4.89	4.57	3.04	2.77	1.42	1.07	1.28	1.01	1.14	1.05
± SD	± 0.44	± 0.64	± 0.62	± 0.63	± 0.33	± 0.13	± 0.21	± 0.11	± 0.46	± 0.15
p value (A vs B)	<0.05		<0.05		<0.01		<0.01		<0.05	

Group II	LVMi (g/m^2)		SV (ml)		HR (bpm)		CO (l/min)		CI (l/min/m^2)	
(n = 7)	A	B	A	B	A	B	A	B	A	B
I. Z.	167	85.7	156.4	90.6	62	86	9.70	7.80	4.45	2.91
J. V.	165.3	125.6	102.2	104.4	77	68	7.87	7.10	5.24	4.49
C. L.	274.5	99.4	100.7	60.2	92	98	9.27	5.90	5.48	3.53
J. S.	192.1	103.6	98	65.7	85	76	8.33	5.00	5.04	3.01
A. D.	141.9	85.1	90.2	72.8	121	92	10.92	6.70	7.37	4.52
J. M.	162.1	97.3	87	59.1	90	115	7.83	6.80	4.23	3.15
L. V.	176.5	152.1	107.9	94.4	75	72	8.09	6.80	4.42	3.73
Mean	182.7	106.9	106	78.1	86	86.7	8.85	6.58	5.34	3.84
± SD	± 43.1	± 24**	± 23.3	± 18.1	± 18.5	± 16.5	± 1.15	± 0.89	± 1.03	± 0.65
All (n = 15)										
Mean	210.7	139	101.2	79.5	85	84.6	8.78	6.60	5.48	3.97
± SD	± 48.3	± 50	± 31.6	± 19.3	± 15.7	± 17.7	± 2.07	± 1.49	± 1.54	± 0.94
p value (A vs B)	<0.05		<0.05		NS		<0.001		<0.001	

LVEDD: left ventricular end-diastolic diameter. LVESD: left ventricular end-systolic diameter. IVST: interventricular septum thickness. LVPWT: left ventricular posterior wall thickness. LVMi: left ventricular mass index. SV: stroke volume. HR: heart rate. CO: cardiac output. CI: cardiac index.

Group I (n = 8): patients taking antihypertensive drugs. Group II (n = 7): patients normotensive without drugs. Situation A: before rhEPO. Situation B: after a year of rhEPO.

*: p <0.05 A vs B (Group I), p <0.05 A (Group I) vs A (Group II) and p <0.025 B (Group I) vs B (Group II).

**: p <0.01 A vs B (Group II).

lar mass (LVM) was calculated with the following formula:

$$LVM\ (grams) = 1.05\ ([LVEDD + IVST + LVPWT]^3 - [LVEDD]^3)$$

A correlation between LVM and BSA is present in healthy subjects [Henry et al. 1978]. In order to compare means among different groups, LVM has been corrected for the BSA of each patient, and therefore the results are expressed as the LVM index (LVMi), in g/m^2. The upper normal level of LVMi in our laboratory is 125 g/m^2, in accordance with studies in normal populations [Casale et al. 1986] and HD patients [Silberberg et al. 1989]. The diagnosis of ASH was made with IVST >1.2 cm, LVPWT >1.1 and IVST/LVPWT >1.3.

Statistics

Data are reported as mean ± SD. Statistical methods used were the paired Student's test for comparison of two means and chi-square test to assess differences for categorical variables. Values of $p < 0.05$ were considered as significant.

Results

Clinical and biochemical data

Data concerning clinical and biochemical changes observed before and a year after treatment with rhEPO are summarized in Table 1. Correction of anemia was attempted in a slow fashion, without significant increase of rhEPO dosage in any patient. Mean maintenance dosage was 165 IU/kg/week at the end of the study period. In this way, hemoglobin and hematocrit were 9.1 ± 1.1 g/dl and 26.4 ± 3.3% respectively at 2 months and 10.3 ± 1 g/dl and 31 ± 3.6% at four months, values maintained after a year. Five patients from group I needed further increasing of antihypertensive dosage. After a year of rhEPO, blood pressure was below basal values in both groups. iPTH levels did not change in patients with normal values before rhEPO and increased in patients with elevated basal values, although the difference did not reach significance (Table 1).

Hemodynamic and myocardial parameters

The individual courses of hemodynamic and myocardial parameters after a year of rhEPO treatment are given in Table 2. CI, previously elevated in all patients, decreased significantly after treatment as a result of reduction of SV. LVMi was elevated in all patients before starting rhEPO. After a year, all patients had diminished their LVMi in variable amounts (mean, 33%). Six out of the 15 patients had LVMi below upper normal limit (<125 g/m^2), other 4 within 126 and 150 g/m^2 and the rest above this value. Three patients had finally marked LVH, with LVMi of 200, 212 and 235 g/m^2, respectively. LVMi reduction was achieved by means of significant decrease in LVEDD, LVESD, IVST and LVPWT. IVST and LVPWT achieved similar mean values. Thus, a moderately elevated IVST/LVPWT ratio was corrected after a year of rhEPO.

Before starting rhEPO, LVMi was higher in group I than in group II (235.2 ± 40 vs 182.7 ± 43.1, $p < 0.05$). LVMi had decreased by 28.5% in group I and 41.4% in group II after a year. In spite of this difference, LVMi was higher in group I than in group II at the end of the study (168 ± 50.9 vs 106.9 ± 24, $p < 0.025$).

LVMi was similar in patients with elevated or normal serum iPTH levels before rhEPO (209.4 ± 48.3 vs 212.2 ± 52 pg/ml, respectively). Reduction of LVMi was higher after one year of rhEPO in the group of patients with normal iPTH values than in patients with elevated ones, but this difference was not statistically significant (159.3 ± 51.3 vs 116.9 ± 24 g/m^2, $t = 1.76$, $0.1 < p > 0.05$).

Discussion

The present prospective evaluation of myocardial effects of rhEPO treatment indicates that regression of LVH is noticeable after one year of partial correction of anemia with rhEPO in HD patients. We had previously observed a marked reduction of CI in all HD patients treated with rhEPO during 4 months, achieving values within control range in 8 of the 12 patients analyzed [Teruel et al. in press]. After such limited follow-up, no significant variations in LV diameters and LVM could be observed. Our results confirm the only previous study in which LV dimensions correlated well with anemia in HD patients [London et al. 1987] and agree with a previous evaluation of evolution of LVM after rhEPO treatment [London et al. 1989]. In this work, London and his colleagues showed a decrease of 17% in LVM after 10 to 35 weeks of rhEPO treatment, with echocardiograms performed just when hemoglobin had reached target values. Thus, we were not surprised regarding the more significant decrease observed in our patients (33% of LVMi), with an echocardiogram made after a year of follow-up and a longer period of stabilized correction of anemia.

LVMi decrease was related to both LVEDD and ventricular wall thickness. In several retrospective studies, LVEDD and degree of anemia were correlated [Mehta et al. 1983, Huting et al. 1989, London et al. 1987], and diminution of both LVESD and LVEDD was demonstrated after partial correction of anemia with rhEPO [London et al. 1989, Tutsui et al. 1989, Low et al. 1989]. In our patients, both IVST and LVPWT were also reduced after rhEPO. This aspect, precociously observed by London et al. [1989] is highly interesting, as it has been scarcely observed in HD patients: in only 3 out of the 84 patients studied by Parfrey et al. [1990], a decrease in ventricular wall thickness could be demonstrated after 3 to 5 years of follow-up. Therefore, partial correction of anemia achieved following rhEPO administration is able to invert the tendency to progressive increase in LVH recently observed in patients on maintenance HD

[Deligliannis et al. 1984, Huting et al. 1988, Parfrey et al. 1990].

An ASH pattern has been described in HD patients [Huting et al. 1988, Huting et al. 1989, Deligliannis et al. 1984]. LV septum is subjected to greater systolic stress than free wall, resulting in a higher enlargement and ASH [Heng et al. 1985]. rhEPO administration modified this pattern: after a year of treatment we have demonstrated a decreased IVST/LVPWT ratio and correction of ASH. Then, hemodynamic conditions associated with severe anemia are one responsible factor for development of ASH, an unknown aspect thus far.

Hypertension has been always considered among the contributing factors in LVH of HD patients. Several authors have correlated LV enlargement with increase of blood pressure [Mehta et al. 1983, Harnett et al. 1988, London et al. 1987], while others have not [Huting et al. 1989, Kramer et al. 1986]. In prospective studies a higher progression of LVH in hypertensive patients could not be demonstrated [Huting et al. 1988, Parfrey et al. 1990], nor could the benefit of lowering blood pressure in LVH be observed [Huting et al. 1988]. In our study, before starting rhEPO, LVMi was significantly higher in hypertensive patients. Theoretically the described hypertensive effect of rhEPO [Eschbach et al. 1989, Pollok et al. 1989] could counteract the possible decrement of LVM after correction of anemia. However, LVMi had decreased after a year in all patients, with more intense decrease in the normotensive group (41%) than in the patients taking drugs (28%). At the end of the study period, LVMi continued higher in hypertensive patients, confirming the relative importance of hypertension in the genesis and maintenance of LVH.

Blood pressure control was very good in patients under antihypertensive therapy with exquisite adjustments of drugs to avoid well-described complications [Eschbach et al. 1987, Winearls et al. 1986]. Surprisingly, we have observed lower blood pressure levels after a year of rhEPO in normotensive patients without the need of drugs. We have no explanation for this evolution and to our knowledge, such delayed effect of rhEPO is not described. Although the increase of blood pressure [Hory et al. 1990] and the augmentation of antihypertensive therapy in the majority of series of patients treated with rhEPO have been reported [Eschbach et al. 1987, Winearls et al. 1986, Casati et al. 1987], the need for initiation is less frequent with such therapy in previously normotensive ones. The increase in hematocrit during rhEPO treatment was very slow, approximately 0.1% per day, minimizing the impact of a rapid correction of anemia on blood pressure. In any case, the slight reduction in blood pressure during a year of rhEPO in our patients could be related to some reduction in LVM as it is described in nonuremic patients [Rowlands et al. 1982, Nakashima et al. 1984].

Treatment with rhEPO has partially allowed to know the real influence of secondary hyperparathyroidism in the development of LVH. The relationship between hyperparathyroidism and LVH is a matter of controversy. It has been suggested that PTH could be trophic to heart muscle and contribute to its hypertrophy in HD patients [Harnett et al. 1988]. However, other authors could not establish a positive correlation between hyperparathyroidism and cardiac hypertrophy [Mehta et al. 1983] or, moreover, correlation was even negative in another work [London et al. 1987]. Surprisingly enough, an initial relationship between LVH and iPTH [Harnett et al. 1988] was not evolutively confirmed by the same authors [Parfrey et al. 1990]. Before rhEPO, we did not observe any relationship between iPTH levels and LVH. Of interest, after partial correction of anemia, LVMi was higher in patients with hyperparathyroidism. This less pronounced reduction of LVMi could be explained by the inclusion of more hypertensive patients in the subgroup of elevated iPTH (5/8 vs 3/7). However, this slight predominance of hypertensive patients in the subgroup of elevated iPTH also was present before rhEPO, when no LVMi differences could be seen regarding iPTH levels. Therefore, we suppose that iPTH has effects on myocardium which remain "occult" because of the more intense effect of anemia and are only evident after improvement of hematocrit.

The impressive decrement in LVMi observed in all our patients is probably related to maintained partial correction of anemia, and we may point out anemia as the critical factor in the development of LVH in HD patients. In our previous prospective study of regression of LVH after kidney transplantation we suggested that this reduction was mainly due to the improvement in anemia and correction of fluid overload [Teruel et al. 1987]. Similarly to transplant patients, LVMi was lower in HD patients treated with rhEPO who were normotensive in comparison to those who were hypertensive. Also similarly, reduction of LVMi after a year was less pronounced in hypertensive patients.

The use of Doppler-determined LV outflow to calculate SV and CO has been well validated [Lewis et al. 1984]. Similarly, echocardiographic measurements of LV wall and internal dimensions as well as derived estimates of LVM closely correspond to similar measurements determined by ventriculography [Troy et al. 1972]. Certain inaccuracies are inherent to the echocardiographic method of determining LVM since myocardial thickness is nonuniform and applied geometric models only approximate the shape of LV. Nevertheless, echocardiographically measured LVM has recently been compared to the true anatomic mass with excellent results [Devereux et al. 1977]. The strongest correlation (r = 0.96) was observed when mass was based on an average of both IVST and LVPWT rather than LVPWT alone [Devereux et al. 1977]. The reported accuracy and reproducibility of this method compares favorably with other invasive techniques [Devereux et al. 1977, Lewis et al. 1984]. We performed all hemodynamic and echocardiographic studies immediately after midweek HD, when the patients were on theoretical dry weight. In this way, we avoided fluctuations in CO secondary to progressive circulatory volume overload during the interdialytic period. This is an important aspect that should be taken into consideration in hemodynamic studies performed in HD patients [Tomson et al. 1990].

Considering these data we conclude that LVMi reduction is obtained after partial correction of anemia with rhEPO; previous hypertension and current need for antihypertensive treatment have also a significant effect in the development of LVMi. Beneficial effects of rhEPO have almost only been restricted to quality of life and exercise capacity [Wolcott et al. 1988, Mayer et al. 1988]; regression of LVM is another obvious effect. Whether this reduction could improve outcome in ESRD patients remains to be established.

REFERENCES

Bernardi D, Bergini L, Cini G, Geri AB, Urti DA, Bonechi I 1985 Asymmetric septal hypertrophy in uremic-normotensive patients on regular hemodialysis. An M-mode and two-dimensional echocardiographic study. Nephron *39:* 30–35

Blake JW, Solangi KB, Herman MV, Goodman AA, Meggs LG 1989 Left ventricular response to exercise and autonomic control mechanisms in end-stage renal disease. Arch Intern Med *149:* 433–436

Bullock RE, Hussein AA, Simpson I, Ward MR, Wall RJC 1984 Cardiac abnormalities and exercise tolerance in patients receiving renal replacement therapy. Br Med J *289:* 1479–1484

Casale PN, Devereux RB, Milner M, Zullo G, Harshfield GA, Pickering TG, Laragh JA 1986 Value of echocardiographic measurement of left ventricular mass in predicting cardiovascular morbid events in hypertensive men. Ann Intern Med *105:* 173–178

Casati S, Passerini P, Campise MR, Graziani G, Cesana B, Perisic M, Ponticelli C 1987 Benefits and risks of protracted treatment with human recombinant erythropoietin in patients having hemodialysis. Br Med J *295:* 1017–1020

Degoulet P, Legrain M, Reach I, Aime F, DeVries P, Rojas P, Jacobs C 1982 Mortality risk factors in patients treated in chronic hemodialysis. Nephron *31:* 103–110

Deligliannis A, Paschalidou E, Sakellariou G, Vargemezis V, Geleris P, Kontopoulos A, Papadimitrou M 1984 Changes in left ventricular anatomy during hemodialysis, continuous ambulatory peritoneal dialysis and after renal transplantation. Proc Eur Dial Transplant Assoc *21:* 185–189

Devereux RB, Reichek N 1977 Echocardiographic determination of left ventricular mass in man. Anatomic validation of the method. Circulation *55:* 613–618

Eschbach JW, Downing MR, Egrie JC, Browne JK, Adamson JW 1989 USA multicenter clinical trial with recombinant human erythropoietin. Results in hemodialysis patients. Contrib Nephrol *76:* 160–165

Harnett JD, Parfrey PS, Griffiths SM, Gault MH, Barre T, Guttmann RD 1988 Left ventricular hypertrophy in end stage renal disease. Nephron *48:* 107–115

Heng MK, Janz RF, Jobin J 1985 Estimation of regional stress in the left ventricular septum and free wall: An echocardiographic study suggesting a mechanism for asymmetric septal hypertrophy. Am Heart J *110:* 84–91

Henry WL, Ware J, Gardin JM, Hepners SI, McKay J, Weiner M 1978 Echocardiographic measurements in normal subjects. Growth related changes that occur between infancy and early adulthood. Circulation *57:* 278–284

Himelman RB, Landzberg JS, Simonson JS, Amend W, Bouchard A, Merz R, Schiller NB 1988 Cardiac consequences of renal transplantation: Changes in left ventricular morphology and function. J Am Coll Cardiol *12:* 915–923

Hory K, Onoyama K, Iseki K, Fujimi S, Fujishima M 1990 Hemodynamic and volume changes by recombinant human erythropoietin (rHuEPO) in the treatment of anemic hemodialysis patients. Clin Nephrol *33:* 293–298

Huting J, Kramer W, Shutterle S, Wizemann V 1988 Analysis of left ventricular changes associated with chronic hemodialysis. A non invasive follow-up study. Nephron *49:* 284–290

Huting J, Kramer W, Charra B, Laurent G, Wizemann V, Shutterle G 1989 Asymmetric septal hypertrophy and left atrial dilatation in patients with end-stage renal disease on long-term hemodialysis. Clin Nephrol *32:* 276–283

Kramer W, Wizemann V, Thormann J, Kindler M, Mueller K, Schlepper M 1986 Cardiac dysfunction in patients on maintenance hemodialysis. Contrib Nephrol *52:* 97–107

Levy D, Garrison RJ, Savage DD, Kannel WB, Castelli WP 1990 Prognostic implications of echocardiographically determined left ventricular mass in the Framingham heart study. N Engl J Med *322:* 1561–1566

Lewis JF, Kuo LC, Nelson JC, Limacher MC, Quiñones MA 1984 Pulsed Doppler echocardiographic determinations of stroke volume and cardiac output: clinical validations of two new methods using the apical window. Circulation *70:* 425–431

London GM, Fabiani F, Marchais SJ, deVernejoul MC, Guerin AP, Safar ME, Metivier E, Llach F 1987 Uremic cardiomyopathy: an inadequate left ventricular hypertrophy. Kidney Int *31:* 973–980

London GM, Zins B, Pannier B, Nared C, Berthelot JM, Jacquot C, Safar M, Drueke TP 1989 Vascular changes in hemodialysis patients in response to recombinant human erythropoietin. Kidney Int *36:* 878–882

Low I, Grutzmacher P, Bergmann M, Schoeppe W 1989 Echocardiographic findings in patients on maintenance hemodialysis substituted with recombinant human erythropoietin. Clin Nephrol *31:* 26–30

Mayer G, Thum J, Coda EM, et al. 1988 Working capacity is increased following recombinant human erythropoietin therapy. Kidney Int *34:* 525–528

Mehta BR, Ireland MA, Shin MF 1983 Echocardiographic evaluation of cardiac size and function in dialysis patients. Clin Nephrol *20:* 61–66

Nakashima Y, Fouad FM, Tarazi RC 1984 Regression of left ventricular hypertrophy from systemic hypertension by enalapril. Am J Cardiol *53:* 1044–1050

Parfrey PS, Harnett JD, Griffiths SM, Taylor R, Hand J, King A, Barre PE 1990 The clinical course of left ventricular hypertrophy in dialysis patients. Nephron *55:* 114–120

Pollok M, Bommer J, Gurland HJ, Koch KM, Schoeppe W, Scigalla P, Baldamus CA 1989 Effects of recombinant human erythropoietin treatment in end-stage renal disease patients. Results of a multicenter phase II/III study. Contrib Nephrol *76:* 201–211

Rostand SG, Sanders C, Kirk KA, Rutsky EA, Fraser RG 1988 Myocardial calcification and cardiac dysfunction in chronic renal failure. Am J Med *85:* 651–657

Rowlands DB, Glover DR, Ireland MA, McLeay RAB, Stallard TJ, Watson RDS, Littler WA 1982 Assessment of left ventricular mass and its response to antihypertensive treatment. Lancet *i:* 467–470

Sahn DJ, DeMaria A, Kisslo J, Weyman A 1978 Recommendations regarding quantitation in M mode echocardiography: Results of a survey of echocardiographic measurements. Circulation *58:* 1072–1083

Silberberg JS, Barre PE, Prichard SS, Sniderman AD 1989 Impact of left ventricular hypertrophy on survival in end-stage renal disease. Kidney Int *36:* 286–290

Teruel JL, Rodriguez Padial L, Quereda C, Yuste P, Ortuño J 1987 Regression of left ventricular hypertrophy after renal transplantation. A prospective study. Transplantation *43:* 307–309

Teruel JL, Pascual J, Jiménez M, Liaño F, Rivera M, Martínez J, Moya JL, Ortuño J 1990 Hemodynamic changes in hemodialyzed patients during treatment with recombinant human erythropoietin. Nephron (in press)

Tomson CRV 1990 Echocardiographic assessment of systolic function in dialysis patients. Nephrol Dial Transplant *5:* 325–331

Troy BL, Pombo J, Rackley CE 1972 Measurement of left ventricular wall thickness and mass by echocardiography. Circulation *45:* 602–611

Tutsui N, Suzuki M, Hirasawa Y 1989 Renewed cardiovascular dynamics induced by recombinant erythropoietin administration. Nephrol Dial Transplant 4 *(Suppl):* 146–150

Winearls CG, Oliver DO, Pippard MJ, Reid C, Downing MR, Cotes PM 1986 Effect of human erythropoietin derived from recombinant DNA on the anemia of patients maintained on chronic hemodialysis. Lancet *ii:* 1175–1178

Wolcott DL, Marsh JT, La Rue A, Carr C, Nissenson AR 1989 Recombinant human erythropoietin treatment may improve quality of life and cognitive function in chronic hemodialysis patients. Am J Kidney Dis *14:* 478–485

LETTERS TO THE EDITOR

Uric acid calculus in renal transplant patients treated with cyclosporine

Sir, – The development of uric acid calculi in transplanted kidneys has been reported as an unusual phenomenon [1–2]. Recently, an incrase in uric acid urolithiasis in renal graft recipients has been observed, suggesting a relationship with the use of the immunosuppressor cyclosporine [3].

Of 365 kidney transplants performed by our group, 3 per cent developed lithiasis in the graft. This percentage is identical whether patients receive azathioprine or cyclosporine. However, we observed a different calculus composition in the two groups. In the azathioprine group all calculi contained calcium compounds, whereas in the cyclosporine group 60 per cent of graft lithiases were made up of uric acid. No uric lithiasis was detected before renal transplantation.

This study included 223 renal transplant recipients with stabilized renal function and serum creatinine below 2.5 mg/dl. One hundred and eleven were treated with cyclosporine and 112 received azathioprine. In both groups, we measured serum creatinine, serum uric acid, urinary urate excretion, urate clearance, fractional uric acid clearance and urine pH. The results are shown in Table 1. In the cyclosporine-treated group, 66.4% of the azathioprine-treated patients. Uric acid lithiasis appeared at 6.3 ± 1.5 months. In cyclosporine-treated patients, compared to the azathioprine group, we found: higher serum creatinine and uricemia, lower urate clearance and urate excretion fraction ($p < 0.01$), higher urinary urate concentration ($p = 0.07$) and decreased (acid) urinary pH ($p < 0.01$). All these parameters were studied as well as their relationship under diuretic treatment and, unlike the reports of other authors, no statistical differences were found.

In all renal transplant recipients in this study, uric acid stone formation appeared only in patients treated with cyclosporine. This group also had a slightly abnormal renal function, probably secondary to cyclosporine use, as other authors have reported previously [4–5]. The association with elevated urinary urate concentration and urinary acid pH can contribute to lithiasis formation.

M. C. Cantarell, L. Capdevila, M. Morlans and L. Piera
Servicio de Nefrologia, Hospital General Vall D'Hebron, Paseo Vall D'Hebron S/N, 08035 Barcelona, Spain

REFERENCES

[1] *Hayes JM, Streem SB, Graneto D, Steinmuller DR, Novick AC* 1989 Urolithiasis after renal transplantation. Transplant Proc *21(1):* 1960–1961

[2] *Motayne GG, Jindal SL, Irvine AH, Abele RP* 1984 Calculus formation in renal patients. J Urol *132:* 448–449

[3] *Dieckmann KP, Schwarz A, Klan R, Offermann G* 1988 Uric acid calculus complicating renal transplantation. Clin Transpl *2:* 211–213

[4] *Versalius DJ, Wenting GJ, Jeekel J, Weimar W* 1988 The influence of cyclosporine A on proximal tubular function in renal allografts. Transplant Proc 20 (3) *suppl 3:* 686–690

[5] *Kahan BD* 1989 Cyclosporine. New Engl J Med *321(5):* 1725–1738

Table 1 Clinical characteristics of renal-allograft recipients taking cyclosporine or azathioprine.

Characteristic	Urolithiasis – group (3/111)	Cyclosporine – group (111)	Azathioprine – group (112)
Creatinine	2.4 ± 0.1**	1.6 ± 0.4	1.4 ± 0.5 mgrs/dl*
Serum uric acid	9.5 ± 0.7	8.3 ± 1.4	6.2 ± 1.9 mgrs/dl*
Urinary urate excretion	673 ± 347	626 ± 160	617 ± 122 mgrs/24 h
Urate clearance	4.7 ± 2	4.6 ± 1.5	6.6 ± 3.2 ml/min*
Fractional uric acid clearance	12.6 ± 3.7	10 ± 4.7	12.7 ± 8.3%*
Urinary pH	5.1 ± 0.3	5.1 ± 0.3	5.7 ± 0.7*

* = $p < 0.01$ for the comparison with the cyclosporine and azathioprine group
** = $p < 0.01$ for the comparison of the urolithiasis group with the cyclosporine and azathioprine group

Author index

Abuelo JG 78
Ahlberg M 270
Akutsu Y 184 (letter)
Albonico G 176
Andrassy K 139
Arakawa M 134 (letter)
Arcasoy A 135 (letter)
Asano Y 66

Bailie GR 88 (letter)
Banner B 6
Bárány P 270
Barbe MC 89 (letter)
Barber E 130
Baretto S (letter) 235
Barrillon D 137 (letter)
Barrish A 234 (letter)
Baskan S 135 (letter)
Bateman JM 148
Bazzi C 176
Bergstralh EJ 52
Bergström J 270
Bianchi AM 98
Böhler J 243
Boisclair MD 26
Borel JF S23
Bourgeois V 187
Bouteiller G 183 (letter)
Brodehl J S8
Broneer D S37
Browning MC 47
Broyer M S31
Brummer-Korvenkontio M 233 (letter)
Burden RP 252
Burden SH 198

Caillette A 235 (letter)
Cameron JS 263
Cantarell MC 288 (letter)
Capdevila L 288 (letter)
Carney S 44 (letter)
Cassuto-Viguier E 137 (letter)
Cattran DC S43
Cavdar AO 135 (letter)
Cervellati M 59
Chagnac A 24
Chan MK 207
Chantler C 263
Charmes JP 183 (letter)
Chazan JA 78
Cheng IKP 207
Cirami C 98
Coad NAG 10
Condamin MC S37
Cotton RE 252
Coulange C 89 (letter)
Cunningham J 182 (letter)
Curtis JR 26
Cy C 207

D'Amico GD 176, 237
D'Elia F 59
Davenport A 151
Davies PM 263
Davison AM 151
Dawborn JK 227
Defferari G 39
Delaney V 45 (letter)
Depierreux M 187
Descombes E 171
Dessibourg CA 171
Dohi K 1
Drouet M 183 (letter)
Ducobu J 187
Ducros J 89 (letter)
Duley JA 263
Duplay H 137 (letter)
Dupont P 187

Ekin M 135 (letter)
Endoh M 93
Erb A 139

Fang GX 207
Farrell PC 198
Feddersen A 255
Fellay G 171
Fellin G 176, 237
Fornarelli G 59
Fujishima M 134 (letter)
Funai M 105

Gaiter A 39
Garcia R 213
Gentile MG 237
Ghabra N 6
Gillies A 20, 44 (letter)
Gimenez E 235 (letter)
Gotti E 237
Granadillo VA 213
Grazi G 98
Greenberg A 6
Grotz W 243

Habib R S31
Hallett MD 198
Harrison NA 148
Hemingway J 88 (letter)
Hichens M 234 (letter)
Hirakata H 134 (letter)
Hirano T 1
Hirayama T 1
Hoffmann L 190
Hone PW 198
Hong JH 45 (letter)
Horii Y 1
Hosni N 235 (letter)
Hoyer J 255
Hultman E 270

Ido K 66
Imagawa A 105
Innes A 252
Ireland HA 26
Ishikawa H 1
Ishitsuka T 134 (letter)
Iskandar SS 47
Itami N 184 (letter)
Iwano M 1

Jambou P 137 (letter)
James EM 52
Jiménez-Mena M 280
Jonas L 190
Jones B 44 (letter)

Kagami S 105
Kamouchi M 134 (letter)
Kawaguchi Y 72
Kawahito S 105
Kawamoto C 66
Kaye M 130
Keller E 243
Kimura K 66
Kimura Y 72
King J 123
Kishimoto T 1
Klein B 190
Koderisch J 139
Korzets A 24
Kravaritis A 224
Kumplainen T 190
Kuriyama S 72
Kuroda Y 105
Kusunoki Y 184 (letter)
Kwan JTC 182 (letter)

Labeuuw M 235 (letter)
Lai KN 218
Lake N 20
Lane DA 26
Law E 218
Ledingham JGG 148
Lee GSL 184 (letter)
Lee SMK 123
Leondi A 224
Leroux-Robert C 183 (letter)
Leung AKC 119
Leung JKC 218
Levi J 24
Li PKT 218
Liano F 86 (letter), 280
Libbey NP 78
London MR 78
Lorentz WB 47
Lui SF 218

Mallick NP S3
Malone M 88 (letter)
Manna G 237
Manno C 59
Marco-Franco JE 52
Marshall T 10
Maschio G 237
Massarino F 39
Mathur R 17
McBride MB 263
McCarthy JT 52
McMahon LP 227
Mecca G 237
Meyrier A S37
Mingarelli M 59
Miura M 93
Miyazaki M 93
Morgann RG 47
Morlans M 288 (letter)
Moro F 263
Moya JL 280
Muraguchi A 1
Murai K 134 (letter)
Mustonen J 233 (letter)
Muto S 66

Nagano M 35
Nakayama M 72
Nanikvell BJ 20
Nanra R 44 (letter)
Navarro JA 213
Neusy AJ 110
Niaudet P S31
Nicholls MG 218
Nixon DE 52
Nomoto Y 93
Nortier J 187
Nube MJ 165

Ogawa S 1
Ogg CS 263
Ohtani M 66
Okada K 105
Okamura K 134 (letter)
Okomoto T 105
Oldrizzi L 237
Onoyama K 134 (letter)
Ori Y 24
Ortuno J 86 (letter), 280
Otabe S 66

Pagani C 176
Palla R 98
Panichi V 98
Papadakis JT 224
Papakostas K 224
Parrini M 98
Pascual J 86 (letter), 280
Passerini P S16
Pasternack A 233 (letter)
Patrikarea A 224
Peter HH 243
Pettersson E 270

Piera L 288 (letter)
Piraino B 6
Pono L 78
Ponticelli C S16
Pontremoli R 39
Poole-Warren LA 198
Puvaneswary M 44 (letter)

Radford J 227
Rampal M 89 (letter)
Remuzzi G 237
Rhinehart R 158
Ritz E 139
Robaudo C 39
Robson WLM 119
Rodríguez-Iturbe B 213
Rohrbach R 243
Romero RA 213
Rosansky SJ 158
Roux C 137 (letter)
Rowe B 10
Rowe PA 252
Rugiu C 237
Rush JE 234 (letter)

Sack K 255
Saha H 233 (letter)
Saingra S 89 (letter)
Saito H 35
Sakai H 93
Sakai O 72
Salgado O 213
Saradi S 224
Sato H 134 (letter)
Sato K 66
Schena FP 59
Schollmeyer R 243
Shade R 158
Shiki H 1
Simmonds HA 263
Simpson LO 183 (letter)
Smith R 148
Snyder DL 234 (letter)
Sommer BG 45 (letter)
Sorgato G 176
Spargo BH 123
Steinhoff J 255
Stella M 59
Suga T 93
Sumrani N 45 (letter)
Sureda A 86 (letter)
Suzuki S 134 (letter)

Tagawa H 35
Taylor CM 10
Teruel JL 86 (letter), 280
Thompson E 26
Tibi T 137 (letter)
Ton That H 183 (letter)
Torres VE 52
Trevillian P 44 (letter)
Tsuji H 134 (letter)
Tümer N 135 (letter)

Umezu M 35

Vafiadis S 224
Valeri A 110
Van Geelen JA 165
Vasilevsky M 130
Verzetti G 89 (letter)

Waldherr R 139
Wanner C 243
Warren J 17
Watanabe S 72
Wei D 207
Wiffen P 88 (letter)
Will EJ 151
Wilson DM 52
Woo KS 218
Woo KT 184 (letter)
Wood WG 255

Yamakado M 35
Yano I 105
Yasoshima K 184 (letter)
Yu L 207

Zevin D 24
Zuurbier PA 165

Subject index

acetate dialysate 224
acquired cystic kidney disease 52
AIDS 110
allopurinol 263
amoxicillin 187
amyloidosis 182 (letter)
anemia 207, 270, 280
antineutrophil cytoplasmic antibodies 139
atrial natriuretic peptide 218
autoimmunity S23

beta thromboglobulin 26
biochemical parameters 78
bone pathology 78

CAPD 20, 24, 198, 207, 213, 218
carbonic anhydrase 190
chlorambucil S8, S16
cholelithiasis 86 (letter)
chronic renal failure 218
cirrhosis 6
complement 198
corticosteroids S16
CT Scan 123
cyclophosphamide S8
cyclosporin A S23, S31, S37, S43, S48
– –, animal experiments S23
cyclosporin 255, 288
–, patient's knowledge 88 (letter)

desferrioxamine B 213
dialysate 198
dialysis 52
–, phosphate deficiency 130
–, related amyloidosis 227
diet 237

ECG 35
EEG 171
electrophysiology 176
empyema thoracis 17
endothelin 218
erythrocyte transketolase activity 171
erythropoietin 165, 270
–, recombinant 207
–, recombinant human 35, 280
exit site infection 198
exploratory excisions 190

familial gout 263
Fanconi syndrome 148
fibrin degradation products 26
fibrinopeptide A 26
fractional urate clearance 263

G6PD deficiency 89 (letter)
glomerular hyperfiltration 59
glomerulonephritis 6, 183 (letter), S43
–, crescentic 243
–, IgA 139
–, membranoproliferative 47
–, mesangiocapillary 47
–, minimal-change S37, S48
–, rapidly progressive 2, 139
glomerulosclerosis, focal-segmental S3, S37, S48
gouty nephropathy 263

hemodialysis 26, 35, 158, 165, 171, 176, 224, 270, 280
–, chronic 76
–, iron deficiency 87 (letter)
hemodynamics 35
hemolytic uremic syndrome 10, 86 (letter), 119
– anemia 89 (letter)
heparin measurement 26
hepatocellular carcinoma 66
human IgG 98
hypercalcemia 182 (letter)
hyperlipidemia 237
hyperreninemic hypoaldosteronism 66
hypersensitivity reactions 224
hypertension 35
–, accelerated 39
–, severe 39
hyperuricemia 263
hypophosphatemic osteomalacia 148
hypozincemia 135 (letter)

IgA 6
– nephritis 44 (letter)
– nephropathy 1
– neuropathy 184 (letter)
IgM S3
immune-complexes 47
immunoglobulins 198
immunohistochemical detection 190
immunometric assays 255
immunosuppression S23
immunosuppressive therapy S16
infectious mononucleosis 137 (letter)
interleukin 6 1
intracerebral pressure 151
intrauterine device 24

kidney donors 59
– biopsies S48

liver transplantation 6
– failure 151

MCNS 93
mesangial cell 1
mesangioproliferative disease S3
metal removal 213
microalbuminuria 59
minoxidil 39
mycobacterial avium-intracellulare infection 45 (letter)

naproxen 187
nasal carriage 198
nephritis S23
–, acute interstitial 184 (letter), 187
–, tubulointerstitial 105
nephropathia epidemica 233
nephropathy, AIDS-associated 110
–, IgA 134 (letter)
–, membranous 98, S16, S43
–, minimal-change S3
nephrotic syndrome 47, 93, 98, 187, 237
–, idiopathic S16
–, –, adult S37
–, –, children S31
–, minimal-change S8
–, therapy 98
neutrophil count 10
nutrition 270

obesity 123
osmolality 158
oxalate 52

peritonitis 198
–, pneumococcal 24
–, recurrent bacterial 20
pharmacokinetics 72
plasmapheresis 119
platelet factor 4 44 (letter)
precocious gout 263
prednisone S8
primary biliary cirrhosis 134 (letter)
prostacyclin 151
proteinuria 255

renal allograft 45 (letter)
– biopsy, percutaneous 44 (letter), 123
– dysfunction S48
– failure, acute 105, 110, 119
– –, glomerular 148
– –, progression 39
– osteodystrophy 78
– transplant 288
– transplantation 255
– vasculitis 252
renin activity 218
reno-cutaneous fistula 17
rheumatoid factor 93

shoulder ultrasound 227
sickle cell disease 47
silicon 52
sodium ferric gluconate complex 87 (letter)
staphylococcal vaccination 198
Staphylococcus aureus 198
– epidermis 20
sterile pyuria 87 (letter)
streptokinase 20
symptomatic-asymptomatic 227

thiamine deficiency 171
thrombin-antithrombin complex 26
thrombocytopenia 119
trace metals 213
transplant rejection 255
tubulointerstitial disorders 134 (letter)

urate oxidase 89 (letter)
urea kinetics 165
uremia 270
uremic cardiomyopathy 218
– polyneuropathy 176
uric acid calculus 288
urine pH 190

vanadium 52
vasoactive hormones 218
vasopressin 158
ventricular hypertrophy 280
verocytotoxin producing Escherichiae coli 10
vitamin D3 72

Wegener's granulomatosis 139, 243
Wernicke's encephalopathy 171

xanthogranulomatous pyelonephritis 17

Yersinia pseudotuberculosis 105

B 21852 E
Sondernummer

clinical nephrology

Cyclosporin A (Sandimmun®) in Nephrotic Syndrome

Guest Editor: C. Ponticelli

Vol. 35, Supplement No. 1, 1991

Dustri-Verlag
Dr. Karl Feistle
München-
Deisenhofen

Preface

In spite of extensive experimental and clinical investigation, the treatment of primary glomerulonephritis remains largely unsatisfactory. Most therapeutic approaches are based on the administration of corticosteroids and/or alkylating agents. These drugs can produce remission of proteinuria in most patients who have minimal-change nephropathy, but the treatment of either frequently relapsing or steroid-dependent patients remains a difficult task for the nephrologist. The role of corticosteroids and of alkylating agents in focal-segmental glomerulosclerosis and membranous nephropathy is still controversial. The main limitation in using these drugs to treat a chronic disease is their low therapeutic index; the toxic threshold is very close to the clinically effective dose in the treatment of glomerulonephritis.

The recent development of cyclosporin A (CyA, Sandimmun®) had made available new possibilities for the treatment of patients with idiopathic nephrotic syndrome. A number of studies have shown that CyA produces remission of proteinuria in most steroid-sensitive patients. However, the results are less exciting in those who are steroid-resistant. Nevertheless, a proportion of these cases may attain partial or complete remissions with CyA. Unfortunately, most patients experience early relapse of the nephrotic syndrome on stopping CyA. On the other hand, prolonged administration of the drug carries a theoretical risk of progressive nephrotoxicity.

Thus, there are many questions in the use of CyA that are still unanswered: What are the correct indications for CyA in idiopathic nephrotic syndrome? What is the optimal dosage? What is the safe duration of treatment with CyA? Is it better to give CyA alone or in association with low-dose prednisone? What clinical parameter is the best indicator of early nephrotoxicity? These and other aspects were the main subjects of discussion at a seminar/workshop, Cyclosporin A in Nephrotic Syndrome*, held on November 5, 1990, in Nice, France.

This supplement to *Clinical Nephrology* is a report of the proceedings** of that meeting. The first part focuses on the natural course of idiopathic nephrotic syndrome and the effects of conventional therapy. The second part is entirely devoted to the possible role of CyA in the treatment of the disease. The mechanisms of action of the drug, its therapeutic results and the drug-related side-effects have been thoroughly reviewed by some of the most distinguished experts in this field. I would like to extend my thanks to all those who attended this meeting for their active participation and contributions to this important area of ongoing research.

Claudio Ponticelli

* The meeting was sponsored by Sandoz Pharma Ltd, Basel, Switzerland.

** These proceedings were prepared for publication by CCT Presentations Ltd, London, UK.

Epidemiology and natural course of idiopathic nephrotic syndrome

N. P. Mallick

Department of Renal Medicine, The Royal Infirmary, Manchester, M13 9WL, UK

Abstract. The term "idiopathic nephrotic syndrome" is poorly defined and is used to refer to a variety of glomerular lesions. This article seeks to clarify the situation by considering the case for treating minimal-change nephropathy, focal and segmental glomerulosclerotic lesions, and mesangioproliferative lesions with predominantly IgM deposition as separate disease entities. In children, nephrotic syndrome has a pattern different from that in adults, in whom a wider pathogenetic spectrum is seen. There is support for the use of prospective clinicopathological data as the basis of identifying those patients with nephrotic syndrome who will progress to end-stage renal failure. Very heavy, persisting proteinuria is one marker of such progression and is also an indicator of metabolic complications, such as cardiovascular disease, which further increase the risks of mortality and morbidity in this group of patients.

Key words: minimal-change nephropathy – focal and segmental glomerulosclerosis – IgM – mesangioproliferative disease

This article discusses three questions: What is the idiopathic nephrotic syndrome? Is minimal-change nephropathy an entity distinct from focal and segmental glomerulosclerosis and IgM mesangial proliferative disease, both of which are controversial entities? What is the natural history of the nephrotic syndrome in general?

Definition of nephrotic syndrome

The term "idiopathic nephrotic syndrome" must first be defined. The term is very widely used, but its definition varies. On reviewing the literature of the last two or three years, the idiopathic nephrotic syndrome has been described, by authoritative sources, as including cases in which the renal biopsy shows no change on light microscopy, IgM mesangial proliferation, mesangiocapillary changes, and membranous nephropathy as well as focal glomerulosclerosis. Some have included all of these conditions, others only some of them. Those reporting on children have a distinctive concept of this syndrome. The term "steroid-sensitive nephrotic syndrome" is widely used, sometimes interchangeably with and sometimes distinct from "idiopathic nephrotic syndrome" but, again, this is imprecise. A wide variety of histopathological lesions can respond to steroids, but neither predictably nor reliably. Use of the term to infer the biopsy findings, which therefore requires inference of the pathogenetic mechanisms, is inexact. It is time that we, as a specialist medical community, made our working definitions more precise.

As regards a clinical definition of the nephrotic syndrome, the current vogue is to ascribe significance to proteinuria greater than 3.5 g/day; this is incorrect. For a complete description of nephrotic syndrome, in addition to the proteinuria, there should be hypoalbuminemia and edema, if the patient is a well-nourished adult; proteinuria of at least 5 g/day (equivalent to 40 mg/m^2/h in a child) is the threshold beyond which the metabolic and clinical consequences of nephrotic syndrome become evident [Mallick et al. 1987].

Figure 1 shows that, while a "snapshot" of proteinuria is not helpful, the longer-term regular assessment of daily protein loss is an aid to prognosis. Regular assessment of proteinuria over a mean period of eight years showed that, for those patients in whom values were never greater than 5 g/day, there were no sinister consequences. If, however, proteinuria which was initially below 5 g/day rose above this level, which was often the case, the prognosis was less certainly benign. If proteinuria persists at levels $>$10 g/day, the metabolic and clinical consequences are severe.

Reprint requests to Professor N. P. Mallick.

INFLUENCE OF REMISSION ON DEVELOPMENT OF RENAL FAILURE

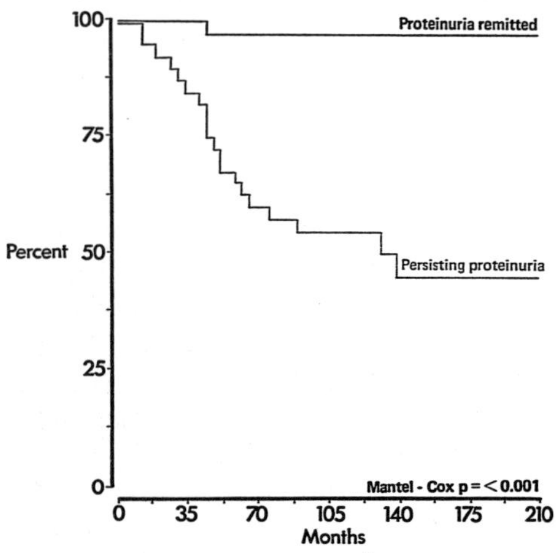

Fig. 1 Effect of remission on the development of renal failure: as soon as remission occurs, renal function is maintained.

Definition of minimal-change disease

Is minimal-change disease a separate entity? Review of the literature on children reveals that the terms "idiopathic nephrotic syndrome", "steroid-sensitive nephrotic syndrome", and "minimal-change nephropathy" have been used interchangeably so often that there is no clear definition of this disease. Furthermore, is focal and segmental glomerulosclerosis a separate disease entity? These two clinical patterns predominate in the nephrotic syndrome of childhood.

In Manchester, together with our pediatric department, we studied 61 patients (male to female ratio 3.5:1) who had steroid-responsive, biopsy-proven minimal-change nephropathy [Lewis et al. 1989]. All had presented with the disease in childhood at least 10 years earlier. The mean duration of follow-up was 14 years (range 10–21 years). None of these patients were hypertensive at the end of the follow-up period (defined as a blood pressure greater than the 97th percentile of that considered normal for age) and none had a reduced glomerular filtration rate (GFR). Furthermore, none of these patients had developed focal and segmental glomerulosclerosis.

During the last five years, there have been reports, including ours, of a total of 291 children with biopsy-proven minimal-change disease. None of these children developed end-stage renal failure, and none appeared to have transformed into focal and segmental glomerulosclerosis. Of these children, who were followed for a mean duration of 17 years, 95% have relapsed. Over the same period of time, there have been two reports of adults with minimal-change nephropathy. One of these was a multicenter review of 265 cases by Coggins et al. [1985]. Only two of these patients developed what was considered end-stage renal failure. Bearing in mind the multicenter nature of this trial, occasional diagnostic uncertainty is inevitable. Therefore, it would appear that minimal-change nephropathy is a distinct entity with an excellent clinical prognosis when treated with steroids, although death may occur because of secondary metabolic and other consequences of the illness especially if treatment is initiated too late.

It is important to differentiate the diagnosis of "no change on light microscopy" from minimal-change nephropathy on the basis of a combination of the histopathology, clinical pattern, response to steroids and natural history. In a series of over 400 biopsied patients at our own institution [Mallick et al. 1987], followed for a mean duration of eight years, 33 were easily diagnosed to have minimal-change nephropathy. All presented with a nephrotic syndrome and all responded promptly to therapy. However, among other patients who showed no change on light microscopy, some had a nephrotic syndrome which was, at best, only partly responsive to steroids, and the remainder had various other presentations. None of those who had minimal-change nephropathy developed renal impairment or focal and segmental glomerulosclerosis, whereas such changes were observed in some of the other cases. Therefore, a diagnosis should not be established on the basis of the histopathology alone.

Focal and segmental glomerulosclerosis

This histopathological appearance is found in many experimental models of glomerulopathy. Recent work on the progression of renal failure has shown that this appearance develops in the remnant kidney. In the Zucker rat, it is seen in relation to the hyperlipidemic state of these animals. Recently, it has been seen in patients with human immunodeficiency virus (HIV) disease, both in affected adults and in their children; thus, experimentally and clinically, this histopathological pattern can arise as a secondary phenomenon. There are, however, many patients who do not manifest any of the above-mentioned problems, yet develop focal and segmental glomerulosclerosis and the nephrotic syndrome.

There has been some debate as to whether or not minimal-change disease progresses to focal and segmental glomerulosclerosis. If care has been taken in the diagnosis of minimal-change disease, such progression does not appear to occur. However, some, but not all, patients with focal and segmental glomerulosclerosis may by steroid-responsive, as are some patients with other nephropathies. A recent report by Fogo et al. [1990] analyzed a series of biopsies from patients who showed no change on light microscopy. They found that, in those who had minimal-change disease – defined as in this article – the glomeruli were of similar size compared with those of the controls whereas, in those patients who were eventually diagnosed as having focal and segmental glomerulosclerosis, the glomeruli were larger than either those of the controls or those with minimal-change disease (Figure 2). It may well be that there is now a convergence of the experimental evidence of secondary focal and segmental glomerulosclerosis and the idiopathic disease as seen in humans; there are similar early changes in the glomeruli, and many of these patients are not steroid-responsive.

Overall, patients with focal and segmental glomerulosclerosis have a poor response to prednisolone – a few will respond to steroids while most will remit spontaneously; some will relapse. In the recent literature, approximately 15 to 20% progressed to end-stage renal failure. Magil and Cohen [1989] have recently reported that foam cells – lipid-laden cells characteristic of, for example, lesions in the Zucker rat – tend to develop with time in focal and segmental glomerulosclerosis. These may be indicative of progressive renal damage, and the hyperlipidemia produced by an aggressive and persisting nephrotic syndrome may itself contribute to the progression of the disease; thus, this may be an important feature to note in the late natural history of the disease.

IgM mesangioproliferative disease

Another controversial lesion, which is often confused with minimal-change disease, and focal and segmental glomerulosclerosis, is IgM mesangioproliferative disease. There is still much debate as to whether this is related to the two lesions previously discussed, or whether it is a separate disease entity. Two papers, one by Bhasin [1978] and another by Cohen et al. [1978] drew attention to the possibility that there may be a glomerular lesion, affecting adults in particular, in which IgM was the predominant immunoglobulin accompanied by mesangial expansion. Our own experience was published two years later [Lawler et al. 1980]. In a further review, to be published in the *Quarterly Journal of Medicine* [O'Donoghue et al. 1991], of 77 patients diagnosed as having IgM mesangioproliferative disease, the histopathology has remained true in all cases rebiopsied; 40% of these patients have gone into remission vs 26% who have progressed to end-stage renal failure. However, 15% have relapsed, including some who are responsive to steroids.

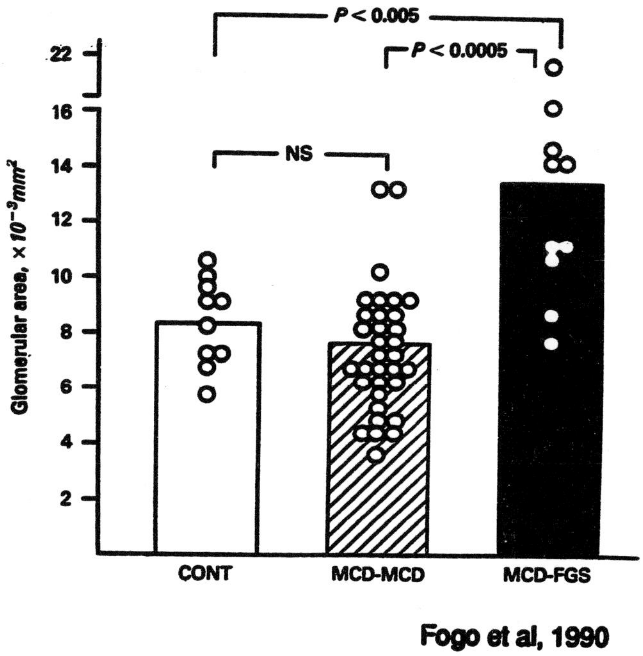

Fig. 2 In a comparative series of renal biopsies, the mean glomerular area was higher in focal and segmental glomerulosclerosis (FGS) than in minimal-change nephropathy (MCD) or controls (CONT). With permission from *Fogo et al.* 1990 Kidney Int. 38: 115–123.

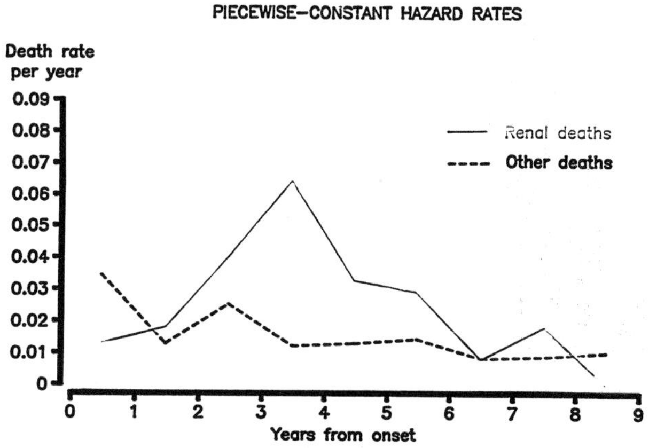

Fig. 3 The risk of developing end-stage renal failure (ESRF) peaks within four to five years of glomerular disease onset. The late development of ESRF may involve secondary mechanisms, such as hypertension, hyperlipidemia or diet-associated factors.

Table 1 Patients (%) with proteinuria according to levels of plasma creatinine at disease onset and after one year

	Plasma creatinine (mmol/l)		
	<0.12	0.12–0.19	≥0.20
At disease onset (n = 77)	53	29	18
After one year (n = 139)	55	28	17

Table 2 Retrospective analysis of patients according to level of proteinuria

	At 4 months	At 12 months	At 24 months
State 1 (5–10 g/day)	2.1 ± 0.62 (8)	1.3 ± 0.79 (4)	1.9 ± 0.72 (6)
	***	***	***
State 2 (>10 g/day)	3.0 ± 0.57 (20)	3.0 ± 0.62 (20)	2.7 ± 0.66 (15)

***p <0.001
( ) = Factor of risk for renal failure

Table 3 Retrospective analysis using likelihood ratios of patient risk for renal failure according to state of proteinuria

	At 12 months
State 0 (Plasma creatinine <0.2 mmol/l, ratio <4)	–
State 1 (Plasma creatinine <0.2 mmol/l, ratio ≥4)	2.8 ± 1.1*** (17)
State 2 (Plasma creatinine ≥0.2 mmol/l, ratio <4)	4.0 ± 1.2*** (54)
State 3 (Plasma creatinine ≥0.2 mmol/l, ratio ≥4)	4.9 ± 1.1*** (130)

***p <0.001 vs State 0 (baseline)
Figures are given as coefficients ± s.e.; ( ) = relative risk

Thus, once again, steroid responsiveness cannot be a diagnostic criterion. The overall presentation of IgM mesangial proliferation is very different from minimal-change disease, and resembles focal and segmental glomerulosclerosis and other glomerulopathies in its progression. In proteinuric illnesses, the diagnosis should be based on the biopsy, clinical presentation, natural history, and response to treatment in order to define clearly the disease.

Summary

There is now little doubt that, in patients presenting with an idiopathic proteinuric illness, minimal-change disease, focal and segmental glomerulosclerosis, and IgM mesangioproliferative disease are three separate entities, the first with its well-known good prognosis, and the latter two with the same prognosis as other causes of the nephrotic syndrome.

The nephrotic syndrome in the adult is usually self-limiting. Only in a minority does renal failure develop and, in those cases, relatively quickly. How can we identify these patients, and is the renal biopsy useful in this regard? Our own studies show that, of 242 patients followed for a median duration of seven years (range 11 weeks to 33 years), 158 (66%) were alive, mainly in remission and using their own functioning kidneys, and 44 (18%) had progressed to end-stage renal failure [Hunt et al. 1988]. However, Table 1 shows that the percentages of patients with plasma creatinine levels < 0.12, 0.12 – 0.19 and ≥ 0.20 mmol/l, measured at disease onset (n = 77) and after one year (n = 139), were similar in each of the three groups.

Another method of analyzing the data, as this was a large series, was to start at the endpoint and review the data retrospectively (Table 2). On selecting those patients who had proteinuria of 5–10 g/day (State 1) and > 10 g/day (State 2), and using renal failure as the index point, it was found that the relative risk for patients with State 1 proteinuria was higher than for those with levels ≤5 g/day, but it was very much higher for patients with State 2 (Table 2).

A similar time-lag exercise for four states (0, 1, 2, 3) of serum creatinine (Table 3) showed that patients in State 3 (heavy proteinuria and raised serum creatinine) had a relative risk, 12 months previously, of 130. As these patients tend to progress to renal failure very quickly – within three or four years of onset (Figure 3) – the "window of opportunity" for therapy is very small. Furthermore, although there is a small possibility that those patients who are likely to progress to renal failure can be identified, renal biopsy findings – as evaluated in these forward or time-lag models, with the possible exception of mesangiocapillary disease – were not accurate indicators for identifying patients at greatest risk of renal failure.

The patients who progress to renal failure later than four years after onset may have different, and less common, causes of disease progression and eventual death. On the other hand, renal failure is not always the only cause of death in patients who develop the nephrotic syndrome; a significant minority develop, or die because of, ischemic heart disease. In an overall series of 242 relatively young patients (median age

36 years), there were 15 deaths in total. On evaluating the morbidity in this group of patients, approximately 10% developed ischemic heart disease, which is a very high proportion for such a young patient group.

Thus, careful definition of the disease and of the patient group involved is essential for the correct diagnosis and treatment of nephrotic syndrome as well as the possible prevention of its secondary metabolic and other consequences.

REFERENCES

Bhasin HK, Abuelo JG, Nayak R, Esperaza AR 1978 Mesangial proliferative glomerulonephritis. Lab Invest *39:* 21–29

Coggins CH, and the Collaborative Study 1985 Adult minimal change nephropathy: Experience of the Collaborative Study of glomerular disease. Trans Am Clin Climatol Assoc *97:* 18–26

Cohen AH, Border WA, Glasock RJ 1978 Nephrotic syndrome with glomerular mesangial IgM deposits. Lab Invest *38:* 610–619

Fogo A, Hawkins EP, Berry PL, Glick AD, Chiang ML, MacDonell RC Jr et al. 1990 Glomerular hypertrophy in minimal change disease predicts subsequent progression to focal gomerular sclerosis. Kidney Int *38:* 115–123

Hunt LP, Short CD, Mallick NP 1988 Prognostic indicators in patients presenting with the nephrotic syndrome. Kidney Int *34:* 382–388

Lawler W, Williams G, Tarpey P, Mallick NP 1980 IgM associated primary diffuse mesangial proliferative glomerulonephritis. J Clin Pathol *33:* 1029–1038

Lewis MA, Davis N, Postlethwaite RJ, Baildom EM, Houston IB 1989 Nephrotic syndrome: From toddlers to twenties. Lancet *ii:* 255–259

Magil AB, Cohen AH 1989 Monocytes and focal glomerulosclerosis. Lab Invest *61:* 404–409

Mallick NP, Short CD, Hunt LP 1987 How far since Ellis?: The Manchester Study of glomerular disease. Nephron *46:* 113–124

O'Donoghue DJ, Lawler W, Hunt LP, Acheson JA, Mallick NP 1991 IgM associated primary diffuse mesangial proliferative glomerulonephritis: Natural history and prognostic indicators. Q J Med (in press)

Clinical Nephrology, Vol. 35. Suppl. No 1 – 1991 (pp. S. 8–15)

Conventional therapy for idiopathic nephrotic syndrome in children

J. Brodehl

Kinderklinik, Medizinische Hochschule Hannover, Postfach 61 01 80, W-3000 Hannover 61, Germany

Abstract. In children, the most frequent type of idiopathic nephrotic syndrome is the minimal-change nephrotic syndrome (MCNS). Its treatment is aimed at inducing remission, preventing relapses and avoiding side-effects. Minimal-change disease is responsive to immunosuppressive therapy. The conventional treatment consists of glucocorticosteroids and the most widely used derivative is prednisone. Initial treatment should be intensive, for example, prednisone for 12 weeks, in order to reduce the risk of subsequent relapse. Treatment of relapses should be standardized in order to categorize the patient's disease for further treatment. If a frequent relapser develops signs of steroid toxicity, alkylating drugs should be prescribed: cyclophosphamide or chlorambucil for eight weeks for frequent relapsers who are not steroid-dependent; cyclophosphamide for 12 weeks for those who are. In steroid-resistant cases, a renal biopsy is indicated and treatment should be administered according to histological changes.

Key words: minimal-change nephrotic syndrome – prednisone – cyclophosphamide – chlorambucil

Introduction

The idiopathic nephrotic syndrome (NS) is produced by a variety of glomerular diseases which lead to severe selective proteinuria, mainly of albumin, followed by hypoalbuminemia and dysproteinemia. The International Study of Kidney Disease in Children [ISKDC, 1978] has defined the syndrome in children as proteinuria exceeding 40 $mg/m^2/h$ (approximately equivalent to 1 $g/m^2/day$) and serum albumin below 25 g/l. The clinical picture is characterized by hypovolemia, edema, hypercoagulability and an increased susceptibility to infections.

Idiopathic NS is not a lone pathomorphological entity, but is associated with various glomerular lesions. Children may have the same diseases as adults, although the frequency distribution of the histological lesions will be different (Table 1) [Glassock et al. 1981]. In children, the so-called minimal-change nephrotic syndrome (MCNS) predominates while all other histological categories are rare. In contrast, MCNS in adults makes up only 21% of cases, and membranous glomerulopathy and endocapillary proliferative glomerulonephritis are the most frequent findings.

Reprint requests to Professor Dr. Johannes Brodehl.

Thus, in pediatrics, the term idiopathic NS is often used interchangeably with MCNS – which is not correct – and the clinical approach of a pediatrician to a child with NS is the same as if the child had MCNS. On this basis, a child with a primary NS does not usually undergo renal biopsy, but is treated initially as an MCNS patient. Only if there is a non-response to treatment is the renal biopsy indicated; this usually reveals histological changes other than those of MCNS.

Minimal-change nephrotic syndrome (MCNS)

This syndrome is a clinical entity which, in brief, is defined as a NS of unknown etiology. It has a characteristic clinical picture, including: responsiveness to glucocorticoids, alkylating agents and cyclosporin A (CyA, Sandimmun®); a high tendency to relapse; an absence of progressive renal deterioration; and a minimal morphological finding on light and immunofluorescence microscopy. There is much evidence that the disease is of pathoimmunological origin [Schnaper 1989], but the exact pathogenetic mechanism is as yet undetermined.

The treatment of MCNS has a threefold objective: 1. Remission of NS should be induced as soon as possible, as the nephrotic state is associated with a high rate of dangerous and possibly fatal complications, such as infections, thromboembolism and vascular collapse [Hoyer et al. 1986, Krensky et al. 1982]; 2. Relapses of NS should be prevented as much as possible, as each relapse endangers the patient by new complications and treatment side-effects; 3. Side-effects should be avoided as much as possible, as the disease can run a long relapsing course which may potentiate side-effects such as osteoporosis, dwarfism, cataracts and psychoemotional disturbances [Chesney et al. 1978, Lam and Arneil 1968, Rees et al. 1988].

Glucocorticosteroids have been used for more than 40 years in the treatment of MCNS and are generally considered to be the drug of choice for the initial treatment. The steroid derivative most widely used is prednisone. There are no convincing data available to claim that other derivatives of glucosteroids are more advantageous than prednisone or prednisolone; therefore, the following refers exclusively to these steroids.

Initial treatment

The initial attack of MCNS is very responsive to prednisone, as indicated in the data from the International Study of Kidney Disease in Children (ISKDC) [1981 a]. Ninety-three percent of cases with MCNS responded to an eight-week course of prednisone, which suggests that nearly 72% of all children with NS are steroid-responsive (Table 2). Of all the other histological categories of NS, only focal-global glomerulosclerosis (FGGS) exhibited a similarly high response rate; all other categories did not respond to prednisone, but remained steroid-resistant.

The response to prednisone is not prompt. There is a delay of one to two weeks before a urinary remission can be observed [Arbeitsgemeinschaft für Pädiatrische Nephrologie (APN) 1988]. In the cooperative studies of the APN, urinary remission was defined as the disappearance of significant proteinuria (< 4 mg/m^2/h) for at least three consecutive days. On this basis, 50% of cases had a urinary remission with prednisone after eight days of treatment, and the great majority after 14 days [APN 1988]. A complete remission was defined as the normalization of serum albumin (≥ 35 g/l). This followed the urinary remission after a further two weeks of prednisone treatment. Thus, a complete remission of the NS in children with MCNS – which is the primary aim of treatment – could be achieved after four weeks of prednisone treatment.

However, the question which remains is whether four weeks of prednisone as the initial treatment is enough to achieve the second aim of the treatment, the prevention of subsequent relapses. In order to test the efficacy of the initial treatment, the APN compared three types of initial treatment in randomized trials: a short regimen vs the standard regimen [APN 1988]; and the standard regimen vs a long regimen [APN 1990]. The duration and dosage of prednisone in these studies are shown in Table 3. It was observed that, after the short initial regimen, 81% of patients experienced a relapse within the first 12 months after

Table 1 Comparison of histopathological lesions of idiopathic nephrotic syndrome in adults and children

	Prevalence (%) Children (n = 1066)	Adults (n = 428)
Minimal-change disease	66	21
Mesangioproliferative GN	3	2
Focal glomerulosclerosis	8	8
Membranous glomerulopathy	4	32
Membranoproliferative GN	9	5
Endocapillary proliferative GN	6	30
Other chronic GN	4	2

GN = glomerulonephritis [Glassock et al. 1981]

Table 2 Steroid response in children with idiopathic nephrotic syndrome

Histopathological category	N	Responders n (%)	% of $\geqq$ N
MCNS	363	338 (93.1)	71.8
FGGS	8	6 (75.0)	1.3
DMH	9	5 (55.6)	1.1
FSGS	37	11 (29.7)	2.3
Prolif GN	12	3 (25.0)	0.6
MPGN	29	2 (6.9)	0.4
Miscellaneous	13	3 (23.0)	0.6

[ISKDC 1981 a]

MCNS = Minimal-change nephrotic syndrome; FGGS = Focal-global glomerulosclerosis; DMH = Diffuse mesangial hypercellularity; FSGS = Focal-segmental glomerulosclerosis; Prolif GN = Proliferative glomerulonephritis; MPGN = Membranoproliferative glomerulonephritis

Table 3 Duration (days) of initial prednisone treatment in children with nephrotic syndrome

	Continuous (60 mg/m^2/day)	Alternate-day (40 mg/m^2/48 h)
Long	42	42
Standard	28	28
Short	14+6	16+8

[APN 1988, 1990]

cessation of continuous prednisone [APN 1988] compared with 61% receiving the standard regimen, and 36% receiving the long regimen (Table 4). Furthermore, the number of patients who relapsed, as well as the number of relapses which occurred, was highest after the short, compared with the standard and long, treatments as suggested by the percentage of patients defined as infrequent (less than two relapses within six months) and frequent (two or more relapses within six months) relapsers. More than twice as many patients were frequent relapsers after the short, compared with the long, therapy (Table 4). Thus, the risk of becoming a frequent relapser is much higher after four, compared with 12, weeks of prednisone as the initial treatment.

Table 4 Relapses within 12 months of stopping continuous initial prednisone therapy

Regimen	Total N	Infrequent relapsers	Frequent relapsers	Both
Long (12 w)	33	21%	15%	36%
Standard (8 w)	66	44%	17%	61%
Short (4 w)	32	47%	34%	81%

w = weeks [APN 1988, 1990]

From the results of these studies, it is obvious that the intensity of the initial treatment has a decisive influence on the subsequent rate of relapse – the more aggressive the initial prednisone treatment, the lower the relapse rate thereafter, and the longer lasting the subsequent remission. Comparable results were obtained recently in a Japanese study by Ueda et al. [1988] and, from the early days of treatment when steroids were given for prolonged periods, by Lange et al. [1958], and Arneil and Lam [1966]. Thus, the second aim of MCNS treatment, the prevention of relapses, is best approached with intensification of the initial treatment.

However, before a definitive recommendation for the initial treatment can be declared, one has to evaluate the side-effects of the treatment according to the third objective of treatment, the avoidance of side-effects. It is evident that the side-effects of steroids increase with increases in the dosage and length of treatment. Well known side-effects of steroids are a cushingoid appearance, striae, hypertension, osteoporosis, cataracts, growth retardation and psychosocial disturbances. In the above-mentioned studies by the APN, the side-effects of the long regimen were assessed in comparison to those of the standard treatment [APN 1990]. The results showed that the side-effect risk with a 12-week course of prednisone was not greater than that with an eight-week course [Brodehl 1991]. The APN, therefore, decided that the advantages of a prolonged initial prednisone treatment outweighed the risks and, accordingly, have recommended a 12-week course of prednisone as initial treatment.

Treatment of relapse

A characteristic feature of MCNS is the recurrence of heavy proteinuria and a relapse of the NS. According to the original data of the ISKDC [Barnett et al. 1978], only 36% of children did not relapse within six months of stopping the initial treatment compared with 18% who were infrequent relapsers and 39% who were frequent relapsers. Unfortunately, there are no serological, laboratory or morphological criteria available to allow a prospective of the course of the disease in terms of rate of subsequent relapses [APN 1988]. One way to compensate for this would be to classify the patient according to the severity of the disease, follow a standardized relapse protocol and register the rate of relapse with the treatment [Brodehl et al. 1982, ISKDC 1982].

The relapse is usually as steroid responsive as the initial attack of MCNS. In the APN study, the mean duration of prednisone treatment to achieve a urinary remission was the same for the initial attack and the first or second relapse [APN 1988]. However, in contrast to the initial attack, the intensity of the treatment for the relapse had no further influence on the subsequent relapse rate. Thus, the duration of remission after the first relapse does not depend on the dosage of the prednisone treatment, whether of short or standard duration [APN 1988]. This finding is in accordance with the results of a therapeutic trial of the ISKDC [1979] in which an intensified (tapering) prednisone regimen was compared with a standard relapse regimen in children after the first relapse. There were no differences in subsequent relapse rate between these two regimens.

From these observations, it is unlikely that the standard relapse treatment regimen, as proposed by the APN [Brodehl et al. 1982], requires modification. According to this, the standard relapse treatment comprises prednisone 60 mg/m^2/day (maximum 80 mg/day) in three divided doses until the urine is protein-free for three consecutive days; this is then followed by four weeks of alternate-day prednisone (40 mg/m^2/48 h) as a single morning dose every other day.

Treatment should be started when a relapse is incipient, as indicated by an increased proteinuria (> 4 mg/m^2/h) on three out of seven days. If treatment is delayed, allowing full-blown NS to develop – which may be rapid – the risk of complications is greatly increased. Although studies have shown that a certain percentage of incipient relapses may remit spontaneously [Wingen et al. 1985], it is not possible to predict this future course of the disease in any given patient. It is therefore recommended that the patient/parents perform a routine check of the urine for proteinuria using dip-sticks. If a proteinuria of more than 2 to 3 mg persists for three days, relapse treatment should be initiated. In cases of infrequent relapse (< two relapses in six months), the standard relapse therapy should be repeated. Usually, the NS will remain steroid-responsive.

Frequent relapsing and steroid-dependent MCNS

The rate at which children with MCNS become frequent relapsers or steroid-dependent is partially determined by the initial treatment as described above. There are no criteria available by which to predict the future development of the disease. Therefore, decisions concerning further treatment, especially those involving the use of cytotoxic drugs, should be based on careful evaluation of the course of the disease, using stringent criteria which are only applicable if a standard relapse regimen has been used for any previous relapses. On the basis of this criterion, a frequent relapser is defined as a patient who is initially responsive to prednisone, but who has two relapses within six months of his initial response, or four relapses within a one-year period [APN 1982]. Steroid dependency is defined as when two consecutive relapses occur during the standard relapse therapy, or within 14 days after cessation of steroid therapy – which then is called a "fast relapse" – or when two out of four relapses in a six-month period are fast relapses.

Children with frequent relapses usually remain steroid-responsive [APN 1979, 1981] and can be treated with either standard relapse therapy repeatedly or long-term alternate-day prednisone. So far, comparison of these two forms of therapy, in terms of efficacy, side-effects and cost of treatment, has not been investigated in randomized trials. Our preference is for the repeated standard relapse regimen which allows precise evaluation of the course of the disease.

If the disease persists for months and years, prolonged steroid treatment carries the risk of severe steroid toxicity, including osteoporosis, growth retardation, cataract and psychoemotional disturbances. Review of the literature revealed that more than 5% of children treated for glomerulopathies with steroids for prolonged periods of time had died because of drug-induced side-effects and not renal disease [Brodehl 1972]. Thus, in these cases, the need for an alternative immunosuppressive treatment is mandatory.

It has been known for many years that alkylating agents such as nitrogen mustard (mechlorethamine hydrochloride) [Schoeneman et al. 1983, West 1958], cyclophosphamide [Chiu and Drummond 1974, Etteldorf et al. 1967, ISKDC 1974] and chlorambucil [Baluarte et al. 1978, Grupe et al. 1976] are more effective than steroids in MCNS. On the other hand, azathioprine has failed to show any significant effect in preventing relapses of MCNS [Abramowicz et al.

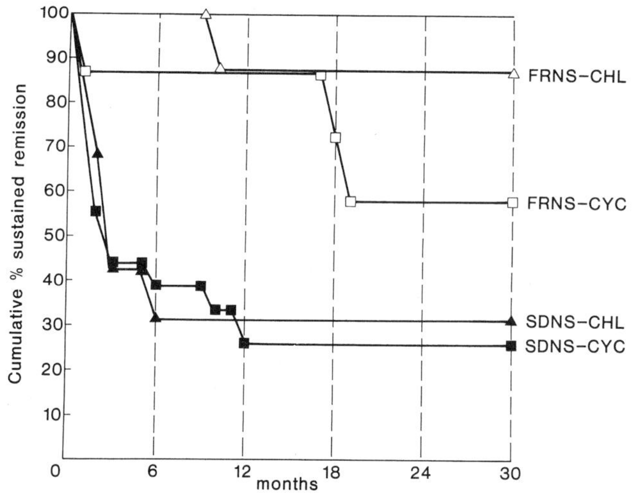

Fig. 1 Cumulative percentage of sustained remissions in patients who were frequent relapsers without steroid dependency (FRNS) and in those who were steroid-dependent (SDNS) treated with chlorambucil (CHL) or cyclophosphamide (CYC). With permission from Brodehl et al. [1982].

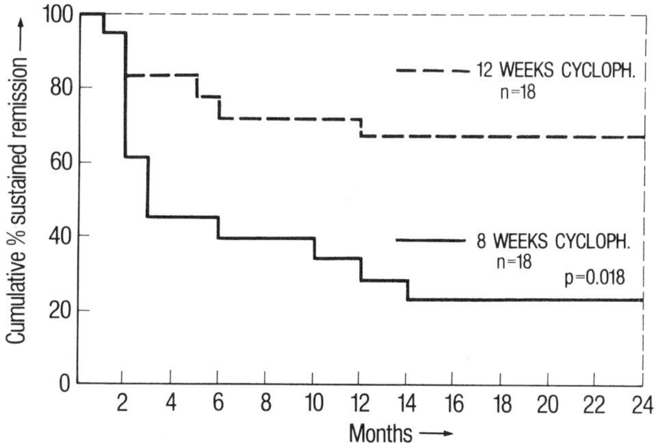

Fig. 2 Cumulative percentage of sustained remissions in steroid-dependent minimal-change nephrotic syndrome: comparison of eight-week and 12-week treatments with cyclophosphamide after two years. With permission from APN [1987].

Table 5 Primary non-response to steroid treatment in children with idiopathic nephrotic syndrome

Histopathological category	N	Non-responders n	n/N (%)	n/≧ N (%)
MCNS	363	25	6.9	5.3
FGGS	8	2	25.0	0.4
FSGS	37	26	70.3	5.5
DMH	9	4	44.4	0.8
Prolif GN	12	9	75.0	2.0
MPGN	29	27	93.1	5.7
Miscellaneous	13	10	77.0	2.1

For abbreviations, see Table 2 [ISKDC 1981 b]

Table 6 Steroid resistance in children with MCNS: percentage of total cases according to histology

Histological subcategory	Weeks after initial prednisone 8	26	52	104 (n)
Nil	4.7	1.4	0.9	0.9 (2)
FGO	7.8	3.3	2.2	2.2 (2)
MMT	6.3	6.3	0.0	0.0 (0)
FTC	14.3	10.7	3.6	0.0 (0)
MMH	14.8	14.8	7.4	7.4 (2)
DMH	45.5	18.2	9.1	9.1 (1)
Total	31/383 (8.1%)	16/383 (4.2%)	8/383 (2.1%)	7/383 (1.8%)

[ISKDC 1981 b]

Nil = Nil disease; FGO = Focal-global obsolescence; MMT = Mild mesangial thickening; FTC = Focal-tubular changes; MMH = Mild mesangial hypercellularity; DMH = Diffuse mesangial hypercellularity

1976, Barratt et al. 1977]. The use of alkylating drugs, however, is limited by their toxic side-effects, primarily affecting the gonads [Etteldorf et al. 1976, Guesry et al. 1978, Trompeter et al. 1981], bone marrow [Palmer et al. 1984] and oncogenicity [Baker et al. 1987, Kinlen et al. 1979, Wall and Klausen 1975].

To determine the optimal aklyating drug and dosage to be used in children with steroid-toxic MCNS, the APN conducted controlled therapeutic trials comparing the efficacy and safety of cyclophosphamide (2 mg/kg/day) and chlorambucil (0.15 mg/kg/day) [APN 1982]. The children were frequent relapsers with or without steroid dependency. Each drug was administered for eight weeks after remission of relapse had been achieved with prednisone, and each was given in combination with tapering doses of prednisone. The cumulative dose of cyclophosphamide was 112 mg/kg, which is below the known gonadal toxicity threshold (>300 mg/kg) [Etteldorf et al. 1976, Trompeter et al. 1981, Watson et al. 1985], and that of chlorambucil was 8.4 mg/kg, which is very close to its known gonadal toxicity threshold (8–10 mg/kg) [Callis et al. 1980]. The dosages of both alkylating agents were approximately equivalent in efficacy. Children with frequent relapses and without steroid dependency benefited from the treatment; 70% remained in subsequent prolonged remission. However, of those children with steroid dependency, only 30% remained in such prolonged remission (Figure 1).

A later study was carried out to determine whether children with steroid-dependent MCNS would gain more benefit from prolonged cytotoxic treatment [APN 1987]. As prolongation of treatment would exceed the maximum safe gonadal dose of chlorambucil, only cyclophosphamide was used (cumulative dosage 168 mg/kg). After 12 weeks of cyclophosphamide treatment, the percentage of patients with long-lasting remission increased to 70%, with no serious side-effects occurring either during or after treatment (Figure 2). For steroid-dependent MCNS, therefore, treatment with cyclophosphamide for 12 weeks is recommended in order to achieve long-lasting remission.

Those children who again relapsed after cytotoxic drug treatment are usually frequent relapsers. They respond well to prednisone and may again become steroid-dependent. In general, however, we do not recommend repeat cytotoxic drug treatment as the efficacy is equivocal and the toxicity is cumulative. Our preference would be to use CyA, which has a proven efficacy in steroid-sensitive MCNS [Brodehl et al. 1988]. However, as this drug is not part of the conventional treatment of NS in children, it is not discussed in this article.

Steroid-resistant MCNS and other glomerulopathies

Initial steroid resistance of MCNS is rare [APN 1988, ISKDC 1981b]. Table 5 shows that 22% of all children with an idiopathic NS do not respond to an eight-week prednisone regimen. Renal biopsies of these cases indicate that approximately one-fourth each are MCNS, focal-segmental glomerulosclerosis (FSGS) and membranoproliferative glomerulonephritis (MPGN). The remaining one-fourth are rare miscellaneous entities. In cases of MCNS, even if there is no remission after eight weeks of prednisone, it is still possible that a prolonged treatment with prednisone and/or the addition of a cytotoxic agent will produce a final remission [ISKDC 1981b]. Almost all subcategories of MCNS responded to treatment after two years, and only seven out of 383 cases remained unresponsive to treatment (Table 6). It is, therefore, our policy in histologically proven cases of MCNS to continue the immunosuppressive treatment, either with a combination of alternate-day prednisone plus 12 weeks of cyclophosphamide, or alternate-day prednisone plus six to 12 months of CyA. To our knowledge, there are as yet no controlled studies comparing these two treatment regimens in terms of efficacy and safety.

In cases of FSGS, only 25% respond initially to prednisone, but these often relapse and become steroid-resistant after the first or second relapse ("subsequent non-responder"). The majority of cases develop a progressively downhill course and reach end-stage renal disease after two to 15 years [Habib 1973, Arbus et al. 1982]. Those who respond initially to prednisone appear to fare better than those who have an initial steroid-resistant course. The efficacy of cytotoxic drugs on FSGS is still unconvincing although, recently, Mendoza et al. [1990] claimed that combination of prolonged pulsed methylprednisolone with an alkylating agent had a beneficial effect in the majority of children with FSGS. Cyclosporin A was also found to be effective in some cases [Brodehl et al. 1988].

In cases of MPGN, the prognosis is doubtful and the therapeutic approach still controversial [Habib et al. 1973, Cameron et al. 1983]. Cases showing severe NS and crescents in the histology appear to have a more rapid deterioration of renal function than others. It has been postulated that treatment with alternate-day prednisone over years may alter the downhill course of the disease and even lead to a remission [West 1986]. Controlled studies, however, are not available to confirm this claim. Other treatment modalities, such as immunosuppressive drugs plus anticoagulants or plasmapheresis, have also failed to establish convincing efficacy. Our approach, therefore, is to treat children with steroid-resistant MPGN only symptomatically.

Conclusions

The idiopathic NS in children is most probably MCNS which responds to steroids. The therapeutic approach of the pediatrician, therefore, includes:

1. The initial attack should be an intensive steroid regimen, such as continuous prednisone 60 mg/m^2/day (not more than 80 mg/day) divided into three doses, for six weeks followed by alternate-day prednisone 40 mg/m^2/48 h for six weeks.
2. Relapse should be met with a standardized treatment, such as continuous prednisone 60 mg/m^2/day (not more than 80 mg/day) until urine is protein-free for three consecutive days, followed by alternate-day prednisone 40 mg/m^2/48 h for four weeks.
3. Further relapses should be treated with a standard relapse regimen (see 2).
4. Frequent relapsers without steroid dependency but with signs of steroid toxicity should receive alkylating drugs for eight weeks, such as cyclophosphamide 2 mg/kg/day or chlorambucil 0.15 mg/kg/day combined with alternate-day tapering prednisone.
5. Steroid-dependent MCNS with signs of steroid toxicity should receive cyclosphosphamide 2 mg/kg/day for 12 weeks combined with alternate-day tapering prednisone.
6. Frequent relapsing and steroid-dependent MCNS after alkylating drugs have failed should be treated with CyA 100 to 150 mg/m^2/day for six to 12 months or more.

REFERENCES

Abramowicz M, Arneil GC, Barnett HL, et al. 1976 Controlled trial of azathioprine in children with nephrotic syndrome. Lancet *i:* 959

Arbeitsgemeinschaft für Pädiatrische Nephrologie 1979 Alternate-day versus intermittent prednisone in frequently relapsing nephrotic syndrome. Lancet *i:* 401

Arbeitsgemeinschaft für Pädiatrische Nephrologie 1981 Alternate-day prednisone is more effective than intermittent prednisone in frequently relapsing nephrotic syndrome. Eur J Pediatr *135:* 229

Arbeitsgemeinschaft für Pädiatrische Nephrologie 1982 Effect of cytotoxic drugs in frequently relapsing nephrotic syndrome with and without steroid dependence. N Engl J Med *306:* 451

Arbeitsgemeinschaft für Pädiatrische Nephrologie 1987 Cyclophosphamide treatment of steroid-dependent nephrotic syndrome: comparison of eight weeks with 12 weeks course. Arch Dis Childh *62:* 1102

Arbeitsgemeinschaft für Pädiatrische Nephrologie 1988 Short versus standard prednisone therapy for initial treatment of idiopathic nephrotic syndrome in children. Lancet *i:* 380

Arbeitsgemeinschaft für Pädiatrische Nephrologie 1990 Minimal-change nephrotic syndrome (MCNS): long prednisone versus standard prednisone therapy (Abst). Pediatr Nephrol *4 (C):* 60

Arbus GS, Poucell S, Bacheyie GS, Baumal R 1982 Focal-segmental glomerulosclerosis with idiopathic nephrotic syndrome: three types of clinical response. J Pediatr *101:* 40

Arneil GC, Lam CN 1966 Long-term assessment of steroid therapy in childhood nephrosis. Lancet *ii:* 819

Baker GL, Kahl LE, Zee BC, Stolzer BL, Agarwal AK, Medsger TA 1987 Malignancy following treatment of rheumatoid arthritis with cyclophosphamide. Long-term case-control follow-up study. Am J Med *83:* 1

Baluarte HJ, Hiner L, Gruskin AB 1978 Chlorambucil dosage in frequently relapsing nephrotic syndrome: A controlled clinical trial. J Pediatr *92:* 295

Barnett HL, Schoeneman M, Bernstein J, Edelmann CM 1978 Minimal-change nephrotic syndrome. In: *Edelmann CM* (ed). Pediatric Kidney Disease. Boston, Little, Brown and Co., p 695

Barratt M, Cameron JS, Chantler C, Counahan R, Ogg CS, Soothill JF 1977 Controlled trial of azathioprine in treatment of steroid-responsive nephrotic syndrome of childhood. Arch Dis Childh *52:* 462

Brodehl J 1972 Steroide oder Zytostatika beim kindlichen nephrotischen Syndrom. Klin Pädiat *184:* 241

Brodehl J 1991 Steroids and cytotoxic drugs in treatment of minimal-change nephrotic syndrome. Proceedings of the XI. International Congress of Nephrology, 1990. Tokyo, Springer-Verlag (in press)

Brodehl J, Brandis M, Helmchen U, et al. 1988 Cyclosporin A treatment in children with minimal-change nephrotic syndrome and focal-segmental glomerulosclerosis. Klin Wochenschr *66:* 1126

Brodehl J, Krohn HP, Ehrich JHH 1982 The treatment of minimal-change nephrotic syndrome (lipoid nephrosis): cooperative studies of the Arbeitsgemeinschaft für Pädiatrische Nephrologie (APN). Klin Pädiat *194:* 162

Callis L, Nieto J, Vila A, Rende J 1980 Chlorambucil treatment in minimal-lesion nephrotic syndrome: A reappraisal of its gonadal toxicity. J Pediatr *97:* 653

Cameron JS, Turner DR, Heaton J, et al. 1983 Idiopathic mesangiocapillary glomerulonephritis. Comparison of types I and II in children and adults and long-term prognosis. Am J Med *74:* 175

Chesney RW, Mazess RB, Rose P, Jax DK 1978 Effect of prednisone on growth and bone mineral content in childhood glomerular disease. Am J Dis Child *132:* 768

Chiu J, Drummond KN 1974 Long-term follow-up of cyclophosphamide therapy in frequent-relapsing minimal-lesion nephrotic syndrome. J Pediat *84:* 825

Etteldorf JN, Roy S, Summitt RL, Sweeney NJ, Wall HP, Berton WM 1967 Cyclophosphamide in the treatment of idiopathic lipoid nephrosis. J Pediatr *70:* 758

Etteldorf JN, West CD, Pitcock JA, Williams DL 1976 Gonadal function, testicular histology, and meiosis following cyclophosphamide therapy in patients with nephrotic syndrome. J Pediatr *88:* 206

Glassock RJ, Cohen AH, Bennett CM, Martinez-Maldonado M 1981 Primary glomerular diseases. In: *Brenner DG, Rector FC* (eds). The Kidney. Philadelphia, WB Saunders, p 1351

Grupe WE, Makker SP, Ingelfinger JR 1976 Chlorambucil treatment of frequently relapsing nephrotic syndrome. N Engl J Med *295:* 746

Guesry P, Lenoir R, Broyer M 1978 Gonadal effects of chlorambucil given to prepubertal and pubertal boys for nephrotic syndrome. J Pediatr *92:* 299

Habib R 1973 Focal-glomerular sclerosis. Kidney Int *4:* 355

Habib R, Kleinknecht C, Gubler MC, Levy M 1973 Idiopathic membranoproliferative glomerulonephritis in children. Report of 105 cases. Clin Nephrol *1:* 193

Hoyer PF, Gonda S, Barthels M, Krohn HP, Brodehl J 1986 Thromboembolic complications in children with nephrotic syndrome. Risk and incidence. Acta Paediatr Scand *75:* 804

International Study of Kidney Disease in Children 1974 Prospective controlled trial of cyclophosphamide therapy in children with the nephrotic syndrome. Lancet *ii:* 423

International Study of Kidney Disease in Children 1978 Nephrotic syndrome in children: prediction of histopathology from clinical and laboratory characteristics at time of diagnosis. Kidney Int *13:* 159

International Study of Kidney Disease in Children 1979 Nephrotic syndrome in children. Randomized trial comparing 2 prednisone regimens in steroid-responsive patients who relapse early. J Pediatr *95:* 239

International Study of Kidney Disease in Children 1981a The primary nephrotic syndrome in children. Identification of patients with minimal-change nephrotic syndrome from initial response to prednisone. J Pediatr *98:* 561

International Study of Kidney Disease in Children 1981b Primary nephrotic syndrome in children: Clinical significance of histopathologic variants of minimal-change and of diffuse mesangial hypercellularity. Kidney Int *20:* 765

International Study of Kidney Disease in Children 1982 Early identification of frequent relapsers among children with minimal-change nephrotic syndrome. J Pediatr *101:* 514

Kinlen LJ, Sheil AGR, Peto J, Doll R 1979 Collaborative United Kingdom-Australasian study of cancer in patients treated with immunosuppressive drugs. Br Med J *2:* 1461

Krensky AM, Ingelfinger JR, Grupe WE 1982 Peritonitis in childhood nephrotic syndrome. Am J Dis Child *136:* 732

Lam CN, Arneil GC 1968 Long-term dwarfing effects of corticosteroid treatment of childhood nephrosis. Arch Dis Childh *43:* 589

Lange K, Wassermann E, Slobody LB 1958 Prolonged intermittent steroid therapy for nephrosis in children and adults. JAMA *168:* 377

Mendoza SA, Reznik VM, Griswold WR, Krensky AM, Yorgin PD, Tune BM 1990 Treatment of steroid-resistant focal-segmental glomerulosclerosis with pulse methylprednisolone and alkylating agents. Pediatr Nephrol *4:* 303

Palmer RG, Dore CJ, Denman AM 1984 Chlorambucil-induced chromosome damage to human lymphocytes is dose-dependent and cumulative. Lancet *i:* 246

Rees L, Greene SA, Adlard P, et al. 1988 Growth and endocrine function in steroid-sensitive nephrotic syndrome. Arch Dis Childh *63:* 484

Schnaper HW 1989 The immune system in minimal-change nephrotic syndrome. Pediatr Nephrol *3:* 101

Schoeneman MJ, Spitzer A, Greifer I 1983 Nitrogen mustard therapy in children with frequent-relapsing nephrotic syndrome and steroid toxicity. Am J Kidney Dis *5:* 526

Trompeter RS, Evans PR, Barratt TM 1981 Gonadal function in boys with steroid-responsive nephrotic syndrome treated with cyclophosphamide for short periods. Lancet *i:* 1177

Ueda N, Chihara M, Kawaguchi S, et al. 1988 Intermittent versus long-term tapering prednisolone for initial therapy in children with idiopathic nephrotic syndrome. J Pediatr *112:* 122

Wall RL, Klausen KP 1975 Carcinoma of the urinary bladder in patients receiving cyclophosphamide. N Engl J Med *293:* 271

Watson AR, Rance CP, Bain J 1985 Long-term effects of cyclophosphamide on testicular function. Br Med J *291:* 1457

West CD 1958 Use of combined hormone and mechlorethamine (nitrogen mustard) therapy in lipoid nephrosis. Am J Dis Child *95:* 498

West CD 1986 Childhood membranoproliferative glomerulonephritis: An approach to management. Kidney Int *29:* 1077

Wingen AM, Müller-Wiefel DE, Schärer K 1985 Spontaneous remissions in frequently relapsing and steroid-dependent idiopathic nephrotic syndrome. Clin Nephrol *23:* 35

Clinical Nephrology, Vol. 35, Supl. No. 1–1991 (pp. S. 16–21)

Conventional treatment of idiopathic nephrotic syndrome and membranous nephropathy in adults

C. PONTICELLI and P. PASSERINI

Division of Nephrology and Dialysis, Istituto Scientifico Ospedale Maggiore, via Commenda 15, I-20122 Milano, Italy

Abstract. This article is a review of the results of corticosteroid and immunosuppressive treatment in adults with idiopathic nephrotic syndrome. Adults with minimal-change nephropathy usually require a prolonged administration of corticosteroids to achieve remission which, in itself, carries the risk of severe and even life-threatening complications. Therefore, intravenous high-dose steroid pulses, alternate-day prednisone, short courses with cytotoxic agents and long-term administration of azathioprine have been suggested as alternatives to the classical prolonged corticotherapy. While most patients with focal-segmental glomerulosclerosis do not respond to short-term prednisone, almost half of the patients with nephrotic syndrome will attain remission with a more prolonged administration of corticosteroids and/or cytotoxic agents. A six-month course of methylprednisolone and chlorambucil preserves renal function and reduces the proteinuria in many patients with membranous nephropathy, even in the presence of initial renal insufficiency. Thus, there is growing evidence that corticosteroids and/or immunosuppressive agents can favorably alter the natural course of disease in many patients with idiopathic glomerulonephritis. However, these agents have a low therapeutic index. Further studies are needed to find more effective and less toxic treatment approaches in patients with primary glomerulonephritis.

Key words: idiopathic nephrotic syndrome – membranous nephropathy – corticosteroids – immunosuppressive therapy – chlorambucil

Introduction

The term "idiopathic nephrotic syndrome" includes at least two subgroups of glomerulonephritis, namely, minimal-change nephropathy (MCN) and focal-segmental glomerulosclerosis (FSGS), which probably represent different evolutionary stages of the same disease. In spite of some overlapping, however, many clinicians still prefer to consider these two diseases as separate entitites as they differ in histological appearances, clinical presentations, natural courses and responses to therapy.

Minimal-change nephropathy

Approximately 25 to 30% of adults with nephrotic syndrome (NS) show a pattern of minimal-change nephropathy at renal biopsy [Coggins 1981, Sharpstone et al. 1969]. There is a slight male predominance among patients. The clinical presentation is similar in adults and children, consisting of edema, hypoalbuminemia, hyperlipidemia and massive proteinuria. However, severe hypertension and diminished renal function are more frequent in adults, particularly in those aged over 60 years [Nolasco et al. 1986]. The renal outcome is generally favorable with less than 1% of patients progressing to renal failure [Coggings 1981]. Patients with poor renal outcomes are generally those who failed to show even a partial response to corticosteroids [Idelson et al. 1977]. Acute anuric renal failure is a relatively frequent complication [Raij et al. 1976, Imbasciati et al. 1981] and has occurred in up to 10% of patients in some series [Cameron et al. 1974]. This complication may resolve spontaneously and usually within a few days but, on occasions, after many months of oligoanuria [Imbasciati et al. 1981]. In a few cases, the anuria may be irreversible [Imbasciati et al. 1981, Raij et al. 1976].

Adults with MCN have a slower response to corticosteroids than children. While 93% of children enter complete remission of proteinuria within eight weeks of treatment [ISKDC 1974, ISKDC 1978,

Reprint requests to Professor C. Ponticelli.

ISKDC 1981], only 50 to 60% of adults become free of proteinuria over the same duration of corticosteroid treatment. However, if corticosteroid administration is prolonged to up to 28 weeks, a complete remission may be obtained in 81 to 91% of adults [Nolasco et al. 1986, Korbet et al. 1988]. While Nolasco et al. [1986] did not find any relationship between response to treatment and age at disease onset, Korbet et al. [1988] reported that patients aged over 40 years responded significantly more slowly than those under 40 years of age. This slower response of older adults to corticosteroids has been attributed to the fact that the initial doses of prednisone in adults (approximately 1 mg/kg/day) are lower than those given to children (60 mg/m^2/day) [Nolasco et al. 1986]. After the first episode, approximately 70% of adults show multiple relapses [Korbet et al. 1988]. As with children, the optimal treatment for adults who are frequent relapsers remains controversial.

In order to reduce the side-effects of corticosteroids, a short course of three consecutive intravenous methylprednisolone pulses followed by moderate doses of prednisone was given for six months. As the results obtained in a preliminary study were good [Ponticelli et al. 1980], a multicenter controlled trial was begun. Patients with MCN were randomized to either a conventional treatment regimen with prednisone (1 mg/kg/day for adults, 60 mg/m^2/day for children, gradually tapered off over six months), or to three pulses of methylprednisolone followed by prednisone at doses which were half the amount given in the other arm of the study. No differences were seen in the number of responders, mean time to respond, number of relapses and mean time free of relapse. However, the number of corticosteroid-related side-effects was significantly lower in patients assigned to methylprednisolone pulses than in those given the conventional treatment [Imbasciati et al. 1985].

A different approach has been attempted by Simon and Meyrier [1988]. Of 56 adults with MCN, 28 were treated with prednisone 1 mg/kg/day for three months with progressive tapering of the dose over the ensuing nine months. The remaining 28 patients received a regimen of prednisone administered on alternate days. Except for the three steroid-resistant patients in each group, the initial remission rate was similar between the two groups. However, there were significantly more relapses in those treated with the short-term prednisone. Tolerability was excellent in patients assigned to alternate-day therapy. Furthermore, because of the smaller number of relapses, the cumulative dosage of prednisone in this group of patients was also smaller.

Immunosuppressive agents have been used in adults who are frequent relapsers, or steroid-dependent or -resistant. Approximately 60% are free of proteinuria within eight weeks of treatment with cyclophosphamide and 20% may enter complete remission if cyclophosphamide is given for 28 weeks. Such a response is more likely when cyclophosphamide is given in combination with prednisone [Nolasco et al. 1986]. The duration of remission is longer after cyclophosphamide than after corticosteroids, and 50 to 60% of patients remain free of proteinuria for up to 15 years [Al-Khader et al. 1979, Nolasco et al. 1986]. Azathioprine given for three to six months has been found to be ineffective in MCN [Abramowicz et al. 1970], but very prolonged treatment with this antimetabolite has proved to be helpful in the management of adults with idiopathic NS. Cade et al. [1986] gave azathioprine for a mean period of four years to 13 adults who had steroid-resistant NS (nine with MCN and four with focal glomerulosclerosis). A progressive reduction of proteinuria was seen in all patients and all achieved complete remission within three years. After a follow-up period of three to 15 years, only one patient relapsed; this patient had stopped taking azathioprine and, on reintroduction of the drug, re-entered complete remission.

In summary, adults with MCN respond to corticosteroids more slowly and perhaps less completely than children. This may be due to the lower doses of prednisone used in adults. The conventional eight-week course of cyclophosphamide may induce remission in only approximately 60% of patients while the prolonged administration of cyclophosphamide or azathioprine is able to maintain most patients without proteinuria. Thus, longer-term administration of corticosteroids and/or immunosuppressive agents is required in adults to attain remission of proteinuria.

The main problem, especially for older patients, is related to the toxicity of prolonged treatments. Coggings [1981] reported 21 deaths in 202 adults with MCN followed for a mean duration of 48 months. At least half of these deaths were considered to be related to the corticosteroid treatment. This present author, therefore, has cautioned against aggressive therapy in adults with NS. On the other hand, Nolasco et al. [1986] reported severe complications of the NS in 19 of 84 adults with MCN. Moreover, there is now evidence that a prolonged nephrotic condition significantly increases the risk of cardiovascular disease [Ordonez, et al. 1989]. In view of the risk of counteractive side-effects of corticosteroids in older patients, regimens such as intravenous methylprednisolone or alternate-day prednisone are preferential for repeated or prolonged treatments. In frequent relapsers and steroid-dependent patients, a trial using cyclophosphamide, which is able to obtain stable remission in a good proportion of patients, should be given, although it is recommended that this treatment should not be given for more than 12 to 16 weeks to avoid severe side-effects.

Focal-segmental glomerulosclerosis

Focal-segmental glomerulosclerosis (FSGS), a primary glomerular disease commonly associated with NS, can arise at any age. The prognosis for patients with FSGS is generally poor, although those with non-nephrotic proteinuria have a milder clinical course [Beaufils et al. 1978, Cameron et al. 1978, Korbet et al. 1986]. Treatment with corticosteroids or immunosuppressive agents is generally considered to be ineffective in most patients with FSGS, and adults have been considered even less likely to respond to therapy than children [Newman et al. 1976].

In a retrospective analysis of the literature, it appears that less than 2% of untreated patients enter complete remission of proteinuria, a proportion only slightly smaller than the 6% observed in patients receiving short-term prednisone. In patients treated with immunosuppressive agents, the rate of remission was somewhat higher at approximately 15% [Ponticelli et al. 1986]. On the basis of this poor response, most clinicians are reluctant to treat patients with FSGS.

However, some studies in children have reported that aggressive and prolonged treatment with corticosteroids and immunosuppressive agents may favor remission and may considerably improve the long-term prognosis [Mongeau et al. 1981, Geary et al. 1984, Mendoza et al. 1990].

Good results with prolonged corticotherapy have also been obtained in adults. Korbet et al. [1986] observed a complete remission of proteinuria in 30% and a partial remission in 20% of nephrotic adults with FSGS after an average prednisone-treatment period of 3.7 months (60 mg/day). None of the responders progressed to renal failure. Pei et al. [1987] observed the complete disappearance of proteinuria in 39% of nephrotic adults with FSGS treated with prednisone for at least six months. The 10-year kidney survival rate was 96% in responders, while nearly all of the non-responders or untreated patients progressed to renal failure. Banfi et al. [1988] treated 60 adults with FSGS and NS either with prolonged corticotherapy (21 patients; mean treatment period 9.3 ± 7.4 months) or with long-term cytotoxic therapy (39 patients; mean treatment period 12.8 ± 8.8 months). After a mean follow-up time of 68 ± 52 months, 27 patients were in complete remission, six were in partial remission, 12 were still nephrotic and 15 had progressed to renal insufficiency. Again, the renal prognosis was good in responders. Only one of 36 patients who had initially responded to therapy developed renal failure, while 65% of non-responders showed renal dysfunction within 10 years. Finally, Nanra et al. [1990] treated 41 nephrotic patients with corticosteroids and cyclophosphamide for approximately two years. Proteinuria was reduced in 35 patients, and the 10-year survival rate was 86%.

In summary, there is growing evidence to suggest that aggressive treatment with corticosteroids and/or cytotoxic agents can obtain complete remission of proteinuria in a consistently good proportion of nephrotic patients. The renal prognosis is excellent in responders, suggesting a protective effect of therapy. Unfortunately, the available data are from non-controlled studies. Prospective, randomized trials are needed to identify the patient who is most likely to respond to therapy in order to determine the most effective therapeutic regimen and to balance the potential benefits of the chosen treatment against its possible side-effects.

Membranous nephropathy

Idiopathic membranous nephropathy (MN) is the most common cause of NS in adults, but is rarely seen in children. The natural course of the disease is variable; some patients show fluctuations of proteinuria and even complete remission, while others remain nephrotic and eventually progress to end-stage renal disease. There are differing opinions regarding the long-term prognosis of untreated patients. Some investigators report a 10-year patients' survival rate ranging from 75 to 80% [Donadio et al. 1988, Wehrmann et al. 1989, Murphy et al. 1988] but, in other series, approximately half of the patients presenting with NS were either dead or on chronic dialysis within 10 years of the clinical onset [Row et al. 1975, MacTier et al. 1986, Zucchelli et al. 1987]. These apparent variations in the natural course of the disease complicate evaluation of the various treatment regimens available.

A two-month course of high-dose prednisone taken every other day proved to be effective in producing a transient remission of proteinuria while preserving renal function in a prospective controlled trial [American Collaborative Study 1979]. However, these results have not been confirmed by a randomized study organized by the Medical Research Council (MRC) in the United Kingdom [Cameron et al. 1989]. One hundred and three patients with MN and NS were randomized to receive either placebo or prednisone 125 mg every other day for two months. Patients were followed for at least three years. No differences were observed between treated and untreated patients in either the mean proteinuria or mean plasma creatinine at any time during the study.

In another controlled study in Toronto, Canada, there were no differences between untreated patients and patients receiving prednisone 45 $mg/m^2/48$ h for six months in the number of complete or partial responses nor in the number of patients showing deterioration of renal function [Cattran et al. 1989]. A more aggressive approach was used in the treatment of MN in the form of a six-month course of corticosteroids, beginning with three intravenous methylprednisolone pulsed followed by oral prednisone 0.5 mg/kg/day, and chlorambucil 0.2 mg/kg/day on alternate months. After a median follow-up period of five years, 66% of treated patients and 23% of untreated controls were free of NS. Excluding three patients who died (one receiving treatment and two in the control group), 9% of treated patients vs 44% of the untreated controls showed an increase in plasma creatinine of at least 50% over their baseline values [Ponticelli et al. 1989]. It appears, therefore, that methylprednisolone and chlorambucil given monthly alternately for six months may improve the chances of remission of NS and retard the progression of MN. These conclusions have been confirmed by other investigators [Altieri et al. 1986, Przechera et al. 1990], although a study group in Greece was unable to reproduce these results [Vosnides et al. 1986].

Until recently, patients with MN and renal insufficiency have received only symptomatic treatment. Some studies, however, have shown that aggressive therapy may reverse renal dysfunction and reduce proteinuria in some patients who are renal insufficient. The regimens which have proved to be of most benefit to patients with renal insufficiency include high-dose intravenous methylprednisolone followed by prednisone either alone [Short et al. 1987] or in combination [Williams and Bone 1989] with azathioprine, the prolonged administration of cyclophosphamide [West et al. 1987], and a six-month course with methylprednisolone and chlorambucil [Mathieson et al. 1989].

On the basis of these results, some clinicians prefer to postpone treatment until renal insufficiency appears in order to spare patients who may yet undergo spontaneous remission of NS of a potentially toxic treatment regimen. It must be pointed out, however, that immunosuppressive agents are more dangerous and less well tolerated by uremic patients than those who have normal kidney function [Ponticelli 1986, Mathieson et al. 1989]. Moreover, when tubulointerstitial lesions appear, the likelihood of a response to therapy is significantly reduced [Ponticelli et al. 1989] and the risk of progression to end-stage renal disease is significantly increased [Wehrmann et al. 1989].

Finally, the mechanisms leading to renal insufficiency in MN may be multiple. Treatment is likely to be of value in patients who have a reduced kidney function if renal biopsy shows recent immune-complex deposition and a mild-to-moderate glomerulosclerosis and/or interstitial fibrosis. It is difficult, however, to imagine that any form of treatment will have an effect in patients with advanced chronic lesions. This may explain why immunosuppressive therapy does not produce an improvement in some patients with MN and renal insufficiency [Wetzels et al. 1989].

In summary, there is some clinical data to suggest that the natural course of MN can be altered by therapy. A therapeutic response is more likely in patients without tubulointerstitial lesions and, therefore, suggests the early treatment of nephrotic patients; this, however, may have the disadvantage of treating a (small) proportion of patients who may otherwise undergo spontaneous remission. On the other hand, early treatment may provide protection of renal function and may encourage the remission of NS, a condition which in itself exposes the patient to life-threatening complications. At present, a six-month regimen of methylprednisolone and chlorambucil appears to offer the best results with limited side-effects. However, the search for the optimal drugs or treatment schedules with better therapeutic indices would be most welcome.

REFERENCES

Abramowicz M, Arneil GC, Barnett HL, Barron BA, Edelmann CM, Gordillo G et al. 1970 Controlled trial of azathioprine in children with the nephrotic syndrome. Lancet *i:* 959–961

Al-Khadar AA, Lien JWK, Aber GM. 1979 Cyclophosphamide alone in the treatment of adult patients with minimal-change glomerulonephritis. Clin Nephrol *11:* 26–30

Altieri P, Manca O, Bolasco PG, Bolasco F, Barracca A, Cadeddu M et al. 1986 Trattamento della nefropatia membranosa idiopatica. G Ital Nefrol *2:* 183–186

Banfi G, Moriggi M, Sabatini E, Ferrario F, Pozzi C, Bissoli F et al. 1988 Decorso clinico della glomerulosclerosi focale con sindrome nefrosica dell'adulto. Studio retrospettivo e collaborativo di 60 casi trattati con steroidi e/o citostatici. G Ital Nefrol *5:* 9–16

Beaufils H, Alphonse JC, Guedon J, Legrain M. 1978 Focal glomerulosclerosis: natural history and treatment. Nephron *21:* 75–85

Cade R, Mars D, Privette M, Thompson R, Croker B, Peterson J et al. 1986 Effect of long-term azathioprine administration in adults with minimal-change glomerulonephritis and nephrotic syndrome resistant to corticosteroids. Arch Intern Med *147:* 737–741

Cameron JS, Chantler C, Ogg CS, White RHR. 1974 Long-term stability of remission in nephrotic syndrome after treatment with cyclophosphamide. Br Med J *4:* 7–11

Cameron JS, Healy MJR, Adu D. 1990 The Medical Research Council Trial of short-term high-dose alternate-day prednisolone in idiopathic membranous nephropathy with nephrotic syndrome in adults. Q J Med *74:* 113–156

Cameron JS, Turner DR, Ogg CS, Chantler C, Williams DG. 1978 The long-term prognosis of patients with focal-segmental glomerulosclerosis. Clin Nephrol *10:* 213–218

Cattran DC, Delmore T, Roscoe J, Cole E, Cardella C, Charron R et al. 1989 A randomized controlled trial of prednisone in patients with idiopathic membranous nephropathy. N Engl J Med *4:* 210–215

Coggins CH. 1981 Minimal-change nephrosis in adult. In: *Zurukzoglu W (ed).* Proceedings of the 8th International Congress of Nephrology. Karger, Basel, pp 336–344

Collaborative Study of the Adult Idiopathic Nephrotic Syndrome. 1979 A controlled study of short-term prednisone treatment in adults with membranous nephropathy. N Engl J Med *301:* 1301–1306

Donadio JV, Torres VE, Velosa JA, Wagoner RD, Holley KE, Okamura M et al. 1988 Idiopathic membranous nephropathy: the natural history of untreated patients. Kidney Int. *33:*708–715

Geary DF, Farine M, Thorner P, Baumal R. 1984 Response to cyclophosphamide in steroid-resistant focal-segmental glomerulosclerosis: a reappraisal. Clin Nephrol *22:* 109–113

Idelson BA, Smithline N, Smith GW, Harrington JT. 1977 Prognosis in steroid-treated idiopathic nephrotic syndrome in adults. Arch Intern Med *137:* 891–896

Imbasciati E, Ponticelli C, Case N, Altieri P, Bolasco F, Mihatsch MJ et al. 1981 Acute renal failure in idiopathic nephrotic syndrome. Nephron *28:* 186–191

Imbasciati E, Gusmano R, Edefonti A, Zucchelli P, Pozzi C, Grassi C et al. 1985 Controlled trial of methylprednisolone pulses and low dose oral prednisone for the minimal change nephrotic syndrome. Br Med J *291:* 1305–1308

International Study of Kidney Disease in Children. 1974 Prospective controlled trial of cyclophosphamide therapy in children with the nephrotic syndrome. Lancet *ii:* 423–427

International Study of Kidney Disease in Children. 1978 Prediction of histopathology from clinical and laboratory characteristics at the time of diagnosis. Kidney Int. *13:* 159–165

International Study of Kidney Disease in Children. 1981 The primary nephrotic syndrome in children. Identification of patients with minimal-change nephrotic syndrome from initial response to prednisone. J Pediatr. *98:* 560–564

Korbet SM, Schwartz MM, Lewis E. 1986 The prognosis of focal-segmental glomerular sclerosis of adulthood. Medicine *65:* 304–311

Korbet SM, Schwartz MM, Lewis EJ. 1988 Minimal-change glomerulopathy of adulthood. Am J Nephrol *8:* 291–297

MacTier R, Boulton-Jones JM, Payton CD, MacLay A. 1986 The natural history of membranous nephropathy in the West of Scotland. Q J Med *60:* 793–802

Mathieson PW, Turner AN, Maidment GGM, Evans DJ, Rees A. 1988 Prednisolone and chlorambucil treatment in idiopathic membranous nephropathy with deteriorating renal function. Lancet *ii:* 869–872

Mendoza SA, Reznik VM, Griswold WR, Krensky AM, Yorgin PD, Tune BM. 1990 Treatment of steroid-resistant focal glomerulosclerosis with pulse methylprednisolone and alkylating agents. Pediatr Nephrol *4:* 303-307

Mongeau JG, Corneille L, Robitaille P, O'Regan S, Pelletier M. 1981 Primary nephrosis in childhood associated with focal glomerular sclerosis. Is long-term prognosis that severe? Kidney Int. *20:* 743–746

Murphy BF, Kincaid-Smith PS, Fairley KF. 1988 Idiopathic membranous glomerulonephritis: long-term follow-up in 139 cases. Clin Nephrol *30:* 175–181

Nanra RS, Jones BF, Trevillian PR. 1990 Primary focal glomerular sclerosis (PFGS). Factors influencing outcome in 89 patients. Proceedings of the XIth International Congress of Nephrology, Tokyo, pp 6A

Newman WJ, Tisher CC, McCoy RC, Gunnells JC, Krueger RP, Clapp JR et al. 1976 Focal-glomerular sclerosis: contrasting clinical patterns in children and adults. Medicine *55:* 67–87

Nolasco F, Cameron JS, Heywood EF, Hicks J, Ogg C, Williams DG. Adult-onset minimal-change nephrotic syndrome: a long-term follow-up. Kidney Int *29:* 1215–1223

Ordonez JD, Hiatt R, Killebrew E, Fireman B. 1990 The risk of coronary artery disease among patients with the nephrotic syndrome. (Abst) Kidney Int *37:* 243

Pei Y, Cattran D, Delmore T, Katz A, Lang A, Rance P. 1987 Evidence suggesting under-treatment in adults with idiopathic focal-segmental glomerulosclerosis. Am J Med *82:* 938–944

Ponticelli C. 1986 Prognosis and treatment of membranous nephropathy. Kidney Int *29:* 927–940

Ponticelli C, Fogazzi GB, Passerini P. 1986 Pharmacological treatment of chronic primary glomerulonephritis. In: *Bertani T, Remuzzi C, Garattini S (eds).* Drugs and Kidney. Raven Press, New York, pp 221–234

Ponticelli C, Imbasciati E, Case N, Zucchelli P, Cagnoli L, Pasquali S. 1980 Intravenous methylprednisolone in minimal-change nephrotic syndrome. Br Med J *280:* 685–687

Ponticelli C, Zucchelli P, Passerini P, Cagnoli L, Cesana B, Pozzi C et al. 1989 A randomized trial of methylprednisolone and chlorambucil in idiopathic membranous nephropathy. N Engl J Med *320:* 8–13

Przechera M, Mündlein E, Weber A, Heering P, Zäuner I, Müller G et al. 1990 Idiopathische membranöse Glomerulonephritis mit nephrotischem Syndrom (MGN). Immunosuppressive Therapie im Vergleich. (Abst) Nier Hochdruck *19:* 407

Raij L, Keane WF, Leonard A, Shapiro FL. 1976 Irreversible acute renal failure in idiopathic nephrotic syndrome. Am J Med *61:* 207–214

Row PG, Cameron JS, Turner DR, Evans DJ, White RHR, Ogg CS et al. 1975 Membranous nephropathy: long-term follow-up and association with neoplasia. Q J Med *44:* 207–239

Sharpstone P, Ogg CS, Cameron JS. 1969 Nephrotic syndrome due to primary renal disease in adults: a survey of incidence in South East England. Br Med J *2:* 533–535

Short CD, Solomon LR, Gokal R, Mallick NP. 1987 Methylprednisolone in patients with membranous nephropathy and declining renal function. Q J Med *247:* 929–940

Simon P, Meyrier A. 1989 One-year alternate-day dosage, corticosteroid Rx reduces rate of further relapses in adult minimal-change nephrosis. (Abst) Kidney Int. *35:* 201

Vosnides G, Edipidis K, Sotsiou F, Papadakis G, Siakotos M, Lemoniatou H et al. 1987 Poor response of idiopathic membranous glomerulonephritis to alternate courses of steroids and chlorambucil. (Abst) Nephrol Dial Transplant. *1:* 75

Warwick G, Boulton-Jones JM. 1988 Immunosupression for membranous nephropathy. Lancet *ii:* 1361

Wehrmann M, Bohle A, Bogenschutz O, Eissele R, Freislederer A, Ohlschlegel C et al. 1989 Long-term prognosis of chronic idiopathic membranous glomerulonephritis; an analysis of 334 cases with particular regard to tubulointerstitial changes. Clin Nephrol *31:* 67–76

West ML, Jindal KK, Bear RA, Goldstein MB. 1987 A controlled trial of cyclophosphamide in patients with membranous glomerulonephritis. Kidney Int. *31:* 579–584

Wetzels JFM, Hoitsma AJ, Koene RAP. 1989 Chlorambucil in steroid-resistant idiopathic membranous glomerulonephritis. (Abst) Kidney Int. *36:* 510

Williams PS, Bone JM. 1989 Immunosuppression can arrest progressive renal failure due to idiopathic membranous glomerulonephritis. Nephrol Dial Transplant. *4:* 181–186

Zucchelli P, Ponticelli C, Cagnoli L, Passerini P. 1987 Long-term outcome of idiopathic membranous nephropathy with nephrotic syndrome. Nephrol Dial Transplant *2:* 73–78

Discussion: Summary

This discussion focused on the identification of factors that may be predictive of the long-term renal outcome for patients with membranous nephropathy. There was a consensus that the presence of glomerular stages 3 and 4 (according to the Ehrenreich and Churg classification) and, even more so, severe tubulointerstitial lesions at renal biopsy are good indicators of a poor prognosis. The clinical pattern of the disease is also of great importance. A heavy persisting proteinuria of more than 15 g/day is almost invariably associated with a negative outcome. A consistent and persistent increase in plasma creatinine was also considered to be an indicator of a poor renal outcome. It must be borne in mind, however, that variations in volemia related to the nephrotic syndrome may have an effect on the levels of plasma creatinine.

There was general agreement among the delegation that patients with membranous nephropathy and asymptomatic proteinuria do not require "specific" treatment; however, how and when to manage nephrotic patients was more controversial. Some were in favor of early treatment with methylprednisolone and chlorambucil in order to prevent the development of irreversible renal lesions, while others suggested that not every patient with a nephrotic syndrome should be treated immediately, as spontaneous remission can occur in some patients. For those in favor of this latter policy, the persistence of heavy proteinuria for one year or more may be considered a good indication for starting treatment. Most participants agreed that withholding treatment until there was a sustained increase in plasma creatinine was likely to be too late. Serial measurements of the membrane attack complex in the patients' urine may be useful parameter for monitoring the activity of membranous nephropathy. Unfortunately, experience with this technique is, as yet, very limited.

Some aspects of the Italian treatment regimen of methylprednisolone and chlorambucil were clarified. In particular, the difficulty in assessing when treatment should be considered a failure was discussed. Indeed, many patients respond late to treatment, as long as several months after the therapy has been stopped. Such late responses may be due to either the slow release of chlorambucil, which tends to accumulate in the fatty tissues, or to the severity of the renal lesions which may take more time to recover, or to spontaneous remission. On re-treatment, patients who have relapsed respond in a manner similar to their first course of treatment. Patients who entered remission after six months of methylprednisolone and chlorambucil usually remit on re-treatment while those who did not respond to the first course generally were also refractory to the second course of treatment.

The use of cyclophosphamide and chlorambucil was also discussed. A controlled study carried out in Germany several years ago of children with minimal-change nephrotic syndrome showed that a dose of 2 mg/kg/day of cyclophosphamide compares well with 0.15 mg/kg/day of chlorambucil. However, gonadal toxicity is much more likely to occur with chlorambucil. This drug is also considered to have greater mutagenicity, although studies in rheumatic patients have shown that cyclophosphamide produces more chromosomal abnormalities than chlorambucil. Bladder toxicity is more frequent and more severe with cyclophosphamide. Therefore, the suggestion is that chlorambucil be used as the initial treatment of oliguric patients requiring an alkylating agent.

Finally, there was agreement that approaching the mangement of the nephrotic syndrome (whatever its etiology) only in terms of preventing end-stage renal failure is a limited view. Because of the correlation between the amount and duration of proteinuria and chronic ischemic heart disease, treatment which provides some degree of cardioprotection is recommended. Hypolipidemic, antiproteinuric and antiplatelet agents may be of benefit to patients with prolonged nephrotic syndrome, especially those who are refractory to "specific" treatments.

Clinical Nephrology, Vol. 35, Suppl. No. 1–1991 (pp. S. 23–30)

Mechanism of action of cyclosporin A and rationale for use in nephrotic syndrome

J. F. Borel

Department of Preclinical Research, Sandoz Pharma Ltd., Lichtstrasse 35, CH-4002 Basel, Switzerland

Abstract. Cyclosporin A (CyA, Sandimmun®) is the forerunner of a new generation of immunosuppressive drugs. It is highly effective in both antibody- and cell-mediated immunity and in inhibiting chronic inflammatory reactions. Cyclosporin A is, therefore, widely used to prevent rejection in clinical organ transplantation and appears to be very promising in the treatment of several autoimmune diseases. Cyclosporin A is not only effective when given at the time of sensitization (prevention of disease), but also when administered therapeutically during an immune response, such as during the active course of an autoimmune disease. The most important aspect of its immunosuppressive mechanism is the inhibition of lymphokine production secreted by activated T cells. The pharmacological effects of CyA are rapid in onset, dose-dependent and often quickly reversible when treatment is stopped.

Key words: animal experiments – nephritis – autoimmunity – cyclosporin A – immunosuppression

Introduction

Cyclosporin A (CyA, Sandimmun®) is a cyclic undecapeptide isolated from *Tolypocladium inflatum Gams.* The compound has several N-methylated amino acids and one novel C_9-amino acid. The peptide is neutral, rich in hydrophobic amino acids, and insoluble in water, but soluble in lipids and in many other organic solvents. Studies have revealed that it is effective in inhibiting both humoral and cell-mediated immune responses. Its effect is reversible and specific for T lymphocytes. Hemopoietic tissues are not affected in immunosuppressed animals.

The efficacy of a drug to modify the course of an autoimmune disease can be tested in two ways: preventively, that is, its ability to inhibit the primary event of sensitization; or therapeutically, its ability to alleviate the symptoms of the ongoing disease after sensitization.

Although data from animal models help us to understand autoimmunity, extrapolation to the human condition must be made with caution. These experimental models of autoimmune disease have the disadvantage that many are artificially induced, and correlation with the human counterpart of even the genetic models remains in dispute. Thus, both the induced and spontaneous models of uveitis and nephritis are susceptible to CyA treatment. In contrast, only the induced, but not the spontaneous, form of thyroiditis responds to therapy. Similarly, streptozocin- and virus-induced diabetes are refractory to CyA whereas spontaneously developing diabetes, in both bio-breeding (BB) rats and non-obese diabetic (NOD) mice, promptly react to prophylactic treatment with CyA [for review see Borel, 1989].

Reprint requests to Professor J. F. Borel.

Experimental models of immunological nephritis

There are several methods of experimentally inducing immune-mediated nephritis, usually in mice, rats and rabbits (Table 1). Glomerular proliferation in acute serum sickness (ASS) nephritis in rabbits is predominantly the result of an influx of monocytes into the glomerulus and is associated with proteinuria. Serum sickness was induced in rabbits by a single injection of bovine serum albumin with *Escherichia coli* endotoxin. When CyA (15 or 25 mg/kg/day) was injected intramuscularly, starting either two days before or at time of induction of ASS, proteinuria was profoundly reduced and glomerular proliferation was inhibited, indicating that T cells may play a role in mediating the ASS nephritis. Even when rabbits were treated with CyA (25 mg/kg/day) five days after the induction of nephritis, proteinuria and glomerular proliferation were similarly inhibited [Neild et al. 1983]. In those animals, it was subsequently observed that these treatment regimens led to the development of glomerular capillary thrombosis and cortical infarc-

Table 1 Summary of results obtained with cyclosporin A in autoimmune nephritis model in rodents

Autoimmune models	Species	Preventive/ therapeutic treatment	References
Acute serum sickness nephritis	Rabbit	+/+	Neild et al. 1983 Neild et al. 1984 b
Chronic serum sickness nephritis	Rat	+/+	Neild et al. 1986 Shigematsu & Koyama 1988
Antibody-induced glomerulonephritis	Mouse Rat	+/ND +/–	Schrijver et al. 1988 Tipping & Holdsworth 1985 Tipping et al. 1985 Wood et al. 1988 Thaiss et al. 1986
Heymann's nephritis	Rat	+/–	de Heer et al. 1985 Cattran 1988
Interstitial nephritis	Rat	+/+	Thoenes et al. 1987 Giménez et al. 1987 Shih et al. 1988
Mercuric chloride-induced autoimmune glomerulonephritis	Rat	+/+	Aten et al. 1988 Baran et al. 1986
Murine autoimmune systemic lupus erythematosus	NZB/W mouse	+/+[a]	Israël-Biet et al. 1983 Jones et al. 1983, 1985 Gunn & Ryffel 1986 a, b Gunn 1986 Okudaira et al. 1987
Murine autoimmune lpr disease	MRL/lpr mouse	+/+	Gozes et al. 1982 Berden et al. 1986 Mountz et al. 1987 Gunn & Hiestand 1988

+ = beneficial CyA effect; – = detrimental CyA effect; ND = experiment not done

[a] Relapse of symptoms on stopping CyA treatment

tion, lesions which are not usually seen in unmodified ASS, but are reminiscent of the pathological appearances found in hemolytic-uremic syndrome. The signs of this renal injury include hematuria, transient proteinuria, glycosuria and oliguria, all of which appear during the rapid phase of antigen elimination when immune complexes are being formed [Neild et al. 1984 a].

Further investigations have shown that muscular arteries of the heart and splanchnic organs develop an arterial injury in which there is extensive fibrinoid necrosis of the vessel wall, but little or none of the mononuclear cell reaction that is usually associated with the arteritis of ASS. A microvascular injury also occurs which leads to interstitial hemorrhage in the gastric mucosa, and multifocal necrosis in the heart and liver. These lesions were seen with equal frequency in all groups of rabbits with ASS who received CyA irrespective of whether they also received endotoxin [Neild et al. 1984 b].

A model of chronic serum sickness (CSS) can be established in rats by intraperitoneal injection of bovine serum albumin five days/week. Albuminuria increased gradually over the first 80 days and persisted thereafter. On day 146, the animals were given CyA 25 mg/kg/day intraperitoneally for three days; the albuminuria fell from 1.7 to 0.45 mg/ml. On examination of the renal histology on day 150, the glomeruli showed no significant abnormalities. A striking feature of this model was the abrupt onset of microscopic hematuria with CyA treatment [Neild et al. 1986].

The suppressive effect of CyA (20 mg/kg/day intramuscularly) on the development of CSS nephritis in the rat was also demonstrated by another group.

When CyA was taken during the pre-immunization stage, neither induction of glomerulonephritis nor a specific antibody response was observed. In contrast, when CyA was administered during the stage of continuous sensitization (one month later), mild CSS nephritis as well as specific antibody response developed [Shigematsu et al. 1988].

Another type of experimental glomerulonephritis producing glomerular injury and proteinuria can be induced by injection of antiglomerular basement-membrane antibody or immune complexes. Using a mouse model of passive antiglomerular basement-membrane nephritis, it was shown that preventive CyA therapy (75 mg/kg/day orally on days 1 to 4) had a profound antiproteinuric effect. It was suggested that this effect was not related to immunosuppression but, rather, was mediated by a reduction of the glomerular filtration rate (GFR) and probably also by a change in glomerular permselectivity [Schrijver et al. 1988].

Development of autologous or active antiglomerular basement-membrane glomerulonephritis requires two events: production of an antigen-specific immmune response, and triggering of an inflammatory response within the glomeruli. The effects of antibody-induced glomerulonephritis in the autologous rat model have been shown to be mediated by macrophages. The T-cell infiltrate consisted mainly of T helper (T_H) cells, reached its maximum at 24 hours after induction of disease and clearly preceded the peak of macrophage influx and glomerular damage. The use of CyA (25 mg/kg/day subcutaneously beginning on the day prior to immunization) to suppress T-cell function prevented T-cell accumulation and the subsequent macrophage-induced damage [Tipping et al. 1985].

However, treatment which commenced after the antibody response was established failed to alter antibody production, its deposition in the glomeruli or the outcome of the disease. Treatment had no effect on passive (heterologous) glomerulonephritis, which occurs 24 hours after intravenous administration of sheep anti-rat glomerular basement-membrane globulin to unimmunized rats. Thus, CyA is able to block the disease by preventing an active antibody response, but has no effect when the antibody response is established or when glomerular injury is passively induced [Tipping and Holdsworth 1985].

Another similarly designed study reported that CyA, when given prior to or at the onset of immunological insult, induced extensive glomerular infiltration by polymorphonuclear leukocytes and glomerular thrombosis, lesions which are not seen in unmodified nephritis or in rats receiving CyA alone [Wood et al. 1988]. The reasons for these contradictory results remain unclear.

The influence of CyA on the development of renal injury in the in-situ immune-complex glomerulonephritis in rats was examined. Cyclosporin A (15 or 25 mg/kg/day orally in two divided daily doses) inhibited proteinuria without affecting immune-complex deposition, or glomerular cell accumulation and proliferation. On stopping CyA, proteinuria either appeared or increased, indicating that cellular and tissue-damaging inflammatory processes were not irreversibly prevented, but only suppressed in the presence of CyA [Thaiss et al. 1986].

Single footpad immunization of rats with crude preparations of renal epithelium together with Freund's complete adjuvant (FCA) leads to a membranous type of chronic glomerulonephritis known as Heymann's nephritis, which has lesions similar to those of human membranous glomerulonephritis. Treatment with CyA (15 mg/kg/day intramuscularly from day 0 to 14) markedly inhibited the development of disease to a subsequent nephritogenic challenge. This tolerance, however, could not be transferred by lymphoid cells from CyA-treated rats, but was transferable by lymphocytes derived from the thymus or spleen of high antigen dose-tolerant rats, suggesting that CyA prevented the occurrence of a suppressor cell (CD8) that is responsible for high dose-tolerance [de Heer et al. 1985].

The effects of CyA treatment (8 mg/kg/day subcutaneously) on active Heymann's nephritis were studied at different time intervals after disease induction. When given at the time of antigen injection, CyA blocked both free antibody and circulating immune-complex formation. Immunopathology and renal function tests remained normal despite a rise in both these parameters to control values after CyA was discontinued. When CyA was given at a later stage of the disease process, there was no evidence of amelioration of any pathological and functional changes despite a limited suppression of both antibody and immune-complex formation [Cattran 1988].

In a rat model of a similarly induced tubulointerstitial nephritis, CyA (10 mg/kg/day orally), when given before or at the time of disease-onset, completely inhibited the expression of nephritis in spite of autoantibodies against tubular basement membranes persisting in the circulation and in the kidney [Thoenes et al. 1987]. These results were essentially corroborated by another group [Giménez et al. 1987]. In addition, these authors showed that a delay in CyA treatment (20 mg/kg/day subcutaneously) until day 10 after immunization – when antibody response is established – was still able to reduce drastically the levels of serum antitubular basement-membrane IgG and to abrogate the interstitial inflammatory cell response in spite of persistent kidney-bound antibodies [Giménez et al. 1987]. This therapeutic effect of CyA in interstitial nephritis in rats has also been confirmed by other workers. [Shih et al. 1988] found that administration of CyA (6 mg/kg/day subcutaneously) after the development of interstitial nephritis (from day 15 to 36 after immunization) arrested the progression of the histological lesions.

The mercuric chloride-induced autoimmune glomerulonephritis in rats is biphasic and characterized by lymphoid hyperplasia and glomerulonephritis. All manifestations of mercuric chloride-induced disease were prevented in rats treated concurrently with CyA at doses of either 7 or 10 mg/kg/day orally. The initial phase of nephritis was completely suppressed by a short, 15-day course of CyA. The later phase of the disease was tempered by CyA therapy, starting on day 10 after the first mercuric chloride injection and continuing for 60 days. Cyclosporin A appears to interfere with the polyclonal activation of B cells in mercuric chloride-induced autoimmune nephritis, which accounts for the drug's striking preventive and curative effect in this model [Baran et al. 1986].

Treatment with CyA (20 mg/kg/day orally from day 0 to 10) during mercuric chloride administration completely prevented the autoimmune phenomena of glomerulonephritis; moreover, a prolonged unresponsiveness to mercuric chloride was induced which lasted for at least a further five weeks. This unresponsiveness was not adoptively transferable by peripheral lymphoid cells from CyA-treated rats (in contrast to the case with untreated donors in remission), but could be overcome by reconstitution with naive lymphocytes.

These results suggest that the tolerogenic effect of CyA in mercuric chloride-induced autoimmunity is not mediated by active suppression; instead, the observed unresponsiveness may be due to direct functional deletion of autoreactive T lymphocytes [Aten et al. 1988]. A dissociation between the development of proteinuria and synthesis of anti-glomerular basement-membrane autoantibodies has been demonstrated, thereby suggesting that a CyA-sensitive cellular effector mechanism may be involved in the induction of proteinuria in this disease model [Aten et al. 1988].

In summary, treatment with CyA was effective in both preventing the development of nephritis in all models tested and improving the symptoms of established nephritis in most models, with the exception of Heymann's nephritis and antibody-induced glomerulonephritis. It appears that the drug interferes mainly with the cellular effector mechanisms involved in proteinuria, as a rapid reversal of proteinuria was obtained in several instances despite the persistence of autoantibodies and circulating immune complexes. However, preventive CyA treatment was also effective in suppressing autoantibody formation. Interestingly, CyA treatment induced a state of unresponsiveness in two conditions, Heymann's nephritis and mercuric chloride-induced glomerulonephritis. In both cases, tolerance could not be transfered by lymphocytes derived from CyA-treated animals, although this was possible with cells from appropriate control donors. In several of these nephritis models, CyA was successfully used as a probe to elucidate a T-cell involvement at some stage of their development. These various experimental models are thought to bear some relevance to clinical nephrotic diseases.

Spontaneous autoimmune lupus models in mice

The New Zealand black/white (NZB/W) hybrid mouse spontaneously develops an autoimmune disease with characteristics that resemble systemic lupus erythematosus (SLE) in humans. By two to three months of age, a systemic (non-organ-specific) immune-complex disease develops with nephritis and proteinuria. This follows a predictable course leading to chronic renal failure with a 50% mortality rate by the time the mice are eight to nine months of age. Chused et al. [1987] have analyzed and published the multigenic basis of autoimmune disease in New Zealand mice (see also Theofilopoulos and Dixon [1985]).

In an initial experiment, we observed that CyA (60 mg/kg/day in the feed), administered at 24 weeks and continued through to 75 weeks of age, failed to prolong survival of NZB/W hybrid mice. However, CyA at this dosage markedly reduced the proteinuria to the same extent as CyA 50 mg/kg over 10 days intraperitoneally; this reduction was maintained throughout the 75-week observation period [Borel 1981 a].

Another early study reported a dramatic diminution of anti-DNA antibody level in old (56-week-old) NZB/W hybrid mice which remained low throughout CyA therapy (approximately 120 mg/kg/day orally, five times/week) and persisted for seven weeks after drug withdrawal. Glomerular deposits were decreased compared with that in control mice [Israël-Biet et al. 1983].

A third and last early study showed that CyA (100 mg/kg/day orally) significantly prolonged the life span of female NZB/W hybrid mice and reduced the levels of anti-dsDNA autoantibody. It also prevented glomerular damage and renal failure despite the similar degree of cellular infiltration, and immunoglobulin (Ig) and complement deposition in the glomeruli, as seen in control mice [Jones et al. 1983]. These latter investigation were pursued and extended but, essentially, the earlier findings were confirmed [Jones et al. 1985]. Surprisingly, the levels of rheumatoid factors were found to be increased in CyA-treated mice.

More in-depth studies were performed in our laboratory by Gunn [1986], Gunn and Ryffel [1986 a, b], and Borel [1981 b].

Autoimmune NZB/W hybrid mice were treated with CyA (100 mg/kg/day orally five times/week) for 12 weeks. Young (12-week-old) and old (36-week-old) mice were used to assess the prophylactic and therapeutic effects of the drug in these two mice populations, respectively. Cyclosporin A proved to be effective in preventing autoantibody production (anti-DNA and anti-SE antibodies) in the young population and markedly reduced the autoantibody titers in the old mice.

These findings clearly establish that autoantibodies, at least in this murine lupus model, can be controlled pharmacologically [Gunn, 1986]. Moreover, CyA prevented the deposition of immune complexes in the kidneys, and the subsequent development of glomerulonephritis and proteinuria in young mice, and also exerted a therapeutic effect in old mice by reducing proteinuria even in those exhibiting an advanced stage of glomerular damage [Gunn and Ryffel 1986 a, b]. On renal histology, the glomeruli appeared to be almost normal with only minimal residual lesions after 12 weeks of treatment (at 48 weeks of age) [Borel 1981 b, Gunn and Ryffel 1986 a].

Further experiments revealed that another CyA congener, (Nva^2)-CyA, thought to possess a reduced nephrotoxicity in rats, is also very successful in suppressing a strong ongoing immune response in the NZB/W hybrid mouse [Gunn et al. 1986]. Similar results were obtained by Okudaira et al. [1987] when eight-month-old NZB/W hybrid mice were treated with CyA (50 mg/kg/day orally, six times/week). Cyclosporin A significantly depressed blood urea nitrogen (BUN) levels and clearly prolonged the animals' life span. Deposition of IgG and C3 was remarkably decreased, but the concentrations of anti-DNA antibodies and circulating immune complexes in the serum were not affected. Histological examination indicated a much milder glomerulonephritis in the CyA-treated mice than in the untreated controls [Okudaira et al. 1987].

The MRL/lpr mouse strain spontaneously develops glomerulonephritis, marked lymphoid hyperplasia, arteritis and chronic polyarthritis, and has a 50% mortality at approximately five months of age [Kyogoku et al. 1987; Theofilopoulos et al. 1985]. An initial report mentioned that short-term in-vivo treatment of three-month-old SLE lpr/lpr mice using CyA (200 mg/kg/day intraperitoneally over 10 days) significantly reduced serum levels of anti-DNA antibodies, but had no effect on the spontaneous massive T-cell proliferation seen in this strain [Gozes et al. 1982].

A similar treatment regimen, but using a CyA dose of 60 mg/kg/day, administered to MRL/lpr mice, only modestly suppressed IgM levels and anti-DNA antibodies, but markedly reduced mesenteric lymph node weight [personal communication Theofilopoulos AN, La Jolla, CA]. MRL/lpr mice were treated with CyA (25 mg/kg/day orally) from six to 22 weeks of age. Blood levels of CyA lying within the therapeutic range were obtained. Treatment with this low dose slightly increased serum IgG levels, but did not alter autoantibody titers, and had no effect on glomerulonephritis and glomerular proliferation. There were, however, reductions in the amount of mesangial IgG deposition, the extent of interstitial and perivascular infiltration, and the frequency and severity of necrotizing arteritis in the kidneys of CyA-treated MRL/lpr mice. The most prominent effect of CyA was an obvious reduction in lymphoproliferation in these mice [Berden et al. 1986]. The same CyA regimen, when given to BXSB mice [Theofilopoulos et al. 1985], had no apparent effect on any of the parameters measured [Berden et al. 1986]. As the major abnormality in MRL/lpr mice appears to reside in the T_H circuit while, in BXSB mice, the site appears to be the B-cell circuit, these results, using a clearly suboptimal dose of CyA for modulating antibody production, were not unexpected.

The lymphadenopathy of the MRL/lpr mouse strain is primarily due to the expansion of an unusual $CD4^-$, $CD8^-$, $6B2^+$ T-cell population. Treatment with CyA (40 mg/kg/day intraperitoneally) in mice aged from four to 18 weeks prevented lymphadenopathy and expansion of this unusual T-cell population in the peripheral lymph nodes as well as in the thymus. The increased expression of the *c-myb* and T-cell receptor β-chain genes associated with these unusual cells was also checked. The finding of increased numbers of $CD4^-$, $CD8^-$, $6B2^+$ thymocytes in untreated mice suggests abnormal intrathymic differentiation in lpr/lpr mice, a defect that was corrected by CyA [Mountz et al. 1987]. The CyA-treated mice also showed a marked decrease in arthritis and glomerulonephritis, and significantly prolonged survival duration. These beneficial effects of CyA occurred despite a lack of reduction in anti-DNA antibodies, circulating immune complexes, rheumatoid factor titers, or Ig concentrations. These results demonstrate that the B-cell hyperactivity of MRL/lpr mice can proceed in association with the T-cell proliferative disease [Mountz et al. 1987].

In conclusion, CyA exerts profound prophylactic as well as therapeutic effects in the different murine spontaneous SLE models. An interesting feature is

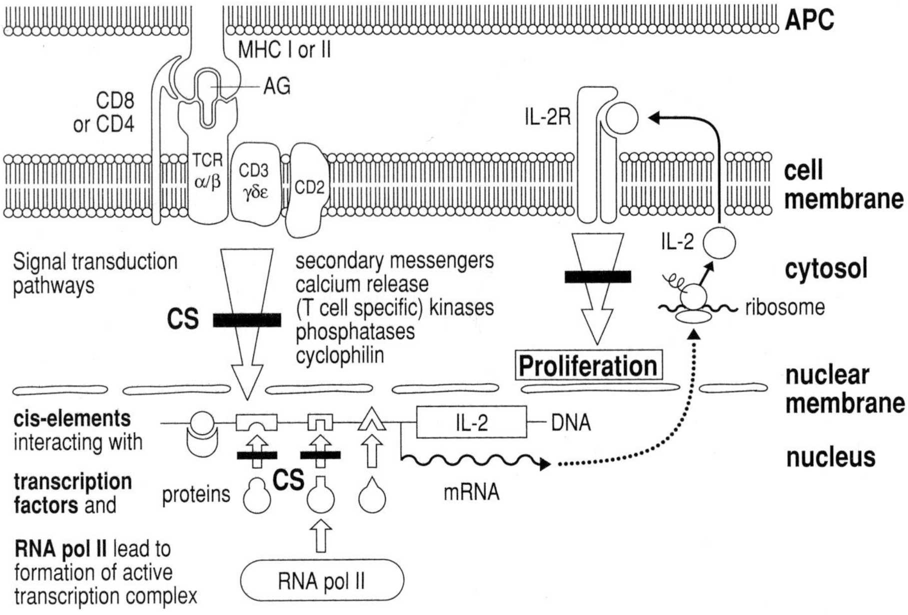

Fig. 1 Hypothetical mechanism of cyclosporin A (CS) action and its effects on T-cell activation. Il-2 = interleukin 2; mRNA = messenger RNA; APC = antigen-presenting cell; MHC = major histocompatibility complex; AG = antigen; IL-2R = Il-2 receptor; RNA pol II = RNA polymerase II.

that symptomatic improvement is not necessarily associated with a concurrent reduction in autoantibody levels.

Mechanism of action of cyclosporin A in autoimmune diseases

Effect at the cellular level

Most, if not all, of the immunosuppressive effects of CyA are the consequence of the inhibition of interleukin 2 (IL-2) and other lymphokine secretion by activated T cells. At a cellular level, this implies that cytotoxic and other effector T cells that destroy the target cells by interaction with the antigen are inhibited. In autoimmune diseases, this prevents tissue destruction. The lymphocytic subpopulation of T_H cells no longer produces and secretes IL-2 or the lymphokines necessary to activate B cells and their maturation into antibody-secreting (therefore autoantibody-producing) plasma cells. Inflammatory effector mechanisms cease to function in the absence of other delayed-type hypersensitivity (DTH) T-lymphocyte-derived (T_{DTH}) lymphokines, such as macrophage-activating factor, interferons and colony-stimulating factors. In autoimmune diseases, this inhibits the inflammatory process.

These effects are all rapid in onset, dose-dependent and often quickly reversible on stopping treatment. Other CyA effects on the immune system are less well defined and more controversial, including: inhibition of IL-I production; possible inhibition of interleukin-2 receptor (IL-2R) expression on membranes; failure to affect T-suppressor cell function; and direct inhibition of activated cytotoxic T cells. It is noteworthy that CyA does not affect the main macrophage and granulocyte functions, such as phagocytosis, chemotaxis and the release of most monokines, as this suggests that the drug has a greater selectivity than other immunosuppressant drugs currently in use.

Effect at the subcellular level

Certain clinical benefits of CyA can only be explained by assuming an effect of the drug at a specific site on the chromosomes associated with lymphokine production. Cyclosporin A most probably manifests its immunosuppressive effects by inhibiting the synthesis of IL-2 and other lymphokine messenger RNAs (mRNAs) during the process of T-cell activation. Effects on other events of the activation process, such as IL-2R expression, cannot be excluded. The detailed molecular events involved in CyA inhibition of mRNA synthesis are as yet not known, but it is likely that the drug prevents transduction of the mitogenic signal from the cell surface to the nucleus at a time subsequent to the rise in intracellular calcium generated by the mitogenic signal. Its immunosuppressive action may also be related to the binding of an intracellular receptor protein, cyclophilin, a major cytosolic constituent of most cells. The normal physiological function of this protein and its involvement in T-cell activation, if any, are not yet known. The hypothetical mechanisms of CyA action at the subcellular level is illustrated in Figure 1.

The following is a summary of the hypothetical knowledge of the effects of CyA on T-cell activation thus far. Cyclosporin A does not inhibit recognition of antigen by the T-cell receptor, and has no effect on transmembranous signalling. Mitogen- or antigen-induced activation of protein kinase C, and phosphoinositol turnover with the subsequent rise in intracellular calcium levels are not inhibited. It is most likely that CyA diffuses passively through the cell membrane and is concentrated intracellularly. One potential target in the cytoplasm is the major high-affinity binding protein cyclophilin, an enzyme which catalyzes a rate-determining isomerization in protein folding *in vitro*. In murine and human cell lines, and in normal lymphocytes, CyA has been found to inhibit transcription of mRNA for a variety of lymphokines. However, it does not inhibit the bulk of the mitogen-induced protein synthesis. Cyclosporin A affects binding of transcription factors to the IL-2 promoter at concentrations paralleling its immunosuppressive activity *in vitro*. It inhibits the synthesis of IL-2R only at high concentrations. Synthesis of other activation antigens and expression of major histocompatibility-complex gene products are significantly reduced by CyA. The effects of high concentrations of CyA on antigen-presenting cell functions such as the processing and presentation of antigen to T cells, and Il-I production, is still controversial.

Conclusions

Cyclosporin A is a potent immunosuppressive compound that is effective in prolonging allograft survival and in the treatment of many autoimmune syndromes. Its pharmacological effects on both antibody- and cell-mediated immunity are rapid in onset, dose-dependent and quickly reversible. Its suppressive action is primarily directed towards activated T-cell functions, particularly secretion of lymphokines. Large series of experimental studies have revealed that its mechanism of action *in vivo* may differ from and is more complex than that observed under straightforward in-vitro conditions.

Cyclosporin A has shown remarkable efficacy in numerous animal models of autoimmunity when given both prophylactically and therapeutically. On the basis of the vast experience gained with transplant patients, many clinical studies of autoimmune diseases have been performed or are still ongoing. Pilot studies, often conducted in therapy-resistant patients, have been followed-up by randomized controlled trials with a shift towards patients with less advanced disease and frequently involving multiple centers for adequate statistical power.

REFERENCES

Aten J, Bosman CB, de Heer E, Heodemaeker PJ, Weening JJ 1988 Cyclosporin A induces long-term unresponsiveness in mercuric chloride-induced autoimmune glomerulonephritis. Clin Exp Immunol *73:* 307–311

Baran D, Vendeville B, Vial MC, Cosson C, Bascou C, Teychenne P, Druet P 1986 Effect of cyclosporine A on mercury-induced autoimmune glomerulonephritis in the Brown Norway rat. Clin Nephrol *25 (Suppl 1):* 175–180

Berden JHM, Faaber P, Assmann KJM, Rijke TPM 1986 Effects of cyclosporin A on autoimmune disease in MRL/lpr and BXSB mice. Scand J Immunol *24:* 405–411

Borel JF 1981 a Cyclosporin A: Present experimental status. Transplant Proc *13:* 344–348

Borel JF 1981 b From our laboratories: Cyclosporin A. Triangle *20:* 97–105

Borel JF 1989 Pharmacology of cyclosporine (Sandimmune). IV. Pharmacological properties in vivo. Pharmacol Rev *41:* 318–339

Cattran DC 1988 Effect of cyclosporin on active Heymann's nephritis. Nephron *48:* 142–148

Chused TM, McCoy KL, Lal RB, Brown EM, Baker PJ 1987 Multigenic basis of autoimmune disease in New Zealand mice. Concepts Immunopathol *4:* 129–143

de Heer E, Daha MR, van Es LA 1985 The autoimmune response in active Heymann's nephritis in Lewis rats is regulated by T-lymphocyte subsets. Cell Immunol *92:* 254–264

Giménez A, Leyva-Cobián F, Fierro C, Rio M, Bricio T, Mampaso F 1987 Effect of cyclosporin A on autoimmune tubulointerstitial nephritis in the Brown Norway rat. Clin Exp Immunol *69:* 550–556

Gozes Y, Theofilopoulos AN, Park CH, Slack JH, Balderas RS, Dixon FJ 1982 Effects of cyclosporin A on in vitro and in vivo Ig and anti-DNA autoantibody production by splenocytes of autoimmune and normal mice. (Abst 1619) Fed Proc *41:* 547

Gunn HC 1986 Successful treatment of autoimmunity in (NZB × NZW) F_1 mice with cyclosporin and (Nva^2)-cyclosporin. I. Reduction of autoantibodies. Clin Exp Immunol *64:* 225–233

Gunn HC, Hiestand PC 1988 Cyclosporin A and G enhance IgG rheumatoid factor production in MRL/lpr mice. Transplant Proc *20 (Suppl 4):* 238–242

Gunn HC, Ryffel B 1986 a Glomerulonephritis in NZB/W mice: therapeutic effect of cyclosporine. Clin Nephrol *25 (Suppl 1):* 198 S – 192 S

Gunn HC, Ryffel B 1986 b Successful treatment of autoimmunity in (NZB × NZW) F_1 mice with cyclosporin and (Nva^2)-cyclosporin. II. Reduction of glomerulonephritis. Clin Exp Immunol *64:* 234–242

Gunn HC, Ryffel B, Hiestand PC, Borel JF 1986 The effects of (Nva^2)-cyclosporine on autoimmunity in the NZB/W mice. Transplant Proc *18:* 667–668

Israël-Biet D, Noël LH, Bach MA, Dardenne M, Bach JF 1983 Marked reduction of DNA antibody production and glomerulopathy in thymulin (FTS-Zn) or cylosporin A-treated (NZB × NZW) F_1 mice. Clin Exp Immunol *54:* 359–365

Jones MG, Harris G 1985 Prolongation of life in female NZB/NZW (F_1) hybrid mice by cyclosporin A. Clin Exp Immunol *59:* 1–9

Jones MG, Harris G, Cowing G 1983 Respone of murine autoimmune disease to cyclosporine and thiols. Transplant Proc *15 (Suppl 1):* 2904–2908

Kyogoku M, Nose M, Sawai T, Miyazawa M, Tachiwaki O, Kawashima M 1987 Immunopathology of murine lupus – Overview, SL/Ni, and MRL/Mp-lpr/lpr-. In: Animal Models: Assessing the Scope and Their Use in Biomedical Research. Alan R. Liss, New York, pp 95–130

Mountz JD, Smith HR, Wilder RL, Reeves JP, Steinberg AD 1987 CS – A therapy in MRL-lpr/lpr mice: Amelioration of immunopathology despite autoantibody production. J Immunol *138:* 157–163

Neild GH, Ivory K, Hiramatsu M, Williams DG 1983 Cyclosporin A inhibits acute serum sickness nephritis in rabbits. Clin Exp Immunol *52:* 586–594

Neild GH, Ivory K, Williams DG 1984a Glomerular thrombosis and cortical infarction in cyclosporin-treated rabbits with acute serum sickness. Br J Exp Pathol *65:* 133–144

Neild GH, Ivory K, Williams DG 1984b Severe systemic vascular necrosis in cyclosporin-treated rabbits with acute serum sickness. Br J Exp Pathol *65:* 731–743

Neild GH, Ivory K, Williams DG 1986 Effect of cyclosporine on proteinuria in chronic serum sickness in rats. Clin Nephrol *25 (Suppl 1):* 186 S – 188 S

Okudaira H, Terada E, Okudaira K 1987 Animal models utilised in the research of autoimmune disease control: experimental therapy of glomerulonephritis in NZB/W F_1 mice. Prog Clin Biol Res *229:* 157–174

Schrijver G, Wetzels JFM, Robben JCM, Assmann KJM, Koene RAP, Berden JHM 1988 Antiproteinuric effect of cyclosporine A in passive antiglomerular basement membrane nephritis in the mouse. Transplant Proc *20 (Suppl 4):* 304–308

Shigematsu H, Koyama A 1988 Suppressive effect of cyclosporin A on the induction of chronic serum sickness nephritis in the rat. Acta Pathol Jap *38:* 11–19

Shih W, Hines WH, Neilson EG 1988 Effects of cyclosporin A on the development of immune-mediated interstitial nephritis. Kidney Int *33:* 1113–1118

Thaiss F, Mihatsch MJ, Batsford S, Vogt A, Schollmeyer P 1986 Effect of cyclosporine on in situ immune complex glomerulonephritis. Clin Nephrol *25 (Suppl 1):* 181 S – 185 S

Theofilopoulos AN, Dixon FJ 1985 Murine models of systemic lupus erythematosus. Adv Immunol *37:* 269–390

Thoenes GH, Umscheid T, Sitter T, Langer KH 1987 Cyclosporin A inhibits autoimmune experimental tubulointerstitial nephritis. Immunol Lett *15:* 301–306

Tipping PG, Holdsworth SR 1985 Effect of cyclosporin A on antibody-induced experimental glomerulonephritis. Nephron *40:* 201–205

Tipping PG, Neale TJ, Holdsworth SR 1985 T lymphocyte participation in antibody-induced experimental glomerulonephritis. Kidney Int *27:* 530–537

Wood A, Adu D, Birtswistle RJ, Brewer DB, Michael J 1988 Cyclosporin A and antiglomerular basement membrane antibody glomerulonephritis in rats. Br J Exp Pathol *69:* 189–195

Clinical Nephrology, Vol. 35, Suppl. No. 1 – 1991 (pp. S. 31–36)

Treatment of idiopathic nephrotic syndrome with cyclosporin A in children

P. NIAUDET, M. BROYER and R. HABIB

Department of Pediatric Nephrology and INSERM U 192, Hôpital Necker-Enfants Malades, 149 rue de Sèvres, F-75015 Paris, France

Abstract. Cyclosporin A (CyA, Sandimmun®) was given to 71 children with idiopathic nephrotic syndrome, 45 of whom were steroid-dependent with signs of steroid toxicity, and 23 who were steroid-resistant. Cyclosporin A was effective in 80% of the steroid-dependent patients, allowing cessation of corticosteroid treatment. However, most of these patients relapsed when CyA was tapered or withdrawn. In these patients, CyA may be required for long periods of time. Conversely, CyA was less effective in steroid-resistant patients; only 7% achieved remission with CyA alone. Cyclosporin A in association with prednisone may be an effective alternative as 8 out of 14 patients entered remission with this treatment combination. Serial renal biopsies were performed in 43 patients to evaluate the potential nephrotoxicity of the treatment. Eighteen patients developed significant tubulointerstitial lesions which were attributable to CyA nephrotoxicity. The risk of developing chronic nephrotoxicity appears to be higher in steroid-resistant patients, and was not related to the duration of treatment. Cyclosporin A nephrotoxicity can develop in patients with normal renal function.

Key words: cyclosporin A – nephrotoxicity – children – steroid-responsive – steroid-resistant – steroid-dependent

Introduction

Idiopathic nephrotic syndrome is defined as the combination of nephrotic syndrome and minimal-change glomerular disease (MCD) without immune-complex deposition [Habib and Kleinknecht 1971]. In some cases, diffuse mesangial proliferation (DMP) [Waldherr et al. 1978] or focal-segmental glomerulosclerosis (FSGS) [Habib 1973] may be seen on light microscopy, and IgM deposits may be present on immunofluorescence microscopy [Cohen et al. 1978]. The clinical significance of these various morphological features have been the subject of numerous studies. Although morphological anomalies carry prognostic features, they do not allow the identification of distinct and specific diseases [Habib and Churg 1984, Habib et al. 1988]. Response to steroids carries a greater prognostic weight than the histological features seen on initial biopsy. Thus, it would appear to be advisable to distinguish the two types of idiopathic nephrotic syndrome according to the response to steroids: as steroid-responsive and steroid-resistant [Niaudet et al. 1988].

The vast majority of children (90%) are steroid-responsive, but more than half relapse on withdrawal of steroid therapy or when the dosage is decreased. These patients are steroid-dependent and the side-effects of steroid therapy lead to the use of other drugs, such as alkylating agents, which are themselves not without risk [Cameron et al. 1974, McDonald et al. 1974, Williams et al. 1989, Grupe 1982, Guesry et al. 1978]. These patients may benefit from cyclosporin A (CyA, Sandimmun®) therapy [Meyrier et al. 1986, 1988, Brodehl et al. 1988, Niaudet et al. 1987, Tejani et al. 1988].

In 10% of cases, the nephrotic syndrome is resistant to steroid therapy. The severity of these cases lies essentially in the risk of developing end-stage renal failure, which occurs in up to 50% of cases. The treatment of steroid-resistant nephrosis with alkylating agents has been studied in a number of trials, but the results have often been contradictory [Geary et al. 1984, Siegel et al. 1975, White and Glasgow 1971, Tejani et al. 1983, Baluarte et al. 1980, Williams et al. 1989]. Despite this, however, it is clear that some patients do benefit from such treatment. Cyclosporin A has also been administered in these cases, but the results have been difficult to interpret [Waldo and Kohaut 1987, Brandis et al. 1988, Maher et al. 1988, Garin et al. 1988, Niaudet et al. 1988].

This is a report of our experience with CyA in 71 children who have idiopathic nephrotic syndrome including the side-effects of the drug and its eventual nephrotoxicity, as assessed by repeat renal biopsies of 43 patients.

Reprint requests to Professor P. Niaudet.

Patients and methods

Patients

Seventy-one children with idiopathic nephrotic syndrome (NS) whose disease had not been well controlled by other forms of therapy were treated with CyA. The diagnosis of idiopathic NS was based on the presence of a nephrotic syndrome and the results of renal biopsy. All children received daily prednisone (60 mg/m^2) for one month, followed by three intravenous boluses of methylprednisolone (1 g/ 1.73 m^2) in case of persistent proteinuria at the end of the prednisone treatment. Subsequently, prednisone, starting at a dose of 60 mg/m^2, was given as a single dose on alternate days for two months, and the dosage was reduced by 15 mg/m^2 every two weeks. Patients who relapsed during the tapering period were treated with an alternate-day prednisone regimen for several months at the lowest remission-maintaining dose.

After the steroid therapy, 45 children entered complete remission, but all experienced several relapses with serious therapy-related side-effects. These 45 patients are here referred to as "steroid-dependent". Patients who did not respond to initial steroid therapy (n = 23) were considered "early non-responders". Three further patients, who had initially responded to steroid therapy, failed to respond after a subsequent relapse; these were considered "late non-responders". These 26 patients are here referred to as "steroid-resistant".

Renal biopsies

All patients but one, a late non-responder, underwent at least one biopsy before CyA treatment. A second biopsy was performed in 43 patients two to 19 months after the initiation of CyA treatment. A third biopsy was obtained in 13 patients after 11 to 37 months of CyA treatment.

Cyclosporin A therapy

Cyclosporin A treatment was initiated after informed consent of the parents was obtained. Patients who had either a creatinine clearance below 50 ml/ min/1.73 m^2 or impaired liver function, and those who had received immunosuppressive agents within the past two months were excluded from the study.

Patients received an initial CyA dose of 6 mg/kg body weight in two daily oral doses; the dose was adjusted to maintain trough plasma levels between 50 and 150 ng/ml, as measured by polyclonal radioimmunoassay (RIA) or trough whole blood levels between 100 and 200 ng/ml using the monoclonal RIA. Regular evaluation of renal and liver function was performed. Cyclosporin A was given at full dose for periods ranging from two to eight months. In steroid-responsive patients, prednisone treatment was tapered and stopped within one to four months after initiation of CyA therapy. In steroid-resistant patients, CyA was given alone or in combination with prednisone 30 mg/m^2/day for one month, and on alternate days for five months thereafter.

Results of cyclosporin A treatment

Steroid-dependent patients

Examination by light microscopy of the renal biopsies obtained at various times after onset of the disease and before initiation of CyA therapy gave the following results: 40 were classified as MCD, two as DMP and three as FSGS.

The 45 steroid-responsive cases had last relapsed while receiving alternate-day prednisone within the three months preceding CyA treatment. They received CyA for periods of at least three months. Fifteen patients were receiving daily prednisone and 27 were taking alternate-day prednisone when CyA therapy was started. Three patients were no longer receiving prednisone.

Thirty-six of the 45 patients either entered remission or remained relapse-free while receiving full-dose CyA despite the fact that prednisone had been withdrawn. Of these 36 patients, three were protein-free when last examined, but all were still receiving CyA. Thirty-three patients relapsed: 23 while CyA was tapered to doses ranging from 0.7 to 6.6 mg/kg, and 10 at seven to 120 days after withdrawal of CyA treatment. Cyclosporin A was ineffective in two patients who relapsed upon starting alternate-day prednisone therapy. The remaining seven patients relapsed on withdrawal of prednisone treatment, but the association of CyA with low-dose prednisone allowed remission to be maintained. The responses to CyA treatment according to histology are shown in Table 1.

Of the 33 children who had relapsed on tapering or withdrawal of CyA, 29 received another course of the drug. An increase of CyA dosage induced remission in 10 patients whereas, in 15 further patients, remission was achieved with a combination of CyA and prednisone. In four children, CyA combined with prednisone failed to induce remission. Interestingly, in three of these cases, CyA, when given several months later, was again effective.

Of the 25 patients who responded to CyA after the first relapse, in 10 cases the treatment was with-

Table 1 Response to cyclosporin A in steroid-responsive idiopathic NS according to histology

	Complete remission	Relapse on prednisone withdrawal	No response
Minimal-change disease	31	6	2
Diffuse mesangial proliferation	2	–	–
Focal-segmental glomerulosclerosis	3	1	–
Total	36	7	2

Table 2 Response to cyclosporin A in steroid-resistant idiopathic NS according to histology

	Complete remission	Partial remission	No response
Minimal-change disease	–	1	4
Diffuse mesangial proliferation	–	–	2
Focal-segmental glomerulosclerosis	–	3	3
No biopsy	1	–	–
Total	1	4	9

drawn nine to 30 months later after further relapses. The remaining 15 patients who were still in remission after seven to 40 months had received CyA (2–6 mg/kg body weight) alone or in combination with alternate-day prednisone (0.15–1 mg/kg).

Steroid-resistant patients

No renal biopsy was performed in one patient who was a late non-responder. The remaining 25 patients were classified on the basis of light microscopy: 12 MCD; 11 FSGS; and 2 DMP.

Fourteen patients were given CyA as monotherapy; these included 11 early non-responders and three late non-responders (Table 2). Only one patient, a late non-responder, went into complete remission within the first month of CyA treatment. This patient was still in remission one year after stopping treatment. Four patients achieved partial remission with a significant decrease in proteinuria, but this returned to pretreatment levels on stopping CyA. The remaining nine patients failed to respond to CyA.

When CyA was given together with prednisone to 14 patients, eight entered complete remission (Table 3). Of interest was one patient who achieved remission with the combination, but relapsed on withdrawal of the drugs. The relapse was steroid-responsive, and the patient was still in complete remission one year after stopping treatment.

Side-effects

Renal function

Impaired renal function was observed in 10 patients. Of four steroid-dependent patients who showed transient increases in serum creatinine levels, the increases occurred during a relapse in three patients who had low CyA trough levels. In the fourth patient, the increases in creatinine levels were completely reversed on withdrawal of CyA. Six steroid-resistant patients had impaired renal function, which was transient; four of these patients recovered completely. In one patient, the renal function impairment was only partially reversed. In the remaining patient, renal function was impaired after two months of treatment and deteriorated further within one year of stopping CyA. It should be noted that nephrotoxicity

Table 3 Response to cyclosporin A and prednisone in steroid-resistant idiopathic NS according to histology

	Complete remission	Partial remission	No response
Minimal-change disease	5	–	3
Focal-segmental glomerulosclerosis	3	2	1
Total	8	2	4

Table 4 Response to cyclosporin A in steroid-responsive idiopathic NS

Authors	No. of patients	Remission after prednisone withdrawal
Capodicasa et al. [1986]	6	5
Tejani et al. [1988]	13	11
Brodehl et al. [1988]	6	6
Mentser et al. [1988]	6	6
Kitano et al. [1990]	17	17
Niaudet et al. [present series]	45	36
Total	93	81

Table 5 Response to cyclosporin A in steroid-resistant idiopathic NS

Authors	No. of patients	Response to CyA Partial	Complete
Capodicasa et al. [1986]	4		2
Brandis et al. [1988]	4		4
Waldo & Kohaut [1987]	6	1	
Brodehl et al. [1988]	7	2	
Tejani et al. [1988]	7		3
Niaudet et al. [1987]	13	4	1
Total	41	7	10

was related to high plasma trough levels in only two patients.

Hypertension

Blood pressure (BP) was moderately elevated in 16 patients, 11 of whom were receiving prednisone therapy. One patient was hypertensive before receiving CyA in spite of the absence of prednisone. Three patients whose BPs were normal on initiation of treatment developed hypertension while receiving CyA. In these patients, the BP returned to normal values after CyA withdrawal.

Other side-effects

Hypertrichosis was frequently observed (n = 50) whereas moderate gingival hyperplasia was seen in 37 patients. Liver function test results, including determinations of serum transaminase and bilirubin levels, showed no changes. Hyperkalemia occurred in only one patient in conjunction with impaired renal function. Another patient developed seizures while taking CyA and prednisone.

Cyclosporin A nephrotoxicity

A prospective study was conducted to assess the potential nephrotoxicity of CyA at a starting dose of 6 mg/kg body weight/day in children who had idiopathic NS. Forty-three patients (10 girls and 33 boys), aged 1.4 to 12.3 years at onset of the disease, were entered into the study. Thirty-seven patients were steroid-dependent and had had two to 29 relapses, and six were steroid-resistant. Duration of the disease before CyA therapy ranged from 0.3 to 13.9 years. All patients were biopsied at least twice, once before starting CyA, and again after two to 20 months of CyA treatment. Thirteen patients were biopsied for a third time after 11 to 37 months of CyA therapy.

The initial biopsies showed: 34 MCD (32 steroid-dependent, two steroid-resistant); two DMP (both steroid-dependent); six FSGS (two steroid-dependent, four steroid-resistant); one focal-global fibrosis (FGF; steroid-dependent) patient. Cyclosporin A was effective in 33 steroid-dependent and three steroid-resistant patients (29 MCD, two DMP, four FSGS, one FGF).

The lesions observed on the first post-treatment biopsy were classified according to the severity of tubulointerstitial damage, considered to be the best indicator of chronic CyA nephrotoxicity. Grade 0 (n = 16) indicated no modification of renal parenchyma; Grade I (n = 11) indicated scattered atrophic tubules; Grade II (n = 11) indicated several foci of atrophic tubules within stripes of interstitial fibrosis; and Grade III (n = 5) indicated confluent or extensive areas of interstitial fibrosis with atrophic and/or collapsed tubules. The second post-therapy biopsy, performed in 13 patients, revealed extension of the tubulointerstitial lesions in seven patients, two progressing from Grade 0 to Grade I, three from Grade I to Grade II, and three from Grade II to Grade III. Persistent impairment of renal function occurred in only one patient.

Discussion

Cyclosporin A was given to 71 children with idiopathic NS who either were at risk of steroid toxicity because of multiple relapses (steroid-responsive/steroid-dependent, n = 45), or had failed to respond to steroids (steroid-resistant, n = 23). This treatment was effective in 36 out of the 45 steroid-responsive children who did not relapse during CyA treatment in spite of prednisone withdrawal. However, most of these patients relapsed when CyA treatment was tapered or stopped. Cyclosporin A reduced the prednisone requirement in seven patients and was ineffective in two. A review of the literature including our cases [Brodehl et al. 1988, Tejani et al. 1988, Capodicasa et al. 1986, Mentser et al. 1988, Kitano et al. 1990] of 93 children who had steroid-dependent NS indicates that CyA treatment resulted in a high rate of response: 81 (87%) either achieved remission, if the patient had been in relapse, or maintained remission, thus allowing withdrawal of prednisone (Table 4).

By contrast, only one of the 14 steroid-resistant patients entered complete remission with CyA whereas a partial response was observed in four patients and no response in nine. The combination of CyA with prednisone induced remission in eight out of 14 patients. Review of the pediatric literature [Brodehl et al. 1988, Tejani et al. 1988, Waldo and Kohaut 1987, Capodicasa et al. 1986] indicates that, of 41 steroid-resistant patients treated with CyA, only 14 entered complete remission and a further six achieved a transient remission (Table 5).

On the basis of these results and data from other studies, we conclude that the response to CyA in patients with idiopathic NS is better correlated to their initial steroid-responsiveness than their histopathological classification. Of the children treated with CyA in the pediatric series, 60 were classified as MCD, 75% of whom responded to treatment; of 37 patients who showed lesions of FSGS on renal biopsy, 35% responded to CyA treatment.

The important side-effect of CyA is nephrotoxicity. In our series, the drug was well tolerated in steroid-responders; only four of these patients experienced a transient impairment of renal function and this occurred during a relapse in three cases. In contrast, seven of the 14 steroid non-responders had impaired renal function (which was reversed in four cases) either during CyA treatment (n = 6) or after stopping CyA (n = 1). Lesions of nephrotoxicity, characterized by stripes of fibrosis containing atrophic tubules, were observed in four out of six steroid-resistant patients after two to 13 months of CyA and in only four out of 37 steroid-dependent patients after 12 to 32 months of CyA treatment.

This study showed that: 1. Cyclosporin A nephrotoxicity is not related to the duration of treatment; 2. The risk of developing chronic nephrotoxicity appears to be higher in steroid-resistant than in steroid-dependent patients; 3. Histological signs of nephrotoxicity can develop in patients with normal glomerular filtration rate. Renal biopsy appears, therefore, to be the surest method of detecting patients who develop CyA nephrotoxicity.

In conclusion, CyA is a good alternative to steroids in the treatment of idiopathic NS, especially in steroid-dependent patients at risk of developing steroid toxicity. Cyclosporin A alone is less effective in steroid-resistant patients in whom the risk of CyA nephrotoxicity is higher. Low-dose steroids in combination with CyA may be a better approach in such patients. Because of the high incidence of relapses on withdrawal of CyA, it appears that the drug needs to be administered for longer periods of time than was initially believed, thus increasing the risk of nephrotoxicity. Consequently, renal function should be monitored frequently, although the results of our serial biopsies show that lesions of nephrotoxicity may arise in the absence of any signs of renal function impairment.

REFERENCES

Baluarte HJ, Gruskin AB, Polinski MS, Prebis JW, Rosenblum H 1980 Chlorambucil therapy in the nephrotic syndrome. In: *Gruskin AB, Norma HE* (eds). Pediatric Nephrology: Proceedings of the 5th International Pediatric Nephrology Symposium. Martinus Nijhoff, The Hague, pp 423–429

Brandis M, Burghard R, Leititis J, Zimmerhackl D, Hildebrandt F, Helmchen U 1988 Cyclosporine A for treatment of nephrotic syndrome. Transpl Proc *20 (Suppl 4):* 275–279

Brodehl J, Hoyer PF, Oemar BS, Helmchen U, Wonigeit K 1988 Cyclosporine treatment of nephrotic syndrome in children. Transpl Proc *20 (Suppl 4):* 269–274

Capodicasa G, De Santo NG, Nuzzi F, Giordano C 1986 Cyclosporine A in nephrotic syndrome of childhood: A 14-month experience. Int Pediatr Nephrol *7:* 69–72

Cameron JS, Chantler C, Ogg CS, White RHR 1974 Long-term stability of remission in nephrotic syndrome after treatment with cyclophosphamide. Br Med J *4:* 7–14

Cohen AH, Border WA, Glassock RJ 1978 Nephrotic syndrome with glomerular mesangial IgM deposits. Lab Invest *38:* 610–619

Garin EH, Orak JK, Hiott KL, Sutherland SE 1988 Cyclosporine therapy for steroid-resistant nephrotic syndrome. A controlled study. Am J Dis Child *142:* 985–988

Geary DF, Farine M, Thorner P, Baumal R 1984 Response to cyclophosphamide in steroid-resistant focal-segmental glomerulosclerosis. A reappraisal. Clin Nephrol *22:* 109–113

Grupe WE 1982 Cytotoxic drugs for nephrotic syndrome. N Engl J Med *307:* 313

Guesry P, Lenoir G, Broyer M 1978 Gonadal effects of chlorambucil given to prepubertal and pubertal boys for nephrotic syndrome. J Pediatr *92:* 299

Habib R 1973 Focal-glomerular sclerosis. Kidney Int *4:* 355–361

Habib R, Churg J 1984 Minimal-change disease, mesangial proliferative GN and focal sclerosis; individual entities or a spectrum of disease. In: *Robinson R* (ed) Nephrology today: Proceedings of the 9th International Congress on Nephrology, Los Angeles. Springer, New York – Berlin – Heidelberg, pp 634–644

Habib R, Girardin E, Gagnadoux MF, Hinglais N, Broyer M 1988 Immunopathological findings in idiopathic nephrosis: Clinical significance of glomerular "immune deposits". Pediatr Nephrol 2: 402–408

Habib R, Kleinknecht C 1971 The primary nephrotic syndrome of childhood. Classification and clinicopathologic study of 406 cases. Pathol Ann *6:* 417–474

Kitano Y, Yoshikawa N, Tanaka R, Nakamura H, Nimomiya M, Ito H 1990 Cyclosporin treatment in children with steroid-dependent nephrotic syndrome. Pediatr Nephrol *4:* 474–477

Maher ER, Sweny P, Chappel M, Varghese Z, Moorhead JF 1988 Cyclosporin in the treatment of steroid-responsive and steroid-resistant nephrotic syndrome in adults. Nephrol Dial Transpl *3:* 728–732

McDonald J, Murphy AV, Arneil GC 1974 Long-term assessment of cyclophosphamide therapy for nephrosis. Lancet *ii:* 980–982

Mentser M, Shannon B, Mahan JD 1988 Cyclosporine treatment of frequently relapsing minimal-change nephrotic syndrome in children. Response to therapy and evidence for a T-cell abnormality. Kidney Int *33:* 329

Meyrier A, Simon P, Perret G, Condamin-Meyrier MC 1986 Remission of idiopathic nephrotic syndrome after treatment with cyclosporine A. Br Med J *292:* 789–793

Meyrier A, Condamin MC, Simon P 1988 Treatment with cyclosporine of adult idiopathic nephrotic syndrome resistant to corticosteroids and other immunosuppressants. Transpl Proc *20 (Suppl 4):* 259–261

Niaudet P, Habib R, Gagnadoux MF, Tete MJ, Broyer M 1988 Treatment of severe childhood nephrosis. Adv Nephrol *17:* 151–172

Niaudet P, Habib R, Tete MJ, Hinglais N, Broyer M 1987 Cyclosporine in the treatment of idiopathic nephrotic syndrome in children. Pediatr Nephrol *1:* 566–573

Niaudet P, Tete MJ, Broyer M, Habib R 1988 Cyclosporine and childhood idiopathic nephrosis. Transpl Proc *20 (Suppl 4):* 265–268

Siegel NC, Gur A, Krassner LS 1975 Minimal lesion nephrotic syndrome with early resistance to steroid therapy. J Pediatr *87:* 377–380

Tejani A, Nicastri AD, Sen D 1983 Long-term evaluation of children with nephrotic syndrome and focal-segmental glomerulosclerosis. Nephron *35:* 225–232

Tejani A, Butt K, Trachtman H, Suthanthiran M, Rosenthal CJ, Khawar MR 1988 Cyclosporine A-induced remission of relapsing nephrotic syndrome in children. Kidney Int *33:* 729–734

Waldherr R, Gubler MC, Levy M, Broyer M, Habib R 1978 The significance of pure diffuse mesangial proliferation in idiopathic nephrotic syndrome. Clin Nephrol *10:* 171–179

Waldo FB, Kohaut EC 1987 Therapy of focal-segmental glomerulosclerosis with cyclosporine A. Pediatr Nephrol *1:* 180–182

White RHR, Glasgow EF 1971 Focal glomerulosclerosis. A progressive lesion associated with steroid-resistant nephrotic syndrome. Arch Dis Childh *46:* 877–886

Williams SA, Makker SP, Ingelfinger JR, Grupe WC 1989 Long-term evaluation of chlorambucil plus prednisone in idiopathic nephrotic syndrome of childhood. N Engl J Med *302:* 929–933

Clinical Nephrology, Vol. 35, Suppl. No. 1–1991 (pp. S. 37–42)

Treatment of adult idiopathic nephrotic syndrome with cyclosporin A: Minimal-change disease and focal-segmental glomerulosclerosis

A. Meyrier[a], M.-C. Condamin, D. Broneer[b], and The Collaborative Group of the French Society of Nephrology

Hôpital Avicenne, Bobigny Medical School, Paris North University, Bobigny, France

Abstract. Two open studies were conducted to determine the efficacy and tolerance of cyclosporin A (CyA, Sandimmun®) 5 mg/kg/day. Sixty-four patients received CyA as monotherapy, and efficacy was assessed at three months; in 48 other patients, CyA was given with prednisone 12–15 mg/kg/day, and efficacy was assessed at six months. Of these 112 patients, 14 withdrew prematurely because of adverse events or other reasons, and a further nine patients were excluded for protocol violation. The remaining 98 patients were considered valid for the evaluation of efficacy (52 with minimal-change disease [MCD] and 46 with focal-segmental glomerulosclerosis [FSGS]; 37/98 were steroid-dependent [SD], and 61/98 were steroid-resistant [SR]). The remission: failure rate depended on histology (36:16 in MCD, 11:35 in FSGS) and steroid response (25:12 in SD, 22:39 in SR). The rate of remission was highest in SD MCD (71%) and lowest in SR FSGS (20%; chi square = 18.6, p <0.001). Tolerance was assessed by serum creatinine and, in 36 cases, by repeat renal biopsy at six to 42 months. Serum creatinine was remarkably stable in MCD. Rising creatinines were observed mostly in cases of SR FSGS, particularly those who had pretreatment interstitial lesions; this was considered due to both an increase of interstitial lesions and progression of the glomerular lesions of FSGS. We conclude that: 1. The best indication of CyA, in terms of efficacy and tolerance, is SD MCD; 2. Cyclosporin A may be used in SR FSGS only if renal function is normal and the pretreatment biopsy shows no interstitial lesions; 3. CyA-responsive patients are CyA-dependent, and its long-term (> one year) tolerance is yet to be determined.

Key words: cyclosporin A – minimal-change disease – focal-segmental glomerulosclerosis – steroid toxicity

Introduction

Nephrosis with minimal glomerular changes (minimal-change disease; MCD) or complicated by lesions of focal-segmental glomerulosclerosis (FSGS) is by far the predominant cause of idiopathic nephrotic syndrome (NS) in children. It also remains a significant problem in adults. Adult idiopathic NS may be due to persistence of the disease after age 15 or may supervene later, even in the elderly. Its frequency among other etiologies of NS is approximately 40% at age 40 and 30% subsequently [Cameron 1987]. Adult MCD is steroid-responsive in approximately 80% of cases [Meyrier and Simon 1988], but this apparently favorable figure should not obscure the fact that many patients undergo a multirelapsing course, and that steroid-sensitive forms may also be steroid-dependent. In such instances, repeated or continuous courses of corticosteroid treatment inevitably lead to the well-known complications of glucocorticoid toxicity. Idiopathic NS accompanied by lesions of FSGS responds to corticosteroid treatment in only 20% of cases, and a lack of response is highly predictive of eventual progression to end-stage renal failure [Korbet et al. 1986, Meyrier and Simon 1988]. Steroid dependency, steroid resistance and a multirelapsing course are recognized indications for a course of cytotoxic drugs. However, alkylating agents in themselves entail numerous risks, and failures of such treatment represent more than 60% of cases with FSGS.

Some investigators have reported that, in children [Capodicasa et al. 1986, Hoyer et al. 1986, Brodehl et al. 1988, Niaudet et al. 1988, Tejani et al. 1988] as well as in adults [Lagrue et al. 1986, Meyrier et al. 1986, 1989], treatment with cyclosporin A (CyA; Sandimmun®) obtained remissions in cases

---

Reprint requests to Professor Alain Meyrier.

[a] Study Coordinator; [b] Study Coordination Monitor.

considered failures both of corticosteroid and of cytotoxic regimens. Thus, for the first time since 1949, a new form of treatment of nephrosis has become available.

In 1986, the French Society of Nephrology undertook a large-scale collaborative study to assess the efficacy and tolerance of CyA in adult idiopathic NS, using a protocol in which the drug was used alone for three months [Meyrier et al. 1989]. A second protocol was designed two years later in which CyA was associated with low-dose prednisone to determine whether such a combination would increase the efficacy of the immunosuppressive regimen. Thus far, more than 100 adult patients have been included in the two studies. Some have been treated continuously for five years. Description of this population and of the results observed in terms of both efficacy and tolerance form the basis of this report.

Patients and study design

Study 1

Patients were enrolled on the basis of idiopathic NS; steroid resistance or dependency, or contraindication to corticosteroid treatment; and MCD or FSGS proven by recent renal biopsy. Patients with blood pressure >180/100 mmHg, creatinine clearance <50 ml/min, liver disease, pregnancy or infection were excluded.

After an 18-day placebo period, CyA (in oily solution) was started at an initial dosage of 5 mg/kg/day (in two divided doses, 12 hours apart), subsequently titrated for target whole-blood trough levels of 200–800 ng/ml (12 hours post-dose, polyclonal radioimmunoassay [RIA]). The main goals of the study were to assess the efficacy of treatment at three months, and the incidence of relapses after discontinuation – CyA dependency. In cases of relapse, investigators were free to resume treatment as monotherapy or with additional corticosteroids.

This study comprised 64 patients (including eight who had been randomized against cyclophosphamide), with a mean age of 31.8 ± 14 years (range 14–67 years); 41 (64%) patients were steroid-resistant and 23 (36%) were steroid-dependent. Nephrotic syndrome had evolved 54 ± 63 months before the trial. At some time, 27 patients had been treated with conventional immunosuppressive drugs. Twenty-nine patients were classified as MCD and 35 as FSGS. In the MCD group, two-thirds were steroid-dependent; in the FSGS group, 27 (82%) were steroid-resistant. Before treatment, serum creatinine was 104 ± 45 μmol/l and creatinine clearance was 92 ± 35 ml/min. Five patients withdrew before Month 3 (one because of a coronary event, three due to intercurrent infection, one because of a rapidly rising serum creatinine).

Study 2

Cyclosporin A was given in the form of soft gelatine capsules together with low-dose prednisone. Patients were enrolled basically on the same criteria as in Study 1; the differences were: 1. More stringent inclusion criteria as regards renal function; 2. More rigid monitoring of renal toxicity: Patients were withdrawn from the study if serum creatinine rose by 30% over their own baseline values and remained elevated despite two successive dose reductions; 3. More accurate definitions of "complete remission", "partial remission" and "failure". Results were assessed at six months as: Complete remission = proteinuria <0.5 g/24 h and serum albumin >3 g/dl; partial remission = proteinuria between 0.51 and 3.0 g/24 h and serum albumin >3 g/dl; failure = proteinuria >3 g/24 h irrespective of serum albumin levels. Thus, patients who showed a definite improvement in clinical status, and a rise in serum albumin to over 3 g/dl (including cases where it returned to normal), but whose proteinuria remained in excess of 3 g/24 h were considered failures whereas, in Study 1, they were assessed as partial remissions.

The study design varied according to previous response to corticosteroids. Prednisone was tapered to 0.2 mg/kg/day in the steroid-resistant group. Treatment with CyA was started at a dose of 5 mg/kg/day and subsequently modified for target whole-blood trough levels of 100–200 ng/ml (specific monoclonal

Table 1 Results of the French Society of Nephrology studies of adult patients with idiopathic nephrotic syndrome treated with CyA.

	Steroid-dependent (n = 37)		Steroid-resistant (n = 61)	
	Remissions[a]	Failures	Remissions[a]	Failures
Minimal-change disease (n = 52)	22	9	14	7
Focal-segmental glomerulosclerosis (n = 46)	3	3	8	32

[a] As the definitions of complete vs partial remission varied only slightly between Studies 1 and 2, data from both have been pooled under this heading

RIA) 12 hours post-dose. Full-dose treatment was given for six months, at the end of which time those in partial or complete remission received treatment for a further three months, followed by tapering to a stop for a final three months (total 12 months). This tapering was adopted in order to assess CyA dependency in responsive patients.

This study comprised 48 patients, with a mean age of 34.9 ± 15.2 years (range 17–65 years), including 29 (60%) who were steroid-resistant and 19 (40%) who where steroid-dependent. Nephrotic syndrome had developed 39 ± 64 months before the trial (range 3–300 months). Half of the patients had, at some time, been treated with conventional immunosuppressive drugs. Twenty-nine patients were classified as having MCD and 19 as FSGS. In the MCD group, 17/29 (59%) were steroid-dependent and, in the FSGS group, 17/19 (90%) were steroid-resistant. Before treatment, serum creatinine was 94 ± 28 µmol/l and creatinine clearance was 110 ± 39 ml/min.

Nine patients withdrew before Month 6 (two due to uncontrollable hypertension, four because of rapidly rising serum creatinine and three who defaulted).

Results

Due to the similarity between patients and protocols in Study 1 and Study 2, and despite the fact that initial assessment was made at three months in Study 1 and at six months in Study 2, the results are presented as pooled data.

Of a total of 112 patients enrolled, five patients in Study 1 and nine in Study 2 withdrew prematurely. A further nine patients in Study 2 were excluded (inclusion error in eight and protocol violation in one). Thus, 98 patients were considered valid for assessing treatment efficacy. However, of the nine exclusions for protocol violation, eight had been treated for at least six months and were considered valid for the assessment of tolerance (n = 106).

Efficacy

Remission at six months

The success rate was clearly dependent on two factors, namely, glomerular histology (MCD vs FSGS), and previous response to corticosteroid therapy (steroid dependency vs steroid resistance; Table 1). The previous response to steroids was of greater predictive value than the type of glomerular lesion, at least for patients with MCD. This was less apparent in patients with FSGS, the majority of whom

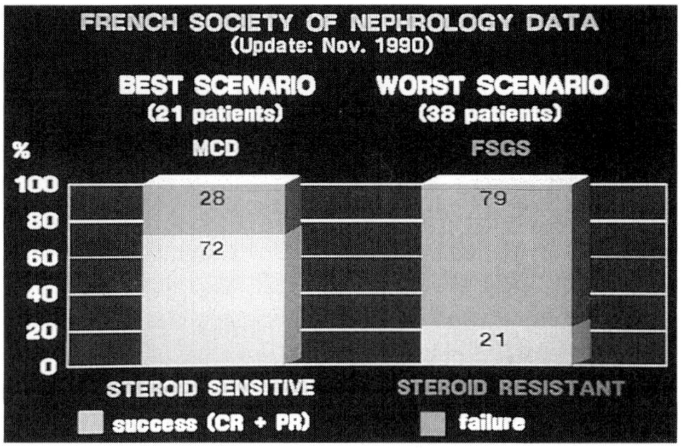

Fig. 1 Results of the French Society of Nephrology studies show a best case/worst case relationship when considering patients on the basis of a combination of steroid responsiveness and glomerular histology.

were steroid-resistant. Taking steroid responsiveness and glomerular histology together led to a best scenario/worst scenario relationship (Figure 1). A patient with steroid-dependent MCD had a 72.4% chance of remission with CyA while a patient with steroid-resistant FSGS had a 79% chance of not responding to such treatment.

Maintenance of remission and CyA dependency

Recurrence of proteinuria during dose-tapering was extremely frequent. This was deliberately tested in 11 patients in Study 2, for which the protocol included dose-tapering from month 9 onwards if complete remission was achieved by that time. Of these 11 cases, six remained in complete remission after tapering. The longest follow-up of these patients was 24 months, and the longest stable remission after stopping CyA was 12 months. In the five patients who relapsed after tapering, proteinuria recurred within a minimum of two weeks and a maximum of nine months. In three of these patients, increasing the dose induced a second remission. In the remaining two cases, returning to their previous doses did not achieve remission and these patients were considered secondary failures.

Long-term efficacy

Of 27 patients who where treated with CyA for at least one year, the longest observation was of a 30-year-old black woman in Study 1. This patient has been maintained in stable remission since 1985 with CyA at 360 mg (5 mg/kg/day) plus prednisone 10 mg/day. The 12-hour post-dose whole-blood trough CyA levels are extremely low – approximately 30 ng/ml. However, all attempts to reduce the dosage of either prednisone of CyA led to an immediate relapse of proteinuria, thus necessitating that the previous dosages be resumed.

Short-term tolerance

Minor side-effects

Minor side-effects (those not requiring stopping treatment) were numerous, most frequently gastrointestinal discomfort, tremor and hypertrichosis. Hypertension, either elicited or aggravated by CyA, was common, but easily controlled by antihypertensive treatment. Interestingly, gastrointestinal side-effects were less frequent in Study 2 than in Study 1, perhaps because of the improved presentation of CyA in soft gelatine capsules.

Major side-effects

A total of 10 patients withdrew prematurely due to major side-effects: five with rapidly rising serum creatinine; three with intercurrent infection; and two with incontrollable hypertension. Nine of these 10 patients had FSGS.

Long-term tolerance

Renal

Renal tolerance was assessed by comparison of the pre-CyA and endpoint serum creatinine, and the initial and final histologies in patients treated for at least six months. Initial mean serum creatinine was 96.5 ± 42.4 μmol/l (range 49–210 μmol/l) and, at the final evaluation, 96.6 ± 43.6 μmol/l (range 50–239 μmol/l).

Repeat biopsies were carried out in 36 cases, 25 of whom had an initial diagnosis of MCD. In eight patients, lesions of FSGS became apparent, accompanied by moderate-to-severe interstitial fibrosis. In two cases who progressed to FSGS and who initially were diagnosed as MCD, interstitial or vascular lesions were already present on the initial biopsy. In the other 11 patients, the inital diagnosis was FSGS, and interstitial and/or vascular lesions were already present in 10 of them before CyA treatment. On repeat biopsy, both glomerular and interstitial/vascular lesions had become clearly more severe.

Non-renal

The only late withdrawals not due to treatment failure or renal side-effects as described above were three patients with malignancy, discovered after more than a year of CyA treatment. One was a 62-year-old man with FSGS who achieved partial remission with CyA. He had previously received several courses of various immunosuppressive regimens, including cytotoxic drugs, over several years. After 13 months of CyA treatment, squamous cell lung carcinoma was discovered and the patient died of metastases after surgery. The second late withdrawal was a 60-year-old woman who was found to have pelvic carcinoma (presumably endocervical) after 14 months of CyA treatment and who died shortly thereafter. In both cases (especially in this age group), an association between malignancy and CyA treatment cannot be ruled out.

Finally, a 22-year-old man with MCD was found to have Hodgkin's lymphoma. On the basis of various lines of argument, the investigators in charge of this patient concluded that the nephrotic syndrome had probably heralded the Hodgkin's disease rather than favoring the hypothesis of lymphoma complicating immunosuppression [Fouque et al. 1990].

Discussion

Since 1949, the treatment of idiopathic nephrotic syndrome has rested on steroids and, in cases of failure to respond, on alkylating agents (or, rarely, purine analogues) [Meyrier and Simon 1988]. With such therapies, the nephrologist must essentially weigh up the complications of nephrosis against the complications of the treatment in managing the patient. In this respect, CyA is no exception. Therefore, its value in the treatment of nephrotic syndrome must be evaluated in terms of both efficacy and tolerance.

Efficacy

Is CyA an advance in the treatment of adult nephrosis? The answer is yes, and the data in support of this have been consistent. Most of the patients included in our study were considered failures or, in some instances, had a contraindication to conventional treatments. Approximately half had already been unsuccessfully treated with steroids as well as alkylating agents and, in some instances, purine analogues. This indicates that CyA is not just another immunosuppressive agent but, in the treatment of nephrotic syndrome, is endowed with a mode of action distinct from those of cyclophosphamide, chlorambucil and azathioprine.

What is this mode of action? The currently accepted hypothesis is that MCD is due to lymphokine(s) secretion by activated T cells; the trigger is, as yet, not known [Lagrue et al. 1975, Levin et al. 1985, Meyrier et al. 1986, Ooi et al. 1974, Shalhoub 1974]. Impairment of lymphokine secretion by CyA has been amply documented [Borel 1991]. On this basis, remission of nephrotic proteinuria is likely to be more specific with CyA than with alkylating agents, which indiscriminately alter the DNA of virtually all cells in the body, thus leading to the attendant hazards of such cytotoxicity.

On the other hand, CyA exerts non-specific vasoconstrictive effects on renal circulation [Puschett et al. 1990], and it can be argued [Zietse et al. 1989] that the disappearance of proteinuria with CyA treatment is mostly due to vasoconstriction and functional renal insufficieny, and may even be the forerunner of further vascular and interstitial damage. This may indeed be the case when CyA only decreases, rather than eliminates, proteinuria while renal function declines and blood pressure rises. In other words, so-called partial remission may, in such cases, be attributable to a non-immunological side-effect of the drug. However, this is not tenable in cases where: 1. Cyclosporin A induces complete remission with the total elimination of proteinuria; 2. Renal function remains stable; and 3. Remission is delayed after starting treatment and relapse of proteinuria does not occur until several weeks after stopping treatment. Such a beneficial and specific effect of CyA is particularly seen in steroid-dependent MCD which represents the best indication for CyA of the various forms and etiologies of idiopathic nephrotic syndrome [Meyrier 1989].

Another difference between CyA and alkylating agents is the frequently observed CyA dependency, manifested by relapse on dose-tapering or stopping of CyA treatment [Meyrier 1989]. This phenomenon suggests that CyA inhibits, rather than cures, the process(es) responsible for the massive proteinuria of nephrotic syndrome. The drawback of CyA dependency is that the majority of patients in remission must remain under continuous treatment. Conversely, the advantages of CyA are that it has a very limited potential to encourage opportunistic infections and that it has no toxic effect on the germinal line.

Tolerance

Does the risk-benefit ratio warrant the paradoxical prescription of a potentially nephrotoxic drug in renal disease? In our overall experience, as with that of others [Clasen et al. 1988], renal function remained remarkably stable in cases of CyA-induced complete remission (virtually all patients with MCD). In contrast, the glomerular filtration rate (GFR) declined in treatment failures (mostly those with FSGS). However, whether treatment was a success or failure was determined within a mean period of 10 weeks, with a maximum time of six months. Therefore, in cases of treatment failure, the drug can be stopped early enough to entail no significant insult to the renal tissue. Furthermore, the cases involving deterioration of renal function were almost invariably those with glomerular lesions of FSGS (usually steroid-resistant). Moreover, in most of these patients, pre-CyA renal biopsy had already disclosed vascular and/or interstitial lesions which could not be ascribed to CyA.

The question of whether these lesions worsen because of CyA or because it is an expression of the natural course of the primary renal disease is unsettled. However, the experience acquired in other indications, particularly renal transplantation, suggests that the nephrotoxic potential of CyA is influenced by preexisting renal lesions [Mihatsch et al. 1988, Puschett et al. 1990], thus indicating the importance of careful examination of the renal biopsy – carried out as recently as possible – before deciding to embark on CyA treatment. The presence of conspicuous interstitial lesions should be a strong argument against use of this regimen.

However, pediatricians have observed long-term renal lesions on repeat biopsies, even when the initial biopsy was considered normal [Niaudet 1991]. Therefore, in adults, despite the overall good renal tolerance of CyA, it was deemed advisable to carry out a repeat renal biopsy after a maximum of one year of treatment before continuing, or not, with the regimen. This policy not only permitted the detection of interstitial lesions, but also allowed a second examination of the glomerular histology. Indeed, there were some cases of failure or sluggish partial remission in which the repeat biopsy disclosed FSGS, although the preinclusion biopsy had shown only minimal glomerular changes.

Cyclosporin A was well tolerated, not only because of the relatively low dose used, but also due to careful initial monitoring of whole-blood trough levels [Moyer et al. 1988]. There were cases wherein the initial dosage of 5 mg/kg/day induced unpredictable rises in the 12-hour post-dose trough levels – to more than 800 ng/ml. In such instances, rapid titration was required to maintain whole-blood levels at less than 500 ng/ml. The most important measure was the meticulous monitoring of serum creatinine levels with immediate dosage reduction whenever serum creatinine increased by more than 30% over the patient's own baseline values.

These precautions emphasize that the safe use of CyA in the treatment of idiopathic NS largely rests on the commitment and expertise of the medical team. Experience has taught us that CyA should not be prescribed indiscriminately in each and every form of steroid-resistant nephrosis; its successful use depends equally on correct indication, meticulous surveillance and early discontinuation in cases of failure.

In conclusion, CyA represents a major advance in the treatment of those patients who have idiopathic NS with contraindications to, and failure or severe complications with the conventional modes of therapy.

REFERENCES

Borel JF 1991 Mechanism of action of cyclosporin A and rationale for use in nephrotic syndrome. Clin Nephrol (this supplement)

Brodehl J, Brandis M, Helmchen U, Hoyer PF, Burghard R, Ehrich JHH et al. 1988 Cyclosporin A treatment in children with minimal-change nephrotic syndrome and focal-segmental glomerulosclerosis. Klin Wochenschr *66:* 1126–1137

Cameron JS 1987 The nephrotic syndrome and its complications. Am J Kidney Dis *10:* 167–171

Capodicasa G, DeSanto NG, Nuzzi F, Giordano C 1986 Cyclosporin A in nephrotic syndrome of childhood. Intern J Pediatr Nephrol *7:* 69–72

Clasen A, Kindler J, Mihatsch MJ, Sieberth HG 1988 Long-term treatment of minimal-change nephrotic syndrome with cyclosporin: A control biopsy study. Nephrol Dial Transplant *3:* 733–737

Fouque D, Laville M, Colon S, French M, Berger F, Labeeuw M et al. 1990 Cyclosporin A-sensitive nephrotic syndrome preceding Hodgkin's disease by 32 months. Clin Nephrol *34:* 1–4

Hoyer PF, Krull F, Brodehl J 1986 Cyclosporin in frequently relapsing minimal-change nephrotic syndrome. Lancet *ii:* 335

Korbet SM, Schwartz MM, Lewis EJ 1986 The prognosis of focal-segmental glomerular sclerosis of adulthood. Medicine *65:* 304–311

Lagrue G, Laurent J, Belghiti D, Robeva R 1986 Cyclosporin and idiopathic nephrotic syndrome. Lancet *ii:* 692–693

Lagrue G, Xheneumont S, Branellec A, Hirbec G, Weil B 1975 Lymphokines and nephrotic syndrome. Lancet *i:* 271

Levin M, Smith C, Walter MSD, Gascoine P, Barratt TM 1985 Steroid-responsive nephrotic syndrome; a generalised disorder of membrane negative charge. Lancet *ii:* 239–242

Meyrier A 1989 Treatment of glomerular disease with cyclosporin A. Nephrol Dial Transplant *4:* 923–931

Meyrier A, Collaborative Group of the Société de Néphrologie 1989 Cyclosporin in the treatment of nephrosis – Minimal-change disease and focal segmental glomerulosclerosis. Am J Nephrol *9 (Suppl 1):* 65–71

Meyrier A, Simon P 1988 Treatment of corticoresistant idiopathic nephrotic syndrome in the adult: Minimal-change disease and focal-segmental glomerulosclerosis. In: *Grünfeld JP* (ed) Advances in Nephrology. Yearbook, Chicago, pp 127–150

Meyrier A, Simon P, Perret G, Condamin-Meyrier MC 1986 Remission of idiopathic nephrotic syndrome after treatment with cyclosporin A. Br Med J *292:* 789–792

Mihatsch MJ, Steiner K, Abeywickrama KH, Landmann J, Thiel G 1988 Risk factors for the development of chronic cyclosporin nephrotoxicity. Clin Nephrol *29:* 165–175

Moyer TP, Post GR, Sterioff S, Anderson CF 1988 Cyclosporine nephrotoxicity is minimized by adjusting dosage on the basis of drug concentration in blood. Mayo Clin. Proc. *63:* 241–247

Niaudet P 1991 Treatment of nephrotic syndrome with cyclosporin A in children. Clin Nephrol (this supplement)

Niaudet P, Tete MJ, Broyer M, Habib R 1988 Cyclosporin and childhood idiopathic nephrosis. Transpl Proc *20 (Suppl 4):* 265–268

Ooi BS, Orlina AR, Masmaitis L 1974 Lymphocytotoxins in primary renal disease. Lancet *ii:* 1348–1350

Puschett JB, Greenberg A, Holley J, McCauley J 1990 The spectrum of cyclosporin nephrotoxicity. Am J Nephrol *10:* 296–309

Shalhoub R 1974 Pathogenesis of lipoid nephrosis: a disorder of T-cell function. Lancet *ii:* 556–560

Tejani A, Butt K, Trachtman H, Suthantiran M, Rosenthal C, Khawar M 1988 Cyclosporin A-induced remission of relapsing nephrotic syndrome in children. Kidney Int *33:* 729–734

Zietse R, Wenting GJ, Kramer P, Mulder P, Schalekamp MA, Weimar W 1989 Contrasting response to cyclosporin in refractory nephrotic syndrome. Clin Nephrol *31:* 22–25

Clinical Nephrology, Vol. 35, Suppl. No. 1–1991 (pp. S. 43–47)

Current status of cyclosporin A in the treatment of membranous, IgA and membranoproliferative glomerulonephritis

D. C. Cattran

CCRW3-884, 101 College Street, Toronto, Ontario M5G 1L7, Canada

Abstract. The effects of cyclosporin A (CyA, Sandimmun®) therapy in various types of primary glomerular diseases are discussed. In membranous nephropathy, the data strongly support a positive effect in this disorder, but there have been no control trials thus far to indicate the risk-benefit ratio, the need for adjunctive therapy such as steroids, or what to expect in terms of time to response or duration of response. The risk of nephrotoxicity needs to be more precisely quantitated both from a functional and pathological perspective. Proper prospective controlled trials are needed to establish the safety and efficacy of CyA in this disease. In both IgA and membranoproliferative glomerulonephritis, the data are more sparse. Although isolated studies have suggested a benefit in both these categories, the risks are also evident and more careful pilot studies are indicated before any further conclusions can be drawn as regards the use of this agent in these disorders.

Key words: cyclosporin A – glomerulonephritis – membranous nephropathy

Introduction

This article is a summary of the current status of cyclosporin A (CyA, Sandimmun®) treatment in patients with membranous glomerulonephropathy, and IgA and membranoproliferative glomerulonephritis.

Membranous glomerulonephropathy

Idiopathic membranous glomerulonephropathy is characterized by a wide variability in the natural history with most reports indicating a 25 to 35% spontaneous remission rate. This factor, combined with the lack of correlation between both initial renal function, and pathological grade and outcome, should be borne in mind when assessing the results of any therapeutic intervention.

Zietse et al. [1988, 1989] described a non-randomized study which included six patients with biopsy-proven membranous nephropathy. All had stopped taking any other immunosuppressive therapy for at least four weeks prior to starting CyA treatment, and all had previously demonstrated resistance to steroid therapy and/or other cytotoxic agents, although the doses and duration of these treatments were not specified. At entry, creatinine clearance levels averaged 82 ml/min (range 32–132 ml/min) and urine protein averaged 12 g/day (range 3.6–16.9 g). Cyclosporin A was given at 6 mg/kg and plasma trough levels of the drug were between 50 and 150 ng/ml. The duration of treatment was 12 weeks.

All six patients responded, as defined by a reduction of proteinuria of ≥30% compared to entry values and, although five patients showed a decrease in creatinine clearance, this averaged only 6% by the end of the trial period. Fractional excretion of protein [proteinuria corrected for changes in glomerular filtration rate (GFR)] also improved significantly ($p < 0.05$). A major concern, however, was that all six patients returned to their pre-CyA treatment levels of proteinuria within one month of discontinuation of the drug. Another concern, on review of this study, was their definition of response, as none of the patients became protein-free. It is debatable whether a 30% reduction of proteinuria is sufficient to justify exposing patients to such a potentially nephrotoxic agent as CyA, particularly if the drug is required on a permanent basis, as suggested by the 100% relapse rate on discontinuation.

An earlier study by De Santo et al. [1987] reported on the effects of CyA plus prednisone in five patients who had failed to respond to the Italian protocol of alternating monthly treatment with steroid and chlorambucil over a six-month period [Ponticelli et al. 1989]. After a two-month wash-out

Reprint requests to Dr. D. C. Cattran.

period during which no therapy was given, CyA plus steroids were initiated and maintained for six months. Four of the five patients had a complete remission between the second and fourth months of treatment which was maintained during the rest of the therapeutic trial. It has been suggested that the no-drug wash-out period was of insufficient duration, and that the response may have been due to the earlier drug regimen; however, the response was dramatic and was temporally related to CyA therapy.

A more recent letter in the Lancet by Rostoker et al. [1989] reported a retrospective, uncontrolled study of 15 patients with longstanding steroid- or steroid/cytotoxic-resistant membranous nephropathy who were treated with CyA. The mean duration of their disease prior to entry was 68 months (range 9–360 months). The initial treatment regimen was CyA at 4 mg/kg for a maximum of six months. If a response was noted, as defined by proteinuria of less than 2 g/day, the dose of the drug was reduced. The five patients who received this treatment all responded within two to four months, but all relapsed on rapid withdrawal of the drug.

The authors therefore changed the protocol for the next 12 patients (including two of the above-mentioned group). Although the same initial dose of CyA was used, they aimed for a whole blood trough level [by monoclonal radioimmunoassay (RIA)] of 100 to 250 ng/ml, which was to be maintained for four to six months, and followed by slow tapering of the drug dose over the next eight to 12 months. Five patients showed no significant improvement in proteinuria, three had a partial remission (<2 g/day) and four had a complete remission (<0.2 g/day). There was no clear predictor of the type of response, but those patients with Stage 3 lesions on histopathology and those whose initial creatinine values were >150 μmol/l were more frequently among the non-responders. Results indicated that there was no deterioration in renal function in any of the patients, including those in the non-responsive group.

In our initial report [Cattran et al. 1985] of patients with membranous nephropathy, CyA treatment appeared to have a beneficial effect. The patients were selected not only on the basis of steroid resistance but, in addition, all had impaired creatinine clearance at entry; furthermore, during the four-month run-in period when no therapy was allowed, patients had to demonstrate a progressive deterioration in renal function.

These patients were treated with CyA for a minimum of four months and were followed for an average of 12 months. Nine of our initial 20 patients with primary glomerular disease had the membranous variant. At entry, these nine had creatinine clearances ranging from 26 to 65 ml/min and their mean proteinuria was 7.4 g/day (range 3–19 g/day). The mean decline in creatinine clearance during their four-month pre-drug period was 20 ml/min. One of the patterns observed before, during and after CyA treatment is shown in Figure 1. In this example, there appeared to be a prolonged benefit in both proteinuria and rate of decline in creatinine clearance after the drug was withdrawn compared with the pre-drug period.

Figure 2 shows a different pattern of only a partial initial response in proteinuria and complete relapse on withdrawal of the drug. The creatinine

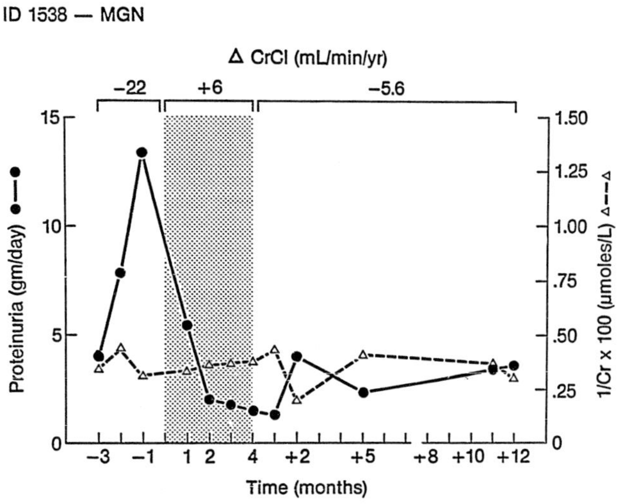

Fig. 1 Effects on proteinuria and creatinine clearance suggest a benefit with CyA lasting 12 months after discontinuation of the drug.

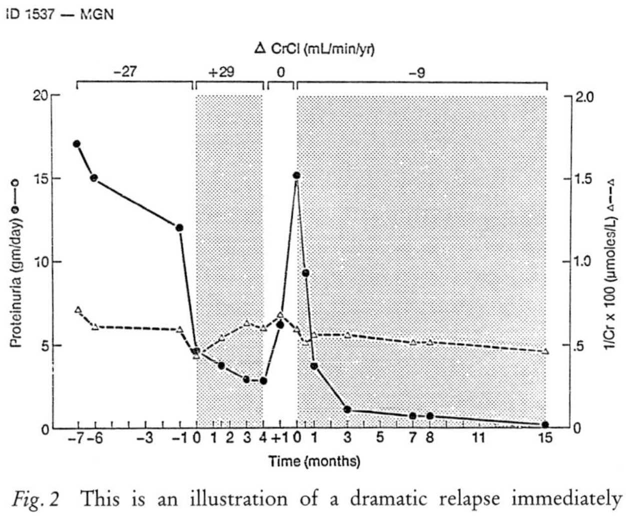

Fig. 2 This is an illustration of a dramatic relapse immediately post-CyA. The improvement when CyA was reintroduced indicates that some patients may require constant drug treatment in order to maintain a response.

clearance improved during the CyA treatment, but returned toward baseline after stopping the drug. When treatment was reinstated, the patient had a complete remission in proteinuria, but the creatinine clearance continued to deteriorate slowly. This may suggest that, even among patients who have a complete remission, there may be problems; for example, the nephrotoxicity of CyA may cause a further decline in renal function, or the drug-related improvement in proteinuria may not be parallelled by stabilization of the GFR.

Overall, after 16 weeks of treatment with CyA, the patients with membranous nephropathy showed an improvement in proteinuria, creatinine clearance and fractional excretion of protein (Table 1). Adverse effects were as expected except in the patients who had the most severe disease (the lowest creatinine clearance at entry). These patients had more gastrointestinal symptoms with CyA than the average reported in the literature. All of these patients were followed for up to 26 months, and stabilization of long-term function, in terms of both creatinine clearance (Table 2) and fractional excretion of protein (Table 3), has been observed in these patients compared to their pre-CyA treatment values.

In summary, these studies suggest that, in patients with membranous glomerulonephropathy, there may be a benefit to short-term CyA therapy. Adverse effects, however, appeared more frequently in patients whose creatinine clearance rates were <40 ml/min, and the rate of relapse within six months of stopping the drug has been reported to be as high as 100%. However, although these uncontrolled short-term trials suggest that CyA may benefit patients with severe membranous nephropathy, the true response rate, optimal dose and duration of action of the drug, and the risk-benefit ratio of this therapy require the results of well designed prospective, randomized trials.

IgA nephropathy

IgA nephropathy is now the most commonly recognized type of nephritis which progresses to end-stage renal disease [D'Amico 1987]. The only published randomized, placebo-controlled trial of this disease using CyA was reported by Lai et al. [1988]. All of these patients had significant disease at entry, as demonstrated by an average creatinine clearance of 77 ml/min and a urinary protein excretion rate of at least 1.5 g/day. Other characteristics of this group of patients at entry are shown in Table 4.

Cyclosporin A was given for 12 weeks, starting at a dose of 5 mg/kg; no other immunosuppressive therapy was allowed. The target trough level, as measured in plasma by polyclonal RIA, was 50 to 100 ng/ml. The mean values of both plasma IgA and proteinuria were significantly improved in the treatment group, but creatinine clearance worsened when compared with controls. In all 10 of the patients receiving treatment, creatinine clearance values returned to baseline within two months of discontinuation of the therapy (Figure 3); however, one patient

Table 1 Changes in parameters of renal function in nine patients with severe membranous nephropathy after 16 weeks of cyclosporin A

	Mean	Range	p value
Proteinuria (g/day)	−4.5	−10.9 to −1.5	0.001
Creatinine clearance (ml/s/mo)	0.03	0.12 to −0.01	0.009
$\frac{\text{Proteinuria}}{\text{(Creatinine clearance + 1)}}$	−2.6	−8.4 to −0.3	0.007

Table 2 Changes in creatinine clearance (ml/s/mo) during and after cyclosporin A treatment of membranous nephropathy

	Mean ± SD	Significance
Before treatment	−0.044 ± 0.02	** (vs. during); * (vs. total follow-up)
During treatment	0.01 ± 0.02	**
One year post-treatment	−0.002 ± 0.02	
During total follow-up (mean 26 mo)	−0.007 ± 0.009	*

* p = 0.005; ** p = 0.013

Table 3 Changes in fractional excretion[a] of protein with cyclosporin A treatment of membranous nephropathy

	Mean ± SD	Significance
Before treatment	6.83 ± 2.8	** (vs. during); *** (vs. after)
During treatment	4.21 ± 2.9	**
After treatment	4.69 ± 3.15	***

** p = 0.013; *** p = 0.04

[a] $\frac{\text{Protein (g/day)}}{\text{[Creatinine clearance (ml/s) + 1]}}$

Table 4 Patient characteristics on entry into a trial of cyclosporin A treatment of IgA nephropathy

	Cyclosporin A	Placebo
Gender (male/female)	4/8	7/5
Plasma creatinine (μmol/l)	99 ± 12	118 ± 9
Corrected creatinine clearance (ml/min)	77 ± 6	70 ± 3
Proteinuria (g/day)	3.9 ± 0.8	2.5 ± 0.2
Serum IgA (g/l)	3.9 ± 0.3	2.9 ± 0.3

Lai et al. 1988

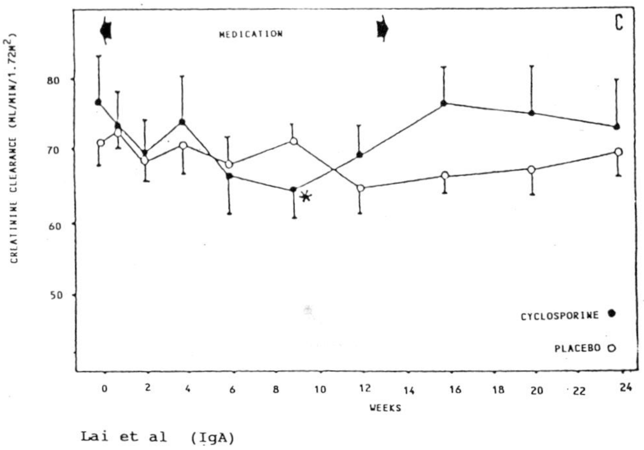

Fig. 3 Cyclosporin A significantly depresses creatinine clearance, but the effect is small and reversible after the drug is discontinued. With permission from Lai et al. 1988 Transpl. Proc. *20 (Suppl 4)*: 297–303

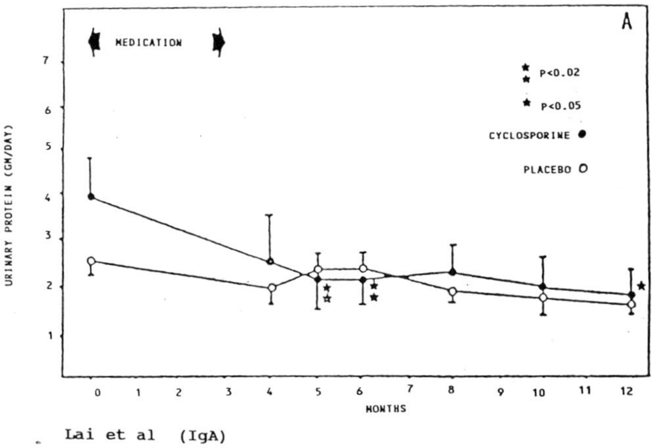

Fig. 4 Effect of CyA (cyclosporine) in patients with severe IgA nephropathy. The beneficial effects on proteinuria are apparent for up to six months post-therapy. With permission from Lai et al. 1988 Transpl. Proc. *20 (Suppl 4)*: 297–303

in the CyA-treated group subsequently developed malignant hypertension and progressed to end-stage renal failure over a period of several months. There was a significant improvement in proteinuria in the CyA group, as measured at six and 12 months post-drug compared with pretreatment levels, although there were no significant differences between the control and treatment groups at these time points (Figure 4).

The results of this study suggest the possibility that the potential of CyA to induce nephrotoxicity or hypertension may be higher in IgA nephropathy in comparison to other types of glomerulonephritis, but this may be counterbalanced by a long-term benefit in control of proteinuria. However, the value of CyA in IgA nephropathy is as yet not confirmed and further evaluations, probably in the form of pilot studies in patients with established severe disease, are required.

Membranoproliferative glomerulonephritis

Published studies of CyA in the treatment of membranoproliferative or mesangiocapillary glomerulonephritis have been sparse. The therapeutic rationale, especially in Type I disease, appears to be that the disorder is immune complex-mediated. The largest study so far was carried out by Erbay et al. [1988]. Twelve of the 16 patients in their report had membranoproliferative histopathology. Although it was stated that all of these patients were steroid- and cytostatic-resistant, the dosage and duration of their therapies were not included. The mean creatinine value in the total study population at entry was 1.2 ± 0.6 mg/dl with a creatinine clearance of 93 ± 33 ml/min. All patients were nephrotic with a mean protein excretion rate of 7.7 g/day.

The pertinent results from the entire study population are shown in Table 5. The report states that the two patients who showed no improvement with CyA had membranoproliferative glomerulonephritis, suggesting that the other 10 responded to treatment. Three patients developed hepatotoxicity with elevated liver enzymes, but all returned to normal levels on reduction of the CyA dose. The mean levels of serum creatinine and creatinine clearance did not deteriorate during the study period (Table 5). It must be recognized, however, that these values are not the ideal

Table 5 Results of a trial (n = 16) of cyclosporin A treatment including 12 patients with membranoproliferative glomerulonephropathy

Day	Proteinuria (g/day)	BUN (mg/dl)	Serum creatinine (mg/dl)	Creatinine clearance (ml/min)
Initial	7.7 ± 4.2	21.9 ± 13	1.2 ± 0.6	93.1 ± 33
15	3.7 ± 2.8	22.7 ± 10	1.3 ± 0.2	80.1 ± 34
30	1.6 ± 1.5	20.1 ± 8	1.0 ± 0.1	103 ± 22
60	1.0 ± 1.1	18.6 ± 7	1.1 ± 0.2	98 ± 27
90	0.8 ± 0.8	17.7 ± 5	1.0 ± 0.3	101 ± 31

Erbay et al. 1988

parameters for following renal function, especially in patients who are receiving potentially nephrotoxic agents such as CyA [Myers et al. 1988]. Furthermore, the study was neither randomized nor controlled, and patients continued to take prednisone during the entire 90-day study period. In addition, it is not possible to assess the duration of response, as all patients were given cyclophosphamide immediately upon completion of the course of CyA. Only a few other isolated case reports are available regarding CyA treatment of this type of glomerulonephritis; any conclusions concerning the effects of CyA in this disorder must await further studies.

REFERENCES

Cattran DC, Dossetor J, Halloran PF 1985 Cyclosporin in glomerulonephritis – a pilot study. In: *Schindler R (ed).* Cyclosporin in autoimmune disease. Springer-Verlag, Heidelberg, p 311

D'Amico G 1987 The commonest glomerulonephritis in the world: IgA nephropathy. Q J Med *245:* 709

DeSanto NG, Capodicasa G, Giordano C 1987 Treatment of idiopathic membranous nephropathy unresponsive to methylprednisolone and chlorambucil with cyclosporin. Am J Nephrol *7:* 74

Erbay B, Karatan O, Duman N, Ertug AE 1988 The effect of cyclosporine in idiopathic nephrotic syndrome resistant to immunosuppressive therapy. Transpl Proc *20 (Suppl 4):* 292

Lai KN, Mac-Moune Lai F, Vallance-Owen J 1988 A short-term controlled trial of cyclosporine A in IgA nephropathy. Transpl Proc *20 (Suppl 4):* 297

Myers BD, Sibley R, Newton L, Tomlanovich SJ, Boshkos C, Stinson E et al 1988 The long-term course of cyclosporin-associated chronic nephropathy. Kidney Int *33:* 590

Ponticelli C, Zucchelli P, Passerini P, Cagnoli L, Cesana B, Pozzi et al 1989 A randomized trial of methylprednisolone and chlorambucil in idiopathic membranous nephropathy. N Engl J Med *320:* 7

Rostoker G, Ben Maadi A, Sandreux T, Chevet D, Lang P, Toro L et al 1989 Cyclosporin in idiopathic steroid-resistant membranous glomerulonephritis. Lancet *ii:* 975

Zietse R, Wenting GJ, Kramer P, Mulder P, Schalekamp MA, Weimar W 1989 Contrasting response to cyclosporin in refactory nephrotic syndrome. Clin Nephrol *31:* 22

Zietse R, Wenting GJ, Kramer P, Schalekamp MADH, Weimar W 1988 Fractional excretion of protein: a marker of the efficacy of cyclosporin A treatment in nephrotic syndrome. Trans Proc *20:* 280

Clinical Nephrology, Vol. 35, Suppl. No. 1 – 1991 (pp. S. 48 – 60)

Safety and tolerability of cyclosporin A (Sandimmun®) in idiopathic nephrotic syndrome

Collaborative Study Group of Sandimmun® in Nephrotic Syndrome*

Department of Clinical Research/Immunology, Sandoz Pharma AG, CH-4002 Basel, Switzerland

Abstract. The safety and tolerability of cyclosporin A (CyA, Sandimmun®) in idiopathic nephrotic syndrome were analyzed in 661 patients enrolled in 10 clinical studies. The majority had minimal-change nephropathy (MCN, 34%) or focal-segmental glomerulosclerosis (FSGS, 33%). The safety experience covered 435 patient years of CyA exposure. The initial CyA dose averaged 5 mg/kg/day in adults and 6 mg/kg/day in children, and was further titrated according to efficacy or adverse reactions. Relevant CyA-induced renal dysfunction occurred almost exclusively in patients (mostly FSGS) who had abnormal baseline renal function. Renal tolerability was better in patients who had complete remission of nephrotic syndrome than in those who did not respond to treatment. However, in the latter, the risk was still relatively low if CyA treatment was stopped after three to four months of treatment. Sixty-nine patients had a renal biopsy performed after one to three years of continuous CyA therapy, and CyA-associated nephropathy, especially interstitial fibrosis, was seen in a few of these patients. Kidney biopsies may therefore be advisable in MCN patients treated successfully for one to two years and in whom further CyA therapy is indicated. Hypertension occurred in approximately 10% and was usually well controlled with conventional antihypertensive therapy. There were a few infectious complications, but the course of these was not unusual. Malignancies developed in five patients, including Hodgkin's lymphoma in two. Overall, adverse reactions resulted in CyA treatment discontinuation in 7.4% of patients, half of them because of renal dysfunction.

Key words: cyclosporin A – minimal-change disease – focal-segmental glomerulosclerosis – renal dysfunction – kidney biopsies – adverse reactions

Introduction

The efficacy of cyclosporin A (CyA, Sandimmun®) in inducing remission of idiopathic nephrotic syndrome has been demonstrated in several studies, as reviewed in Meyrier [1989]. In steroid-dependent nephrotic syndrome – mostly minimal-change nephropathy (MCN) – CyA induced a complete remission in 70 to 80% of the patients. With steroid-resistant disease – mostly focal-segmental glomerulosclerosis (FSGS) – complete remission was obtained in approximately 20%. Remission occurred quickly, the majority within one or two months of starting treatment. However, the majority of patients relapsed within a few months of stopping CyA treatment. Hence, continuous therapy appears to be necessary for maintaining remission, at least during the first year of treatment.

The safety experience in single studies was usually limited to a relatively small number of patients, as only those who were steroid-resistant and steroid-dependent were treated with CyA. Larger populations than those available in single studies were deemed necessary for assessment of the adverse reactions, especially those of low incidence, and for defining subgroups of patients with special risk.

The aim of this work was to analyze the adverse reactions in a population pooled from several studies and corresponding to an overall sample of 435 patient years. Because of the risk of CyA-associated kidney abnormalities, special attention was paid to the evaluation of kidney function and morphology.

Reprint requests to Dr. G. Feutren.

*Writing committee: B. von Graffenried, G. Feutren, W. Schiess, C. Rohrmann (Sandoz Pharma Ltd., Basle); J. Brodehl (Hanover); A. Meyrier (Bobigny); P. Niaudet (Paris); C. Ponticelli (Milan). Data management/statistics: E. Nüesch, C. Leininger, C. Miller (Sandoz Pharma Ltd., Basle).

Patients and methods

Patients

Since 1985, there have been five non-controlled and four randomized controlled studies, sponsored and monitored by Sandoz, including 270 patients treated with CyA. In addition to patients studied within these prospectively planned trials, other patients have been treated without the involvement of Sandoz. The results of these patients, however, have been presented at meetings and published, but often without details of the individual patients [Meyrier 1989]. In order to enlarge the database for a structured analysis, details of 391 patients were collected retrospectively (termed "Retrospective Data Collection"). In total, safety data for CyA were available in 661 patients treated in 132 centers worldwide. Of these patients, 398 were adults (aged >15 years) and 263 were children. The safety experience covers 435 patient years of CyA exposure, including 165 patients treated for 7 to 12 months, 68 patients for between one and two years, and 24 patients for more than two years (Table 1).

Table 1 Duration of exposure to cyclosporin A

Duration of exposure	No. of patients	No. of patients (cumulative)
0 – 3 months	173	661
> 3 – 6 months	231	488
> 6 – 12 months	165	257
> 12 – 14 months	68	92
≥ 24 months	24	24

The characteristics of the patient population are summarized in Table 2. The majority had either MCN (n = 225, 34%) or FSGS (n = 215, 33%). Patients included in the study were those considered to be most in need of alternative treatment. With few exceptions, the patients were either steroid-resistant or, if steroid-responsive, steroid-dependent (or frequently relapsing) with signs of steroid toxicity. Many had already received cytostatic agents and either had subsequently relapsed or had been unsuccessfully treated.

Table 2 Patient's characteristics

	All patients	Adults	Children
Number of patients	661	398	263
Age (years)	24.7 ± 0.7	34.8 ± 0.8	6.9 ± 0.3
Male/female (n)[1]	432/226	253/142	179/84
Disease duration (mo)	47 ± 2	48 ± 3	45 ± 3
Steroid sensitivity			
Steroid-resistant	357	247	110
Steroid-dependent	205	92	113
Frequent relapsers	61	24	37
No previous steroids	38	35	3
Histology			
Focal-segmental glomerulosclerosis	215	131	84
Minimal-change nephropathy	225	112	113
Membranous GN**	77	74	3
Mesangioproliferative GN	43	23	20
Mesangiocapillary GN	28	23	5
IgM nephropathy	11	4	7
Lupus nephritis	6	6	0
Alport's syndrome	3	3	0
IgA nephropathy	12	12	0
No biopsy done	41	10	31
Pretreated with cytostatics	318	166	152

[1] Gender of three patients not documented.

GN = glomerulonephritis.

All figures are mean ± SEM.

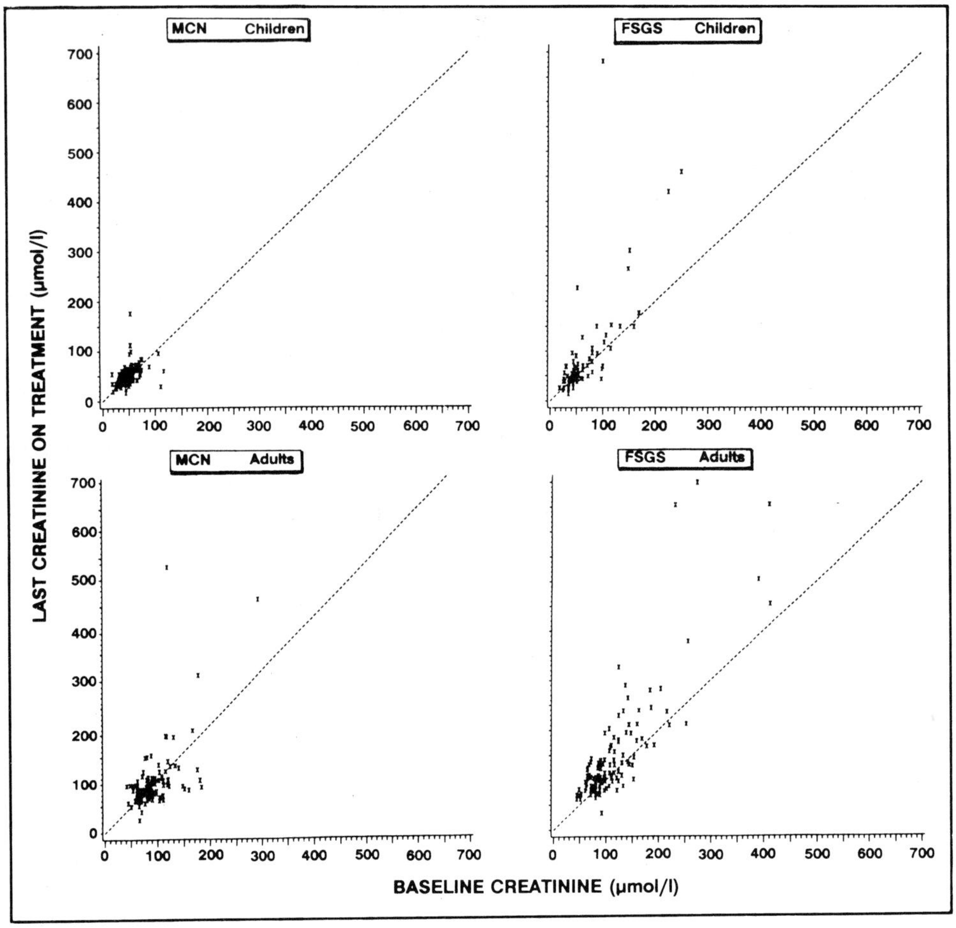

Fig. 1. Serum creatinine (µmol/l): value at baseline vs last value with CyA treatment in children or adults with minimal-change disease (MCN) or focal-segmental glomerulosclerosis (FSGS). Each symbol represents one patient.

Treatment

The initial CyA doses were usually 4 to 6 mg/kg/day. The idea was to apply the highest CyA dose which, in other diseases, had been shown to be well tolerated, and to taper the doses, depending on adverse events or, in some studies, excessive CyA levels. This led to mean CyA doses up to remission or failure of 4.8 mg/kg/day (MCN) and 4.6 mg/kg/day (FSGS) in adults, and 6.1 mg/kg/day (MCN) and 5.9 mg/kg/day (FSGS) in children. The lowest effective dose was estimated from the dose at which patients relapsed during a systematic tapering-off procedure. On average, this was 2.5 mg/kg/day, although this varied considerably.

Cyclosporin A levels

Trough (pre-dose) CyA concentration was measured by non-specific polyclonal radioimmunoassay [Donatsch et al. 1981] in whole blood (n = 178) or in plasma (n = 90). A small number of patients had CyA concentration measured by high-performance liquid chromatography (HPLC) and were not included in this analysis. Specific monoclonal radioimmunoassay was not yet available at the time of the clinical trials included in this evaluation.

Results

Renal adverse events

Cyclosporin A treatment was discontinued in 25 patients (3.8% of all CyA-treated patients) because of renal dysfunction. Most of these patients had steroid-resistant nephrotic syndrome, mainly FSGS. Their most important risk factor was abnormal renal function before starting CyA.

Renal function

The main parameter for evaluating renal function was serum creatinine, which was regularly measured in all patients. In carefully studied CyA-treated patients with autoimmune diseases, it was shown that changes in serum creatinine correlate well with changes in the glomerular filtration rate [Mason and Moore 1990]. Conclusions on renal function based on serum creatinine are therefore valid as long as patients do not have severely impaired renal function. Nevertheless, creatinine clearance was also measured in some patients.

Minimal-change nephropathy (MCN)

In MCN, the highest creatinine level ever measured was moderately, but significantly, increased in both children and adults, in comparison to baseline. The last value measured at the end of CyA therapy was not, however, significantly increased above baseline for adults (Figure 1). In children, this increase was slight (median increase 6.7%), but significant and, at that time, only a few patients had values outside of the normal range. The results in the subgroup with at least 12 months of therapy were very similar. The last creatinine value in these patients treated with long-term CyA was virtually unchanged in adults, and only insignificantly higher than at baseline in children. This slight increase in creatinine in children may be related to the natural increase of plasma creatinine in growing children which is approximately 5% per year [Schwartz et al. 1976].

In the subgroup of patients whose creatinine values were available after stopping treatment, renal dysfunction was reversible in most (Figure 2), and there were no significant differences from baseline. There were, however, three patients who developed end-stage renal failure despite stopping CyA; these patients are included in Figure 2. All three were considered cases of steroid-resistant MCN which may, in fact, have been FSGS that was misdiagnosed at biopsy. Cyclosporin A had no beneficial effects on the nephrotic syndrome in any of these patients.

Focal-segmental glomerulosclerosis (FSGS)

In FSGS, the changes were more pronounced in both children and adults. At the end of therapy (before stopping CyA), the median percentage

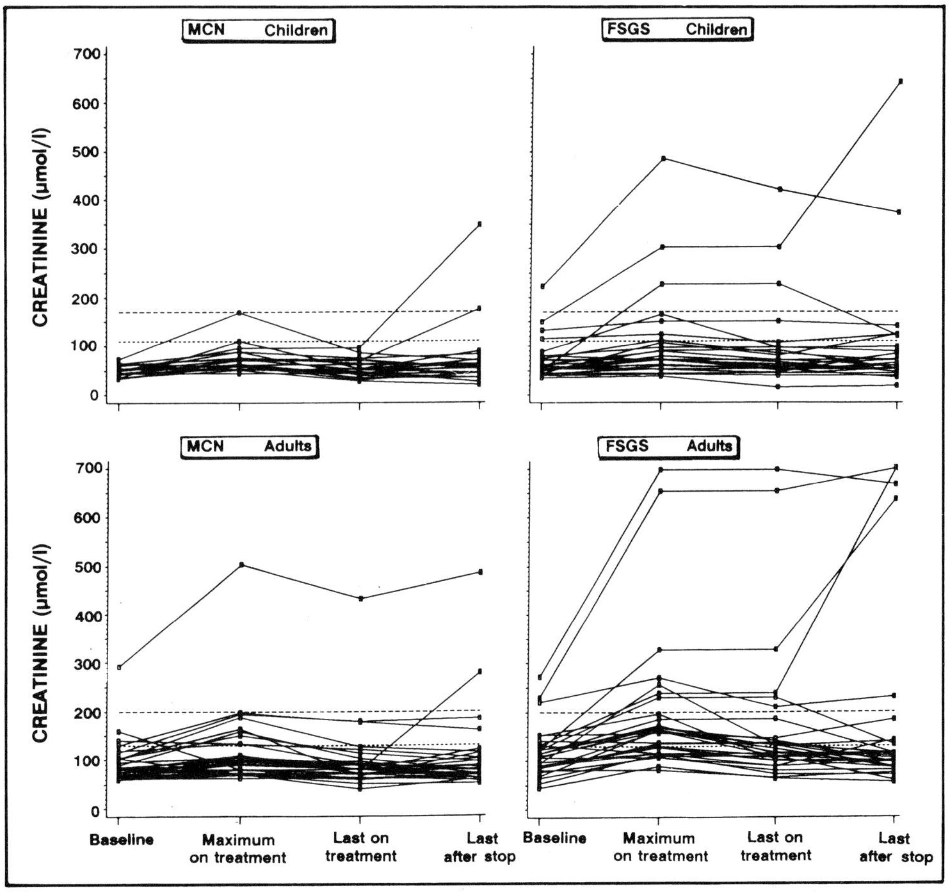

Fig. 2. Time course of serum creatinine before, during and after CyA treatment in individual patients: children or adults with minimal-change disease (MCN) or focal-segmental glomerulosclerosis (FSGS). Dotted lines represent the upper limit of normal values and the limit for clinically relevant abnormalities.

Table 3 Creatinine clearance (ml/min/1.73 m^2) with cyclosporin A treatment

	Baseline	Last on treatment
Minimal-change nephropathy		
Children (n = 36)	131 ± 9	135 ± 9
Adults (n = 36)	92 ± 10	96 ± 9
Focal-segmental glomerulosclerosis		
Children (n = 37)	114 ± 7	96 ± 6
Adults (n = 46)	88 ± 7	73 ± 6

Values are mean ± SEM.

Table 4 Serum creatinine (μmol/l) at baseline and at outcome: complete remissions vs failures

	Minimal-change nephropathy; Baseline/outcome	Focal-segmental glomerulosclerosis; Baseline/outcome
Children		
Complete remission	50.0/ 53.0 (25 – 116)/(25 – 80)	51.4/ 44.6 (30 – 100)/(27 – 71)
Failure	44.2/ 47.5 (18 – 73)/(27 – 177)	44.2/ 70.0 (25 – 248)/(15 – 683)
Adults		
Complete remission	84.0/ 82.0 (53 – 217)/(53 – 157)	88.7/ 97.6 (44 – 411)/(44 – 369)
Failure	97.0/100.0 (44 – 914)/(50 – 997)	106.1/120.5 (44 – 409)/(63 – 699)

Values are median (range).

increase of creatinine over baseline was 16% in children and 22% in adults (Figure 1). These increases were significant. The proportion of patients with creatinine values outside the normal range at the end of therapy was higher than that at baseline. For adults, for instance, a creatinine value above 130 μmol/l was detected in 25% of FSGS patients at baseline and in 42% at the end of CyA therapy. The data in the subset of patients treated for one year or more were similar. After stopping CyA, there was a decrease in creatinine in most patients, but the difference from baseline was no longer significant in children and of only borderline significance in adults (Figure 2). As can be seen from Figures 1 and 2, however, six patients developed end-stage renal failure. Most of these patients had abnormal renal function at baseline, which is a definite risk factor for the development of further functional impairment, be it CyA-induced, an expression of disease progression, or a combination of both. None of these six patients had a remission of nephrotic syndrome with CyA.

Membranous and other glomerulonephritides

The results in membranous glomerulonephritis (MGN) are very similar to those in FSGS. There were significant increases of creatinine over baseline at the end of therapy (median percentage increase of 18%), and reversibility was incomplete in those who had abnormal baseline creatinine values. The creatinine changes in the other histologies (mainly mesangioproliferative and mesangiocapillary glomerulonephritides) were less pronounced. The increases over baseline at the end of therapy were not significant and not clinically relevant. After stopping CyA, reversibility was seen in all but three patients, all of whom showed increased values before starting therapy.

Creatinine clearance

The results of the creatinine clearance measurements are shown in Table 3. They are similar to the serum creatinine data described above.

Abnormal serum creatinine at baseline

In 38 patients (44 treatment courses), serum creatinine was clearly abnormal at baseline (>200 μmol/l in adults, n = 30; <140 μmol/l in children, n = 8). Seventeen (45%) of these patients had FSGS, three (8%) were MCN, including one patient with IgM nephropathy, 10 (26%) had MGN, three (8%) had mesangioproliferative glomerulonephritis and five (13%) had mesangiocapillary glomerulonephritis. In 19 (43%) of the 44 treatment courses, substantial increases in serum creatinine until outcome were observed. The outcomes of these 19 courses were 11 failures, five partial remissions and three complete remissions. In the 25 treatment courses without relevant increases in creatinine, the outcomes were five failures, 16 partial remissions and four complete remissions.

Abnormal renal function before starting CyA treatment was the most important risk factor for development of end-stage renal failure (whether due to CyA, to the natural course of the disease, or to a combination of these). This was especially true in patients with steroid-resistant nephrotic syndrome (mostly FSGS).

Changes in serum creatinine and outcome

The proportion of patients with relevant increases in creatinine was higher in those who failed compared with those who entered remission, espe-

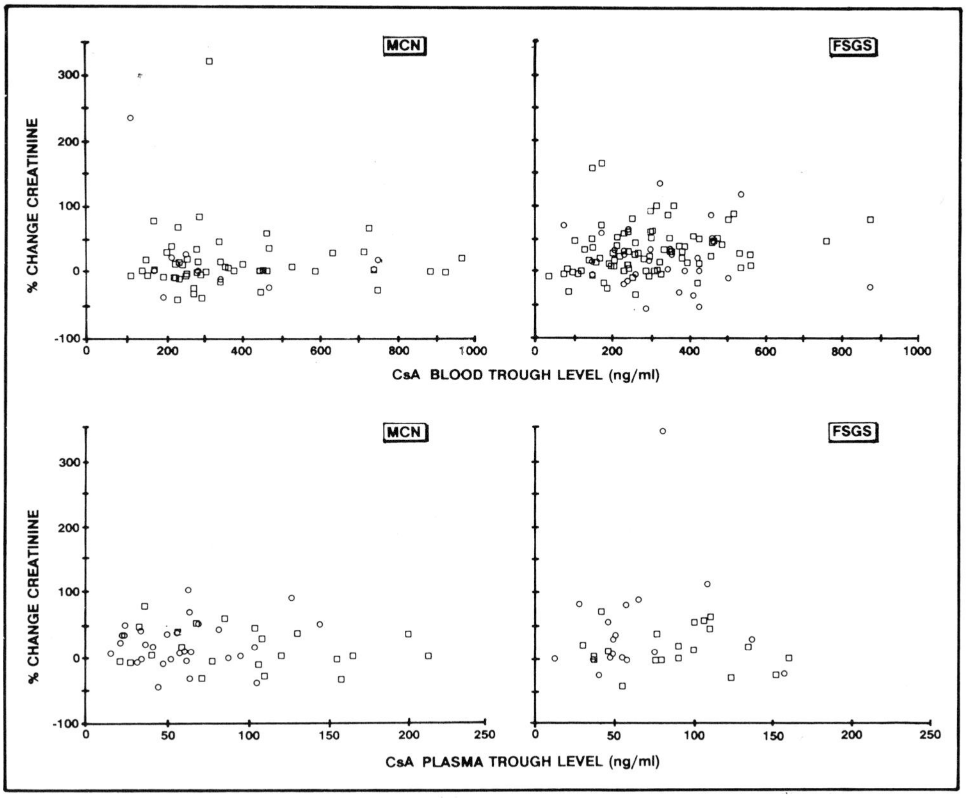

Fig. 3. Percent change of serum creatinine from baseline to outcome vs CyA trough level (mean until outcome) measured in whole blood (upper) or plasma (lower) by non-specific polyclonal radioimmunoassay in patients with minimal-change disease (MCN) or focal-segmental glomerulosclerosis (FSGS). Each symbol represents one patient: circle = child, square = adult.

cially in FSGS. Similarly, at outcome, no significant increase of serum creatinine was detected in the group of patients in complete remission in contrast to those who had failed with CyA (Table 4).

Serum creatinine and CyA blood levels

The results of repeated CyA trough level measurements were available for 268 patients. Trough levels were measured in whole blood (n = 178) and in serum plasma (n = 90). There was no relevant or significant correlation between the mean CyA levels until outcome and changes in serum creatinine at outcome. This applied to all histologies, for adults and children, and measurements in whole blood or plasma. The absence of a relationship is shown graphically for whole blood and plasma levels in MCN and FSGS (Figure 3).

Kidney biopsies

Methodology

Documentation of renal biopsies performed after CyA therapy was available for 69 patients (68% children). On the basis of biopsies taken at an average of 17 months before starting CyA treatment, patients were diagnosed as 50 MCN, 17 FSGS and two MGN (Table 5). Detailed reports of biopsies performed before starting treatment were available in 52 patients, and these were compared with the post-CyA biopsies.

Table 5 Characteristics of patients with renal biopsy after cyclosporin A (CyA) treatment

	All	MCN	FSGS	MGN
n	69	50	17	2
Adults/children	22/47	16/34	5/12	1/1
Male/female (n)	46/23	33/17	12/5	1/1
Steroid sensitivity (n)				
Resistant	23	8	13	2
Dependent	45	42	3	
Not determined	1		1	
CyA dosage (mg/kg/day)[1]				
Initial	5.1 ± 0.2	5.4 ± 0.2	4.5 ± 0.4	2.5; 6.0
Mean till biopsy	5.4 ± 0.3	5.4 ± 0.3	5.4 ± 0.6	8.6; 6.2

MCN = minimal-change nephropathy; FSGS = focal-segmental glomerulosclerosis.
[1] Mean ± SEM.

For most of these patients, reports by the local pathologist were available. In addition, many biopsies were analyzed by a review pathologist (Professor M. Mihatsch, Institute of Pathology, Basle, Switzerland) who has evaluated, according to a standardized procedure, a large number of biopsies of CyA-treated patients (renal transplant and non-renal transplant) over recent years.

Minimal-change nephropathy

In seven (14%) MCN patients, FSGS was diagnosed in the post-CyA biopsies. The mean interval between the pre- and post-CyA biopsies in these patients was 82 months (range 14–108 months) and was substantially longer than in patients who remained MCN. In all of these cases, minimal or slight interstitial fibrosis was present in the post-CyA biopsies for the first time.

No relevant increase in obsolescent glomeruli and no significant arteriolopathy were observed. Interstitial fibrosis and tubular atrophy of moderate intensity were detected in three (6%) patients, in one of whom the post-CyA diagnosis and changed from MCN to FSGS, which may explain the new occurrence of interstitial fibrosis. In none was arteriolopathy apparent. It is also important to note that "moderate" and "severe" fibrosis was also seen in pre-CyA biopsies, in one patient each, respectively. Tubular calcifications were observed in two post-CyA biopsies.

Focal-segmental glomerulosclerosis

There was a slight increase in the proportion of obsolescent glomeruli after, in comparison to before, CyA. Eleven of the 12 patients on pre-CyA biopsy had less than 10% obsolescent glomeruli compared with 10 out of 16 on post-CyA biopsy. This is compatible with natural progression of the disease during the interval between biopsies (mean 27 months). There was, however, no increase in the number of glomeruli showing FSGS.

In two (12%) patients, moderate arteriolopathy was recorded. Their biopsies also showed slight or moderate interstitial fibrosis and tubular atrophy.

The frequency of slight and moderate interstitial fibrosis, and tubular atrophy among post-CyA biopsies was higher than in those taken before starting treatment (71% vs 33%), and tubular calcifications were observed in two post-CyA biopsies. In an additional case, tubular calcification was already apparent on the pretreatment biopsy. As tubulointerstitial changes in FSGS are known to progress over time, interpretation of the possible pathogenetic role of CyA is difficult.

Membranous glomerulonephritis

No relevant changes were seen in the biopsies of the two patients who had MGN.

Hypertension

Elevated blood pressure

Elevated blood pressure was defined according to the World Health Organization (WHO) in adults [Gross et al. 1984], and the British Hypertension Society in children [de Swiet et al. 1989]. Hypertension was identified when antihypertensive therapy was being given, or when patients not receiving antihypertensive therapy showed persistently elevated blood pressure, or when hypertension was mentioned by the investigator as a concomitant disease.

Preexisting hypertension

Preexisting hypertension was observed in 163 patients and elevated blood pressure at baseline in an additional 65 patients out of the 661 treated with CyA. The incidence of definite preexisting hypertension was lower in children (14.8%) than in adults (31.2%), and higher in patients with FSGS, MGN and other histologies compared with MCN.

On starting CyA treatment, 108 of the 228 patients with either preexisting hypertension or elevated blood pressure were already receiving antihypertensive therapy whereas antihypertensive therapy was begun in 38 patients after starting CyA. In 154 (68%) of the 228 patients, blood pressure was adequately controlled. There was no difference in rates of adequate control of hypertension among the different histologies: MCN (71%); FSGS (63.3%); MGN (73.3%); other (64.9%). Four patients discontinued CyA because of worsening of preexisting hypertension.

Newly developed hypertension

Hypertension developed in 59 patients (8.9% of all CyA-treated patients). The incidence of definite newly developed hypertension was lower in children ≤6 years (4.6%) than in older children (8.6%) or adults (10.1%). Patients with FSGS had a higher risk of developing definite hypertension (12%) compared

Table 6 Malignancies with cyclosporin A therapy (n = 661)

Tumor	Age (years)	Renal disease	Duration of NS before CyA (mo)	CyA dose (mg/kg/day)	CyA duration (mo)
Hodgkin's lymphoma	21	FSGS	10	5	22
Hodgkin's lymphoma	20	FSGS	2	4 – 5	3
Renal adenocarcinoma	38	MGN	6	4 – 6	16
Bronchus squamous cell carcinoma	61	FSGS	60	5 – 1	12
Uterus adenocarcinoma[1]	63	MCN	–	3 – 5	16

NS = nephrotic syndrome, FSGS = focal-segmental glomerulosclerosis, MGN = membranous glomerulonephritis, MCN = minimal-change nephropathy.
[1]Spontaneous report: Patient not included among the 661.

Table 7 Incidence of clinical adverse reactions (%)

Adverse event	Total (n = 661)	Clinical trials (n = 270)	Retrospective Data Collection (n = 391)
Hypertrichosis	18	31	9
Gingival hyperplasia	16	27	8
Gastrointestinal symptoms	11	18	6
Hypertension	9	14	5
Paresthesias	6	12	2
Tremor	4	6	3
Headache	3	6	2

to patients with other histologies. Antihypertensive therapy was started in 42 patients, and blood pressure adequately controlled in 26 (62%). Cyclosporin A therapy was not discontinued or temporarily interrupted because of newly occurring hypertension.

Infections

In 51 patients, including 14 children (7.7% of all CyA-treated patients), 58 infectious complications arose during treatment. Ten cases were rated as severe, 28 as moderate, 19 as mild and, in one patient, no severity rating was given. Severe infections occurred predominantly in steroid-resistant patients who concomitantly received steroids. Of the 58 infections, 17 were caused by a virus and nine were bacterial. The etiology of the other infections was unknown. Therapy was discontinued because of an infectious complication in seven patients, five of whom had a serious infection: tuberculosis (n = 2), pulmonary abscess, pneumonia and meningitis. All recovered after specific therapy.

Malignancies

Malignancies occurred during CyA treatment in five patients: Hodgkin's lymphoma (n = 2), and bronchial, renal and uterine carcinomas (Table 6). All had steroid-resistant disease and CyA had a satisfactory therapeutic effect on the nephrotic syndrome. The patient with carcinoma of the bronchus had several risk factors for developing cancer: nicotine abuse, previous history of tuberculosis and previous therapy with cytotoxic agents. In the two patients with Hodgkin's lymphoma, remission of the nephrotic syndrome was maintained despite discontinuation of CyA treatment after remission of the malignancy had been obtained by chemotherapy.

One patient (63 years old), who had received three courses of chlorambucil over a period of 20 years because of MCN, developed a refractory anemia (pre-leukemic syndrome) after a total of 31 months of CyA therapy (maximum dose of 4.8 mg/kg/day).

Other clinical adverse reactions

Adverse events (Table 7) included the most typical and well-known clinical adverse reactions of CyA, such as hypertrichosis, gingival hyperplasia, hypertension, paresthesia, gastrointestinal complaints, tremor and headache. The incidence of adverse reactions was much higher in formal clinical trials than in the Retrospective Data Collection, perhaps because adverse reactions were systematically searched for in the former whereas only those that were prominent were recorded in the latter.

Table 8 Treatment discontinuation because of adverse events (n = 661)

Reason for discontinuation	n (%)
Renal dysfunction	25 (3.7)
Infection	7 (1.1)
Gastrointestinal system	5 (0.8)
Malignancies	5 (0.8)
Hypertension	4 (0.6)
Myocardial infarction	1 (0.2)
Hypertrichosis	1 (0.2)
Total	48 (7.3)

Laboratory safety data

There was a significant fall in hemoglobin within the first month, which did not progress thereafter. The extent of change was small (mean fall in hemoglobin 0.4 mmol/l). There were no patients in whom the degree of anemia was regarded as sufficiently clinically relevant to merit either discontinuing CyA or reducing the dosage.

A small, but significant, increase of serum bilirubin was seen within the first month. Mean values remained well within the normal range, and there was no progressive change. The percentage of abnormally high values increased from 0.5% to a maximum of 4%. Clinically relevant increases necessitating a change in CyA dose occurred in five patients. In all five, bilirubin normalized after reduction of dose. No patient discontinued CyA because of bilirubin increase. There were no systematic changes in serum glutamic-oxaloacetic transaminase (SGOT) or serum glutamic-pyruvic transaminase (SGPT).

Relatively marked increases were seen in alkaline phosphatase. The effect was apparent after the first month and reached a maximum at month 6. The percentage of patients with abnormally high values increased from 11% at baseline to 35% at month 6. Mean values remained within the normal range. The clinical relevance is unclear. The effect may be partly explained by increased alkaline phosphatase of bone origin associated with "catching-up" growth in children as a result of remission of the nephrotic syndrome and "weaning" from steroids.

Mild, but significant, increases in serum potassium and uric acid, and a decrease in serum magnesium were observed, presumably as an expression of the effect of CyA on renal tubular function. The relevance of these non-progressive changes, which remained mostly within the normal range is doubtful; no cases of gout were reported, for instance. Cyclosporin A was discontinued in one patient because of hyperkalemia and, in another patient, the CyA dose was reduced because of hyperuricemia.

Treatment discontinuations because of adverse reactions

A total of 48 patients stopped taking CyA (7.3% of all CyA-treated patients) because of adverse reactions. The reasons for discontinuation are summarized in Table 8, the most common being renal dysfunction.

An additional 13 patients interrupted CyA treatment temporarily for one to three months because of infection (n = 7), renal dysfunction (n = 4) and nausea (n = 2).

Discussion

In general, the adverse events with CyA in nephrotic syndrome were similar to those in all non-transplant indications. These have recently been summarized in the context of a general review of CyA experience in autoimmune disease [von Graffenried et al. 1989]. The most frequent adverse events in studies of nephrotic syndrome were renal dysfunction, hypertrichosis, gingival hyperplasia, tremor and paresthesia, gastrointestinal symptoms (nausea, loss of appetite) and hypertension. The most relevant events are those which lead to discontinuation of therapy. This was the case in 48 patients (7.3% of all CyA-treated patients), and the most frequent reason for discontinuation was renal dysfunction (n = 25).

As regards CyA in nephrotic syndrome, renal dysfunction and hypertension are of special concern. The adverse effects of CyA on the kidney affect both function and structure [Mason 1990 a, b]. Dose-dependent and reversible reduction of glomerular filtration rate is due to arteriolar vasoconstriction and results in a rise of serum creatinine and urea. Tubular dysfunction is expressed primarily as a decrease in serum magnesium, and a mild increase in serum potassium and uric acid.

Arteriolopathy, striped interstitial fibrosis and tubular atrophy have been described as structural changes (CyA nephropathy) which may be irreversible [Mihatsch et al. 1983, Palestine et al. 1986, Mihatsch et al. 1988]. The incidence and risk factors of CyA nephropathy have been analyzed in 192 patients treated with CyA for various autoimmune diseases not affecting the kidney and who had a kidney biopsy while taking CyA [Feutren 1990]. The overall conclusion was that the risk of CyA nephropathy is dose-dependent and closely correlated with the extent of the functional (reversible) renal dysfunction as measured by the increase of serum creatinine. The risk of developing unacceptable structural changes can be minimized by limiting the initial CyA dosage to a maximum of 5 mg/kg/day (in adults) and by titrating the dosage according to serum creatinine, for example, to reduce the dose by 0.5 to 1 mg/kg/day whenever serum creatinine increases by more than 30% over the patient's own baseline value.

Patients with nephrotic syndrome are far from ideal subjects for a study of the renal adverse effects of CyA. Changes in renal function may have multiple causes. Hypoalbuminemia and edema can affect glomerular perfusion, and the status of nephrotic syndrome (remission/relapse) will therefore influence serum creatinine. Concomitant therapy, such as with diuretics and antihypertensives, may also influence the levels of creatinine, potassium, magnesium and uric acid. During long-term therapy, changes in renal function cannot be automatically attributed by CyA, but may be due to the natural progression of the basic disease. The interpretation of changes in renal biopsies can also be difficult, for example, in FSGS, in which interstitial fibrosis may be CyA-induced as well as a result of the disease [Churg et al. 1970, Cameron 1979].

Analyses of renal function have been carried out mainly on the basis of serum creatinine. In most studies, creatinine clearance was also measured, although less often; the clearance results were in concordance with the serum creatinine levels. Indeed, a strong correlation has been found between changes in serum creatinine and inverse changes in glomerular filtration rates in carefully studied CyA-treated patients with autoimmune diseases [Mason and Moore 1990]. Hence, measuring changes in serum creatinine gives an appropriate estimate of changes in glomerular filtration, at least in patients who do not have severely impaired renal function.

The main conclusion of the various analyses on renal safety of CyA in nephrotic syndrome is that, in the vast majority of patients, the benefit achieved with CyA is obtained without the development of unacceptable impairment of renal function. In patients with normal baseline renal function who achieved remission, serum creatinine remained unchanged. There was a trend towards an increased serum creatinine in patients not entering remission, especially with FSGS. This is not to suggest that CyA treatment is contraindicated in patients with FSGS or, more generally, with steroid-resistant disease; a substantial proportion of such patients benefited from CyA and achieved remission. However, because steroid-resistant patients have a greater risk of developing renal dysfunction, CyA treatment should be stopped in the absence of satisfactory clinical response, which can be assessed after not more than three or four months.

In most patients, renal dysfunction was reversible, as is the usual pattern in all autoimmune diseases. There is, however, one group of patients with nephrotic syndrome at an increased risk of developing excessive, and sometimes irreversible, creatinine increase, namely, those with impaired renal function at baseline. Most of the patients in whom CyA had to be discontinued because of renal adverse reaction (n = 25) belonged to this category. The majority were FSGS patients at an advanced stage of the disease. In some patients, renal dysfunction was reversible but, in nine, renal function worsened progressively after stopping CyA. It is impossible to know to what extent CyA was responsible for this unsatisfactory outcome, and to what extent it represents the natural course of the disease [Cameron 1979, Glassock et al. 1988]. The message, however, is clear: patients with impaired renal function are at an increase risk of further deterioration. If it is decided to treat such patients, the initial dose should be low (2.5 mg/kg/day), and should be slowly increased only if frequent measurements of creatinine (initially weekly, then bi-weekly and monthly if stable) do not indicate a problem.

Perhaps more important than the data on creatinine are the results of renal biopsies performed in 69 patients after a mean exposure of 16 months to CyA. In MCN, typical CyA arteriolopathy was not detected. Three patients (6%), however, developed moderate interstitial fibrosis and tubular atrophy. This has also been described in some patients undergoing long-term treatment [Niaudet et al. 1990]. These changes may be CyA-related, but that they may represent the natural course of the disease cannot be excluded. In this respect, it is important to note that, in seven MCN patients, FSGS was diagnosed in the post-CyA biopsies. The number of obsolescent glomeruli did not increase to any relevant extent, and serum creatinine at the time of biopsy was not increased over baseline. If at any time during CyA treatment there were episodes of renal dysfunction, these did not reflect structural changes and thus were reversible. The interpretation of biopsies in FSGS is more difficult as tubulointerstitial lesions are frequently seen in FSGS, and the disease is progressive in nature [Churg et al. 1970]. Doses and blood levels of CyA did not correlate with the extent of histological changes. The main predictive factor for the development of CyA nephropathy in patients with autoimmune diseases other than nephrotic syndrome is the extent of the presumably CyA-induced and reversible creatinine increase [Feutren 1990]. Such a relationship cannot be shown in patients with nephrotic syndrome as creatinine increase can have, as described earlier, many causes other than CyA. In order to be safe, it may be advisable to perform a biopsy after one to two years of continuous CyA therapy in MCN patients in whom the clinical assessment of risk/benefit justifies continuation of therapy.

With any type of immunosuppressant drug, the question of increased incidence of infections and malignancies will arise [Penn 1988]. Unlike steroids, CyA does not interfere with the neutrophil or "natural-killer" functions [Janco and English 1983, Kasaian and Biron 1990]. This feature may explain why infections are not an especial problem in nephrotic syndrome, nor in other autoimmune diseases treated with CyA [Feutren et al. 1986, The Multiple Sclerosis Study Group 1990]. In all cases, either spontaneous recovery was observed, or CyA was discontinued (in a total of seven patients), and/or adequate antibacterial or antiviral therapy permitted rapid control of the adverse events.

Malignancies occurred in five patients during CyA treatment, corresponding to a crude incidence of 0.6%. On the one hand, an increased incidence of malignancies, especially skin cancer and lymphoma, has been reported during immunosuppressive therapy, including CyA [Cockburn and Krupp 1989]. On the other hand, there is an association between nephrotic syndrome and malignant neoplasia [Glassock et al. 1986].

Different mechanisms have been suggested: the malignancy may induce glomerular damage and nephrotic syndrome; the renal disease may lead to the emergence of malignant cell clones; treatment with cytostatic agents may induce malignancy through direct mutagenic effects. The latter mechanism may have been operative in one patient, a smoker, who developed carcinoma of the bronchus, and in another patient who had a pre-leukemic syndrome, as the development of leukemias is known to occur years after chlorambucil treatment [Cameron 1977]. Membranous glomerulonephritis (MGN) is the most common morphological pattern observed in patients who develop nephrotic syndrome in association with carcinomas [Eagen and Lewis 1977]. Such was the case in a patient (taking CyA) whose renal adenocarcinoma was diagnosed 22 months after the onset of nephrotic syndrome. Although it was a long interval, it does not preclude the possibility that the tumor preceded the MGN.

Association of Hodgkin's lymphoma and nephrotic syndrome have been described, mostly with MCN, but also with FSGS, as in the case of two patients treated with CyA. The incidence of nephrotic syndrome in Hodgkin's lymphoma is approximately 10 times that in non-Hodgkin's lymphoma [Ma et al. 1978]. Nephrotic syndrome associated with Hodgkin's lymphoma is usually steroid-resistant and remits when the tumor is removed. This was the case for these patients in whom the nephrotic syndrome remained in remission after successful therapy of Hodgkin's disease. Although it is clear from the above that the type of tumors observed in CyA-treated patients is not unusual in nephrotic syndrome, it is not possible to draw any conclusions as to their frequency or the possible contribution of immunosuppression by CyA to the development of these malignancies. The other adverse events have been similar to those previously reported by CyA-treated patients [von Graffenried et al. 1989].

In summary, the adverse reactions observed with CyA in nephrotic syndrome appear to be manageable as long as a few simple rules are adhered to: 1. The dose should not exceed 5 mg/kg/day in adults or 6 mg/kg/day in children; 2. Doses should be reduced by 0.5 to 1.0 mg/kg/day whenever serum creatinine consistently increases by more than 30% over the patient's own baseline value; 3. The initial dose should not be greater than 2.5 mg/kg/day in patients with abnormal baseline creatinine; 4. Treatment should not be administered for more than three months in the absence of satisfactory clinical response.

REFERENCES

Cameron JS 1977 Chlorambucil and leukemia. N Engl J Med *296:* 1065

Cameron JS 1979 The natural history of glomerulonephritis. In: *Black D, Jones NF* (eds) Renal disease, 4th ed. Blackwell Scientific Proceedings, Oxford, pp 329–382

Churg J, Habib R, White RHR 1970 Pathology of the nephrotic syndrome in children. A report for the international study of kidney disease in children. Lancet *i:* 1299–1302

Cockburn ITR, Krupp P 1989 The risk of neoplasms in patients treated with cyclosporine A. J Autoimmun *2:* 723–731

de Swiet M, Dillon JJ, Littler W, O'Brien EO, Padfield PL, Petrie JC 1989 Measurement of blood pressure in children. Br Med J *299:* 497

Donatsch P, Abisch E, Homberger M, Traber R, Trapp M, Voges R 1981 A radioimmunoassay to measure cyclosporin A in plasma and serum samples. J Immunoassay *2:* 19–32

Eagen JW, Lewis EJ 1977 Glomerulopathies of neoplasia. Kidney Int *11:* 297–309

Feutren G 1990 Risk factors associated with cyclosporine A nephropathy in patients treated for autoimmune diseases. J Am Soc Nephrol *1:* 610

Feutren G, Papoz L, Assan R, et al. 1986 Cyclosporin increases the rate and length of remissions in insulin-dependent diabetes of recent onset. Lancet *ii:* 119–124

Glassock RJ, Adler SG, Ward HJ, Cohen AH 1986 Primary glomerular disease. In: *Brenner B, Rector F* (eds) The kidney. WB Saunders, Philadelphia, pp 929–1013

Glassock RJ, Adler SG, Ward HJ, Cohen AH 1988 Primary glomerular diseases. In: *Brenner B, Rector F* (eds) The kidney, 3rd ed. WB Saunders, Philadelphia, pp 961–1013

Graffenried B von, Friend D, Shand N, Schiess W, Timonen P 1989 Cyclosporin A (Sandimmun®) in autoimmune disorder: In: *Thomson AW* (ed) Cyclosporin, mode of action and clinical applications. Kluwer Academic Publishers, Boston, pp 213–251

Gross F, Pisa Z, Strasser T, Zanchetti A 1984 Management of arterial hypertension. World Health Organization, Geneva

Janco RL, English D 1983 Cyclosporine and human neutrophil function. Transplantation *35:* 501–503

Kasaian MT, Biron CA 1990 Cyclosporin A inhibition of Interleukin 2 gene expression, but not natural killer cell proliferation, after interferon induction in vivo. J Exp Med *171:* 745–762

Ma KW, Golbus SM, Kaufman R, Staley N, Londer H, Brown DC 1978 Glomerulonephritis with Hodgkin's disease and herpes zoster. Arch Pathol Lab Med *102:* 527–529

Mason J 1990 a Renal side-effects of cyclosporin A. Br J Dermatol *122 (Suppl 36): 71–77*

Mason J 1990 b The pathophysiology of Sandimmune (cyclosporine) in man and animals. Pediatr Nephrol *4:* 554–574

Mason J, Moore LC 1990 Indirect assessment of renal dysfunction in patients taking cyclosporin A for autoimmune diseases. Br J Dermatol *122 (Suppl 36):* 79–84

Meyrier A 1989 Treatment of glomerular disease with cyclosporin A. Nephrol Dial Transpl *4:* 923–931

Mihatsch MJ, Bach JF, Coovadia HM, et al. 1988 Cyclosporine-associated nephropathy in patients with autoimmune diseases. Klin Wochenschr *66:* 43–47

Mihatsch MJ, Thiel G, Spichtin HP, et al. 1983 Morphological findings with kidney transplants after treatment with cyclosporine. Transpl Proc *4 (Suppl 1):* 2821–2835

Niaudet P, Broyer M, Habib R 1990 Evaluation of nephrotoxicity by sequential biopsies in 38 children with idiopathic nephrosis treated with cyclosporin A (CsA). Kidney Int *37:* 260

Palestine AG, Austin HA, Balow JE, et al. 1986 Renal histopathologic alterations in patients treated with cyclosporine for uveitis. N Engl J Med *314:* 1293–1298

Penn I 1988 Cancer is a long-term hazard of immunosuppressive therapy. J Autoimmun *1:* 545–558

Schwartz GJ, Haycock GB, Spitzer A 1976 Plasma creatinine and urea concentration in children: Normal values for age and sex. J Pediatr *88:* 828–830

The Multiple Sclerosis Study Group 1990 Efficacy and toxicity of cyclosporine in chronic progressive multiple sclerosis: a randomized, double-blinded, placebo-controlled clinical trial. Ann Neurol *27:* 591–605

Participants

Collaborative group of the Société Française de Néphrologie:
A Meyrier (Bobigny, Coordinator), PY Zech (Lyon), D Cordonnier (Grenoble), P Simon (Saint-Brieuc), JM Suc (Toulouse), P Duhoux (Luxembourg), J Guenel (Nantes), F Schillinger (Troyes), P Vanhille (Valenciennes), M Legrain (Paris), JP Ryckelynck (Caen), G Touchard (Poitiers), JL Bacri (Dieppe), P Bagros (Tours), D Chevet (Rennes), P Deteix (Clermont-Ferrand), B François (Pierre-Bénite), D Fries (Le Kremlin-Bicêtre), P Gautier (Metz), JJ Haultier (Merlebach), JM Idatte (Paris), H Jahn (Strasbourg), G Janin (Maçon), O Kourilsky (Evry), P Lebon (Le Mans), P Lesavre (Paris), J Moret (Chambéry), J Potier (Cherbourg), G Rifle (Dijon), JL Tual (Boulogne-Billancourt).

Italian multicenter study group:

C Ponticelli, A Edefonti (Milan, main investigators), G Rizzoni (Rome), R Gusmano (Genoa), P Altieri (Cagliari), V Andreucci (Napoli), G Zacchello (Padova), GA Cinotti (Rome), E Lusvarghi (Modena), L Minetti (Milano), A Castellani (Brescia), P Zuchelli (Bologna), E Imbasciati (Sondrio), F Locatelli (Lecco), R Maiorca (Brescia), G Maschio (Verona), G Mecca (Bergamo).

Study group of the French Club of Pediatric Nephrology:

P Niaudet, M Broyer (Paris, main investigators), L David (Lyon), M Foulard (Lille), H Nivet (Tours), JL André (Vandoeuvre), R Dumas (Montpellier), MT Freycon (Saint-Priest-en-Jarez), C Loirat (Paris), JB Palcoux (Clermont-Ferrand).

Japanese multicenter study group:

S Tojo (Tsukuba, chairman), H Itoh, T Miyahara, T Nagasawa (Tokyo), N Yoshikawa (Kobe), S Maki (Osaka), H Ishikawa (Nara), M Narita (Tsukuba).

Other studies (main investigators):

G Lagrue (Créteil, France), A Tejani (New York, USA), RK Kuehn, J Brodehl (Hanover, Germany), W Schulz (Bamberg, Germany), B Erbay (Ankara, Turkey), W Weimar (Rotterdam, Netherlands), W Clasen (Aachen, Germany), P Sweny (London, UK), K Olgaard (Copenhagen, Denmark), I Simon (Valencia, Spain), JRT Gabriel (London, UK), R Confalonieri (Milan, Italy).

Other investigators:

Australia: JR Burke (Brisbane), AR Clarkson (Adelaide); Austria: P Balcke (Vienna), P Koenig (Innsbruck); Belgium: W Proesmans (Leuven); Canada: J Klassen (Calgary), S O'Regan (Montreal), BT Steele (Hamilton); Germany: B Grabensee (Düsseldorf), K Schaerer (Heidelberg); India: KV Dakshinamurty (Vellore); Netherlands: RJ Hene (Utrecht), BD Wolff (Rotterdam), JP van Hoff (Maastricht); South Africa: HM Coovadia (Durban); Spain: V Gutierrez-Millet, N Gallego, JML Gomez, A Gonzalo, R Muley-Alonso, M Navarro-Torres (Madrid), MA de Frutos Sanz (Malaga), MR Sanchez (Cadiz), M Valles-Prats, L Garcia Garcia, R Poveda, J Aubia, AM Castello, T Gonzales Alverez (Barcelona), J Arrietta

(San Sebastian), S Malapa (Oviedo), JAM Carrasco, D Pons Grau (Valencia); Sweden: AB Bohlin (Huddinge); United Kingdom: AGP Chandler, MA Mansell, A Rees, R Baratt, G Clark, B Hulme, ABD Palmer (London), R Wilkinson (Newcastle), D Adu (Birmingham), GRD Catto (Aberdeen), M Majid (Coventry), PS Williams (Liverpool), FW Ballardie, RJ Postlethwaite (Manchester), M McHugh (Sunderland), AV Murphy, M Boulton-Jones (Glasgow), JR Cove-Smith (Cleveland), P Harrison (Bristol), P Naish (Stoke-on-Trent); Yugoslavia: M Macanovic (Sarajewo).

Trial organization and monitoring (Sandoz):

B von Graffenried, C Miller, W Schiess, C Rohrmann, A Jan ten Tige, G Feutren (Basle, Switzerland), A Lallemand, D Sumar, C Bon, D Bronner (France), G Corbetta, O Della Casa-Alberighi (Italy), H Adam (Germany), T Arvidsson (Sweden), G Berger (Austria), N Børresen (Denmark), J De Juan (Spain), P Dekayser (Belgium), R Dierdorf (CH), G Murphy (Canada), T Poole (UK), D Solbu (Norway), J Stockvis (NL), K Sasaki (Japan).

Final discussion: Summary

The main objective of this discussion was to establish a set of guidelines for the use of cyclosporin A (CyA, Sandimmun®) in idiopathic nephrotic syndrome. It was agreed that the starting dose should not exceed 5 mg/kg/day in adults, but that this problem is more complicated in children. Pediatricians recommended that the dosage be calculated according to body surface area rather than body weight. The initial dose should be 150 mg/m^2/day and the maximum dose should not exceed 200 mg/m^2/day; renal side-effects should then be minimal. In those patients with focal-segmental glomerulosclerosis whose renal biopsies showed tubulointerstitial lesions even before starting CyA therapy, the nephrotoxic effects of CyA may be accentuated.

The importance of measuring blood levels of CyA as part of patient monitoring remained a controversial issue. Some investigators rely more on the CyA dosage than on the blood levels. Examples were given of patients who had had their CyA doses increased to 7–8 mg/kg/day because the blood levels were below the suggested therapeutic level; some of these patients developed unquestionable signs of nephrotoxicity in spite of the low cyclosporinemia. Thus, low blood levels of the drug are not a guarantee against adverse reactions.

On the other hand, the measurement of blood levels offers several advantages. It allows verification of patient compliance to the prescribed therapy, and dosage adjustment when drugs that interfere with the metabolism of CyA are given concomitantly; for example, ketoconazole, erythromycin, particular calcium antagonists and other drugs tend to increase CyA blood levels whereas barbiturates, rifampicin and isoniazid tend to decrease blood levels. The bioavailability of the drug, which may vary considerably from one subject to another, can also be assessed. The final consensus was that both the dosage and the blood levels are important. As a general rule, in cases of high whole blood levels (more than 150–160 ng/ml by the monoclonal specific radioimmunoassay method), it is safer to decrease the CyA dose. Conversely, if blood levels are low, but the dose is over 5 mg/kg/day in adults or 200 mg/m^2/day in children, there is still an increased risk of increasing adverse effects with increasing the dose.

Should CyA be used as monotherapy or in association with corticosteroids? Retrospective cumulative analysis (Sandoz data on file) shows that the combination of CyA with prednisone – even at low doses – appears to improve the chance of remission. It was agreed that the combination of the two drugs was probably more effective than CyA as monotherapy in steroid-resistant patients. In most steroid-dependent patients, CyA alone may be sufficient to maintain remission. Whether to associate the drug with low-dose prednisone (thus allowing a reduction of the CyA dose) or not (thus allowing corticosteroid washout) may depend upon the clinical indications of the patient. For children still in the growing stages who show severe signs of steroid toxicity, the avoidance of corticosteroids should be considered.

There was some debate concerning the optimal indicator of renal function for monitoring the possible development of CyA-related renal toxicity. Some doubts were expressed as to the value of measuring creatinine clearance, as CyA may increase the tubular secretion of creatinine, thus resulting in an overestimation of renal function. However, in a study by Professor Meyrier of patients treated with CyA, a good correlation was found between inulin and creatinine clearances. Professor June Mason has reviewed a series of 140 CyA-treated patients, who had various autoimmune disorders, whose serum creatinine and inulin or DTPA clearances had been measured simultaneously. The results of this analysis showed clearly that measuring changes in serum creatinine is just as good a way of measuring a change in glomerular filtration rate (GFR), provided that the GFR does not decrease by more than 50% of its initial value. Thus, from a practical point of view, repeated measurements of serum creatinine can be considered a reliable indicator of renal function in CyA-treated patients.

When it has been established that serum creatinine has increased in an adult patient, the CyA dose should be reduced. Some investigators suggest dosage decrease in steps of 0.5–1 mg/kg/day. Others recommend greater dosage decreases (30 to 50% reductions, for example). In patients with focal-segmental glomerulosclerosis – in whom a differential diagnosis between CyA toxicity and natural progression of the disease is difficult – it was suggested that CyA treatment be temporarily withheld. A rapid improvement of renal function would indicate CyA toxicity whereas the persistence of renal dysfunction would suggest that either the disease is following its natural course, or the CyA toxicity has resulted in irreversible organic scarring.

The problem of treatment-related toxicity is more complicated in children. Indeed, fluctuations of serum creatinine can spontaneously occur in pediatric patients. Pediatricians conclude that, although serum creatinine clearance can be considered the best available parameters, more sensitive parameters of assessing CyA renal effects should be sought and identified.

Finally, there was much discussion of the need for repeat renal biopsies to monitor the effects of long-term CyA administration. Most investigators recommend a control biopsy after one year of treatment, as a number of patients may show interstitial fibrosis on histology in spite of unchanged serum creatinine levels. However, for patients with focal-segmental glomerulosclerosis, it may be difficult to determine whether the interstitial lesions are a consequence of CyA toxicity or part of the natural progression of the renal disease. A reasonable compromise was to repeat a renal biopsy after approximately one year in patients who have minimal-change disease and, if no interstitial changes are apparent and serum creatinine levels have not changed over that time, then CyA treatment may be continued without further biopsy provided that the CyA dose has not been increased. A further renal biopsy should also be considered if the duration of treatment exceeds three years.

clinical nephrology

Volume 36 – 1991

Dustri Verlag
Dr. Karl Feistle
München-
Deisenhofen

clinical nephrology

clinical nephrology

Clinical Nephrology appears monthly and publishes reviews, editorials, original papers, case reports, letters, book reviews and current information. The editors reserve the right of selection from submitted manuscripts (after consulting at least two reviewers) and the right to make stylistic changes or abridgements. The manuscripts may not be offered elsewhere for printing or publication; following acceptance the publisher acquires all copyrights. Rejected manuscripts are returned to the authors, the copies being sent under separate cover as printed matter, air mail.

This journal is regularly listed in Current Contents and Index Medicus.

PUBLISHER:
DUSTRI-VERLAG Dr. Karl Feistle,
Bahnhofstraße 9, Postfach 49,
W-8024 München-Deisenhofen, Germany
Telefon München (089) 613861-0
Teletex 897156 = DUSTRI
Telefax (089) 6135412

EDITOR-IN-CHIEF (responsible):
Prof. Dr. med. K. M. Koch,
Medizinische Hochschule Hannover,
Zentrum für Innere Medizin,
Konstanty-Gutschow-Straße 8,
W-3000 Hannover 61, Germany

MANAGING EDITOR:
Dr. Joyce Mayer
DUSTRI-VERLAG Dr. Karl Feistle,
Bahnhofstraße 9, Postfach 49,
W-8024 München-Deisenhofen, Germany
Telephone Munich (089) 613861-23

Printed in West Germany
by Mayr Miesbach,
Am Windfeld 15,
W-8160 Miesbach, Germany
ISSN 0301-0430

ADVERTISING:
Representatives in USA:
M. J. Mrvica Associates, Inc.
155 S. White Horse Pike
Berlin, NJ 08009, USA
Telephone (609) 768-9360

Germany:
H. P. Eckardt
DUSTRI-VERLAG Dr. Karl Feistle

Volumes 35 and 36 (6 issues per volume) will be published in 1991.
Published monthly.
Subscription price for 1991: DM 312.–, US $ 154.– plus postage (air mail only): Europe: $ 8.50; USA: $ 15.–; Japan/Brazil: $ 24.–; Australia: $ 28.–.
Single copies:
DM 28.–, US $ 15.– plus postage.
Parallel editions in microfiche can be purchased. Prices on order.
Available from all booksellers or direct from the publishers.

Second Class postage rate paid at Jamaica, NY 11431, USA.
U.S. Postmaster: Send address changes to CLINICAL NEPHROLOGY, Publications Expediting Inc., 200 Meacham Avenue, Elmont, NY 11003, USA.
Air freight and mailing in the US by Publications Expediting, Inc.
200 Meacham Ave., Elmont, NY 11003, USA.
Subscriptions are automatically canceled at the end of the year and recommence only with renewal. Prepayment is required on all orders.

Contents for Volume 36

Volume 36 No. 1 1991
July

C4A deficiency and poor prognosis in patients with IgA nephropathy 1
R. J. Wyatt, B. A. Julian, S. Y. Woodford, C. Wang, J. Roberts, J. S. Thompson, M. J. Christenson and R. H. McLean

Pattern of proteinuria in IgA nephritis by SDS-PAGE: clinical significance 6
K. T. Woo, Y. K. Lau, Grace S. L. Lee, S. S. Wei and C. H. Lim

Autoreactive lymphocytotoxic IgM antibodies in highly sensitized dialysis patients waiting for a kidney transplant: identification and clinical relevance 12
S. Barocci, U. Valente, R. Gusmano, F. Perfumo, S. Cantarella, A. Leprini, A. Icardi and A. Nocera

Abnormal diastolic left ventricular filling by pulsed Doppler echocardiography in patients on continuous ambulatory peritoneal dialysis 21
J. Hüting, W. Kramer, J. Reitinger, K. Kühn, G. Schütterle and V. Wizemann

An analysis of ten-year trends in infections in adults on continuous ambulatory peritoneal dialysis (CAPD) 29
J. Bernardini, J. L. Holley, J. R. Johnston, J. A. Perlmutter and B. Piraino

Pharmacokinetics of vancomycin in patients undergoing hemodialysis with polyacrylonitrile 35
J. Torras, C. Cao, M. C. Rivas, M. Cano, E. Fernandez and J. Montoliu

Acute thrombosis of the renal transplant artery: a case report and review of the literature 42
G. C. Groggel

Diffuse mesangial sclerosis in a fetus 46
G. S. Spear, K. A. Steinhaus and A. Quddusi

Announcements 49

Letters to the editor 50

Volume 36 No. 2 1991
August

The impact of prolonged immunosuppression on the outcome of idiopathic focal-segmental glomerulosclerosis with nephrotic syndrome in adults. A collaborative retrospective study 53
G. Banfi, M. Moriggi, E. Sabadini, G. Fellin, G. D'Amico and C. Ponticelli

Effects of triple therapy in IgA nephritis: a follow-up study 5 years later 60
K. T. Woo, G. S. L. Lee, Y. K. Lau, G. S. C. Chiang and C. H. Lim

Intraglomerular lipid deposition in routine biopsies 67
H. S. Lee, J. S. Lee, H. I. Koh and K. W. Ko

The kidney disease of Crow-Fukase (POEMS) syndrome: a clinico-pathological study of four cases 76
A. Fukatsu, H. Tamai, K. Nishikawa, W. Matsukawa, F. Yoshida, S. Matsuo, A. Takeda, K. Kodera, K. Morozumi, Y. Ito, K. Miyakawa, T. Toriyama, H. Kawahara and H. Shigematsu

Pulmonary and renal toxicity of intravenous immunoglobulin 83
R. Rault, B. Piraino, J. R. Johnston and A. Oral

Correlation of renal organic anion and cation transport with blood pressure in SHR 87
N. Gharib, C. Y. Gao, J. L. Areas, M. El Zein and H. G. Preuss

Renal vasoconstriction after low and high osmolar contrast agents in ischemic and non ischemic canine kidney 93
G. Deray, B. Baumelou, F. Martinez, G. Brillet and C. Jacobs

Intragastric long-term pH-metry in hemodialysis patients. A study with famotidine 97
U. Gladziwa, S. Wagner, K. V. Dakshinamurty, B. Bechtel, H. Mann and H.-G. Sieberth

Announcements 103

Letters to the editor 104

Volume 36 No. 3 1991
September

Prognostic implication of anti-neutrophil cytoplasmic autoantibodies with myeloperoxidase specificity in anti-glomerular basement membrane disease 107
X. Bosch, E. Mirapeix, J. Font, X. Borrellas, R. Rodríguez, A. López-Soto, M. Ingelmo and L. Revert

Immune material processing by phagocyte cell system in cryoglobulinemia 114
D. Roccatello, G. Mazzucco, R. Coppo, G. Piccoli, F. Malavasi, G. Cavalli, G. Martina, M. C. Amprimo, M. G. Guerra, A. Amore, G. Quattrocchio, A. Molino, S. Maffei, G. Picciotto and L. M. Sena

Immunohistological localization of apolipoproteins in the glomeruli in renal disease: specifically apoB and apoE 127
H. Sato, S. Suzuki, H. Kobayashi, S. Ogino, A. Inomata and M. Arakawa

FSGS-like lesions in pre-eclampsia 134
Y. Nagai, H. Arai, Y. Washizawa, Y. Ger, M. Tanaka, M. Maeda and S. Kawamura

Clinical significance of serum and urinary neopterins in patients with chronic renal disease 141
K. Godai, J. Uemasu and H. Kawasaki

Myocardial revascularization in patients on renal replacement therapy 147
M. De Meyer, W. Wyns, R. Dion, G. Khoury, Y. Pirson and C. van Ypersele de Strihou

Letters to the editor 152

Volume 36 No. 4 1991
October

Foreward 159
J. Rosenthal

The heart in hypertension 160
E. D. Frohlich

Hypertension in pregnancy: advances and controversies 166
M. D. Lindheimer and A. I. Katz

Diagnostic procedure in renovascular hypertension 174
A. Distler and K.-P. Spies

Renin inhibitors in hypertension 181
R. R. Luther, H. N. Glassman and R. S. Boger

SCH 34826: an overview of its profile as a neutral endopeptidase inhibitor and ANF potentiator 187
E. J. Sybertz

Predictive value of thallium-201-dipyridamole myocardial stress scintigraphy in chronic hemodialysis patients and transplant recipients 192
K. Derfler, K. Kletter, P. Balcke, G. Heinz and R. Dudczak

Intercellular adhesion molecule-1 expression in human kidneys with glomerulonephritis 203
G. A. Müller, J. Markovic-Lipkovski and C. A. Müller

Letters to the Editor 209

Volume 36 No. 5 1991
November

Morphologic findings in "zero-hour" biopsies of renal transplants 215
E. Curschellas, J. Landmann, M. Dürig, B. Huser, M. Kyo, V. Basler, G. Thiel and M. J. Mihatsch

A membranous nephropathy associated with adult polycystic kidney disease 223
K. Shikata, H. Makino and Z. Ota

Urine kallikrein excretion in relation to renal sodium handling in minimal change nephrotic syndrome 228
N. Ueda, Y. Niinomi and T. Nonoda

Repeated albumin infusions do not lower blood pressure in preeclampsia 234
P. Stratta, C. Canavese, M. Dogliani, L. Gurioli, M. C. Porcu, T. Todros, O. Fianchino, C. Benedètto, M. Massobrio and L. Balbi

Renal failure and cholesterol crystal embolization: a report of 4 surviving cases and a review of the literature 240
C. K. Mannesse, P. J. Blankestijn, A. J. Man in 't Veld and M. A. D. H. Schalekamp

Once weekly versus twice weekly subcutaneous administration of recombinant human erythropoietin in patients on continuous ambulatory peritoneal dialysis 246
S. F. Lui, C. B. Law, S. M. Ting, P. Li and K. N. Lai

Effect of recombinant human erythropoietin (rHuEpo) on the hemostatic system in chronic hemodialysis patients 252
S. Huraib, A. K. Al-Momen, A. M. A. Gader, A. Mitwalli, F. Sulimani and H. Abu-Aisha

Iatrogenic hypercalcemia in hemodialysis patients 258
M. A. Muhammedi, B. Piraino, R. Rault, J. R. Johnston and J. B. Puschett

Letters to the editor 262

Book reviews 266

Volume 36 No. 6 1991
December

Interleukin-1 production by monocytes from patients with glomerulonephritis after stimulation in vitro with soluble immune complexes 267
K. Matsumoto

Do limited changes in phosphate intake modulate $1,25(OH)_2D_3$ levels in early renal failure? 274
A. Seidel, G. Stein, S. Schneider, H. Schmidt-Gayk and E. Ritz

Lithium clearance in patients with chronic renal diseases 281
N. Clericetti and C. Beretta-Piccoli

Uremic autonomic dysfunction evaluated by pattern recognition analysis 290
G. Vita, P. Princi, V. Savica, G. Bellinghieri, R. M. Puglisi, L. Marabello and C. Messina

Experience of pain after subcutaneous administration of different preparations of recombinant human erythropoietin: a randomized, double-blind crossover study 294
C. Granolleras, W. Leskopf, S. Shaldon and J. Fourcade

Surgical treatment of massive hydrothorax complicating continuous ambulatory peritoneal dialysis 299
S. M. Allen and H. R. Matthews

X-ray microanalysis of the fingernails of uremic patients treated by hemodialysis 302
D. Zevin, T. Weinstein, J. Levi and M. Djaldetti

Letters to the editor 305

Announcements 310

Clinical Nephrology, Vol. 36 No. 1 – 1991 (1–5)

C4A deficiency and poor prognosis in patients with IgA nephropathy

R. J. Wyatt[1], B. A. Julian[2], S. Y. Woodford[3], C. Wang[1], J. Roberts[4], J. S. Thompson[3], M. J. Christenson[5] and R. H. McLean[5]

[1] *Division of Nephrology, Department of Pediatrics, University of Tennessee, Memphis,* [2] *Division of Nephrology, Department of Medicine, University of Alabama, Birmingham,* [3] *Department of Medicine, University of Kentucky College of Medicine, Lexington;* [4] *Department of Biology, California State University, Chico, CA and* [5] *Division of Pediatric Nephrology, Department of Pediatrics, the Johns Hopkins University School of Medicine, Baltimore, MD, USA*

Abstract. IgA nephropathy (Berger's disease) is an important cause of end-stage renal failure in persons of Asian and European descent. We performed C4 phenotyping on plasma from 123 patients with IgA nephropathy who resided in several different parts of the United States. All of these patients underwent diagnostic renal biopsy in adulthood. Six patients had a total deficiency for the C4A protein and all six had chronic renal insufficiency (serum creatinine concentration higher than 1.4 mg/dl at last follow-up). In contrast, 47% of the patients without C4A deficiency had chronic renal insufficiency ($p = 0.001$). The C4 gene defect was due to deletion of both C4A genes in only two individuals, whereas three patients were heterozygous for the C4A gene deletion. We speculate that the functional alteration of the complement system related to C4A deficiency might lead to expression of clinically severe disease in an individual with a genetic susceptibility to IgA nephropathy.

Key words: glomerulonephritis – IgA nephropathy – C4A – complement deficiency

Introduction

IgA nephropathy (Berger's disease) is the most common form of chronic glomerulonephritis in persons of Asian and European descent [D'Amico 1987, Levy and Berger 1988]. In some regions this condition accounts for up to 10% of the individuals progressing to end-stage renal failure [Berger et al. 1980]. The only markers of a poor prognosis accepted by all investigators are pathological or clinical: severity of renal histologic changes, older age at apparent onset, presence of hypertension and magnitude of proteinuria [Clarkson et al. 1977, D'Amico et al. 1985]. Although immunogenetic markers for prognosis have been identified for patients from some regional centers [Le Petit et al. 1981, Rambausek et al. 1982, Kashiwabara et al. 1982, Beukhof et al. 1984, Berthoux et al. 1988], there is no consensus for a such marker for patients from diverse geographical regions or ethnic backgrounds [Wyatt et al. 1987b].

The fourth component of complement, C4, is encoded by two loci (C4A and C4B) in the major histocompatibility complex (MHC) [O'Neill et al. 1978, Awdeh and Alper 1980]. In vitro studies of immune precipitates provide strong support for the concept that C4A deficiency might reduce solubilization and/or clearance of potentially nephritogenic immune complexes [Law et al. 1984, Schifferli et al. 1986].

We have extended previous work on C4 phenotypes in children and adults from Kentucky with Henoch-Schoenlein purpura or IgA nephropathy [McLean et al. 1984] with the identification of six adult patients with IgA nephropathy and C4A deficiency. The six affected patients were ascertained since our initial report and all have chronic renal insufficiency.

Methods

The diagnosis of IgA nephropathy was based upon the demonstration by direct immunofluorescence of IgA as the dominant or co-dominant immunoglobulin in a primarily mesangial deposition and the absence of any systemic disease or infection

Received December 14, 1990; February 13, 1991.

Reprint requests to Dr. R. J. Wyatt, Pediatric Research, Room B310, 956 Court Ave., Memphis, TN 38163, USA.

[Wyatt et al. 1984]. Patients were included in the study if they were Caucasian and over age 18 at the time of the biopsy. Patients diagnosed in childhood were not included in the study because a much longer follow-up period would be required to determine outcome for such patients as compared to patients identified in adulthood. Patients were followed at five locations (number of patients shown in brackets): Lexington, KY (83), Birmingham, AL (21), Chico, CA (8), Chattanooga, TN (7), and Tupelo, MS (4). All subjects from these centers with suitable EDTA-plasma samples submitted for C4 phenotyping prior to January 1, 1989 were entered into the study.

A serum creatinine concentration at last follow-up greater than 1.4 mg per deciliter was the criterion for chronic renal insufficiency. Only patients with persistence of the elevation of the serum creatinine concentration were considered to have chronic renal insufficiency. Clinical follow-up included ascertainment of macroscopic hematuria. Some patients without macroscopic hematuria at clinical presentation subsequently experienced an episode. Chronic renal insufficiency occurred in a high percentage of patients from each location: Chico, CA (63%), Lexington, KY (51%), Birmingham, AL (43%), Chattanooga, TN (29%), and Tupelo, MS (25%).

Plasma drawn into EDTA-containing tubes was stored in aliquots at −70° C until the assays were performed. Factor B (Bf) phenotyping was performed by low voltage agarose electrophoresis followed by immunofixation with a monospecific antiserum to factor B [Alper et al. 1972]. C4 phenotyping of plasma specimens was performed by the combined analysis of immunofixation [Awdeh and Alper 1979] and crossed-gel electrophoresis for detection of single null alleles [Awdeh et al. 1979]. Sodium dodecyl sulfate-polyacrylamide gel electrophoresis (SDS-PAGE) and Western blotting of immunoprecipitated C4 was used to analyze C4 alpha-chain mobility in the subjects with C4A deficiency [Ross et al. 1982]. Nomenclature used in this manuscript concurs with that proposed at the IVth International Workshop for the Genetics of Complement [Mauff et al. 1983].

Taq 1 DNA fragments were separated by agarose electrophoresis and transferred to nylon membranes as previously described [McLean et al. 1988]. Restriction fragment length polymorphisms were determined by hybridization with a 0.6 kilobase (kb) BamHI/KPN 1 fragment of the pAT-A cDNA C4 probe (kindly provided by Dr. Michael C. Carroll, Boston, MA). The probe hybridizes to the 5′ end of both the C4A and C4B genes. Four Taq 1 digestion fragments (7.0 kb, 6.4 kb, 6.0 kb and 5.4 kb) are produced. The 7.0 kb fragment corresponds to the end of the C4A gene. The presence of a 6.4 kb fragment indicates the deletion of the C4A gene and the presence of a "short" C4B gene. With rare exceptions [McLean et al. 1988, Palsdottir et al. 1987] the 6.0 kb fragment represents a portion of the 22 kb "long" C4B gene and the 5.4 kb RFLP is a portion of the 16 kb "short" C4B gene.

HLA typing was performed by standard techniques. Statistical analysis of differences between patient groups for outcome was done by a Fisher's exact test. The differences between groups for mean age at onset and biopsy and length of follow-up was analyzed by a two-tailed Student's t test. Significance was set at the 0.05 level.

Results

Six of the 123 (4.9%) adult patients with IgA nephropathy available for study had C4A deficiency. These patients lived in different geographical locations and none was known to be related to another patient with IgA nephropathy [Wyatt et al. 1987b]. Two of the patients with C4A deficiency lived in Alabama and one each in Kentucky, West Virginia, Tennessee and California.

The molecular patterns for C4 genes and HLA studies done for these patients suggested that more than one mechanism was responsible for the C4A deficiencies and that no extended MHC haplotype was common to all of the affected patients (Table 1). Five of the patients with C4A deficiency had DNA available for molecular studies. Only two of the five were homozygous for a deleted C4A gene, as indicated by homozygosity for the 6.4 kb fragment. Three patients had one apparent C4A gene fragment present and one deleted C4A gene as indicated by the 7.0 kb, 6.4 kb RFLP phenotype. All six patients with C4A deficiency had HLA A, B and DR phenotyping performed (Table 1). Three of the six patients had all three HLA alleles (A1, B8, DR3) which belong to the extended haplotype most often associated with a deleted C4A gene [Garlepp et al. 1986]. The HLA B60 allele was detected in three of the patients, but was not present in the patients who were homozygous for a deleted C4A gene.

SDS-PAGE of plasma from the C4A deficient patients showed that all patients except patient 3 lacked the 96 kilodalton (KD) alpha chain which characterizes C4A allotypes. Patient 3 had a weak 96 KD alpha chain by SDS-PAGE but this fragment lacked Rogers 1 antigen by Western blotting. This suggests the presence of a hybrid C4 gene with characteristics of both C4A (e.g. 96 KD alpha chain) and C4B (absent Rogers 1 antigen and C4B mobility in agarose). Probing of DNA digests with C4A and C4B specific oligonucleotides would be required to detect conversion of C4A to C4B [Braun et al. 1990].

Table 1 Major histocompatibility complex phenotypes in patients with C4A deficiency

Pt no.	Bf	C4B	5′ C4 probe*	HLA A	HLA B	HLA DR
1	S, S	1, –	6.4	1, 2	8, 9	3, 4
2	F, S	1, –	7.0, 6.4, 5.4	1, 2	8, 44	7, 10
3	S, S	2, 3	not done+	2, –	51, 60	2, 4
4	F, S	1, 2	7.0, 6.4, 5.4	3, 24	8, 60	6, 8
5	S, S	1, 2	7.0, 6.4, 5.4	1, 2	8, 60	3, 6
6	S, S	1, –	6.4	1, 2	8, 39	3, –

* Restriction enzyme Taq I
+ Patient expired – DNA not available

Table 2 Association between renal function and C4 deficiency states

	Renal function at last follow-up normal	Chronic renal insufficiency
C4 isotype deficiency		
C4A	0	6*
C4B	5	4
No C4 isotype deficiency		
C4A single null	11	11
C4B single null	12	11
No apparent C4 null	36	27

* Comparison of prevalence of chronic renal insufficiency for patients with and without C4A deficiency, p = 0.011

All patients with C4A deficiency had chronic renal insufficiency; one had normal renal function at time of apparent onset and three have progressed to end stage disease (Table 2). The patients with C4A isotype deficiency were much more likely to have chronic renal insufficiency than those without C4A deficiency ($p = 0.011$). Patients with C4B deficiency or single null alleles for C4A or C4B had a 44 to 50% prevalence of with progressive disease which was similar to that of 43% found in patients with no apparent C4 null allotypes.

The patients grouped according to C4 phenotype could not be distinguished from each other by clinical features, including sex or a history of macroscopic hematuria (Table 3). Age at apparent clinical onset, age at biopsy and years of follow-up after biopsy did not differ significantly between the groups.

Discussion

C4A deficiency has been observed in 1 to 2.4% of healthy Caucasian individuals [Alper et al. 1979, McCluskey et al. 1983, Mijovic et al. 1985, Julian et al. 1988]. In the present study C4A deficiency was detected in 4.9% of 123 patients with IgA nephropathy and in 10.1% of the 59 patients with progressive renal disease. Several studies have found C4A deficiency in approximately 10% of white patients with systemic lupus erythematosus (SLE) [Fielder et al. 1982, Howard et al. 1986, Kemp et al. 1987]. Patients with SLE and C4A deficiency usually show a homozygous C4A gene deletion [Kemp et al. 1987]. The molecular basis of the C4A deficiency in the patients with IgA nephropathy and renal insufficiency is not homozygous. Only 40% (2/5) were homozygous for deletion of C4A genes whereas three have a combination of one C4A gene deletion and one presumed non-functioning C4A gene. Non-functioning C4A genes may be due to gene conversion (C4A to C4B) or to true pseudogenes [Braun et al. 1990]. C4 genes from patient 3 could not be studied, but analysis of the serum C4 is compatible with a hybrid gene product [Roos et al. 1984]. Alternatively, this patient could have a poorly antigenic C4A gene product [Ghanem et al. 1988].

Table 3 Clinical data for patients with IgA nephropathy

	Sex (M:F)	Macroscopic hematuria	Age at apparent onset (mean ± SE)	Age at biopsy (mean ± SE)	Years since biopsy* (mean ± SE)
C4 isotype deficiency					
C4 deficiency	5: 1	33%	36.9 ± 3.9	41.3 ± 3.9	3.0 ± 1.3
C4B deficiency	5: 4	67%	30.6 ± 5.7	35.2 ± 5.0	7.1 ± 1.2
No C4 isotype deficiency					
C4A single null	15: 7	64%	32.1 ± 2.5	35.5 ± 2.4	4.6 ± 0.8
C4B single null	20: 3	48%	33.0 ± 3.2	36.1 ± 3.3	4.4 ± 0.7
No apparent C4 null	44:19	43%	29.7 ± 1.7	34.1 ± 1.7	5.0 ± 0.4

* Time until last visit or initiation of dialysis

Studies from several regional centers have proposed immunogenetic markers for prognosis in patients with IgA nephropathy. In an attempt to explain data on prognostic indicators in Dutch patients with IgA nephropathy, IgA nephropathy was suggested to represent at least two distinct disease entities with differing outcomes [Beukhof et al. 1984]. HLA-DR blank phenotypes (DR alleles which are homozygous, non-expressed or untypeable) and the absence of macroscopic hematuria occurred in patients having a poor clinical outcome. Patients with the other "disease entity" had a history of macroscopic hematuria and maintenance of normal renal function. The HLA B35 allele has been associated with poor outcome in French patients [Berthoux et al. 1988]. The complement phenotypes, C3F and BfF, have been associated with severe disease for German and Dutch patients [Rambausek et al. 1987]. Our previous data from Kentucky did not show an association between poor outcome and either history of macroscopic hematuria or the presence of the following immunogenetic markers: DR blank phenotype, HLA-B35 allele, C3F phenotype or BfF phenotype [Wyatt et al. 1987a]. In the present study the history of macroscopic hematuria is not of prognostic importance.

We hypothesize that a disease susceptibility allele(s) for IgA nephropathy exists. We have found that at least 60% of the patients with IgA nephropathy from Kentucky are related to other patients with the disease and that the ancestors of the related patients are clustered in distinct geographical regions [Wyatt et al. 1987b]. The best explanation for this findings is a "Founder Effect" whereby an allele conveying susceptibility to IgA nephropathy was carried into eastern Kentucky by one or more of the early settlers. The C4A deficiency is not likely to be associated with a disease susceptibility allele. Rather, the functional alteration of the complement system related to the deficiency might lead to expression of clinically severe disease in an individual having the genetic predisposition to the development of IgA nephropathy.

The ability to identify consistent markers of prognosis for patients with IgA nephropathy will be an important early step in the eventual control of the disease. Data from the present study suggests that intact function of the complement system is important for maintenance of normal renal function in patients with IgA nephropathy.

Acknowledgements

We are indebted to Drs. Richard Baehler, John Cox, Thomas Ferguson, Frank Miller, Greg McMorrow, Adel Shenouda, Joseph Wattlington, Thomas Wooldridge and Jackson Yium for allowing us to perform these studies on their patients and for providing clinical follow-up, to Dr. John Phillips for isolating and storing DNA on the subjects with C4A deficiency, to Ms. Trudie Patterson for assistance in data management, and to Thomas LaRosa for technical assistance.

We were supported by grants from the American Kidney Fund, the Dialysis Clinics, Inc., Nashville, TN, Lexington, KY. branch, the LeBonher Children's Medical Center, Memphis, TN and the National Institutes of Health (R01-31920 and N01-A1-82686).

This article was presented at the annual meeting of the American Federation for Clinical Research, Washington, D.C., May 1, 1989.

REFERENCES

Alper CA, Boenisch T, Watson L 1972 Genetic polymorphism in human glycine-rich beta-microglobulin. J Exp Med *135:* 68

Awdeh ZL, Raum D, Alper CA 1979 Genetic polymorphism of human complement C4 and detection of heterozygotes. Nature *282:* 205

Awdeh ZL, Alper CA 1980 Inherited structural polymorphism of the fourth component of complement. Proc Natl Acad Sci USA *77:* 3576

Berger J, Yaneva H, Crosnier J 1980 La glomérulonéphrite á dépots mésangiaux d'IgA: une cause fréquente d'insuffisance rénale terminale. Nouv Presse Med *9:* 219

Berthoux FC, Alamartine E, Pommier G, Le Petit JC 1988 HLA and IgA nephropathy revisited 10 years later: HLA-B35 antigen as a prognostic factor (letter). N Engl J Med *319:* 1609

Beukhof JR, Ockhuizen TH, Halie LM, Westra J, Beelen JM, Donker AJM, Hoedemaeker PhJ, van der Hem GK 1984 Subentities within primary adult IgA-nephropathy. Clin Nephrol *22:* 195

Braun L, Schneider PM, Giles CM, Bertrams J, Rittner C 1990 Null alleles of human complement C4. Evidence for pseudogenes at the C4A locus and for gene conversion at the C4B locus. J Exp Med *171:* 129

Clarkson AR, Seymour AE, Thompson SJ, Haynes WDG, Chan YL, Jackson B 1977 IgA nephropathy: a syndrome of uniform morphology, diverse clinical features and uncertain prognosis. Clin Nephrol *8:* 459

D'Amico G, Imbiasciati E, Barbiano Di Belioioso G, Bertoli S, Fogazzi F, Ferrario F, Fellin G, Ragni A, Colasanti G, Minetti L, Ponticelli C 1985 Idiopathic IgA mesangial nephropathy. Clinical and histological study of 374 patients. Medicine *64:* 49

D'Amico G 1987 The commonest glomerulonephritis in the world: IgA nephropathy. Quart J Med *245:* 709

Fielder AHL, Walport MJ, Batchelor JR, Rynes RI, Black CM, Dodi IA, Hughes GRV 1983 Family studies of the major histocompatibility complex in patients with systemic lupus erythematosus: importance of null alleles of C4A and C4B in determining susceptibility. Br Med J *286:* 425

Garlepp MJ, Wilton AN, Dawkins RL, White PC 1986 Rearrangement of 21-hydroxylase genes in disease-associated MHC supratypes. Immunogenet *23:* 100

Ghanem N, Uring-Lambert B, Abbal M, Hauptmann G, LeFranc MP, LeFranc G 1988 Polymorphism of MHC class III genes: definition of restriction fragment linkage groups and evidence for frequent deletions and duplications. Hum Genet *79:* 209

Howard PF, Hochberg MC, Bias WB, Arnett FC, Jr, McLean RH 1986 Relationship between C4 null genes, HLA-D region antigens, and genetic susceptibility to systemic lupus erythematosus in Caucasian and black Americans. Am J Med *81:* 187

Julian BA, Woodford SY, Baehler RW, McMorrow RG, Wyatt RJ 1988 Familial clustering and immunogenetic aspects of IgA nephropathy. Am J Kidney Dis *12:* 366

Kashiwabara H, Shishido H, Tomura S, Tuchida H, Miyajima T 1982 Strong association between IgA nephropathy and HLA-DR 4 antigen. Kidney Int *22:* 377

Kemp ME, Atkinson JP, Skanes VM, Levine RP, Chaplin DD 1987 Deletion of C4A genes in patients with systemic lupus erythematosus. Arthritis Rheum *30:* 1015

Law SKA, Dodds AW, Porter RR 1984 A comparison of the properties of the two classes, C4A and C4B, of the human complement component C4. Eur Mol Biol Org J *3:* 1819

Le Petit JC, van Loghem EV, de Lange GD, Berthoux FC, Capius-Cellier C, Serre JL 1981 GM, AM, PI, KM markers in mesangial IgA nephropathy. J Immunogenet *8:* 415

Levy M, Berger J 1988 Worldwide perspective of IgA nephropathy. Am J Kidney Dis *12:* 340

Mauff G, Alper CA, Awdeh Z, Batchelor JR, Bertrams J, Bruun-Peterson G, Dawkins RL, Demant P, Edwards J, Grosse-Wilde H, Hauptman G, Klouda P, Lamm L, Mollenhauer E, Nerl C, Olaisen B, O'Neill G, Rittner C, Roos MH, Skanes V, Teisberg P, Wells L 1983 Statement on the nomenclature of human C4 allotypes. Immunobiology *154:* 184

McCluskey J, McCann VJ, Kay PH, Zilko PJ, Christiansen FT, O'Neill JG, Dawkins RL 1983 HLA and complement allotypes in type 1 (insulin-dependent) diabetes. Diabetologia *24:* 162

McLean RH, Wyatt RJ, Julian BA 1984 Complement phenotypes in glomerulonephritis: increased frequency of homozygous null C4 phenotypes in IgA nephropathy and Henoch-Schoenlein purpura. Kidney Int *26:* 855

McLean RH, Donohoue PA, Jospe N, Bias WB, van Dop C, Migeon CJ 1988 Restriction fragment analysis of duplication of the fourth component of complement (C4A). Genomics *2:* 76

Mijovic C, Fletcher J, Bradwell AR, Harvey T, Barnett AH 1985 Relation of gene expression (allotypes) of the fourth component of complement to insulin dependent diabetes and its microangiopathic complications. Br Med J *291:* 9

O'Neill GJ, Yang SY, Dupont B 1978 Two HLA-linked loci controlling the fourth component of human complement. Proc Natl Acad Sci USA *75:* 5165

Palsdottir A, Aranson A, Fossdal R, Jensson O 1987 Gene organization of haplotypes expressing two different C4A allotypes. Hum Genet *76:* 220

Rambausek M, van den Wall Bake AWL, Schumacher-Ach R, Spitzenberg R, Rother U, van Es LA, Ritz E 1987 Genetic polymorphism of C3 and Bf in IgA nephropathy. Nephrol Dial Transplant *2:* 208

Roos MH, Mollenhauer E, Demant P, Rittner C 1982 A molecular basis for the two locus model of human complement C4. Nature *298:* 854

Roos MH, Giles CM, Demant P, Rittner C 1984 Rogers (Rg) and Chido (Ch) determinants on human C4: characterization of the two C4B5 subtypes, one of which contains Rg and Ch determinants. J Immunol *133:* 2634

Schifferli JA, Steiger G, Paccaud J-P, Sjoholm AG, Hauptman G 1986 Difference in the biological properties of the two forms of the fourth component of human complement (C4). Clin Exp Immunol *63:* 473

Wyatt RJ, Julian BA, Bhathena DB, Mlitchell BL, Holland NH, Malluche HH 1984 IgA nephropathy: presentation, clinical course and prognosis in children and adults. Am J Kidney Dis *4:* 192

Wyatt RJ, Julian BA, Woodford SY, McLean RH, Thompson JS 1987a Immunogenetic markers as prognostic features in patients from Kentucky with IgA nephropathy. Sem Nephrol *7:* 389

Wyatt RJ, Rivas MR, Julian BA, Quiggins PA, Woodford SY, McMorrow RG, Baehler RW 1987b Regionalization in hereditary IgA nephropathy. Am J Hum Genet *41:* 36

Clinical Nephrology, Vol. 36 No. 1 – 1991 (6–11)

Pattern of proteinuria in IgA nephritis by SDS-PAGE: clinical significance

K.T. Woo, Y. K. Lau, Grace S. L. Lee, S. S. Wei and C. H. Lim

Department of Renal Medicine, Singapore General Hospital, Singapore – 0316, Republic of Singapore

Abstract. Of sixty patients with IgA nephritis, none had CRF at first examination, 13 developed CRF with creatinine above 1.6 mg/dl within 6 years. Among these patients who had analysis of proteinuria by sodium dodecyl sulphate polyacrylamide gel electrophoresis (SDS-PAGE), 31 patients had middle molecular weight (MMW) proteinuria alone (pattern 1), 10 had MMW and Low MW (LMW) or tubular proteinuria (pattern 2), 10 had high MW (HMW) and MMW proteinuria (Pattern 3) and 9 had HMW, MMW and LMW proteinuria (Pattern 4). At the end of a follow up period of 6 years (1983–1989) patients with mixed proteinuria had a higher incidence of chronic renal failure (CRF), 11/29 (38%) compared to those with pattern 1 proteinuria, 2/31 (6%) ($\chi^2 = 8.7$, $p < 0.005$). Based on the glomerular selectivity index (GSI), 19 patients had nonselective proteinuria but they did not have a higher incidence of CRF. By the selectivity index (SI), 18 patients had nonselective proteinuria and they showed a significantly higher incidence of CRF. Compared to the 41 patients who did not have LMW proteinuria, 19 patients with LMW proteinuria had more severe proteinuria. After a follow-up period of 6 years, patients with LMW proteinuria had a higher incidence of CRF (10% versus 47%, $p < 0.001$). The presence of LMW proteinuria indicates a less favourable outcome and the pattern of proteinuria as assessed by the SDS-PAGE appears to be a better prognostic index in IgA nephritis than the SI and the GSI.

Key words: pattern of proteinuria – glomerular selectivity index – selectivity index – low molecular weight proteinuria – tubular proteinuria

Introduction

Most studies in IgA nephritis [D'Amico et al. 1986, Woo et al. 1986, Kobayashi et al. 1987] have shown that severe proteinuria is associated with a poor prognosis. Several colleagues, including ourselves [Beukhof et al. 1984, Woo et al. 1986, Nagy et al. 1987, Woo et al. 1989] have shown that those patients with selective proteinuria tend to have a better outcome when compared to those with nonselective proteinuria. Molecular weight related urinary protein analysis has been found to be a valuable diagnostic tool in nephrology [Balant et al. 1974, Lison et al. 1989]. This study analyses the pattern of proteinuria in patients with IgA nephritis based on molecular weight using sodium dodecyl sulphate polyacrylamide gel electrophoresis (SDS-PAGE) in an attempt to classify the various types of protein found in the urine of these patients to determine the value of urinary protein pattern as a prognostic index.

Received September 10, 1990; in revised form February 11, 1991.

Reprint requests to Dr. K. T. Woo

Patients and methods

Sixty patients with biopsy proven IgA nephritis had their proteinuria evaluated using SDS-PAGE to establish the pattern of proteinuria. The diagnosis of IgA nephritis was based on the demonstration of IgA as the predominant immunoglobulin in the mesangium on immunofluorescence and exclusion of systemic diseases such as systemic lupus erythematosus, Henoch-Schoenlein purpura, cirrhosis of the liver or systemic vasculitis. All patients had significant proteinuria (urinary protein >150 mg per day) and a normal renal function (serum creatinine $\leq = 1.6$ mg/dl) at the beginning of the study.

Renal biopsy

Specimens were fixed in Dubosq-Brazil solution and 2 micron sections were cut and stained with hematoxylin and eosin, periodic acid-Schiff and silver-Masson's trichrome. Immunofluorescence studies were performed on 6 micron cryostat sections using FITC-conjugated antisera against IgA, IgG and IgM,

C1q, C3 and fibrinogen (Behring, Germany). The percentage of sclerosed glomeruli (segmental and global) was obtained by dividing the number of sclerosed glomeruli by the total number of glomeruli per section and multiplied by 100. Specimens containing less than 10 glomeruli per section were excluded.

Clinical data

Data from 1983 to 1989 were extracted from the patient record and these included blood pressure, micro- or macro-hematuria, total urinary protein, serum creatinine and creatinine clearance (Ccr). Hypertension was defined as BP exceeding 150/90 and renal impairment as serum creatinine of >1.6 mg/dl. Total urinary protein and the creatinine concentrations in serum and urine samples were determined using the Biuret Reagent Kit and the Alkaline Picrate Reagent Kit (Roche, Switzerland) and Ccr calculated from the measured 24-hour urine volume.

SDS-PAGE

This was performed on the PhastSystem (Pharmacia, Sweden) which comprises a gel electrophoresis unit and an automated staining unit. The small precast gels (43 × 50 mm), gradient 8–25% of acrylamide, were used together with PhastGel SDS Buffer strips. Urine (24-hour collection with thymol crystals as preservative) was applied without further treatment. Eight samples in 1 microlitre aliquots were applied to each gel and electrophoresis was programmed to run at 150 volt, 6 milliamp, 1.8 watt, 15° C and 90 accumulated volt hour. The process took about 1 hour. After the electrophoresis run, the gel was transferred to the automated staining unit for staining in 0.1% PhastGel Blue R (Coomassie R 350 stain) in acetic acid/methanol/aqueous solution (1 : 3 : 6 vol) for 8 minutes at 50° C and subsequent destaining to give a sufficiently clear background. This process usually took another hour. The gel was then dried in the oven at 60° C for 15 minutes and mounted in super-slide mount (Gepe, 40×40×2 mm) with anti-Newton glasses for storage and subsequent quantitation by densitometry.

Densitometry

Semi-quantitation was done by scanning in the Appraise Densitometer (Beckman, USA) in the absorbance test mode (optical density measurement) using a 2 mm slit length and the interference filter 520 nm. Printout was in relative percentage of the total area for each area under an individual peak (protein band).

Identification of proteins on SDS-PAGE gels

After electrophoresis, the gel was left in-situ and a piece of pure nitrocellulose membrane (0.45 micron pore size, Bio-Rad, USA) (cut to size and pre-wetted in distilled water for at least 5 minutes) was layered onto it. The gel bed was then heated to 37° C and transfer of protein bands by diffusion was allowed to take place for 20 minutes. The membrane was then lifted off, blocked in 3 gm% gelatin in TBS (Tris buffered saline: 20 mM Tris, 500 mM NaCl, pH 7.5) for 30 minutes, rinsed in TBST (TBS plus 0.05% Tween 20) before cutting into individual strips for separate incubation with specific rabbit antisera to human albumin and transferrin (diluted 1 : 100 in TBST containing 1 gm% gelatin). After 2 hours of incubation on a rotator, the membrane was washed thoroughly in TBST before reacting with Protein G-Gold (Bio-Rad, USA) diluted 1 : 25. The colloidal gold produced a distinctive rose-red color for visualizing membrane bound antigens reactive to the primary antisera in 15 minutes to 4 hours, depending on the antigen concentrations.

The pattern of proteinuria

Protein bands were classified as high molecular weight (HMW), low (LMW) and middle (MMW) as per definition of Beukhof et al. [1984]: HMW > transferrin (90 kD); LMW < albumin (69 kD); LMW < MMW < HMW. The pattern of proteinuria was then categorized by inspection as:
pattern 1: middle MW (MMW) proteinuria
pattern 2: MMW + low MW (LMW) or tubular proteinuria
pattern 3: high MW (HMW) + MMW proteinuria
pattern 4: HMW + MMW + LMW proteinuria

Glomerular selectivity index (GSI)

This index of proteinuria was based on the ratio, MMW/HMW [Nagy et al. 1987]. The amount of MMW or HMW in the urine was derived by densitometry. As the HMW proteins were absent in 41 patients, division by zero gave incalculably large GSI in these instances. For statistical analysis, these cases were given the arbitrary value of GSI = 200 as the highest calculable GSI value was 193. According to Nagi et al. [1987] proteinuria was regarded as selective if GSI ≥ = 8 and based on this cutoff point

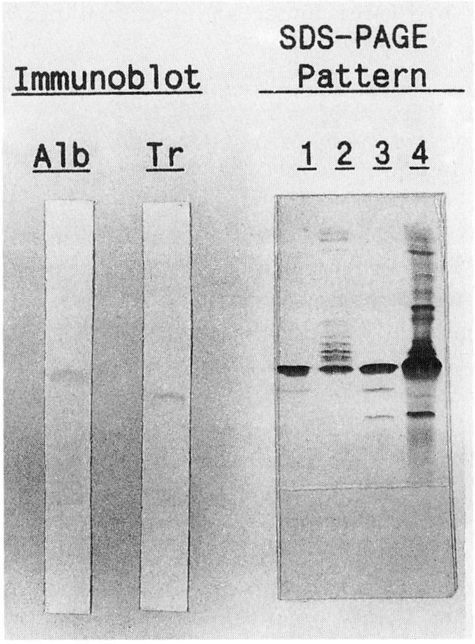

Fig. 1 Identification of the albumin and transferrin bands and the 4 patterns of proteinuria. Protein bands are transblotted onto pure nitrocellulose membrane by simple diffusion and identified with monospecific rabbit antisera to human albumin (Alb, 69 kD) and transferrin (Tr, 90 kD) and Protein G-Gold (Bio-Rad, USA). Patterns of proteinuria are obtained by SDS-PAGE. Middle molecular weight proteins (MMW) are defined as proteins inclusive of the albumin and transferrin and bands that run between them in the SDS-PAGE. Low molecular weight (LMW) proteins are defined as proteins smaller than albumin (69 kD) and are bands that run above the albumin band. High molecular weight (HMW) proteins are defined as larger than transferrin (90 kD) and are bands that run below the transferrin band. Patterns of proteinuria are classified as:
pattern 1 – MMW proteins only
pattern 2 – MMW proteins + LMW proteins
pattern 3 – MMW proteins + HMW proteins
pattern 4 – MMW proteins + HMW proteins + LMW proteins

we would have only 2 patients in the non-selective group, insufficient for statistical comparison. In order to be able to further investigate GSI as an index of prognosis in our experience here, we compared patients with no detectable HMW protein or selective proteinuria (GSI = 200) against patients with detectable HMW proteins or nonselective proteinuria (GSI < 200).

Selectivity Index (SI)

This was based on the simple ratio of the clearance of IgG over the clearance of transferrin (Tr) as described by Cameron and Blandford [1966]. Serum and urinary IgG and Tr concentrations were measured by radial immunodiffusion technique with monospecific antisera (Behring, Germany). As the volume and time values were equal, the index was calculated using the formula: SI = (urine IgG/serum IgG)/(urine Tr/serum Tr). A SI value $\leq = 0.2$ indicates selective proteinuria while a value > 0.2 indicates non-selectivity. When IgG and Tr were not measurable in the urine and a SI value not calculable, then SI = 0 as albumin was always measurable in urine with significant proteinuria of >150 mg protein/day.

Time schedule of investigations

Patients were seen between 1981 and 1983. Biopsies were performed during this period. Sampling of urine and blood for investigations were performed in 1983 and 1989.

Statistics

Results were expressed as mean ± SD. Statistics were performed using Student's t-test, the chi-square test and Pearsons's correlation analysis. Samples of blood and urine required for proteinuria studies were obtained at the same time as those required for serum creatinine, Ccr and total urinary protein. After 6 years (1989), patients were studied with respect to outcome in relation to the pattern of protein excretion as a prognostic marker.

Table 1 Comparison of outcome between patients with selective and nonselective proteinuria as based on the pattern of proteinuria, glomerular selectivity index (GSI), selectivity index (SI) and the absence or presence of low molecular weight (LMW) bands (at an average of 6 years after presentation).

Indices	Stable renal function	Chronic renal failure	χ^2	Probability
Pattern				
1	29	2 (2/31 = 6%)		
2, 3, 4	18	11 (11/29 = 38%)	8.7	<0.005
GSI				
= 200	34	7 (7/41 = 17%)		
< 200	13	6 (6/19 = 32%)	1.6	NS
SI				
≤ = 0.2	37	5 (5/42 = 12%)		
> 0.2	10	8 (8/18 = 44%)	7.9	<0.005
LMW bands				
without	37	4 (4/41 = 10%)		
with	10	9 (9/19 = 47%)	10.8	<0.001

Results

Pattern of protein excretion

All 60 patients had a pathological proteinuria at the first examination (1.6 ± 1.6 g/d) in 1983. At follow up in 1989, proteinuria was 1.6 ± 2.5 g/d. Figure 1 shows the positions of the albumin and transferrin bands and the four patterns of proteinuria on SDS-PAGE. Patients with pattern 1 proteinuria were the only group with a homogeneous protein fraction whereas those with the other 3 patterns had a mixed protein pattern. Proteinuria in the 60 patients could be categorized as:

	1983	1989
Pattern 1: MMW proteinuria alone	31	24
Pattern 2: MMW + LMW	10	2
Pattern 3: HMW + MMW	10	21
Pattern 4: HMW + MMW + LMW	9	13

Comparison of outcome based on indices of proteinuria

Table 1 examines the incidence of chronic renal failure at an average of 6 years after presentation. Thirty-one patients with pattern 1 were compared with 29 patients with mixed pattern (pattern 2, 3, 4). Patients with mixed pattern had a significantly higher incidence of chronic renal failure (CRF), 11/29 (38%) compared to 2/31 (6%) among patients with pattern 1, $\chi^2 = 8.7$, $p < 0.005$. The GSI separated the 60 patients into two groups. There were 41 patients with GSI = 200 (selective proteinuria) and 19 with GSI <200 (nonselective proteinuria). A comparison of the two groups (selective and nonselective proteinuria) showed the incidence of chronic renal failure (CRF) after a 6-year follow up was not significantly different, 7/41 (17%) versus 6/19 (32%). When the clearance of IgG exceeded 20% that of the clearance of transferrin (SI >0.2), proteinuria is considered nonselective. Based on this criterion, proteinuria was shown to be selective in 42 and nonselective in 18 patients. Significantly, the rate of chronic failure was higher among patients with nonselective proteinuria, 8/18 (44%) versus 5/42 (12%) among patients with selective proteinuria ($\chi^2 = 7.9$, $p < 0.005$). Analyses by SDS-PAGE showed that there were 19 patients with LMW proteinuria and 41 patients with no LMW proteinuria in the urine. There was a higher incidence of CRF in the final outcome among patients with LMW proteinuria. Forty-seven percent among those with LMW proteinuria compared to 10% among those with no LMW proteinuria ($\chi^2 = 10.8$, $p < 0.001$) had chronic renal failure.

Correlation between the various indices of proteinuria

Table 2 shows the correlations between the pattern of protein excretion, GSI, SI and LMW bands. There were very good correlations between pattern and the other 3 indices of proteinuria. In contrast, there was no correlation among the indices of GSI, SI and LMW bands. In addition the pattern of proteinuria was significantly correlated with tubular atrophy and tubulointerstitial lesions (r = 0.30, p <0.025) as well as medial hyperplasia of blood vessels (r = 0.26, p <0.05).

Table 2 Correlation between various indices of proteinuria and with tubular atrophy and tubulointerstitial lesion (TA); medial hyperplasia of blood vessels (Med. Hyp.)

n = 60	Index	Correlation coefficient (r)	Statistical significance (p)
1. Pattern of proteinuria (1, 2, 3, 4)	Pattern		
	GSI	−0.81	<0.001
	SI	0.39	<0.002
	LMW bands	0.51	<0.001
	TA	0.30	<0.025
	Med. Hyp.	0.26	<0.05
2. Glomerular selectivity index (GSI)	Pattern		
	GSI	−0.81	<0.001
	SI	−0.24	NS
	LMW bands	−0.21	NS
	TA	−0.34	<0.01
	Med. Hyp.	−0.21	NS
3. Selectivity index (SI)	pattern		
	GSI	0.39	<0.002
	SI	−0.25	NS
	LMW bands	0.10	NS
	TA	0.09	NS
	Med. Hyp.	0.06	NS
4. LMW bands	Pattern		
	GSI	0.51	<0.001
	SI	−0.21	NS
	LMW bands	0.10	NS
	TA	0.08	NS
	Med. Hyp.	0.11	NS

Table 3 Comparison of patients with pattern 1 and patterns 2, 3, 4

Parameter	Pattern 1	Patterns 2, 3, 4	t-test
Number	31	29	
Age (years)	26 ± 7	27 ± 7	NS
Sex (m/f)	21 / 10	25 / 4	NS
Duration FU. months	84 ± 62	83 ± 41	NS
Presentation:			
Asymptomatic haematuria /proteinuria	25	23	NS
Gross haematuria /proteinuria	6	6	NS
Hypertension	5/31 (16%)	11/29 (38%)	NS
Proteinuria (gm/day)			
(1983)	1.0 ± 0.6	2.2 ± 2.0	p <0.005
(1989)	1.1 ± 1.0	2.2 ± 3.3	NS
Se Creat (mg/dl)			
(1983)	1.1 ± 0.2	1.3 ± 0.2	p <0.005
(1989)	1.2 ± 0.3	2.1 ± 2.0	p <0.05
Ccr (ml/min)			
(1983)	92 ± 27	85 ± 24	NS
(1989)	76 ± 33	66 ± 32	NS
Histology:			
Segmental sclerosis %	12 ± 15	12 ± 10	NS
Global sclerosis %	15 ± 16	18 ± 12	NS
Crescents %	3.5 ± 6.9	2.1 ± 3.9	NS

Table 4 Comparison of patients with and without low molecular weight proteinuria

Parameter	Without LMW	With LMW	t-test
Number	41	19	
Age (years)	26 ± 7	26 ± 7	NS
Sex (m/f)	30 / 11	16 / 3	NS
Duration FU. months	82 ± 59	85 ± 40	S
Presentation:			
Asymptomatic haematuria /proteinuria	33	15	NS
Gross haematuria /proteinuria	8	4	NS
Hypertension	10/41 (24%)	6/19 (32%)	NS
Proteinuria (gm/day)			
(1983)	1.2 ± 1.3	2.5 ± 1.8	p <0.005
(1989)	1.5 ± 2.8	1.8 ± 1.6	S
Se Creat (mg/dl)			
(1983)	1.1 ± 0.2	1.3 ± 0.2	p <0.05
(1989)	1.3 ± 0.3	2.4 ± 2.5	p <0.01
Ccr (ml/min			
(1983)	86 ± 26	94 ± 25	NS
(1989)	73 ± 31	68 ± 36	NS
Histology:			
Segmental sclerosis %	12 ± 13	13 ± 11	NS
Global sclerosis %	17 ± 16	16 ± 10	NS
Crescents %	3.2 ± 6.3	2.0 ± 4.1	NS

Comparison of patients with pattern 1 and patterns 2, 3, 4

Table 3 shows the profile of the 31 patients with pattern 1 compared to the 29 patients with mixed pattern (patterns 2, 3, 4). There were no significant differences between their age, sex, duration of follow up, mode of presentation or incidence of hypertension. However, patients with mixed pattern had more severe proteinuria when compared to those with type 1 pattern. Patients with mixed pattern also had higher serum creatinine values at presentation as well as at final follow up (1989). Comparison of the renal biopsy features at presentation revealed no differences in the distribution of glomerulosclerosis and crescents.

Comparison of patients with and without LMW proteinuria

Table 4 shows profiles of the 2 groups of patients with and without low molecular weight proteinuria. There were no differences in their age, sex, duration of follow up, presentation and incidence of hypertension. However, patients with LMW proteinuria had more severe proteinuria and higher serum creatinine levels compared to those with no LMW proteinuria. There was no significant difference in the various histological indices.

Discussion

Proteinuria in patients with IgA nephritis can be classified into 4 patterns: MMW proteinuria alone or pattern 1 proteinuria as opposed to those with a mixed pattern (patterns 2, 3, 4). Patients with pattern 1 proteinuria have a better outlook than those with mixed patterns because the mixed pattern contain either LMW or HMW protein, both associated with a poorer outcome. The present data on analysis of the pattern of proteinuria in IgA nephritis based on MW related urinary protein excretion confirms Lison's

[1989] observation regarding the clinical value of studying the pattern of protein excretion.

The GSI was not as good a prognostic guide compared to the pattern of proteinuria as its calculation based on the ratio of MMW/HMW does not take into consideration the presence of LMW protein which is a prognostic index of poor outcome. The present data is in agreement with those of Lison et al. [1989] which showed that classification of proteinuria by visual inspection of the pattern was just as good as a classification based on the GSI which was more tedious as it involved densitometric scanning of the protein bands. A visual scanning by examination of the protein bands in relation to the HMW and LMW bands and the relative position of albumin (thickest band) and transferrin also obviates the need to purchase a densitometer.

Nagy et al. [1987] reported an incidence of 62% nonselective proteinuria in patients with IgA nephritis. Beukhoff et al. [1984] reported 25% and our data show 48% (mixed pattern). The present data also confirm our earlier studies using SI (selectivity index) based on the clearance ratio of IgG over transferrin as measured by the immunodiffusion method which showed that the SI was a useful prognostic index [Woo et al. 1989]. In the present study, the SI was positively correlated with the pattern of protein excretion and a value >0.2 indicates nonselective proteinuria and a less favourable outcome. However, using SI which is based on immunodiffusion, a less expensive methodology, it is not always possible to determine the SI especially when proteinuria is less than about 1.5 gm/day or when there is very little transferrin or IgG in the urine and only albumin is measurable. The SDS-PAGE method on the other hand allows the pattern of proteinuria to be more easily determined even in patients with mild proteinuria. The SDS-PAGE also allows the identification of specific groups of proteins, especially LMW or tubular proteins which have a particularly poor prognosis.

LMW proteinuria appears to be a better prognostic marker than the GSI. After 6 years of follow up, patients with LMW proteinuria had a 47% incidence of developing CRF compared to only 10% ($\chi^2 = 10.8$, $p < 0.001$) among patients with no LMW proteinuria. These observations confirmed earlier reports by Nagy et al. [1987] who recorded an incidence of 64% of tubular protein in patients with IgA nephritis and that those patients with LMW proteinuria do worse compared to those who do not have LMW proteinuria. In our study the incidence of LMW proteinuria was 32% (19/60). There was a positive correlation between the pattern of proteinuria and the degree of tubular atrophy and tubulointerstitial lesions, that is, pattern 1 (only MMW proteins) had lesser degree of tubular atrophy and interstitial lesions whereas patients with patterns 2, 3, 4 who have LMW and or HMW proteins in increasing order of severity have more severe tubular atrophy and interstitial lesions. Our findings are consistent with Nagy's [1987] report in which he suggested that in patients with IgA nephritis, in additional to the glomerular lesion, there were also morphological and functional tubulointerstitial damages which are related to the progression of the disease.

Acknowledgement

This work was supported by grants from the Department of Clinical Research and the Medical Research Council, Ministry of Health, Singapore.

REFERENCES

Balant L, Mulli JC, Fabre J 1974 Urinary protein analysis with sodium dodecylsulphate polyacrylamide gel electrophoresis – a comparison with other analytical techniques. Clin Chim Acta *54:* 27

Beukhof JR, Ockhuizen T, Fleuren GJ, et al. 1984 Relationship between proteinuria and morphology in IgA nephropathy. Contr Nephrol *40:* 228

Cameron JS, Blandford G 1966 The simple assessment of selectivity in heavy proteinuria. Lancet *2:* 242

D'Amico G, Minetti L, Ponticelli C, et al. 1986 Prognostic indicators in idiopathic IgA mesangial nephropathy. Q J Med *59:* 363

Ghiggeri GM, Ginevri F, Candiano G, et al. 1987 Characterization of cationic albumin in minimal change nephropathy. Kidney Int *32:* 547

Ginevri F, Ghiggeri GM, Candiano G, et al. 1989 Endogenous albumin as a marker of renal selectivity in steroid-unresponsive nephrotic syndrome. Nephron *52:* 133

Jackson PJ, Sampson CJ, Cooper EH, et al. 1988 Analysis of proteinuria using a commercial system for automated electrophoresis and isoelectric focusing. Ann Clin Biochem *25:* 319

Kobayashi Y, Hiki Y, Fuji K, et al. 1987 IgA nephropathy: Heterogeneous clinical pictures and steroid therapy in progressive cases. Semin Nephrol *7:* 382

Lison AE, Doedt E, Meyer E 1989 Automatic microdisc electrophoresis for urinary protein analysis: a comparison with standard analysis. Clin Nephrol *32:* 40

Nagy J, Milteny M, Dobos M, et al. 1987 Tubular proteinuria in IgA glomerulonephritis. Clin Nephrol *27:* 76

Woo KT, Edmondson RPS, Wu AYT, et al. 1986 The natural history of IgA nephritis in Singapore. Clin Nephrol *25:* 15

Woo KT, Wu AYT, Lee EJC, et al. 1986 Protein Selectivity in IgA Nephropathy. Nephron *42:* 236

Woo KT, Lau YK, Yap HK, et al. 1989 Protein Selectivity: A prognostic index in IgA nephritis. Nephron *52:* 300

Clinical Nephrology, Vol. 36 No. 1 – 1991 (12–20)

Autoreactive lymphocytotoxic IgM antibodies in highly sensitized dialysis patients waiting for a kidney transplant: identification and clinical relevance

S. Barocci, U. Valente[1], R. Gusmano[2], F. Perfumo[2], S. Cantarella, A. Leprini[3], A. Icardi[4] and A. Nocera

Departments of Immunology, Transplant Surgery[1], Anatomy[3] and Nephrology[4], S. Martino Hospital and University of Genoa, Viale Benedetto XV, 10, I-16132 Genoa and Department of Pediatric Nephrology[2], G. Gaslini Institute, Via 5 Maggio, 39, I-16148 Genoa, Italy

Abstract. The contribution of different families of lymphocytotoxic antibodies in the serologic reactivity of 45 highly sensitized dialysis patients (HSDP) (panel reactivity antibody value-PRA >80%) was assessed by analyzing patients' sera for the presence of auto- and alloreactive IgM and alloreactive IgG antibodies. A total of 220 sera was screened at different incubation temperatures, before and after treatment with the reducing agent dithiothreitol, against a large variety of cell targets by means of complement dependent cytotoxicity (CDC) and antiglobulin augmented (AHG) CDC assays. The results allowed to subdivide the HSDP under study into four groups: Group 1 consisted of 13 untransplanted patients and 14 patients with a prior failed graft whose PRA values did not change following DTT treatment. Alloreactive IgG antibodies alone, with anti-HLA specificity, were present in the sera of this patient group. Group 2 consisted of 3 untransplanted patients whose sera did not contain any autolymphocytotoxic antibody but appeared completely unreactive to panel lymphocytes following DTT treatment, thus confirming the presence of alloreactive IgM only endowed with antiHLA reactivity. Group 3 consisted of 4 untransplanted and 4 patients with a prior failed graft whose sera were found to contain in addition to autoreactive IgM also alloreactive IgG antibodies. Their PRA values declined after DTT treatment on average from 96.2% to 45% and from 95% to 52.5%, respectively. Group 4 consisted of 6 untransplanted patients whose PRA reactivity to both autologous and panel lymphocytes completely disappeared following DTT treatment, thus indicating that their sera contained exclusively autolymphocytotoxic IgM antibodies. The presence of autoreactive IgM antibodies appeared to be also correlated with an increased frequency of HLA-DR1 antigen. Four patients belonging to group 4 were successfully transplanted with a first kidney graft (two from cadaver donors, one from a living related haploidentical donor and the other one from a living unrelated donor) in the presence of a current-negative peak-positive T- and B-cell crossmatch, that became negative following DTT treatment.

Key words: highly sensitized dialysis patients – lymphocytotoxic antibodies – pretransplant crossmatch – dithiothreitol treatment – kidney allograft

Introduction

One of the major problems in renal transplantation is represented by the accumulation on the waiting lists of highly sensitized dialysis patients (HSDP) whose sera generally react against more then 80% of a random panel of allogenic peripheral blood lymphocytes. This patient category has a low possibility of receiving a compatible kidney graft with a negative crossmatch (Xmatch) because of the presence in patients' sera of alloreactive lymphocytotoxic antibodies directed against a large number of HLA public and private specificities. In the last years, increasing evidence has been provided that not all HSDP have graft-damaging antibodies [Ettenger et al. 1981, Cardella et al. 1982, Ettenger et al. 1983, Ayoub et al. 1983, Ting and Morris 1983, Barger et al. 1989]. In fact, lymphocytotoxic preformed antibodies in such

Received March 16, 1990; in revised form January 12, 1991.

Reprint requests to Dr. Arcangelo Nocera, Department of Immunology, S. Martino Hospital and University of Genoa, Viale Benedetto XV, 10, I-16132 Genoa, Italy.

patients can be classified into different families according to Ig class (IgG, IgM) [Chapman et al. 1986, Taylor et al. 1987, Iwaki et al. 1988], antigenic specificity (anti-HLA, anti-non HLA, alloreactive and autoreactive) [Chapman et al. 1986, Taylor et al. 1987, Iwaki et al. 1988, Mohanakumar et al. 1981, Ahern et al. 1982, Barocci et al. 1988, Ting 1989] and effect on renal allograft survival (not harmful, detrimental) [Ettenger et al. 1981, Cardella et al. 1982, Ettenger et al. 1983, Ting and Morris 1983, Barger et al. 1989, Vaidya and Ruth 1989, Mohanakumar et al. 1981, Ahern et al. 1982, Ayoub et al. 1983, Ting 1989]. Autoreactive lymphocytotoxic antibodies generally belong to IgM class, are found alone or together in a certain proportion of HSDP patients and when present alone do not seem to have a damaging effect on renal graft [Ettenger et al. 1983, Ting and Morris 1983, Barger et al. 1989, Ting 1989, Vaidya and Ruth 1989]. In fact recent studies have shown that renal transplants performed in the presence of a positive crossmatch due to IgM lymphocytotoxic autoantibodies (AT-IgM Ab) have a good allograft survival with a low risk of hyperacute or acute rejection [Ettenger et al. 1983, Ting and Morris 1983, Barger et al. 1989, Ting 1989, Vaidya and Ruth 1989]. The present study was aimed at the identification in our series of those patients in which no other lymphocytotoxic Ab other than AT-IgM Ab were present.

Materials and methods

Patients

Fourty-five dialysis patients from the 307 (14.6%) on our waiting list, whose sera showed a high reactivity (PRA >80%) against a random peripheral blood lymphocyte panel were studied. Twenty-seven patients were on a waiting list for a first kidney transplant and 18 had a prior failed graft and were on the waiting list for a second transplant. All the patients received blood transfusions with filtered blood or packed red cells (range number: 1 to >50) either for clinical needs or pretransplant immune conditioning policy or both. Serum samples from HSDP were collected at bimonthly intervals or more frequently following blood transfusions and screened at room temperature (r.t.) against an extended panel of thirty allogeneic HLS-typed PBL by means of a long incubation two-stage NIH microcytotoxicity technique (CDC). Sera showing PRA values <80% against the above extended cell panel were selected for a reanalysis that was aimed at the detection of lymphocytotoxic auto- and alloreactive IgM antibodies (AT-IgM Ab, AL-IgM ab) and alloreactive IgG Ab (AL-IgG Ab). A total of 220 sera, selected as above, were screened at different incubation temperatures (4° C, 22° C) against a large variety of cell targets before and after treatment with the reducing agent dithiothreitol (DTT) with both CDC and antiglobulin augmented (AHG) CDC assays.

DTT treatment

Recipients' sera were treated with DTT as previously described [Pirofsky and Rosner 1974]. Briefly, serum samples were divided into two 90 µl aliquots to which 10 µl of 50 mM DTT (final concentration: 5 mM) or 10 µl of phosphate-buffered saline (PBS) were added respectively. Both the aliquots were incubated for 30 min at 37° C and cooled at 22° C before being added to target cells. Briefly, 1 µl of DTT treated sera was mixed with 1 µl of target cells and incubated for 30 min at 22° C. After washing twice, 5 µl of rabbit complement were added to the mixture that was incubated at 22° C for 90 min before the addition of eosin as dye [Barger et al. 1989].

AHG augmented CDC assay

AHG augmented CDC assays were performed as previously described [Fuller et al. 1982].

Cell targets

The following cell targets were utilized for CDC assays: i) Allogeneic PBL. These targets were prepared by Ficoll-Hypaque (F-H) density gradients from peripheral blood of thirty HLA-A, B, C, and DR typed healthy subjects and used at concentration of 4×10^6/ml; ii) Autologous PBL. These cells were prepared as above from each patient under study. iii) EBV-induced autologous B-lymphoblasts. These cells were obtained following transformation of autologous PBL with Epstein-Barr virus containing supernatants prepared from B 95-8 marmoset cell line [Bird et al. 1981] and used at the concentration of 2×10^6/ml; iv) phytohemagglutin (PHA) induced autologous T-lymphoblasts. These cells were established by in vitro PHA activation (Difco, Detroit Michigan) (1 µg/ml) of patients' autologous PBL and subsequent expansion with recombinant IL-2 (Hoffman-La Roche, Nutley, N.J.) (5 U/ml) [Nocera et al. 1986]. PHA T-lymphoblasts were used at the concentration of 2×10^6/ml; v) K562 cell line. K562 cells, which do not express HLA antigens, were grown in RPMI 1640 medium supplemented with 10% FCS, 2 mM L-glutamine, 100 U/ml penicillin and 100 µg/ml streptomycin. Cells were harvested in the growth phase, resuspended in RPMI-1640 10% FCS and used at the concentration of 2×10^6/ml [Deierhoi et al. 1984].

The above allogeneic and autologous targets as well as K562 cells were used to differentiate anti-HLA antibodies (IgM, IgG) from autoreactive IgM antibodies.

Absorption and precipitation procedures for AT-IgM removal

AT-IgM from selected HSDP sera were absorbed with different cell preparations. Different aliquots of the same serum were absorbed either with autologous PHA induced T-lymphoblasts or EBV transformed B-lymphoblasts or K562 cells. Briefly, absorption procedures were performed using a two-stage technique. In the first stage, 200 µl of serum were incubated with 30 × 10^6 absorbing cells for 2 hrs at 37° C. After this first incubation, serum was centrifuged twice and incubated a second time with the same amount of absorbing cells overnight at 4° C [Barocci et al. 1988].

Precipitation procedures with polyethylenglicol (PEG) were also used for AT-IgM Ab removal. PEG precipitation was performed by mixing 2 ml of serum with an equal volume of 8% PEG (6000 M.W.). The mixture was incubated for 16 hrs at 4° C and then centrifuged 1 hr at 20,000 rpm. After decanting the supernatant, the precipitate was washed with a 3.5% PEG solution and redissolved in 0.1 M NaOH. The protein concentration was measured by the absorbance at 280 nm [Digeon et al. 1977]. After the above procedures sera were tested against autologous and allogeneic PBL for evaluating the residual autolymphocytotoxic activity. A long incubation two-stage microcytotoxicity, performed at 22° C, was used for both cell targets.

Pre-transplant Xmatches

Final Xmatches between renal allograft recipients' sera and potential donor cells or autologous lymphocytes were performed with a long incubation CDC technique, using DTT untreated and treated

Table 1 Antibody reactivity against different cell targets of untreated and dithiothreitol (DTT) treated sera from 27 highly sensitized dialysis patients in waiting list for a first kidney graft

Patient	Age	Sex	Untreated sera Reactivity against extended[1] PBL Panel	autologous[2] PBL	autologous[1] EBV B-cell lines	autologous[2] PHA T-cell lines	K562[1]
R. G.	58	M[5]	90	Neg.	Neg.	Neg.	Neg.
B. S.	21	M	100	Pos.	Pos.	Pos.	Pos.
C. C.	57	F[6]	85	Neg.	Neg.	Neg.	Neg.
R. R.	54	F	100	Neg.	Neg.	Neg.	Unc.[4]
B. E.	52	F	100	Pos.	Pos.	Unc.	Pos.
F. G.	50	F	80	Neg.	Neg.	Neg.	Pos.
G. R.	52	F	100	Neg.	Neg.	Neg.	Neg.
G. G.	54	M	85	Neg.	Neg.	Neg.	Unc.
L. A.	32	F	80	Neg.	Neg.	Neg.	Neg.
O. E.	51	F	100	Pos.	Pos.	Pos.	Pos.
P. S.	4	F	100	Pos.	Pos.	Pos.	Pos.
R. D.	52	F	95	Neg.	Neg.	Neg.	Neg.
R. C.	40	F	85	Neg.	Neg.	Neg.	Neg.
R. N.	48	M	90	Pos.	Pos.	Pos.	Pos.
S. C.	55	F	80	Pos.	Pos.	Pos.	Pos.
S. G.	60	F	100	Neg.	Neg.	Neg.	Neg.
S. C.	51	F	90	Neg.	Neg.	Neg.	Neg.
S. A.	42	F	100	Neg.	Neg.	Neg.	Neg.
S. R.	54	F	100	Neg.	Neg.	Neg.	Neg.
B. L.	51	F	85	Neg.	Neg.	Neg.	Neg.
B. E.	4	M	85	Neg.	Neg.	Neg.	Neg.
S. L.	6	M	85	Neg.	Neg.	Neg.	Neg.
R. G. F.	54	M	100	Pos.	Pos.	Pos.	Pos.
P. A.	62	M	100	Pos.	Pos.	Pos.	Pos.
D. M.	52	M	100	Pos.	Pos.	Pos.	Pos.
B. F.	24	F	90	Pos.	Pos.	Pos.	Pos.
G. S.	50	F	90	Neg.	Neg.	Neg.	Neg.

representative peak sera and current sera. Sera giving a positive Xmatch were reanalyzed after DTT treatment.

T- and B-cell purification for pre-transplant Xmatches

Columns prepared with scrubbed nylon wool (Fenwall Laboratories, Illinois) were utilized for obtaining enriched T- and B-cell suspension from donor peripheral blood, lymph nodes and spleen, respectively. T-lymphocytes were recovered in the non adherent fractions whereas B-lymphocytes were recovered after eluting the adherent cell fraction. Purified T and B cells were utilized as targets in pretransplant Xmatch assays.

HLA-DR typing

Patients and healthy controls were typed for HLA-DR antigens by standard technique using a battery of sera specific for the DR specificities recognized by the X Histocompatibility Workshop.

Results

Control sera

To check that DTT treatment was effective in our panel studies we used an anti HLA-DQW2 mAb (MP1) and an anti HLA-B7 mAb, both of IgM class (a generous gift of Dr. G. B. Ferrara, Istituto per la

Table 1 Continued

Patient	Age	Sex	DTT Treated sera Reactivity against extended[1] PBL Panel	autologous[2] PBL	autologous[1] EBV B-cell lines	autologous[2] PHA T-cell lines	K562[1]	Conclusion Antibody class	Antigenic specificity
R. G.	58	M[5]	90	NT[3]	NT	NT	Neg.	IgG	HLA
B. S.	21	M	0	Neg.	Neg.	Neg.	Neg.	IgM	auto (non HLA)
C. C.	57	F[6]	80	NT	NT	NT	Neg.	IgG	HLA
R. R.	54	F	100	NT	NT	NT	Pos.	IgG	HLA
B. E.	52	F	0	Neg.	Neg.	Neg.	Neg.	IgM	auto (non HLA)
F. G.	50	F	80	NT	NT	NT	Pos.	IgG	HLA
G. R.	52	F	100	NT	NT	NT	Neg.	IgG	HLA
G. G.	54	M	85	NT	NT	NT	Neg.	IgG	HLA
L. A.	32	F	80	NT	NT	NT	Neg.	IgG	HLA
O. E.	51	F	0	Neg.	Neg.	Neg.	Neg.	IgM	auto (non HLA)
P. S.	4	F	50	Neg.	Neg.	Neg.	Neg.	IgM + IgG	auto (non HLA) + HLA
R. D.	52	F	90	NT	NT	NT	Neg.	IgG	HLA
R. C.	40	F	85	NT	NT	NT	Neg.	IgG	HLA
R. N.	48	M	40	Neg.	Neg.	Neg.	Neg.	IgM + IgG	auto (non HLA) + HLA
S. C.	55	F	0	Neg.	Neg.	Neg.	Neg.	IgM	auto (non HLA)
S. G.	60	F	0	NT	NT	NT	Neg.	IgM	HLA
S. C.	51	F	0	NT	NT	NT	Neg.	IgM	HLA
S. A.	42	F	0	NT	NT	NT	Neg.	IgM	HLA
S. R.	54	F	100	NT	NT	NT	Neg.	IgG	HLA
B. L.	51	F	85	NT	NT	NT	Neg.	IgG	HLA
B. E.	4	M	80	NT	NT	NT	Neg.	IgG	HLA
S. L.	6	M	85	NT	NT	NT	Neg.	IgG	HLA
R. G. F.	54	M	0	Neg.	Neg.	Neg.	Neg.	IgM	auto (non HLA)
P. A.	62	M	0	Neg.	Neg.	Neg.	Neg.	IgM	auto (non HLA)
D. M.	52	M	50	Neg.	Neg.	Neg.	Neg.	IgM + IgG	auto (non HLA) + HLA
B. F.	24	F	70	Neg.	Neg.	Neg.	Neg.	IgM + IgG	auto (non HLA) + HLA
G. S.	50	F	0	NT	NT	NT	NT	IgM	HLA

[1] Complement dependent cytotoxicity assays were performed only at 22° C incubation temperature, [2] complement dependent cytotoxicity assays were performed at 4° C and 22° C incubation temperature with the same results, [3] NT: not tested, [4] Unc: uncertain, [5] M: Male, [6] F: Female

Ricerca sul Cancro, Genoa Italy) that were tested against DQW2^{+} and B7^{+} EBV transformed B-cell lines by CDC assay, respectively. DTT treatment completely inactivated the reactivity of these mAbs against their specific EBV target cells.

Antibody reactivity studies with and without DTT

Three peak sera or more (when available) from 27 HSDP waiting for a first graft and from 18 HSDP with a prior failed graft were tested, before and after DTT treatment, at different temperatures against a variety of cell targets as detailed under *Materials and methods* (Tables 1 and 2). The differential reactivity pattern displayed by patients' sera against various target cell types, allowed to subdivide HSDP into four groups according to the class and antigen specificity of the antibodies present in their sera (Tables 1 and 2). Group 1 consisted of 13 patients (28.8%) waiting for a first graft and 14 patients with a prior failed graft (31.1%) whose sera contained AL-IgG Ab alone having anti-HLA antigen specificity. For these patients PRA values did not change following DTT treatment. Group 2 consisted of 4 patients (8.8%) waiting for a first graft whose sera did not contain any autolymphocytotoxic antibody but were found to become completely unreactive to panel lymphocytes following DTT treatment. Alloreactive IgM only with anti-HLA specificity were present in these sera.

Group 3 consisted of 4 patients (8.8%) waiting for a first graft and 4 patients (8.8%) with a prior failed graft whose sera were found to contain in addition to autoreactive non HLA IgM Ab also alloreactive IgG Ab endowed with anti-HLA reactivity. PRA values of these sera declined after DTT treatment from 95.0% ± 5.7 to 52.5% ± 12.5 and from 96.2% ± 7.5 to 45.0% ± 12.9 respectively (mean ± S.D.). Group 4 consisted of 6 patients (13.3%) waiting for a first graft whose sera were found to become completely unreactive to both autologous and panel lymphocytes as well as to K562 cells following DTT treatment, thus indicating that these sera contained very likely only autolymphocytotoxic IgM antibodies. These results are summarized in Table 3. It is worth mentioning that, as previously reported (Deierhoi et al. 1984], K562 cells appeared a suitable target for the detection of AT-IgM. In fact, the large majority of sera containing AL-IgG ab did not show any reactivity with this cell line. Sera from only three patients (R. R., G. G. and F. O.), showing AL-IgG Ab, were found to give a very weak reaction with K562 cells (Tables 1 and 2).

Table 2 Antibody reactivity against different cell targets of untreated and dithiothreitol (DTT) treated sera from 18 highly sensitized dialysis patients in waiting list for a second kidney graft

Patient	Age	Sex	Untreated sera Reactivity against extended[1] PBL Panel	autologous[2] PBL	autologous[1] EBV B-cell lines	autologous[2] PHA T-cell lines	K562[1]
L. D.	19	M[5]	80	Neg.	Neg.	Neg.	Neg.
C. G.	48	M	100	Pos.	Pos.	Pos.	Pos.
P. R.	52	M	90	Neg.	Neg.	Neg.	Neg.
G. M.	55	F[6]	100	Neg.	Neg.	Neg.	Neg.
O. D.	53	M	100	Pos.	Pos.	Pos.	Pos.
S. S.	32	M	85	Pos.	Pos.	Pos.	Pos.
V. O.	41	F	90	Neg.	Neg.	Neg.	Neg.
F. D.	17	M	90	Neg.	Neg.	Neg.	Neg.
C. S.	24	F	100	Neg.	Neg.	Neg.	Neg.
C. I.	22	F	100	Neg.	Neg.	Neg.	Neg.
G. S.	4	M	85	Neg.	Neg.	Neg.	Neg.
F. O.	8	M	80	Neg.	Neg.	Neg.	Unc.[4]
O. B.	35	F	100	Neg.	Neg.	Neg.	Neg.
D. M.	25	F	100	Pos.	Pos.	Pos.	Pos.
B. C.	56	M	80	Neg.	Neg.	Neg.	Neg.
A. F.	55	M	85	Neg.	Neg.	Neg.	Neg.
F. C.	21	F	100	Neg.	Neg.	Neg.	Neg.
P. R.	50	M	80	Neg.	Neg.	Neg.	Neg.

AT-IgM removal

In another set of experiments sera containing autoreactive IgM, obtained from the 14 patients belonging to group 3 and 4, were analyzed in order to evaluate the efficacy of different procedures such as cell target absorption, PEG precipitation and DTT treatment in removing AT-IgM. The results (Table 4) showed that DTT treatment appeared to be the most reliable procedure for AT-IgM removal (mean residual autoreactivity: 5%) and for discriminating between AT-IgM Ab and AL-IgG Ab. Other methods

Table 2 Continued

Patient	Age	Sex	DTT Treated sera Reactivity against extended[1] PBL Panel	autologous[2] PBL	autologous[1] EBV B-cell lines	autologous[2] PHA T-cell lines	K 562[1]	Conclusion Antibody class	Antigenic specificity
L. D.	19	M[5]	80	NT[3]	NT	NT	Neg.	IgG	HLA
C. G.	48	M	50	Neg.	Neg.	Neg.	Neg.	IgM + IgG	auto (non HLA) + HLA
P. R.	52	M	85	NT	NT	NT	Neg.	IgG	HLA
G. M.	55	F[6]	100	NT	NT	NT	Neg.	IgG	HLA
O. D.	53	M	30	Neg.	Neg.	Neg.	Neg.	IgM + IgG	auto (non HLA) + HLA
S. S.	32	M	40	Neg.	Neg.	Neg.	Neg.	IgM + IgG	auto (non HLA) + HLA
V. O.	41	F	90	NT	NT	NT	Neg.	IgG	HLA
F. D.	17	M	90	NT	NT	NT	Neg.	IgG	
C. S.	24	F	100	NT	NT	NT	Neg.	IgG	HLA
C. I.	22	F	100	NT	NT	NT	Neg.	IgG	HLA
G. S.	4	M	85	NT	NT	NT	Neg.	IgG	HLA
F. O.	8	M	80	NT	NT	MT	Unc.	IgG	HLA
O. B.	35	F	100	NT	NT	NT	Neg.	IgG	HLA
D. M.	25	F	60	Neg.	Neg.	Neg.	Neg.	IgM + IgG	auto (non HLA) + HLA)
B. C.	56	M	80	NT	NT	NT	Neg.	IgG	HLA
A. F.	55	M	85	NT	NT	NT	Neg.	IgG	HLA
F. C.	21	F	100	NT	NT	NT	Neg.	IgG	HLA
P. R.	50	M	80	NT	NT	NT	Neg.	IgG	HLA

[1] Complement dependent cytotoxicity assays were performed only at 22° C incubation temperature, [2] complement dependent cytotoxicity assays were performed both at 4° C and 22° C incubation temperature with the same results, [3] NT: not tested, [4] Unc: uncertain, [5] M: Male, [6] F: Female

Table 3 Autoreactive IgM (AT-IgM), alloreactive IgM (AL-IgM) and alloreactive IgG (AL-IgG) lymphocytotoxic antibody incidence in 45 highly sensitized dialysis patients (PRA >80%)

Patient Category	Patients positive for Alloreactive IgG (HLA) n°	Alloreactive IgM (HLA) n°	Autoreactive IgM (non HLA) n°	Alloreactive IgG (HLA) plus Autoreactive IgM (non HLA) n°
Highly sensitized dialysis patients in waiting list for a first kidney graft (NTP) (N° 27)	13	4	6	4
Highly sensitized dialysis patients in waiting list for a second kidney graft (PFG) (N° 18)	14	0	0	4

Table 4 IgM autoantibody removal from highly sensitized dialysis patients sera by means of different procedures

	Cell absorption with K562	autologous EBV B-cell lines	autologous PHA T-cell lines	PEG precipitation	DTT treatment
Residual reactivity against autologous PBL	32 ± 10[1]	20 ± 9[2]	25 ± 12[2]	50 ± 8[3]	5 ± 0.9[3]

[1] Mean ± S. E.: 10 sera were tested
[2] Mean ± S. E.: 5 sera were tested
[3] Mean ± S. E.: 33 sera were tested

such as absorption with K562, EBV transformed or PHA induced autologous lymphoblasts were not found as efficient as DTT treatment in removing AT-IgM Ab (range of residual autoreactivity: 20–32%). PEG precipitation represented the least effective treatment (mean residual autoreactivity: 50%).

HLA-DR phenotyping

The 14 patients showing AT-IgM together or alone with AL-IgG were typed for HLA-DR antigens and compared with 157 healthy unrelated individuals of the same ethnic background. HLA-DR1 antigen appeared to have an increased frequency in AT-IgM patients (8/14; 57.1%) when compared to controls (25/157; 15.9%) (χ^2 with Yates' correction: 11.5 $p < 0.001$) (data not shown). This difference remained significant also after multiplying the significance value by the number of the 10 DR alleles tested [Grumet et al. 1971] ($p < 0.01$).

Pre-transplant Xmatches

Since December 1987, four patients showing in their sera AT-IgM Ab only were transplanted with a first kidney graft. In particular two of them received a cadaveric (CAD) transplant, a third patient was transplanted with an haploidentical kidney from a living related donor whereas the fourth with a kidney from a living unrelated donor (his wife). At the time of transplantation all four recipients had a negative Xmatch against donor B- and T-lymphocytes with the current serum. In contrast their historic peak sera gave positive crossmatches that became negative following DTT treatment (Table 3). No hyperacute rejection was observed and there was an immediate allograft function with the only exception of one case of acute tubular necrosis (patient O. E.). The kidney survival for the four patients has reached now 33, 27, 15 and 8 months respectively with an excellent graft function.

Discussion

It has become evident in the last years that a positive T- + B- or T-cell crossmatch in renal transplant recipients may not be a contraindication, providing that the antibody responsible for the positive Xmatch belongs to IgM class. Therefore it is important to know which types of preformed antibodies are present in sera of potential renal allografts recipients. In our series of 45 HSDP, 18 patients (40%) were found to show DTT sensitive IgM lymphocytotoxic antibodies alone or together with IgG lymphocytotoxic Ab.

A detailed analysis showed that IgM were directed at non auto HLA structures in 4 cases (alloreactive IgM) and at autologous non HLA membrane target structures in 14 cases (autoreactive IgM). In 8 of the above 14 patients autoreactive IgM Ab were found together with alloreactive IgG Ab, whereas in the remaining six autoreactive IgM Ab represented very likely the only lymphocytotoxic antibody type. However, in these latter patients it was not possible to exclude absolutely that some AL-IgM Ab could be present in addition to AT-IgM Ab; to date there are to our knowledge no technical approaches, in addition to those used in this paper, to answer definitely this question. Considering the total number of our local transplant candidates, AT-IgM Ab were detected as the only lymphocytotoxic Ab type in 6/45 highly sensitized dialysis patients (13.3%) with a global incidence of 1.9% considering the number (306) of our local transplant candidates. These percentages were very similar to those reported by some studies from North American centers [Ettenger et al. 1981, Barger et al. 1989, Vaidya 1989] but lower than those found by other authors [Lobo 1981; Ting 1989]. For instance autoreactive IgM Ab have been reported by Ting in Oxford's series [Ting 1989] to occur in about 10% of patients waiting for a first graft and up to about 50% in those with a prior failed graft. Several factors such as the methods used for detection, the composition of patients' series as well as the characteristic pattern of appearance and disappearance from patients' sera of

Table 5 Pre-transplant crossmatches[1] against donor specific purified T-lymphocytes (TL) performed with dithiothreitol (DTT) untreated and treated sera from four highly sensitized dialysis patients

Patient	Sex	Graft	HLA-A, B mismatches	HLA-DR mismatches	Crossmatches against autologous PBL		T-lymphocytes[2]		Graft outcome
					Peak	Current	Peak	Current	
O. E.	F[3]	1CAD[5]	3	1	+[8]	–[9]	+[8]	–[9]	Good at 33 months
R. G.	M[4]	1CAD	4	1	+[8]	–[9]	+[8]	–[9]	Good at 27 months
B. S.	M	1LRD[6]	2	1	+[8]	–[9]	+[8]	–[9]	Good at 15 months
P. A.	M	1LUD[7]	2	1	+[8]	–[9]	+[8]	–[9]	Good at 8 months

[1] Crossmatches were performed by means of complement dependent cytotoxicity. [2] T-lymphocytes were purified from lymph nodes of cadaver donors and from peripheral blood lymphocytes of living donors. Similar results were obtained against spleen and peripheral blood purified B-lymphocytes obtained from cadaver and living donors, respectively. [3] Female. [4] Male. [5] 1CAD: First transplant from a cadaver donor. [6] 1LRD: First transplant from a living related donor. [7] 1LUD: First transplant from a living unrelated donor. [8] The peak sera tested were 3 for patient O. E., 6 for patient R. G., 4 for patient B. S. and 6 for patient P. A. These sera became completely unreactive against both autologous-PBL and donor derived T- and B-lymphocyte targets after DTT treatment. [9] In addition to current serum negative crossmatch, auto and donor T and B negative crossmatch were also obtained with sera collected during the 4 months prior to transplantation for patient O. E., the 10 months for patient R. G., the 20 months for patient B. S. and the 20 months for patient P. A.

AT IgM antibodies are very likely responsible for the discrepancies in the incidence rates of AT IgM antibodies among different centers. Four of the above six patients having autoreactive IgM Ab only were transplanted in our center across a peak positive current negative crossmatch with no evidence of hyperacute rejection. All the grafts have shown until now an excellent function; unfortunately the other two patients could not be transplanted because they died during their permanence on the waiting list. In agreement with a previous report [Barger et al. 1989] patients of our series showing AT-IgM Ab alone were only found in the non-transplant category, whereas AT-IgM Ab together with AL-IgG were found both in the non-transplant patients and in those with a prior failed graft. This observation may indicate that a number of transplant unrelated events (e.g. blood transfusions, pregnancies and viral infections) in association with immunoreactivity-related individual factors are responsible, in selected patients, for the induction of AT-IgM Ab only. In this study AT-IgM appearance appeared to be significantly correlated to HLA-DR1 phenotype but not to any particular cause of end-stage renal disease. This latter finding is an agreement with a previous study [Barger et al. 1989] showing that the presence of AT-IgM Ab in renal allograft recipients was correlated to the black ethnic background, to an increased frequency of DR1 phenotype and to systemic lupus erythematosus as cause of ESRD. To our knowledge, our report is the first one in the literature showing the presence of an association between DR1 phenotype and AT-IgM production also in a caucasoid renal transplant candidate population. DR1 phenotype has been previously associated with low immunological responsiveness and increased allograft survival [Cicciarelli 1987]. In this regard, the increased presence of non-harmful AT-IgM might be one of the mechanisms responsible for an improved graft survival in DR1$^+$ kidney graft sensitized recipients.

The results here reported together with those from other groups [Cardella et al. 1982, Ettenger et al. 1983, Goeken 1985] can be useful to explain previous conflicting reports about the possibility to transplant safely in the presence of a current-negative, peak-positive Xmatch as reviewed in [Ting and Morris 1983, and Cardella et al. 1982, Ayoub et al. 1983, Goeken 1985]. In this respect, only patients with a peak-positive Xmatch due to DTT sensitive autoreactive IgM antibodies should be considered as suitable candidates for receiving a safe transplant, as opposed to those with a peak-positive Xmatch due to AL-IgG or to a mixture of AT-IgM and AL-IgG Ab. Unfortunately also these latter HSDP, represented in our waiting list by 8 out of 44 (18.1%), despite the presence of AT-IgM Ab do not represent a category susceptible of having, by means of this strategy, an increased chance of a safe transplant. Four patients waiting for a first graft were found to display in their sera anti-HLA AL-IgM alone. AL-IgM have been previously reported to appear without any apparent stimuli in dialysis patients [Tongio and Mayer 1985] and in transplanted patients under immunosuppression [Stocker et al. 1969]. At present the exact role played by AL-IgM in allograft survival has not yet been well characterized, even if it has been previously reported [Ting 1989] that also transplants, performed across a T-cell peak positive current negative Xmatch due to this ab type, can have an acceptable success rate (67% at 1 year). More patients with these characteristics should be studied in the future to solve this problem. All the above results underline the necessity of clarifying individually which antibody category is responsible for patient sensitization and may have a practical importance in order to increase the possibility of a safe transplant for those HSDP having a donor specific positive peak and/or current Xmatch because of the presence in their sera of AT-IgM Ab alone. The recognition strategy of different antibody families might also be useful for a correct definition of inclusion criteria in international kidney exchange trials that should therefore be limited to hyperimmunized dialysis patients having alloreactive lymphocytotoxic antibodies.

Acknowledgements

We wish to thank Dr. T. C. Fuller (Histocompatibility Laboratory Massachusetts General Hospital, Boston MA, USA) for providing us with reagents for AHG-CDC assays. This work has been partially supported by grants n° CN.89.00233.PF.703 and n° 89.00179.70 (P. F. Biotecnologie e Biostrumentazione) from Consiglio Nazionale delle Ricerche, by grants from Ministero della Pubblica Istruzione (quote 40 and 60%) and by NATO grant 0135/88.

REFERENCES

Ahern AT, Artruc SB, Della Pelle P, Cosimi AB, Russell PS, Colvin RB, Fuller TC 1982 Hyperacute rejection on HLA-AB-identical renal allografts associated with B-lymphocyte and endothelial reactive antibodies. Transplantation *33:* 103

Ayoub GM, Terasaki PI, Tonai RJ 1983 Improvements in detection of sensititation. Transpl Proc *15:* 1202

Barger B, Shroyer TW, Hudson SL, Deierhoi MH, Barber WH, Curtis JJ, Julian BA, Luke RG, Diethelm AG 1989 Successful renal allografts in recipients with crossmatch-positive, dithioerythritol-treated negative sera. Transplantation *47:* 240

Barocci S, Valente U, Carozzi S, Mantero D, Fontana I, Cantarella S, Millo R, Gusmano R, Nocera A 1988 Characterization of different patterns of antibody reactivity in highly sensitized dialysis patients. Transpl Proc *20:* 951

Bird AG, Mc Lachlan SM, Britton S 1981 Cyclosporin A promotes spontaneous outgrow in vitro of Epstein-Barr virus-induced B-cell lines. Nature *289:* 300

Cardella CJ, Falk JA, Nicholson MJ, Harding M, Cook GT 1982 Successful renal transplantation in patients with T-cell reactivity to donor. Lancet, *2:* 1240

Chapman JR, Taylor CJ, Ting A, Morris PJ 1986. Immunoglobulin class and specificity of antibodies causing positive T-cell crossmatches. Relationship to renal transplant outcome. Transplantation *42:* 608

Cicciarelli J 1987 HLA-DR1 is a low responsiveness antigen in human kidney transplant recipients. In: *Terasaki PI,* ed. Clinical Transplants. Los Angeles: UCLA Tissue Typing Laboratory, 381.

Deierhoi MH, Ting A, Morris PJ 1984 Reactivity of lymphocyte cytotoxic autoantibodies from renal patients with cell line K562. Transplantation *38:* 557

Digeon M, Laver M, Riza J, Bach JF 1977 Detection of circulating immune complexes in human sera by simplified assays with polyethylene glycol. J Immunol Methods *16:* 165

Ettenger RB, Jordan S, Fine RN 1981 Autolymphocytotoxic antibodies in patients on dialysis awaiting renal transplantation. Transplantation *32:* 248

Ettenger RB, Jordan SC, Fine RN 1983 Cadaver renal transplant outcome in recipients with autolymphocytotoxic antibodies. Transplantation *35:* 429

Fuller TC, Phelan D, Gebel HM, Rodey GE 1982 Antigenic specificity of antibody reactive in the antiglobulin-augmented lymphocytotoxicity tests. Transplantation *34:* 24

Goeken NE 1985 Outcome of renal transplantation following a positive crossmatch with historical sera: The second analysis of the ASHI survey. Transplant Proc *17:* 2443

Grumet FC, Coukell A, Bodmer JG, Bodmer WF, McDevitt HO 1971 Histocompatibility (HL-A) antigen associated with systemic lupus erythematosus. A possible genetic predisposition to disease. New Engl J Med *285:* 193

Iwaki Y, Law M, Terasaki PI 1988 Successful transplants across T-warm-positive crossmatches due to IgM antibodies. Clin Transplant *2:* 81

Lobo PI 1981 Nature of autolymphocytotoxins present in renal hemodialysis patients. Transplantation *32:* 233

Mohanakumar T, Rhodes C, Mendez-Picon G, Goldman M, Moncure C, Lee H 1981 Renal allograft rejection associated with presensitization to HLA-DR antigens. Transplantation *31:* 93

Nocera A, Barocci S, Valente U, Carozzi S, Burastero S, Zicca A, Cadoni A, Dessì V, Celada F 1986 In vitro characterization of a donor-specific cytolytic T-cell line established from human lymphocytes homing in a rejected kidney allograft. Transplantation *41:* 135

Pirofsky B, Rosner E 1974 DTT- test: A new method to differentiate IgM and IgG erytrocyte antibodies. Vox Sang. *27:* 480

Stocker JW, McKenzie IFC, Morris PJ 1969 IgM activity in human lymphocytotoxic sera after renal transplantation. Nature *222:* 483

Taylor CJ, Chapman JR, Fuggle SV, Ting A, Morris PJ 1987 A positive B-cell crossmatch due to IgG anti-HLA-DQ antibody present at the time of transplantation in a successful renal allograft. Tissue Antigens *30:* 104

Ting A 1989 Positive crossmatches: when is it safe to transplant. Transplant Int *2:* 2

Ting A, Morris PJ 1983 Successful transplantation with a positive T- and B-cell cross-match due to autoreactive antibodies. Tissue antigens *21:* 219

Tongio MM, Mayer S 1985 Naturally occurring HLA antibodies. Transplant Clin Immunol *17:* 45

Vaidya S, Ruth J 1989 Contribution and clinical significance of IgM and autoantibodies in highly sensitized renal allograft recipients. Transplantation *47:* 956

Clinical Nephrology, Vol. 36 No. 1 – 1991 (21–28)

Abnormal diastolic left ventricular filling by pulsed Doppler echocardiography in patients on continuous ambulatory peritoneal dialysis

J. Hüting [1], W. Kramer [1], J. Reitinger [2], K. Kühn [2], G. Schütterle [1] and V. Wizemann [1]

[1] *Center of Internal Medicine, Justus-Liebig University, Gießen, and* [2] *Dept. of Nephrology, Klinikum Karlsruhe, Germany*

Abstract. To determine characteristics of diastolic left ventricular (LV) function in patients on continuous ambulatory peritoneal dialysis (CAPD), two groups of CAPD patients without (n = 23; group 1) vs with (n = 25; group 2) LV hypertrophy (>13 mm) were compared with a group of untreated non-renal hypertensive patients with LV hypertrophy (n = 11; group 3) using Doppler-echocardiography. Age and body surface area were comparable in all three groups, mean CAPD-duration (32 ± 28 vs 26 ± 23 months; p = NS) was comparable in renal patients. LV systolic function in echocardiography (LVEF: 62 vs 64 vs 63%) and systolic time intervals were normal and comparable in all three groups. Atrial maximum filling velocities (96 ± 25 vs 91 ± 25 vs 67 ± 8 cm/s) were comparably increased, the ratio of maximal early/atrial filling velocities was comparably decreased (0.73 ± 0.25 vs 0.77 ± 0.21 vs 0.99 ± 0.05) in both groups of renal patients as compared to group 3 (p <0.05–0.01). Atrial filling fractions were increased in all three groups, more pronounced in group 1 than in group 3 (50 ± 11 vs 40 ± 7%; p <0.05). The normal correlation of Doppler parameters with age and with LV radius/thickness ratio was altered in renal patients such that high patient age tended to have an additional negative influence on LV diastolic function of hypertrophied, but not of normal myocardium. Isovolumic relaxation time was prolonged in all three groups (134 ± 38 vs 131 ± 34 vs 116 ± 17 ms; p = NS). We conclude that in patients on CAPD, diastolic LV filling is impaired both in normal and hypertrophied myocardium. High age is a factor that further attributes to diastolic dysfunction of hypertrophied myocardium in CAPD.

Key words: continuous ambulatory peritoneal dialysis – diastolic left ventricular function – pulsed Doppler echocardiography

Introduction

High cardiovascular morbidity and mortality account for more than half of the deaths of patients with end-stage renal disease (ESRD), the average 10-year patient survival being as low as 45% [Wing et al. 1984]. A high prevalence of left ventricular (LV) hypertrophy and associated problems has been described both for hemodialysis [Cohen et al. 1987, Hüting et al. 1988, Niwa et al. 1985, Chazan et al. 1987, Mc Lenachan et al. 1987] and CAPD patient [Eisenberg et al. 1987, Leenen et al. 1985]. While LV systolic function has been found mostly normal in both groups [Alpert et al. 1986, Cohen et al. 1987, Eisenberg et al. 1987, Hüting et al. 1990], abnormalities of diastolic LV filling have been described with high prevalence for patients on hemodialysis both during the dialysis procedure [Ritz et al. 1987] and in the dialysis-free interval using invasive [Kramer et al. 1986] and non-invasive [Ruffmann et al. 1990] methods of determination.

The importance of diastolic LV filling in dialysis patients has been documented by Himelman et al. [1988]: they found diastolic LV dysfunction rather than LV hypertrophy or parameters of LV systolic performance to be associated with high perioperative mortality during renal transplantation in patients on chronic hemodialysis.

Therefore, to obtain parameters indicative of the risk of diastolic heart failure especially during interventions such as operations and acute changes of hydration, we analyzed characteristics of diastolic LV filling in a group of 48 patients on CAPD and related our hemodynamic findings to cardiac structure [Sartori et al. 1987, Maron et al. 1987, Pearson et al. 1988, Phillips et al. 1987, Snider et al. 1985], age [Sartori et al. 1987, Bryg et al. 1987, Kuo et al. 1987], blood pressure [Pearson et al. 1988, Phillips et al. 1987,

---

Received October 31, 1990; in revised form November 13, 1990.

Reprint requests to Dr. J. Hüting, Center of Internal Medicine, University of Gießen, Klinikstraße 36, W-6300 Gießen, Germany

Snider et al. 1985] and parameters of blood purification. These findings were compared to those from a group of 11 non-renal hypertensive patients. The possible role of metabolic and structural abnormalities of the myocardium in dialysis is discussed [Silberbauer et al. 1988, Zazgornik et al. 1987, Mall et al. 1990].

Patients and methods

Patients

The study group consisted of 48 patients on an outpatient program coming for a routine consultation. None of the patients had signs of acute cardiopulmonary decompensation. The patients were examined in the left lateral recumbent position after a 15 minute rest period and with no intraperitoneal dialysis solution installed. Blood pressure values were obtained from the last two weeks before the examination.

Patients on CAPD were divided in two subgroups without (group 1) vs. with (group 2) LV hypertrophy. For the purpose of this study, LV hypertrophy was defined as a thickness of either the septum or the LV free wall of >13 mm. Doppler echocardiographic findings of these patients were compared to those of a group of 11 patients with untreated essential hypertension (group 3).

Echocardiography

Echocardiographic and Doppler-echocardiographic determinations were performed with a Hewlett Packard 77 020 A echo and Doppler imaging system using a 2.5 MHz transducer. Simultaneous phonocardiograms, electrocardiograms and indirect carotid pulse tracings were recorded on a Panasonic 6300 video cassette recorder and as paper prints for later analysis. Echocardiographic measurements were made according to the standards of the American Society of Echocardiography [Sahn et al. 1978].

Doppler-echocardiography

Pulsed Doppler examinations of the LV inflow tract were performed under 2-D guidance from the apical four chamber view. The sample volume was positioned at the level of the tips of the mitral valve leaflets and aligned so that the angle between the ultrasound beam and the blood flow vector as determined from the color flow image was as close to zero as possible. An average of five consecutive cycles was taken from the following measurements: (1) peak velocity of early and late left ventricular filling (peak E, peak A) and their ratios [Rokey et al. 1985, Friedman et al. 1986, Miyatake et al. 1984]; (2) E and A acceleration and deceleration rates [Pearson et al. 1988, Friedman et al. 1986]; (3) early and atrial time velocity integrals and their ratios including atrial filling fraction [Rokey et al. 1985; Pearson et al. 1988, Spirito et al. 1986]; (4) peak early and atrial filling velocities normalized for mitral stroke volume [Bowman et al. 1988].

The following time intervals were determined: (1) isovolumic relaxation period from aortic valve closure in carotid pulse tracing to beginning of mitral inflow in Doppler; (2) total filling period from beginning to end of mitral inflow in Doppler; (3) duration of early and atrial filling periods and their ratios in Doppler; (4) time to peak early (atrial) filling from the onset of early LV filling in Doppler to peak early filling; (5) isovolumic contraction from cessation of LV inflow in Doppler to aortic valve opening in carotid pulse tracing; (6) pre-ejection period from beginning of electrocardiographic systole to aortic valve opening in carotid pulse tracing.

Statistics

Data are expressed as mean ± standard deviation. For correlation studies, Pearson's correlation coefficient for linear regression analysis was determined. A correlation coefficient was considered significant for a probability that the observed correlation is due to chance $p < 0.05$. The significance of differences was determined with Student's t-test for unpaired data.

Results

Clinical patient data

Clinical data are summarized in Table 1. Mean patient age was comparable between the three groups, total dialysis duration was comparable between the two groups of renal patients.

A history of hypertension before the start of CAPD therapy, usually a period of elevated blood pressure for 3–6 months, was known for 77% of renal patients. Blood pressure for these patients during that pre-dialysis period averaged 183 ± 32 mmHg (range: 110–240 mmHg) systolic, 99 ± 21 mmHg (range: 70–150 mmHg) diastolic and 127 ± 23 mmHg (range: 87–200 mmHg) mean (Table 1). At the time of the study, blood pressure for renal patients averaged 136 ± 19 mmHg (range: 80–180 mmHg) systolic, 78 ± 11 mmHg (range: 40–100 mmHg) diastolic, and 97 ± 12 mmHg (range: 53–117 mmHg) mean. Comparable to values of CAPD patients before treatment, mean arterial blood pressure was 126 ± 9.8 mmHg for patients with essential hypertension.

Antihypertensive medication was taken by 47 patients (= 84%) on CAPD, the average number of cardiovascular drugs per patient being 1.17 ± 1.13 (range: 0–4). The most frequently used antihypertensive drugs were calcium antagonists (26 patients), clonidine (9 patients), β-receptor blocking agents (7 patients), angiotensin converting enzyme inhibitors (2 patients) and dihydralazine (2 patients). None of the patients had relevant mitral or aortic stenosis or regurgitation as evaluated by color flow Doppler analysis.

Non-renal patients were studied before the institution of antihypertensive medication. None of these patients had signs of impaired renal function.

Table 1 Clinical characteristics of patients on CAPD (groups 1 and 2) and non-renal hypertensives (group 3). In all tables, the significance of differences and correlations is marked as: *: p <0.05, **: p <0.01, ***: p <0.001

Parameter	Dimension	CAPD-patients Normal LV Muscle mass Mean ± S.D.		LV Hypertrophy Mean ± S.D.		Non-renal hypertensives Mean ± S.D.		t-values 1 vs 2	1 vs 3	2 vs 3
Number		25 (16F)		23 (7F)		11 (M)				
Age	years	59.68	9.18	55.3	12.14	54.1	7.9	1.45	0.8	0.31
Body surface area	M^2	1.71	0.15	1.77	0.22	1.76	0.22	1.14	0.82	0.13
CAPD duration	months	33.28	27.89	25.74	23.28	–		1.03	–	–
Antihypertensive drugs		0.85	0.77	1.52	1.02	0	0	2.64*		
Mean arterial blood pressure:										
before start of CAPD	mmHg	123.6	22.9	130.9	18.6	–		1.23	–	–
at time of study	mmHg	97.5	10.5	96.4	13.3	126	9.8	0.33	7.87**	6.76***

Biochemical data

Biochemical parameters of CAPD patients are summarized in Table 2. Mean hemoglobin, creatinine and urea concentrations were comparably altered in the two groups of CAPD patients. These parameters were in the normal range in non-renal hypertensive patients.

Table 2 Blood chemistry in patients on CAPD. Parameters of non-renal patients were in normal range

Parameter	Dimension	Normal LV Muscle mass Mean ± S.D.		LV Hypertrophy Mean ± S.D.	
Hemoglobin	g/dl	10.08	1.8	9.31	1.84
creatinine	mg/dl	8.81	2.5	10.37	3.3
urea	mg/dl	9.98	2.88	11.16	3.03

Statistical significance in tables:

	Group:	1 vs 2	1 vs 2	2 vs 3
Group 1 = CAPD without hypertrophy	p <0.05	*	+	$
Group 2 = CAPD with hypertrophy	p <0.01	**	++	$$
Group 3 = non-renal hypertensives	p <0.001	***	+++	$$$

Echocardiographic parameters

Echocardiographic characteristics are summarized in Table 3. In all three groups, the following parameters were in the normal range: LV enddiastolic and endsystolic dimensions, LV ejection fraction, fractional shortening, velocity of circumferential fibre shortening, and cardiac index. Mean left atrial diameters were comparably increased in all three groups. Corresponding to the study design, mean LV muscle mass was higher in groups 2 and 3 than in group 1 (p <0.001), due both to thickening of the interventricular septum and of the LV posterior wall.

Doppler parameters

Doppler measurements are summarized in Table 4. Peak and mean velocities of atrial filling were greater, the ratios of early/atrial peak and mean filling velocities were smaller in either group of CAPD patients than in non-renal hypertensives.

The ratios of peak early/atrial filling velocities were inversely correlated with age in CAPD patients with LV hypertrophy, but not in the other two groups (Figure 1). A correlation with age was also found for peak early filling velocity normalized for total mitral inflow volume (Figure 2). No correlation with patient age or radius/thickness ratio was found for peak early and atrial filling velocities in any of the three patient groups.

Atrial filling fractions were increased in all three groups over normal values. Atrial time-velocity integrals and atrial filling fractions were greater in CAPD patients without LV hypertrophy than in non-renal hypertensives. A direct correlation between atrial filling fractions and age was found only in CAPD patients with LV hypertrophy, but not in the other groups (Figure 3). No correlation of atrial filling fractions was observed with radius/thickness ratio in either group. Parameters of blood purification in CAPD patients were not related to any of the analyzed Doppler parameters.

Table 3 Echocardiographic characteristics of the three patient groups

Parameter	Dimension	CAPD-Patients Normal LV Muscle mass Mean ± S.D.		LV Hypertrophy Mean ± S.D.		Non-renal hypertensives Mean ± S.D.		p (1 vs 2)
Heart rate	min^{-1}	81	12	77	12	73.3	9.7	
LV Diameter (D)	mm	51.2	6.9	52.8	5.7	54.1	3.1	
LV Diameter (S)	mm	31.9	8.1	31.8	7.2	32.9	3.8	
LA Diameter	mm	41.2	6.6	40.7	7.8	39.0	3.7	
IVS Thickness (D)	mm	10.9	1.4	15.2	1.6	15.1	2.6	***
LVPW Thickness (D)	mm	7.7	1.1	8.9	1.2	9.7	1.8	***
IVS/LVPW Thicknesses		1.44	0.24	1.74	0.27	1.60	0.33	***
LV Muscle mass	g	216	52.3	324	73	349	73	***
LV Muscle mass index	g/m^2	127	29.9	185	46.7	182	40.0	***
Cardiac index	$l/(m^2*min)$	5.02	1.12	5.26	1.42	4.76	0.77	
Ejection fraction	%	62.1	10.9	64.0	13.3	63.0	6.9	
VCF	circ/s	1.53	0.34	1.61	0.46	1.42	0.24	

Table 4 Doppler parameters of LV diastolic filling

Parameter	Dimension	CAPD-Patients Normal LV muscle mass Mean ± S.D.		With LV Hypertrophy Mean ± S.D.		Non-renal hypertensives Mean ± S.D.	
Peak velocity:							
E-Wave	cm/s	67.48	21.75	69.51	26.26	65.84	17.45
A-Wave	cm/s	95.50	24.6++	90.62	24.72$ $	66.54	8.36
PFR-E (Normal)	l/s	4.28	1.8	3.84	0.97	4.31	0.38
PFR-A (Normal)	l/s	6.09	1.7++ $	5.14	1.23	4.5	0.64
Peak E/A		0.73	0.25++	0.77	0.21$ $	0.99	0.05
E-Deceleration	cm/s^2	407	306	352	189	446	238
TVI:							
E-Wave	cm	8.74	4.51	10.20	4.57	9.31	2.58
A-Wave	cm	8.05	2.67+	8.15	2.27$ $	5.93	0.65
TVI Ratios:							
E/A	%	1.10	0.44++	1.29	0.52	1.60	0.34
E/Total	%	0.50	0.11+	0.54	0.10	0.60	0.07
A/Total	%	0.50	0.11+	0.46	0.10	0.40	0.07

Systolic and diastolic time intervals are summarized in Table 5. Pre-ejection periods, LV ejection times and their ratios, and isovolumic contraction periods were comparable in all three groups. Isovolumic relaxation periods were comparably increased in all three groups. The mean ratio of early/atrial filling duration was greater in both patient groups on CAPD than in non-renal patients, the duration of atrial filling was shorter in renal than in non-renal patients.

Discussion

Patient characteristics

To characterize the influence of end-stage renal failure on LV diastolic mechanics, we analyzed parameters of LV filling in CAPD patients with and without LV hypertrophy. These data are compared to those from a group of untreated non-renal hypertensives and to normal controls from the literature.

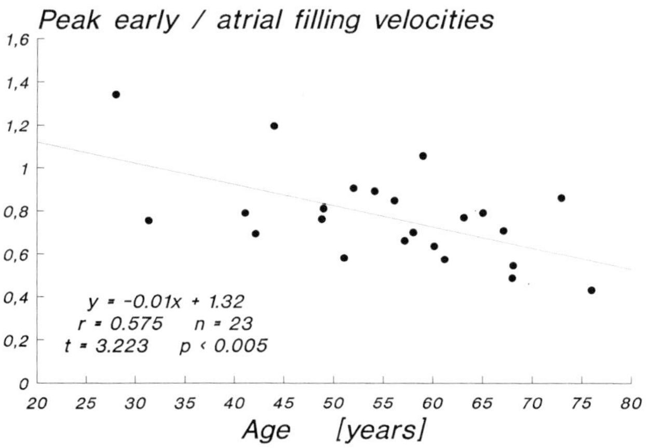

Fig. 1 In CAPD patients with LV hypertrophy, the ratios of peak early/atrial filling velocities were inversely correlated with age.

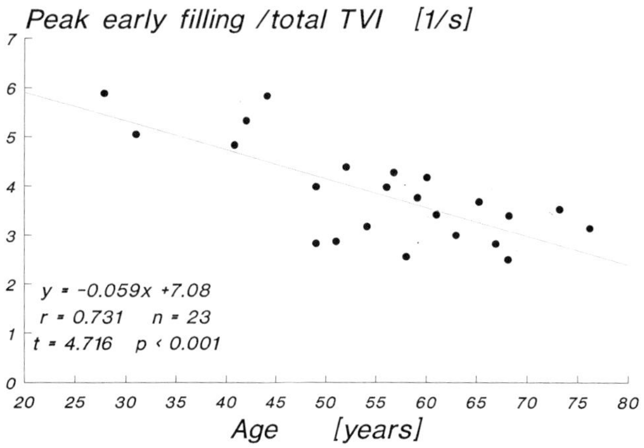

Fig. 2 Peak early filling velocities normalized for total time-velocity integral (TVI) were inversely correlated with age in CAPD patients with LV hypertrophy.

Since LV diastolic filling is characteristically altered and impaired in patients with LV hypertrophy, we defined subgroups of CAPD patients on the basis of this criterion to determine

- whether and to what degree LV diastolic mechanics are altered in renal patients without LV hypertrophy, and
- what additional influence LV hypertrophy may exert on diastolic LV function.

Doppler parameters

Left ventricular hypertrophy in non-renal patients is associated with characteristic changes of LV filling in pulsed Doppler as compared to normal controls [Sartori et al. 1987, Maron et al. 1987, Pearson et al. 1988, Phillips et al. 1987, Snider et al. 1985]: Both maximal filling velocities and filling fractions of the atrial wave are increased in LV hypertrophy, maximal early filling velocities and filling fractions are decreased.

Our data indicate that LV diastolic filling is impaired in both groups of CAPD patients and in our group of non-renal hypertensives: Philips et al. [1987] found an E/A ratio of 1.1 ± 0.4 in hypertensive hypertrophy, Maron et al. [1987] report a ratio of 1.4 ± 0.8 in a comparable group. Spirito et al. [1986] found E/A ratio range for this age group to be normal at 2.6, Wind et al. [1984] report a normal value of 1.5. Both our groups of CAPD patients had considerably lower E/A ratios (with hypertrophy: 0.77 ± 0.21; without hypertrophy: 0.73 ± 0.25) indicating severely altered diastolic LV filling. Our data are comparable to those of Ruffmann et al. [1990], who found an E/A ratio of 0.66 ± 0.2.

While mean values of peak early filling velocities were comparable in the three groups, we found a tendency of individual values to decrease with increasing age only for CAPD patients with LV hypertrophy (Figure 2). This finding suggests an influence of patient age on LV filling in renal patients with LV hypertrophy, while the amount of LV hypertrophy itself does not directly determine the amount of diastolic LV dysfunction as could be expected. Therefore, other factors such as electrolyte shifts, metabolic alterations or cellular edema may play a major role for diastolic myocardial relaxation in these patients.

Characteristics of diastolic LV function are most reliably reflected in the amount of atrial contribution of LV filling [Maron et al. 1987, Pearson et al. 1988], with normal values of atrial filling fraction being in the range of 26 ± 7 to 43 ± 8% [Sartori et al. 1987, Miyatake et al. 1984]. The atrial portion of LV filling is increased in LV hypertrophy: Pearson et al. [1988] found an atrial filling fraction of 49 ± 12% in these patients. This value is comparable both to the 46 ± 10% atrial contribution found in our renal patients

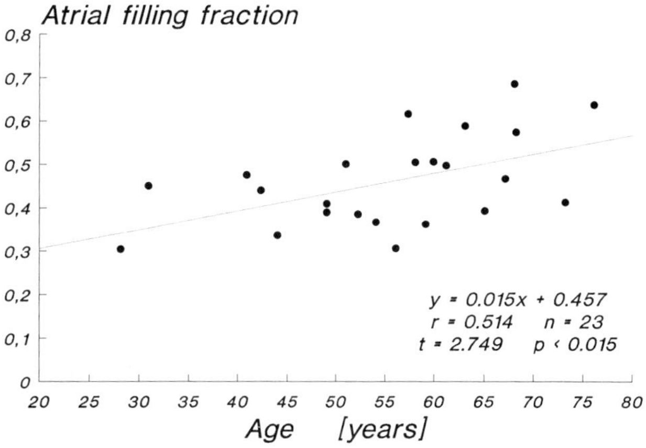

Fig. 3 Atrial filling fractions were directly related to age in CAPD patients with LV hypertrophy.

Table 5 Diastolic and systolic time intervals

Parameter	Dimension	CAPD-Patients Normal LV Muscle mass Mean ± S.D.		With LV Hypertrophy Mean ± S.D.		Non-renal hpertensives Mean ± S.D.	
IVR	ms	134	38	130	3	116	17
IVC	ms	71	15	72	2	76	7
PEP	ms	112	20	125	2	121	15
LVET	ms	253	44	252	3	273	24
PEP/LVET		0,45	0,08	0,50	0,1	0,45	0,08
IVC/IVR		0,57	0,22	0,57	0,2	0,67	0,13

Abbreviations:
IVR = isovolumic relaxation period, IVC = isovolumic contraction period, PEP = pre-ejection period, LEVT = left ventricular ejection time

with hypertrophy and to the 50 ± 11% atrial filling fraction in our patients with normal LV muscle mass.

Atrial filling velocities in our CAPD patients were also considerably altered: The normal range of atrial filling velocities is 46 ± 13 to 69 ± 17 cm/s [Maron et al. 1987, Pearson et al. 1988, Wind et al. 1987]. Pearson et al. [1988] found increased peak atrial filling velocities of 100 ± 20 cm/s in patients with LV hypertrophy. This is comparable to the maximal atrial filling velocities of 91 ± 25 cm/s in patients with LV hypertrophy and 96 ± 25 cm/s for CAPD patients without hypertrophy in our study.

It is an obvious limitation of the presented data, that no invasive hemodynamic measurements were performed to support our data of severely impaired diastolic filling in CAPD patients. Yet, although we did not measure left atrial or pulmonary capillary wedge pressures, there was no reason to assume that our patients had highly increased left atrial pressures, which would alter the LV diastolic filling pattern, making it difficult or impossible to attribute changes of filling to abnormal diastolic LV mechanics [Appleton et al. 1988]. Studies were performed before the bag-exchange procedure, hence in a state of relative volume constancy. Also, since a beneficial effect on LV diastolic mechanics has been described for several of the antihypertensive drugs used in both groups of CAPD patients, we have reason to assume that alterations of diastolic LV filling would be even more pronounced without that medication.

Correlation of Doppler parameters with age and radius/thickness ratios

The presented data demonstrate that in patients on CAPD with normal systolic LV function, LV diastolic filling is comparably impaired both in patients with and without septal hypertrophy. No significant differences in Doppler parameters were found between these two groups of renal patients. The direct relation of maximal early/atrial filling velocities and atrial filling fractions with age described for non-renal patients without LV hypertrophy by Kuo et al. [1987] was not found in our group of CAPD patients with normal septal thickness. However, high age was related to more severely disturbed diastolic LV function in CAPD patients with LV hypertrophy in Doppler analysis. One important factor contributing to these functional abnormalities may be the increased myocardial fibre content found in dialysis patients [Zazgornik et al. 1987, Mall et al. 1990]: Since LV relaxation is an active, energy consuming myocardial process, it can easily be impaired by alterations of myocardial structure.

Time intervals

Average isovolumic relaxation period was considerably prolonged in all three groups suggesting diastolic LV dysfunction: Normal values for this parameter are in the range of 70–80 ± 10–15 ms (Maron et al. 1987; Miyatake et al. 1984, Wind et al. 1987]. This parameter was even more increased in both groups of CAPD patients (134 ± 38 vs 131 ± 34 ms) than in non-renal hypertensives (116 ± 17 ms). Our data for non-renal hypertensive patients are in good agreement with those of Maron et al. [1987] (98 ± 24 ms).

LV ejection time has been found shorter in LV hypertensive hypertrophy than in normal subjects: Pearson et al. [1988] found it to be 264 ± 55 ms in hypertensive hypertrophy and 308 ± 3 ms in normal controls. In all three of our groups, systolic time intervals were in normal range.

Significance of findings

In summary, we found left ventricular diastolic function in patients on CAPD to be disturbed not only in patients with LV hypertrophy, but also in patients with normal LV muscle mass. This is paralleled by invasive findings of LV diastolic dysfunction from our group [Kramer et al. 1986] in patients on intermittent hemodialysis using conductance catheter and from Ruffmann et al. [1990] using Doppler. Therefore, LV diastolic dysfunction appears not to be related to a special method of blood purification, but seems to be a characteristic finding of the heart in uremia.

Ruffmann found abnormal LV filling in Doppler to be associated with clinical occurrence of diastolic decompensation (hypotensive episodes). Himelman et al. [1988] report perioperative pulmonary edema during renal transplantation in 13 of 19 patients with altered preoperative diastolic LV function, as compared with only 1 of 9 patients with normal function. Other preoperative echocardiographic parameters, such as LV muscle mass, LV volume/mass ratio or cardiac output were not predictive of pulmonary edema. LV parameters indicating disturbed LV diastolic filling did not correlate with LV muscle mass or systolic performance. Therefore, Doppler analysis is necessary to determine which individual patient is at risk of diastolic LV dysfunction. The amount of hypotensive episodes cannot be easily determined in CAPD patients for lack of controlled episodes of acute volume depletion, which on the other hand makes this method best suitable for patients with diastolic LV dysfunction.

Realizing the additional negative influence both of age and LV hypertrophy on LV diastolic function in CAPD patients, therapeutic efforts must be made to reduce the amount of LV hypertrophy and avoid situations of acute changes of volume loading, which may have deleterious effects for these patients.

REFERENCES

Alpert MA, Van Stone J, Twardowski ZJ, Ruder MA, Whiting RB, Kelly DL, Madsen BR 1986 Comparative cardiac effects of hemodialysis and continuous ambulatory peritoneal dialysis. Clin Cardiol *9:* 52–60

Appleton CP, Hatle LK, Popp RL 1988 Relation of transmitral flow velocity pattern to left ventricular diastolic function: New insights from a combined hemodynamic and Doppler echocardiographic study. J Am Coll Cardiol *12:* 426–440

Bowman LK, Lee FA, Jaffe CC, Mattera J, Wackers FJ, Zaret BL 1988 Peak filling rate normalized to mitral stroke volume: a new Doppler echocardiographic filling index validated by radionuclide angiographic techniques. J Am Coll Cardiol *12:* 937–943

Bryg RJ, Williams GA, Labovitz AJ 1987 Effect of aging on left ventricular diastolic filling in normal subjects. Am J Cardiol *59:* 971–974

Chazan JA, Pono LM 1987 Sudden death in patients with chronic renal failure on hemodialysis. Dial Transplant *16:* 447–448

Choong CY, Herrmann HC, Weyman AE, Fifer MA 1987 Preload dependence of Doppler-derived indexes of left ventricular diastolic function in humans. J Am Coll Cardiol *10:* 800–808

Cohen JL, Barooah B, Segal K, Batuman V 1987 Two-dimensional echocardiographic findings in patients on hemodialysis for more than six months. Am J Cardiol *60:* 743–745

Devereux RB, Reichek N 1977 Echocardiographic determination of left ventricular mass in man. Anatomic validation of the method. Circulation *55:* 613–618

Diver DJ, Royal HD, Aroesty JM, McKay RG, Ferguson JJ, Warren SE, Lorell BH 1988 Diastolic function in patients with aortic stenosis: Influence of left ventricular load reduction. J Am Coll Cardiol *12:* 642–648

Eisenberg M, Prichard S, Barre P, Patton R, Hutchinson T, Sniderman A 1987 Left ventricular hypertrophy in end-stage renal disease on peritoneal dialysis. Am J Cardiol *60:* 418–419

Finkelhor RS, Hanak LJ, Bahler RC 1986 Left ventricular filling in endurance-trained subjects. J Am Coll Cardiol *8:* 289–293

Friedman BJ, Drinkovic N, Miles H, Shih WJ, Mazzoleni A, DeMaria AN 1986 Assessment of left ventricular diastolic function: Comparison of Doppler echocardiography and gated blood pool scintigraphy. J Am Coll Cardiol *8:* 1348–1354

Himelman RB, Landzberg JS, Simonson JS, Amend W, Bouchard A, Merz R, Schiller NB 1988 Cardiac consequences of renal transplantation: Changes in left ventricular morphology and function. J Am Coll Cardiol *12:* 915–923

Hüting J, Kramer W, Schütterle G, Wizemann V 1988 Analysis of left ventricular changes associated with chronic hemodialysis. Nephron *49:* 284–290

Hüting J, Kramer W, Reitinger J, Kühn K, Wizemann V, Schütterle G 1990 Cardiac structure and function in continuous ambulatory peritoneal dialysis: Influence of blood purification and hypercirculation. Am Heart J *119:* 344–352

Kramer W, Wizemann V, Lämmlein G, Thormann J, Kindler M, Schlepper M, Schütterle G 1986 Cardiac dysfunction in patients on maintenance hemodialysis. Contr Nephrol *52:* 110–124

Kuo LC, Quinones MA, Rokey R, Sartori M, Abinader EG, Zoghbi WA 1987 Quantification of atrial contribution to left ventricular filling by pulsed Doppler echocardiography and the effect of age in normal and diseased hearts. Am J Cardiol *59:* 1174–1178

Leenen FHH, Smith DL, Khanna R, Oreopoulos DG 1985 Changes in left ventricular hypertrophy and function in hypertensive patients started on continuous ambulatory peritoneal dialysis. Am Heart J *110:* 102–106

Mall G, Huther W, Schneider J, Lundin P, Ritz E 1990 Diffuse intermyocardiocytic fibrosis in uraemic patients. Nephrol Dial Transplant *5:* 39–44

Maron BJ, Spirito P, Green KJ, Wesley YE, Bonow RO, Arce J 1987 Noninvasive assessment of left ventricular diastolic function by pulsed Doppler echocardiography in patients with hypertrophic cardiomyopathy. J Am Coll Cardiol *10:* 733–742

McLenachan JM, Henderson E, Morris KI, Dargie HJ 1987 Ventricular arrhythmias in patients with hypertensive left ventricular hypertrophy. N Engl J Med *317:* 787–792

Miyatake K, Okamoto M, Kinoshita N, Owa M, Nakasone I, Sakakibara H, Nimura Y 1984 Augmentation of atrial contribution to left ventricular inflow with aging as assessed by intracardiac Doppler flowmetry. Am J Cardiol *53:* 586–589

Niwa A, Taniguchi K, Ito H, Nakagawa S, Takeuchi J, Sasaoka T, KanayamaM 1985 Echocardiographic and Holter findings in 321 uremic patients on maintenance hemodialysis. Jap Heart J *26:* 403–411

Pearson AG, Goodgold H, Labovitz AJ, Ratcliff J 1988 Comparison of pulsed Doppler echocardiography and radionuclide angiography in the assessment of left ventricular filling. Am J Cardiol *61:* 446–454

Pearson AC, Gudipati CV, Labovitz AJ 1988 Systolic and diastolic flow abnormalities in elderly patients with hypertensive hypertrophic cardiomyopathy. J Am Coll Cardiol *12:* 989–995

Phillips RA, Coplan NL, Krakoff LR, Yeager K, Ross RS, Gorlin R, Goldman ME 1987 Doppler echocardiographic analysis of left ventricular filling in treated hypertensive patients. J Am Coll Cardiol *9:* 317–322

Ritz E, Ruffmann K, Rambausek M, Mall G, Schmidli 1987 Dialysis hypotension – is it related diastolic left ventricular malfunction? Nephrol Dial Transplant *2:* 293–297

Rokey R, Kuo LC, Zoghbi WA, Limacher MC, Quinones MA 1985 Determination of parameters of left ventricular diastolic filling with pulsed Doppler echocardiography: comparison with cineangiography. Circulation *71:* 543–550

Ruffmann K, Mandelbaum A, Bommer J, Schmidli M, Ritz E 1990 Doppler echocardiographic findings in dialysis patients. Nephrol Dial Transplant *5:* 426–31

Sahn DJ, DeMaria A, Kisslo J, Weyman A 1978 The committee on M-mode standardization of the American Society of Echocardiography: Recommendations regarding quantitation in M-mode echocardiography: Results of a survey of echocardiographic measurements. Circulations *58:* 1072–1083

Sartori MP, Quinones MA, Kuo LC 1987 Relation of Doppler-derived left ventricular filling parameters to age and radius/thickness ratio in normal and pathologic states. Am J Cardiol *59:* 1179–1182

Silberbauer K, Juhasz M, Ohrenberger G, Hess C 1988 Noninvasive assessment of left ventricular diastolic function by pulsed Doppler echocardiography in young alcoholics. Cardiology *75:* 431–439

Snider AR, Gidding SS, Rocchini AP, Rosenthal A, Dick M, Crowley DC, Peters J 1985 Doppler evaluation of left ventricular diastolic filling in children with systemic hypertension. Am J Cardiol *56:* 921–926

Spirito P, Maron BJ, Verter I, Merrill JS 1988 Reproducibility of Doppler echocardiographic measurements of left ventricular diastolic function. European Heart J *9:* 879–886

Spirito P, Maron BJ, Bellotti P, Chiarella F, Vecchio C 1986 Noninvasive assessment of left ventricular diastolic function: Comparative analysis of pulsed Doppler ultrasound and digitized M-Mode echocardiography. Am J Cardiol *58:* 837–843

Teichholz LE, Kreulen T, Herman MV, Gorlin R 1976 Problems in echocardiographic volume determinations: Echocardiographic-angiographic correlations in the presence or absence of asynergy. Am J Cardiol *37:* 7–11

Wind BE, Snider R, Buda Aj, O'Neill WW, Topol EJ, Dilworth LR 1987 Pulsed Doppler assessment of left ventricular diastolic filling in coronary artery disease before and immediately after coronary angioplasty. Am J Cardiol *59:* 1041–1046

Wing AJ, Brunner FP, Brynger H, Jacobs C, Kramer P, Selwood NH, Gretz N 1984 Cardiovascular-related causes of death and the fate of patients with renovascular disease. Contr Nephrol *41:* 306–311

Woythaler JN, Singer SL, Kwan O, Meltzer RS, Reubner B, Bommer W, DeMaria A 1983 Accuracy of echocardiography versus electrocardiography in detecting left ventricular hypertrophy: comparison with postmortem mass measurements. J Am Coll Cardiol *2:* 305–311

Zarich SW, Arbuckle BE, Cohen LR, Roberts M, Nesto R 1988 Diastolic abnormalities in young asymptomatic diabetic patients assessed by pulsed Doppler echocardiography. J Am Coll Cardiol *12:* 114–120

Zazgornik J, Balcke P, Biesenbach G, Kaiser W, Stockenhuber F 1987 Myocardial calcinosis associated with hemodialysis. Am J Cardiol *60:* 421–422

Clinical Nephrology, Vol. 36 No. 1 – 1991 (29–34)

An analysis of ten-year trends in infections in adults on continuous ambulatory peritoneal dialysis (CAPD)

J. Bernardini, J. L. Holley, J. R. Johnston, J. A. Perlmutter and B. Piraino

Renal Electrolyte Division of the University of Pittsburgh and the Veterans Administration Medical Center, Pittsburgh, PA

Abstract. Infectious complications are the Achilles heel of CAPD. To determine trends in these events, we analyzed the CAPD related infections of 303 adults on CAPD at a single university center between 1979 and 1989. During this decade the percentage of insulin-dependent diabetics increased from 14% to 39% ($p < 0.005$). Peritonitis rates fell from 2.4 episodes/y in 1979 to 0.8 episodes/y in 1989. The proportion of patients with multiple episodes of peritonitis decreased (40% of the patients in 1979–1982 vs 15% in 1983–1989, $p = 0.0001$) while the proportion of patients with no episodes of peritonitis increased during the same periods (29% vs 49%, $p = 0.005$). The proportion of peritonitis episodes due to *S. aureus* rose over the 10-year period ($p = 0.005$), while those due to *S. epidermidis* decreased ($p < 0.10$). The overall incidence of *S. aureus* peritonitis remained unchanged. Catheter infection rates initially increased and then fell during the decade; *S. aureus* remained the predominant cause. The proportion of peritonitis episodes associated with catheter infection rose (13% in 1982 vs 24% in 1989, $p = 0.025$), and in 1989, 80% of these episodes were caused by *S. aureus.* Catheter loss was also primarily due to *S. aureus* infections in 1989 (80%). Infections due to *P. aeruginosa* were a persistent problem. The proportion of patients transferring to hemodialysis each year paralleled catheter loss rates, which in turn appeared to be more related to catheter infection rates than to peritonitis rates. We conclude that control of *S. aureus* and *P. aeruginosa* will be the key to future reductions in the infectious complications of CAPD patients.

Key words: CAPD infections – peritonitis – S. aureus – S. epidermidis – P. aeruginosa

Introduction

Since the introduction of CAPD [Popovich et al. 1976], use of this technique has grown such that over 13,000 end-stage renal disease patients in the United States are currently maintained on CAPD [Nolph et al. 1988]. Technical improvements such as plastic containers for dialysis solutions and disconnect systems have been instrumental in reducing infectious complications associated with CAPD [Nolph et al. 1988] yet peritonitis and catheter infections remain the most important causes of CAPD failure [Piraino et al. 1987]. Reports of long-term CAPD experience do not consider infectious complications in detail or have small numbers of patients [Nolph et al. 1985, Kurtz et al. 1983, Ramos et al. 1983, Chan et al. 1981, Segoloni et al. 1984]. We examined CAPD related infections from 1979–1989 in 303 adult patients followed in a university center dialysis program. Trends in patient demographics, organisms causing peritonitis and catheter infections, relationships between catheter infections and peritonitis, and the outcome of such infections are detailed.

Received July 23, 1990; in revised form January 30, 1991

Reprint requests to J. Bernardini, 1191 Scaife Hall, University of Pittsburgh, Pittsburgh, PA 15261.

Methods

Patients

Between August 1979 and August 1989, data were collected on 392 CAPD patients. Eighty-nine of these patients were excluded from the present analysis: those younger than 18 years of age when starting CAPD, those trained at another center, and those on automated PD. The remaining 303 adult patients constituted the study group. Time on CAPD was recorded from the beginning of training until the patient discontinued CAPD, or until August 1989, whichever occurred first. Time on temporary intermittent peritoneal dialysis and hemodialysis was excluded as were events preceding the first day of CAPD training. Data recorded for each patient (prospectively since 1982) included time on dialysis, catheter removals and the reasons for such, and the occurrence and culture results of all peritoneal dialysis related infections.

All patients were trained and followed in one of two centers which comprise the University of Pittsburgh CAPD Program. The Presbyterian University Hospital Peritoneal Dialysis Program was established in 1979 and trained 229 of the patients included in the study. The Oakland Veterans Administration Hospital Peritoneal Dialysis Program was established in 1982. Seventy-four of the patients included in this study were trained and followed at this center. The head nurse of each CAPD program remained the same but individual nurses working in the CAPD programs of each center have varied.

From 1979 through 1986, the standard spike system for performing CAPD was used by most patients. In 1987, a disconnect system (the Y-set without disinfectant) was offered to patients. Most of the patients beginning CAPD after its introduction chose the Y-set, and by the end of the study period, 82% of patients were using the Y-set. During the 10 years of the study, other exchange methods used included the ultraviolet device (18 patients), a spike-assist device (13 patients), a luer-lock connection (16 patients), and the sterile connection device (5 patients).

Definitions and catheters

Four hundred forty six catheters were inserted in 303 patients during the 10 years. The exit site and tunnel of the peritoneal catheters were examined at each clinic visit and whenever the patient reported any catheter-related problem. An exit site infection was defined as pericatheter erythema and/or drainage. Any subsequent exit site infection in a patient was considered to be a new infection if the patient had not taken antibiotics in the previous 2 weeks, and the exit site had been examined in the interval and found to be normal. Catheter infection data prior to 1982 were unreliable and therefore were not included in this analysis. A peritoneal catheter tunnel infection was defined as erythema, edema, and/or tenderness over the subcutaneous catheter pathway. Since there was sometimes an overlap between exit site and tunnel infections, these two catheter related infections are combined for statistical purposes and called "catheter infections". Cases of simultaneous tunnel and exit site infections were recorded as one catheter infection. Peritonitis was defined as cloudy dialysate with more than 100 leukocytes/uL, more than 50% of which were polymorphonuclear cells.

Catheter infections (exit site or tunnel infections or both) and peritonitis were considered to be associated if 1) the two infections occurred simultaneously or 2) peritonitis followed the catheter infection within 2 weeks of antibiotic therapy. Moreover, the organisms cultured from the infections had to be the same, or one or both cultures had to be sterile.

Peritoneal catheters were inserted through either a midline or a lateral incision by members of the Surgical Department of the University of Pittsburgh. The vast majority of catheters were double-cuff Tenckhoff catheters. The inner cuff was embedded in the rectus muscle; the outer cuff was placed approximately 2 cm from the exit site. Generally no suture was placed around the catheter at the exit site. The exit site was superior to the tunnel which followed a downward direction in most patients. CAPD training began usually no less than 2 weeks after catheter insertion. Patients were often placed on intermittent peritoneal dialysis or temporary hemodialysis before CAPD training. Postoperative exit site care consisted of daily cleaning with povidone-iodine solution followed by hydrogen peroxide or isopropyl alcohol. For the first week the exit site was covered by sterile gauze. Since 1987, a clear occlusive dressing covered the exit site and was not removed for routine cleaning for the first week after catheter insertion. When the incision was well-healed, daily soap and water washing of the exit site while showering was recommended. After initiation of CAPD, individual patient preference determined exit site covering and anchoring of the catheter. Patients chose either a gauze or adhesive dressing or left the exit site uncovered.

Infectious reasons for removal of a peritoneal catheter were 1) intractable peritonitis that did not resolve after 5–10 days of appropriate antibiotic therapy, 2) persistent catheter infection that did not resolve after multiple (at least two) courses of antibiotics, 3) catheter infection associated with peritonitis that did not respond to antibiotic therapy, and 4) fungal peritonitis. Catheters removed for mechanical reasons were recorded separately.

Cultures and treatment

Any exit site drainage was cultured following standard microbiologic techniques [Am Soc Microbiology 1988]. Sixty-five (12.5%) of the catheter infections had no drainage and thus could not be cultured. Twenty-nine (5.6%) were cultured but were sterile. From 1979 to 1984, peritoneal fluid was cultured by a direct plate inoculation technique of a

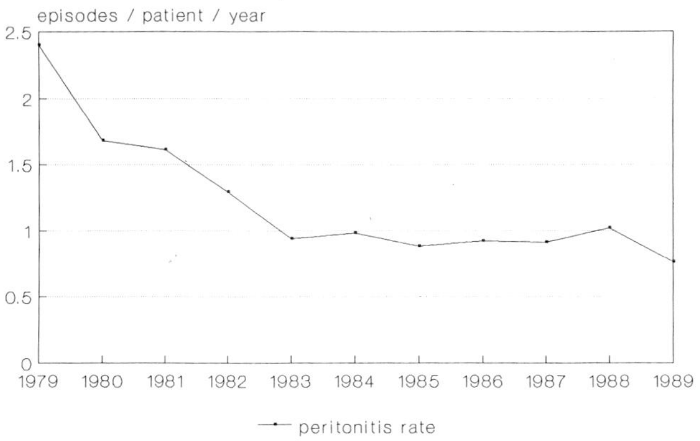

Fig. 1 Trends in the rate of peritonitis in adults on CAPD.

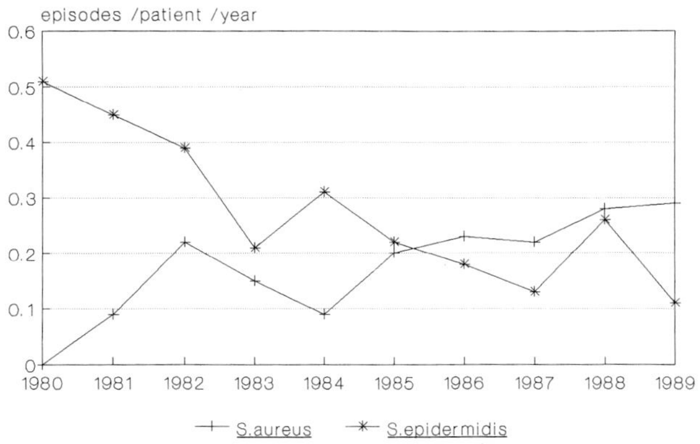

Fig. 2 Trends in the rate of peritonitis due to *S. aureus* and *S. epidermidis.*

centrifuged specimen. Beginning in 1985, peritoneal fluid was cultured in Bactec bottles which were inoculated directly by the nurse evaluating the patient for peritonitis. Ninety-three (21%) of the peritonitis episodes had sterile cultures. In two episodes, the dialysate was not cultured.

Antibiotic therapy for exit site infections was variable. Oral antibiotics (usually cephalexin or, recently, ciprofloxacin) were usually given for 10–14 days. A two-week course of parenteral antibiotics (vancomycin, cefazolin, or occasionally, gentamicin depending on culture results) was usual for tunnel infections. Peritonitis was treated with intraperitoneal antibiotics (vancomycin, a cephalosporin, or an aminoglycoside as directed by culture results) for a minimum of 4 days. Ten days of therapy was completed with either continuation of intraperitoneal antibiotics or a course of oral antibiotics. Antibiotics were adjusted as necessary depending upon the results of sensitivity testing and the response to treatment.

Statistical analysis

Data are presented as mean values plus or minus the standard deviation. Chi square analysis with Yates' correction was used to compared proportions involving demographic data. Chi squared with Goodness of Fit was used to compared trends in organisms over time. Infection rates (peritonitis and catheter infections) were calculated as total number of infections for all patients in a group divided by total time on continuous peritoneal dialysis. Sterile cultures and those instances in which cultures were not obtained were excluded from analysis.

Table 1 Proportion of patients with 0, 1, 2, or 3 or more peritonitis episodes

	1979 – 1982	1983 – 1989	p
no peritonitis	29% (22/75)	49% (111/228)	0.005
1 episode	17% (13/75)	21% (47/228)	ns
2 episodes	13% (10/75)	16% (36/228)	ns
3 or more episodes	40% (30/75)	15% (34/228)	0.0001

Results

The 303 adult patients trained between 1979 and 1989 had a total of 454 patient years on CAPD, with a range of 0.1 to 83 patient months, and a mean of 18 patient months. Over the ten years, insulin dependent diabetics have accounted for an increasing number of our patients, from 14% in 1980 to a current 39% (chi square = 30.7, $p < 0.005$). The mean patient age has remained stable at 55 ± 14 years, as has the ratio of male (53%) to female (47%), and black (23%) to white patients (77%). No differences were seen among diabetics and nondiabetics in peritonitis rate (0.98/y for diabetics and 0.97 y/ for nondiabetics) or *S. aureus* infections.

Four hundred forty-one episodes of peritonitis occurred over the 10-year period. The rates of peritonitis fell from 2.4 episodes/patient/year in 1979 to 0.9 in 1983 and remained stable until 1989 when it decreased to 0.8 episodes/patient/year (Figure 1). Between 1981 and 1989, 436 patients were treated for peritonitis (18 in 1981, 46 in 1982, 57 in 1983, 74 in 1984, 67 in 1985, 56 in 1986, 49 in 1987, 48 in 1988, and 21 in 1989). The proportion of patients developing multiple, single, or no episodes of peritonitis while on CAPD were compared during the program's first three years, when peritonitis rates were high, to the last 7 years, when rates had fallen (Table 1). The percentage of patients with no peritonitis episodes rose from 29% during the first three years to 49%

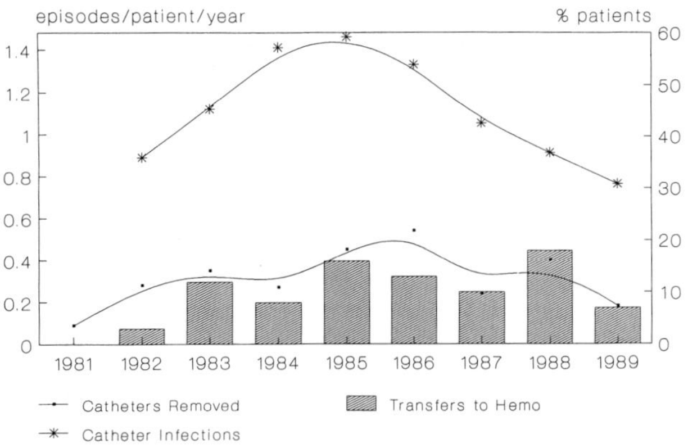

Fig. 3 Trends in the rate of catheter infections, catheter loss, and the percentage of patients transferring to hemodialysis.

during the more recent period (p=0.005). The percentage of patients with 3 or more peritonitis episodes fell from 40% in the early years to 15% in the later years (p = 0.0001).

The most common organism causing peritonitis for the first 5 years of the study was *S. epidermidis* (Figure 2). Since 1987, however, *S. aureus* has been the most common cause of peritonitis. The proportion of peritonitis due to *S. aureus* increased over the years (chi square = 32.5, p = 0.005), while the proportion due to *S. epidermidis* decreased (p <0.10). The overall incidence of *S. aureus*, however, was unchanged. The

Table 2 Infecting organisms causing peritonitis and catheter infections

	# of Episodes of P	# of Episodes of CI
Gram Positive	268	292
S. epidermidis	102	41
S. aureus	74	140
Streptococcus	31	3
Enterococcus	6	1
All Others	42	19
Multiple Gram$^+$	13	88
Gram Negative	61	65
Pseudomonas aeruginosa	24	40
Acinetobacter	7	0
E. Coli	6	2
Klebsiella	4	3
All Others	15	16
Multiple Gram$^-$	5	4
Mixed Gram$^+$ and Gram$^-$	12	69
Fungus	5	0
Sterile	93	29
No Culture	2	65
Total	441	520

percentage of peritonitis caused by other organisms has remained fairly constant (Table 2). *P. aeruginosa* accounted for 4 to 11% of peritonitis episodes per year and other Gram negative organisms 5 to 17% per year.

A total of 520 catheter infections occurred during the 10-year period. Catheter infection rates increased in the middle of the decade and then fell (Figure 3). These infections were most commonly caused by *S. aureus* throughout the study period, averaging to 49% of all positive cultures. The rates of catheter infections due to *S. aureus* ranged from 0.2 (1982) to 0.6 episodes/patient/year (1986). In 1989 this organism was responsible for 83% of such infections. *P. aeruginosa* catheter infection rates were less variable, averaging 0.1 episodes/patient/year (range 0.1 to 0.2).

The percentage of peritonitis episodes preceded by a catheter infection rose from 13% in 1982 to 24% in 1989 (chi square=5.2, p=0.025). The annual mean rate of catheter infection-associated peritonitis (0.15 episodes/patient/year) did not vary over time. In 1982, 40% of peritonitis episodes complicated by catheter infections were caused by *S. epidermidis,* a percentage which gradually fell to zero in 1989. *S. aureus* was the causative organism in 20% of peritonitis episodes associated with catheter infections in 1982, compared with 83% in 1989 (chi square = 17.2, p <0.025). *P. aeruginosa* was cultured in nearly 21% of these infections each year.

One hundred eighty six (42%) catheters were removed. The mean rate of catheter loss due to infections was 0.25/patient/year but fluctuated from year to year (chi square = 32.8, p <0.005, Figure 3). *S. aureus* was the responsible organism in 34% and *P. aeruginosa* in 17% of infections resulting in catheter removal. In 1989, *S. aureus* infections accounted for 80% of all catheters removed for infectious reasons.

The percentage of patients who transferred to hemodialysis (mean 10.9%/year) was highest during 1985, 1986, and 1988 (Figure 3). During these years, catheter loss due to infections peaked.

Discussion

We analyzed CAPD related infections over a 10-year span at a university dialysis center. The rates of peritonitis fell and the proportion of organisms causing these infections changed. *S. epidermidis,* once the most common cause of peritonitis, has been supplanted by *S. aureus* in more recent years.

These results confirm those reported elsewhere, but add a new trend of the rising incidence of *S. aureus* infections. In early reports, peritonitis rates were high and Gram positive organisms, mostly *S. epidermidis,* were identified as the most common pathogens [Nolph et al. 1985, Segoloni 1984, Prowant et al. 1986]. Recent reports have described a progressive decline in peritonitis rates [Bint et al. 1987, Tarchini et al. 1988, Pollock et al. 1989, Ataman et al. 1988]. This trend can be attributed in part to the "flush before fill" disconnect systems that probably decreases peritonitis caused by touch contamination [Piraino et al. 1990a, Canadian CAPD Clinical Trials Group 1989]. As a result, peritonitis caused by *S. epidermidis* has become less common, and *S. aureus* is now the most commonly cultured organism [Canadian CAPD Clinical Trials Group 1989].

We began using a disconnect system in 1987 and by 1989 82% of our CAPD patients were using the system. Thus, the use of the disconnect system is a likely explanation for the most recent fall in *S. epidermidis* peritonitis at our center [Piraino et al. 1990a]. As a consequence, increasing numbers of patients had no episodes of peritonitis and fewer numbers of patients had multiple episodes.

In contrast to peritonitis rates, rates of catheter infections initially increased in the middle of the decade and declined in the last few years. Catheter infection rates in 1989 were similar to those reported in the National CAPD Registry. The initial rise in catheter infections at our center may have been due to increased interest in such infections, and thus closer attention to the exit site and tunnel appearance at each patient visit.

There are several possible explanations for the most recent decline in the catheter infections rates. Starting in 1987 an occlusive dressing was used during the first post-operative week after catheter insertion. This may have promoted exit-site healing and reduced the incidence of early catheter infections. Likewise, the increased use of disconnect systems since 1987 may have contributed to the fall in catheter infections by decreasing exit site trauma [Piraino et al. 1990a].

Despite an overall decline in catheter infection rates since 1985, *S. aureus* catheter infections have not decreased. Episodes of peritonitis [Sewell et al. 1982] and catheter infections [Zimmerman et al. 1988, Luzar et al. 1990b) caused by *S. aureus* have been firmly linked to *S. aureus* nasal carriage. Data on nasal carriage are not available in the present study as such cultures were obtained beginning in 1989. Other than *S. aureus* nasal carriage, no other factors conclusively contribute to catheter infections. Body size [Piraino et al. 1990b] and catheter location [Piraino et al. 1989], for example, have little influence on catheter infections. A practice of covering the exit-site and cleaning with povidone iodine has been shown to be associated with fewer exit-site infections than soap and water cleaning, without a dressing [Luzar et al. 1990a]. However, *S. aureus* catheter infections were not reduced by the former protocol and still accounted for 83% of catheter infections, a percentage the same as at our center in 1989. Similarly, disconnect systems have not resulted in a fall in *S. aureus* catheter infections despite being associated with lower catheter infection rates [Piraino et al. 1990a].

Episodes of peritonitis without catheter infection have declined but peritonitis with catheter infection has remained constant. Thus, the proportion of peritonitis episodes due to catheter infection has risen from 13% in 1982 to 24% in 1989. *S. aureus* accounted for 83% of these infections in 1989.

By the end of the decade, *S. aureus,* more than any other organism, was also responsible for more of the catheters removed for infectious reasons. In 1989, 80% of the catheters removed for CAPD related infection were infected with *S. aureus.*

The rates at which catheters were removed peaked in 1985 and 1986, years in which the catheter infection rates were also very high (Figure 3). Paradoxically, this was a period when peritonitis rates were low. In 1989 when catheter infection rates had fallen to 0.8 episodes/patient/year, there was a fall in the catheter removal rate to 0.2 catheters/patient/year. Thus, catheter removal tended to parallel catheter infection rather than peritonitis.

The percentage of patients transferring to hemodialysis fluctuated from year to year (Figure 3). In general, the percentage of patients transferring to hemodialysis in a given year paralleled rates of catheters removed for infectious reasons.

Several important trends emerged from this analysis. The rates of *S. epidermidis* peritonitis have declined. Infections due to *P. aeruginosa* remain a persistent problem. *S. aureus,* always a major cause of catheter infections [Piraino et al. 1987, Zimmerman et al. 1988, Abraham et al. 1988], has become the leading cause of peritonitis and catheter loss. With declining rates of peritonitis, catheter infections are becoming an even more important factor in the success of CAPD [Copley 1987]. Continued investigation into technique and patient factors responsible for catheter infections, especially *S. aureus* and *P. aeruginosa,* may further reduce the impact of this complication on CAPD.

Acknowledgements

We have already published this article in abstract form in the Journal of The American Society of Nephrology 1990; 1: 387.

We are grateful to Dr. Michael Sorkin who designed and implemented the CAPD data bank, and to our CAPD nurses, Carol

Dacko, Mary Bird, and Jean Miller, without whom we would not have a successful peritoneal dialysis program. Particular help was also given by Dr. Richard Day and Ada Owens in assisting with the statistical analysis, and by Dr. R. Samuel Arthur in reviewing the manuscript.

REFERENCES

Abraham G, Savin E, Ayiomamitis A, Izatt S, Vas SI, Mathews RE, Oreopoulos DG 1988 Natural history of exit-site infection (ESI) in patients on continuous ambulatory peritoneal dialysis (CAPD). Perit Dial Int *8:* 211–216

American Society of Microbiology. Manual of Clinical Microbiology. 4th Edition 1988, Washington, DC.

Ataman R, Burton PR, Gokal R, Brown CB, Marsh FP, Walls J 1988 Long-term CAPD – some UK experience. Clin Neph *30:* S71–S75

Bint AJ, Finch RG, Gokal R, Goldsmith HJ, Junor B, Oliver D 1987 Diagnosis and management of peritonitis in continuous ambulatory peritoneal dialysis. Lancet *2:* 845–849

Canadian CAPD Clinical Trials Group 1989 Peritonitis in continuous ambulatory peritoneal dialysis (CAPD): A multicentre randomized clinical trial comparing the Y-connector disinfectant system to standard systems. Perit Dial Int *9:* 159–163

Chan MK, Baillod RA, Chuah P, Sweny P, Raftery MJ, Verghese Z, Moorhead JF 1981 Three years' experience of continuous ambulatory peritoneal dialysis. Lancet *1:* 1409–1412

Copley JB 1987 Prevention of peritoneal dialysis catheter-related infections. Am J Kid Dis *10:* 401–40

Kurtz SB, Wong VH, Anderson CF, Vogel JP, McCarthy JT, Mitchell JC, Kumar R, Johnson WJ 1983 Continuous ambulatory peritoneal dialysis: Three years' experience at the Mayo Clinic. Mayo Clin Proc 58: 633–639

Luzar MA, Brown CB, Balf D, Hill L, Issad B, Monnier B, Moulart J, Sabatier J-C, Wauquier J-P, Peluso F 1990a Exit-site care and exit-site infection in continuous ambulatory peritoneal dialysis (CAPD): results of a randomized multicenter trial. Periton Dial Int *10:* 25–29

Luzar MA, Coles GA, Faller B, Slingeneyer A, Dah Dah G, Briat C, Wone C, Knefati Y, Kessler M, Peluso FL 1990 Staphylococcus S. aureus nasal carriage and infection in patients on continuous ambulatory peritoneal dialysis. N Engl J Med *322:* 505–509

Nolph KD, Cutler SJ, Steinberg SM, Novak JW 1985 Continuous ambulatory peritoneal dialysis in the United States: A three year study. Kidney Int *28:* 198–205

Nolph KD, Lindblad AS, Novak JW 1988 Continuous ambulatory peritoneal dialysis. N Engl J Med *318:* 1595–1600

Piraino B, Bernardini J, Sorkin M 1987 A five-year study of the microbiologic results of exit site infections and peritonitis in continuous ambulatory peritoneal dialysis. Am J Kid Dis *10:* 281–286

Piraino B, Bernardini J, Johnston JR, Sorkin MI 1989 Exit-site location does not influcence peritoneal catheter infection rate. Perit Dial Int *9:* 127–129

Piraino B, Bernardini J, Sorkin MI 1990a The effects of the Y-set on catheter infection rates in CAPD patients. Am J Kid Dis *16:* 46–50

Piraino B, Bernardini J, Centa PK, Johnston JR, Sorkin MI 1990b Effect of body weight on CAPD related infections and catheters loss. Perit Dial Int *1:* 64–68

Pollock CA, Ibels LS, Caterson RJ, Mahony JF, Wough DA, Cocksedge B 1989 Continuous ambulatory peritoneal dialysis: eight years experience at a single center. Medicine *68:* 293–308

Popovich RP, Moncrief JW, Decherd JF, Bomar JB, Pyle WK 1976 The definition of a portable-wearable equilibration peritoneal technique (Abst). Kidney Int *5:* 64

Prowant B, Nolph D, Ryan L, Twardowski Z, Khanna R 1986 Peritonitis in continuous ambulatory peritoneal dialysis: analysis of an 8-year experience. Nephron *43:* 105–109

Ramos JM, Gokal R, Siamopoulos K, Ward MK, Wilkinson R, Kerr DNS 1983 Continuous ambulatory peritoneal dialysis: Three years' experiences. Q J Med *206:* 165–186

Segoloni GP 1984 Evaluation of the clinical and organizational impact of CAPD in the three year period from 1980–1983; the experience of 21 centers. Intern J Artif Organs *7:* 73–75

Sewell CM, Clarridge J, Lacke E, Weinman EJ, Young EJ 1982 Staphylococcal nasal carriage and subsequent infection in peritoneal dialysis patients. JAMA *248:* 1493–1495

Tarchini R, Segoloni GP, Gentile MG, Lupo A, Cancarini G, Salomone M, D'Amico G, Mioli V, Vercellone A, Zucchelli 1988 Long-term results of CAPD in Italy: a report from the Italian CAPD study group. Clin Neph *30:* S68–S70

Zimmerman SW, O'Brien M, Wiedenheoft FA, Johnson CA 1988 Staphylococcus Aureus peritoneal catheter-related infections: a cause of catheter loss and peritonitis. Perit Dial Int *8:* 191–194

Clinical Nephrology, Vol. 36 No. 1 – 1991 (35–41)

Pharmacokinetics of vancomycin in patients undergoing hemodialysis with polyacrylonitrile

J. Torras[1], C. Cao[2], M. C. Rivas[2], M. Cano[3], E. Fernandez[1] and J. Montoliu[1, 4]

[1] Nephrology and [2] Biochemical Services, Hospital Arnau de Vilanova, Lleida, [3] Pharmacy, L'Aliança Mataronina, Mataro and [4] Dept. of Medicine and Surgery, Estudi General de Lleida, U. B., Catalonia, Spain

Abstract. The pharmacokinetics of vancomycin in patients undergoing dialysis with cuprophane membranes are well known, however little has been reported of the use of polyacrylonitrile membranes in dialysis. We studied, in a crossover design, eigth dialysis patients (7 men, 1 woman) aged 30 to 66 years who prospectively received 1 gram of vancomycin i. v. before first dialysis and were subsequently hemodialyzed with cuprophane every second day for a total of three times. A month later trial was repeated using polyacrylonitrile. A mono-compartment model was used to calculate pharmacokinetic parameters. Mean ± standard deviation of vancomycin clearance varied from 5.2 ± 2.1 ml/min in the interdialysis period to 9.7 ± 2.7 ml/min during dialysis with cuprophane and to 58.4 ± 15.6 ml/min during dialysis with polyacrylonitrile ($p < 0.001$). Vancomycin half-life varied from 71.5 ± 23.0 to 35.9 ± 9.8 and to 6.1 ± 1.4 hours, respectively ($p < 0.001$). Fractional removal of vancomycin increased from 4% using the cuprophane dialyzer to 34% using the polyacrylonitrile dialyzer ($p < 0.001$). Serum vancomycin levels at 100 and 168 hours were higher with cuprophane than with polyacrylonitrile (7.0 ± 2.2 vs 3.9 ± 1.2 µg/ml) ($p < 0.001$). Moreover, the mean levels at 100 hours were suboptimal on polyacrylonitrile. Approximately 208 ± 53 mg of vancomycin were removed during one polyacrylonitrile dialysis. Thus, those patients who undergo dialysis with polyacrylonitrile and are treated with vancomycin may need supplementary doses post dialysis or to lessen dosage intervals than those traditionally used for dialysis patients since clearance of the drug is significantly higher than with cuprophane dialyzers. Continuous monitoring of vancomycin levels is also recommended.

Key words: vancomycin – pharmacokinetics – polyacrylonitrile – hemodialysis

Introduction

Glycopeptidic vancomycin was introduced as an antibiotic in 1956 [McCormick et al. 1956]. The drug is a bacterial antibiotic highly effective against all strains of staphylococci and some strains of hemolytic streptococci, streptococci viridans, pneumococci, corynebacteria and clostridia [Cook and Farrar 1978]. Vancomycin is excreted primarily by the kidneys and its mean half-life is 6 hours in patients with normal renal function [Matzke et al. 1986]. In these patients, it is considered as a second or third choice antibiotic after penicillins or cephalosporins, which are cheaper and less toxic. The volume of distribution of vancomycin ranges from 0.39 to 0.45 l/kg [Matzke et al. 1986] and the protein binding from 10 to 44% [Lindholm and Murray 1986, Cutler et al. 1984].

In patients with renal disease, serum vancomycin half-life is prolonged and there is a strong correlation between vancomycin clearance and creatinine clearance [Matzke et al. 1984]. In patients with end-stage renal disease, the half-life is approximately 140 or 160 hours and therefore vancomycin can be administered once a week [Eykyn et al. 1970, Lindholm and Murray 1966]. Moreover, the cellulose membranes used classically produce only negligible clearance of the drug [Matzke et al. 1986]. Thus, vancomycin has become the first choice antibiotic in the treatment of the dialysis access site suffered by these patients.

As the trend is towards the use of newer high permeability membranes with better clearance of urea (cellulose acetate) or middle molecules (polyacrylo-

Received April 2, 1990; in revised form March 6, 1991.

Reprint requests to Dr. J. Montoliu, Nephrology Service, Hospital Arnau de Vilanova, Rovira Roura, 80, ES-25006 Lleida, Spain nitrile, polysulfone...), the pharmacokinetics of vancomycin with these dialyzers should be studied and the vancomycin dosage schedule redefined accordingly.

Removal of a drug by dialysis depends on certain factors: the physicochemical and kinetic properties of the drug, membrane properties, and dialysis specific factors [Lee and Marbury 1984]. Vancomycin has a molecular weight of 1,448 in the middle molecule range, and therefore higher clearance with polyacrylonitrile dialyzers can be expected [Pfeiffer 1981]. Vancomycin also has in its structure six groups capable of ionizing differently, at different pH, with a net molecule charge variation of +2 to −4 [Pfeiffer 1981]. The polyacrylonitrile dialyzer has its surface negatively charged and may, therefore, interact with charged molecules.

The aim of this study was to determine the elimination kinetics of vancomycin during hemodialysis with polyacrylonitrile and to compare them to kinetics with cuprophane.

Patients and methods

Patients

After informed consent was obtained, vancomycin pharmacokinetics were studied in eight patients with end-stage renal failure. None of the patients had any evidence of infection or received any other antimicrobial agent before or during the study and none had congestive heart failure, hepatic dysfunction or drug allergy. The patients were studied in a paired fashion, with each patient being studied on each dialyzer membrane, therefore serving as his own control. The patients suffered from a variety of renal diseases and two were diabetics.

Table 1 shows the main clinical characteristics. There were seven men and one woman. Patients were aged between 30 and 66 years (mean 53.9 years). Five patients had anuria. A further two had residual creatinine clearance of less than 3 ml/min (patients 6 and 7). One patient had residual diuresis of 1000 ml/24 hours and creatinine clearance was 3.2 ml/min (patient 5).

Dosing, sampling and hemodialysis

1 gram of vancomycin was diluted in 100 ml of saline serum and injected into a forearm vein for a period of 75 minutes (13 mg/min). Immediately after vancomycin infusion ended the dialysis session was started. The patients were hemodialyzed every second day for a total of three times with cuprophane dialyzer (Izasa, AM 160, hollow fibre, membrane surface area 1.6 m^2). Blood samples were obtained from arterial lines of the artificial kidney at the following hours post vancomycin infusion: 0,5, 4 (first dialysis), 48, 49, 50, 51, 52 (second dialysis), 96, 100 (third dialysis) and 168 (a week), and from venous lines at 49 hours.

A month later the same protocol was applied using the polyacrylonitrile dialyzer (Hospal, Filtral 16, AN 69 hollow fibre, membrane surface area 1.6 m^2).

Unless otherwise stated, dialysis characteristics were maintained for all patients with respect to a blood flow rate of 250 ml/min and a conventional acetate dialysate at a flow rate of 500 ml/min. The duration of each dialysis session was 4 hours. Blood flow was measured by bubble transit time utilizing the formula and the suggestions of Gotch [Gotch 1976].

Assay

Blood samples were collected and centrifuged, and the serum separated and frozen at −70° C until assayed. The vancomycin concentration of serum samples was determined by fluorescence polarization immunoassay (TDx, Abbot Diagnostics, Irving, Texas, USA). The intra-assay coefficient of variation was 7.2% on replicate samples.

At 49 hours post vancomycin infusion the following biochemical parameters from arterial and venous lines were calculated: hematocrit, total protein, urea and creatinine, using the routine methods at our hospital.

Kinetic analysis

All the kinetics analyses were calculated at the second dialysis (48, 49, 50, 51, 52 hours post vancomycin administration) when steady state was already obtained.

Dialyzer creatinine clearance was calculated according to the following formula:

$$C_{Cr} = Q_B\ (A - V)/A$$

where Q_B refers to blood flow and A and V to arterial and venous serum creatinine concentrations, respectively. Ultrafiltration rates were not included in these calculations.

For kinetic analysis of vancomycin, data were processed by an IBM personal computer using the PKCALC programme [Schumaker 1986] applied to a mono-compartment model.

The intradialytic ($T_{1/2\ D}$) and interdialytic ($T_{1/2\ ID}$) biologic half-life of vancomycin was calculated from the following relationships:

$$T_{1/2\ D} = 0.693/K_D \text{ and } T_{1/2\ ID} = 0.693/K_{ID}$$

Table 1 Clinical and pharmacokinetic characteristics

Patient nº	Age (yr)	Sex	Weight (kg)	Hct (%)	Plasma total protein (g/dl)	Residual creatinine clearance (ml/min)	Renal diagnosis	Vancomycin dosage (mg/kg)	Vd (l/kg)	Inter HD vancomycin clearance (ml/min)	Inter HD vancomycin $T_{1/2}$ (h)
1	56	M	88.5	23	6.8	0	Nephrosclerosis	11.4	0.33	7.1	50.5
2	60	F	52.0	18	6.7	0	Chronic glomerulonephritis	19.2	0.44	2.2	111.6
3	30	M	60.5	25	7.2	0	Chronic glomerulonephritis	16.5	0.43	3.4	92.3
4	58	M	72.0	29	7.2	0	Chronic glomerulonephritis	13.9	0.36	3.7	81.2
5	57	M	66.5	23	7.1	3.2	Diabetic nephropathy	15.0	0.48	8.6	39.8
6	51	M	54.0	19	7.9	1.0	Diabetic nephropathy	18.5	0.68	6.5	67.5
7	53	M	47.5	30	7.4	1.3	Systemic sclerosis	21.0	0.64	5.5	62.3
8	66	M	91.5	25	7.2	0	Chronic pyelonephritis	10.9	0.31	4.3	67.1
Mean	53.9							15.8	0.46	5.2	71.5
SD	10.6							3.7	0.13	2.1	23.0

Table 2 Serum vancomycin concentration at different times in patients on hemodialysis with cuprophane (μg/ml)

Patient	Hours post vancomycin administration						
	First HD		Second HD		Third HD		
	0.5	4	48	52	96	100	168
1	30.1	17.0	9.3	9.3	8.0	6.7	5.9
2	40.6	20.5	15.6	12.2	11.0	9.9	8.8
3	36.6	22.4	16.1	14.7	10.9	9.9	–
4	35.9	20.2	14.0	13.2	11.4	9.8	8.6
5	29.9	15.5	7.2	6.2	4.6	3.5	2.3
6	25.8	15.4	9.8	9.7	9.4	7.6	7.6
7	31.0	16.8	10.3	8.2	8.2	7.6	6.0
8	34.3	16.7	10.6	9.4	8.4	7.9	7.0

Table 3 Serum vancomycin concentration at different times in patients on hemodialysis with polyacrylonitrile (μg/ml)

Patient	Hours post vancomycin administration						
	First HD		Second HD		Third HD		
	0.5	4	48	52	96	100	168
1	28.8	11.2	10.4	3.7	3.6	2.6	2.7
2	34.8	13.6	11.0	3.5	3.8	3.4	3.8
3	35.6	17.3	14.0	6.7	7.6	4.9	4.7
4	31.2	12.6	11.2	6.1	7.1	4.9	4.7
5	24.5	10.2	5.3	3.0	3.2	0.6	1.5
6	25.1	12.9	10.8	6.1	7.2	4.3	4.8
7	27.0	12.8	10.7	6.0	7.6	4.7	4.9
8	26.3	11.2	8.5	5.1	6.2	3.6	3.9

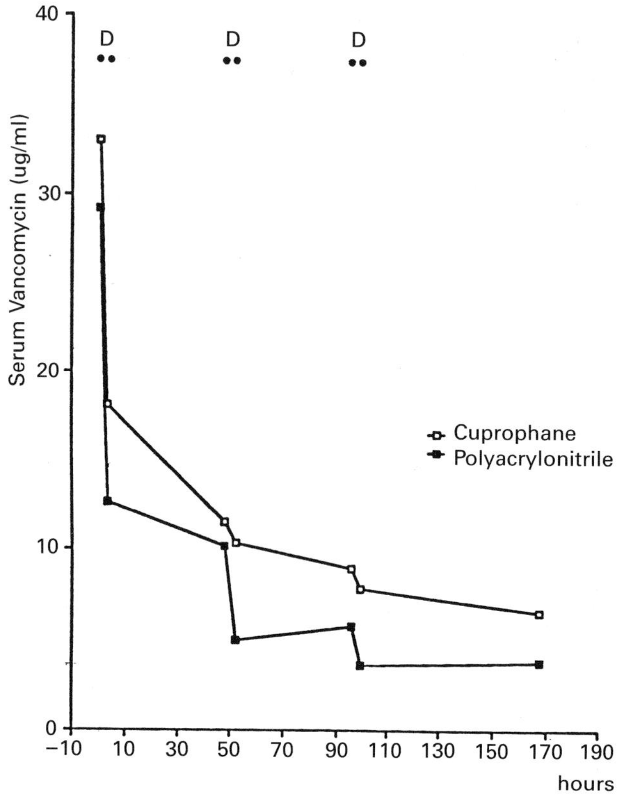

Fig. 1. Mean serum concentration-time profiles for both dialyzers (see text). D = four-hour dialysis

where K_D and K_{ID} are, respectively, the elimination rate constants of vancomycin determined by non-linear regression analysis using serum concentration-time profiles on a semi-logarithmic scale in both periods. The apparent volume of distribution (Vd) was obtained by dividing the amount of drug administered by the serum vancomycin value extrapolated at time zero.

The area under the semi-logarithmic serum concentration-time curve during hemodialysis (AUC_T) and during the interdialytic period (AUC_{ID}) was determined by the trapezoidal rule. Total vancomycin clearance during dialysis (C_T) and during the interdialytic period (C_{ID}) was calculated by the formula:

$$C_T = \text{vancomycin dosage}/AUC_T$$
$$C_{ID} = \text{vancomycin dosage}/AUC_{ID}$$

Dialyzer vancomycin clearance (C_d) was calculated from the following:

$$C_D = C_T - C_{ID}$$

The fractional removal of vancomycin during a dialysis session (Fr) was calculated according to the relationship:

$$Fr = (K_{ID}/K_D) \cdot (1 - e^{-K_{ID}t})$$

where t is duration of dialysis in hours. The amount of vancomycin in milligrams removed during dialysis (RD) was determined by:

$$RD = Vd \cdot C \cdot Fr$$

where C is the mean value of serum vancomycin measurements evaluated during dialysis.

Statistics

Statistical analysis was performed by Student's t-test for paired data. Results are expressed as mean ±

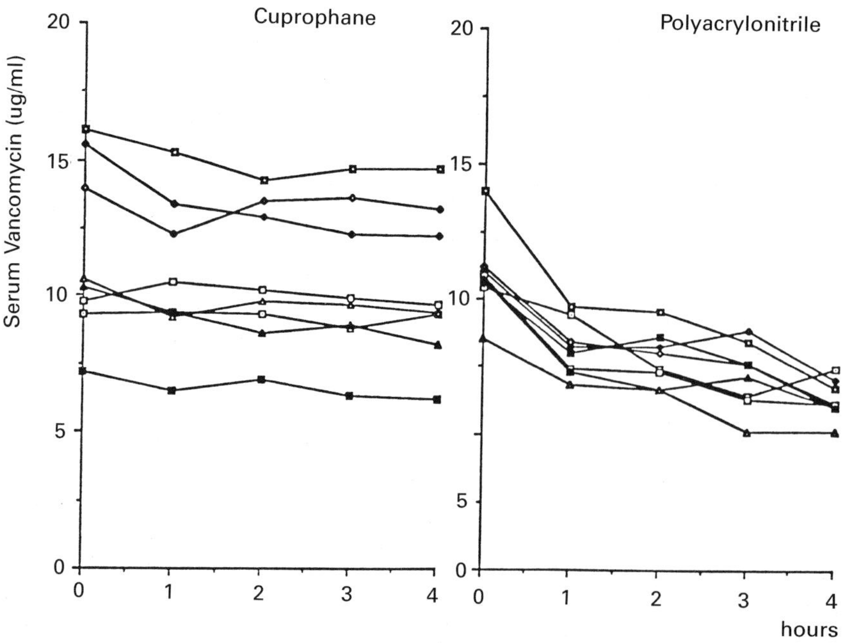

Fig. 2. The hourly change in serum vancomycin levels during hemodialysis with both dialyzers. Individual symbols represent the same patient dialyzed on the two different membranes

Table 4 Pharmacokinetics of vancomycin during dialysis with cuprophane and with polyacrylonitrile. Calculations were done at second dialysis (from 48 to 52 hours post endovenous administration of 1 gram of vancomycin)

	Net fluid removal (kg)	Dialyzer creatinine clearance (ml/min)	Dialyzer vancomycin clearance (ml/min)	Total vancomycin clearance (ml/min)	$T_{1/2}$ (h)	Fractional drug removal (%)	Vancomycin removed (mg)
Cuprophane							
Mean	2.9	121.3	4.5	9.7	35.9	4.0	
SD	1.2	10.0	2.4	2.7	9.8	2.0	
Polyacrylonitrile							
Mean	3.1	123.2	53.2	58.4	6.1	34.0	208
SD	1.1	12.5	14.8	15.6	1.4	7.0	53
p	NS	NS	<0.001	<0.001	<0.001	<0.001	

standard deviation. P values less than 0.05 were considered significant.

Results

Table 1 shows the main pharmacokinetic vancomycin parameters for the eight patients interdialysis: interdialysis vancomycin clearance 5.2 ± 2.1 ml/min, interdialysis vancomycin $T_{1/2}$ 71.5 ± 23.0 hours, and the volume of distribution of vancomycin 0.46 ± 0.13 l/kg. Vancomycin dosage varied from 11.4 to 21.0 mg/kg, with a mean value of 15.8 mg/kg. Hemodialyses were well tolerated. There was no difference in ultrafiltration rate with both membranes.

Tables 2 and 3 show serum vancomycin concentration values for each patient with both membranes throughout the study. Figure 1 shows mean serum vancomycin concentration-time profiles for both dialyzers. Serum vancomycin levels at 100 hours (cuprophane 7.9 ± 2.2 versus polyacrylonitrile 3.6 ± 1.5 μg/ml) and at 168 hours (cuprophane 7.0 ± 2.2 versus polyacrylonitrile 3.9 ± 1.2 μg/ml) were higher with cuprophane than with polyacrylonitrile ($p < 0.001$). Moreover, patients on polyacrylonitrile had suboptimal vancomycin levels at 100 and 168 hours. Of note, two patients (25%) on polyacrylonitrile (patients 1 and 5) already had absolute subtherapeutic levels at 100 hours if we accept 3.1 μg/ml as the upper limit of minimum inhibitory concentration for staphylococci.

Only one patient (patient 5) on cuprophane had a subtherapeutic vancomycin level, and at 168 hours. It is remarkable that this patient had non-negligible residual creatinine clearance.

When we examined the change in serum vancomycin levels during one hemodialysis (second hemodialysis) with both membranes (Figure 2) we found a higher reduction of serum vancomycin with polyacrylonitrile than with cuprophane ($p < 0.01$). The cuprophane dialyzer resulted in a minimal decrease from a mean value of 11.6 ± 3.2 to 10.4 ± 2.8 μg/ml during four hours of dialysis. However, polyacrylonitrile dialyzer produced a marked reduction in serum vancomycin from a mean value of 10.2 ± 2.5 to 5.0 ± 1.4 μg/ml. Pharmacokinetic parameters with both membranes calculated from the above data at second dialysis are shown in Table 4. Dialyzer urea (data not shown) and creatinine clearance were similar with both membranes (p NS).

The fractional removal of vancomycin increased from 4.0% using the cuprophane dialyzer to 34.0% using the polyacrylonitrile dialyzer ($p < 0.001$). Using the cuprophane dialyzer, the intradialytic $T_{1/2}$ of vancomycin was 35.9 ± 9.8 hours, while the polyacrylonitrile dialyzer showed a markedly reduced intradialytic $T_{1/2}$ of 6.1 ± 1.4 hours ($p < 0.001$).

Vancomycin clearance varied from 5.2 ± 2.1 ml/min during the interdialytic period to 9.7 ± 2.7 ml/min during hemodialysis with cuprophane or to 58.4 ± 15.6 ml/min during hemodialysis with polyacrylonitrile ($p < 0.001$). The contribution of dialyzers to vancomycin clearance was 4.5 ± 2.4 and 53.2 ± 14.8 ml/min respectively ($p < 0.001$). Approximately 208 ± 53 mg of vancomycin were removed during one hemodialysis with polyacrylonitrile (calculated at second dialysis).

Finally, to determine the effect of blood flow rate on vancomycin clearance with the polyacrylonitrile dialyzer, this pharmacokinetic parameter was calculated at two different blood flows (250 and 300 ml/min, measured by bubble transit time) in four patients (patients 1, 2, 3 and 5) (Figure 3). Vancomycin clearance increased significantly over the two blood flows studied ($p = 0.05$). The mean values were 58.2 ±

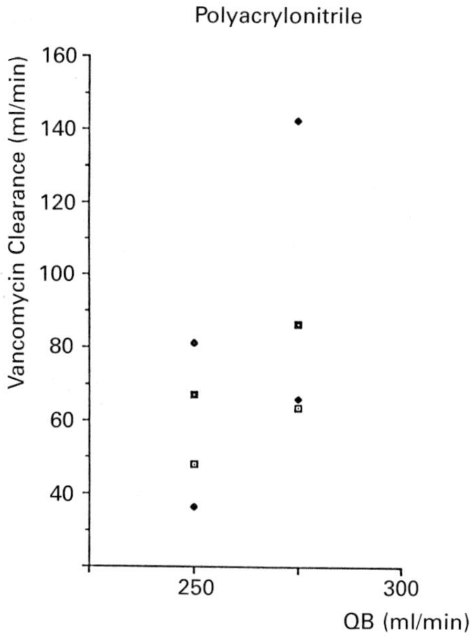

Fig. 3. The effect of blood flow (Q_B) on serum vancomycin clearance using polyacrylonitrile, evaluated in four patients. Data for individual patients are designated by different symbols for each patient. Mean values are statistically different (p = 0.05)

19.8 ml/min at blood flow of 250 ml/min and 89.7 ± 36.7 ml/min at 300 ml/min.

There were no side-effects from vancomycin throughout the study.

Discussion

Vancomycin is an antibiotic widely used in the treatment of systemic or shunt infections in hemodialysis patients. For the most part, the microorganisms that cause these infections are very susceptible to vancomycin with a minimum inhibitory concentration (MIC) ranging from 0.1 to 3.1 μg/ml [Geraci 1977, Sande and Mandel 1980] for Staphylococcus aureus and from 0.4 to 3.1 μg/ml [Geraci 1977, Sande and Mandel 1980] for Staphylococcus epidermidis. Higher values for MIC in these [Wilcox et al. 1985] and other microorganisms may occur, particularly with enterococci.

There do not appear to be any data relating to how long serum vancomycin concentrations remain above MIC to clinical cures [Edwards and Pancorbo 1987]; nevertheless, some empiric dosing schedules have been proposed in order to obtain peak concentrations 10- to 20-fold higher than usual MIC values and to maintain concentrations in excess of the MIC value throughout the entire dosage interval [Edwards and Pancorbo 1987].

Matzke suggested peak vancomycin concentrations of 30 μg/ml and trough concentrations of 7.5 μg/ml as desirable for optimal therapy [1984]. With cuprophane dialyzers, this has been successfully accomplished with 1 gram of intravenous vancomycin once a week [Eykyn et al. 1970]. Our results with cuprophane confirm this, with mean peak and trough concentrations of 33.0 and 7.0 μg/ml, respectively. Nevertheless, when dialysis was performed using polyacrylonitrile, the mean peak concentration was 29.2, sufficiently high, but the mean trough concentration (at 168 hours) was 3.9 μg/ml, clearly suboptimal. Moreover, at 100 hours the mean serum vancomycin level was already suboptimal.

Vancomycin kinetic properties include a small volume of distribution [Matzke et al. 1986] and protein binding between 10 and 44% [Lindholm and Murray 1966, Cutler et al. 1984]. Therefore, its clearance during dialysis is primarily a function on the permeability of the dialysis membrane.

In 1986, Matzke et al. first reported the disposition of vancomycin during hemofiltration using a polyamide hemofilter. Their results showed vancomycin clearance as high as 152.6 ± 21.5 ml/min and a vancomycin removal of approximately 400 mg in one session. It is noteworthy that the mean blood flow used was excessively high (567 ± 69 ml/min) and that it is rarely used in routine hemodialysis. Later, Bastani claimed in an incomplete study [1988] the vancomycin clearance in hemodialysis being higher using cellulose acetate and polyacrylonitrile membranes, resp. as compared to the cuprophane membrane. Matzke and Bastani suggested the need for careful monitoring of vancomycin and shorter dosing intervals when a patient is being dialyzed with these kinds of membrane.

Recently other authors have reported their pharmacokinetic data on hemodialysis or hemofiltration with high permeability membranes [Lanese et al. 1989, De Bock et al. 1989] with results quite similar to ours. Nevertheless, none of them studied the kinetics of vancomycin with polyacrylonitrile.

In the present study in patients undergoing dialysis with polyacrylonitrile, the elimanation half-life was markedly reduced from 71.5 hours during the interdialytic period to 6.1 hours during the dialysis session. In parallel, vancomycin clearance increased approximately ten-fold, from 5.2 ml/min to 58.4 ml/min. These changes were the effect of the increased elimination of vancomycin via the artificial kidney during hemodialysis since 34% of the drug was removed by dialysis. On the other hand, vancomycin clearance experienced few changes when hemodialysis was performed with cuprophane (5.2 in the interdialytic period versus 9.7 ml/min during hemodialysis).

Finally, as blood flow increases, so does vancomycin clearance with polyacrylonitrile.

Mean plasma levels of vancomycin rose after the second and third hemodialysis when using polyacrylonitrile. As some authors have reported [De Bock et al. 1989, Matzke et al. 1986], this could more likely represent delayed intercompartmental equilibration with a concentration rebound post dialysis. Thus, some of our calculations may be partially erroneous. Nevertheless as it has been shown above, mean trough vancomycin concentration at 168 hours was clearly suboptimal when using polyacrylonitrile.

It was calculated at the second dialysis that approximately 208 mg of vancomycin (131 to 302 mg) were eliminated through polyacrylonitrile. As mean serum vancomycin was at suboptimal therapeutic levels at the end of the third dialysis with polyacrylonitrile, we suggest administration of the next 1 gram of vancomycin dose every third hemodialysis, at the end of the session, when using this membrane.

In a recent paper, it was proposed to administer vancomycin at the beginning of dialysis instead of at the end in order to avoid an additional stay of two hours in the dialysis unit [Edell et al. 1988]. As our results suggest, we should only accept this when using cuprophane membranes but never when using polyacrylonitrile membranes.

In conclusion, those patients who undergo hemodialysis with polacrylonitrile and are treated with vancomycin may need supplementary doses post hemodialysis or to lessen dosage intervals than those traditionally used for hemodialysis patients since clearance of the drug is significantly higher than with cuprophane dialyzers. Continuous monitoring of vancomycin levels is also recommended.

Acknowledgements

We are indebted to Conxa Fonayet and the entire medical and nursing staff at the Nephrology Service of the Hospital Arnau de Vilanova, Lleida, Spain for their cooperation in conducting this study and to Cristine O'Hara for preparation and translation of the manuscript.

We thank Abbot Diagnostics for providing the TDx kit for vancomycin assay.

REFERENCES

Bastani B, Spyker DA, Minocha A, Cummings R, Wetervelt FB 1988 In vivo comparison of three different haemodialysis membranes for vancomycin clearance: cuprophan, cellulose acetate, and polyacrylonitrile. Dial Transplant *17:* 527–543

Cook FV, Farrar WE 1978 Vancomycin revisited. Ann Intern Med *88:* 813–818

Cutler NR, Narang PK, Lesko LJ, Nimos M, Power M 1984 Vancomycin disposition: the importance of age. Clin Pharmacol Ther *36:* 803–810

De Bock V, Verbeelen D, Maes V, Sennesael J 1989 Pharmacokinetics of vancomycin in patients undergoing hemodialysis and hemofiltration. Nephrol Dial Transplant *4:* 635–639

Edwards DJ, Pancorbo S 197 Routine monitoring of serum vancomycin concentrations: waiting for proof of its value. Clin Pharm *6:* 252–254

Edell LS, Westby GR, Gould SR 1988 An improved method of vancomycin administration to dialysis patients. Clin Nephrol *29 (2):* 86–87

Eykyn S, Phillips I, Evans J 1970 Vancomycin for staphylococcal shunt site infections in patients on regular hemodialysis. Br Med J *3:* 80–82

Geraci JE 1977 Vancomycin. Mayo Clin Proc *52:* 631

Gotch FA 1976 Hemodialysis: technical and kinetic considerations. In: *Brenner BM, Rector FC* (eds). The kidney. Saunders, Philadelphia, p 1676

Lanese DM, Alfrey PS, Molitoris BA 1989 Markedly increased clearance of vancomycin during haemodialysis using polysulfone dialysers. Kidney Int *35:* 1409–1412

Lee ChC, Marbury TC 1984 Drug therapy in patients undergoing haemodialysis. Clinical pharmacokinetic consideration. Clin Pharmacokinet *9:* 42–66

Lindholm DD, Murray JS 1986 Persistence of vancomycin in the blood during renal failure and its treatment by haemodialysis. New Eng J Med *274:* 1047–1051.

Matzke GR, McGory RW, Halitenson CE 1984 Pharmacokinetics of vancomycin in patients with various degrees of renal function. Antimicrob Agents Chemother *25:* 433–7

Matzke GR, Zhanel GG, Guay DRP 1986 Clinical pharmacokinetics of vancomycin. Clin Pharmacokinet *11:* 257–282

Matzke GR, O'Connel MB, Collins AJ, Keshaviah PR 1986 Disposition of vancomycin during haemofiltration. Clin Pharmacol Ther *40:* 425–430

McCormick MH, Stark WM, Pittenger GE, Pittenger RC, McGuire JM 1956 Vancomycin, a new antibiotic. Chemical and biologic properties. Antibiot Annu *56:* 606–611

Pfeiffer RR 1981 Structural features of vancomycin. Rev Infect Dis *(Suppl) 3:* S 205 – S 209

Sande MA, Mandel GL 1980 Antimicrobial Agents. In: *Gilman AG, Goodman LS, Gilman A* (eds). Goodman and Gilman's the Pharmacological Basis of Therapeutics. 6th edn. McMillan Publishing Co., p 1230

Schumaker B 1986 PKCALC: a basic interactive computer program for statistical pharmacokinetics analysis of data. Drug Metabol Rev *17:* 331–348

Wilcox MH, Edwards R, Finch RG 1985 Laboratory studies on coagulase-negative staphilococci from CAPD-associated peritonitis. Jour Antimicrob Chemother 15: 297–303.

Clinical Nephrology, Vol. 36 No. 1 – 1991 (42–45)

Acute thrombosis of the renal transplant artery: a case report and review of the literature

G. C. Groggel

Department of Medicine, College of Medicine, University of Vermont, Burlington, Vermont 05405

Abstract. Acute thrombosis of the renal transplant artery is a known but unusual complication of renal transplantation usually occurring in the first month. Reported here is a case of acute renal artery thrombosis in a well functioning long-term renal allograft in which there was clear angiographic evidence of a normal renal artery two years earlier.

Key words: thrombosis – kidney – allograft – transplant – vascular

Introduction

Acute thrombosis of the renal transplant artery is a known vascular complication of renal allografts [Belzer et al. 1988]. Incidence of this complication varies between 0.5% and 3.5% [Jones et al. 1988, Jordan et al. 1982, Lee et al. 1977, Nerstrom et al. 1972, Palleschi et al. 1980, Rigotti et al. 1986, Rijksen et al. 1986, Rao et al. 1976, Vidne et al. 1976]. This complication usually occurs within the first month after transplantation. Beyond this period of time, this complication is distinctly uncommon except in a rejected kidney. Reported here is the case of a patient with a well functioning kidney transplant when he suffered acute thrombosis of his renal transplant artery and lost his allograft.

Case report

The patient was a 30-year-old white male with end-stage renal disease secondary to reflux nephropathy. He had been on long-term hemodialysis since December 1983. He was hypertensive with a blood pressure of 150/100. In April 1984 he underwent a four antigen match, living-related kidney transplant from his sister at the University of Utah Medical Center. He had immediate function of his graft and left the hospital with a serum creatinine of 1.5 mg/dl (133 µmol/l) on an immunosuppressive regimen of cyclosporine and prednisone.

In November 1986, he was admitted to the University of Utah Medical Center with a blood pressure of 200/120 after discontinuing his antihypertensives five months earlier. A renal arteriogram was performed during the admission and demonstrated in multiple views a normal renal transplant artery (Figure 1A). No renal vein renins were collected. He was discharged on cyclosporine, prednisone, azathioprine, clonidine, captopril and propranolol. Serum creatinine was 1.2 mg/dl (106 µmol/l) with a creatinine clearance of 90 ml/min. In December of 1986 cyclosporine was discontinued without a change in the blood pressure. He was hospitalized at the University of Utah Medical Center in February 1988 with a serum creatinine of 6.9 mg/dl (610 µmol/l) which was felt to be secondary to volume depletion. He underwent a renal biopsy during that admission which was normal except for mild interstitial fibrosis. Discharge creatinine was 1.7 mg/dl (150 µmol/l) and medications included azathioprine, prednisone, furosemide, propranolol, clonidine and hydralazine. In April 1988 the serum creatinine was 1.3 mg/dl (115 µmol/l).

On December 15, 1988 he was admitted to his local hospital for a total hip replacement on the right because of aseptic necrosis of the femoral head. His admission laboratory examination revealed a hematocrit of 43.6%, a WBC of 7,100, a platelet count of 216,000. The prothrombin time was 10.9 (control 11.6), partial thromboplastin time was 20.8 (control 26.7), bleeding time 6.3 minutes and erythrocyte sedimentation rate 27 mm per hour. The serum creatinine was 1.4 mg/dl (124 µmol/l), blood urea nitrogen was 19 mg/dl (6.8 mmol/l), serum cholesterol was 229 mg/dl (5.92 mmol/l) and serum electrolytes were normal. His urinalysis showed a trace of protein and 0–2 white blood cells per high power field. His medications at the time of admission

Received September 10, 1990; in revised form February 11, 1991.

Reprint requests to Dr. G. C. Groggel, Nephrology Unit, University of Vermont, D305 Given Building, Burlington, VT 05405.

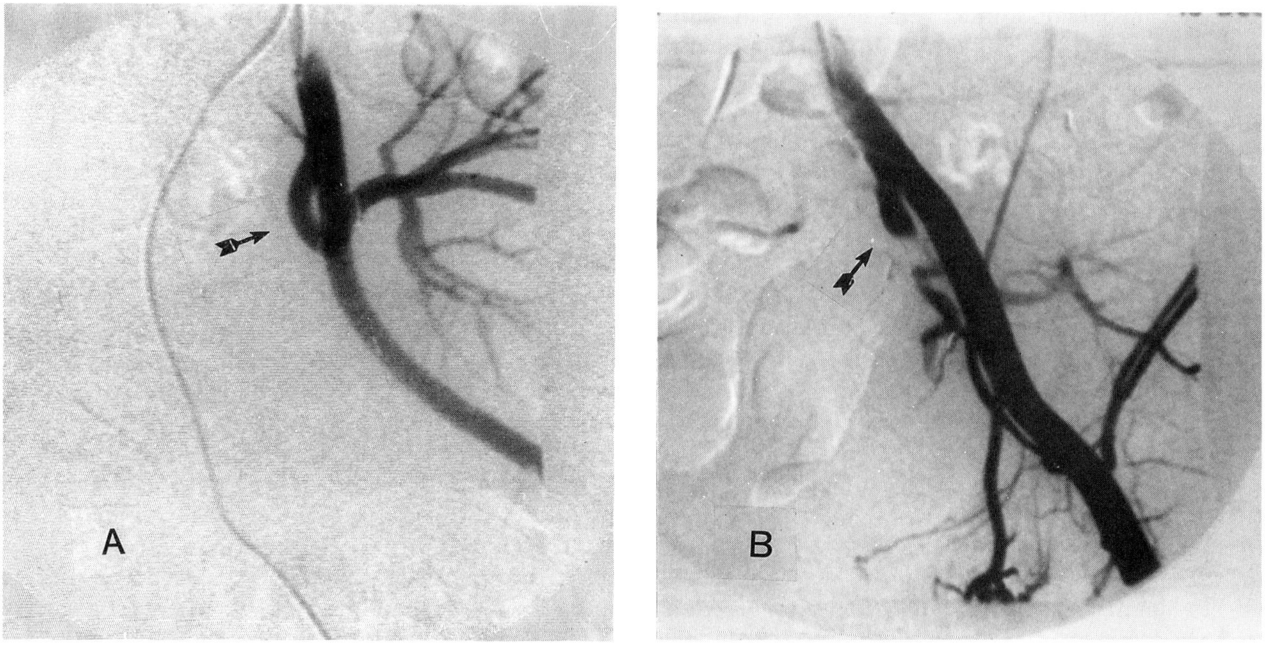

Figure 1. Figure 1A is a renal arteriogram performed 2 years previously demonstrating a normal renal transplant artery with an end-to-end anastomosis to the hypogastric artery. Figure 1B is a renal arteriogram demonstrating complete occlusion of the renal artery at the anastomosis site with the hypogastric artery. Arrow points to the renal artery.

included furosemide 10 mg twice a day, propranolol 40 mg twice a day, clonidine 0.3 mg twice a day, hydralazine 100 mg twice a day, azathioprine 100 mg once a day, and prednisone 5 mg once a day. His pre-operative blood pressure was 190/120. During the surgery his blood pressure rose to a high of 240/140 mmHg and dropped to a low of 158/100 mmHg. He was treated with intravenous hydralazine throughout surgery. Approximately four hours after surgery he became and remained anuric. During this immediate post-operative period his blood pressure dropped to a low of 106/64. By 8 p.m. on the 15th of December, his blood urea nitrogen had risen to 33 mg/dl (11.8 mmol/l) and serum creatinine to 2.9 mg/dl (256 µmol/l). By the next morning his blood urea nitrogen was 41 mg/dl (14.6 mmol/l) and serum creatinine 4.5 mg/dl (398 µmol/l). The hematocrit was 34.1% and platelets 145,000.

He was transferred to the University of Utah Medical Center. On arrival, he had a blood urea nitrogen of 51 mg/dl (18.2 mmol/l), serum creatinine 7.0 mg/dl (619 µmol/l), serum sodium 140 mEq/l, serum potassium 5.4 mEq/l, serum chloride 108 mEq/l, and a serum bicarbonate of 15 mEq/l. His blood pressure on arrival was 250/150. The blood pressure was controlled with intravenous nitroprus-

Table 1. Summary of acute thrombosis of renal transplant artery

Investigator	N Transplant	N with Thrombosis	Time post-Tx	Graft Lost	Outcome Death
Jones [1988]	110	2 (1.8%)	0–54 days	2	
Jordan [1982]	341	12 (3.5%)	0–27 days	12	1
Lee [1977]	345	5 (1.4%)	0.5–45 months	3	1
Nerstrom [1972]	155	3 (1.9%)	1–47 months	3	2
Palleschi [1980]	600	5 (0.8%)	0–16 days	4	
Rigotti [1986]	325	6 (1.8%)	4–12 days	6	
Rijksen [1986]	400	7 (1.8%)	1–28 days	7	
Venkatesara [1976]	100	2 (2%)	7–64 days	2	1
Vidne [1976]	202	4 (2%)		4	
Totals	2,578	46 (1.8%)		43 (92%)	5 (11%)

side. He immediately underwent a renal scan which showed no flow or function in the transplanted kidney. This was followed by a renal angiogram. The angiogram demonstrated complete occlusion of the renal artery at the anastomosis site to the hypogastric artery (Figure 1B). Three days later, because of difficulty in controlling his blood pressure, he underwent a transplant nephrectomy. The patient subsequently returned to chronic hemodialysis. An echocardiogram was performed to look for an embolic source and was normal. Pathologic examination of the kidney showed an edematous completely necrotic kidney. The renal artery was completely occluded with clot without evidence of stenosis.

Discussion

In summary, a patient who had a well functioning kidney transplant for more than four and one-half years suffered acute thrombosis of his renal artery related to undergoing hip surgery. To our knowledge this is only the fourth case reported of this complication occurring in a patient with a long-term well functioning renal allograft. The patient clearly was severely hypertensive at the time of his surgery and then developed a relative hypotension episode in the immediate post-operative period which may have been related to the acute thrombosis of the renal artery.

What also makes this case unique is the fact that 2 years earlier the patient had a completely normal renal arteriogram. This is the only case in which there is documented anatomic evidence of a normal renal artery in a renal transplant patient later developing acute thrombosis of the renal artery.

In the only other reports of patients with long-standing renal transplants who developed acute thrombosis, very little information is available [Lee et al. 1977, Nerstrom et al. 1972, Swanson and Sullivan 1976]. One patient was a white female who had a functioning renal allograft for 4 years and developed acute thrombosis of the hypogastric-renal artery associated with an acute myocardial infarction [Swanson and Sullivan 1976]. The second case was a 39-year-old white female with a renal tranplant for 3½ years who had underlying renal artery stenosis and developed occlusion of the renal artery associated with sepsis and respiratory failure [Lee et al. 1977]. The third case of acute occlusion occurred 47 months after transplantation in a patient with severe hypertension [Nerstrom et al. 1972]. No further information was available. In two of these three reported cases the acute thrombosis was associated with significant other acute medical problems and death. Thus this report is only the second case of acute thrombosis in an otherwise healthy patient.

In a review of the literature the incidence of this complication varies between 0.8% and 3.5% as shown in Table 1. Frequently this complication has been associated with acute rejection, technical problems or renal artery stenosis. Most commonly this occurs within the first month after transplantation. In a review of over 2,500 transplants there were 46 cases reported for an overall incidence of 1.8% (Table 1). Of these, 80% occurred within the first month after transplantation and 93% within the first year.

The incidence of this complication is felt to be increased with the use of cyclosporine. Rigotti found an incidence of 1.8% with cyclosporine and no cases in patients treated with azathioprine and prednisone [Rigotti et al. 1986]. The Canadian Multicenter Transplant Study Group [1983] found an incidence of renal artery thrombosis or stenosis of 7% with cyclosporine and 1% with conventional therapy. There are a variety of effects cyclosporine might have but most likely it is the effect of cyclosporine on endothelial cells to decrease prostacycline production which predisposes to thrombosis.

The two most common types of arterial anastomosis are end-to-end of the renal artery to the hypogastric artery and end-to-side to the external iliac artery [Flye 1989]. The most common type of anastomosis is probably the former because it is easier and faster to perform and will not compromise the circulation to the leg. But it has a higher incidence of stenosis than the end-to-side anastomosis.

The patient presented here was no longer on cyclosporine and had evidence for no other risk factors. He also had a normal arteriogram two years earlier but did have the end-to-end anastomosis which has a higher incidence of stenosis. But significant hypertension which this patient had may be a risk factor for thrombosis.

Almost invariably this complication results in loss of the allograft, frequently requiring nephrectomy (Table 1). There have been isolated case reports of successful revascularization of acute thrombosis with up to 12 hours of occlusion, and the recommendation has been made to attempt revascularization within 12 hours of the occlusion [Lee et al. 1977, Gerard et al. 1982]. There has been one report of successful therapy with streptokinase in acute thrombosis [Zajko et al. 1982]. But if any form of therapy is going to be successful, the diagnosis of acute thrombosis must be established immediately. In any patient developing anuria, a diagnosis of acute renal artery occlusion should be considered.

In summary we report only the second case of acute thrombosis of the renal transplant artery in a patient with a long-standing well functioning renal allograft without other significant medical problems. This is the only case of acute thrombosis in which the patient had previous evidence of a normal renal artery.

REFERENCES

Belzer FO, Glass N, Sollinger H 1988 Technical complications after renal transplantation. In: *Morris PJ (ed)*: Kidney Transplantation. Principles and Practice. Saunders, Philadelphia, p 511

The Canadian Multicentre Transplant Study Group 1983 A randomized clinical trial of cyclosporine in cadaveric renal transplantation. New Engl J Med *309:* 809

Flye MW 1989 Renal Transplantation. In: *Flye ME* (ed): Principles of Organ Transplantation. Saunders, Philadelphia, p 264

Gerard DF, Devin JB, Halasz NA, Collins GM 1982 Transplant renal artery thrombosis. Revascularization after 5½ hours of ischemia. Arch Surg *117:* 361

Jones RM, Murie JA, Ting A et al. 1988 Renal vascular thrombosis of cadaveric renal allografts in patients receiving cyclosporine, azathioprine and prednisolone triple therapy. Clinical Transplantation *2:* 122

Jordan JL, Cook GT, Cardella CJ 1982 Ten years of experience with vascular complications in renal transplantation. J Urology *128:* 689

Lee HM, Mendez-Picon G, Pierce JC, Hume DM 1977 Renal artery occlusion in transplant recipients. Am Surg *43:* 186

Nerstrom B, Ladefoged J, Lund FL 1972 Vascular complications in 155 consecutive kidney transplantations. Scan J Urol Nephrol; suppl 15, *6:* 65

Palleschi J, Novick AC, Braun WE, Magnusson MO 1980 Vascular complications of renal transplantation. Urology *16:* 61

Rao KV, Smith EJ, Alexander JW et al. 1976 Thromboembolic disease in renal allograft recipients. Arch Surg *111:* 1086

Rigotti P, Flechner SM, Van Buren CT et al 1986 Increased incidence of renal allograft thrombosis under cyclosporine immunosuppression. Int Surg *71:* 38

Rijksen JFVB, Koolen MI, Walaszewski JE et al. 1986 Vascular complications in 400 consecutive renal allotransplants. J Cardiovas Surg *23:* 91

Swanson DA, Sullivan MJ 1976 Thromboendarterectomy for anuria 4½ years post-renal transplant: A case report. J Urology *116:* 799

Vidne BA, Leapman SB, Butt KM, Kountz SL 1976 Vascular complications in human renal transplantation. Surgery *79:* 77

Zajko AB, McLean GK, Grossman RA et al. 1982 Percutaneous transluminal angioplasty and fibrinolytic therapy for renal allograft arterial stenosis and thrombosis. Transplantation *33:* 447

Clinical Nephrology, Vol. 36 No. 1 – 1991 (46–48)

Diffuse mesangial sclerosis in a fetus

G. S. Spear[1], K. A. Steinhaus[2] and A. Quddusi[1]

Department of [1]Pathology and [2]Pediatrics, California College of Medicine, University of California Irvine, Irvine, CA USA

Abstract. An 18-week fetus was born following termination of pregnancy by prostaglandin induction. Pregnancy was terminated because of elevated maternal serum alpha-fetoprotein and ultrasonographic evidence of severe oligohydramnios, intrauterine growth retardation, non-visualization of the bladder, dolichocephaly and possible mild hydrocephalus. Pathologic examination disclosed diffuse mesangial sclerosis and histologic evidence of the nephrotic syndrome. To our knowledge this is the first reported example of ante-natal diffuse mesangial sclerosis; of fetal congenital nephrosis other than Finnish type; and of fetal congenital nephrosis with prominent glomerular lesions.

Key words: diffuse mesangial sclerosis – fetus – congenital nephrotic syndrome

Introduction

Diffuse mesangial sclerosis (DMS) is a distinctive form of infantile nephrotic syndrome which has a poor prognosis [Habib and Bois 1973, Sibley et al. 1989, Habib et al. 1989, 1990]. We describe a fetus with DMS, to our knowledge the first reported example of ante-natal DMS; the first recorded example of fetal congenital nephrosis not of Finnish type; and the first report of fetal congenital nephrosis with prominent glomerular lesions.

Case report

This female fetus was the product of an 18-week gestation in a 23-year-old mother who was gravida 2 para 1, blood type B positive, RPR non-reactive and rubella immune. The husband was also 23 years old. The couple's 10-month-old daughter was in apparently good health. Consanguinity was denied. There was no family history of renal disease, birth defects or mental retardation. Two weeks prior to delivery prenatal screening disclosed a maternal serum alpha-fetoprotein level of 5.99 multiples of the median (normal is less than 2.5). Four days before delivery ultrasonography disclosed a mean gestational age of $17^{5}/_{7}$ weeks, marked oligohydramnios, intrauterine growth retardation, non-visualization of the bladder, dolichocephaly and possible mild hydrocephalus. Pregnancy was terminated by prostaglandin induction.

Pathologic examination revealed a female fetus weighing 231 grams with measurements and organ weights compatible with a gestational age of 18–20 weeks with the exception of splenomegaly. The head circumference was 16.0 cm. External examination disclosed low set ears and possibly mild micrognathia. The pleural and pericardial cavity contained minimal fluid, and the abdominal cavity 1cc of clear fluid. The genitourinary tract was normal. There were no thrombi in renal or other veins. Whole body x-rays were normal. The brain was autolyzed but appeared normal; the ventricles were not dilated. Cultured liver tissue revealed a normal female karyotype and there was no evidence of 11p deletion. The placenta weighed 85 grams and approximately 10% of the maternal surface was infarcted.

Microscopic examination of the placenta revealed intervillous thrombosis and focal infarction. The spleen disclosed deficiency of white pulp. Microscopic examination of the ovaries and remaining tissues was normal with exception of the kidneys. There was no evidence of congenital infection.

The kidneys manifested notable histopathologic findings affecting tubules, interstitium and glomeruli. There were many microscopic cysts up to 0.5 mm in diameter in the mid-cortex, especially in the deep cortex, and rarely in the medulla (Figure 1). Predominantly distal and occasionally collecting tubules were affected; proximal tubules were not affected. Variably, cysts were empty or contained hyaline or granular substance and cysts were lined by cuboidal or

---

Received December 26, 1990; in revised form February 11, 1991.

Reprint requests to: Dr. G. S. Spear, Department of Pathology, University of California Irvine Medical Center, 101 City Drive South, Orange, CA 92668, USA

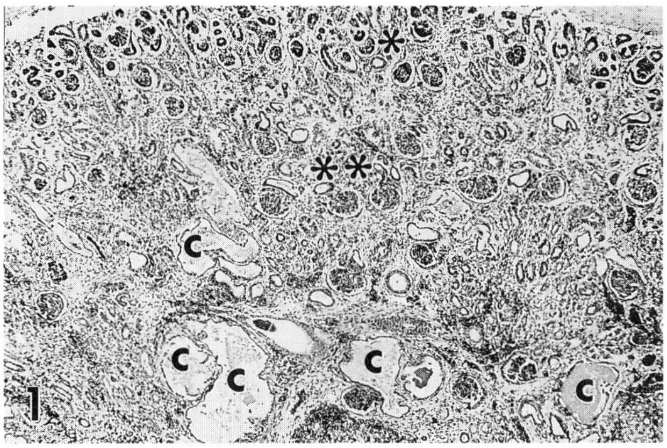

Fig. 1 Overview of renal parenchyma. Subcapsular zone of glomerulogenesis and immediately subjacent glomeruli are normal (asterisk). Deeper glomeruli are abnormal (double asterisk). Many cortical cysts (c). (×48).

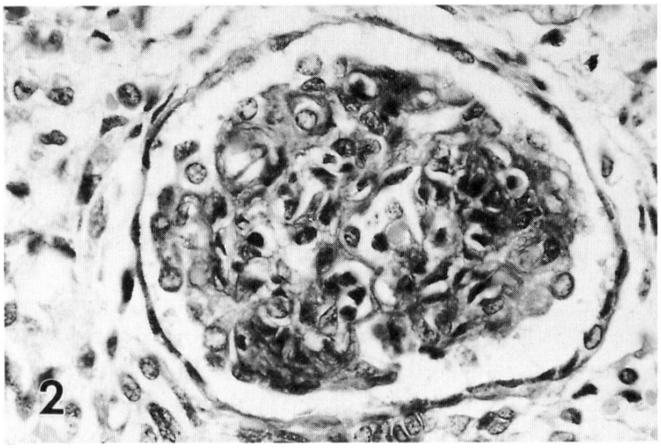

Fig. 2 Typical deep glomerulus consolidated by sclerosis, hypercellularity and (on the left) extracapillary epithelial proliferation. (×600).

flat epithelium. Glomerular cysts were uncommon. Proximal tubules were scarce in areas with cysts. Elsewhere, epithelium of proximal tubules displayed numerous colloid droplets. The architecture of the medulla was disturbed by disproportionate interstitial connective tissue. There was no interstitial inflammation. Subcapsular parenchyma was not atrophic and glomeruli immediately beneath the zone of nephrogenesis were normal (Figure 1). Deeper glomeruli manifested global or segmental sclerosis and/or hypercellularity (Figures 1, 2). Sclerotic glomeruli manifested excessive mesangial matrix, solidification, bloodlessness and sporadic thickening of glomerular capillary walls, at times with double contours. Hypercellularity was both endo- and extra-capillary. Endocapillary hypercellularity comprised both circulating cells and proliferation of indigenous cells. Extracapillary hypercellularity was severe and widespread and consisted of marked epithelial proliferation in Bowman's space, often with crescents. Uncommonly, Bowman's space was dilated. Colloid droplets were observed in visceral epithelium. The kidney exhibited no microscopic evidence of thrombosis or infection. Immunoperoxidase studies for immunoglobulins, complement, albumin and alpha-fetoprotein were inconclusive. Similar studies for Tamm-Horsfall protein confirmed disordered architecture in the medulla: thick ascending limbs were few and disorderly and reacted weakly in comparison with controls. Electron microscopic studies of glomeruli were limited to formalin fixed necropsy tissue. Interpretation, particularly of cytoplasmic changes, was constrained, therefore, by artifacts. Nevertheless there was segmental: hypertrophy and hyperplasia of mesangial matrix; mesangial hypercellularity; thickening and layering of glomerular basement membranes accompanied by particles and granular precipitate; and circumferential mesangial interposition. Extracellular electron dense deposits of immune complex character were not identified.

Discussion

Infantile nephrotic syndrome and congenital nephrotic syndrome may be associated with many histopathological lesions [Sibley et al. 1989]. DMS is a distinctive glomerular lesion observed in the congenital and infantile nephrotic syndromes which manifests between birth and 42 months of age and is associated with a poor prognosis [Habib and Bois 1973, Sibley et al. 1989, Habib et al. 1989, 1990]. The pathogenesis of DMS is unknown. Seelig and co-workers suggested a role for immune complexes [Seelig et al. 1975] but Rumpelt and Bachmann hypothesized a disturbance in the development of glomerular basement membrane [Rumpelt and Bachmann 1980] and Habib et al. have proposed an ante-natal dysgenetic process [Habib et al. 1985, 1989], specifically an anomaly in the biochemical composition of glomerular basement membrane [Habib et al. 1990]. Habib et al. also have emphasized an intimate relationship to the Drash syndrome [Habib et al. 1985, 1989]. Frequently reported in siblings, it has been suggested that DMS is inherited as an autosomal recessive trait [Sibley et al. 1989, Habib et al. 1989].

The present case demonstrates that well developed glomerular lesions of DMS are evident by 18 weeks of gestation. The glomerular lesions were compatible with DMS both by light and electron microscopy. However, the three cortical zones described by Habib et al. [1985, 1990] were not apparent. In particular, there was no subcapsular zone of atrophy. In fact, the subcapsular zone of glomerulogenesis and immediately subjacent glomeruli were unaffected. At this phase of development, at least, this does not support the theory [Habib et al. 1985] that subcapsular atrophy in DMS may be due to sclerosis of immature glomeruli which were developmentally arrested in fetal life.

Like congenital nephrotic syndrome of Finnish type (CNF), this fetus came to clinical attention because of elevated alpha-fetoprotein in maternal serum. The pathogenesis of the latter is similar to that in CNF: the severe proteinuria of the nephrotic syndrome transfers excessive alpha-fetoprotein into the amniotic fluid from which alpha-fetoprotein gains access to the maternal circulation. Microscopic examination of the kidney attested to the severe proteinuria: numerous colloid droplets were present in epithelium of proximal tubules.

Congenital nephrotic syndrome has been reported previously in fetuses. To our knowledge all have been CNF and DMS has not been reported in a fetus. Our fetus differs from CNF in that no fetus with CNF has manifested DMS, or even manifested prominent glomerular lesions.

Despite undoubted severe proteinuria, the present fetus did not manifest anasarca or edema. Similarly, insofar as we can judge, no fetus with CNF has been described with anasarca or edema.

In light of the association of DMS with pseudohermaphroditism and Wilms' tumor [Habib et al. 1985, 1988, 1990] it should be noted that the present fetus did not have a nephroblastoma, the ovaries and external genitalia were normal, the karyotype was 46XX and there was no evidence of 11p deletion.

Acknowledgement

The authors wish to thank Dr. R. Habib for review of the kidney sections and confirmation of the diagnosis.

REFERENCES

Habib R, Bois E 1973 Hétérogénéité des syndromes néphrotiques à début précoce du nourrisson (syndrome néphrotique "infantile") Etude anatomo-clinique et génétique de 37 observations. Helv Paediat Acta *28:* 91–107

Habib R, Loirat C, Gubler MC, Niaudet P, Bensmau A, Levy M, Broyer M 1985 The nephropathy associated with male pseudohermaphroditism and Wilms' tumor (Drash syndrome): a distinctive glomerular lesion – report of 10 cases. Clin Nephrol *24:* 269–278

Habib R, Gubler MC, Niaudet P, Gagnadoux MF 1989 Congenital/infantile nephrotic syndrome with diffuse mesangial sclerosis: relationship with Drash syndrome. In: *Bartsocas CS* (ed). Genetics of kidney disorders. Alan R Liss Inc, New York, pp 193–197

Habib R, Gubler MC, Antignac C, Loirat C, Gagnadoux MF 1990 Syndrome néphrotique congénital ou infantile avec sclérose mésangiale diffuse. Ann Pédiatr (Paris) *37:* 73–77

Rumpelt HJ, Bachmann HJ 1980 Infantile nephrotic syndrome with diffuse mesangial sclerosis: a disturbance of glomerular basement membrane development? Clin Nephrol *13:* 146–150

Seelig HP, Seelig R, Schärer K 1975 Immunhistologische Untersuchungen bei der diffusen mesangialen Sklerose mit nephrotischem Syndrom im Säuglingsalter. Z Kinderheilk *120:* 111–120

Sibley RK, Striegel J, Melvin T 1989 Nephrotic syndrome in the first year of life. In: *Tisher CC, Brenner BM* (eds). Renal pathology with clinical and functional correlations. JB Lippincott Co, Philadelphia, pp 1214–1232

ANNOUNCEMENTS

The **XXVIIIth Congress of the European Dialysis and Transplant Association – European Renal Association** (EDTA/ERA) will be held in Belgrade, Yugoslavia from September 1 to 4, 1991.

For further information, contact the Organizing Secretariat: Yugotours, Congress, Incentive & Exhibition Department, Djure Djakovića 31, Y-11000 Belgrade, Yugoslavia. Tel.: 3811/763-028, 764-622; Telex: 11000, 12902; Fax: 3811/766-447.

The **22nd Annual Congress of the Nephrology Society** will take place from September 15–18, 1991 in Heidelberg, Germany.

The Nephrology Society will be awarding a prize for the best doctoral thesis dealing with a nephrological theme. Eligible theses and further inquiries should be sent to the following address: Dr. M. Walla, c/o Prof. Ritz, Med. Univ. Clinic/Section of Nephrology, Bergheimerstr. 56a, W-6900 Heidelberg.

The **Second Seminar on Renal Involvement in Systemic Vasculitis** will take place September 21, 1991 in Vimercate, a city near Milan in Italy. Contemporary issues relating to immunopathology of Systemic Lupus Erythematosus, with special regard to anti-endothelial and anti-cardiolipin antibodies, clinicopathological correlations and treatment will be discussed.

For further information please contact Dr. Adalberto Sessa, Unità Operativa di Nefrologia e Dialisi, Ospedale di Vimercate, I-20059 Vimercate/Milan, Italy, Tel.: 39/6654/544 or /672 or /327 or /481; Fax: 39/669079.

The **Third Roma Nephrology Conference** will be held in Fiuggi (Rome), Italy on September 27–28, 1991. The main topic will be "The Glomerular Mesangium: From Cell Biology to Clinics".

For further information contact Prof. Giulio A. Cinotti, Cattedra di Nefrologia, 2a Clinica Medica, Policlinico Umberto I, Viale del Policlinico, I-00161 Rome, Italy. Tel.: 39/6/445-7130, Fax: 39/6/445-7735.

The **Seventh International Symposium of Nephrology at Montecatini,** October 14–16, 1991. The title of the symposium is "Kidney, Proteins and Drugs". Advances in protein hormones research, proteinuria, proteins and progression of kidney disease and nephrotoxicity of drugs will be discussed.

For further information please contact Dr. Claudio Bianchi, Unita di Nefrologia, Clinica Medica 2, University of Pisa, I-56100 Pisa, Italy. Tel.: 050–592573.

A **Festakt in honor of Priscilla Kincaid-Smith** will be held on November 5–8th, 1991 in Melbourne, Australia. Events will include state of the art lectures and symposia.

For further information contact The Festschrift Organizing Committee, c/o Department of Nephrology, The Royal Melbourne Hospital, Victoria 3050, Australia.

The **International Meeting on Molecular Approaches to Nephrology Prospect in Diagnosis and Management** will take place on March 19–21, 1992 in Bari, Italy.

For further information please contact Prof. F. P. Schena, Chair and Division of Nephrology, Polyclinic, I-70124 Bari, Tel.: 39/80/271237 or 271232.

The **IIIrd International Conference on SLE** will be held in the Queen Elizabeth II Conference Centre, Westminster, London, April 13–15, 1992.

For further details, please contact Dr. Graham Hughes or Mrs. Denzil Fletcher, Rheumatology Department, St. Thomas' Hospital, London SE1 7EH. Tel. and Fax: 0163394 22.

The **XXIXth Congress of the European Dialysis and Transplant Association** – European Renal Association (EDTA – ERA) will be held at the Palais des Congrès in Paris, France on June 28 – July 1, 1992. For further information contact Prof. C. Jacobs, Congress President, Service de Néphrologie, Hôpital de la Pitié, 83 bd de l'Hôpital, 75013 Paris, France (Fax: 33144 239984) or the organizing Secretariat: Convergences – EDTA 1992, 120 av. Gambetta, 75020 Paris, France (Fax: 3314030 0165).

The **Third Symposium on Uroradiology** (Imaging and Intervention) will take place August 24–27, 1992 at Herlev Hospital, University of Copenhagen, Denmark.

For further information, please contact Dr. Henrik S. Thomsen, Department of Diagnostic Radiology 54E2, Herlev Hospital, Herlev Ringvej 75, DK-2730 Herlev, Denmark. Tel.: 4544/535300, Ext. 278; Fax: 4544/535332.

The **VIth Congress of the International Society for Peritoneal Dialysis** will take place October 1–4, 1992 in Thessaloniki, Greece.

For additional information write to the First Department of Internal Medicine, AHEPA University Hospital, 54636 Thessaloniki, Greece. Tel. and Fax: (3031) 214606.

LETTERS TO THE EDITOR

Peritonitis caused by *Candida lusitaniae* in patient on continuous ambulatory peritoneal dialysis (CAPD)

Sir, – Fungal peritonitis is a rare complication in patients on continuous ambulatory peritoneal dialysis (CAPD). Amongst the fungi, *Candida genus* is most commonly isolated, meanly *C. albicans* (Kerr et al. 1983 Ann Intern Med *99:* 334–336, Rubin et al. 1987 Am J Kidney Dis *10:* 361–368). We present a case of peritonitis in a 79-year-old male, with end-stage renal failure, without serious underlying disorder, had been maintained on CAPD during the last two years, he was admitted to the Cádiz Hospital with abdominal signs, peritoneal fluid markedly turbid and intestinal evaluation difficulties. He had presented three processes of bacterial peritonitis caused by *Staphylococcus epidermidis, Staphylococcus intermedius* and *Klebsiella pneumoniae,* which were treated with usual antibiotics included in our protocol. Physical examinations revealed a fever of 38° C, abdominal pain, positive Blumberg sign and slow peritoneal drainage. The cloudy peritoneal dialysate contained 540 white blood cells (WBC) per mm^3 with 50% neutrophils. The Gram stain and microbiological cultures resulted negative. A non-bacterial peritonitis was suspected, associated with a local infection of the Tenckhoff catheter or tunnel, and his catheter was removed and replaced. New cultures was solicited from the dialysate and dialysis catheter tip to the investigation of unusual microorganisms. *Candida lusitaniae* were isolated from peritoneal fluid and catheter after three days of incubation of the cultures. Antifungal therapy was promptly initiated with intraperitoneal 5-fluorocytosine at a dosis of 200 mg every 6 hours, for three days, decreasing the dosage to 100 mg/6 hours afterwards. Ketoconazole was simultaneously given at a dosis of 400 mg/day orally, this being substituted by intraperitoneal myconazole, 100 mg/6 hours. The peritonitis evolved slowly with significant variances of total peritoneal fluid cell counts (ranging between 60–500 leukocytes per mm^3); *C. lusitaniae* was repetitively isolated from control cultures of peritoneal fluid despite continuous peritoneal lavages. One month later the cultures became negative and dialysates achieved normal aspect. Within ten days the patient aggravated, presenting a febrile episode with temperatures ranging from 39° to 40° C, shivering, leukocytosis of 13,000 cells per mm^3 and neutrophilia of 75 per cent, plus general physical deterioration. Bilateral pleural effusion was appreciated in the thorax X-ray. He became progressively worsened and died from cardiorespiratory failure two months after his admission.

An increase of peritonitis caused by fungi, mainly yeast of genus *Candida,* has been observed in the last years in patients on CAPD (Bastani and Westervelt 1986 Am J Kidney Dis *8:* 265–266, Tzamaloukas and Avasthi 1987 Int J Artif Organs *10:* 301–303). These infections are related to long-term use of broad-spectrum antibiotics, which may help to produce fungal overgrowth on the skin areas next to the catheter orifice, through which fungi can reach the peritoneum. In our casuistic from 1982 to 1989, fungal etiology only represents a 1.3% of the total peritonitis. The diasease usually remained localized intra-abdominally and rarely is disseminated, as it happened in our case.

Several factors predisposing to the development of fungal peritonitis concurred in the patient presented here: namely, age, indwelled peritoneal catheter, recent episodes of bacterial peritonitis treated with broad-spectrum antibiotics, plus the impairment of the defense mechanisms secondary to chronic renal insufficiency. The presence of fever, peritoneal signs, turbid dialysate and positive peritoneal culture, constitute the clinical evidence of peritonitis. The microbiological diagnosis presents some difficulty due to the fact that direct Gram stain shows low sensitivity. Catheter substitution, together with systemic and intraperitoneal antifungal treatment are the basis for the resolution of the infectious process; the only administration of antifungal agents has proved to be useless on many cases (Eisenberg et al. 1986 Rev Infect Dis *8:* 309–321). Though mortality by fungal peritonitis is not excessively high when a correct treatment is administrated, the death by other causes is frequent in these patients.

Candida lusitaniae has recently been implicated in human infections, especially on immunocompromised patients, but this species has not been notified in peritonitis (Merz 1984 J Clin Microbiol *20:* 1194–1195).

P. García-Martos[1], J. Díaz[1], M. Castaño[1], M. Pérez[2], P. Marín[1].

[1]Microbiology and [2]Nephrology Services, Cádiz Hospital, Ana de Viya, 21, ES-11009 Cádiz, Spain

Treatment of Nephrotic Hyperlipidemia with Lovastatin

Sir, – Lipid and lipoprotein abnormalities in patients with nephrotic syndrome (NS) are common [Chopra et al. 1971] and contribute to the increased incidence of ischemic heart disease [Mallick and Short 1981]. Morever, hyperlipidemia may also play a pathogenic role in the developement of focal and segmental glomerulosclerosis [Diamond and Karnovsky 1988], while lipid lowering therapy reduces the incidence of glomerulosclerosis in animals [Kasiske et al. 1988] and possibly in humans [Rabelink et al. 1990].

Lovastatin, a competitive inhibitor of the enzyme HMG-CoA reductase has been shown to be a safe and efficient antilipemic drug [Grundy 1988]. To our knowledge there are four studies in which HMG-CoA reductase drugs (lovastatin – simvastatin) were used in the treatment of nephrotic hyperlipidemia [Vega and Grundy 1988, Rabelink et al. 1988, Golper et al. 1989, Kasiske et al. 1990]. However, in these studies the beneficial effect of the drugs is limited by the short duration of the studies.

In this study we evaluated the long-term efficacy and safety of lovastatin in 16 patients (7 male – 9 female) aged 21–67 years with nephrotic hyperlipidemia. The disease duration was more than 6 months in all patients. The etiology of NS was membranous glomerulonephritis in 10 patients, focal glomerulosclerosis in 3 patients, mesangial glomerulonephritis in 1 patient, lupus

Table Laboratory investigation before and after treatment with lovastatin

Parameters	Before drug therapy	End of the study	p
Serum creatinine (mg/100 ml)	1.22 ± 0.54	1.58 ± 1.13	NS
Creatinine clearance (ml/min)	75.75 ± 23.30	69.40 ± 27.30	NS
Serum albumin (g/100 ml)	3.08 ± 0.38	3.20 ± 0.80	NS
Proteinuria (g/24 h)	4.00 ± 1.00	3.20 ± 1.70	NS
SGOT (IU/L)	24.00 ± 6.00	23.00 ± 4.00	NS
SGPT (IU/L)	17.00 ± 5.00	17.00 ± 6.00	NS
CPK (IU/L)	120.00 ± 15.00	130.00 ± 20.00	NS

nephritis in 1 patient. In one patient no biopsy was performed due to single kidney. None of the patients had a family history of primary hyperlipidemia, diabetes mellitus or severe renal failure. All patients were on a diet poor in cholesterol (<300 mg/day) and saturated fatty acids for at least 6 months previously to the study and had hyperlipidemia (serum total cholesterol concenctration >280 mg/100 ml and LDL cholesterol >200 mg/100 ml). The same diet was continued during the study. All patients were receiving small doses of furosemide (20–40 mg per day) while 3 patients were on nifedipine or methyldopa. Pulses of cyclophosphamide and small doses of methylprednisolone were also given to the patient with lupus nephritis. In all patients lovastatin 20 mg per os was started. Blood samples were obtained after a 14 hours overnight fast for determination of lipid parameters, muscle and liver enzymes as well as for creatinine and albumin before treatment, two and four months later and at the end of the study (12 months). Twenty-four-hour urine protein and creatinine were also measured at the same intervals. At each visit physical examination was performed and the patients were questioned about adverse experiences.

Changes in the concentration of plasma lipid parameters are shown in the Figure. Baseline plasma cholesterol decreased significantly from 357 ± 65 to 241 ± 45 mg/100 ml ($p < 0.001$) after 2 months of treatment with a further significant reduction (190 ± 21 mg/100 ml) at the end of the study. Similarly, the mean baseline LDL cholesterol decreased significantly from 263 ± 62 to 162 ± 40 mg/100 ml ($p < 0.001$) after 2 months of treatment with a further reduction (118 ± 24 mg/100 ml) at the end of the study. Plasma HDL cholesterol decreased slightly but these changes did not achieve a statistical significance. Plasma triglycerides declined during the course of lovastatin treatment from 243 ± 87 to 185 ± 88, 198 ± 93, 152 ± 61 mg/100 ml at 2, 4 and 12 months after treatment respectively.

Lovastatin was uniformly well tolerated and as it is shown in the Table, muscle and liver enzymes remained within normal levels. Serum creatinine, Ccr and albumin concentrations as well as proteinuria remained stable over the entire course of treatment.

It has recently been reported that the HMG-CoA reductase inhibitor simvastatin may induce a partial remission in nephrosis without affecting the renal function [Rabelink et al. 1990].

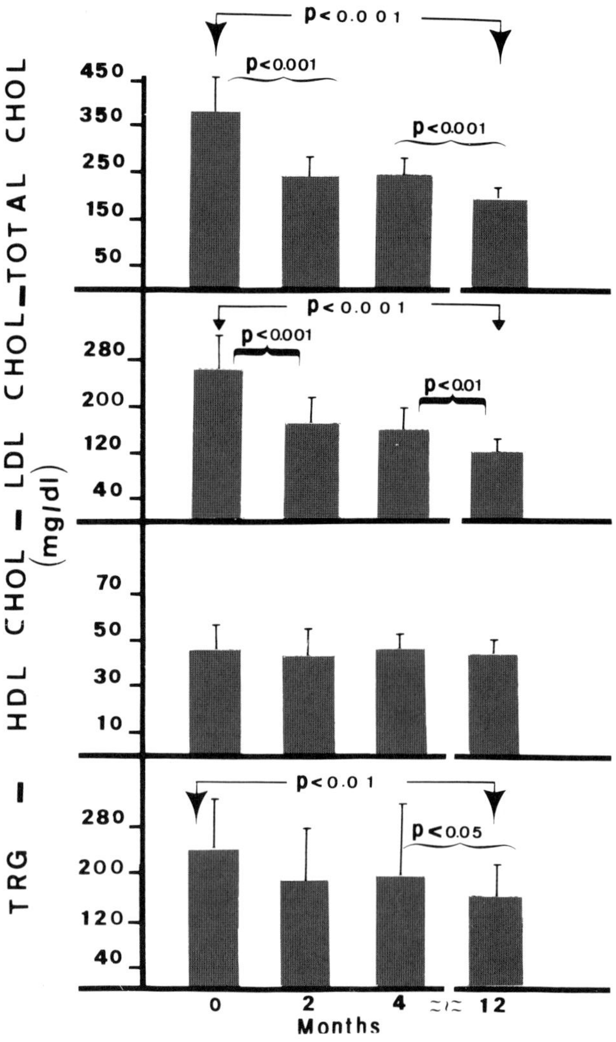

Profile of lipid parameters before, during and at the end of treatment with lovastatin

Although the results of this uncontrolled study were critisized correctly [Thomas and Moorhead 1990], our data support the beneficial effect of lovastatin administration in nephrosis. At the latest follow-up there was a reduction in proteinuria with a slight reduction in the renal function of our patients. However, these changes did not achieve a statistical significance and the deterioration of the serum creatinine and Ccr mean values at latest follow-up were mainly due to one patient's worsening of renal function, which could also be ascribed to the evolution of his primary nephropathy.

We conclude that long-term treatment with lovastatin in small doses is an effective, safe and well tolerated drug in treating nephrotic hyperlipidemia.

M. Elisaf, M. Dardamanis, M. Pappas, G. Sferopoulos and K. C. Siamopoulos
Department of Internal Medicine, School of Medicine, University of Ioannina, Ioannina, Greece

Correspondence address:

K. C. Siamopoulos, Associate Professor of Medicine/Nephrology, School of Medicine, University of Ioannina, 451 10 Ioannina, Greece, Tel.: 0651-92945, Fax: 0651-92944

REFERENCES

Chopra JS, Mallick NP, Stone MC 1971 Hyperlipoproteinemias in nephrotic syndrome. Lancet *i:* 317–321

Diamond JR, Karnovsky MJ 1988 Focal and segmental glomerulosclerosis: analogies to atherosclerosis. Kidney Int *33:* 917–924

Golper TA, Illingworth DR, Morris CD, Bennett WM 1989 Lovastatin in the treatment of multifactorial hyperlipidemia associated with proteinura. Am J Kidney Dis *13 (4):* 312–320

Grundy SM 1988 HMG-CoA reductase inhibitors for treatment of hypercholesterolemia. N Engl J Med *39:* 24–33

Kasiske BL, O'Donnell MP, Garvis WJ, Keane WF 1988 Pharmacologic treatment of hyperlipidemia reduces glomerular injury in rat 5/6 nephrectomy model of chronic renal failure. Circ Res *62:* 367–374

Kasiske BL, Velosa JA, Halstenson CE, LaBelle P, Langendorfer A, Keane WF 1990 The effects of lovastatin in hyperlipidemic patients with the nephrotic syndrome. Am J Kidney Dis *15:* 8–15

Mallick NP, Short CD 1981 The nephrotic syndrome and ischemic heart disease. Nephron *27:* 54–57

Rabelink AJ, Hene RJ, Erkelens DW, Joles JA, Koomans HA 1988 Effects of simvastatin and cholestyramine on lipoprotein profile in hyperlipidaemia of nephrotic syndrome. Lancet *ii:* 1335–1338

Rabelink AJ, Hene RJ, Erkelens DW, Joles JA, Koomans HA 1990 Partial remission of nephrotic syndrome in patient on long-term simvastatin. Lancet *335:* 1045–1046

Thomas M, Moorhead JF 1990 Nephrotic syndrome and simvastatin. Lancet *335:* 1344–1345

Vega GL, Grundy SM 1988 Lovastatin therapy in nephrotic hyperlipidemia: Effects on lipoprotein metabolism. Kidney Int *33:* 1160–1168

Post partum renal failure in systemic lupus erythematosus associated with circulating lupus anticoagulant and anticardiolipin antibody

In 1988 we reported renal thrombotic microangiopathy identical with that seen in post partum renal failure in a series of 12 patients [Kincaid-Smith et al. 1988] four of whom had serological evidence of systemic lupus erythematosus, but only two of whom had histological features of lupus nephritis. All patients had a circulating lupus anticoagulant demonstrated and 8 of 10 in whom it was tested also had an anticardiolipin antibody in the serum. Renal function was impaired in 6 patients and some patients had typical severe post partum renal failure. In 10 of the 12 patients the thrombotic microangiopathy developed during or immediately after pregnancy. We suggested that in patients presenting with post partum renal failure lupus anticoagulant should be sought as it may be a precipitating cause.

It seems that the two patients described by Dinour et al. [Dinour, Yinnon, Slotki et al. 1990] are very similar to those which we described, however, they appear to have overlooked our publication and do not comment on the presence or absence of lupus anticoagulant.

Like those reported by Dinour et al., the majority of our cases were different from those described by Kant et al., [Kant, Pollak, Weiss, Glueck, Miller, Hess, 1981] because only two of our cases had associated lupus nephritis.

The microangiopathic anemia and thrombocytopenia which Dinour described were also present in our patients with impaired renal function and raised fibrin degradation products were also demonstrated in the serum.

Since our publication, further references have been made to the association between acute and chronic vascular lesions of thrombotic microangiopathy and lupus anticoagulant [Neild 1989, Dnillon, Snaith, 1989, Kleinknecht, Borbrie, Meyer, Noel, Callard, Ramdane 1989 and Editorial 1989 Lancet 2].

Sera may still be available from the cases described by Dinour et al., and if antiphospholipid antibodies were demonstrated, this would strengthen our view that lupus anticoagulant may be a causal factor in the thrombotic microangiopathy of post partum renal failure.

Professor Priscilla Kincaid-Smith, Director Department of Nephrology, Royal Melbourne Hospital, Melbourne, Victoria, 3050, Australia.

REFERENCES

Dinour D, Yinnon AM, Slotki IN et al. 1990 Postpartum renal failure in systemic lupus erythematosus. Clin Nephrol *34:* 152–156

Dnillon VB, Snaith ML, Isenberg DA 1989 Lupus nephritis: A review. Postgrad Med J *65:* 336–343

Editorial 1989 Lupus nephritis and pregnancy. Lancet *2:* 82–83

Kant KS, Pollak VE, Weiss MA et al.: 1981 Glomerular thrombosis in systemic lupus erythematosus: prevalence and significance. Medicine *60:* 71–86

Kincaid-Smith P, Fairley KF, Kloss M 1988 Lupus anticoagulant associated with renal thrombotic microangiopathy and pregnancy-related renal failure. QJM *69:* 795–815

Kleinknecht D, Bobrie G, Callard P et al. 1989 Recurrent thrombosis and renal vascular lesions in patients with a lupus anticoagulant. Nephrol Dial Transplant *4:* 854–858

Neild GN 1989 Role of vascular injury in lupus nephritis (abstract). Postgrad Med J *65:* 341

Clinical Nephrology, Vol. 36 No. 2 – 1991 (53–59)

The impact of prolonged immunosuppression on the outcome of idiopathic focal-segmental glomerulosclerosis with nephrotic syndrome in adults. A collaborative retrospective study

G. Banfi [1], M. Moriggi [1], E. Sabadini [2], G. Fellin [2], G. D'Amico [2] and C. Ponticelli [1]

[1] *Division of Nephrology, Ospedale Maggiore and*
[2] *Division of Nephrology, Ospedale S. Carlo Borromeo, Milan, Italy*

Abstract. In this retrospective study we report the outcome of 59 adults with idiopathic focal-segmental glomerulosclerosis (FSGS) and nephrotic syndrome (NS) treated with corticosteroids and/or immunosuppressive drugs. Twenty-seven patients were initially treated with corticosteroids alone for 9.3 ± 8 months; nineteen patients received corticosteroids and immunosuppressive agents associated or every other month for 5.5 ± 4 months; thirteen patients received either azathioprine or cyclophosphamide alone for 25 ± 27 months. At the end of a mean follow-up of 75 ± 51 months, 35 patients (60%) were in complete (CR) or partial (PR) remission, 6 (10%) were stable and 18 (30%) had either chronic renal failure (CRF) or end-stage renal failure (ESRF). Out of 36 patients (61%) initially responsive to therapy, 30 (83%) obtained CR, 4 (11%) PR, one (2.7%) developed CRF and one (2.7%) ESRF. Only 10 of the responders (28%) attained remission within 8 weeks of treatment. Out of the 23 (39%) patients originally resistant to therapy, only one (4%) had CR, 6 (26%) remained unchanged, 6 (26%) developed CRF and 10 (43%) ESRF. The presence at initial renal biopsy of interstitial fibrosis was the only feature which could predict a poor renal outcome. These data show that prolonged treatment of FSGS can obtain sustained remission of the disease and improved renal survival in a consistent proportion of adult patients which would be considered refractory to a two-month course with corticosteroids.

Key words: focal-segmental glomerulosclerosis – nephrotic syndrome – corticosteroids – immunosuppressive drugs

Introduction

Idiopathic focal-segmental glomerulosclerosis (FSGS) is a frequent cause of nephrotic syndrome and often carries a bad prognosis, indeed some 50% of patients presenting with nephrotic syndrome progress to uremia within 10 years [Cameron 1979]. The majority of patients with FSGS are considered to be resistant to treatment with corticosteroids and/or cytotoxic agents. On reviewing the literature we found that only 6% of patients treated with corticosteroids alone (generally given for not more than 8 weeks) attained a complete recovery from proteinuria, a response only marginally better than the 1.5% of remissions that occur spontaneously. When cytotoxic agents were employed, either alone or in combination with corticosteroids, the rate of remission increased to 16% [Ponticelli et al. 1986]. Thus, although some patients with FSGS may obtain stable remission of proteinuria with therapy, there is a tendency to not treat patients, especially adults who are considered to be even more refractory to treatment than children [Newman et al. 1976]. On the other hand, a 40–60% rate of remission for nephrotic adults has been reported by several investigators who administered corticosteroids alone or combined with cytotoxic agents for several months [Saint-Hillier et al. 1975, Banfi et al. 1983, Korbet et al. 1986, Pei et al. 1987]. There is therefore the suspicion that the poor responses to therapy observed in many studies reflect undertreatment of the disease rather than true resistance to treatment.

In order to evaluate the effect of prolonged treatment on the outcome of FSGS in adults with nephrotic syndrome, we retrospectively reviewed the clinical courses of 59 adult patients treated with corticosteroids and/or immunosuppressive drugs and followed for a mean of 75 months after renal biopsy.

Received November 12, 1990; in revised form February 20, 1991.

Reprint requests to Dr. G. Banfi, Division of Nephrology, Ospedale Maggiore, Via Commenda, 15, I-20122 Milano, Italy.

Table 1 Patient characteristics at presentation. (All patients and single treatment groups)

	All patients	(A)	(B)	(C)	P value §
No. of patients	59	27	19	13	
Age (years)	35 ± 15	32 ± 17	36 ± 15	38 ± 13	ns
Male/female	35 / 24	13 / 14	12 / 7	10 / 3	
Duration of nephropathy before biopsy (months)	15 ± 30	21 ± 36	13 ± 27	13 ± 16	ns
Proteinuria (g/24 h)	6.8 ± 3.8	6.7 ± 3.5	6.5 ± 3.6	7.5 ± 4.8	ns
Serum creatinine (mg/dl)	1.1 ± 0.3	1.0 ± 0.3	1.3 ± 0.3	1.0 ± 0.3	ns
Microscopic hematuria (%)	59	56	59	66	ns
Hypertension	36	33	42	31	ns
Follow-up (months)	75 ± 51	57 ± 45	65 ± 35*	127 ± 51	<0.000

§ A vs B, A vs C, B vs C.
* C vs B and C vs A

Patients and methods

Among the adult patients with nephrotic syndrome submitted to renal biopsy between 1970 and 1987, fifty-nine showed the characteristic histological features of FSGS according to accepted pathologic criteria [Churg and Sobin 1982]. For these patients secondary causes of FSGS, such as reflux nephropathy, partial nephrectomy, obesity, i.v. drug abuse, previous history of pre-eclampsia, hereditary nephritis could be excluded.

Renal biopsy, after routine preparation for light microscopy were stained with HE, PAS, Masson thricrome, AFOG and silver methenamine. They were examined by two independent pathologists unaware of the patient's clinical history. Two patients had diagnoses made by immunofluorescence (IF) and electron microscopy (EM) because of a lack of representative tissue in the LM specimen. Fifty-seven biopsies were analyzed semiquantitatively analysis. The following morphologic features were evaluated: the proportion of obsolescent glomeruli, the proportion of glomeruli showing segmental sclerosis; the presence of diffuse mesangial hypercellularity; the degree of interstitial fibrosis and of arteriolar sclerosis, both scored from 0 to 2+. Reports of IF studies were reviewed in order to exclude other conditions associated with FSGS and to evaluate the incidence of diffuse staining of glomeruli with IgM. EM was performed to confirm the diagnoses for doubtful cases or for the few cases for whom no IF study was performed.

Patients were divided into three groups according to treatment: (A) twenty-seven patients were given corticosteroids for a mean duration of 9.3 ± 8 months (2 to 48; median 6 months). Fourteen patients were given oral prednisone at an initial dose of 1 mg/kg/day for at least 8 weeks, then gradually tapered; thirteen patients were given i.v. methylprednisolone pulses, 1 g/day for three consecutive days followed by oral prednisone, 0.5 mg/kg/day, for 8 weeks then gradually tapered. Most patients continued corticotherapy in decreasing doses for several months. (B) Nineteen patients were given corticosteroids and immunosuppressive agents for a mean duration of 5.5 ± 4 months (1 to 12; median 5 months). Eight patients were given oral prednisone by the same modality and dosage as group A plus an oral cytotoxic drug (chlorambucil 0.1–0.2 mg/kg/day or cyclophosphamide or azathioprine 2 mg/kg/day). Eleven patients were given monthly courses of i.v. methylprednisolone pulses, 1 g/day for three consecutive days followed by prednisone 0.5 mg/kg/day alternated with oral cyclophosphamide, 2 mg/kg/day, or chlorambucil, 0.1–0.2 mg/kg/day every other month. (C) Thirteen patients were given azathioprine or cyclophosphamide at the same dosage as group B, associated with small doses of prednisone (0.1–0.2 mg/kg/day) in some cases, for a mean duration of 25 ± 27 months (2 to 110, median 19 months).

No specific criteria led to the different forms of treatment; they merely reflected different approaches adopted by the two renal units participating in the study. Hypertensive patients received anti-hypertensive medications. The drugs most commonly used were: beta-blockers, hydralazine, clonidine, usually associated to diuretics. Eight patients with severe renal failure needed calcium-antagonist agents and only two of them had to be switched to converting enzyme inhibitors to control blood pressure. Salt restriction was the only dietary intervention in the majority of nephrotic and/or hypertensive patients. Low-protein diet was given only to four patients with terminal renal failure.

Definitions. Nephrotic syndrome was defined as daily proteinuria equal to or greater than 3.5 g, microscopic hematuria as the presence of more than 2 erythrocytes per hpf, arterial hypertension as supine blood pressure values higher than 150/90 mmHg in at least three different measurements before any treatment was started. Complete remission was defined as daily proteinuria of less than 200 mg with stable serum creatinine of less than 1.5 mg/dl (132 mmol/l). Remission was considered to be partial whenever non-nephrotic proteinuria persisted in the absence of hypoalbuminemia (defined as less than 2.5 g/l) and of chronic renal insufficiency. Patients were defined as responders whenever they attained at any time either a complete or a partial remission. Chronic renal insufficiency was defined by a serum creatinine persistently equal to or higher than 1.5 mg/dl (132 mmol/l), whatever the amount of proteinuria. Renal death was defined as the need for dialysis or transplantation.

Statistics. The data were analyzed by the Student's two-tailed test for means and the chi-square test for correlations. Renal survival was calculated by the Kaplan-Mayer actuarial method.

Results

The clinical characteristics at presentation are shown in Table 1. They were comparable in the three treatment groups except that the mean follow-up was significantly longer in group C. The histologic features at biopsy are reported in Table 2. Arteriolosclerotic lesions were more frequent in patients of group B than in the other patients.

Cumulative outcome (Table 3). Thirty-six patients (61%) initially responded to medication. Fourteen of them had a total of 25 episodes of relapses, 23 of which were reversible with treatment and 2 were refractory. At the end of follow-up, 30 of the

Table 3 Clinical status at the end of follow-up in patients responders and non-responders to the initial therapy

	Responders	Non-responders	Total (%)
Complete remission	30	1	31 (52.5)
Partial remission	4	0	4 (7)
Nephrotic syndrome	0	6	6 (10)
Renal failure	2	16	18 (30.5)
	36 (61%)	23 (39%)	

* Complete + partial remissions vs nephrotic syndrome + renal failure. Chi-square test: $p < 0.000$

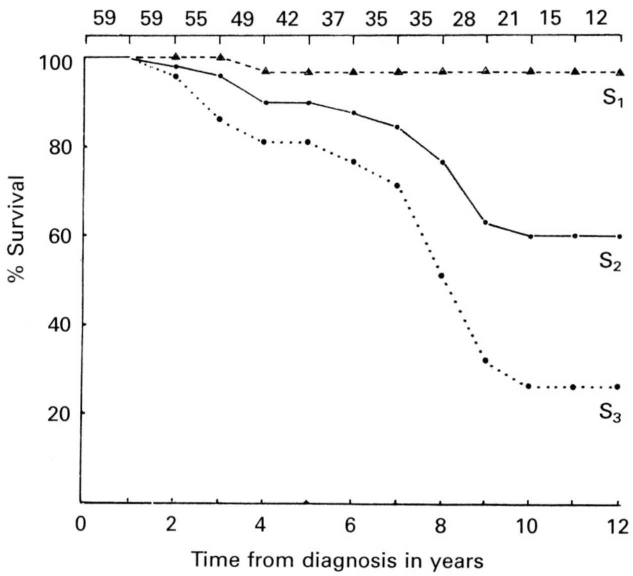

Fig. 1 Renal actuarial survivals for all patients (S_2) and for patients who had either partial or complete remission (S_1) versus those who were refractory to initial treatment (S_3). (S_1 vs S_3 $p < 0.001$)

Table 2 Pathology

	All patients (%)	(A) (%)		(B) (%)	(C) (%)	P value
Light microscopy						
Segmental sclerosis						
>25% of glomeruli	53	63		33	54	ns
Global sclerosis						
>10% of glomeruli	35	34		33	38	ns
Diffuse mesangial						
hypercellularity	37	38		39	31	ns
Interstitial fibrosis (≥1+)	39	31		44	46	ns
Arteriolosclerosis (≥1+)	35	19	*	61	31	<0.001
Fluorescent microscopy						
Diffuse IgM	38	43		25	37	ns

* B vs A

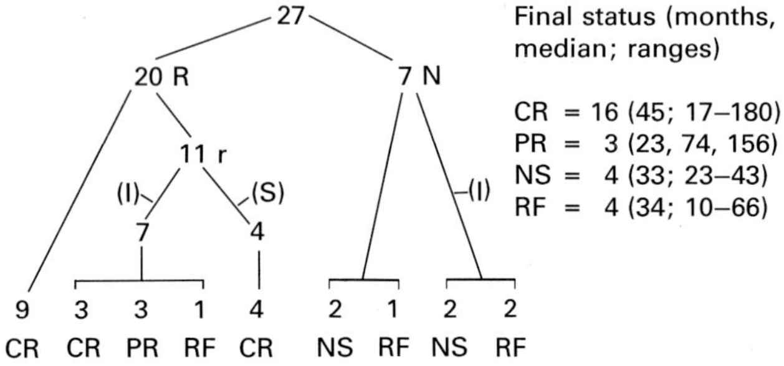

R responder, N non-responder, r relapser, CR complete remission, PR partial remission, NS nephrotic syndrome, RF renal failure, (S) steroids, (I) immunosuppressive drugs.

Fig. 2 Outcome of patients treated with corticosteroids as first therapeutic trial. (Group A)

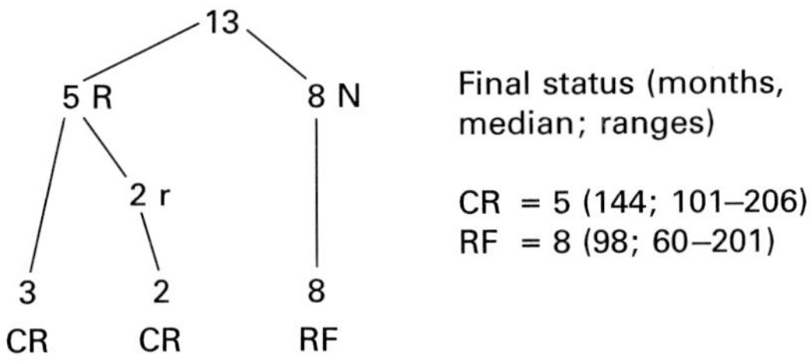

For abbreviations see Figure 2.

Fig. 3 Outcome of patients treated with corticosteroids and immunosuppressive drugs. (Group B)

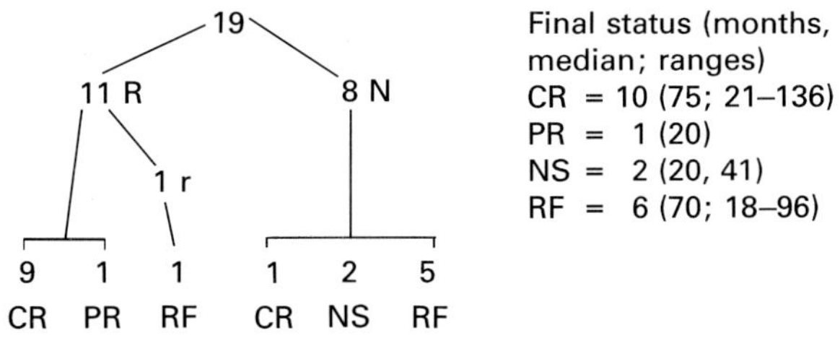

For abbreviations see Figure 2.

Fig. 4 Outcome of patients treated with immunosuppressive agents. (Group C)

responders were in complete remission (two died of neoplasia), four were in partial remission, one had nephrotic syndrome and moderate renal insufficiency (plasma creatinine: 1.8 mg/dl) and one was on dialysis. Twenty-nine patients with complete remission were off therapy for 60 ± 45 months, and three patients with partial remission were off therapy 17, 18 and 96 months. Patients who experienced either sustained or temporary remission obtained it after a median period of treatment of 5 months (0.5 to 72, mean 13 ± 17.5 months). Proteinuria cleared within 8 weeks of therapy in only ten patients (28%).

At the end of observation, among patients originally resistant to treatment, only one was in complete remission 115 months after diagnosis. Six patients had nephrotic syndrome and normal renal function, six had renal insufficiency (one died of myocardial infarction), ten had been on dialysis, 32 ± 9, 91 ± 65 and 76 ± months after diagnosis.

The rate of remissions (either complete or partial) versus failures (persistence of nephrotic syndrome or renal insufficiency) was significantly higher for patients initially responsive to treatment than for the refractory ($p > 0.000$). Even limiting the observation to 36 patients with 5 years of follow-up, the incidence of renal insufficiency was still significantly higher in non-responders (10/14 vs 1/22 $p < 0.000$). The kidney survival rate was significantly better in responders than in non-responders ($p > 0.001$) (Figure 1).

Group A (27 patients) (Figure 2). Twenty patients had complete remission of proteinuria after a mean of 5.8 + 3 months (2 to 10 months) of corticotherapy. Only nine of them achieved complete remission within 8 weeks of treatment; in the others proteinuria cleared 3 to 24 months after starting therapy (mean 9.6 ± 7.5) and four of them some months (1 to 14 months) after having stopped it. Nine patients were still in complete remission 56 ± 44 months after diagnosis (17 to 115 months). Eleven patients had 1 to 4 relapses each (total 21 episodes). Four of these were again given corticosteroids for a mean of 16 ± 12 months and attained complete remission within 1 to 6 months. Seven patients were given alkylating agents combined with prednisone, or on an every other month schedule for a mean period of 12 ± 11 months. Three of them had complete and three partial remission within 1 to 12 months of therapy and one became resistant and developed end-stage renal failure. Two patients who were in complete remission died during follow-up. One developed pulmonary neoplasia 6 years after stopping therapy. He had been treated with corticosteroids for 22 months and subsequently with azathioprine for 44 months. The other patient developed mesothelioma 24 months after diagnosis and 12 months after stopping treatment. He had taken steroids for 6 months and chlorambucil for the next 2 months. At the last follow-up, fourteen patients were in complete remission after a mean of 63 ± 48 months, three were in partial remission 84 ± 67 months after biopsy, and one was on dialysis 36 months after diagnosis.

Seven patients did not respond to the original treatment with prednisone given for 2 to 7 months (mean 3.5 ± 2). Four of them were subsequently given alkylating agents (cyclophosphamide to three and chlorambucil to one) for 2 to 16 months (mean 5.5 ±

6), without benefit. When last seen, four had nephrotic syndrome and normal renal function 30 ± 16 months after presentation, one had moderate renal insufficiency (plasma creatinine: 2.5 mg/dl) and two were on dialysis, 66, 10 and 34 months after diagnosis. One nephrotic patient with rapidly progressive renal insufficiency developed irreversible arterial thrombosis of the leg 6 months after starting therapy. One patient with refractory nephrotic syndrome had recurrent episodes of bronchopneumonia 12 months after stopping medication. No other important complications or side effects of therapy were observed in the remaining patients.

Group B (19 patients) (Figure 3). Eleven patients were initially responsive to treatment protracted for 4.5 ± 1.8 months. Nine achieved complete and stable remission and two partial remissions 2 to 60 months after starting therapy (mean 17 ± 23). One of the patients who had a partial remission after a 6-month course of therapy had a relapse 6 months after stopping medication and was refractory to a further course of treatment.

Seven patients did not show any response to treatment given for 5 ± 3.5 months, and five of them developed renal insufficiency. The last patient, resistant to a 3-month course of medication, became free of proteinuria 18 months after stopping therapy. At the last observation, ten patients were in complete remission 77 ± 34 months after diagnosis and one was in partial remission 20 months after diagnosis. Two patients were nephrotic with normal renal function 20 and 41 months after presentation. Two had renal insufficiency (plasma creatinine: 1.7 mg/dl) 95 and 31 months after diagnosis and four were on dialysis 66 ± 34 months after diagnosis.

During follow-up, one patient with persistent nephrotic syndrome, moderate hypertension and renal insufficiency (plasma creatinine 1.7 mg/dl), developed hemiparesis one month after starting treatment. Another patient, who attained complete remission, developed hemorrhagic cystitis which healed after cyclophosphamide was stopped.

Group C (13 patients) (Figure 4). Five patients who had therapy for 37.5 ± 41 months (2 to 110), attained complete remission 8 to 72 months after starting therapy. Two of them had relapses but responded again to therapy protracted for 6 and 35 months. When last seen, 150 ± 42 months after presentation, all these five patients were in complete remission. Eight patients did not show any response to 18.5 ± 10.5 months of treatment. Four of them had renal insufficiency (plasma creatinine 3.5 ± 2.3 mg/dl) and four were on dialysis, 112 ± 61 and 100 ± 78 months after presentation.

During follow-up, one patient, aged 48, with advanced renal insufficiency (plasma creatinine 5 mg/dl) died of myocardial infarction, 88 months after diagnosis and 86 months after stopping therapy. Another patient in complete remission while on cyclophosphamide for 18 months developed diabetes 28 months and renal calculosis 48 months after presentation.

Table 4 Clinical features at presentation. Comparison of patients with different renal outcome

	CR & PR	NS & RF	P value
No. of patients	35	24	
Follow-up (months)	80 ± 52	67 ± 49	ns
Male/female	18/17	17/7	ns
Age (years)	37 ± 16	33 ± 15	ns
Duration of nephropathy before biopsy (months)	16 ± 30	18 ± 28	ns
Microscopic hematuria (%)	58.5	62.5	ns
Hypertension (%)	34	37.5	ns
Serum creatinine (mg/dl)	1.0 ± 0.3	1.1 ± 0.4	ns
≥1.5 mg/dl (%)	17	21	ns
Proteinuria (g/24 h)	6.2 ± 3.1	7.7 ± 4.5	ns
≥10 g/24 h (%)	11.5	29	ns

CR complete remission, PR partial remission, NS nephrotic syndrome, RF renal failure

Table 5 Histologic features at presentation. Comparison of patients with different renal outcome

	CR & PR	NS & RF	P value
No. of patients	33	24	
Global sclerosis >10% of glomeruli (%)	36.5	33.5	ns
Segmental sclerosis >25% of glomeruli	45.5	62.5	ns
Diffuse mesangial hypercellularity	39.5	33.3	ns
Interstitial fibrosis (≥1+)	21	62.5	<0.004
Arteriolosclerosis (≥1+)	27	46	ns
Diffuse IgM	39	35.5	ns

Abbreviations as Table 4

Prognostic factors (Tables 4 and 5). Univariate analysis was used to evaluate the possible influence of different parameters on the final outcome (complete or partial remission versus nephrotic syndrome or renal insufficiency). The following parameters at presentation were examined: age, sex, mean duration of renal disease before biopsy, duration of renal disease longer than 6 months, mean serum creatinine, serum creatinine exceeding 1.5 mg/dl, mean daily proteinuria, daily proteinuria exceeding 10 g, the presence of microscopic hematuria, arterial hypertension, more than 10% obsolescent glomeruli, segmental sclerosis in more than 25% of glomeruli and, of whatever degree, diffuse mesangial hypercellularity, diffuse glomerular IgM staining, interstitial fibrosis and arteriosclerosis. The only feature which was associated with a poor prognosis was the presence of interstitial fibrosis ($p > 0.004$).

Discussion

Surveys of the literature have shown that only 10 to 20% of patients with focal-segmental glomerulosclerosis obtain sustained remission with therapy [Ponticelli et al. 1986, Cameron 1989]. However, most studies were not controlled and based on a small number of patients, most of them treated with prednisone for not more than 8 weeks. The few studies in which patients were treated for more prolonged periods showed that some 40–60% of patients can enter sustained remissions [Saint-Hillier et al. 1975, Banfi et al. 1983, Korbet et al. 1986, Pei et al. 1987]. Furthermore, aggressive treatment with repeated methylprednisolone pulses and alkylating agents has been shown recently to produce complete remission in 50% of steroid-resistant children with FSGS (Mendoza et al. 1990]. Responders only exceptionally progressed to chronic renal failure while many among non-responders or untreated patients either died or developed end-stage renal failure.

This study was based on one of the largest numbers of treated adults with nephrotic syndrome. The clinical characteristics at presentation were comparable to those reported in other studies. The prevalence of arterial hypertension though similar to that of other series [Saint-Hillier et al. 1975, Cameron et al. 1978, Arbus et al. 1982] was lower than that observed by other authors [Newman et al. 1976, Korbet et al. 1986, Pei et al. 1987].

After a mean follow-up of 75 months, 52% of the patients were in complete and 7% were in partial remission. The majority of them had been without therapy for a mean of 58 months. Only 5.5% of the patients originally responsive to treatment versus 70% of those initially refractory developed renal failure.

Because the study was retrospective and based on heterogeneous treatments, the results of treatment in each group could not be compared by statistical analysis, but they still deserve some comment. The rates of remission in the three groups were comparable. The proportion of responders tended to be higher in patients originally treated with corticosteroids alone, but they developed relapses more frequently than those given immunosuppressive agents. This would support previous observations that cytotoxic drugs may induce more stable remission [Saint-Hillier et al. 1975, Geary et al. 1984]. Immunosuppressive agents, however, did not give any advantage to cortico-resistant patients. This is in agreement with some reports [Cameron et al. 1978, Mongeau et al. 1981, Arbus et al. 1982, Tejani et al. 1983], but, at least for children, others have reported a favorable response to these agents in a considerable number of cortico-resistant cases [Geary et al. 1984, Trompeter 1987, Mendoza et al. 1990].

According to previous data [Saint-Hillier et al. 1975, Korbet et al. 1986, Trompeter 1987, Pei et al. 1987], the time required to achieve complete remission was extremely variable, the median value being 5 months. Several patients who had only partial remission by the end of treatment became free of proteinuria only some months after stopping therapy. It must be pointed out that fewer than one third of the patients obtained complete remission within 8 weeks. Therefore, if the classical two-month course of prednisone had been the only modality of therapy only a small proportion of responders would have been identified. These data show that the duration of treatment can influence the rate and stability of remission and may explain the unsatisfactory results obtained when immunosuppression is given for short periods [Newman et al. 1976, Cameron et al. 1978, Lim et al. 1981, Tejani et al. 1983, SPNSG 1985].

It is well known that prolonged administration of either corticosteroids or cytotoxic agents increases the risk of severe side effects. However, during follow-up, none of our patients had severe side effects attributable to corticotherapy. The only patient who developed diabetes had been treated with cyclophosphamide and, of the three patients who had severe vascular complications, one had an extremely severe nephrotic syndrome with rapid progression towards uremia and two showed diffuse signs of atherosclerosis before the onset of nephropathy. In addition, all these three patients had been given mainly immunosuppressive drugs. Both alkylating agents and purine analogues have a low therapeutic index and their potential toxicity must be balanced against the expected benefits. Bone marrow depression; bladder, liver and gonadal toxicity and neoplasia are the most severe complications. Severe bone marrow toxicity was never observed in our series, while in some cases reversible leukopenia developed during cyclophosphamide or chlorambucil administration. Two patients died of neoplasia and an enhancing role of the immunosuppressive treatment cannot be excluded, although one of these patients had been treated with chlorambucil for only two months. It should be pointed out that in several patients given prolonged immunosuppressive treatment the observation period was relatively short for a neoplastic disease to become manifest. So, a more protracted follow-up of these patients is needed to evaluate the incidence of such a complication.

In conclusion, this study shows that prolonged treatment of FSGS can obtain sustained remission of the disease in about half of the patients who would be considered refractory to treatment after only a two-month course of corticosteroids. Most patients who responded to therapy maintained a normal renal function over time, suggesting that in a good proportion of patients with FSGS the long-term renal outcome may improve by treatment. For this "orphan" disease for which only one controlled trial, published in abstract form has been devoted (ISKDC 1983), optimal therapy is still far from established. Prospective controlled studies are needed to assess the benefits and the risks of prolonged treatment and to indicate which of the potentially active drugs offers the best therapeutical index for this disease.

Acknowledgements

We are endebted to Dr. C. Pozzi (Nephrology Unit Ospedale di Lecco), Dr. F. Bissoli (Nephrology Unit Ospedale di Magenta), Dr. R. Bellazzi (Nephrology Unit Ospedale di Vigevano), Dr. P. Scalia (Nephrology Unit Ospedale di Tradate) for giving us the follow-up data of some patients and to Prof. M. J. Mihatsch (Institute of Pathology University of Basle) for performing the electron microscopy study.

REFERENCES

Arbus GS, Poucell S, Bacheyie GS, Baumal R 1982 Focal segmental glomerulosclerosis with idiopathic nephrotic syndrome: three types of clinical response. J Pediatr *101:* 40

Banfi G, Guerra L, Passerini P, Fogazzi GB, Imbasciati E 1983 Possibilità terapeutiche della glomerulosclerosi focale con sindrome nefrosica dell 'adulto. Efficacia degli steroidi e/o citostatici. In: *Wichtig* (ed) Nefrologia Dialisi Trapianto, p 387

Cameron JS, Turner DR, Ogg CS, Chantler C, Williams DG 1978 The long-term prognosis of patients with focal segmental glomerulosclerosis. Clin Nephrol *10:* 213

Cameron JS 1979 The problem of focal segmental glomerulosclerosis. In: *Kincaid-Smith P, D'apice AJF, Atkins RC* (eds) Progress in Glomerulonephritis. Wiley Medical Publication, New York, p 209

Cameron JS 1989 Treatment of primary glomerulonephritis using immunosuppressive agents. Am J Nephrol 9 *(suppl 1):* 33

Churg J, Sobin LH 1982 Renal disease. Classification and atlas of glomerular diseases. Igaku-Shoin, Tokio – New York

Geary DF, Farine M, Thorner P, Baumal R 1984 Response to cyclophosphamide in steroid resistant focal segmental glomerulosclerosis: a reappraisal. Clin Nephrol *22:* 109

International Study of Kidney Disease in Children 1983 Cyclophosphamide therapy in focal segmental glomerular sclerosis: a controlled clinical trial. Eur J Pediat (Abs) *140:* 149

Korbet SM, Schwartz MM, Lewis EJ 1986 The prognosis of focal segmental glomerulosclerosis of adulthood. Medicine *65:* 304

Lim VS, Sibley R, Spargo B 1974 Adult lipoid nephrosis: clinicopathological correlations. Ann Intern Med *81:* 314

Mendoza SA, Reznik VM, Griswold WR, Krensky AM, Yorgin PD, Tune BM 1990 Treatment of steroid-resistant focal segmental glomerulosclerosis with pulse methylprednisolone and alkylating agents. Pediatr Nephrol *4:* 303

Miyata J, Takebayashi S, Taguchi T, Naito S, Harada T 1986 Evaluation and correlation of clinical and histological features of focal segmental glomerulosclerosis. Nephron *44:* 115

Mongeau JG, Corneille L, Robitaille P, O'Regan S, Pelletier M 1981 Primary nephrosis in childhood associated with focal glomerular sclerosis: is long-term prognosis that severe? Kidney Int *20:* 743

Newman WJ, Tisher CC, McCoy RC, Gunnells JC, Krueger RP, Clapp JR, Robinson RR 1976 Medicine *55:* 67

Pei Y, Cattran D, Delmore T, Katz A, Lang A, Rance P 1987 Evidence suggesting under-treatment in adults with idiopathic focal segmental glomerulosclerosis. Am J Med *82:* 938

Ponticelli C, Fogazzi GB, Passerini P 1986 Pharmacological treatment of chronic glomerulonephritis. In: *Remuzzi G, Bertani T* (eds) Drugs and kidney. Raven Press, New York, p 221

Saint-Hillier Y, Morel-Maroger L, Woodrow D, Richet G 1975 Focal and segmental hyalinosis. Adv Nephrol *5:* 67

Schoeneman MJ, Bennett B, Greifer I 1978 The natural history of focal segmental glomerulosclerosis with and without mesangial hypercellularity in children. Clin Nephrol *9:* 45

Southwest, Pediatric Nephrology Study Group 1985 Focal segmental glomerulosclerosis in children with idiopathic nephrotic syndrome. Kidney Int *27:* 442

Tejani A, Nicastri AD, Sen D, Chen CK, Phadkè K, Adamson O, Butt KMH 1983 Long-term evaluation of children with nephrotic syndrome and focal segmental glomerular sclerosis. Nephron *35:* 225

Trompeter RS 1987 Steroid resistant nephrotic syndrome: a review of the treatment of focal segmental glomerulosclerosis (FSGS) in children. In: *Murakami K, Kitagawa T, Yabuta K* (eds) Recent advances in pediatric nephrology. Excerpta Medica Amsterdam, p 363

Velosa JA, Holley KE, Torres VE, Offord KP 1983 Significance of proteinuria on the outcome of renal function in patients with focal segmental glomerulosclerosis. Mayo Clin Proc *58:* 568

Waldherr R, Gubler MC, Levy M, Broyer M, Habib R 1978 The significance of pure diffuse mesangial proliferation in idiopathic nephrotic syndrome. Clin Nephrol *10:* 171

Wehrmann M, Bohle A, Held H, Schumm G, Kendziorra H, Pressler H 1990 Long-term prognosis of focal sclerosing glomerulonephritis. An analysis of 250 cases with particular regard to tubulointerstitial changes. Clin Nephrol *33:* 115

Clinical Nephrology, Vol. 36 No. 2 – 1991 (60–66)

Effects of triple therapy in IgA nephritis: a follow-up study 5 years later

K. T. Woo, G. S. L. Lee, Y. K. Lau, G. S. C. Chiang and C. H. Lim

Department of Renal Medicine, Singapore General Hospital

Abstract. This study is a 5-year post trial assessment of patients with IgA nephritis who entered a 3-year prospective controlled trial of cyclophosphamide, dipyridamole (D) and low-dose warfarin (W). Patients entered the trial from 1979 to 1981 and the trial ended in 1984 with those in the treatment group having more stable renal function and less proteinuria compared to the control group. Present reassessment of the patients in 1989 showed no difference in the renal function between those in the treatment group (n = 27) and the control group (n = 21). 6 patients in the treatment group and 7 in the control group were in ESRF. At the conclusion of the trial in 1984, among the 27 patients in the original treatment group, 13 patients elected to continue with D + W while the other 14 patients chose to cease therapy and therefore served as the new control group. 5 years later, renal function in the new treatment group (n = 13) was significantly stable compared to the new control group (n = 14), (serum creatinine 1.4 ± 0.7 versus 4.4 ± 3.2 mg/dl, $p < 0.01$). Furthermore, all the 6 patients with ESRF in the original treatment group of 27 patients were from the new control group (n = 14) where treatment with D + W had been ceased. None of the patients still on D + W are in ESRF.

Key words: IgA nephritis – cyclophosphamide – dipyridamole – warfarin – follow-up study

Introduction

Various therapeutic agents have been used in the treatment of IgA nephritis including steroids [Kobayashi et al. 1987], cyclosporin A [Lai et al. 1987], angiotensin converting enzyme inhibitors [Woodroffe et al. 1987], and eicosapentanoic acid [Bennet et al. 1989].

We have previously reported the effects of a combination regimen of cyclophosphamide (6 months), dipyridamole (36 months) and low-dose warfarin (36 months) in patients with diffuse mesangial proliferative glomerulonephritis (GN) including IgA nephritis [Woo et al. 1987] and have shown that the patients in the treatment group had more stable renal function and less proteinuria compared to the control group at the end of 3 years.

This communication reports the status of the patients with IgA nephritis, 5 years after the original triple therapy.

Reprint requests to Dr. K. T. Woo, Department of Renal Medicine, Singapore General Hospital, Singapore 0316.

Received October 11, 1990; in revised form March 4, 1991.

Material and methods

The diagnosis of IgA nephritis was made on the demonstration of IgA deposits as the sole immunoglobulin or in association with other immunoglobulins but with IgA present in equivalent strength in the mesangial area on immunofluorescent study. Liver disease, systemic lupus erythematosus and Henoch Schonlein purpura were excluded in all patients.

Original prospective study

In the original study, patients with mesangial proliferative GN including those with IgA nephritis entered a 3-year prospective controlled trial from 1979 through to 1981. 52 pairs of patients who entered the trial were matched for renal function and the degree of glomerulosclerosis, all having proteinuria exceeding 1 gm/day at the time of biopsy. However, some patients by the time they entered the trial, had proteinuria less than 1 gm/day even though the initial proteinuria at biopsy was more than 1 gm/day. A few patients had to wait, sometimes up to a period of 6 months before a suitable match (renal function and degree of glomerulosclerosis) could be found, by which time the proteinuria had decreased to less than 1 gm/day. 39 patients (27 with IgA nephritis) in the treatment group and 34 patients (21 with IgA nephritis) in the control group completed the trial in 1984.

Creatinine concentrations in serum and urine samples were determined using the alkaline picrate reagent kit (Roche, Switzerland) and creatinine clearance (CCT) calculated from the measured 24-hour urine volume. Total urinary protein was measured by the Biuret reagent kit (Roche, Switzerland).

Follow-up study

At the conclusion of the trial, among the group of 27 patients with IgA nephritis in the original treatment group, 13 patients elected to continue therapy with dipyridamole and warfarin daily, while the other 14 patients chose to stop treatment and therefore served as the control group. These two groups were the treatment subgroup and the control subgroup. The patients in the treatment subgroup continued to receive dipyridamole (100 mg thrice daily) and warfarin to maintain the thrombotest between 30% to 50% and medication for treatment of hypertension. Patients in the control subgroup received only hypotensives when indicated. There were two patients with hypertension in the treatment subgroup at the beginning of the study and they were on propranolol and hydrallazine throughout the trial. In the control subgroup there was only one patient with hypertension at the beginning of the trial and he was also treated with propranolol and hydrallazine.

Each of the group had only one patient with nephrotic syndrome which was defined as edema associated with proteinuria of more than 3 gm/day and hypoalbuminemia of less than 3 gm/L. A few patients in both groups though they had nephrotic range proteinuria were not considered to have the nephrotic syndrome as the serum albumin was more than 3 gm/L.

Renal impairment was defined as serum creatinine of 1.6 mg/dl or > and ESRF as serum creatinine of 10 mg/dl or >. The treatment subgroup

Table 1 Mesangial IgA Nephritis (1979–1989). Comparison of patients in the original prospective trial: reassessment 5 years after the trial in 1989

Patients	Sex	Age (Yrs)	Follow Up (Mths)	Se Creat (mg) Before	Se Creat (mg) After	CCT (ml/min) Before	CCT (ml/min) After	Proteinuria (Gm/Day) Before	Proteinuria (Gm/Day) After	Number with CRF Before	Number with CRF After
Treatment Group	M = 18 F = 9 n = 27	25 ± 6	94 ± 22	1.2 ± 0.3	2.9 ± 2.7	98 ± 23	61 ± 44	2.4 ± 2.5	0.8 ± 0.8	R.I. = 2	R.I. = 6 ESRF = 6
				P <0.005		P <0.001		P <0.005			
Control Group	M = 16 F = 5 n = 21	26 ± 9	86 ± 22	1.1 ± 0.2	3.4 ± 3.1	109 ± 23	61 ± 46	1.7 ± 2.0	2.1 ± 2.0	R.I. = 0	R.I. = 6 ESRF = 7
				P <0.005		P <0.001		NS			

Table 2 Mesangial IgA Nephritis (1979–1989). Comparison of the 27 patients in the original treatment group which had been divided into the treatment subgroup (n = 13) and the control subgroup (n = 14) at entry into the trial from 1979 and at the final assessment in 1989

Patients	Sex	Age (Yrs)	Follow Up (Mths)	Se Creat (mg) Before	Se Creat (mg) After	CCT (ml/min) Before	CCT (ml/min) After	Proteinuria (Gm/Day) Before	Proteinuria (Gm/Day) After	Number with CRF Before	Number with CRF After
Treatment Sub-Group	M = 7 F = 6 n = 13	25 ± 7	104 ± 9	1.1 ± 0.3	1.4 ± 0.7	95 ± 22	69 ± 35	1.7 ± 1.4	0.7 ± 0.5	R.I. = 0	R.I. = 4 *ESRF = 0
				NS		P <0.005		P <0.01			
Control Sub-Group	M = 10 F = 4 n = 14	24 ± 5	84 ± 25	1.3 ± 0.3	4.4 ± 3.2	100 ± 25	53 ± 49	3.1 ± 3.0	0.9 ± 1.0	R.I. = 1	R.I. = 2 *ESRF = 6
				P <0.005		P <0.001		P <0.025		*x^2 = 7.2 (P <0.01)	

had 2 patients with renal impairment while the control subgroup had 3 patients. Treatment with dipyridamole and warfarin was ceased when the serum creatinine approached 7 mg/dl and these patients were considered to have withdrawn from the trial.

Statistical Analyses: Results are expressed as mean ± SD. The Mann Whitney U test and the chi-square test were used to compare the differences between the two groups.

Results

Table 1 compares the patients with IgA nephritis in the original study, 27 patients in the treatment

Table 3 Mesangial IgA Nephritis: Treatment sub-group

	Presentation	Serum Creatinine (mg/dl)			CCT (ml/min)			Proteinuria (gm/day)		
		1979	1984	1989	1979	1984	1989	1979	1984	1989
00001	HP	1.4	1.0	1.2	133	96	111	1.0	0.9	0.5
00002	HP	1.4	1.1	1.5	79	110	68	2.0	0.3	0.3
00003	HP	1.1	1.0	0.9	102	100	116	1.3	1.6	0.3
00004	HP	1.1	1.1	0.9	75	120	72	0.1	0.4	0.2
00005	HP	1.5	1.7	1.9	84	63	31	1.2	0.5	0.5
00006	HP	1.2	1.6	1.5	120	80	98	4.0	0.9	2.0
00007	HP	0.9	0.6	0.6	100	88	127	1.3	0.8	1.0
00008	HP	0.8	0.9	1.1	100	51	33	1.2	1.3	1.2
00009	NS	1.5	1.3	1.3	76	94	41	5.0	0.3	0.1
00010	HP	0.8	0.9	1.6	56	73	41	0.6	1.2	0.5
00011	HP	0.8	0.7	0.8	125	109	76	1.2	3.8	0.9
00012	HP	0.9	1.2	3.4	96	82	30	1.2	3.4	1.0
00013	HP	1.3	1.4	1.9	89	65	51	1.5	1.3	0.5
		1.1 ± 0.3	1.1 ± 0.3	1.4 ± 0.7	95 ± 22	87 ± 20	69 ± 35	1.7 ± 1.4	1.3 ± 1.1	0.7 ± 0.5

HP: asymptomatic hematuria and proteinuria
NS: nephrotic syndrome

Table 4 Mesangial IgA Nephritis: Control sub-group

	Presentation	Serum Creatinine (mg/dl)			CCT (ml/min)			Proteinuria (gm/day)		
		1979	1984	1989	1979	1984	1989	1979	1984	1989
00001	HP	1.6	2.8	2.6	86	54	45	2.4	1.7	1.5
00002	HP	1.5	1.5	7.5*	173	105	12	2.6	3.6	3.6
00003	HP	1.1	1.2	0.8	107	115	72	0.1	0.9	0.8
00004	HP	0.9	1.2	1.2	101	160	142	1.1	0.3	0.3
00005	HP	1.2	1.2	6.8*	97	86	16	2.4	1.8	1.8
00006	HP	0.8	1.9	7.9*	106	64	14	4.2	0.4	0.4
00007	HP	1.0	0.8	0.9	84	90	98	2.3	0.4	0.2
00008	HP	2.0	2.3	7.9*	71	67	12	2.0	1.0	0.2
00009	HP	1.4	1.5	8.1	85	75	13	1.4	0.8	0.8
00010	HP	1.2	0.9	0.9	100	86	146	12.8	0.2	0.3
00011	HP	1.2	0.9	6.5*	88	88	19	1.7	0.5	0.5
00012	NS	0.9	1.2	7.2*	124	101	11	5.3	2.0	2.0
00013	HP	1.4	1.2	1.3	84	73	49	3.9	0.8	0.7
00014	HP	1.4	1.4	1.3	96	86	90	0.8	0.1	0.1
		1.3 ± 0.3	1.4 ± 0.6	4.4 ± 3.2	100 ± 25	89 ± 26	53 ± 49	3.1 ± 3.0	1.0 ± 0.9	0.9 ± 1.0

HP = asymptomatic hematuria and proteinuria
NS = nephrotic syndrome
* patients in ESRF at end of trial with serum creatinine more than 10 mg/dl

group and 21 in the control group, in 1989. There were no longer any significant differences in renal function 5 years after the initial trial. Six patients in the treatment group and 7 in the control group were in end-stage renal failure (ESRF). However, 50% of patients (n = 14) in the treatment group were no longer on therapy since 1984.

Table 2 is a comparison of the 27 patients with IgA nephritis in the original treatment group which had been divided into the treatment subgroup (n = 13) and the control subgroup (n = 14) at entry into the trial from 1979 and at the final analysis in 1989. There was no difference in the sex and age distribution, but the duration of follow-up was significantly shorter in the control subgroup ($p < 0.01$) because of patients who reached ESRF before 1989. In the treatment subgroup, serum creatinine was stable but there was a significant decline in creatinine clearance and decrease in proteinuria. Among those in the control subgroup, there was significant deterioration of serum creatinine with decrease in both creatinine clearance and proteinuria. Tables 3 and 4 show the profile of the two groups with data for 1979, 1984 and 1989.

At the end of the trial there were 4 patients with renal impairment in the treatment subgroup with none in ESRF, but in the control subgroup, there were 2 patients with renal impairment and 6 others in ESRF ($x^2 = 7.2$, $p < 0.01$). The degree of proteinuria was more severe in the control subgroup (3.1 ± 3.0 gm/day) at entry in 1979, compared to 1.7 ± 1.4 gm/day in the treatment subgroup. The difference however, was not statistically significant ($p = 0.1$).

Table 5 compares the patients in the treatment subgroup and the control subgroup in 1984 (when the original triple therapy trial ended and the second phase of the study began) and in 1989 at final analysis. In the treatment subgroup, serum creatinine was stable but there was a significant decrease in creatinine clearance and proteinuria. The control subgroup again showed a significant increase in serum creatinine associated with a decline in creatinine clearance but no change in proteinuria.

Comparison of the degree of proteinuria in 1984 showed no significant difference between the 2 groups (1.3 ± 1.1 gm/day versus 1.0 ± 0.9 gm/day). There were 2 patients with renal impairment (serum creatinine 1.7 and 1.6 mg/dl) before the trial in 1984 and 4 after the trial (1.9, 1.6, 3.4, 1.9 mg/dl) in 1989 in the treatment subgroup. In the control subgroup, there were 3 patients with renal impairment (2.8, 1.9 and 2.3 mg/dl) before the trial and 2 (2.6 and 7.9 mg/dl) after the trial. In addition, there were 6 patients with ESRF in the control subgroup but none in the treatment subgroup ($x^2 = 7.2$, $p < 0.01$) at the end of the trial in 1989. These 6 patients were the same 6 who developed ESRF from among the 27 patients in the treatment group of the original triple therapy. Their respective serum creatinine values at the end of the trial were 16.3 mg/dl (patient 2), 10.5 mg/dl (patient 5), 16.8 mg/dl (patient 6), 12 mg/dl (patient 8), 12.7 mg/dl (patient 11) and 10.8 mg/dl (patient 12). Patients 1 and 9 had renal impairment with serum creatinine levels of 2.6 and 8.1 mg/dl, respectively. None of the patients still on therapy with dipyridamole and warfarin have reached ESRF.

Table 6 shows the blood pressure profile of the patients in the treatment subgroup and the control subgroup. The mean arterial BP of those in the treatment subgroup was 102 ± 11 mmHg before the trial and 108 ± 19 mmHg after the trial. In the control subgroup the mean arterial BP was 103 ± 9 mmHg before and 110 ± 17 mmHg after the trial. There was no significant difference in the incidence or degree of hypertension between the two groups. Hypertension was well controlled and did not pose a management problem in any patient in both groups.

Table 5 Mesangial IgA Nephritis: Controlled trial with Dipyridamole and Warfarin (1984–1989)

Patients	Sex	Age (Yrs)	Follow Up (Mths)	Se Creat (mg) Before	Se Creat (mg) After	CCT (ml/min) Before	CCT (ml/min) After	Proteinuria (Gm/Day) Before	Proteinuria (Gm/Day) After	Number with CRF Before	Number with CRF After
Treatment Sub-Group	M = 7 F = 6 n = 13	25 ± 7	36 ± 3	1.1 ± 0.3	1.4 ± 0.7	87 ± 20	69 ± 35	1.3 ± 1.1	0.7 ± 0.5	R.I. = 2	R.I. = 4 *ESRF = 0
				NS		P <0.01		P <0.01			
Control Sub-Group	M = 10 F = 4 n = 14	24 ± 5	36 ± 2	1.4 ± 0.6	4.4 ± 3.2	89 ± 26	53 ± 49	1.0 ± 0.9	0.9 ± 1.0	R.I. = 3	R.I. = 2 *ESRF = 6
				P <0.001		P <0.001		NS			*$x^2 = 7.2$ (P <0.01)

Table 6

No.	Blood pressure before trial	Blood pressure after trial	Medication	Renal status at onset of trial (1984)	Renal status at end of trial (1989)
	Treatment Sub-Group				
1	110/60	150/100*	Propranolol	Normal	Stable
2	120/80	110/70	–	Normal	Stable
3	120/80	130/80	–	Normal	Stable
4	110/80	110/60	–	Normal	Stable
5	150/100*	150/90	Propranolol, Hydrallazine	Normal	Renal impairment
6	140/100*	110/80	Propranolol, Hydrallazine	Renal impairment	Stable
7	120/70	120/80	–	Renal impairment	Stable
8	120/80	110/70	–	Normal	Stable
9	120/80	120/70	–	Normal	Stable
10	120/80	150/110*	Methyldopa	Normal	Renal impairment
11	120/80	170/105*	Propranolol	Normal	Stable
12	120/80	160/110*	Propranolol, Hydrallazine	Normal	Renal impairment
13	130/90	120/80	–	Normal	Renal impairment
	Mean Arterial BP (mmHg)				
	102 ± 11	108 ± 19			
	Control Sub-Group				
1	140/80	140/100*	Propranolol, Chlortride	Renal impairment	Renal impairment
2	130/90	140/80	–	Normal	ESRF
3	110/60	170/110*	Methyldopa, Chlortride	Normal	Stable
4	130/70	140/80	–	Normal	Stable
5	130/90	150/100*	Propranolol	Normal	ESRF
6	120/80	120/80	–	Renal impairment	ESRF
7	120/80	160/110*	Propranolol	Normal	Stable
8	150/100*	130/90	Propranolol, Hydrallazine	Renal impairment	Renal impairment
9	120/80	100/60	–	Normal	ESRF
10	110/80	140/60	–	Normal	Stable
11	120/80	120/80	–	Normal	ESRF
12	120/80	120/80	–	Normal	ESRF
13	140/80	140/90	–	Normal	Stable
14	120/80	110/70	–	Normal	Stable
	Mean Arterial BP (mmHg)				
	103 ± 9	110 ± 17			

* Hypertension during trial

Discussion

In the original prospective study we reported [Woo et al. 1987] that patients with IgA nephritis treated with dipyridamole and low-dose warfarin seem to have a slower rate of progression to ESRF compared to those not on maintenance therapy.

The main objective of the present continuing study was to answer the question as to how long patients should continue therapy and whether the effects of therapy may be sustained even if therapy had been stopped a few years before. The present data suggest that patients who ceased therapy seem to progress to ESRF at a faster rate (average 3 years) compared to those still on therapy where 5 years later, none have reached ESRF yet.

Referring to Table 1 again, we must emphasize that the reassessment of the patients in 1989 included in the treatment group 50% of patients still on therapy with dipyridamole and warfarin (n = 13) and 50% of patients given no treatment at all (n = 14). And as we have shown in Table 5, none of those in the treatment subgroup (still on therapy) have reached ESRF compared to 6 patients in the control subgroup (not receiving therapy) who have reached ESRF when assessed in 1989.

The weakness of this study lies in the finding that the control subgroup had more severe proteinuria compared to the treatment subgroup in 1979 even though the difference was not significant. It is well-accepted that patients with IgA nephritis with severe proteinuria have a higher incidence of ESRF [Woo et al. 1987]. However, comparison of the proteinuria in the 2 groups in 1984 showed no significant difference. This could of course be explained by increasing glomerulosclerosis resulting in decreased proteinuria at this stage.

A further criticism that could be directed at the present study would be the presence of 2 patients in the treatment subgroup who had milder degrees of renal impairment compared to the 3 patients in the control subgroup, though this difference was also not significant.

This study therefore suffers from the defect of a poorly matched control and treatment group. This was because the present study was not a properly designed prospective trial like the original study. Our intention was to continue a subtrial to help decide whether there would be continuing benefit from previous therapy after ceasing therapy and it would appear that there was none.

In another ongoing trial [Lee et al. 1989] of patients with IgA nephritis with abnormal renal function using only dipyridamole and low-dose warfarin, patients in the treatment group (n = 11) were shown to have more stable renal function and less proteinuria compared to the control group (n = 9) who had significant renal deterioration after a follow-up period of 1 year. Two in the control group are already in ESRF with none in the treatment group.

The rationale for the above regimen is based on our earlier findings with regard to platelet involvement and a thrombogenic tendency in patients with IgA nephritis [Woo et al. 1981, 1985]. Recently, Lee et al. [1989] also demonstrated significant elevation of platelet factor 4 (PF 4) in patients with IgA nephritis compared to patients with other forms of glomerulonephritis. PF 4 is elevated in situations where there is increased platelet activity.

We utilised low-dose warfarin because several studies indicate that therapeutic efficacy could be achieved with prothrombin-time ratios of 1.5 and below with a concomitant diminished incidence of hemorrhage [Francis et al. 1983, Wessler et al. 1984]; though this is below the accepted range of prothrombin-time ratios, a significant antithrombotic effect has been achieved at a ratio of 1.3; data in animals suggested that lower prothrombin-time ratios are effective. Recently, Diamond and Karnovsky [1986, 1988] showed that heparin given in a dose not sufficient to prolong the activated partial thromboplastin time both ameliorated the functional and histologic abnormalities in chronic aminonucleoside nephrosis. They believed that heparin may protect the kidney through an anti-proliferative effect on the mesangial cells.

There is evidence for platelet aggregation and increased thrombosis in glomeruli subjected to raised intraglomerular blood pressure [Diamond and Karnovsky 1986, 1988]. This could occur in the setting of hyperfiltration associated with glomerulosclerosis. It is our surmise that dipyridamole and low-dose warfarin may be useful in this respect. In a previous report [Woo et al. 1987] on the follow up biopsies of patients with IgA nephritis treated with dipyridamole and low dose warfarin, we showed that patients in the control group had significantly higher histological scores, including more severe glomerulosclerosis, compared to patients in the treatment group. The data suggest that therapy with dipyridamole and warfarin may ameliorate the progression of glomerulosclerosis and hence delay the development of ESRF. Whether this is related to a decrease in intraglomerular hypertension or a retardation of mesangial cell proliferation or decrease in mesangial cell contractility will have to await further work on a 5/6 nephrectomised model and culture of mesangial cells which are ongoing. There also appears to be preliminary evidence that dipyridamole may decrease proteinuria through protection of cationic charges in the glomerular capillary wall.

REFERENCES

Bennet WM, Walker RG, Kincaid-Smith F 1989 Treatment of IgA nephropathy with eicosapentanoic acid (EPA): a two-year prospective trial. Clin Nephrol *31:* 128–131

Diamond JR, Karnovsky MJ 1986 Non-anticoagulant protective effects in chronic aminonucleoside nephrosis. Renal Physiol *9:* 366–374

Diamond JR, Karnovsky MJ 1988 Focal and segmental glomerulosclerosis: Analogies to atherosclerosis. Kidney Int *33:* 917–924

Francis CW, Marder VJ, Evarts CM, Yaukoolbodi S 1983 Two-step warfarin therapy: prevention of postoperative venous thrombosis without excessive bleeding. JAMA *249:* 374–378

Kobayashi Y, Hiki Y, Fujii K, Kurokawa A, Kamiyana M, Tateno S 1987 Heterogenous clinical picture and steroid therapy in progressive cases. Seminars in Nephrol *7:* 782–785

Lai KN, Lai FM 1987 Short term controlled trial of Cyclosporin A in IgA nephropathy. Abstract: Second International Symposium on IgA nephropathy, Bari pg 34

Lee GSL, Woo KT, Lim CH 1989 Controlled trial of dipyridamole and low dose warfarin in patients with IgA nephritis with renal impairment. Clin Nephrol *31:* 276

Lee GSL, Woo KT, Lau YK, Lim CH 1991 Platelet Factor 4 in IgA nephritis. Clin Nephrol *35:* 44

Wessler S, Gitel SN 1984 Warfarin: From bedside to bench. New Engl J Med *311:* 645–652

Woodroffe AJ, Bannister KM, Bellon MS, Hale GM, Clarkson AR 1987 Do local hemodynamic alterations mediate injury in IgA nephropathy? Seminars in Nephrol *7:* 341–343

Woo KT, Edmondson RPS, Yap HK, Wu AYT, Chiang GSC, Lee EJC, Pwee HS, Lim CH 1987 Effects of triple therapy on the progression of mesangial proliferative glomerulonephritis. Clin Nephrol *27:* 56–64.

Woo KT, Chiang GSC, Lim CH 1987 Follow up renal biopsies in IgA nephrotic patients on triple therapy. Clin Nephrol *28:* 304–305

Woo KT, Chiang GSC, Lim CH 1987 IgA nephritis in Singapore: Clinical, Prognostic Indices and Treatment. Proc Second International Symposium on IgA nephropathy, Bari. Seminars in Nephrology *7:* 379–381

Woo KT, Tan YO, Yap KH, Lau YK, Lim CH 1981 Beta-Thromboglobulin in mesangial IgA nephritis. Thromb Research *24:* 259–262

Woo KT, Lee EJC, Lau YK, Lim CH 1985 Antithrombin III in mesangial IgA nephritis. Thromb Research *40:* 483–487

Clinical Nephrology, Vol. 36 No. 2 – 1991 (67–75)

Intraglomerular lipid deposition in routine biopsies

H. S. Lee[1], J. S. Lee[1], H. I. Koh[2] and K. W. Ko[1]

[1] *Departments of Pathology, Internal Medicine and Pediatrics, College of Medicine, Seoul National University and*
[2] *Department of Internal Medicine, Paik Hospital, Inje Medical College, Seoul, Korea*

Abstract. Studies have suggested that lipids participate in the pathogenesis of chronic progressive glomerulosclerosis. To examine the frequency of intraglomerular lipid deposition in routine biopsies, renal biopsy material from 631 consecutive patients with glomerular lesions was studied by light, electron, and immunofluorescence microscopy. Fifty-three patients (8.4%) revealed ultrastructurally detectable lipid deposits in nonsclerotic glomeruli. Seven had minimal lesion, 13 focal-segmental glomerulonephritis, two membranous nephropathy, nine membranoproliferative glomerulosclerosis, 11 IgA nephropathy, and 11 other diseases. Ultrastructurally, the lesion affected small segments of glomeruli, with clusters of lipids which exhibited a heterogeneous pattern. A subendothelial accumulation of lipids was observed in 60%, storage of lipids on mesangial matrix in 68%, and intramembranous deposition in 21%. Intracellular accumulation of fat was noted in 23%. Indirect immunofluorescence testing for apolipoprotein B (apo B) and oil red O (ORO) staining were performed in 94 cases. Positive results for apo B and ORO staining in nonsclerotic glomeruli were obtained in 24 patients (26%) and 16 cases (17%), respectively. The distribution of lipids seen in these patients was either in diffuse or focal segmental patterns. The clinical data of 40 patients with glomerular lipid deposition were compared with 80 controls from the residual group of patients matched for age, sex, and disease. Serum creatinine and cholesterol levels, and daily excretion of urinary protein were not significantly different between the two groups. These results suggest that an abnormal accumulation of lipids, mainly of apo B containing lipoprotein, in nonsclerotic glomeruli from routine biopsies is not as rare as previously thought. In addition, factors other than hypercholesterolemia seem to be operative for the glomerular lipid deposition observed in our patients.

Key words: renal biopsy – glomerular lesions – lipid deposition

Introduction

The presence of some lipid droplets in glomeruli and tubules has been regarded as a normal phenomenon [Wolman, 1964]. The storage of lipids is considered abnormal when it occurs in unusually large amounts or involves only a particular parenchymal structure [Faraggiana and Churg 1987]. Abnormal accumulation of lipids in glomeruli can occur in a number of diseases, either because of hereditary enzymatic disorders [Gjone et al. 1974, Faraggiana and Churg 1987] or as a consequence of acquired metabolic alterations, such as cirrhosis of the liver [Hovig et al. 1978] and nephrotic syndrome [Zollinger and Mihatsch 1978, Faraggiana and Churg 1987].

Studies have suggested that chronic progressive glomerulosclerosis may occur through a process analogous to atherosclerosis and that its pathogenesis may include abnormalities in lipid metabolism [Moorhead et al. 1982, Diamond and Karnovsky 1988, Keane et al. 1988].

During the course of an ultrastructural study on 69 renal biopsies diagnosed as having acute postinfectious glomerulonephritis, we observed three patients with clusters of small fat vacuoles in nonsclerotic glomeruli at intramembranous and subendothelial locations [Lee et al. 1990]. The glomerular deposition of lipids in these cases was similar to that noted in lecithin-cholesterol acyltransferase (LCAT) deficiency [Hovig and Gjone 1974] and hepatic glomerulosclerosis [Hovig et al. 1978]. A review of the literature at that time revealed that it is extremely rare to find lipid storage in nonsclerotic glomeruli in routine

Received August 8, 1990; in revised form March 25, 1991.

Reprint requests to Dr. H. S. Lee, Department of Pathology, College of Medicine, Seoul National University, Chongno-gu, Yongon-dong 28, Seoul, Korea.

Table 1 Frequency of ultrastructurally detectable lipid deposition in 631 patients with glomerular lesions

Diagnosis	No. examined	No. of positive cases (%)
Minimal lesion	149	7 (4.7)
Focal-segmental glomerulosclerosis	65	13 (20.0)
Membranous nephrophathy	51	2 (3.9)
Membranoproliferative GN	27	9 (33.3)
IgA nephropathy	181	11 (6.1)
Acute postinfectious GN	18	1 (5.6)
Mild focal nonspecific GN	30	0 (0)
Diffuse sclerosing GN	11	3 (27.3)
Systemic lupus erythematosus	55	4 (7.3)
Henoch-Schoenlein nephritis	21	1 (4.8)
Hereditary nephritis	6	1 (16.7)
Hemolytic uremic syndrome	3	1 (33.3)
Miscellaneous	14	0 (0)
Total	631	53 (8.4)

* Abbreviation is: GN, glomerulonephritis

biopsies [McKenzie and Kincaid-Smith 1969, Saito et al. 1989], although foam cells and lipid deposits are common in the solidified areas of glomeruli in focal segmental glomerulosclerosis (FSGS) [Zollinger and Rohr 1969, Heptinstall 1983, Lee and Spargo 1985].

To define better the relation between glomerular fat deposition and progressive glomerulosclerosis, we initiated a study for investigating two questions: what is the frequency of lipid deposition in nonsclerotic glomeruli in routine biopsies? And what is the significance of fat deposition in glomeruli? Our study of 631 renal biopsies allowed us to address these questions systematically.

Methods

Patients

A total of 631 consecutive patients with glomerular diseases was evaluated at the Department of Pathology, Seoul National University, during the 23-month period ending in May 1990. Four hundred forty-six were adults and 185 were 15 years or younger. For each patient, data were collected concerning age, sex, date of clinical onset, blood pressure, serum creatinine level, serum total protein and albumin concentrations, fasting cholesterol and triglyceride levels, urinalysis and 24-hour urinary protein excretion.

Pathological study

Renal biopsies, all of which contained at least 10 glomeruli, were processed for light, electron, and immunofluorescence microscopy using standard methodologies and are summarized below.

Light microscopy. Biopsy specimens for light microscopy were fixed in Zenker's fixative, embedded in paraffin, serially sectioned and stained with hematoxylin and eosin, and periodic acid-Schiff (PAS). Cryostat sections were stained for neutral lipids with oil red O (ORO).

Table 2 Clinical characteristics of patients with glomerular lipid deposition (lipid +) and controls

	No.	Age, year	Sex, M : F	Serum Cr, mg/dl	Cholesterol, mg/dl	Proteinuria, g/day
Minimal lesion						
Lipid +	7	23.4 ± 6.3	4 : 3	0.7 ± 0.2	658 ± 428	8.7 ± 5.0
Controls	14	24.1 ± 0.3	8 : 6	1.1 ± 0.3	541 ± 197	8.0 ± 5.9
Focal-segmental glomerulosclerosis						
Lipid +	13	22.9 ± 7.1	5 : 8	1.1 ± 0.5	378 ± 202	3.8 ± 3.7
Controls	26	22.5 ± 8.4	10 : 16	1.0 ± 0.5	406 ± 146	5.4 ± 4.1
Membranous nephropathy, lipid +	2	41.0 ± 4.2	2 : 0	1.2 ± 0.2	397 ± 59	11.3 ± 4.5
Membranoproliferative GN						
Lipid +	9	32.1 ± 12.1	7 : 2	1.3 ± 0.6	263 ± 115	3.3 ± 1.2
Controls	18	32.5 ± 10.0	14 : 4	1.1 ± 0.3	315 ± 106	3.8 ± 3.1
IgA nephrophathy						
Lipid +	11	28.5 ± 9.4	5 : 6	1.2 ± 0.6	233 ± 101	2.6 ± 2.5
Controls	22	29.0 ± 8.9	10 : 12	1.2 ± 0.4	203 ± 116	1.5 ± 1.5

Values are mean ± SD except when indicated.

Immunofluorescence. Biopsy specimens for immunofluorescence were embedded in Tissue-Tek O.C.T. Compound (Miles Inc., Elkhart, Indiana) and were snap frozen in liquid nitrogen. All tissue was stored at −70° C until processing. Tissue sections were air-dried, acetone-fixed and then incubated with appropriate dilution of commercially purchased fluoresceinated monospecific antisera to human IgG, IgA, IgM, C3, C1q, and fibrinogen (Dako Corp., Santa Barbara, California). Indirect immunofluorescence testing was carried out for apolipoprotein B (apo B) using the goat anti-apo B (Chemicon, Temecular, California) as the primary antibody. The second reagent was FITC-labeled, rabbit anti-goat IgG (Kallestad, Austin, Texas). To avoid the leaching of lipids, the procedure for acetone fixation was omitted during indirect testing. The amount and extent of fluorescence were graded 0 to 4+. Five biopsies with acute tubular necrosis and three cases with acute tubulointerstitial nephritis were used as controls for apo B, showing all negative staining in the glomeruli.

Electron microscopy. The tissue was fixed in 2.5% glutaraldehyde in phosphate buffer for two hours and post-fixed for one hour in 1% osmium tetroxide. It was processed through graded alcohol and embedded in epon. The glomeruli were selected by light microscopic evaluation of semithin sections stained with toluidine blue. For the purposes of this study, only glomeruli showing no sclerotic lesions were examined. Ultrathin sections were cut on an LKB ultramicrotome and stained with uranyl acetate and lead citrate. One to three glomeruli were examined in each case in a Hitachi electron microscope. The presence of electron-dense proteinaceous material and less electron-dense lipid substances was evaluated according to their location: intramembranous, subendothelial, or mesangial. The amounts of each were graded from 0 to 3+ as follows: ±, trace or questionable deposits; 1+, small but definite deposits; 2+, moderate amounts of deposits; 3+, large amounts of deposits.

Statistical analysis

Differences in the frequency of glomerular lipid deposition between adults and children and between different staining methods were tested using a chi-square test. The significance of the differences between group means was assessed using a Wilcoxon rank sum test. A p value of less than 0.05 was considered statistically significant.

Results

Fifty-three (8.4%) of the 631 patients with glomerular lesions showed ultrastructurally demonstrable accumulations of fat-like vacuoles in the glomeruli. Patients are grouped according to the pathologic diagnosis in Table 1, in which the frequency of lipid deposition is shown.

Clinical characteristics

Of the 53 patients with ultrastructurally detectable lipid deposition, only four (8%) were children:

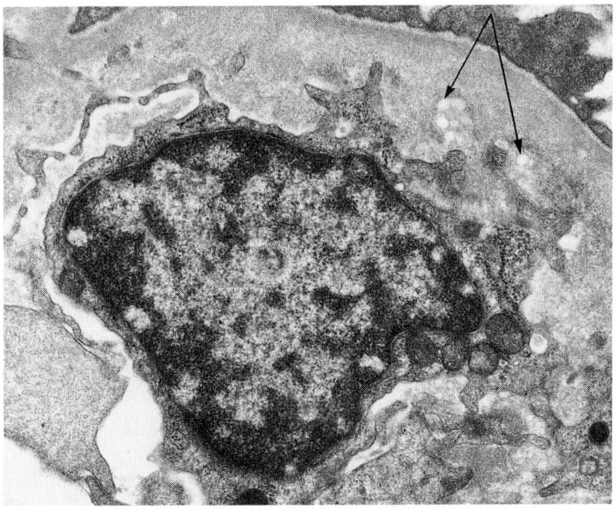

Fig. 1 Minimal lesion. Electron micrograph showing patchy accumulation of lipid vacuoles (arrows) in the subendothelial areas. ×6,480.

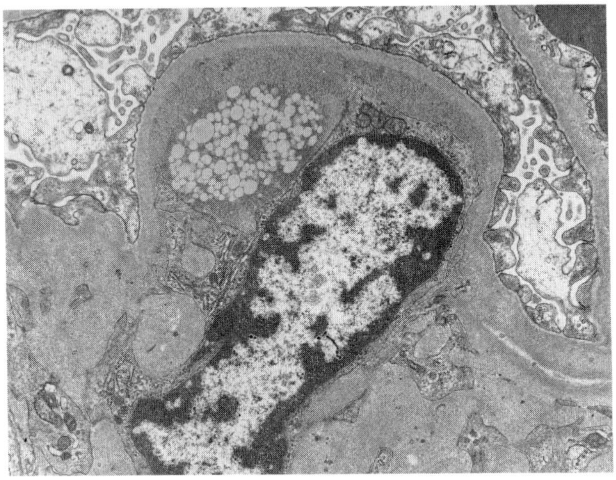

Fig. 2 Focal-segmental glomerulosclerosis. Electron micrograph showing localized accumulation of lipids and electron-dense proteinacous material in the mesangium. ×6,480.

this frequency in children is significantly lower compared with that in adults ($p < 0.01$). Both sexes were affected equally. Twenty-six (49%) had nephrotic range proteinuria ≥3.5 g per day. Hypercholesterolemia, defined as a cholesterol level greater than 260 mg/dl, was noted in 31 cases (58%); 22 of these also showed nephrotic range proteinuria. Renal insufficiency, diagnosed as serum creatinine in excess of 1.5 mg/dl, was observed in 11 patients (21%), mostly to a mild degree.

Clinical data of 42 patients associated with glomerular lipid deposition by electron microscopy are summarized in Table 2. Two controls from the residual group of patients not having demonstrable lipid deposits in glomeruli were matched for age, sex, and disease with each study patient. The 24-hour excretion of urinary protein, along with creatinine and cholesterol levels in patients with lipid deposition, were not significantly different from those in the controls (Table 2).

The response to prednisolone therapy was examined in all patients with minimal lesion and glomerular lipid deposition. Four adults responded well to oral prednisone with complete resolution of their proteinuria within a year. The remaining two adults and one child, however, revealed features of

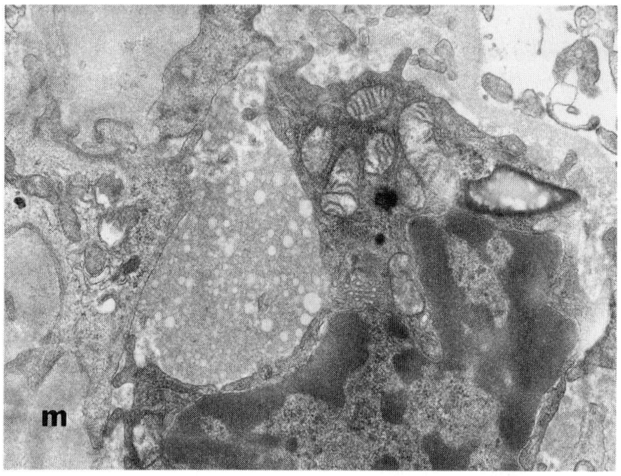

Fig. 3 Focal-segmental glomerulosclerosis. Electron micrograph showing intracellular accumulation of lipids. The cell containing lipids appears to be an activated macrophage in view of the increased numbers of mitochondria and nuclear shape. m = mesangial matrix. ×13,200.

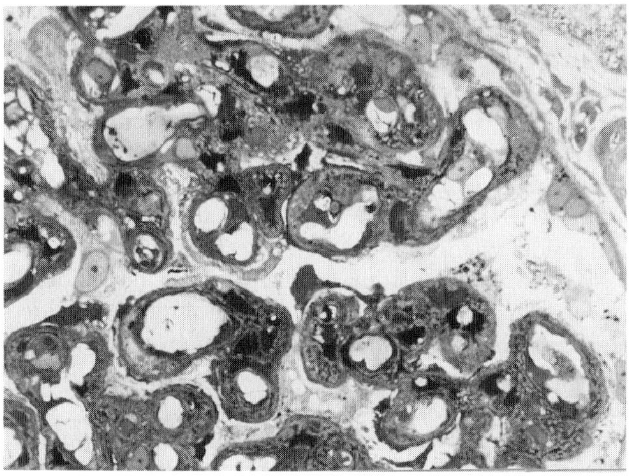

Fig. 5 Membranoproliferative glomerulonephritis, showing considerably thickened capillary loops with some lipid droplets. Plastic embedded toluidine blue stain. ×400.

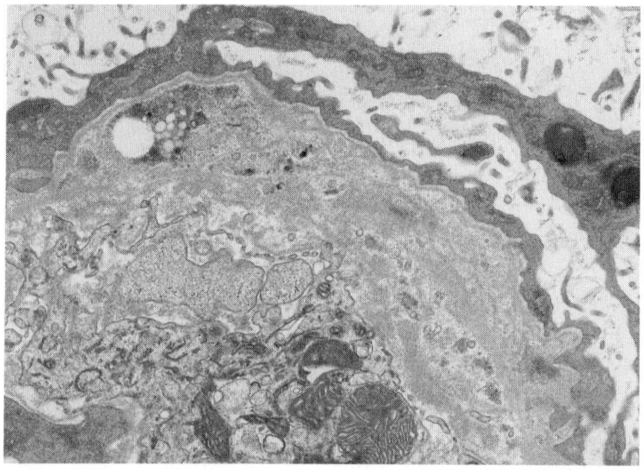

Fig. 4 Advanced membranous nephropathy. Electron micrograph showing an isolated accumulation of lipids within the glomerular basement membrane. The basement membrane is markedly thickened and reticulated. ×7,200.

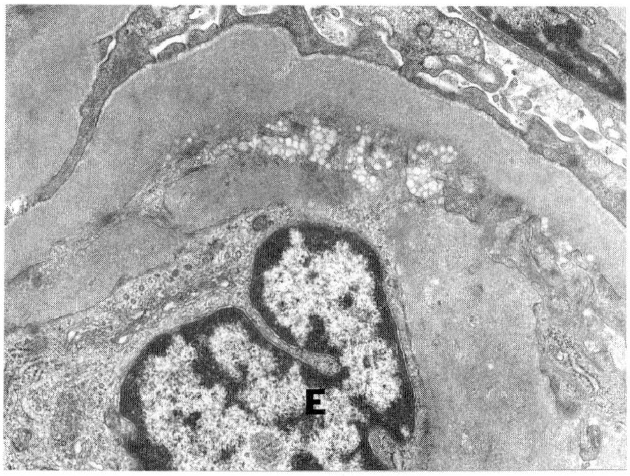

Fig. 6 Electron micrograph of the same case as Figure 5, showing accumulation of lipid droplets in the subendothelial area attached to electron dense-deposits. Mesangial interposition is also seen. E = endothelial cell nucleus. ×9,600.

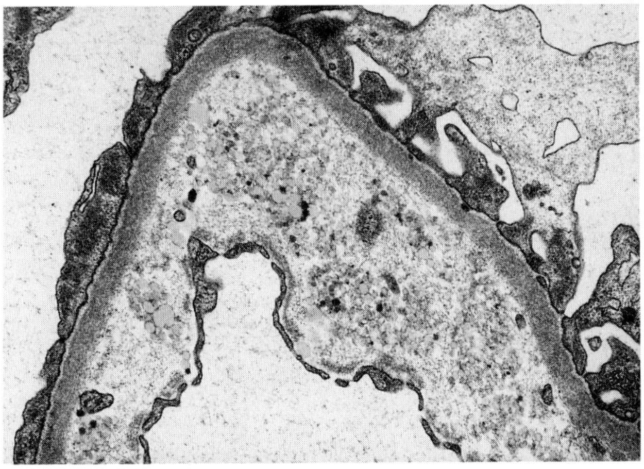

Fig. 7 IgA nephropathy. Electron micrograph showing marked widening of subendothelial space with lipid vesicles. ×9,600.

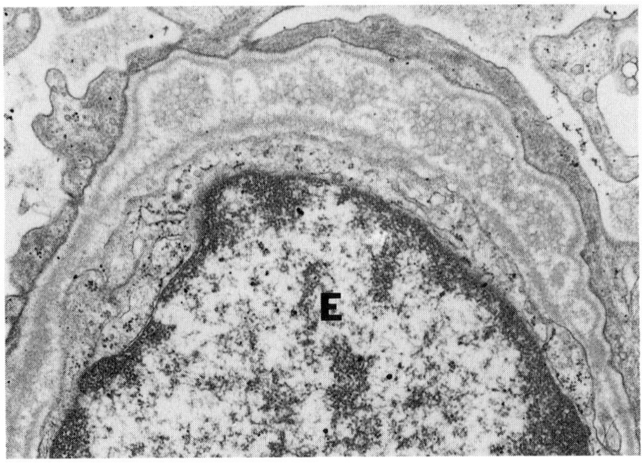

Fig. 8 IgA nephropathy. Electron micrograph showing numerous lipid vacuoles within the glomerular basement membrane. The lamina densa shows splitting and lysis probably related to resorbed deposits. E = endothelial cell nucleus. ×12,960.

frequently relapsing nephrotic syndrome. The proteinuria from the child finally disappeared with cyclophosphamide therapy.

Eight patients with IgA nephropathy (IgAN) and glomerular lipid deposition were followed for longer than a year from the time of renal biopsy. Two patients did not present any urinary abnormalities at the end of the follow-up, of whom one had received steroids for the nephrotic syndrome. Four patients showed stable renal function accompanying varying degrees of hematuria and/or proteinuria. The remaining two patients exhibited deterioration of renal function, of whom one received a renal transplant.

Light and electron microscopy

Minimal lesion (N = 7). Ultrastructurally, two cases exhibited slightly widened subendothelial regions containing small amounts of lucent lipid-like vacuoles with diameters of 35 to 106 nm (Figure 1). In another two cases, the localized widening of subendothelial areas became more pronounced the more they were filled with electron-dense proteinaceous material and lipid droplets. The remaining three cases revealed a mild increase in the mesangium due to accumulation of electron-dense material and fat droplets. Intracellular accumulation of fat was noted in two.

FSGS (N = 13). All biopsies showed focal segmental and/or global sclerosis affecting 6 to 59% of the glomeruli. Ultrastructurally, 11 cases revealed a slight to moderate accumulation of lipid material, mostly in the mesangial matrix (Figure 2) and rarely intracellular (Figure 3). Two of them also showed segmentally widened subendothelial zones containing numerous lipid vacuoles with a diameter of 36 to 160 nm. In the remaining two cases, a mild-to-moderate accumulation of fat was seen confined to the widened subendothelial space.

Membranous nephropathy (N = 2). The first case exhibited a slight accumulation of lipid material in intramembranous, subendothelial and mesangial locations. The second one showed a patchy deposition of lipid vacuoles confined within the glomerular basement membrane which showed a marked distortion and thickening associated with dissolved deposits (Figure 4).

Membranoproliferative glomerulonephritis (N = 9). Six cases exhibited segmental sclerosis involving 8 to 30% of the glomeruli. Semithin sections stained with toluidine blue sometimes demonstrated aggregates of fine lipid droplets in glomeruli (Figure 5). Ultrastructurally, a patchy subendothelial accumulation of dark electron-dense or lucent lipid vesicles with a diameter of 40 to 540 nm was seen in all, frequently attached to subendothelial electron-dense deposits (Figure 6). Six of them also exhibited clusters of lipid droplets on mesangial matrix, and one showed an isolated subepithelial accumulation of fat. Intracellular deposition of fat was observed in three.

IgAN (N = 11). Ultrastructurally, seven cases showed clusters of slightly electron-dense or lucent fat vacuoles with a diameter of 35 to 220 nm in the subendothelial area (Figure 7). One of them also showed an accumulation of lipid droplets in mesangial cell. One patient revealed an isolated accumulation of fat vacuoles in the mesangium. In the remaining three cases, there were patchy intramembranous accumulations of dark or medium electron-dense vacuoles with

Table 3 Ultrastructural features of 53 patients with glomerular lipid deposition

Diagnosis		No. of cases with lipid deposition Extracellular Intramemb	Subendo	MM	Intracellular Endo	MC
Minimal lesion	(N = 7)	0	4	5	1	1
FSGS	(N = 13)	0	3	10	2	4
Membranous nephropathy	(N = 2)	2	1	1	0	0
Membranoproliferative GN	(N = 9)	1	9	6	0	3
IgA nephropathy	(N = 11)	3	7	6	0	1
Acute postinfectious GN	(N = 1)	1	1	0	0	0
Diffuse sclerosing GN	(N = 3)	1	2	3	0	0
Systemic lupus erythematosus	(N = 4)	1	3	3	1	1
Henoch-Schoenlein nephritis	(N = 1)	1	1	1	1	0
Hereditary nephritis	(N = 1)	1	0	0	0	0
Hemolytic uremic syndrome	(N = 1)	0	1	1	1	1
Total	(N = 53)	11	32	36	6	11

* Abbreviation is: FSGS, focal segmental glomerulosclerosis; Intramemb, intramembranous; Subendo, subendothelial; MM, mesangial matrix; Endo, endothelial cell; MC, mesangial cell

Table 4 Results of apolipoprotein B (Apo B) and oil red O (ORO) staining

Diagnosis		No. of positive cases (%) Apo B Nonsclerotic segment	Sclerotic segment	ORO Nonsclerotic segment	Sclerotic segment
Minimal lesion	(N = 12)	4 (33)	0 (0)	3 (25)	0 (0)
Focal-segmental glomerulosclerosis	(N = 12)	2 (17)	7 (58)	2 (17)	5 (42)
Membranous nephropathy	(N = 5)	3 (60)	0 (0)	3 (60)	0 (0)
Membranoproliferative GN	(N = 13)	8 (62)	2 (15)	5 (38)	0 (0)
IgA nephropathy	(N = 32)	5 (16)	8 (25)	2 (6)	4 (13)
Acute postinfectious GN	(N = 1)	0 (0)	0 (0)	0 (0)	0 (0)
Mild focal nonspecific GN	(N = 5)	0 (0)	0 (0)	0 (0)	0 (0)
Diffuse sclerosing GN	(N = 3)	0 (0)	1 (33)	0 (0)	1 (33)
Systemic lupus erythematosus	(N = 5)	1 (20)	0 (0)	0 (0)	0 (0)
Henoch-Schoenlein nephritis	(N = 4)	0 (0)	1 (25)	1 (25)	1 (25)
Hereditary nephritis	(N = 2)	1 (50)	0 (0)	0 (0)	0 (0)
Total	(N = 94)	24 (26)	19 (20)	16 (17)	11 (12)

a diameter of 30 to 260 nm, accompanying severe abnormalities of glomerular basement membrane (Figure 8).

A summary of the main ultrastructural findings is presented in Table 3.

Immunofluorescence and ORO staining

Indirect immunofluorescence testing for apo B and ORO staining were performed in 94 cases (Table 4). Twenty-four patients (26%) showed positive apo B staining in nonsclerotic glomeruli. Positive results for ORO staining in nonsclerotic glomeruli were obtained in 18 cases (19%). The detection rate of lipid deposition by apo B or ORO staining was significantly higher compared with that by ultrastructural examination alone ($P < 0.01$). The distribution of the lipids in nonsclerotic glomeruli detected by apo B or ORO staining was either in diffuse or focal-segmental patterns. Diffuse but occasionally segmental deposits in the mesangial and/or peripheral areas were noted in 58% of the apo B positive cases and 61% of the ORO positive cases, respectively

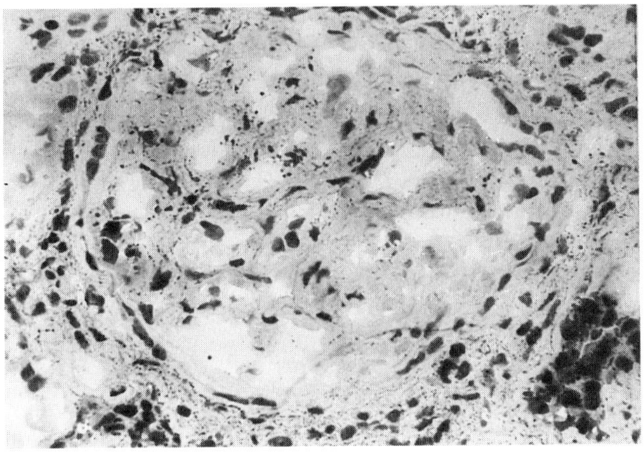

Fig. 9 Oil red O staining in a case with IgA nephropathy, showing positive staining mainly in the mesangium. ×120.

(Figures 9–11). Whereas apo B staining in the sclerotic segments of the glomeruli was almost always accompanied by IgM and C3 staining, the concomitant presence of apo B and IgM in nonsclerotic glomeruli was noted in only six patients (25%). Of the 28 cases with ultrastructurally demonstrable lipid deposition in nonsclerotic glomeruli, 16 biopsies (57%) exhibited positive staining for both apo B and ORO, while none of these two stainings was positive in four cases (14%).

Discussion

The present study was undertaken to examine the frequency of abnormal accumulation of lipids in nonsclerotic glomeruli in various forms of glomerular diseases, correlated to the clinical features. The overall frequency of glomerular lipid deposition seen by electron microscopy in our patients was 8.4%, showing a significantly higher frequency in adults compared with children.

Earlier literature on glomerular lipid deposition mostly emphasized its presence in the damaged or sclerotic glomeruli in cases of chronic glomerulonephritis [Fuller 1941, Simonds and Lange 1941, Wilens et al. 1951] or in cases with diabetes mellitus [Kimmelstiel and Wilson 1936, Wilens et al. 1951]. McKenzie and Kincaid-Smith [1969] reported four cases with glomerular foam cells in their 1400 renal biopsies. Zollinger and Mihatsch [1978] observed isolated endothelial foam cells in 3% of glomerulonephritic diseases and 1.4% of non-glomerulonephritic biopsies. Mesangial foam cells were also demonstrated in 0.6% of glomerulonephritis and 2.8% of renal transplants. Although overall frequency of foam cells in renal diseases was well described, no further information was given on the more frequent form, extracellular accumulation of lipids. Thus, the present study might be the first to demonstrate the frequency and morphologic details of lipid accumulation in glomeruli in routine biopsies. Our frequency of 8.4% even by electron microscopy alone suggests that lipid storage in nonsclerotic glomeruli in routine biopsies is not as rare as previously assumed.

Since lipids are made insoluble by osmium oxidation, a routine electron microscopic method using osmium postfixation of glutaraldehyde fixed tissue allows lipid preservation and morphologic detail [Faraggiana and Churg 1987, Wigglesworth 1988]. The lipid-like nature of the glomerular deposits seen by electron microscopy in this study was confirmed by ORO staining and indirect immunofluorescence

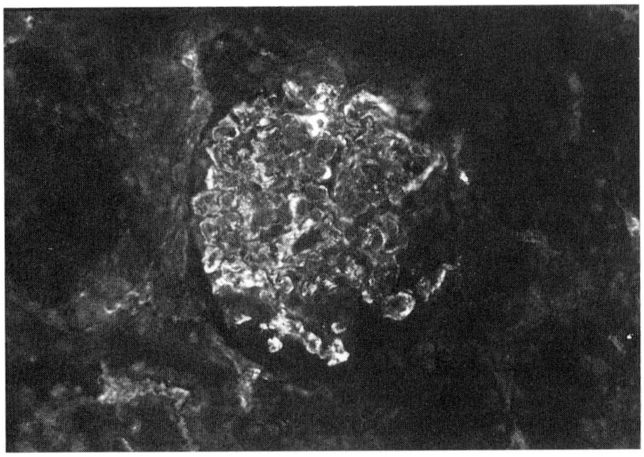

Fig. 10 Immunofluorescence for apo B in a case with focal-segmental glomerulosclerosis, showing positive staining mainly along the capillary walls. ×120.

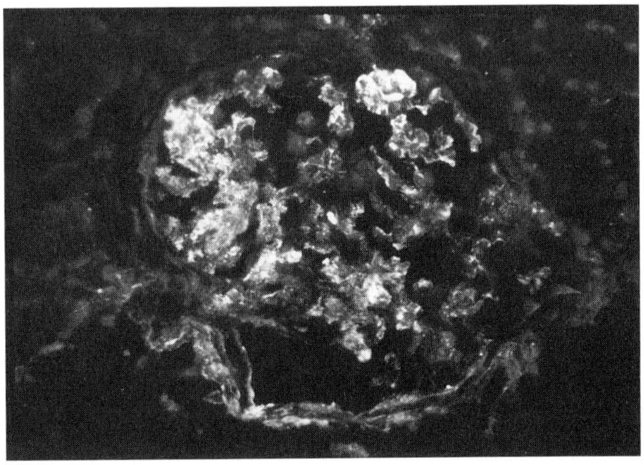

Fig. 11 Immunofluorescence for apo B in a case with IgA nephropathy, showing positive staining partly in the mesangium and partly along the capillary walls. ×120.

with anti-human apo B. The significantly lower rate of detecting lipid material by electron microscopy compared with that by immunofluorescence or ORO staining may be attributed to the much smaller number of glomeruli examined by electron microscopy. The lack of Apo B or ORO staining in four cases with ultrastructurally detectable lipid deposition may be associated with focal segmental distribution of lipids. Although ultrastructural studies of glomerular lesions in our patients revealed a heterogeneous pattern of lipids with some variations in size and electron density, the main component of the deposits appeared to be apo B-containing lipoprotein based on the results of immunofluorescence.

Previous studies have shown that intraglomerular lipid deposition is almost always related to abnormalities in lipid metabolism, in particular hypercholesterolemia. Gjone et al. [1974] suggested that abnormalities in lipid metabolism observed in patients with the rare genetic disorder of LCAT deficiency may be detrimental to glomerular structure and function. In these patients, abnormal low-density lipoprotein (LDL) or apo B was demonstrated in nonsclerotic glomeruli [Gjone et al. 1974, Ohla et al. 1986]. Hovig et al. [1978] also observed intraglomerular lipid deposition in two patients with hepatorenal syndrome and suggested that the mechanisms involved in this lipid deposition may be similar to those occurring in familial LCAT deficiency. Recently, a rare form of dyslipoproteinemia associated with glomerular lipoprotein deposition was described in two Japanese patients [Saito et al. 1989, Watanabe et al. 1989]. It is possible that hypercholesterolemia observed in 58% of our study patients may contribute to the lipid deposition in nonsclerotic glomeruli. Yet, the cholesterol level of the patients with lipid deposition was not significantly higher than that of the controls. The low serum cholesterol level in these may be the result of a very low fat intake: 76% of the calories in the Korean diet comes from starch, 10% from animal foods, and 7% from fat and oils. The average daily intake of fat per person is 24 g in Korea, while that in Japan is 58 g [Tchai and Ju 1987]. Thus, it would appear that factors other than hypercholesterolemia are required to explain the lipid deposition in nonsclerotic glomeruli in these patients.

Endothelial damage associated with the original glomerular injury may induce increased filtration or leakage of plasma lipoproteins in our patients. Even LDL of relatively large size would penetrate through the injured glomerular basement membrane [Moorhead et al. 1982]. Filtered LDL binds to glycosaminoglycans [Iverirus 1972], which are present in glomerular basement membrane and mesangial matrix [Kanwar et al. 1983]. Hoover et al. [1988] demonstrated the binding of LDL to type I collagen. Although the human glomerular basement membrane and mesangium only contain types IV and V collagens by immunohistochemistry [Scheinman et al. 1980], approximately 95% of the total collagen synthesized by cultured mesangial cells is type I [Haralson et al. 1987] suggesting that collagen on mesangial matrix partly binds with LDL. By binding of LDL to mesangial matrix, the passage of LDL may become slow, thus increasing the amount of extracellular lipid. Furthermore, the LDL retained on mesangial matrix could be taken up by mesangial cells through cell receptors [Gupta et al. 1990]. LDL-enriched medium stimulates mesangial cell proliferation in vitro, similar to the pattern observed in vascular smooth muscle cell cultures over a corresponding range of LDL concentrations [Wheeler et al. 1990].

When LDL is trapped for a prolonged period in the injured glomerular basement membrane or in mesangium with decreased perfusion activity, it may undergo oxidative modification due to depletion of antioxidant [Steinberg et al. 1989]. Oxidative changes in the LDL molecule greatly increase its susceptibility to entrapment in the extracellular matrix [Hoover et al. 1988] and in the mesangial cells [Gupta et al. 1990]. Further, oxidatively modified LDL is a chemoattractant for the circulating monocytes, which upon arrival in the subendothelial area become macrophages [Steinberg et al. 1989]. Uptake of oxidized LDL by the macrophage through a scavenger receptor with intracellular delivery of sufficient cholesterol can produce a foam cell [Brown and Goldstein 1983, Steinberg et al. 1989]. The oxidized LDL may trigger the macrophage to secrete cytokines, and further aggravate the endothelial cell injury with the adherence and aggregation of platelets, and the release of growth factors and other mediators that stimulate collagen secretion and promote cell proliferation [Steinberg et al. 1989].

The above considerations lead us to believe that the glomerular lipid deposits become similar to the fatty streaks of atherosclerotic lesions and are injurious to underlying glomerular structures leading to glomerulosclerosis. Although our patients with lipid deposition did not present worse clinical features at time of biopsy when compared to controls, the harmful effect of lipids on glomerular structure and function can be known only through lengthy follow-up. Further investigations will be necessary to evaluate the initiation, evolution and fate of glomerular lipid deposits.

Acknowledgements

We are indebted to Dr. William F. Keane and Dr. Youngki Kim for their helpful comments and suggestions, as well as to all our colleagues who provided us with clinical information. This work was supported by a research grant from Seoul National University Hospital. A preliminary report of this paper was presented at the XIth International Congress of Nephrology, Tokyo, July 1990.

REFERENCES

Brown MS, Goldstein JL 1983 Lipoprotein metabolism in the macrophage: implications for cholesterol deposition in atherosclerosis. Annu Rev Biochem *52:* 223–261

Diamond JR, Karnovsky MJ 1988 Focal and segmental glomerulosclerosis: analogies to atherosclerosis. Kidney Int *33:* 917–924

Faraggiana T, Churg J 1987 Renal lipidoses: A review. Human Pathol *18:* 661–679

Fuller RH 1941 Lipoids in the kidney. Arch Pathol *32:* 556–568

Gjone E, Blomhoff JP, Skarbovik AJ 1974 Possible association between an abnormal low density lipoprotein and LCAT deficiency. Clin Chim Acta *54:* 11–18

Gupta S, Crowley S, Shan Z, Rie J, Schlondorff D 1990 Binding of native and oxidized LDL to rat mesangial cells and matrix (abstr). JASN *1:* 596

Haralson MA, Jacobson HR, Hoover RL 1987 Collagen polymorphism in cultured rat kidney mesangial cells. Lab Invest *57:* 513–523

Heptinstall RH 1983 The nephrotic syndrome. In: Pathology of the kidney (3rd ed), Little, Brown and Co., Boston/Toronto, p 637

Hoover GA, McCormick S, Kalant N 1988 Interaction of native and cell-modified low density lipoprotein with collagen gel. Arteriosclerosis *8:* 525–534

Hovig T, Gjone E 1974 Familial lecithin: cholesterol acyltransferase deficiency. Ultrastructural studies on lipid deposition and tissue reactions. Scan J Clin Lab Invest *33 (suppl 137):* 135–146

Hovig T, Blomhoff JP, Holme R, Flatmark A, Gjone E 1978 Plasma lipoprotein alterations and morphologic changes with lipid deposition in the kidneys of patients with hepatorenal syndrome. Lab Invest *38:* 540–549

Iverius P-H 1972 The interaction between human plasma lipoproteins and connective tissue glycosaminoglycans. J Biol Chem *247:* 2607–2613

Kanwar YS, Rosenzweig LJ, Jakubowski ML 1983 Distribution of de novo synthesized sulfated glycosaminoglycans in the glomerular basement membrane and mesangial matrix. Lab Invest *49:* 216–225

Keane WF, Kasiske BL, O'Donnel MP 1988 Lipids and progressive glomerulosclerosis. Am J Nephrol *8:* 261–271

Kimmelstiel P, Wilson C 1936 Intercapillary lesions in the glomeruli of the kidney. Am J Pathol *12:* 83–98

Lee HS, Spargo BH 1985 Significance of renal hyaline arteriosclerosis in focal segmental glomerulosclerosis. Nephron *41:* 86–93

Lee HS, Choi Y, Oh HY, Koh HI 1990 Abnormalities of glomerular basement membrane in acute postinfectious glomerulonephritis. Clin Nephrol *33:* 220–226

McKenzie IFC, Kincaid-Smith P 1969 Foam cells in the renal glomerulus. J Pathol *97:* 151–154

Moorhead JF, Chan MK, El-Nahas M, Varghese Z 1982 Lipid nephrotoxicity in chronic progressive glomerular and tubulo-interstitial disease. Lancet *ii:* 1309–1311

Ohta Y, Yamamoto S, Tsuchida H, Murano S, Saitoh Y, Tohjo S, Okada M 1986 Nephropathy of familial lecithin-cholesterol acyltransferase deficiency: report of a case. Am J Kidney Dis *7:* 41–46

Saito T, Sato H, Kudo K, Oikawa S, Shibata T, Hara Y, Yoshinaga K, Sakaguchi H 1989 Lipoprotein glomerulopathy: Glomerular lipoprotein thrombi in a patient with hyperlipoproteinemia. Am J Kidney Dis *13:* 148–153

Scheinman JI, Foidart J-M, Michael AF 1980 The immunology of glomerular antigens V. The collagenous antigens of the glomerulus. Lab Invest *43:* 373–381

Simonds JP, Lange JD 1941 Fatty changes in the glomeruli of the kidneys. Am J Pathol *17:* 755–765

Steinberg D, Parthasarathy S, Carew TE, Khoo JC, Witztum JL 1989 Modifications of low-density lipoprotein that increase its atherogenicity. New Engl J Med *320:* 915–924

Tchai BS, Ju JS 1987 The trend of the nutritional status of the Korean, 1969–1984. Wld Rev Nutr Diet (Karger, Basel) *51:* 45–73

Watanabe Y, Ozaki I, Yoshida F, Fukatsu A, Itoh Y, Matsuo S, Sakamoto N 1989 A case of nephrotic syndrome with glomerular lipoprotein deposition with capillary ballooning and mesangiolysis. Nephron *51:* 265–270

Wheeler DC, Persaud JW, Fernando R, Sweny P, Varghese Z, Moorhead JF 1990 Effects of low-density lipoproteins on mesangial cell growth and viability in vitro. Nephrol Dial Transplant *5:* 185–191

Wigglesworth VB 1988 Histological staining of lipids for the light and electron microscope. Biol Rev *63:* 417–431

Wilens SL, Elster SK, Baker JP 1951 Glomerular lipidosis in intercapillary glomerulosclerosis. Ann Int Med *24:* 592–607

Wolman M 1964 Histochemistry of lipids in pathology. In: Handbuch der Histochemie. Gustav Fisher Verlag, Stuttgart, vol V, p 81

Zollinger HU, Rohr HP 1969 Struktur und Bedeutung der renalen Schaumzellen. Virchows Arch Abt A Path Anat *348:* 205–219

Zollinger HU, Mihatsch MJ 1978 Renal pathology in biopsy. Springer-Verlag, Berlin – Heidelberg – New York

Clinical Nephrology, Vol. 36 No. 2 – 1991 (76–82)

The kidney disease of Crow-Fukase (POEMS) syndrome: a clinico-pathological study of four cases

A. Fukatsu[1], H. Tamai[1], K. Nishikawa[1], W. Matsukawa[1], F. Yoshida[1], S. Matsuo[1], A. Takeda[2], K. Kodera[2], K. Morozumi[3], Y. Ito[4], K. Miyakawa[4], T. Toriyama[5], H. Kawahara[5] and H. Shigematsu[6]

[1]The 3rd Department of Internal Medicine, Nagoya University School of Medicine; 65 Tsuruma-cho, Showa-ku, Nagoya 466
[2]The 2nd Nagoya Red Cross Hospital; 2-9 Myoken-cho, Showa-ku, Nagoya 466
[3]The 3rd Department of Internal Medicine, Nagoya City University School of Medicine; 1 Kawasumi, Mizuho-cho, Mizuho-ku, Nagoya 467
[4]The Chubu Rousai Hospital; 1-10-6 Komei, Minato-ku, Nagoya 455
[5]Nagoya Kyoritsu Hospital; 1-172 Hokke, Nakagawa-ku, Nagoya 454 and
[6]The Department of Pathology, Shinshu University School of Medicine, 3-1-1 Asahi, Matsumoto, 390 Japan

Abstract. We studied four cases of Crow-Fukase syndrome with renal dysfunction. Kidney specimens obtained by needle biopsy showed glomerular lesions resembling those seen in conditions characterized by microangiopathy. Common glomerular findings by light microscopy were mesangial expansion and narrowing of the capillary lumina. An enlarged subendothelial space and mesangial area with deposition of amorphous material as well as swelling and vacuolization of endothelial cells were observed by electron microscopy. In an active phase, severe mesangial edema and segmental mesangiolysis, and in a late stage, mesangial cell interposition and sclerosis were seen. Tests by immunofluorescence microscopy for the presence of immunoglobulins A, M, G, λ and κ light chains, C3, and C4 were negative. Decay accelerating factor was found in glomeruli and in the vascular pole. Other findings included lymph node angiosclerosis, peripheral nerve microangiopathy and hemangioma formation with endothelial cell proliferation. These observations suggest that chronic endothelial injury constitutes the basic pathology of Crow-Fukase syndrome. Hemodialysis was required to manage anasarca in three of the patients although serum creatinine levels were below 5.0 mg/dl. Urinalysis revealed mild abnormalities and did not reflect the severity of the glomerular lesion. Corticosteroids given to three of the patients were effective in controlling fever and the lymphadenopathy; in two cases the corticosteroids induced a recovery of renal function. Thus Crow-Fukase syndrome may be due to chronic endothelial injury; the clinical symptoms and renal involvement respond to corticosteroid therapy.

Key words: endothelial injury – glomerulonephritis – Crow-Fukase syndrome – POEMS syndrome

Introduction

Crow-Fukase syndrome [Crow 1956, Shinpo et al. 1968, Driedger et al. 1980] or Takatsuki disease [Takatsuki et al. 1976] is a rare condition characterized by polyneuropathy, organomegaly, endocrinopathy, M-protein, and skin changes, thus also known as POEMS syndrome [Bardwick et al. 1980]. The incidence of this syndrome appears relatively high in Japan [Takatsuki and Sanada 1983, Nakanishi et al. 1984]. Reulecke et al. [1988] found a specific antibody against neuroendocrine tissue. In some cases studies of lymph nodes showed tumor-like changes as found in Castleman's disease [Nakanishi et al. 1984, Tsujimura et al. 1988, Frizzera 1988, Radaszkiewicz et al. 1989]. A role for interleukin 6 (IL-6) in Castleman's disease

Received October 10, 1990; in revised form March 3, 1991.
Reprint requests to A. Fukatsu

has been reported [Yoshizaki et al. 1989]. However, the precise pathogenesis of Crow-Fukase syndrome is not known.

Although renal dysfunction is often recognized [Bardwick et al. 1980, Trentham et al. 1976, Moya-Mir et al. 1986, Talerman and Bateson 1970, Reitan et al. 1980, Fam et al. 1986, Sano et al. 1986, Nakamoto et al. 1989], detailed clinicopathological descriptions are rare [Sano et al. 1986, Viard et al. 1988, Nakamoto et al. 1989]. We recently studied four patients with this syndrome with renal involvement. The patients showed clinical signs of renal disease and had histological abnormalities suggesting primary endothelial pathology.

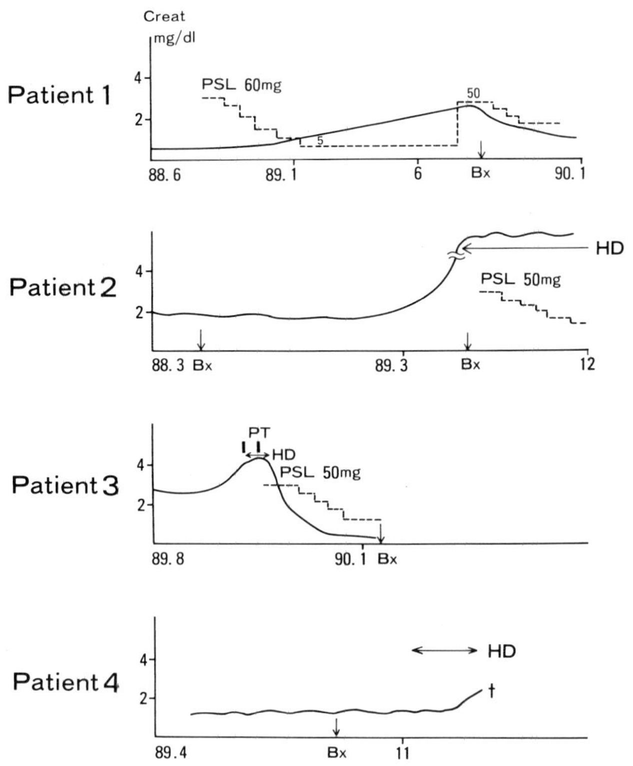

Fig. 1 Serum creatinine level of four patients with Crow-Fukase syndrome and the time of renal biopsies. Creat, serum creatinine level; PSL, prednisolone; Bx, renal biopsy; HD, hemodialysis; PT, pulse therapy methylprednisolone 1 g × 3 days.

Table 1 Symptoms of Crow-Fukase syndrome

Patient	1	2	3	4
Symptoms				
Polyneuropathy	+	+	+	+
Organomegaly	+	+	+	+
Endocrinopathy				
Hypothyroidism	+	+	+	+
Amenorrhea		+	−	+
M-protein	IgG	IgA	IgA	IgA
Skin changes	+	+	+	+
Other				
Peripheral edema	+	+	+	+
Ascites	+	+	+	+
Pleural effusion	+	+	+	+
Fever	−	+	−	−
Renal dysfunction	+	+	+	+
Lymph node swelling	−	+	+	+

Methods

Case reports

The symptoms and the time course of serum creatinine levels are summarized in Table 1 and in Figure 1. Additional features will be summarized below.

Patient 1. A 71-year-old male. Initial corticosteroid therapy was effective to reduce symptoms. Two years later blood examination showed an elevated creatinine level of 1.9 mg/dl with mild proteinuria (0.5–0.9 g/day). A percutaneous renal biopsy was performed. The dose of prednisolone was increased resulting in a reduction of the creatinine level to 0.9 mg/ml. An indirect immunofluorescence microscopy test for circulating anti-pituitary antibodies was positive. His skin had general pigmentation and multiple hemangiomas in the chest and abdominal area. One of about 4 × 4 mm in size, was resected for histological examination. A peripheral nerve biopsy was also performed.

Patient 2. A 47-year-old female. A renal biopsy was performed twice, first when the creatinine level was 2.0 mg/dl and second when hemodialysis was started 12 months after the first biopsy. A biopsy of cervical lymph nodes was also performed. Corticosteroid therapy was effective for the edema and lymphadenopathy, but not for the renal failure.

Patient 3. A 45-year-old female. Renal function declined rapidly and hemodialysis was required temporarily to treat pericardial and pleural effusion. The renal function was restored with corticosteroid therapy. A renal biopsy was performed when serum creatinine had returned to normal.

Patient 4. A 50-year-old female. The patient was suffering from severe anasarca and hemodialysis was introduced to control pericardial and pleural effusion. Serum creatinine had fluctuated around the upper limit of the normal range. Corticosteroids were not administered. The patient died from multi-organ failure as a consequence of sepsis.

In all cases severe anasarca was present without abnormal loss of albumin. The anasarca did not respond to diuretics. Urine abnormalities were mild

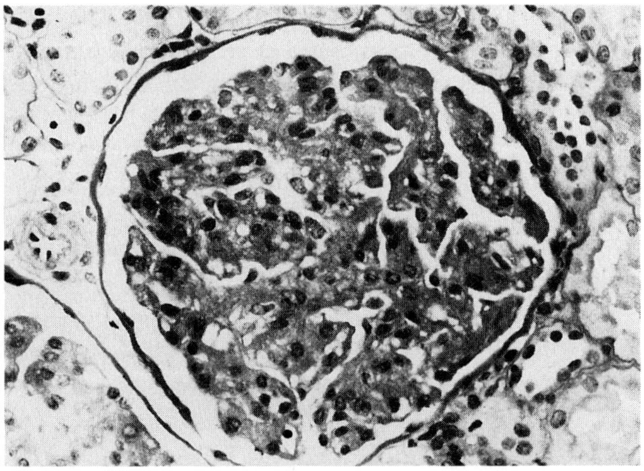

Fig. 2 A light micrograph of a glomerulus of patient 2 showing narrowing of capillary lumina and the expansion of the reticulated mesangial area due to deposition of PAS positive material. PAS × 400.

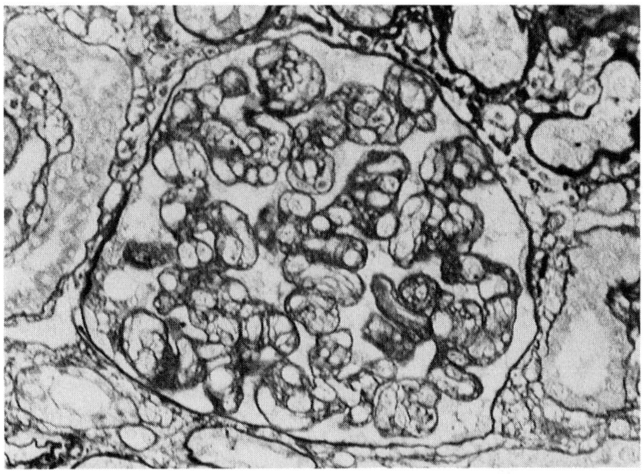

Fig. 3 A glomerulus of the same case as in Figure 2. Duplication of the basement membrane and mild mesangial sclerosis are visible. PAM × 400.

and consisted of proteinuria (less than 1 g/day) and microscopic hematuria.

Histological and immunohistological studies

Kidney tissue obtained by percutaneous needle biopsy was cut into three pieces. One piece was fixed in 10% buffered formalin and embedded in paraffin. Two-micron-thick sections were stained with hematoxylin-eosin (HE), periodic acid-Schiff (PAS), and silver methenamine (PAM). Some sections were stained with Congo-red for the detection of amyloid. The second piece was fixed in 2% glutaraldehyde and processed for electron microscopy. The third part was frozen in liquid nitrogen. Frozen sections were stained for human IgG, IgA, IgM, C3, C4, C1q, fibrinogen, and κ and λ light chains using fluoresceinated antibodies (Behring Institute, Marburg, West Germany). Monoclonal antibody (IgG1) to human decay accelerating factor (DAF) was kindly provided by Dr. Fujita [Fujita et al. 1987]. We used frozen kidney sections of two patients with persistent microscopic hematuria as controls; the kidneys of both patients were normal by light-, electron-, and immunofluorescence microscopy. Frozen sections of the renal specimens of patients with Crow-Fukase syndrome and of the two control patients were first fixed in acetone for 15 min at room temperature, then incubated with the monoclonal antibody to DAF or with non-specific control monoclonal antibody of the same subclass, and then reacted with fluoresceinated goat antibody to mouse IgG (Cappel Laboratories, West Chester, PA).

Detection of specific antibody in patient sera

In an indirect immunofluorescence microscopy test frozen sections of kidney tissue of the control patients and of patients with Crow-Fukase syndrome were incubated first with properly diluted patient sera taken before and after corticosteroid therapy or with properly diluted sera from normal subjects, and then with fluoresceinated goat anti-human IgG antibody.

Results

Histology

Seven to twenty glomeruli were present in the biopsy specimens. In the kidney the main lesions were seen in the glomeruli. The tubules and interstitium were well preserved, even when the serum creatinine level was elevated. The severity of the glomerular changes varied. Common findings by light microscopy are shown in Figures 2 and 3: narrowing of capillary lumina, expansion of mesangial matrix and mild mesangial hypercellularity (Figure 2), and duplication of the basement membrane of the capillary wall (Figure 3) were seen. These findings were observed in patient 3 even after serum creatinine level had returned to normal. The most severe glomerular injury was present in patient 4. The glomeruli showed diffuse mesangial reticulation with segmental mesangiolysis and partial sclerosis (Figure 4), suggesting exacerbation of a chronic process. In addition to the common findings, segmental mesangiolysis and advanced glomerular sclerosis were noticed in the second biopsy specimen of patient 2.

Testing by direct immunofluorescence microscopy for human IgG, IgA, IgM, C3, C4, C1q, and λ and κ light chains was negative. Fibrin(ogen) was seen in a diffuse pattern in glomeruli in all cases. In all patients with Crow-Fukase syndrome, DAF was localized in glomerular cells and in the glomerular vascular pole while it was localized in vascular pole only in the glomeruli of control patients (Figures 5 and 6). Staining for amyloid was negative.

The most striking finding by transmission electron microscopy in all cases was the increase in subendothelial and mesangial space with widespread deposition of amorphous material. In general this material had the same electron density as that in the capillary lumen; however, more electron dense material was also present in the subendothelial space. Mesangial cell interposition associated with newly synthesized extracellular matrix was in evidence (Figure 7). Vacuolization of endothelial cells, infiltrated inflammatory cells, and red blood cells in the subendothelial space were occasionally seen (Figure 8).

A lymph node from patient 2 showed angiofollicular hyperplasia, plasma cell infiltration, and hyalinization of arterioles. Microangiopathy with endothelial cell proliferation and reduplication of basement membrane was found in vasa nervosum of nerve tissue. The skin from patient 1 revealed intravascular papillary endothelial cell hyperplasia.

Serology

By indirect immunofluorescence microscopy, sera from patients with Crow-Fukase syndrome taken in various phases did not contain antibodies reactive with normal kidney tissue or with kidney tissue from patients with Crow-Fukase syndrome.

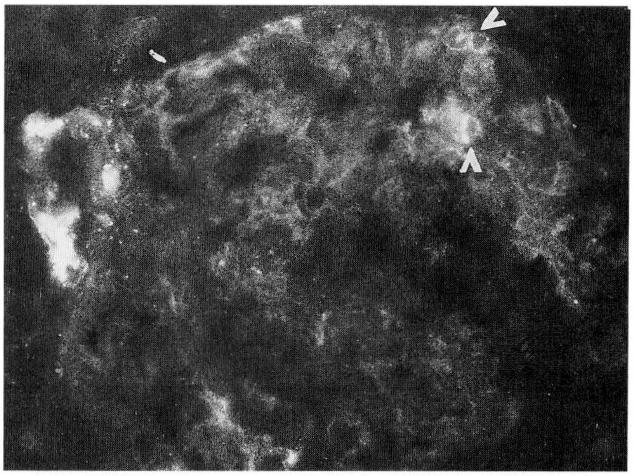

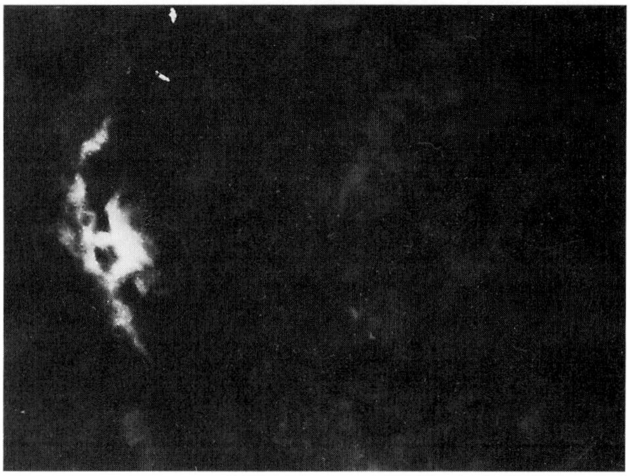

Figs. 5 and 6 Indirect immunofluorescence microscopy for human DAF. DAF is found in the glomerular capillary tuft as well as in the vascular pole of patient 1 (Figure 5), but only in the vascular pole of a glomerulus of a control patient (Figure 6). In some part of the glomerulus DAF is localized in an endothelial pattern (arrow heads). × 400.

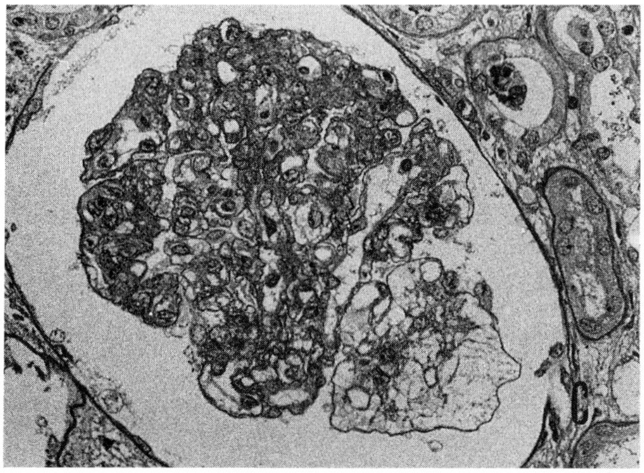

Fig. 4 A glomerulus from patient 4 showing mesangial reticulation and segmental mesangiolysis. A partial sclerotic area is also seen. PAS × 400.

Discussion

The differences in the severity of the renal lesions in our patients with Crow-Fukase syndrome most likely represent various stages of the disease process. The common histological characteristics were: 1) enlargement of the subendothelial and mesangial area with deposition of unknown material, and morphological alterations of endothelial cells, 2) migration of red blood cells and leukocytes into the subendothelial area. These changes were observed in all cases suggesting a chronic, sustained process. In a late stage, duplication of the glomerular basement membrane and mild diffuse mesangial proliferation or sclerosis appeared. In an active stage mesangiolysis was found. Viard et al. reported a case with microangiopathic glomerular lesions compatible to those seen in an active phase in our patients [1988]. The descriptions by Fam et al. [1986], Sano et al. [1986] and Nakamoto et al. [1989] also show certain aspects of a chronic process. The glomerular features are seen in conditions associated with microangiopathy [Churg and Sobin 1982] such as the hemolytic uremic syndrome (HUS) [Shigematsu et al. 1976] and thrombotic thrombocytopenic purpura (TTP). Clinically none of our patients had symptoms or signs of HUS or TTP. Although the cause of HUS may be multifactorial, recently it was reported that patients with HUS in an acute phase had circulating antibodies against normal endothelial cells [Leung et al. 1988]; some of the patients had activated neutrophils that could injure endothelial cells [Forsyth et al. 1989]. These reports support the notion that pathological changes seen in HUS are primarily due to injury to endothelial cells.

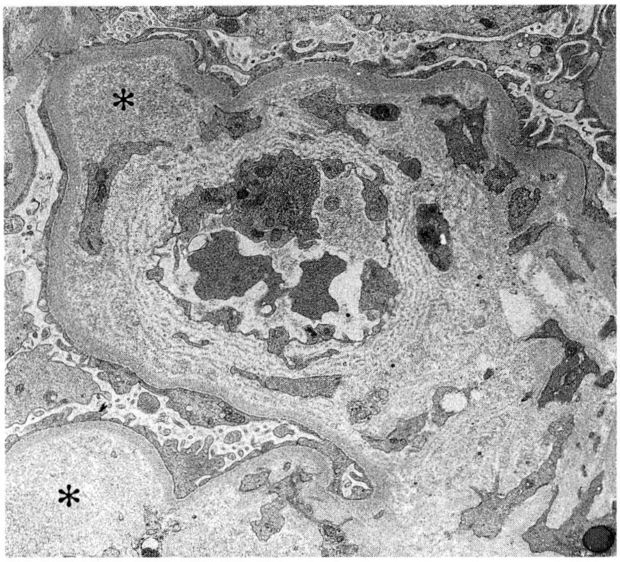

Fig. 7 An electron micrograph of a glomerulus of patient 1 showing widening of the subendothelial and mesangial area with widespread deposition of amorphous material. This material is similar in electron density to that seen in the capillary lumen; in some areas (asterisks) it is more dense. Mesangial and endothelial interposition, and newly formed basement membrane are seen in the capillary wall. × 3,300.

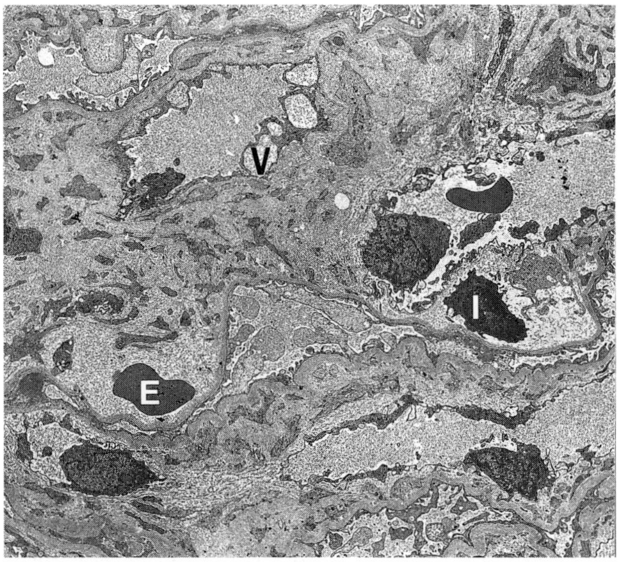

Fig. 8 An electron micrograph of a glomerulus of patient 1. Vacuolization of endothelial cells (V), escape of an erythrocyte (E), and an infiltrating cell (I) into swollen capillary wall are visible. × 3,300.

Based on the above observations a conceivable explanation for the renal pathology of Crow-Fukase syndrome is that chronic endothelial damage, induced by an unknown cause, results in an increased subendothelial space with deposition in this area of plasma-derived material and with infiltration of cells. In an active phase the injury extends beyond endothelial cells and affects the mesangial area causing mesangial edema with segmental mesangiolysis. These stimuli lead to mesangial cell proliferation and interposition, and finally sclerosis. The fact that DAF is expressed in the glomeruli of patients with Crow-Fukase syndrome supports this hypothesis. DAF is localized in blood cells and in various tissue cells including endothelial cells [Kinoshita et al. 1985, Medof et al. 1987, Asch et al. 1986, Cosio et al. 1989]. Cosio et al. [1989] have demonstrated that DAF in normal glomeruli is located only at the vascular pole. By contrast, in diseased glomeruli DAF is also demonstrable in intrinsic glomerular cells [Cosio et al. 1989]. Although the distribution of DAF in diseased glomeruli suggests endothelial localization (Figure 8), it is difficult to state with certainty that DAF is expressed on glomerular endothelial cells because of the limitation of immunofluorescence microscopy. In addition DAF might be present on mesangial [Cosio et al. 1989] as well as on epithelial cells [Quigg et al. 1989].

It is attractive to propose that increased expression of DAF in glomeruli is the result of stimulation of glomerular cells. In a patient with Crow-Fukase syndrome Kato et al. [1989] have demonstrated endothelial cell injury in the liver with deposition of unknown material in Disse's space similar to that seen in subendothelial area of glomeruli in our cases, suggesting that endothelial injury is a generalized phenomenon in this disease. The finding of microangiopathy in lymph nodes and in peripheral nerves is also consistent with generalized endothelial injury.

The pathogenesis of chronic endothelial injury is unknown. We could not detect auto-antibodies reactive with normal or patients' renal structures. Patient 2, whose lymph node showed the Castleman's disease-like pathology, had a M-protein of the IgA class but the bone marrow didn't show myeloma. In none of our cases the deposition of light chains or of amyloid was detected.

The hemangioma of patient 1 with endothelial cell proliferation was histologically compatible to that described by Imayama et al. [1984]. They reported that the hemangioma responded to corticosteroid therapy. It is possible that the endothelial injury is directly or indirectly due to an abnormal activation of endothelial cells.

Pathological activity represented by mesangiolysis did not always correspond to the extent of renal insufficiency. Urinalysis was always mild and did not reflect the severity of renal pathology. Hemodialysis or hemofiltration was often required to manage severe anasarca although serum creatinine levels did not exceed 5.0 mg/dl. It is important from the therapeutical and pathological point of view that the disturbed renal function to a certain degree was reversed by corticosteroid therapy.

In conclusion patients with Crow-Fukase syndrome may have rather typical renal pathology which responds to corticosteroid therapy; it is proposed that the pathology might be due to the chronic injury of endothelial cells.

Acknowledgements

The authors thank Dr. N. Sakamoto (Nagoya Univ.), Dr. J. R. Brentjens (State Univ. of New York at Buffalo) and Dr. H. Okada (Nagoya City Univ.) for their advice. We also thank Mr. N. Suzuki, Mrs. N. Kamei, Miss N. Kuno, and Miss M. Miyawaki for technical assistance. We thank Dr. Fujita for the generous gift of a monoclonal antibody to human DAF.

This work was partly supported by The Monbusho Scientific Research Grants (#63480189) and by Grants from Nagoya Kyoritsu Hospital and Masuko Memorial Hospital.

REFERENCES

Asch AS, Kinoshita T, Jaffe EA, Nussenzweig V 1986 Decay-accelerating factor is present on cultured human umbilical vein endothelial cells. J Exp Med *163:* 221

Bardwick PA, Zvaifler NJ, Gill NJ, Newman D, Greenway GD, Resnick KL 1980 Plasma cell dyscrasia with polyneuropathy, organomegaly, endocrinopathy, M protein and skin changes: the POEMS syndrome – Report on two cases and a review of the literature. Medicine *59:* 311

Churg J, Sobin LH 1982 Hemolytic-uremic syndrome, thrombotic thrombocytopenic purpura and glomerular thrombosis. In: Renal Disease Classification and atlas of glomerular disease, Igaku Shoin, Tokyo, p 198

Cosio FG, Sedmark DD, Mahan JD, Nahman Jr NS 1989 Localization of decay accelerating factor in normal and diseased kidneys. Kidney Int *36:* 100

Crow RS 1956 Peripheral neuritis in myelomatosis. Br Med J *2:* 802

Driedger H, Pruzanski W 1980 Plasma cell neoplasia with peripheral neuropathy: A study of five cases and review of the literature. Medicine *59:* 301

Fam AG, Rubenstein JD, Cowan DH 1986 POEMS syndrome. Study of a patient with proteinuria, microangiopathic glomerulopathy, and renal enlargement. Arthritis Rheumatism *29:* 233

Forsyth KD, Simpsin AC, Fitzpatrick MM, Barratt TM, Levinsky RJ 1989 Neutrophil-mediated endothelial injury in haemolytic-uraemic syndrome. Lancet *II:* 411

Frizzera G 1988 Castleman's disease and related disorders. Seminars in Diag Pathol *5:* 346

Fujita T, Inoue T, Ogawa K, Iida I, Tamura N 1987 The mechanism of action of decay-accelerating factor (DAF). DAF inhibits the assembly of C3 convertase by dissociating C2a and Bb. J Exp Med *166:* 1221

Imayama S, Urabe H 1984 Electron microscope study on the hemangiomas in POEMS syndrome. J Dermatol *11:* 550

Kato A, Toida S, Yasuda H, Takemura T, Kazuhiko M 1989 Electron microscopic study of swelling liver with Takatsuki syndrome. J Clin Electron Microscopy *22:* 323

Kinoshita T, Medof ME, Silber R, Nussenzweig V 1985 Distribution of decay-accelerating factor in the peripheral blood of normal individuals and patients with paroxysmal nocturnal hemoglobinuria. J Exp Med *162:* 75

Leung DYM, Moake JL, Havens PL, Kim M, Pober JS 1988 Lytic anti-endothelial cell antibodies in haemolytic-uraemic syndrome. Lancet *II:* 183

Medof M, Walter EI, Rutgers JL, Knowles DM, Nussenzweig V 1987 Identification of the complement decay-accelerating factor (DAF) on epithelium and glandular cells and in body fluids. J Exp Med *165:* 848

Moya-Mir MS, Martin-Martin F, Barbadillo R et al. 1986 Plasma cell dyscrasia with polyneuritis and dermato-endocrine alterations. Report of a new case outside Japan. Postgrd Med J *56:* 427

Nakamoto Y, Imai H, Yasuda T, Asakura K, Miura AB, Nishimura S 1989 Mesangiolytic glomerulonephritis associated with Takatsuki's syndrome. An analysis of five renal biopsy specimens. Hum Pathol *20:* 243

Nakanishi T, Sobue I, Toyokura Y et al. 1984 The Crow-Fukase syndrome. A study of 102 cases in Japan. Neurol *34:* 712

Quigg RJ, Nicholson-Weller A, Cybulsky AV, Badalamenti J, Salant DJ 1989 Decay accelerating factor regulates complement activation on glomerular epithelial cells. J Immunol *142:* 877

Radaszkiewicz T, Hansmann M-L, Lennert K 1989 Monoclonal and polyclonality of plasma cells in Castleman's disease of the plasma cell variant. Histopathology *14:* 11

Reitan JB, Pape E, Possa SD, Julsrud O-J, Slettnes ON, Solheim OP 1980 Osteosclerotic myeloma with polyneuropathy. Acta Med Scand *208:* 137

Reulecke M, Dumas M, Meier C 1988 Specific antibody against neuroendocrine tissue in a case of POEMS syndrome with IgG gammopathy. Neurol *38:* 614

Sano M, Terasaki T, Koyama A, Narita M, Tojo S 1986 Glomerular lesions associated with the Crow-Fukase syndrome. Virchows Arch A *409:* 3

Shigematsu H, Dikman SH, Churg J, Grishman E, Duffy JL 1976 Mesangial involvement in hemolytic-uremic syndrome. Am J Pathol *85:* 349

Shinpo S, Nishitani H, Tsunematsu T et al. 1968 Solitary plasmacytoma with polyneuritis and endocrine disturbances (Jpn). Nippon Rinsho *26:* 2444

Takatsuki K, Uchiyama T, Sagawa K, Yodoi J Plasma cell dyscrasia with polyneuropathy and endocrine disorder: Review of 32 patients. International Congress Series no. 415, Topics in hematology. Proceeding of the 16th International Congress of Hematology, Kyoto, Japan, p 454

Takatsuki K, Sanada I 1983 Plasma cell neoplasia with peripheral neuropathy and endocrine disorder: Clinical and laboratory features of 109 reported cases. Jpn J Clin Oncol *13:* 543

Talerman A, Bateson EM 1970 Multiple myeloma associated with bone sclerosis and peripheral neuropathy. Br J Radiol *43:* 698

Trentham DE, Masi AT, Marker HW 1976 Polyneuropathy and anasarca: evidence for a new connective tissue syndrome and vasculopathic contribution. Ann Intern Med *84:* 271

Tsujimura T, Kishino B, Itatani H, Aozawa K, Matsumoto K 1988 Plasma cell dyscrasia with polyneuropathy, organomegaly, endocrinopathy, M protein, and skin changes: The POEMS syndrome, associated with preceding polycythemia vera. Acta Pathol Jpn *38:* 1337

Viard J-P, Lesavre P, Boitard C, Noel L-H, Roth A, Said G, Bach J-F 1988 POEMS syndrome presenting as systemic sclerosis. Clinical and pathologic study of a case with microangiopathic glomerular lesions. Am J Med *84:* 524

Yoshizaki K, Matsuda T, Nishimoto N, Kuritani T, Taeho L, Aozasa K, Nakahata T, Kawai H, Tagoh H, Komori T, Kishimoto S, Hirano T, Kishimoto T 1989 Pathological significance of interleukin 6 (IL-6/BSF-2) in Castleman's disease. Blood *74:* 1360

Clinical Nephrology, Vol. 36 No. 2 – 1991 (83–86)

Pulmonary and renal toxicity of intravenous immunoglobulin

R. Rault[1], B. Piraino[1], J. R. Johnston[1] and A. Oral[2]

University of Pittsburgh, Department of Medicine, [1] Renal-Electrolyte Division, [2] Hematology Division, Pittsburgh, PA 15261, USA

Abstract. Three patients treated with intravenous immunoglobulin developed respiratory difficulty and decreased renal function. Previously reported adverse reactions to this class of drugs have included pulmonary toxicity but not, to the best of our knowledge, renal toxicity. Renal dysfunction was mild in one patient but severe in two patients, one of whom required temporary hemodialysis. In all three patients, renal function returned to the pretreatment level after stopping the drug. Urinalysis and urine sodium concentration at the onset of renal failure were consistent with pre renal azotemia although renal biopsy performed later in one patient showed acute tubular necrosis. The exact mechanism of toxicity is unknown, but the fact that all three cases occurred with a particular immunoglobulin preparation would suggest that a contaminant, possibly aggregated IgG might be responsible.

Key words: immunoglobulin – acute renal failure – respiratory failure

Introduction

Intravenous immunoglobulin, consisting mainly of IgG from pooled human plasma, is frequently used in the treatment of primary immunodeficiency syndromes and immune thrombocytopenic purpura [Dwyer 1987, Bussel et al. 1985] and may be of value in preventing infection in the immunocompromised host [Dwyer 1987]. Mild side effects which include fever, chills, headache and back pain occur in 2.5–15% of patients and can often be controlled by slowing the rate of infusion. Severe reactions characterized by hypotension and respiratory failure are considered to be extremely rare [Barandum et al. 1981, Hopkins 1985]. While pulmonary manifestations are well-documented, nephrotoxicity is not a recognized complication of therapy with immunoglobulins, only one previous case having been described [Barton et al. 1987]. In this report we describe three patients who developed pulmonary and renal dysfunction temporally related to intravenous immunoglobulin therapy.

Received November 7, 1990; in revised form March 1991.

Requests for reprints to Dr. R. Rault, Associate Professor of Medicine, University of Pittsburgh, 11431 Presbyterian-University Hospital DeSoto and O'Hara Streets, Pittsburgh, PA 15213, USA.

Case reports

Case 1

A 50-year-old white male with idiopathic thrombocytopenic purpura was admitted to hospital with gastrointestinal bleeding. He had previously been treated with prednisone, vincristine, splenectomy and Danazol without benefit. However, his thrombocytopenia had responded to regular infusions of immunoglobulin (Gamimune®). He also had a history of chronic alcoholism, gastritis and abnormal liver function tests. Eight months before admission, serum creatinine was 0.9 mg/dl. Admission laboratory values were hemoglobin 9.4 g/dl, platelet count 10,000 per mm^3, BUN 36 mg/dl, creatinine 2.3 mg/dl. Urinalysis showed 1+ protein and numerous red blood cells. A renal ultrasound was normal. There was no change in renal function during the first 5 days in hospital suggesting that the rise in creatinine from previous values was chronic rather than acute.

He was initially treated with intravenous immunoglobulin (Gamimune®) 90 g over 6–12 hours for three doses. Serum creatinine remained stable at 2.2 mg/dl and urine output was 2–2½ liters daily. However, on changing to a different immunoglobulin preparation (Sandoglobulin®) 93 g over 6 hours (1 g/kg body weight as a 6% solution), he experienced respiratory distress. During the first infusion he noticed wheezing and shortness of breath. The second infusion was complicated by dyspnea, bronchospasm and arterial hypoxemia (pO_2, 50 mmHg) which resolved on stopping the drug. Blood pressure remained unchanged and the patient's weight was noted to have increased by 2 kg. The chest radiograph showed acute pulmonary edema. During the next two days he became oliguric and serum creatinine rose rapidly to reach a peak of 7.9 mg/dl after 4 days. A renal biopsy was performed. The glomeruli showed mild diffuse mesangial proliferation with neither crescents nor focal necrosis. The proximal tubules showed widespread vacuolization with some cellular degeneration, loss of nuclei and sloughing of cells into the lumen. A few tubular cell mitoses were seen. In addition there was mild interstitial fibrosis with a sparse inflammatory infiltrate consisting of small lymphocytes. There were no eosinophils. On immunofluorescence there was trace granular staining in the mesangium for IgG, IgM, and C_3. These findings were interpreted as showing acute tubular injury superimposed upon chronic glomerular and interstitial disease of unknown etiology.

Before the results of the renal biopsy were available the patient was given methyl prednisolone 1 g intravenously for three days. Recovery of renal function was rapid and the serum creatinine returned to baseline within 2 weeks.

Case 2

A 73-year-old white male with idiopathic thrombocytopenic purpura was admitted for cataract surgery. Past medical history included adult onset diabetes mellitus, and congestive heart failure. Medications were NPH Insulin 48 units, Regular Insulin 5 units once daily, digoxin 0.125 mg once daily, furosemide 40 mg once daily and prednisone 5 mg once daily. He gave a history of allergy to penicillin. Admission laboratory values were hemoglobin 14.7 g/dl, WBC 8,100 per mm^3, platelet count 61,000 per mm^3, BUN 8 mg/dl, creatinine 1.0 mg/dl. Urinalysis was negative for protein and had 5–7 RBC per HPF. He was treated with immunoglobulin (Sandoglobulin®) 35 g (0.4 g/kg body weight as a 3.5% solution) intravenously over 6 hours. During the first infusion, he was noted to have an episode of shortness of breath. During the second infusion he became acutely distressed with wheezing, rigors and cyanosis. Blood pressure decreased from 130/90 to 92/62. Transient oliguria was noted and serum creatinine rose to 1.8 mg/dl. Urinalysis was unchanged. There were no eosinophils in the sediment, but urine sodium was less than 5 mEq/l. He was treated with oxygen, antihistamines and intravenous methyl prednisolone and transferred to the intensive care unit. At this stage a chest radiograph showed acute pulmonary edema, and the arterial pO_2 on 4 liters of oxygen was 72 mmHg. Further treatment included increased oral prednisone and intravenous diuretics. On the second day urine output increased although serum creatinine remained elevated at 1.5 mg/dl, and pulmonary symptoms improved. By the third day, his symptoms resolved and serum creatinine returned to baseline.

Case 3

A 69-year-old white male with chronic lymphocytic leukemia was admitted to the hospital with a history of fever, chills and presumed cellulitis of the chest wall. Medications included prednisone 10 mg p. o. twice daily and ciprofloxacin 750 mg p. o. twice daily. At the time of admission he was febrile with an area of redness and induration measuring 8 cm on the right anterior chest wall and axilla. Laboratory values on admission: hemoglobin 10 g/dl, WBC 1,700 per mm^3, creatinine 1.7 mg/dl, serum calcium 9.8 mg/dl, uric acid 6.6 mg/dl. Urinalysis: trace protein, 40–50 RBC per high power field. Renal ultrasound showed normal sized kidneys with slight increase in echogenicity and no hydronephrosis. He was treated with nafcillin 1 g every 4 hours, aztreonam 1 g every 8 hours, clindamycin 600 mg every 8 hours and continued on prednisone 10 mg twice daily. On the third hospital day, because of persistent leukopenia, he was started on intravenous immunoglobulin (Sandoglobulin®) 55 g over 8 hours (1 g/kg body weight as a 6% solution). The patient received three doses on consecutive days and complained of difficulty in breathing on the third day. On examination there were a few basilar crackles but no wheezing although the patient's weight had increased by 3 kg and a chest radiograph showed bilateral small pleural effusions. However, urine output dropped precipitously to less than 100 cm^3 in 24 hours, and, in retrospect it was clear that the oliguria had started on the second day of intravenous immunoglobulin. Serum creatinine rose to 6.0 mg/dl. Urinalysis showed proteinuria, 20–40 RBC per high power field, 2–4 WBC per high power field but no eosinophils. Urine sodium was less than 6 mEq/l. Both the immunoglobulin and nafcillin were stopped as potential causes of this syndrome and the patient was treated with diuretics and a single dose of methyl prednisolone 1 mg intravenously, followed by oral prednisone 60 mg daily. Renal biopsy could not be performed because of a prolonged bleeding time and the patient required two hemodialyses for volume overload. One week after the onset of oliguria, diuresis occurred and renal function rapidly returned to baseline.

Discussion

The clinical syndrome we observed in these three patients seems to be rather typical. On receiving intravenous immunoglobulin, the patient develops respiratory difficulty which may be mild or severe enough to cause acute respiratory failure. Urine output decreases abruptly but the oliguria is short-lived and urine output usually increases rapidly if the drug is discontinued. However, renal function as judged by serum creatinine, may continue to deteriorate for several days, followed by a return to baseline. There may be a disparity between the severity of the pulmonary and renal manifestations. Whereas both abnormalities were prominent in the first patient, the second patient developed respiratory failure with only mild renal impairment, and the third patient had minimal respiratory difficulty with acute renal failure requiring dialysis. Continued intravenous therapy during the period of oliguria results in fluid overload and radiological changes of acute pulmonary edema. Since we did not perform a systematic study of all patients receiving intravenous immunoglobulin, we are unable to calculate the incidence of this complication.

The close temporal relationship between infusion of the drug and the onset of clinical manifestations is the strongest evidence for a cause and effect relationship. However, no attempt was made to confirm this hypothesis by rechallenging the patients with intravenous immunoglobulin. Two of the patients had mild baseline renal insufficiency but whether this predisposed them to develop acute renal failure is unclear. With regard to the acute renal failure, no other precipitating factor could be identified in cases 1 and 2. Case 3, however, was receiving other drugs capable of causing renal disease, in particular nafcillin. This drug is known to cause acute interstitial nephritis and, in the absence of a renal biopsy, we cannot totally exclude this as the cause of the renal disease. However, there are a number of reasons why acute interstitial nephritis seems unlikely in this patient. Firstly, there was no skin rash, eosinophilia or eosinophiluria. Secondly, the patient did not respond promptly to high-dose prednisone therapy but had persistent acute renal failure for one week. Such a delayed response to intravenous methyl prednisolone makes drug-induced acute interstitial nephritis unlikely.

The mechanism whereby a systemic reaction to intravenous immunoglobulin leads to acute renal failure is obscure. There was no clinical evidence of volume depletion and, although case 2 had a modest decrease in blood pressure, none of the patients became severely hypotensive. In the absence of evident circulatory compromise a direct effect on the kidneys seems most likely. The abrupt onset of oliguria (one patient was anuric for 24 hours), together with the extremely low urine sodium in cases 2 and 3, suggest renal hypoperfusion. A sudden decrease in renal blood flow would explain this initial picture of prerenal or hemodynamically induced renal impairment, followed by acute tubular necrosis as shown on the renal biopsy in case 1 and suggested by the clinical course in case 3. Although renal blood flow is decreased in most types of acute renal failure, the clinical and urinary findings in our patients would suggest an ischemic rather than a nephrotoxic insult to the kidneys. How this decrease in renal blood flow is mediated remains unexplained.

Patients with IgA deficiency treated with intravenous immunoglobulin may develop antibodies to IgA and suffer severe reactions during the infusion [Hopkins 1985]. However, none of the patients described here had IgA deficiency. It is perhaps significant that all three patients reacted to a specific immunoglobulin preparation (Sandoglobulin®). This differs from other immunoglobulins for intravenous use in that it contains a higher proportion of larger molecular weight aggregates (IgG dimers) and such aggregates may be responsible for some of the unpleasant symptoms experienced by patients [Herrera et al. 1989]. The first patient, for example tolerated a different immunoglobulin preparation without difficulty. Large molecular weight aggregates have been shown to activate complement, but in the absence of detailed studies of the complement system in our patients, we cannot say whether this would provide an explanation for the syndrome described. Moreover, the paucity of immunoglobulin deposition in the one renal biopsy sample is evidence against an immunological mechanism and raises the possibility that vasoactive substances present as contaminants acted directly on the renal vasculature.

Some unusual causes of acute renal failure, recognized in recent years, might also be relevant to our observations. Drugs such as mannitol and dextran which raise plasma oncotic pressure are occasionally associated with renal dysfunction [Moran et al. 1987]. It seems unlikely that this mechanism was operative in our patients. The dose of intravenous immunoglobulin (0.4–1 mg/kg body weight) was not excessive and, unlike the agents mentioned above, globulins exert only a modest effect on oncotic pressure. Immunotherapy with interleukin-2 is another recently described cause of transient renal dysfunction [Belldegrun et al. 1987]. Since our patients had both acute renal insufficiency and acute pulmonary edema it is tempting to invoke a lymphokine-mediated effect on vascular permeability. However, there is no evidence that intravenous immunoglobulins cause release of lymphokines and this possibility must be regarded as speculative.

Summary

In summary, we have presented three patients with pulmonary and renal dysfunction closely related to intravenous immunoglobulin therapy. The absence of other potential insults to these systems and the rapid resolution of the syndrome on stopping the immunoglobulin support a casual relationship in these cases. The pathophysiology of these reactions to intravenous immunoglobulin is unclear.

REFERENCES

Barandum S, Morell A 1981 Adverse reactions to immunoglobulin preparations. In: *Nydegger UE* (ed). Immunohemotherapy. A guide to immunoglobulin prophylaxis and therapy. Academic Press, London, pp 223–227

Barton JC, Herrera GA, Galla JH, Bertoli LF, Work J, Koopman WJ 1987 Acute cryoglobulinemic renal failure after intravenous infusion of gamma globulin. Am J Med *82:* 624–629

Belldegrun A, Webb DE, Austin HA III, Steinberg SM, White DE, Linehan WM, Rosenberg SA 1987 Effects of interleukin-2 on renal function in patients receiving immunotherapy for advanced cancer. Ann Intern Med *106:* 817–822

Bussel JB, Cunningham-Rundles C 1985 Intravenous usage of gammaglobulin: humoral immunodeficiency, immune thrombocytopenic purpura, and newer indications. Cancer Invest *3:* 361–366

Dwyer JM 1987 Intravenous therapy with gamma globulin. Adv Intern Med *32:* 111–136

Herrera AM, Saunders NB, Baker JR 1989 Immunoglobulin composition of three commercially available intravenous immunoglobulin preparations. J Allergy Clin Immunol *84:* 556–561

Hopkins SJ 1985 Sandoglobulin®. Drugs Today *21:* 279–282

Moran M, Kapsner C 1987 Acute renal failure associated with elevated plasma oncotic pressure. N Engl J Med *317:* 150–152

Clinical Nephrology, Vol. 36 No. 2 – 1991 (87–92)

Correlation of renal organic anion and cation transport with blood pressure in SHR

N. Gharib, C. Y. Gao, J. L. Areas, M. EL Zein and H. G. Preuss

Georgetown University Medical Center, Department of Medicine, Nephrology Division, Department of Pathology, Washington D. C., USA

Abstract. In 1974, we found that sera from SHR suppressed renal PAH transport (PSEBM 145:97, 1974). Since a "natriuretic factor" depresses PAH as well as Na transport, we proposed that "natriuretic factor" was elevated in SHR. Our current investigation amplifies the previous study. On a given day, one spontaneously hypertensive rat (SHR) and one rat from a normotensive strain [Wistar Kyoto (WKY) or Sprague-Dawley (SD)] were examined together. SHR sera compared to WKY/SD sera significantly depress PAH (organic anion) and TEA (organic cation) uptake by rat renal slices. The ability of SHR sera to depress uptake correlated significantly with the BP: the sera with the greatest depressive influence on renal PAH and TEA uptake came from the SHR with the highest BP (PAH $r = 0.89$, $p < 0.0001$; TEA = $r = 0.76$, $p < 0.01$). Subsequent separation of serum on Sephadex 25 localized the factor to the same fraction as "natriuretic hormone". A similar correlation was found between the ability of the fraction to depress the 2 transports and the height of the BP. The serum factor did not inhibit ATPase activity. In contrast to the serum effects, renal slices removed from SHR showed increased rather than decreased PAH and TEA transport which significantly correlated with the BP. The slices with the highest uptakes came from the SHR with the highest BP. The high uptake of organic ions by the SHR renal slices could be an adaptive response to the serum factor or vice versa. We postulate that a serum factor which depresses PAH and TEA transport and is not "ouabain-like" may play a role in the BP elevation of SHR.

Key words: organic anion-cation transport – transport perturbations – SHR

Introduction

At present, many investigators believe that a circulating factor is important in the pathogenesis of hypertension. In 1969, Dahl, Knudson and Iwai proposed that a circulating substance elevates arterial pressure in salt sensitive rats [Dahl et al. 1969]. However, this proposal was based upon parabiotic studies, which are difficult to control. More direct proof was necessary. Theoretical considerations predict that *in vitro* systems could be used more profitably to associate a circulating humoral substance with hypertension, since they would allow dissociation of the complex physiological changes which accompany parabiotic studies. In 1974, Preuss et al. [1974a] showed via *in vitro* studies that elevated levels of a circulating transport inhibitor exist in spontaneously hypertensive rats (SHR). This work was based on organic anion and cation uptake in incubating rat kidney slices. Compared to renal slices from normotensive rats, SHR renal slices transported more PAH and TEA [Preuss et al. 1974b], but sera from SHR compared to normotensive rats depressed both transport systems [Preuss et al. 1974a]. Since then, many different type experiments have suggested the presence of an inciting factor [Blaustein 1977, Bucklew and Haddy 1989].

The present investigation extends findings from our previous studies, i. e., as a first approximation, we determined how the changes in the organic ion transport systems correlate with the BP and to ascertain if the circulating inhibitors work through ATPase inhibition.

Material and methods

Control normotensive rats, either Wistar Kyoto rats (WKY) or Sprague-Dawley rats (SD), and spontaneously hypertensive rats (SHR) (200–250 g) were studied. All rats received water and Purina Rat Chow *ad libitum.*

Received October 2, 1990; in revised form March 11, 1991.

Reprint requests to Dr. H. G. Preuss, Georgetown University Medical Center, Nephrology Division, Washington, D. C. 200007, USA.

On an experimental day, blood was drawn from the aorta of a normotensive rat (either SD or WKY) and an SHR and stored at 2° C. In some cases, blood pressures (BP) were taken on the paired normotensive and hypertensive rats by tail plethysmography prior to bleeding [Bunag 1973]. Then, the kidneys were removed rapidly and placed in cold isotonic saline. Cortical slices (0.4 mm) were cut with a Stadie-Riggs microtome for assay of transport. The basic incubation medium was that described by Cross and Taggart [1950] and contained Na pyruvate (10 mmol). To this was added ^{14}C-tetraethylammonium bromide (TEA) (1–5 mCi/mmol) and ^{3}H-paraaminohippurate (PAH) (5–15 mCi/mmol) to a concentration of 10 M. To estimate PAH and TEA transport, slices were incubated for 90 min at 24° C on a Dubnoff shaker. Slice weights ranged between 60 and 65 mg, and a minimum of 4 flasks was studied for each rat. Slices were placed in 10% trichloroacetic acid, centrifuged, and the supernate counted. The basic scintillation mixture was composed of Triton X-100 (⅓ volume), Toluene (⅔ volume), 2,5-diphenyloxazole (5.5 g) and 1,4 Bis-(2-4-methyl-5-phenyloxazole) benzene (125 g). Double isotope Beta counting and quench corrections were performed utilizing a Packard Beta Counter.

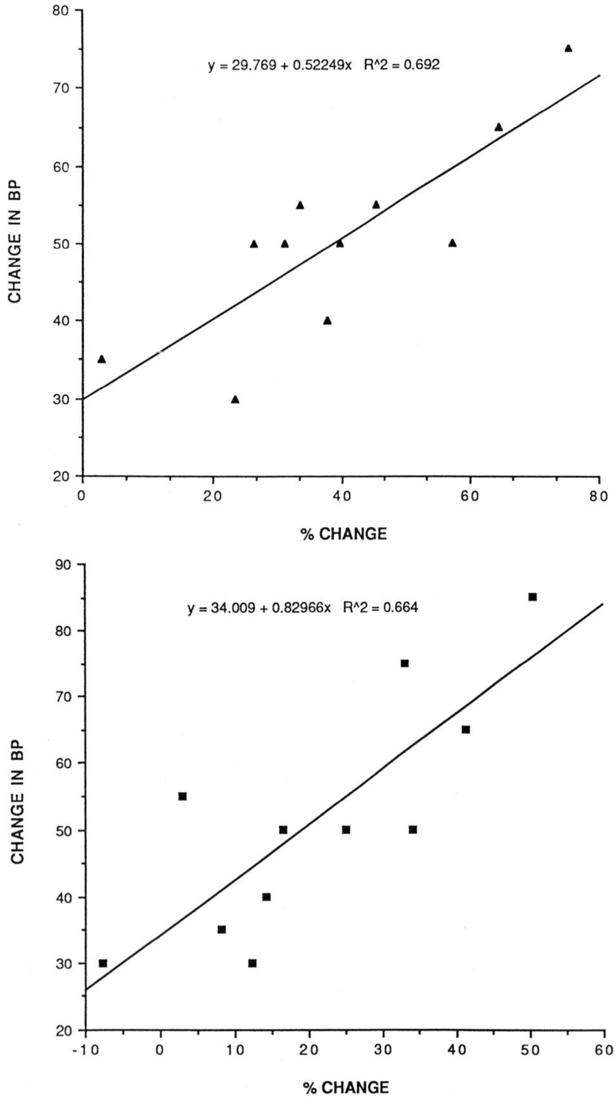

Fig. 1 Comparison of the difference in PAH uptake (upper figure) and TEA uptake (lower figure) in kidney slices from SHR versus kidney slices from SD/WKY

Results of organic ion uptake studies are expressed as S/M ratios, i. e., the ratio of counts per minute per gram of slice weight (S) to the counts per minute per milliliter of incubation medium (M). We expected wide, daily variations in renal slice organic ion transport based on previous experiences [Koishi 1959, Preuss et al. 1974a, Areas et al. 1987]. Therefore, we compared values obtained from a test and control situation on a given day. In one case, kidney slices from a normotensive rat (SD, WKY) and a hypertensive rat (SHR) were arbitrarily paired. Results were expressed as a difference in BP (change in BP) and as an S/M quotient (% of change in the ratio of the test S/M and the control S/M). In the sera studies, a single slice was halved; one half was incubated in the experimental flask containing SHR serum and the other half was incubated in a control flask containing sera from the normotensive rats (SD, WKY). Whether we examined slice function or serum effects, a minimum of 4 flasks were examined and results were averaged. This methodology was first used by Koishi [1959] who originally defined the S/M quotient as the ratio of the S/M of the experimental flask compared to the S/M of the control flask.

To assess how sera from the rat substrains influence ATPase activity, we followed the method described by Finotti and Palatini [1981]. ATPase activity was assessed by the Fiske and Subbarow [1925] phosphate assay. Thirty to 40 µg of enzyme preparation were incubated at 37° C for 10 minutes in 1 ml of medium containing: NaCl, 100 mM; KCl, 20 mM; MgCl, 3 mM; ATP-Tris, 3 mM; Tris-HCl (pH 7.4), 50 mM; EDTA, 0.2 mM; phosphoenolpyruvate, 2 mM; and pyruvate kinase, 30 µg. After equilibration, the reaction was started by the addition of enzyme and stopped by the addition of 0.25 ml of cold 50% trichloroacetic acid. ATPase activity was estimated in the presence of ouabain (O), sera from normotensive rats (NR), sera from hypertensive rats (SHR), or various combinations of these.

Fractions of sera were obtained by methods previously described [Bourgoignie et al. 1971, Preuss et al. 1974]. Sera were applied to Sephadex G-25 in a room with a temperature of 2° C. All pooled fractions were lyophilized and then reconstituted in isotonic saline or water to the original volume of the sera.

Statistics were performed by the paired Student's t-test when 2 columns were present. To analyze differences among more than 2 columns, ANOVA was performed. If the ANOVA showed statistical significance, difference between groups were analyzed by the Scheffe F test. Regression analysis was determined by the least squares method. Statistical significance was determined by a $p < 0.05$.

Results

Tissue PAH and TEA transport

We found a significant increase in PAH uptake by SHR kidney slices incubated in medium (without

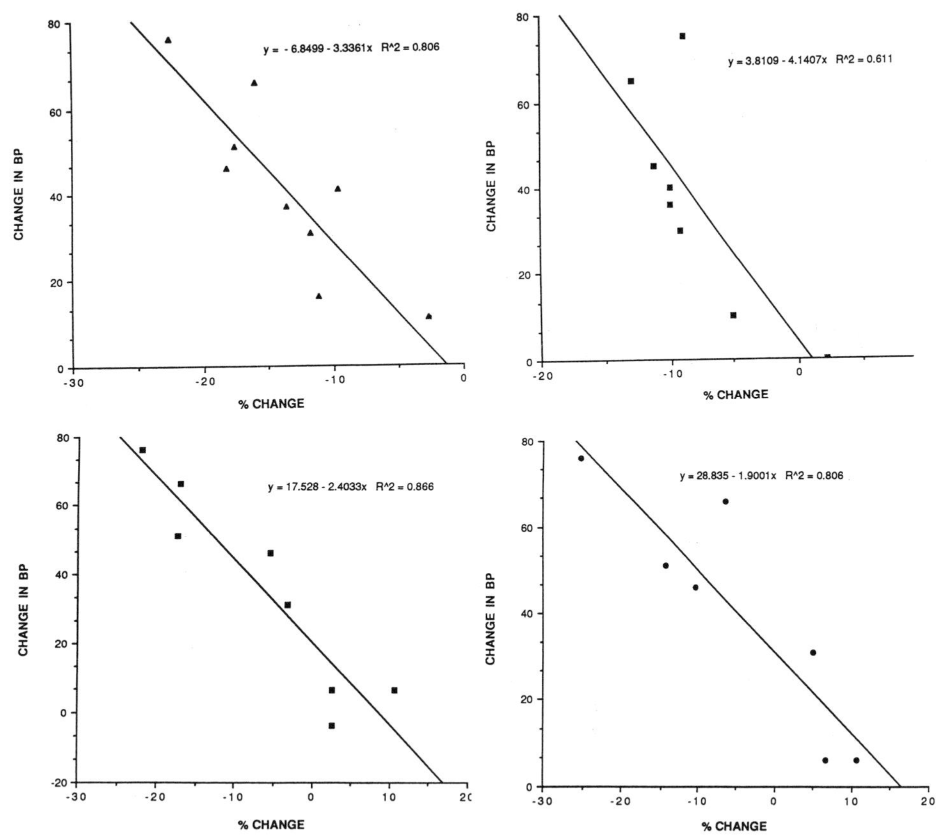

Fig. 2 Depiction of the difference in the depressive effect on renal PAH or TEA uptake of paired SHR sera or fraction 4 of the sera compared to SD/WKY sera or fraction 4 (10% v/v) correlated with the difference in BP between the rats. LUQ = effects of sera on PAH uptake; RUQ = effects of sera on TEA uptake; LLQ = effects of fraction 4 on PAH uptake; RLQ = effects of fraction 4 on TEA uptake.

sera) compared to that from normotensive rats (SD and WKY) incubated under the same conditions (+39.3% + 6.1 [SEM], n = 11, p <0.01). Results were not different whether slices from SD or WKY were used as baseline. These differences between rat pairs studied on a given day, represented as % PAH change of the S/M ratios between the hypertensive and normotensive rats (S/M quotient), showed a linear correlation with the differences in blood pressure (ΔBP) between the pair (Figure 1, top). The slices with the highest uptake came from the SHR with the highest BP. Similarly, TEA transport was increased in SHR compared to kidney slices from normotensive rats (+19% + 5.0 [SEM], n = 11, p <0.01). In addition, we found that this difference in transport (S/M quotient) again showed a linear correlation with ΔBP in the studies where the latter was obtained (Figure 1, bottom).

Effect of sera on PAH and TEA transport

In contrast to the tissue study, sera (10% v/v) from SHR influenced PAH in kidney slices differently. Using slices from SD rats, SHR sera significantly depressed PAH uptake when compared to the effects of sera (10% v/v) from SD or WKY (−11.1% + 3.0 [SEM], n = 20, p <0.01). Importantly, the magnitude of the depression correlated significantly with the difference in BP measured in 8 experiments (Figure 2, LUQ). The sera showing the greatest depression came from the SHR with the highest BP. For TEA transport, the SHR sera also showed a depressive effect on TEA (−9.3% + 2.6% [SEM], n = 20, p <0.01) that correlated with BP (Figure 2, RUQ).

Serum fractions

Based on previous experience, fractions were obtained by passing serum through Sephadex 25 [Bourgoignie et al. 1971, Preuss et al. 1974]. We found that fraction 4 from SD and WKY sera (10% v/v) compared to fraction 4 from SHR sera significantly depressed transport (−11.1% + 3.6% [SEM], n = 11, p <0.01). This depressive effect (% PAH change) correlated significantly with the difference in BP between the rat pairs examined on a given day (Figure 2, LLQ). Similar findings were obtained with TEA transport (−8.3% + 3.5 [SEM], n = 11, p <0.05). We found a significant correlation between % TEA uptake change with fraction 4 from SHR compared to that from SD or WKY sera and with the difference in BP between the rat pairs (Figure 2, RLQ).

To determine the effects of other serum fractions on PAH and TEA transport, we performed similar-type experiments.

Interestingly, we found a significant stimulatory response with fraction 1 from SHR on PAH (29% + 5 [SEM], n = 4, p <0.05) and TEA (69% + 10 [SEM], n = 4, p <0.05) transport compared to that from SD and WKY, while fraction 2 from SHR showed a slight inhibitory effect on PAH and TEA transport compared to that from SD or WKY. Fraction 3 of SHR also showed slight inhibition of PAH, not TEA uptake; and fraction 5 of SHR had a slight stimulatory effect on both PAH and TEA. The differences in fractions 2, 3, and 5 were not significantly different (Figure 3).

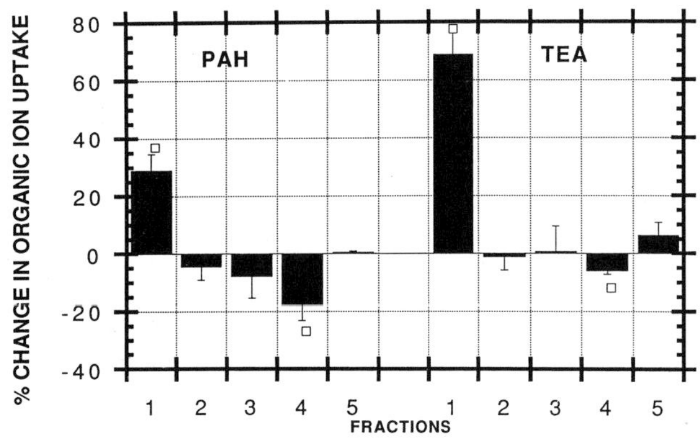

Fig. 3 Depiction of the effects of various serum fractions from SHR compared to the same fraction from WKY/SD on PAH and TEA uptake by kidney slices. Statistically significant difference between SHR and NR

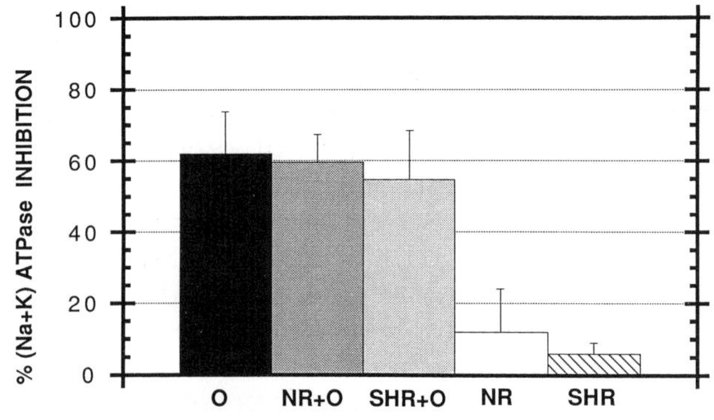

Fig. 4 Inhibition of Na/K ATPase activity by ouabain alone (0); Sera from normotensive SD/WKY + ouabain (NR + 0); sera from SHR + ouabain (SHR + 0); from SD/WKY sera alone (NR); and SHR sera alone (SHR). Amount of sera added was 10% v/v.

Effects on Na-K ATPase activity

To determine how SHR sera (SHR) affect PAH and TEA transport, we tested the influence of SHR and SD sera (NR) (10% v/v) on ATPase activity (Figure 4). We compared the effects of sera to a known cardiac glycoside ATPase inhibitor (ouabain). Serum inhibition was assayed with and without ouabain addition to establish whether a circulating inhibitory factor would show an additive inhibition to ouabain. There was no significant ATPase activity inhibition with SHR sera (−10% + 10 [SEM], n = 4, p = NS) or sera from normotensive rats (NR), (−5.0% + 3.0 [SEM], n = 4, p = NS). Similar results were obtained by replacing whole sera with similar amounts (10% v/v) of fraction 4 from SD and SHR. There was also no inhibition with fraction 4 from SHR or SD (data not shown).

Discussion

Many investigative reports suggest an important role for a circulating factor influencing transport in the regulation of BP [Clarkson et al. 1970, Haddy 1984] presumably through its ability to alter intracellular calcium concentrations [Blaustein 1977, Buckalew and Haddy 1989]. Enhancing this likelihood, high levels of a circulating factor(s) have been found in various forms of experimental [Buckalew and Azer 1984, DeWardener et al. 1981, Haddy 1984] and essential [Devynck 1983, Hamlyn et al. 1982] hypertension. However, the presence of this factor(s) in the spontaneously hypertensive rat of the Okamoto strain (SHR) is still a matter of controversy [Wauquier et al. 1988].

Conflicting results have emanated from *in vivo* work investigating a circulating hypertensive factor in SHR. The early studies of Yamori [1971] on the effects of parabiosis between SHR and Wistar Kyoto rats (WKY) failed to provide evidence for a circulating hypertensive substance in SHR. According to a few reports, however, SHR plasma contains some unidentified substance(s) able to modify the characteristics of vascular smooth muscle. Greenburg et al. [1981] demonstrated that the BP of WKY in parabiosis with SHR increased slowly during the first four weeks of parabiotic union with SHR, then rapidly over the next 3 months, to reach the same pressure levels as those of the SHR strain. Wright [1981] reported that plasma from SHR enhanced the responsiveness of arterial strips to norepinephrine more than did the plasma from WKY or SD rats and that SHR blood contains a substance that produces an elevation of BP in normotensive rats [Wright and McCumbee 1984]. The observation by Murtry et al. [1981] that normotensive rat pups raised by SHR mothers had a sustained elevation in their BP compared with pups left with their natural mothers has been interpreted as a consequence of either the hyperkinetic behavior of the mother or the transmission by the mother's milk of a substance that increases systolic BP in the young normotensive rat.

Many investigators have postulated that the circulating factor produces hypertension through its effects on sodium transport. However, *in vitro* work has not completely clarified this point in SHR. Experiments on cell Na transport did not confirm that active Na transport inhibitors are present in SHR plasma. Studies of plasma-induced changes in Na fluxes from erythrocytes [DeMendoca et al. 1982, Feig et al. 1985], white blood cells, or rat thymocytes [Swales et al. 1984] favor the participation of an inherited membrane defect in SHR, rather than the participation of a plasma substance. Accordingly, circulating factors need not be involved. However, this does not necessarily mean that they are not.

In 1974, Preuss et al. [1974a], using *in vitro* studies, reported that SHR sera contain an inhibitor to PAH transport and raised the possibility that the inhibitor was the previously described natriuretic factor [Bricker and Klahr 1968]. Bricker's group prepared extracts of serum from dialyzed and nondialyzed patients with chronic renal failure, from patients with acute renal failure, and from normal subjects. The natriuretic factor, eluted with 0.01 M ammonium acetate, was found in the fraction emerging after the salt peak from a Sephadex G-25 column. This fraction, labelled 4, inhibited PAH uptake by rabbit renal cortical slices and caused a marked decrease in the Na transport across frog skin or toad bladder. Clarkson et al. [1970] repeated and extended this work. Fragments of rabbit renal tubules were incubated in dog plasma obtained before and after blood volume expansion with equilibrated blood. Bricker's findings were confirmed when the ability of the tubule fragments to concentrate PAH and Na was reduced following incubation in plasma obtained after blood volume expansion (the experimental plasma). It was concluded that this was due to a change in the concentration of a circulating transport inhibitor. We have also found that Na loading of rats results in a depressive factor for PAH transport being present in the blood [Areas et al. 1987].

The studies reported here corroborate our previous work on SHR [Preuss et al. 1974a]. Sera and serum fraction 4 of SHR inhibited both organic anion (PAH) and organic cation (TEA) uptake by incubating renal slices. However, the additional data also show a close correlation between the ability of sera to depress transport and the elevation of BP. Although we presume from previous findings that the substance could be natriuretic as well, the strong parallel between alterations in organic ion transport with BP suggests a role in the pathogenesis whether or not the assumption is correct.

In many ways, our findings concerning tissue uptake of PAH and TEA simulate previous ones dealing with Na transport. Defects in Na transport have been described in various epithelial and nonepithelial cells in animal models of hypertension. For example, various perturbations have been described in erythrocytes [DeMendonca et al. 1982, Feig et al. 1985], in white blood cells or thymocytes [Swales et al. 1984] and, most importantly, in the kidney [Bianchi et al. 1974]. It has been postulated that hypertensive animals possess an increased "leak" of the Na pump in these cells [Haddy and Pamnani 1983]. The latter may be coupled with PAH and TEA transport and cause the relatively enhanced PAH and TEA transport we find in the renal slices of SHR. Accordingly, the serum and tissue effects may be interdependent. It remains to be seen whether the inhibitory effect of sera on transport precedes the enhanced tissue transport or vice versa, i.e., to determine if one adaptation causes the other.

The exact mechanism through which the circulating inhibitor of SHR works is not apparent. Our results suggest that it is not due to an influence on Na/K ATPase. Many have described ouabain-like substances in the blood of essential hypertensives and some animal models of hypertension. With few exception [Wauquier et al. 1988], the majority of reports have failed to show that a ouabain-like factor exists in SHR [Hannaert et al. 1985–86]. In support, the agent canrenone, which competes with ouabain for a common receptor, can decrease BP in models where ouabain-like factors play a significant role, however, it is ineffective in SHR [DeMendonca et al. 1988]. Therefore, we believe the agent affecting organic ion transport in SHR does not work via Na/K ATPase inhibition. Comparing results between SHR and other models of hypertension [DeMendonca et al. 1988] indicates that different circulating factors influencing transport are involved in the pathogenesis of hypertension.

Acknowledgements

Supported by NIH grant AG 06929.

REFERENCES

Areas J, Slemmer D, Balien S, Gao CY, Preuss HG 1987 Effects of sera from uninephrectomized rats on renal slices: PAH and TEA uptake and QO2. Nephron *45:* 59

Bianchi G, Fox U, Di Francesci GF, Giovanetti AM, Pagetti D 1974 Blood pressure changes by kidney cross transplantation between spontaneously hypertensive rats (SHR) and normotensive rats. Clin Sci Mol Med *47:* 435

Blaustein MP 1977 Sodium ions, calcium ions, blood pressure regulation and hypertension: A reassessment and a hypothesis. Am J Physiol *232:* C165

Bourgoignie JJ, Hwang KH, Espinel C, Klahr S, Bricker NS 1977 A natriuretic factor in the serum of patients with chronic uremia. J Clin Invest *51:* 1514

Bourgoignie JJ, Klahr S, Bricker NS 1971 Inhibition of transepithelial sodium transport in the frog skin by a low molecular weight fraction of uremic serum. J Clin Invest *50:* 303

Bricker NS, Klahr S 1968 In-vitro assay for a humoral substance present during volume expansion and uremia. Nature, London *219:* 1058

Buckalew WM, Azer M 1984 Natriuretic and sodium transport inhibitory activity in plasma of volume-expanded dogs. Kidney Int *5:* 12

Buckalew VM, Haddy FJ 1989 The role of digitalis-like factor in the pathophysiology of hypertension. In: *Laragh JH, Brenner BM, Kaplan NM* (eds). Endocrine Mechanisms of Hypertension. Raven Press, New York, NY p 307

Bunag RD 1973 Validation in awake rats of a tail-cuff method for measuring systolic pressure. J Appl Physiol *34:* 279

Clarkson EM, Talner LB, deWardener HE 1970 The effect of plasma from blood volume expanded dogs on sodium, potassium and PAH transport of renal tubule fragments. Clin Sci *38:* 617

Cross LK, Taggart JV 1950 Accumulation of p-aminohippurate by rabbit kidney slices. Am J Physiol *161:* 181

Dahl LK, Knudsen KD, Iwai J 1969 Humoral transmission of hypertension: evidence from parabiosis. Circ Res *1* (Suppl 24, 25): 21

DeMendonca M, Grichois ML, Pernollet MG, Wauquier I, Trouillet-Thorman B, Meyer P, Devynck MA, Garay R 1988 Antihypertensive effect of canrenone in a model where endogenous Ouabain-like factors are present. J Cardiovasc Pharmacol *11:* 75

DeMendonca M, Knorr A, Grichois ML, Ben-Ishay D, Garay R, Meyer P 1982 Erythrocyte sodium ion transport systems in primary and secondary hypertension of the rat. Kid Int *21* (11): 569

Devynck MA, Pernollet MG, Rosenfold JB, Meyer P 1983. Measurement of digitalis-like compound in plasma: application in studies of essential hypertension. Br Med J (Clin Res) *287:* 631

DeWardener HE, MacGregor GA, Clarkson EM 1981 Effect of sodium intake on ability of human plasma to inhibit renal Na+ – K+ adenosine triphosphatase in vitro. Lancet *i:* 411

Feig PU, Mitchell PP, Boylan JW 1985 Erythrocyte membrane transport in hypertensive humans and rats: Effects of sodium depletion and excess. Hypertension *7:* 423

Finotti P, Palatini P 1981 Canrenone as a partial agonist at the digitalis receptor site of sodium-potassium-activated adenosine triphosphatase. J Pharmacol Ex Ther *50:* 303

Fiske CH, Subbarow Y 1925 The colorimetric determination of phosphorus. J Biol Chem *66:* 375

Greenberg S, Gaines K, Sweatt D 1981 Evidence for circulating factors as a cause of venous hypertrophy in spontaneously hypertensive rats. Am J Physiol *241:* H421

Haddy FJ 1984 The role of a numoral Na+ – K+ ATP'ase inhibitor in regulating precapillary vessel tone. J Cardiovasc Pharmacol 6 (Suppl 2): S439

Haddy FJ, Pamnani MB 1983 The role of a humoral sodium-potassium pump inhibitor in low-renin hypertension. Federation Proc *42:* 2673

Hamlyn JM, Ringel R, Schaeffer J, Levinson PD, Hamilton BP, Kowarski AA, Blaustein MP 1982 A circulating inhibitor of Na+ – K+ ATP'ase associated with essential hypertension. Nature *300:* 650

Hanneart P, deMendonca M, Grichois ML, Nazaret C, Abitbol JP, Garay R 1985–86. Involvement of natriuretic hormones and Na+ transport in the antihypertensive action of canrenone. Uremia Investiation 9 (2): 195

Koishi T 1959 Studies on renal tubular transport. 1. Accumulation of p-amino-hippurate by kidney slices. Jap J Pharmacol Exper Therap *8:* 101

Murtry JP, Wright GL, Wexler BC 1981 Spontaneous hypertension in cross suckled rats. Science *211:* 1173

Preuss HG, Grant LD, Parris RC, Zmudka M, Slotkoff LM 1974a Effects of sera and sera fractions from spontaneously hypertensive rats on renal organic anion and cation transport. Proc Soc Exp Bio Med *145:* 397

Preuss HG, Shim PS, Baird K, Gibbings T, Parris R, Grant K, Schreiner GE 1974 PAH in kidney slices from spontaneously hypertensive and normotensive Wistar Rats. Proc Soc Exp Bio Med *147:* 839

Swales JD, Bing RF, Bradlaugh R, El-Ashry A, Godfrey N, Heagerty AM, Thurston H 1984 Cell membrane handling of sodium, sodium balance and blood pressure. J Cardiovasc Pharmacol *6:* S42

Wauquier I, Pernollet MG, Grichois ML, Lacour B, Meyer P, Devynck MA 1988 Endogenous digitalis-like circulation substances in spontaneously hypertensive rats. Hypertension *12:* 108

Wright GL 1981 The vascular sensitizing character of plasma from spontaneously hypertensive rats. Can J Physiol Pharmacol *59:* 1111

Wright GL, McCumbee WE 1984 A hypertensive substance found in the blood of spontaneously hypertensive rats. Life Sci *31:* 1521

Yamori Y 1971 Parabiotic effect on blood pressure in spontaneously hypertensive rats. Jpn Circ J *35:* 821

Clinical Nephrology, Vol. 36 No. 2 – 1991 (93–96)

Renal vasoconstriction after low and high osmolar contrast agents in ischemic and non ischemic canine kidney

G. DERAY, B. BAUMELOU, F. MARTINEZ, G. BRILLET and C. JACOBS

Department of Nephrology, Hôpital de la Pitié, Paris, France

Abstract. We have assessed the effect of contrast media on renal blood flow before and after inducing renal ischemia. Diatrizoate, iopamidol and ioxaglate were injected within 15 seconds at 20 min intervals, at the dose of 1 ml/kg during a control period and 15 min after applying an aortic clamp to reduce the renal perfusion pressure to 70 mmHg. During the control period iopamidol, ioxaglate (17 ± 13%) and diatrizoate (16 ± 2%) induced a comparable decrease in renal blood flow (RBF). During the ischemic period the effects of diatrizoate on renal hemodynamic were dramatically enhanced. Ioxaglate and iopamidol induced a 20 ± 12 and a 32 ± 9% decrease in RBF at 1 minute, respectively. Iopamidol induced an increase in renal vascular resistance (RVR) from 0.8 ± 0.08 to 1.46 ± 0.26 mmHg min/ml ($p < 0.05$). Ioxaglate induced an increase in RVR from 0.8 ± 0.09 to 1.36 ± 0.38 ($p < 0.05$). Diatrizoate induced a 77 ± 10% decrease in RBF and a maximum increase in RVR at 1 minute from 0.9 ± 0.09 to 26 ± 12 mmHg min/ml. There was still a 36 ± 14% and a 23 ± 13% decrease in RBF 10 and 20 min after diatrizoate administration. These changes were significantly higher than those observed with all contrast media during the control period and low osmolar contrast media during the ischemic period. We have thus shown that ischemia potentiates the renal vascular effect of contrast media. This experiment provides substantial support for the thesis according to which contrast media induced renal failure may be primarily caused by renal ischemia. During ischemia low osmolar contrast agents induced less vasoconstriction and may therefore particularly indicated in high risk patients.

Key words: renal ischemia – renal blood flow (RBF) – renal vascular resistance (RVR)

Introduction

Radiographic contrast agent-induced acute renal failure is now a widely recognized clinical event [Cronin 1988, Hou et al. 1983]. The increasing use of diagnostic and interventional radiographic procedures in acutely ill and high-risk patients provides a better understanding of the pathophysiology of this crucial disorder. Multiple factors have been implicated in radiocontrast agent-induced acute renal failure, including renal vasoconstriction, hypertonicity, intratubular precipitation of urinary proteins and direct toxic effects on renal tubular cells [Humes et al. 1987, Tornquist et al. 1985, Talner et al. 1972].

Animal experiments have shown that intravenous or intra-arterial infusion of contrast medium in a clinically acceptable dose produces only minor transient alterations in total renal blood flow (Tornquist et al. 1985, Talner et al. 1972].

However, the renal impairment occurs more frequently in patients with preexisting renal disease, diabetes mellitus, atherosclerosis, severe renal artery stenosis, or cardiac failure [Cronin 1988, Hou et al. 1983].

All these situations have in common alterations in renal hemodynamics leading to ischemic lesions of variable magnitude. It has already been shown that dehydration potentiates the vasoconstrictive effects of contrast media [Larson et al. 1983]. We postulated that in the setting of severe renal ischemia the renal hemodynamic effects of contrast media might be enhanced. Therefore the aim of this study was to assess the renal vasoconstriction induced by contrast media before and after inducing renal ischemia.

Methods

Animal preparation

The study was performed on either male or female adult mongrel dogs weighing 16 to 22 kg

Reprint requests to Dr. G. Deray, Service de Néphrologie, Hôpital de la Pitié, 83, bd de l'Hôpital, F-Paris 75013, France.

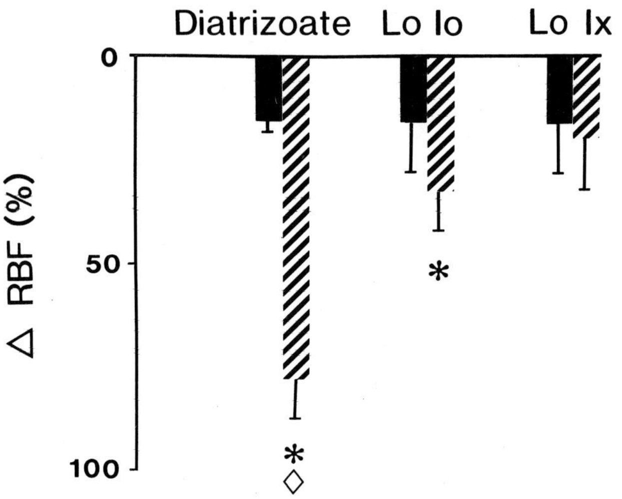

Fig. 1 Maximum decrease in renal blood flow (RBF) after contrast media administration
RBF is expressed as percentage decrease from basal value.
LO: low osmolar contrast média (Ioxaglate and Iopamidol).
IO: Iopamidol, IX: Ioxaglate, ■: Control, ▨: Ischemic period.
*p <0.05 compared with non ischemic period. p <0.05 compared with low osmolar contrast media during the ischemic period.

Table 1 The experimental protocol

Recovery after surgery ↓	Control period	Aortic clamp	↓	↓	↓
60 min	30 min	15 min	20 min	20 min	20 min
		Ischemic period			

↓: Intra renal contrast media administration

(n = 8). Animals were deprived of food and water overnight. On the day of the experiment the animals were anesthetized with vetranquil 0.25 $mg \cdot kg^{-1}$ and pentobarbital sodium 30 $mg \cdot kg^{-1}$, supplemented as needed to maintain surgical anesthesia, intubated, and ventilated by a fixed volume positive pressure respirator on room air. Cannules were placed in the femoral artery for blood pressure recording and blood sampling and in the saphenous vein for drug infusions.

A catheter for renal arteriography was inserted into the right femoral artery and positioned in the right renal artery during contrast medium injection. The right kidney and renal artery were isolated and exposed through an abdominal anterior incision. An electromagnetic flow probe was then placed around the renal artery for determination of renal blood flow (RBF). The electromagnetic flow probe was electronically nulled and zeroed and the zero was checked by momentarilly occluding the renal artery. A Blalock clamp was applied on the aorta just above the origin of the left renal artery such that renal artery perfusion pressure could be controlled during the experiment. At the end of surgery the abdominal cavity was closed and the dogs were allowed to stabilize for 60 minutes.

Experimental protocol

The experimental protocol is shown in Table 1. Eight dogs were studied for 2 periods each. During the first period referred as control and once RBF had stabilized a renal arteriography was performed under fluoroscopic control with an image intensifier (kalliscop CGR Inc.) and television screen during the administration of either meglumine diatrizoate sodium (Radioselectan*) (high osmolar contrast media) (n = 4), iopamidol (iopamiron*) (non ionic low osmolar contrast medium) (n = 2) or ioxaglate (hexabrix*) (ionic low osmolar contrast medium) (n = 2) 1 ml/kg within 15 seconds. The subsequent changes in RBF pulse rate and blood pressure were recorded on a strip recorder for 30 minutes. Then the clamp was applied to obtain a renal perfusion pressure reduced to around 70 mmHg. Fifteen minutes after applying the clamp 3 contrast media administrations were performed at 20 min intervals (n = 8 for each contrast media). The contrast media injected were either diatrizoate, ioxaglate or iopamidol at the dose of 1 ml/kg.

Statistical analysis

The results were analyzed using a one factor analysis of variance. If a significant interaction was detected, the interaction was explored further by using paired Student's t-test. Statistical analysis were performed on an IBM PC using the number crunchers statistical system (Kaysville, UT, USA). All null hypotheses were two-tailed, and the criterion of significance was a level less than 0.05.

Results

The control period

Iopamidol and ioxaglate induced a similar decrease in RBF (Figure 1). The results from these two subgroups being identical were pooled for statistical purpose. The dose of contrast media which was administered was 19 ± 0.7 ml for low osmolar contrast media and 18 ± 0.8 ml for high osmolar contrast media. During this period these 2 low osmolar contrast media induced no change in mean arterial blood pressure (MABP) and pulse rate. The maximum vasoconstriction was observed at 1 min (17 ± 13%) (Figure 1) and was very transient. The decrease in RBF was 4 ± 10% and 5 ± 2%, AT 10 and 20 min, respectively. Renal vascular resistance (RVR) increased from 0.99 ± 0.1 to 1.25 ± 0.1 mmHg min/ml, 1 min after CM administration ($p < 0.05$) and remained significantly elevated for less than 4 minutes.

Diatrizoate induced no change in pulse rate and a slight but significant decrease in MABP from 151 ± 10 to 138 ± 6 mmHg ($p < 0.05$). Diatrizoate induced a 16 ± 2% decrease in RBF ($p < 0.05$) (Figure 1) and a mild increase in RVR from 0.72 ± 0.2 to 0.8 ± 0.2 mmHg min/ml. The decrease in RBF was 13 ± 2% and 8 ± 4% at 10 and 20 min, respectively. These modifications were not different from those observed with low osmolar contrast media.

The ischemic period

During the ischemic period, renal perfusion pressure was 69 ± 3; 69 ± 2 and 68 ± 2 mmHg before diatrizoate, iopamidol and ioxaglate administration, respectively (p = NS). The mean dose of contrast media which was administered, was 18 ± 0.8 ml for diatrizoate; 19 ± 0.6 ml for iopamidol and 18 ± 0.9 ml for ioxaglate (p = NS). MABP was slightly but significantly higher when compared with the control period (163 ± 14 vs 151 ± 10 mmHg) ($p < 0.05$). None of the contrast media induced changes in MABP or heart rate.

Diatrizoate induced a 77 ± 10% decrease in RBF and a maximum increase in RVR at 1 min from 0.9 ± 0.09 to 26 ± 12 mmHg min/ml. There was still a 36 ± 14 and a 23 ± 13% decrease in RBF 10 and 20 min after diatrizoate administration. These changes were significantly higher than those observed with all contrast media during the control period and low osmolar contrast media during the ischemic period. Iopamidol induced a maximum 32 ± 9% decrease in RBF at 1 min (Figure 2) and a maximum increase in RVR at 1 min from 0.8 ± 0.08 to 1.46 ± 0.26 mmHg min/ml ($p < 0.05$). These modifications were significantly higher ($p < 0.05$) than those observed during the control period.

The decrease in RBF was only 13 ± 6% and 3 ± 5%, 10 and 20 min after iopamidol infusion respectively ($p < 0.05$ compared with diatrizoate).

Ioxaglate induced a maximum 20 ± 12% decrease in RBF at 1 min (Figure 1) and a maximum increase in RVR at 1 min from 0.8 ± 0.09 to 1.36 ± 0.38 ($p < 0.05$). These modifications were comparable to those observed during the control period. The decrease in RBF was 12 ± 3% and 10 ± 3%, 10 and 20 min after ioxaglate infusion, respectively ($p < 0.05$) compared with diatrizoate.

Discussion

In this study we found that the renal hemodynamic effects of contrast media are enhanced by ischemia. Moreover, in this setting, low osmolar contrast agents, iopamidol and ioxaglate induced significantly less vasoconstriction.

Because of precarious balance between oxygen supply and demand within the outer medulla, the medullary thick ascending limb, which normally operates on the verge of hypoxia, becomes a prime target for ischemic injury during renal hypoperfusion [Brezis et al. 1984]. Radiocontrast nephropathy regularly develops in the presence of risk factors, which are usually associated with compromised medullary O_2 balance. In preexisting renal failure, one of the most important of these risk factors, the decrease in functioning renal mass leads to an augmented workload per remaining nephron (a condition referred to as tubular hypermetabolism), intensifying mTAL hypoxia.

Based on our observations we suggest that in these patients the renal vasoconstriction induced by contrast media may be greater than in normal kidneys and of major importance in inducing renal failure.

Ischemia causes alteration in the structure of the vascular membranes which leads to an aggregation of red blood cells in the medullary vessel [Wolgast et al. 1982] which will further compromise medullary oxygenation and predispose to contrast nephrotoxicity.

Furthermore it has been shown that diatrizoate has a direct toxic effect on renal proximal tubular cells [Humes et al. 1987]. In this model, diatrizoate also potentiates the degree of cell injury induced by a moderate period of hypoxia. Thus under certain clinical situations of poor renal perfusion, the administration of contrast agents may set a stage for the additive deleterious effects of the potential nephrotoxic contrast medium, and hypoxia after infusion of the dye.

Hypertonicity is a salient feature of all radiocontrast agents. This hypertonicity may be central to its hemodynamic activity, since other hypertonic agents alter renal hemodynamics [Katzerg et al. 1983].

New contrast agents such as ioxaglate and iopamidol have been developed that have lower osmolarity yet retain sufficient iodine to provide satisfactory radiographic visualization. Recent in vitro and in vivo studies suggest that low osmolar contrast agents have a less direct nephrotoxic effect on cells of the proximal renal tubule [Humes et al. 1987, Deray et al. 1990, Messana et al. 1988]. Our study shows that the renal hemodynamic modifications induced by high and low osmolar contrast media are identical in the normal kidney. By contrast the magnitude and the duration of the vasoconstriction appeared to vary directly with the tonicity of the agent used in an ischemic kidney. The more hypertonic the solution, the greater and the more sustained the vasoconstriction. One minute after contrast media infusion the vasoconstriction was slightly but significantly less pronounced with ioxaglate than with iopamidol. This difference may be due to the lower osmolality (600 vs 700 mosm/kg) of ioxaglate.

Although the results recorded in this study do not provide a definitive elucidation of the mechanisms involved in the alteration of renal function caused by contrast agent, they are however well in keeping with several hypotheses currently set forward for explaining the deleterious effects of these iodinated compounds in clinical practice. A possible role for adenosine in causing renal vasoconstriction and ischemic renal failure during these pathological conditions seems likely since tissue, urine and blood levels of adenosine increase markedly during renal ischemia [Larson et al. 1983]. Also in these circumstances angiotensine II levels are elevated and it has been shown that adenosine may be capable of causing sustained renal vasoconstriction of preglomerular vessels when angiotensin II levels are maintained high [Hall et al. 1985, Hall and Granger 1986]. Finally we have recently shown that theophylline and dipyridamole respectively inhibit and enhance the intra renal vasoconstriction induced by contrast media suggesting that endogenous adenosine is essential for the effect of contrast media on renal blood flow [Deray et al. 1990].

In summary, these results demonstrate that ischemia potentiates the renal vascular effects of contrast media. They provide substantial support for the thesis according to which contrast media induced renal failure may be primarily caused by renal ischemia. During ischemia low osmolar contrast agents induced less vasoconstriction and may therefore be useful in high risk patients.

Acknowledgement

This work was supported by a grant in aid from the fonds d'étude du corps médical des Hôpitaux de Paris.

REFERENCES

Brezis M, Rosen S, Silva P, Epstein FH 1984 Selective vulnerability of the medullary thick ascending limb to anoxia in the isolated perfused rat kidney. J Clin Invest *73:* 182–193

Cronin RE 1988 Radiocontrast media-induced acute renal failure. In: Diseases of the Kidney 1301–1317 (Edited by Schrier RW) Fourth edition

Deray G, Dubois M, Martinez F, Baumelou B, Beaufils H, Bourbouze R, Baumelou A, Jacobs C 1990 Renal effects of radiocontrast agents in rats: a new model of acute renal failure. Am J Nephrol *10:* 507–513

Deray G, Martinez F, Cacoub P, Baumelou B, Baumelou A, Jacobs C 1990 A role for adenosine calcium and ischemia in radiocontrast induced intrarenal vasoconstriction. Am J Nephrol *10:* 316–321

Hall JE, Granger JP 1986 Adenosine alter, glomerular filtration control by angiotensin II. Am J Physiol *250:* F917–F923

Hall JE, Granger JP, Hester RL 1985 Interactions between adenosine and angiotensin II in controlling glomerular filtration. Am J Physiol *248:* F340–F346

Hou SH, Bushinsky DA, Wish G et al. 1983 Hospital acquired renal insufficiency: a prospective study. Am J Med *74:* 243–248

Humes HD, Hunt DA, White MD 1987 Direct toxic effect of the radiocontrast agent diatrizoate on renal proximal tubule cells. Am J Physiol *252:* F246–F255

Katzerg RW, Schulman G, Meggs LG et al. 1983 Mechanism of the renal response to contrast medium in dogs. Decrease in renal function due to hypertonicity. Invest Radiol *18:* 74–80

Larson TS, Hudson K, Meretz JI et al. 1983 Renal vasoconstrictive response to contrast medium. The role of sodium balance and the renin angiotensin system. J Lab Clin Med *101:* 385–391

Messana JM, Cieslinski DA, Nguyen VOD, Humes HD 1988 Comparison of the nephrotoxicity of the radiocontrast agents, iopamidol and diatrizoate to rabbit renal proximal tubule cells in vitro. J Pharmacol Exp Ther *244:* 1139–1144

Talner LB, Rushmer HN, Coel MN 1972 The effect of renal artery injection of contrast material on urinary enzyme excretion. Invest Radiol *7:* 311–322

Tornquist C, Almen T, Golman K et al. 1985 Renal function following nephroangiography with metrizamide or iohexol. Acta Radiol Diagnos *26:* 483–489

Wolgast M, Karlberg L, Källskog Ö, Norlen BJ, Nygren K, Öjteg G 1982 Hemodynamic alterations in ischaemic acute renal failure. Nephron *31:* 301–303

Clinical Nephrology, Vol. 36 No. 2 – 1991 (97–102)

Intragastric long-term pH-metry in hemodialysis patients. A study with famotidine

U. Gladziwa[1], S. Wagner[2], K. V. Dakshinamurty[1], B. Bechtel[1], H. Mann[1] and H.-G. Sieberth[1]

[1] *Department of Internal Medicine II, Technical University of Aachen, Pauwelsstr. 30, Aachen, and*
[2] *Department of Gastroenterology and Hepatology, Medizinische Hochschule Hannover, Konstanty-Gutschow-Str. 8, Hannover, Germany*

Abstract. The onset and duration of famotidine action were studied in 14 hemodialysis (HD) patients and 16 healthy controls (control group: CG) who were examined by ambulatory intragastric 24-hour pH-metry. 20 mg famotidine was administered i.v. 90 min after HD in the afternoon (AN; 2 p.m.; n = 8) or evening (E; 8 p.m.; n = 6), followed by a standard meal. Mean onset of action in the AN and E groups of the HD patients was 90.3 ± 28.2 min and 98.8 ± 29.8 min, and in CG patients 36.3 ± 11.9 min and 53.6 ± 22.3 min, respectively ($p < 0.05$). Duration of action in the AN and E groups of the HD patients was 22.7 ± 2.1 h and 21.6 ± 2.6 h, and in CG patients 6.0 ± 1.1 h and 11.4 ± 1.6 h, respectively ($p < 0.05$). Our study showed a retarded and prolonged action of famotidine in HD patients. The time of administration of famotidine had no effect on its action in HD patients. This is in contrast to normal subjects in whom evening administration delays the onset and prolongs the duration of famotidine action in comparison to afternoon administration.

Key words: hemodialysis – long-term pH-metry – pharmacodynamics of famotidine

Introduction

Many authors have repeatedly proved that the increased incidence of peptic ulcer and gastrointestinal bleeding in patients with renal insufficiency is due to hypersecretion of hydrochloric acid and to hypergastrinemia [Goldstein et al., 1967; Ritz et al., 1971; Ventkateswaran et al., 1972; Shepherd et al., 1973; Milito et al., 1983, 1985]. We reported that more than 50% of hemodialysis (HD) patients had gastrointestinal symptoms, and 30% had endoscopically demonstrable peptic ulceration and gastritis [Gladziwa, 1990]. Animal experiments in uremic mice demonstrated a markedly increased parietal cell mass [Ritz, 1978].

Histamine (H_2) receptor antagonists are drugs of choice in the management of acid peptic disease. Famotidine, a relatively new drug, is approximately 6 times more potent than ranitidine and 30 times more potent than cimetidine (on a molar basis) in suppressing acid secretion [Pendleton et al., 1983; Howard et al., 1985; McCallum et al., 1985; Smith et al., 1985]. Renal tubular secretion plays a predominant role in the elimination of famotidine. Its half-life is prolonged in patients with renal failure, and total body clearance depends on renal function [Takabatake et al., 1985; Kroemer & Klotz, 1987].

A 7- to 10-fold prolongation of famotidine's elimination half-life (27.2 ± 8.5 h) was observed in patients with renal failure compared with its half-life (2.6–3.6 h) in subjects with normal renal function, and a dose reduction was recommended [Gladziwa et al., 1988]. By means of ambulatory long-term intragastric pH-metry the course of intragastric pH-profiles and the efficacy of antisecretory drugs can be determined [Fimmel et al., 1985; Walt, 1986]. Using ambulatory intragastric long-term pH-metry we decided to examine the duration of famotidine action in hemodialysis patients and to clarify whether it depends upon the time of administration.

Patients and methods

We studied 30 individuals, 14 HD patients for the study group, 16 patients with normal renal function for the control group (CG) after obtaining their informed consent. The study was in accordance with the declaration of Helsinki (1964) as revised in Tokyo (1975). Both groups were comparable as to age and

Received November 1, 1990; in revised form March 28, 1991.

Reprint requests to Dr. U. Gladziwa, Dept. of Internal Medicine II, Technical University of Aachen, Pauwelsstr. 30, W-5100 Aachen, Germany sex. The clinical characteristics of the patients are shown in Tables 1, 2 and 3. Gastric medication (antacids, H_2-antagonists, prokinetic drugs) was withheld for two weeks before the study.

Intragastric pH was measured by a combined glass electrode (Ingold type 440M4, Ingold AG, Urdorf, Switzerland) connected to a portable solid state recorder (Digitrapper 6200 MII, Synectics Medical, Stockholm, Sweden). The pH measuring unit was calibrated at 37° C using standard buffer solutions of pH 6.70 and 1.11 (Synectics Medical). After each run calibration was repeated to assess the drift of the electrode.

All study subjects were admitted at 2 p.m. for pH-metry one hour after hemodialysis having fasted for three hours. The study was started in the afternoon to enable the patients to have their dinner and to study the effects of dinner on the pH profile. The electrode was fluoroscopically placed in the gastric corpus (8–10 cm below the cardia). Measurements were started immediately and lasted for 24 hours. All subjects were ambulatory. The conditions were standardized as to meal timing and composition (dinner at 6 p.m., breakfast at 8 a.m. and lunch at noon).

Water and unsweetened tea were allowed during meals. No food or liquid was allowed between meals. Normal daily activities were unrestricted. All study subjects noted their activities, meals and special events on a diary card.

Data processing: The pH measurements were stored every 4 sec and the collected data were transferred to an IBM computer (AT 286). The recorded data were analyzed using a commercial computer program (oesophogram Ver. 5.40 and statpHac ver. 2.14, Synectics Medical). Median pH and median hydrogen ion activity and interquartile ranges were calculated for individuals and groups. For graphical presentation the medians of the pH values averaged over 10 min-periods were used because pH values are not normally distributed [Emde et al., 1987; Merki et al., 1988; Savarino et al., 1988; Duroux et al., 1989].

20 mg famotidine was administered i.v. 90 min after hemodialysis to eight patients in the afternoon (AN, at 2 p.m.) and to the other six patients in the evening (E, at 8 p.m.). Two groups of 8 patients each with normal renal function served as control groups. The time of reaching and duration of maintaining an intragastric pH >4 after famotidine were noted.

Non-obligatory t-tests with normally distributed random sampling were used as the method of statistical analysis. Probability values $p < 0.05$ were considered significant in all these tests.

Table 1 Clinical data of the patients studied

	Hemodialysis patients	Control group
Number of patients	14	16
Age (years)	44,9 ± 15,7	41,2 ± 15,6
range	20 – 70	24 – 69
Sex		
Male	9	8
Female	5	8
Duration of hemodialysis treatment (months)	45,6 ± 41,7	–
range	1 – 136	–

Table 2 Demographical characteristics of the hemodialysis patients studied

Patient	Sex	Age (years)	Weight (kg)	Hematocrit (%)	Duration of dialysis (months)	Renal Diagnosis
1. W. S.	(m)	70	60	38	18	Unknown renal disease
2. F. H.	(m)	62	100	38	–	Acute renal failure
3. W. L.	(w)	28	63	33	20	Chronic glomerulonephritis
4. H. H.	(m)	56	82	29	86	Chronic glomerulonephritis
5. R. L.	(w)	52	66	22	3	Analgesic nephropathy
6. U. S.	(w)	24	52	30	69	Chronic glomerulonephritis
7. K. P.	(m)	58	64	29	136	Polycystic kidney disease
8. N. A.	(m)	55	99	32	8	Diabetic nephropathy
9. I. E.	(m)	54	57	25	1	Unknown renal disease
10. M. B.	(w)	20	45	20	1	Chronic glomerulonephritis
11. U. P.	(m)	29	71	44	88	Chronic glomerulonephritis
12. F. P.	(w)	22	55	21	24	Unknown renal disease
13. V. R.	(m)	47	80	29	58	Analgesic nephropathy
14. M. H.	(m)	52	67	28	81	Polycystic kidney disease

Table 3 Clinical characteristics of the hemodialysis patients studied

Patient	Gastrointestinal symptoms/gastric history	Endoscopy	Medication	PTH (mid-region assay) [pmol/l]	Secondary hyperparathyroidism (X-ray: hands[1], acromioclavicular joints[2], sonography[3], CT scan[4] [parathyroid gland], bone biopsy[5])
1. W. S.	Asymptomatic	–	Calcium carbonate	314,4	Normal[1, 2, 3]
2. F. H.	Asymptomatic	–	–	–	–
3. W. L.	Asymptomatic	–	Aluminium hydroxide Calcitriol	>1000	Normal[1, 2] Parathyroid gland hyperplasia[3]
4. H. H.	Heartburn	Erosive gastritis Hiatus hernia	Aluminium hydroxide Magaldrate	320,4	Normal[1, 2, 3, 4]
5. R. L.	Nausea Epigastric pain upper gastrointestinal bleeding (1 episode)	Erosive gastritis	Aluminium hydroxide Calcium lacto-gluconate/-carbonate Metoclopramide	595,3	Normal[1, 2, 3]
6. V. S.	Epigastric pain	Erosive gastritis	Aluminium hydroxide Calcitriol Magaldrate	621,4	Normal[1, 2]
7. K. P.	Heartburn Meteorism	–	Aluminium hydroxide Calcitriol	843,8	Normal[1, 2, 3]
8. N. A.	Heartburn	–	Aluminium hydroxide Calcium lacto-gluconate/-carbonate Magaldrate	486,0	Normal[1, 2]
9. I. E.	Heartburn Epigastric pain Gastric ulcers in the past	Erosive gastritis/ bulbitis	Aluminium hydroxide Calcium lacto-gluconate/-carbonate Ranitidine	691,6	Normal[1, 2]
10. M. B.	Asymptomatic	–	Calcium carbonate	>1000	–
11. U. P.	Heartburn	Reflux esophagitis	Aluminium hydroxide Calcitriol Ranitidine	565,2	Normal[1, 2]
12. F. P.	Asymptomatic	–	Calcium carbonate Calcitriol	970,3	Normal[1, 2]
13. V. R.	Heartburn	Gastritis Hiatus hernia Duodenal diverticulosis	Calcium carbonate Metoclopramide	436,1	Normal[1, 3] Renal osteopathy[2] Aluminium bone disease[5]
14. M. H.	Nausea Epigastric pain	Gastritis Erosive bulbitis	Calcium carbonate Calcitriol Ranitidine	949,9	Normal[1, 2, 3] Renal osteodystrophy[5]

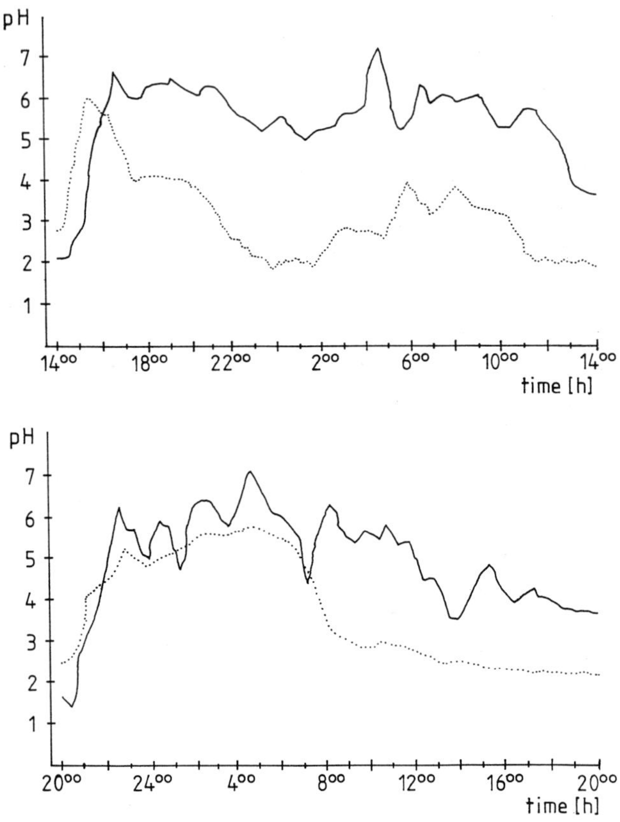

Fig. Median pH values in dialysis patients (——) and in normal subjects (····). a) Famotidine administration in the afternoon (2 p.m.) b) Famotidine administration in the evening (8 p.m.)

Table 4 Pharmacodynamics of famotidine

			Latency of action ($\bar{x} \pm$ SD) (min)	Duration of action ($\bar{x} \pm$ SD) (h)
HD	AN	n = 8	90.3 ± 28.2	22.7 ± 2.1
	E	n = 6	98.8 ± 29.8	21.6 ± 2.6
CG	AN	n = 8	36.3 ± 11.9*	6.0 ± 1.1**
	E	n = 8	53.6 ± 22.3*	11.4 ± 1.6**

$\bar{x} \pm$ SD = mean ± standard deviation; */** $p<0.05$; HD = Hemodialysis patients; CG = Control group; AN = Afternoon (2 p.m.) administration group; E = Evening (8 p.m.) administration group

Results

Table 4 summarizes the results. The pharmacodynamic activity of famotidine showed the following features: the mean onset of action (latency), i.e. to achieve a pH of at least 4, was significantly delayed in the dialysis patients compared to the subjects with normal renal function ($p<0.05$). The latency period was double in the HD patients regarding to CG. But there was no significant difference in the dialysis patients regarding the administration of famotidine in the afternoon or evening ($p>0.05$). In the normal subjects, however, latency was significantly longer in the evening group (54 min vs 36 min, $p<0.05$). The duration of action (maintaining an intragastric pH >4) of famotidine was 22 to 23 hours in the dialysis patients and 6 to 11 hours in those with normal renal function ($p<0.05$) (Fig.).

Discussion

Intragastric long-term pH-metry permits the assessment of intragastric pH profiles and the efficacy of antisecretory drugs. So far, this method of assessment has not been reported in the literature for cimetidine, ranitidine or famotidine in patients with renal insufficiency.

Our study shows that in patients with renal insufficiency the duration of antisecretory action is prolonged in comparison to normal subjects. This is probably due to the reduced elimination of famotidine and higher plasma levels. No clear association between the individual pharmacokinetic and -dynamic data was obvious [Gladziwa et al., 1988]. The fact that the duration of action is less than the elimination half-life in hemodialysis patients but not in healthy individuals can be explained by the higher acid secretion in patients with renal insufficiency [Goldstein et al., 1967; Ritz et al., 1971; Ventkateswaran et al., 1972; Shepherd et al., 1973; Milito et al., 1983 and 1985]. That there was no difference in the duration of action with reference to the administration time in patients with renal failure may be explained by the altered elimination of famotidine. In view of the prolonged action, the dose of famotidine should be reduced to one third of the normal dose. There are several approaches to modify dosage in patients with renal dysfunction. Prolongation of the interval between doses or decreased daily doses during long-term therapy may be followed for the patients with severe renal insufficiency. Lin et al. [1988] have shown that famotidine levels 24 h after i.v. administration of 20 mg famotidine were undetectable in normal young and elderly volunteers, while the famotidine levels following i.v. administration of a 10 mg dose for anuric renal patients were 12.6 ng/ml. Miwa et al. [1984] reported that the plasma concentration of famotidine correlates with the potency of its inhibition of gastric acid secretion, and that the plasma famotidine concentration inhibiting 50% of gastric acid secretion (IC_{50}) is 13 ng/ml. Therefore a lower dose is effective in patients with renal failure.

In patients with normal renal function, the intake of H_2-receptor antagonists in the night [Gledhill et al., 1983; DeGara et al., 1986] and more recently in the early evening [Bauerfeind et al., 1986; Merki et al., 1987a; Merki et al., 1987b] was shown to be more effective than day-time administration. This seems to be due to an interaction of the drug with food [Johnston and Wormsly, 1988]. In contrast to normal subjects, no such difference is found in patients with renal failure. This may be explained by the prolonged action of famotidine masking the effect of food. To patients with renal failure, the drug can therefore be given at any time of the day. To ensure the patient's compliance, however, it may be given in the evening.

The onset of action after famotidine administration is significantly delayed in patients with renal failure compared to subjects with normal renal function. In hemodialysis patients it took twice the time to reach a pH above 4 compared with normal subjects. This may be attributed to the increased gastric acid secretion in renal insufficiency [Ventkateswaran, 1972; Shepherd, 1973; Milito, 1985]. Recently we have shown that patients with renal failure have higher acidity and attenuated alkalinisation by food in comparison to healthy subjects [Gladziwa et al., 1988].

In patients with end-stage renal disease [Daul et al., 1984, Brodde and Daul, 1984] and also in experimental uremia [Mann et al., 1984] an altered sensitivity of adrenergic receptors was observed. This may be explained by a massive spill-over of endogenous adrenergic substances which saturate the corresponding receptor system and lead to loss of sensitivity and diminished receptor response. Similarly it is possible that an accumulation of histamine affects the histamine receptors of dialysis patients. An effect of uremic toxins on the receptor coupling regulatory protein is also possible. This concept may explain the delayed onset of famotidine action in dialysis patients.

In conclusion, in patients with renal insufficiency the onset of famotidine action is delayed and the duration of action is prolonged 2 to 3 times, independent of the time of intake when compared to the control group. A reduction of the normal dose to one third is recommended.

REFERENCES

Bauerfeind P, Cilluffo T, Emde C, Fimmel CJ, Köhler W, Merki H, Gasser T, Blum AL 1986 H_2-antagonists are more effective after early evening intake than after late intake. Gastroenterology 90, no. *5:* 1340

Brodde O-E, Daul A 1984 Alpha- and beta-adrenoceptor changes in patients on maintenance hemodialysis. Contr Nephrol *41:* 99–107

Daul AE, Khalifa AM, Graven N, Brodde O-E 1984 Impaired regulation of β-adrenoceptors in patients on maintenance haemodialysis. Proc EDTA-ERA *21:* 178–183

De Gara CJ, Gledhill T, Hunt RH 1986 Nocturnal gastric acid secretion: its importance in the pathophysiology and rational therapy of duodenal ulcer. Scand J Gastroenterol *21 (Suppl. 121):* 17–24

Duroux PH, Bauerfeind P, Emde C, Koelz HR, Blum AL 1989 Early dinner reduces nocturnal gastric acidity. Gut *30:* 1063–1067

Emde C, Garner A, Blum AL 1987 Technical aspects of intraluminal pH-metry in man: current status and recommendations. Gut *28:* 1177–1188

Fimmel CJ, Etienne A, Cilluffo T, von Ritter C, Gasser T, Rey J-P, Caradonna-Moscatelli P, Sabbatini F, Pace F, Bühler HW, Bauerfeind P, Blum AL 1985 Long-term ambulatory gastric pH monitoring: validation of a new method and effect of H_2-antagonists. Gastroenterology *88:* 1842–1851

Gladziwa U, Klotz U, Krishna DR, Schmitt H, Glöckner WM, Mann H 1988 Pharmacokinetics and -dynamics of famotidine in patients with renal failure. Br J clin Pharmac *26:* 315–321

Gladziwa U 1990 Pharmakokinetik und -dynamik von Histamin-H_2-Rezeptor-Antagonisten bei Niereninsuffizienz. Nieren- und Hochdruckkrankheiten *19:* 457–459

Gledhill T, Howard OM, Buck M, Paul A, Hunt RH 1983 Single nocturnal dose of an H_2 receptor antagonist for the treatment of duodenal ulcer. Gut *24:* 904–908

Goldstein H, Murphy D, Sokol A, Rubini ME 1967 Gastric acid secretion in patients undergoing chronic dialysis. Arch Intern Med *120:* 645–653

Howard JM, Chremos AN, Collen MJ, McArthur KE, Cherner JA, Maton PN, Ciarleglio CA, Cornelius MJ, Gardner JD, Jensen RT 1985 Famotidine, a new, potent, long-acting histamine H_2-receptor antagonist: comparison with cimetidine and ranitidine in the treatment of Zollinger-Ellison syndrome. Gastroenterology *88:* 1026–1033

Johnston DA, Wormsley KG 1988 The effect of food on ranitidine-induced inhibition of nocturnal gastric secretion. Aliment Pharmacol Therap *2:* 507–511

Kroemer H, Klotz U 1987 Pharmacokinetics of famotidine in man. Int J Clin Pharmacol Ther Toxicol *25:* 458–463

Lin JH, Chremos AN, Yeh KC, Antonello J, Hessey II GA 1988 Effects of age and chronic renal failure on the urinary excretion kinetics of famotidine in man. Eur J Clin Pharmacol *34:* 41–46

Mann JFE, Hausen M, Jacobs K-H, Kutter A, Nagel W, Rascher W, Schick M, Sudhoff R, Ritz E 1984 Adrenergic responsiveness in experimental uremia. Contr Nephrol *41:* 108–112

McCallum RW, Chremos AN, Kuljian B, Tupy-Visich MA, Huber PB 1985 MK-208, a novel histamine H_2-receptor inhibitor with prolonged antisecretory effect. Dig Dis Sci *30:* 1139–1144

Merki H, Witzel L, Harre K, Scheurle E, Neumann J, Röhmel J 1987a Single dose treatment with H_2 receptor antagonists: is bedtime administration too late? Gut *28:* 451–454

Merki HS, Witzel L, Walt RP, Neumann J, Scheurle E, Kaufmann D, Mappes A, Heim J, Röhmel J 1987b Comparison of ranitidine 300 mg twice daily, 300 mg at night and placebo on 24-hour intragastric acidity of duodenal ulcer patients. Aliment Pharmacol Therap *1:* 217–223

Merki HS, Fimmel CJ, Walt RP, Harre K, Röhmel J, Witzel L 1988 Pattern of 24 hour intragastric acidity in active duodenal ulcer disease and in healthy controls. Gut *29:* 1583–1587

Milito G, Taccone-Galluci M, Brancaleone C, Nardi F, Fillingeri V, Cesca D, Casciani CU 1983 Assessment of the upper gastrointestinal tract in hemodialysis patients awaiting renal transplantation. American J Gastroenterology *78:* 328–331

Milito G, Taccone-Galluci M, Brancaleone C, Nardi F, Cesca D, Boffo V, Casciani CU 1985 The gastrointestinal tract in uremic patients on long-term hemodialysis. Kidney International 28, suppl *17:* S-157–S-160

Miwa M, Tani N, Miwa T 1984 Inhibition of gastric secretion by a new H_2-antagonist, YM-11170, in healthy subjects. Int J Clin Pharmacol Ther Toxicol *22:* 214–217

Pendleton RG, Torchiana ML, Chung C, Cook P, Wiese S, Clineschmidt BV 1983 Studies on MK-208 (YM-11170) a new, slowly dissociable H_2-receptor antagonist. Arch Int Pharmacodyn *266:* 4–16

Ritz E, Krempien B, Wanke M, Ziegler M, Wesch G, Tomer U 1971 Klinische und experimentelle Untersuchungen zur urämischen Gastritis. Verh Dtsch Ges Inn Med *77:* 220–224

Ritz E 1978 Urämisch bedingte Störungen des Magen-Darmkanals. Symposium "Urämie als Intoxikationszustand", Medical Clinic II, RWTH Aachen, FRG, Beiheft *6:* 125–133

Savarino V, Mela GS, Scalabrini P, Sumberaz A, Fera G, Celle G 1988 24-hour study of intragastric acidity in duodenal ulcer patients and normal subjects using continuous intraluminal pH-metry. Dig Dis Sci *33:* 1077–1080

Shepherd AMM, Stewart WK, Wormsley KG 1973 Peptic ulceration in chronic renal failure. Lancet, June *16:* 1357–1359

Smith JL, Gamal MA, Chremos AN, Graham DY 1985 Famotidine, a new H_2-receptor antagonist. Effect on parietal, nonparietal, and pepsin secretion in man. Dig Dis Sci *30:* 308–312

Takabatake T, Ohta H, Maekawa M, Yamamoto Y, Ishida Y et al. 1985 Pharmacokinetics of famotidine, a new H_2-receptor antagonist, in relation to renal function. Eur J Clin Pharmacol *28:* 327–331

Ventkateswaran PS, Jeffers A, Hocken AG 1972 Gastric acid secretion in chronic renal failure. Br Med J, 7 October: 22–23

Walt R 1986 Twenty-four hour intragastric acidity analysis for the future. Gut *27:* 1–9

ANNOUNCEMENTS

The **XXVIIIth Congress of the European Dialysis and Transplant Association – European Renal Association** (EDTA/ERA) will be held in Belgrade, Yugoslavia from September 1 to 4, 1991.

For further information, contact the Organizing Secretariat: Yugotours, Congress, Incentive & Exhibition Department, Djure Djakovića 31, Y-11000 Belgrade, Yugoslavia. Tel.: 3811/763-028, 764-622; Telex: 11000, 12902; Fax: 3811/766-447.

The **22nd Annual Congress of the Nephrology Society** will take place from September 15–18, 1991 in Heidelberg, Germany.

The Nephrology Society will be awarding a prize for the best doctoral thesis dealing with a nephrological theme. Eligible theses and further inquiries should be sent to the following address: Dr. M. Walla, c/o Prof. Ritz, Med. Univ. Clinic/Section of Nephrology, Bergheimerstr. 56a, W-6900 Heidelberg.

The **Second Seminar on Renal Involvement in Systemic Vasculitis** will take place September 21, 1991 in Vimercate, a city near Milan in Italy. Contemporary issues relating to immunopathology of Systemic Lupus Erythematosus, with special regard to anti-endothelial and anti-cardiolipin antibodies, clinicopathological correlations and treatment will be discussed.

For further information please contact Dr. Adalberto Sessa, Unità Operativa di Nefrologia e Dialisi, Ospedale di Vimercate, I-20059 Vimercate/Milan, Italy, Tel.: 39/6654/544 or /672 or /327 or /481; Fax: 39/669079.

The **Third Roma Nephrology Conference** will be held in Fiuggi (Rome), Italy on September 27–28, 1991. The main topic will be "The Glomerular Mesangium: From Cell Biology to Clinics".

For further information contact Prof. Giulio A. Cinotti, Cattedra di Nefrologia, 2a Clinica Medica, Policlinico Umberto I, Viale del Policlinico, I-00161 Rome, Italy. Tel.: 39/6/445-7130, Fax: 39/6/445-7735.

The **Seventh International Symposium of Nephrology at Montecatini,** October 14–16, 1991. The title of the symposium is "Kidney, Proteins and Drugs". Advances in protein hormones research, proteinuria, proteins and progression of kidney disease and nephrotoxicity of drugs will be discussed.

For further information please contact Dr. Claudio Bianchi, Unita di Nefrologia, Clinica Medica 2, University of Pisa, I-56100 Pisa, Italy. Tel.: 050–592573.

A **Festakt in honor of Priscilla Kincaid-Smith** will be held on November 5–8th, 1991 in Melbourne, Australia. Events will include state of the art lectures and symposia.

For further information contact The Festschrift Organizing Committee, c/o Department of Nephrology, The Royal Melbourne Hospital, Victoria 3050, Australia.

The **International Meeting on Molecular Approaches to Nephrology Prospect in Diagnosis and Management** will take place on March 19–21, 1992 in Bari, Italy.

For further information please contact Prof. F. P. Schena, Chair and Division of Nephrology, Polyclinic, I-70124 Bari, Tel.: 39/80/271237 or 271232.

The **IIIrd International Conference on SLE** will be held in the Queen Elizabeth II Conference Centre, Westminster, London, April 13–15, 1992.

For further details, please contact Dr. Graham Hughes or Mrs. Denzil Fletcher, Rheumatology Department, St. Thomas' Hospital, London SE1 7EH. Tel. and Fax: 0163394 22.

The **XXIXth Congress of the European Dialysis and Transplant Association** – European Renal Association (EDTA – ERA) will be held at the Palais des Congrès in Paris, France on June 28 – July 1, 1992. For further information contact Prof. C. Jacobs, Congress President, Service de Néphrologie, Hôpital de la Pitié, 83 bd de l'Hôpital, 75013 Paris, France (Fax: 33144 239984) or the organizing Secretariat: Convergences – EDTA 1992, 120 av. Gambetta, 75020 Paris, France (Fax: 3314030 0165).

The **Third Symposium on Uroradiology** (Imaging and Intervention) will take place August 24–27, 1992 at Herlev Hospital, University of Copenhagen, Denmark.

For further information, please contact Dr. Henrik S. Thomsen, Department of Diagnostic Radiology 54E2, Herlev Hospital, Herlev Ringvej 75, DK-2730 Herlev, Denmark. Tel.: 4544/535300, Ext. 278; Fax: 4544/535332.

The **VIth Congress of the International Society for Peritoneal Dialysis** will take place October 1–4, 1992 in Thessaloniki, Greece.

For additional information write to the First Department of Internal Medicine, AHEPA University Hospital, 54636 Thessaloniki, Greece. Tel. and Fax: (3031) 214606.

LETTERS TO THE EDITOR

Increased plasma interleukin 6 and renin substrate levels during bacterial peritonitis in CAPD patients

Sir, – Interleukin 6 (IL-6) is a cytokine likely to be an important mediator of the inflammatory response, acting as an endogenous pyrogen and stimulating hepatic acute phase protein synthesis [Kishimoto 1989]. Production of renin substrate (RS), also an acute phase protein produced by the liver [Metsärinne et al. 1988], is stimulated by IL-6 too [Itoh et al. 1989]. Hack et al. [1989] reported increased plasma levels of IL-6 in patients with sepsis and particularly in septic shock.

We studied the effect of acute infectious peritonitis on plasma IL-6 and RS levels in 10 uremic patients on continuous ambulatory peritoneal dialysis (CAPD). The diagnosis of peritonitis was based on 1) fever (temperature above 37 °C), 2) abdominal pain, and 3) an opaque dialysis fluid with a leukocyte count exceeding 100×10^6/l. A positive blood culture *(Escherichia coli)* was obtained in one patient but none of the patients was in septic shock. Plasma RS [Metsärinne et al. 1988] and plasma IL-6 were measured by radioimmunoassay, based on recombinant human IL-6 and polyclonal rabbit anti-human IL-6 (from Genzyme, Boston, MA, USA). This antiserum does not cross-react with interleukin 1α (IL-1α), IL-1β, tumour necrosis factor α (TNFα), TNFβ, interferon α (IFN-α) or IFN-β. Sensitivity of the IL-6 assay was 15 pg/ml.

Increased plasma IL-6 levels were seen during acute infectious peritonitis (Figure 1), with a peak level of 79,2 ng/ml (95% confidence interval 35,9 to 122,5), obtained shortly after admission to the hospital. Plasma IL-6 levels decreased during the next few days and the control value, obtained 2 weeks later, was 6,2 ng/ml (4,5 to 7,9). Plasma RS levels also increased during acute peritonitis (Figure 1), but the peak level, 2725 nmol/l (2225 to 3225) was seen later, on the second day about 30 h after admission. The corresponding control plasma RS concentration was clearly lower, averaging 1286 nmol/l (1048 to 1524).

Increased plasma IL-6 levels in CAPD-patients during bacterial peritonitis were not associated with septic shock. Our data suggest that increased IL-6 production is a cause of rised plasma RS levels. This accords with the concept that IL-6 stimulates production of hepatic acute phase proteins [Kishimoto 1989]. Okamoto et al. [1989] showed that IL-6, but not IL-1 or TNFβ, stimulated RS production *in vitro* in hepatoma cell culture. This study indicates that this may be true also *in vivo*. Whether RS plays a role in inflammation is unknown. RS is structurally related to some serine protease inhibitors [Doolittle 1983], and might possess a similar function in regulating proteolytic activity during acute inflammation. No such functions of RS have been reported, however.

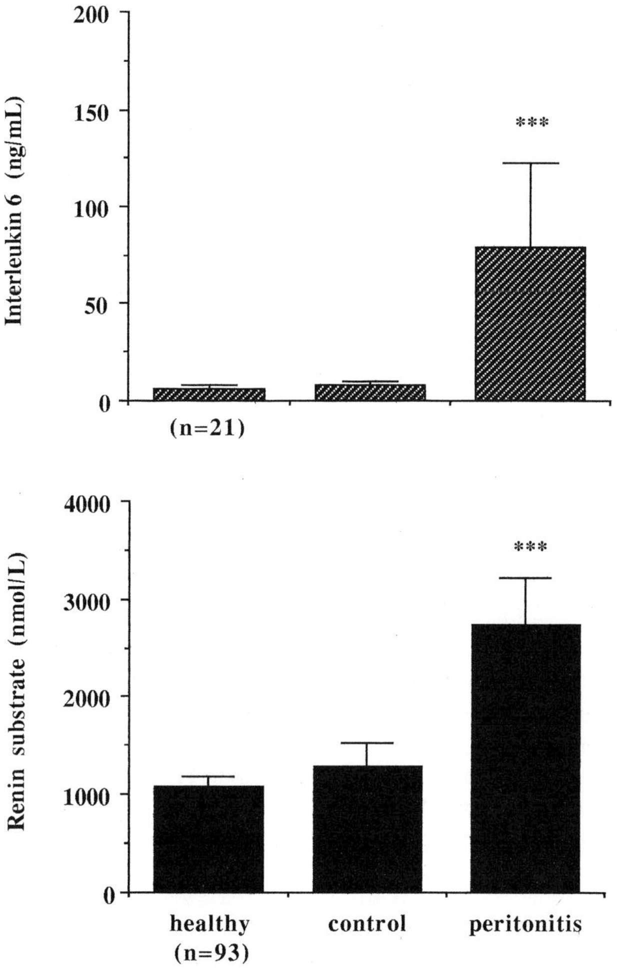

Fig. 1 Plasma interleukin 6 and renin substrate levels in healthy subjects and in 10 CAPD-patients (control and during infectious peritonitis). ***) p <0.001 as compared to control.

K. Metsärinne[1,2], *A.-M. Teppo*[1], *C. Grönhagen-Riska*[1,2], *F. Fyhrquist*[1,2]

IVth Department of Medicine, Helsinki University Central Hospital[1], Unioninkatu 38, SF-00170 Helsinki, Finland and Minerva Foundation Institute for Medical Research[2], Helsinki, Finland.

REFERENCES

Doolittle RF 1983 Angiotensinogen is related to the antitrypsin-antithrombin-ovalbumin family. Science *222:* 417–9

Hack CE, De Groot ER, Felt-Bersma RJF et al 1989 Increased plasma levels of interleukin-6 in sepsis. Blood *74:* 1704–10

Itoh N, Matsuda T, Ohtani R, Okamoto H 1989 Angiotensinogen production by rat hepatoma cells is stimulated by B-cell stimulatory factor 2/interleukin 6. FEBS Lett *244:* 6–10

Kishimoto T 1989 The biology of Interleukin-6. Blood *74:* 1–10

Metsärinne K, Fyhrquist F, Grönhagen-Riska C 1988 Increased levels of immunoreactive plasma renin substrate during infectious peritonitis in patients on CAPD. Clin Sci *75:* 411–4

Comment on "The clinical significance of the glomerular location of segmental lesions in focal glomerulosclerosis"

Sir, – Morita et al. [1990] illustrate and mention parahilar hyaline deposits in glomeruli in children with focal segmental glomerulosclerosis and support the view that such lesions are precursors of hilar focal segmental glomerulosclerosis.

Such parahilar hyaline deposits were described as incidental lesions in the absence of renal disease, diabetes and hypertension in an autopsy study in 1965 [Spear and Kihara 1965]. The patients were aged 5–19. The location, staining characteristics and appearance of the deposits suggested that the lesions represented a variant of the process of hyaline arteriolosclerosis. Similar deposits were subsequently described by Aizawa et al. [1987] who found, in a study of renal biopsies, no relation to age, sex or disease category.

It would seem appropriate, therefore, to exercise caution before concluding that parahilar hyaline deposits are related to focal segmental glomerulosclerosis.

G. S. Spear
Department of Pathology, University of California, Irvine, Califorina College of Medicine, Irvine, California 92717, USA

REFERENCES

Aizawa S, Inomata I, Joh K 1987 A clinicopathological study on vascular pole deposit found in renal biopsy. Abstracts Xth International Congress of Nephrology London, p. 46

Morita M, White RHR, Coad BA, Raafat F 1990 The clinical significance of the glomerular location of segmental lesions in focal segmental glomerulosclerosis. Clin Nephrol *33:* 211–219

Spear GS, Kihara I 1965 "Exudative" lesions in glomeruli of children: a variant of hyaline arteriolosclerosis. Bull Johns Hopkins Hosp *116:* 161–174

Parahilar hyaline deposits and focal segmental glomerulosclerosis

Sir, – I am grateful to Dr. G. S. Spear for drawing attention to the need for caution in interpretating the significance of the parahilar hyaline deposits that we observed in the glomeruli of children with focal segmental glomerulosclerosis [Morita et al. 1990 a]. However, the findings that we have more recently reported on renal biopsies obtained from 24 children and adolescents with reduced renal mass due to reflux nephropathy [Morita et al. 1990 b] add weight to the argument that they are in some way related to FSGS.

Parahilar hyaline deposits were found in 17 out of the 24 biopsies, 8 of which also showed FSGS which was exclusively of hilar origin; moreover all 24 showed the presence of intramural hyaline deposits in the hilar arterioles, which were confirmed by electron microscopy to the located in the subendothelial zone. A similar relationship between hilar hyalinosis and FSGS was noted by Olson et al. [1985] in rats following subtotal nephrectomy.

It is becoming clear that FSGS is a heterogeneous condition. Howie et al. [1989] demonstrated in rats that the lesions resulting from subtotal nephrectomy or high protein feeding were invariably of hilar origin, whereas those associated with puromycin aminonucleoside nephrosis were distributed randomly. The emphasis of our studies is the association of parahilar hyaline deposits with hilar FSGS. I accept that to regard them as immediate precursors of FSGS may not be fully justified by the present evidence, and they may be an extension of the hilar vascular changes which nevertheless appear to precede the development of FSGS in the remnant kidney.

R. H. R. White
Department of Nephrology, The Children's Hospital, Ladywood Middleway, Birmingham, B16 8ET, UK.

REFERENCES

Howie AJ, Kizaki T, Beaman M et al. 1989 Different types of segmental sclerosing glomerular lesions in six experimental models of proteinuria. J Pathol *157:* 141–151

Morita M, White RHR, Coad NAG, Raafat F 1990 a The clinical significance of the glomerular location of segmental lesions in focal segmental glomerulosclerosis. Clin Nephrol *33:* 211–219

Morita M, Yoshiara S, White RHR, Raafat F 1990 b The glomerular changes in children with reflux nephropathy. J Pathol *162:* 245–253.

Olson JL, de Urdaneta AG, Heptinstall RH 1985 Glomerular hyalinosis and its relation to hyperfiltration. Lab Invest *52:* 387–398

Transplantation and nephrectomy in autosomal dominant polycystic disease

Sir, – In response to the article by Rayner et al. [1990], we thought it would be of interest to share our experience with the protocol we have employed since 1980 in patients with end-stage autosomal dominant polycystic kidney disease. Initially, nephrectomy is performed on the more severely affected kidney (determined by larger size or involvement with previous infections) previous to transplantation. 3 to 6 months later, nephrectomy of the remaining native kidney is performed.

This protocol has been followed in 15 patients, 9 men and 6 women, aged from 34 to 64 years (median age: 55 years).

There have been no postoperative mortalities. Morbidity due to 2 surgeries is unusual (1 superficial incisional abscess). Two deaths have occurred in our patients: one 2 years after transplant (rupture of an intracerebral aneurysm), and one 4 months after the graft due to cytomegalovirus infection. In the remaining patients, the graft remains functional, with a posttransplant range from 6 months to 10 years (median: 4 years).

11 patients received cyclosporine alone for immunosuppressive treatment; 4 others received combination therapy with azathioprine and corticosteroids.

Since the advent of the use of synthetic erythropoietin, this "sandwich" technique of transplantation between two nephrectomies is no longer of paramount interest with regard to anemia. However, concerning the patient on hemodialysis, this technique continues to facilitate maintenance of euvolemia while avoiding the inherent complications of polycystic kidneys.

E. Cassuto-Viguier[1], H. Quintens[2], D. Chevallier[2], M. Derrier[1], P. Jambou[1], J. Toubol[2], H. Duplay[1]
[1]Clinique Néphrologique and [2]Service d'Urologie, Hôpital Pasteur, BP 69, F-06002 Nice Cédex, France

REFERENCES

Mendelssohn DC, Harding ME, Cardella CJ, Cook GT, Uldall PR 1988 Management of end-stage autosomal dominant polycystic kidney disease with hemodialysis and transplantation. Clin Nephrol *30:* 315–319
Rayner BL, Cassidy MJD, Jacobsen JE, Pascoe MD, Pontin AR, Van Zyl Smit R 1990 Is preliminary bi-nephrectomy necessary in patients with autosomal dominant polycystic kidney disease undergoing renal transplantation. Clin Nephrol *34:* 122–124

Growth-related changes in echocardiographic measurements

Sir, – Cannella et al. [1990] report the cardiac benefits of erythropoietin (EPO) in a group of anemic dialysed uraemic patients without hypertension. The improvements with EPO are impressive. However when comparing the patients at baseline with a control group they found that several echocardiographic parameters, including the left ventricular end-diastolic diameter (LVEDD) and the interventricular septal thickness (IVS), were not significantly different when the raw data was analyzed but became so when the data were "indexed"; the result of dividing the raw data by the body surface area of the individual. This is clearly only justified if a parameter is known to be directly related to the body surface area. This was previously thought to be the case for most echocardiographic parameters [Epstein et al. 1975] but has subsequently been shown not to be true for several measurements including the LVEDD and the aortic root dimensions which vary in a linear relation to the cube root of the surface area, and the IVS and left ventricular posterior wall thickness which are best related to the square root of the surface area [Henry et al. 1980]. It is however justified for the left ventricular muscle mass and cardiac output which vary directly with the body surface area.

Thus "indexing" will have exaggerated the differences between the patient and control groups since the controls had a larger mean surface area. Instead the relevant raw data should have been divided by the square or cube root of the surface area, as appropriate to the parameter concerned, and then subjected to statistical analysis.

Given the small size of the study it is quite likely that the reported differences are in fact real differences over controls but the method of "indexing" all the variables is not justified.

Kevin Morris, Jon Skinner
Paediatric Nephrology, Paediatric Cardiology

REFERENCES

Cannella G, La Canna G, Sandrini M et al. 1990 Renormalization of high cardiac output and of left ventricular size following long-term recombinant human erythropoietin treatment of anemic dialysed uremic patients. Clin Nephrol *6:* 272–278
Epstein ML, Goldberg SJ, Sahn DJ et al. 1975 Great vessel, cardiac chamber, and wall growth patterns in normal children. Circulation *51:* 1124
Henry WL, Gardin JM, Ware JH 1980 Echocardiographic measurements in normal subjects from infancy to old age. Circulation *62:* 1054–1061

Clinical Nephrology, Vol. 36 No. 3–1991 (107–113)

Prognostic implication of anti-neutrophil cytoplasmic autoantibodies with myeloperoxidase specificity in anti-glomerular basement membrane disease

X. Bosch[1], E. Mirapeix[2], J. Font[1], X. Borrellas[3], R. Rodríguez[2], A. López-Soto[1], M. Ingelmo[1] and L. Revert[2]

Departments of Internal Medicine[1] and Nephrology[2] of the Hospital Clinic i Provincial, Universitat de Barcelona and Department of Nephrology[3] of the Hospital de la Vall d'Hebrón, Universitat Autònoma de Barcelona, Barcelona, Spain

Abstract. Anti-neutrophil cytoplasmic autoantibodies (ANCA) were detected in 12 out of 37 (32%) serum samples from patients with anti-glomerular basement membrane (GBM) disease by an indirect immunofluorescence assay. In 11 cases, ANCA were directed against myeloperoxidase, as revealed employing neutrophils devoid of this enzyme as the test substrate. Patients having both ANCA and anti-GBM antibodies (AGBMA) were considerably older (mean age 59 years) than patients with AGBMA alone (mean age 33 years). In addition, patients with both antibodies had some clinical and pathologic data that suggested an associated systemic vasculitis. This was supported by the fact that among these patients, those with highest ANCA titres recovered renal function despite being initially on hemodialysis, as opposed to those with lowest ANCA titres or AGBMA alone. In patients with both antibodies, there was an inverse relationship between AGBMA and ANCA values ($p = 0.02$). Moreover, the mean AGBMA level tended to be higher for patients with AGBMA alone than for those with both ANCA and AGBMA. These results suggest that, at least in some cases, there may be a contribution of an ANCA-related mechanism in the pathogenesis of anti-GBM disease. Although the exact role of ANCA in this and other diseases remains to be clarified, there is important clinical evidence that in anti-GBM disease ANCA may represent a serologic marker of good prognosis identifying a subset of patients who may recover renal function.

Key words: anti-neutrophil cytoplasmic autoantibodies – anti-glomerular basement membrane antibodies – anti-glomerular basement membrane disease – myeloperoxidase – renal function

Introduction

Autoantibodies against cytoplasmic constituents of neutrophils and monocytes (ANCA) have been detected in sera from patients with systemic vasculitis, especially Wegener's granulomatosis and microscopic polyarteritis [van der Woude et al. 1985, Savage et al. 1987, Nölle et al. 1989, Cohen Tervaert et al. 1989]. Moreover, they have been recently reported in cases of idiopathic and vasculitis-associated necrotizing and crescentic glomerulonephritis [Falk and Jennette 1988, Andrassy et al. 1989, Cohen Tervaert et al. 1990, Falk et al. 1990a]. Two types of these antibodies were first recognized: one with reactivity with myeloperoxidase (MPO) on enzyme-linked immunosorbent assay (ELISA) that produces an artifactual perinuclear immunostaining of ethanol-fixed neutrophils (P-ANCA), and another without reactivity with MPO on ELISA which produces a diffuse cytoplasmic immunostaining (C-ANCA) [Falk and Jennette 1988].

In this report we present data indicating that ANCA are also present in the blood of patients having a diagnosis of anti-glomerular basement membrane (GBM) disease. We further introduce a technical modification for detection of ANCA with specificity for MPO. Thus, anti-MPO antibodies could be identified in all but one patient with both ANCA and anti-GBM antibodies (AGBMA). We give clinical, pathologic and immunological records indicating that

Received November 23, 1990; in revised form March 13, 1991.

Reprint requests to Dr. Xavier Bosch, Servicio de Medicina Interna General, Unidad 1, Hospital Clinic i Provincial, Villarroel, 170, ES-08036 Barcelona, Spain in patients with both antibodies there may be features suggestive of a coexistent systemic vasculitis. In this paper, this is also supported by the evidence that these patients, receiving the same treatment, have a better short-term prognosis (recovery of renal function) than those with AGBMA alone.

Patients and methods

Methods

Detection of AGBMA by radioimmunoassay AGBMA were measured by a solid-phase radioimmunoassay. This assay detects immunoglobulin (Ig) G antibodies that bind to collagenase digests of GBM [Fish et al. 1984].

Preparation of antigens from GBM Human cadaver kidneys were obtained at autopsy within 24 h after death and stored at −70° C until used. The kidneys were partially thawed, the renal corticies dissected away from medullary tissue and the glomeruli isolated from tubules and connective tissue on stainless steel meshes. Glomerular preparations were subjected to ultrasonic disruption in 1 M sodium chloride and washed several times with distilled water, centrifuged and finally lyophilized.

Partial isolation of GBM antigens Lyophilized human GBM was digested using collagenase type IV (Sigma Chemical Co., St. Louis, Missouri). This enzyme was dissolved in distilled water and stored at −70° C. Fifteen mg of GBM were suspended in 0.1 M Tris buffer pH 7.5 (1.5 ml) containing 0.005 M calcium acetate, and 1 mg of collagenase was added. The suspension was stirred for 30 min at 37° C in a water bath, centrifuged at 1000 g for 10 min, and the supernatant heated for 5 min at 60° C to inactivate collagenase. In previous experiments a single digestion for either 60 or 90 min had produced comparable results.

Radioimmunoassay Polypropylene microtiter plates (Dynatech) were coated with 1:100 dilution of the collagen digested GBM in complement fixing diluent (CFD) during 3 h at 37° C and overnight at 4° C. Plates were washed thrice with CFD containing 0.2% Tween 20 (CFDTw) and stored at 4° C until used for assay. Plates were incubated with control (normal and reference positive) and test serum samples (diluted 1:10 in CFDTw) for 1 h at 37° C. After further washing with CFDTw, bound AGBMA were detected with anti-human IgG labelled with iodine 125 in CFDTw at 37° C for 1 h. All volumes were 100 µl. Plates were then washed in CFDTw and counted. Binding of test serum was expressed as a percentage of the reference positive serum sample. Binding of normal serum was 10% of the reference positive serum [Jayne et al. 1990].

Detection of ANCA by indirect immunofluorescence ANCA were tested by an indirect immunofluorescence assay as previously described [Cohen Tervaert et al. 1989], with minor modifications. Briefly, granulocytes from a healthy donor were obtained by dextran sedimentation of heparinized blood and Ficoll-Isopaque (Pharmacia Fine Chemicals, Uppsala, Sweden) centrifugation. After washing the cells, cytocentrifuge preparations were made and fixed for 5 min in absolute ethanol at 4° C. Preparations were stored at −80° C. Test, negative and positive control serum samples were overlaid in 1:20 dilution on the cytopreparations and incubated for 1 h at 37° C. After washing thrice with phosphate-buffered saline (PBS) for 5 min, bound antibody was detected by a fluorescein-isothyocyanate conjugated rabbit antibody against human IgG gamma chains (Dako, Denmark) diluted 1:20 in PBS. Finally, slides were washed again in PBS and mounted in glycerin-PBS for immunofluorescence microscopy.

Identification of ANCA with MPO specificity We developed a simple method to decide, in positive cases, if ANCA were directed against MPO. We used neutrophils from a voluntary donor who was known to have complete and selective inherited deficiency of this enzyme. This rare and otherwise commonly asymptomatic condition consists in the lack of MPO in the azurophil granulations of the neutrophil granulocytes and monocytes [Larrocha et al. 1982]. Such a disorder may be easily detected in routine hematological analysis by automated flow cytochemistry using the Technicon H-1 analyzer (Technicon Instruments Corporation, Tarrytown, New York) which is used to determine the white blood cell differential counting according to the cellular peroxidase activity [Parry et al. 1981]. Sera giving a positive immunofluorescence with normal neutrophils but negative with neutrophils devoid of MPO were considered as possessing anti-MPO antibodies. The procedure was performed twice in all positive cases for confirmation.

Patients

Thirty-seven consecutive patients with a proven diagnosis of anti-GBM disease were included in this study. All sera were collected between March 1988 and April 1990 since our laboratory constitutes a reference center for detection of both AGBMA and ANCA. Several serum samples from each patient were obtained during the entire course of the disease. In all patients, the diagnosis was based on serological and renal biopsy criteria. Renal biopsies were examined

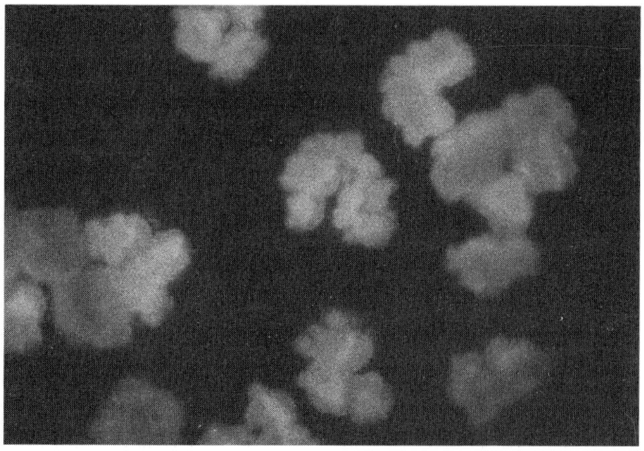

Fig. 1 Immunostaining of neutrophils on immunofluorescence microscopy. Observe the diffuse staining of nuclei with dense endonuclear bands, typical of anti-myeloperoxidase antibodies (× 100).

by light and immunofluorescence techniques. To investigate immunedeposits, fluorescein antibodies with specificity for IgA, IgG and IgM heavy chains, Ig light chains, C3, C4, C1q, and fibrinogen were employed. The clinical data of these 37 patients were reviewed with special attention to clinical presentation, pulmonary and renal involvement, cutaneous vasculitis, peripheral nerve lesions, ocular manifestations, joint involvement, treatment and follow-up. The laboratory data were also reviewed with special attention to the autoimmune profile which mainly included anti-nuclear antibodies screening with HEp-2 cells, anti-native DNA antibodies determination by radioimmunoassay, measure of C3 and C4 complement factors by nephelometry, and total hemolytic complement (CH50) determination by microcomplement consumption test.

Statistical Analysis

The statistical data were analyzed using non-parametric tests. The Mann-Whitney "U" test was performed to compare differences in mean AGBMA levels between groups. The Fisher's exact test was used to compare the clinical outcome in patients with high or low ANCA titres. All p values below 0.05 were considered to indicate statistical significance.

Results

Assays

Of the 37 patients with a proven diagnosis of anti-GBM disease, 25 had AGBMA (group 1) and 12 (32%) had both AGBMA and ANCA (group 2). A rather diffuse nuclear immunostaining pattern with additional dense endonuclear bands was seen in 11 patients of group 2 (Figure 1). In all them, a negative immunofluorescence for ANCA was evident at the minimal dilution (1:20) when neutrophils with deficiency of MPO were used. Conversely, in one case there were no differences of immunostaining between normal neutrophils and those with an absence of MPO at progressive dilutions. In this case, there was a different immunostaining pattern which was clearly perinuclear (Patient No. 5). We then concluded that 11 patients presented ANCA with specificity for MPO, whereas one must have had antibodies to other myeloid antigen or antigens (Table 1).

The mean AGBMA percentage binding tended to be slightly higher for patients of group 1 (44%) than for those of group 2 (36%). In group 2, AGBMA levels were significantly higher for patients with lowest ANCA titres ($\leq$1:80) (50 ± 22: mean ± SD) than for those with highest ANCA ones (>1:80) (26 ± 8), and vice versa (p = 0.02). In addition, a parallel reduction of ANCA and AGBMA values was observed in each case with the treatment of disease.

Clinical and pathologic descriptions of the patients studied

Clinical characteristics At the time of admission, the mean age of patients of group 2 (9 males and 3 females) was 59 years (range 41–80), and the mean age of patients of group 1 (15 males and 10 females) was 33 years (range 18–49). Constitutional symptoms such as weakness and weight loss as well as fever were common in group 2. On admission, serum creatinine was increased in all these patients with a mean value of 1053 µmol/liter (range 707–1414 µmol/liter), 8 being oligoanuric at presentation. Renal function was also impaired in all patients of group 1 (mean serum creatinine 1149 µmol/liter), diuresis being preserved only in 3 who had predominantly pulmonary involvement and mild renal failure (serum creatinine values: 133, 159 and 177 µmol/liter). Microscopic hematuria and proteinuria were commonly present in both groups. The prevalence of pulmonary hemorrhage was 50% for patients of group 2 and 57% for patients of group 1. In group 2 patients, clinical involvement outside the renal and pulmonary systems was present in 5 cases, one having skin rash, 2 arthritis, one sensori-motor polyneuropathy and proximal myositis, and one uveitis (Table 2). Immunological tests were negative or within normal limits in all but one case, which had decreased levels of C3, C4 and CH50 (Patient No. 10).

Table 1 AGBMA levels (radioimmunoassay) and P-ANCA titres (indirect immunofluorescence) at presentation of sera from patients of group 2 (AGBMA plus ANCA)

Case No	AGBMA levels (normal <12%)	P-ANCA titres (positive ≥1:20)	MPO-ANCA
1	22	1:320	+
2	24	1:160	+
3	72	1: 80	+
4	32	1: 40	+
5	28	1:320	–
6	38	1: 80	+
7	20	1:640	+
8	41	1:320	+
9	18	1:320	+
10	76	1: 40	+
11	28	1:640	+
12	32	1: 40	+

AGBMA: anti-glomerular basement membrane antibodies
P-ANCA: anti-neutrophil cytoplasmic antibodies with perinuclear pattern
MPO-ANCA: anti-myeloperoxidase antibodies

Treatment In most cases, it consisted in associating prednisolone (1 mg/kg/day) with cyclophosphamide (1.5–2 mg/kg/day) given over a 4-week period. In addition, azathioprine (1–2 mg/kg/day) was added in patients less than 50 years old. Plasma exchange (3–4 liters of plasma/day during the first week, and subsequently depending on the AGBMA levels) was performed in many patients. According to this protocol, 11 patients of group 2 received immunosuppressive treatment, 10 also having plasma exchange. Furthermore, 11 patients required dialysis (Table 2). In one case, immunosuppressive therapy could not be started as the patient died because of unexplained cardiac arrest at the time of diagnosis while he was on hemodialysis (Patient No. 1). Treatment was similar for patients of group 1, 22 requiring dialysis. In this group, there were 3 patients with mild renal failure who did not require dialysis support.

Clinical Outcome By 3 to 31 months of follow-up, there had been 3 deaths among patients of group 2, one having had an unexplained cardiac arrest before starting treatment (Patient No. 1), one having had septic shock following gram-negative bacteremia (Patient No. 3), and one who died after a lung biopsy a few days after starting treatment (Patient No. 8). In addition, 5 patients, 4 of whom were initially dialysis dependent, had recovered satisfactory renal function with a mean period of 25 days after admission, and remain actually independent of dialysis. The remaining 4 patients presented no response to treatment and are actually maintained on hemodialysis (Table 2). Finally, there had been 9 deaths among patients of group 1, 13 survivors initially dialysis dependent being also dialysis dependent at present. Reasons for

Table 2 Main clinical features of patients of group 2 (AGBMA plus ANCA)

Case No	Age	Sex	Interval before RB	Creatinine at onset*	Diuresis (ml/24 h)	Pulmonary hemorrhage	Other system involvement	Treatment	HD	Outcome**
1	75	M	4 wk	796	preserved	no	none	none	yes	dead
2	53	M	2 mo	707	preserved	no	none	P, Cy, PE	no	recovery (115)
3	80	M	4 wk	1149	<400	yes	skin rash	P, Cy, PE	yes	dead
4	51	M	3 wk	884	<400	no	none	P, Cy, PE	yes	CRF/HD
5	43	M	2 mo	1061	<400	yes	arthritis	P, Cy, Az, PE	yes	recovery (88)
6	69	M	6 wk	972	preserved	yes	arthritis	P, Cy, PE	yes	CRF/HD
7	70	M	4 wk	1061	<400	yes	none	P, Cy	yes	recovery (80)
8	73	M	2 wk	884	preserved	yes	none	P, Cy, PE	yes	dead
9	52	M	5 wk	1238	<400	no	none	P, Cy, PE	yes	recovery (97)
10	41	F	2 mo	1149	<400	yes	polyneuropathy myositis	P, Cy, Az, PE	yes	CRF/HD
11	58	F	5 wk	1326	<400	no	unveitis	P, Cy, PE	yes	recovery (133)
12	45	F	2 wk	1414	<400	no	none	P, Cy, Az, PE	yes	CRF/HD

*: values expressed on µmol/liter; RB: renal biopsy; HD: hemodialysis; P: prednisolone; Cy: cyclophosphamide; Az: azathioprine; PE: plasma exchange; CRF: chronic renal failure
**: creatinine levels at recovery (µmol/liter)

Table 3 Main histologic features in the kidney of patients of group 2 (AGBMA plus ANCA)

Case No	Glomerular necrosis	Crescents*	Other pathologic findings
1	+++	50	small vessel vasculitis
2	++	75	tubular necrosis
3	++	100	none
4	+	75	none
5	+++	25	none
6	+++	50	small vessel vasculitis
7	+++	50	endocapillary proliferation
8	++	100	granulomata, arteriolitis
9	+	75	endocapillary proliferation
10	+	100	none
11	++	100	granulomata, arteriolitis
12	+++	25	small vessel vasculitis

*: approximate percentage; +: mild, ++: moderate, +++: severe (global)

the death in group 1 patients included sudden cardiac arrest in 2, massive gastrointestinal bleeding in 3, and infection in 4.

Renal Pathology A renal biopsy could be performed in all patients. In patients of group 2, there were 5 cases with predominantly necrotizing glomerulonephritis and a percentage of crescents which lay between 25 and 50%. The remaining 7 patients presented with predominantly crescentic glomerulonephritis (75–100% of crescents) with either mild or moderate glomerular necrosis (Table 3). Pathologic findings consistent with renal vasculitis could be observed in 5 patients of this group, 3 having vasculitis involving small arteries, and 2 periglomerular granulomata with additional arteriolitis. Moreover, endocapillary proliferation was present in 2 cases. In patients of group 1, there was no case with predominantly necrotizing form, all them having typical crescentic glomerulonephritis (75–100% of crescents) with absent or only mild glomerular necrosis. Signs suggestive of chronicity such as glomerular sclerosis, fibrous crescents or interstitial fibrosis were absent or insignificant in all patients of both groups. On renal immunofluorescence, there was linear deposition of IgG and occasionally of C3 diffusely along the GBM in all 37 patients. Fibrin-related antigens were found in most patients, chiefly in the crescents and in areas of tuft necrosis.

Clinic – Immunologic Associations

Patients of group 2 who responded to treatment and recovered renal function corresponded to those with highest ANCA titres at presentation (n = 5). On the contrary, patients with no clinical response to treatment were those with lowest ANCA titres (n = 5). There was a significant association between high ANCA titres and a short-term good prognosis (recovery of renal function), and between low ANCA titres and a bad prognosis ($p < 0.005$). Other 2 patients had initially high ANCA titres (1:320) (Patients No. 1 and 8) but their follow-up could not be influenced by treatment, as previously mentioned.

Discussion

According to our results, ANCA can be detected in one third of patients having a diagnosis of anti-GBM disease. In these cases, there are clinical (skin rash, arthritis, polyneuropathy, uveitis) and pathologic (arteriolitis, granuloma formation, necrotizing glomerulonephritis) features as well as prognostic connotations that suggest the coexistence of an ANCA-related systemic vasculitis. In addition, we identify ANCA with MPO specificity as being responsible for most positive cases.

At present, it is accepted that ANCA have two main antigenic specificities, each one associating with different disorders. Thus, C-ANCA mainly correspond to anti-proteinase 3 antibodies which identify most patients with biopsy-proven Wegener's granulomatosis, especially those with sinus and upper respiratory tract involvement [Goldschmeding et al. 1989, Niles et al. 1989, Lüdemann et al. 1990, Falk et al. 1990a]. On the other hand, P-ANCA mainly correspond to anti-MPO antibodies which are strongly associated with pauci-immune necrotizing and crescentic glomerulonephritis with little or no evidence for extra-renal involvement [Falk and Jennette 1988, Cohen Tervaert et al. 1990, Falk et al. 1990a]. Moreover, biopsy-proven renal arteritis can be demonstrated in some patients with anti-MPO antibodies, but it seems to be very rare in patients having anti-proteinase 3 antibodies and Wegener's granulomatosis [Andrassy et al. 1990]. There appears to be, however, a substantial overlap in disease distribution among patients with both antibodies.

In recent studies of ANCA-associated rapidly progressive glomerulonephritis, some patients with anti-GBM disease were occasionally included as a negative control group [Falk and Jennette 1988, Andrassy et al. 1989], whereas in other series they were expressly not included [Cohen Tervaert et al. 1990]. However, O'Donoghue et al. [1989] were the first to claim attention on the presence of ANCA in patients with anti-GBM disease. More recently, in a prospective study which included a large series of patients having a suspected diagnosis of rapidly progressive glomerulonephritis, some of them were found to have both ANCA and AGBMA [Jayne et al. 1990]. The authors concluded that clinical and pathologic data collected from patients with both antibodies suggested the coexistence of a systemic vasculitis. In our work, this is further supported by the evidence that among patients with both antibodies, those with highest titres of ANCA, receiving the same treatment, presented a better clinical response than those with lowest ANCA titres or AGBMA alone. Thus, there were 5 patients with a titre of ANCA between 1:160 and 1:640 who responded to treatment and recovered renal function, despite 4 of them being initially on hemodialysis. On the contrary, no patient with an ANCA titre ≤1:80 or with AGBMA alone had recovered renal function. Furthermore, we have demonstrated that MPO seems to be the antigen involved in these cases.

In anti-GBM disease, some patients have symptoms suggestive of a systemic disorder such as myalgias, arthritic complaints, skin rash and even neurologic disturbances [Glassock et al. 1986, Savage et al. 1986]. On the other hand, there have been some well-documented cases of histologically proven vasculitis reported [Glassock et al. 1986, Wu et al. 1980, Wahls et al. 1987]. Prognosis is generally bad and recovery of renal function, once the patient is dialysis dependent, is unusual in this disease [Jayne et al. 1990, Glassock et al. 1986, Savage et al. 1986]; however, cases of oligoanuric and dialysis dependent patients who recovered sufficient renal function to remain independent of dialysis have been occasionally described in a similar manner that occurs for rapidly progressive glomerulonephritis due to systemic vasculitis [Jayne et al. 1990, Savage et al. 1986] and for ANCA-associated necrotizing and crescentic glomerulonephritis without AGBMA [Falk et al. 1990a]. Therefore, according to these and our results, it may be presumed that an ANCA-related vasculitis could be involved in some of these reported cases.

It is noteworthy that the mean age of our patients with both antibodies was considerably greater than that of our patients with AGBMA alone (59 versus 33). This points out that in anti-GBM disease, ANCA may also identify a subset of patients with a late onset disease.

The central question to be answered is: what is the role of ANCA in anti-GBM disease? Surprisingly, in our study there was an inverse relationship between AGBMA and ANCA values in the group of patients with both antibodies. Moreover, the mean AGBMA level tended to be higher for patients with AGBMA alone than for those with both AGBMA and ANCA. These findings suggest that, at least in some cases, there may be a coexistence of two mechanisms in the pathogenesis of anti-GBM disease: that dependent on AGBMA and a vasculitis mediated by ANCA.

It has been recently demonstrated that ANCA cause neutrophil activation in vitro, thus inducing oxygen and enzymatic release [Falk et al. 1990b]. In crescentic glomerulonephritis, including anti-GBM nephritis, lysosomal enzymes are strongly implicated in the pathophysiological process resulting in GBM degradation [Davies et al. 1978, Johnson et al. 1988a, Lubec et al. 1980]. In addition, the MPO-hydrogen peroxide-halide system seems to be involved in glomerular injury [Johnson et al. 1988b]. It would be attractive to speculate that in some cases of anti-GBM disease, production of ANCA by a unknown factor (infection?) may represent a primary event. Thus, if damage to the GBM by the above mentioned products can uncover new antigenic sites (neoantigens) it could lead to the formation of AGBMA. This hardy hypothesis would be supported by the recent evidence that most AGBMA found in patients with ANCA do not react specifically with the true Goodpasture antigen [Pusey et al. 1990]. In any event, there is important clinical evidence that in anti-GBM disease ANCA may represent a serologic marker of good prognosis identifying a subset of patients who may respond to treatment and recover renal function.

Acknowledgements

Dr. X. Bosch is a Research Fellow sponsored by grants from the Hospital Clinic i Provincial de Barcelona (1990) and the Direcció General d'Universitats de la Generalitat de Catalunya (Formació d'Investigadors 1990). The authors thank Dr. A. De la Sierra for helping with the statistical analysis

REFERENCES

Andrassy K, Koderisch J, Rufer M, Erb A, Waldherr R, Ritz E 1989 Detection and clinical implication of anti-neutrophil cytoplasm antibodies in Wegener's granulomatosis and rapidly progressive glomerulonephritis. Clin Nephrol *32:* 159–167

Andrassy K, Koderisch J, Schäfer A, Waldherr R 1990 Idiopathic rapidly progressive (crescentic) glomerulonephritis with myeloperoxidase antibodies – a new entity linked to female sex? (Letter) Nephron *56:* 99–100

Cohen Tervaert JW, van der Woude FJ, Fauci AS, Ambrus JL, Velosa J, Keane WF, Meijer S, van der Giessen M, The TH, van der Hem GK, Kallenberg CGM 1989 Association between active Wegener's granulomatosis and anti-cytoplasmic antibodies. Arch Intern Med *149:* 2461–2465

Cohen Tervaert JW, Goldschmeding R, Elema JD, van der Giessen M, Huitema MG, van der Hem GK, The TH, von dem Borne AEGK, Kallenberg CGM 1990 Autoantibodies against myeloid lysosomal enzymes in crescentic glomerulonephritis. Kidney Int *37:* 799–806

Davies M, Barret AJ, Travis J, Sanders E, Coles GA 1978 The degradation of human glomerular basement membrane with purified lysosomal proteinases: evidence for the pathogenic role of the polymorphonuclear leukocytes in glomerulonephritis. Clin Sci Mol Med *54:* 233–240

Falk RJ, Jennette JC 1988 Anti-neutrophil cytoplasmic autoantibodies with specificity for myeloperoxidase in patients with systemic vasculitis and idiopathic necrotizing and crescentic glomerulonephritis. N Engl J Med *318:* 1651–1657

Falk RJ, Hogan S, Carey TS, Jennette JC 1990a Clinical course of antineutrophil cytoplasmic autoantibody – associated glomerulonephritis and systemic vasculitis. Ann Intern Med *113:* 656–663

Falk RJ, Terrell RS, Charles LA, Jennette JC 1990b Anti-neutrophil cytoplasmic autoantibodies induce neutrophils to degranulate and produce oxygen radicals in vitro. Proc Natl Acad Sci USA *87:* 4115–4119

Fish AJ, Lockwood MC, Wong M, Price RG 1984 Detection of Goodposture antigen in fractions prepared from collagenase digests of human glomerular basement membrane. Clin Exp Immunol *55:* 58–66

Glassock RJ, Cohen AH, Adler SG, Ward HJ 1986 Secondary glomerular diseases. In: *Brenner BM, Rector FC* (eds) The Kidney. Saunders, Philadelphia: 1032–1036

Goldschmeding R, van der Schoot CE, ten Bokkel Huinink D, Hack CE, van den Ende ME, Kallenberg CGM, von dem Borne AEGK 1989 Wegener's granulomatosis autoantibodies identify a novel diisopropylfluorophosphate – binding protein in the lysosomes of normal human neutrophils. J Clin Invest *84:* 1577–1587

Jayne DRW, Marshall PD, Jones SJ, Lockwood CM 1990 Autoantibodies to GBM and neutrophil cytoplasm in rapidly progressive glomerulonephritis. Kidney Int *37:* 965–970

Johnson RJ, Couser WG, Alpers CE, Vissers M, Schulze M, Klebanoff SJ 1988a The human neutrophil serine proteinases, elastase and cathepsin G, can mediate glomerular injury in vivo. J Exp Med *168:* 1169–1174

Johnson RJ, Guggenheim SJ, Klebanoff SJ, Ochi RF, Wass A, Baker P, Schulze M, Couser WG 1988b Morphologic correlates of glomerular oxidant injury induced by the myeloperoxidase-hydrogen peroxide-halide system of the neutrophil. Lab Invest *58:* 294–301

Larrocha C, Fernández de Castro M, Fontan G, Viloria A, Fernández-Chacón JL, Jiménez C 1982 Hereditary myeloperoxidase deficiency: study of 12 cases. Scand J Haematol *29:* 389–397

Lubec G, Förster O, Coradello H, Maxa E, Pollak A 1980 Proteolytic degradation of the glomerular basement membrane and immunochemical characterization of split products. In: *Lubec G* (ed) The Glomerular Basement Membrane. S. Karger, Basel: 126–132

Lüdemann J, Utecht B, Gross WL 1990 Anti-neutrophil cytoplasm antibodies in Wegener's granulomatosis recognize an elastinolytic enzyme. J Exp Med *171:* 357–362

Niles JL, McCluskey RT, Ahmad MF, Arnaout MA 1989 Wegener's granulomatosis autoantigen is a novel neutrophil serine proteinase. Blood *74:* 1888–1893

Nölle B, Specks U, Lüdemann J, Rohrbach MS, DeRemee RA, Gross WL 1989 Anticytoplasmic autoantibodies: their immunodiagnostic value in Wegener granulomatosis. Ann Intern Med *111:* 28–40

O'Donoghue DJ, Short CD, Brenchley PEC, Lawler W, Ballardie FW 1989 Sequential development of systemic vasculitis with anti-neutrophil cytoplasmic antibodies complicating anti-glomerular basement membrane disease. Clin Nephrol *32:* 251–255

Parry MF, Root RK, Metcalf JA, Delaney KK, Kaplow LS, Richar WJ 1981 Myeloperoxidase deficiency. Prevalence and clinical significance. Ann Intern Med *95:* 293–301

Pusey CD, Turner AN, Gaskin G, Katbamna I, Ryan JJ, Rees AJ 1990 Most anti-GBM antibodies found in patients with ANCA are not directed against the Goodpasture antigen. The 3rd International Workshop on ANCA: November 29–30, Washington, USA

Savage COS, Pusey CD, Bowman C, Rees AJ, Lockwood CM 1986 Antiglomerular basement membrane antibody mediated disease in the British Isles 1980–4. Br Med J *292:* 301–304

Savage CO, Winearls CG, Jones S, Marshall PD, Lockwood CM 1987 Prospective study of radioimmunoassay for antibodies against neutrophil cytoplasm in diagnosis of systemic vasculitis. Lancet *1:* 1389–1393

van der Woude FJ, Rasmussen N, Lobatto S, Wiik A, Permin H, van Es LA, van der Giessen M, van der Hem GK, The TH 1985 Autoantibodies against neutrophils and monocytes: tool for diagnosis and marker of disease activity in Wegener's granulomatosis. Lancet *1:* 425–429

Wahls TL, Bonsib SM, Schuster VL 1987 Coexistent Wegener's granulomatosis and anti-glomerular basement membrane disease. Hum Pathol *18:* 202–205

Wu MJ, Rajaram R, Shelp WD, Beirne GJ, Burkholder PM 1980 Vasculitis in Goodpasture's syndrome. Arch Pathol Lab Med *104:* 300–302

Clinical Nephrology, Vol. 36 No. 3–1991 (114–126)

Immune material processing by phagocyte cell system in cryoglobulinemia

D. Roccatello [1], G. Mazzucco [2], R. Coppo [1], G. Piccoli [1], F. Malavasi [3], G. Cavalli [4], G. Martina [1], M. C. Amprimo [4], M. G. Guerra [5], A. Amore [1], G. Quattrocchio [1], A. Molino [1], S. Maffei [1], G. Picciotto [6] and L. M. Sena [7]

[1] Istituto di Nefro-Urologia, [2] Istituto di Anatomia Patologica e [3] Cattedra di Biologia Cellulare dell'Università di Torino. [4] Laboratorio di Nefrologia e di Immunoematologia dell'Ospedale G. Bosco, [5] Banca del Sangue e [6] Servizio di Medicina Nucleare dell'Ospedale S. Giovanni Battista e della Città di Torino. [7] III Cattedra di Patologia Generale dell'Università di Torino, Turin, Italy

Abstract. An impaired function of splenic macrophages, measured as the clearance rate of erythrocytes coated with IgG (E-IgG), was observed in 7 out of 8 cryoglobulinemic patients with severe urinary abnormalities and systemic symptoms, and in 0 out of 6 patients without urinary symptoms and only mild systemic signs of disease. The E-IgG clearance rate was not related to HLA or Rh phenotype, patients' age or disease duration. Moreover, longitudinal studies showed this parameter to be strictly related to disease activity. To investigate the nature of the defect, five series of analyses were planned using peripheral blood phagocytes (PBP) from 8 patients: a) detection of cell-bound immune material by using the antibody CE59 directed to the Fc fragment of IgG modified by the antibody-antigen reaction; b) cytofluorometric and/or radiometric analyses of the cell surface expression of HLA II, CR1 and FcR structures by means of specific monoclonal antibiodies (MoAbs); c) electron microscopy (EM) examination of diverse combinations of cryoglobulins incubated with PBP from patients and normals; d) analysis of cryoglobulin-induced inhibition of E-IgG phagocytosis; e) measurement of the generation of chemiluminescence (CL) in response to Zymosan, Phorbol Myristate Acetate and n-Formyl-Methyonine-Leucine-Phenilalanine (n-FMLP). Patients' PBP were found to have a higher amount of cell-bound immune material as compared to normals ($p < 0.01$). CR1 and FcR expression was not different from controls, whereas a slight increase in percentage of monocytes bearing HLA II structures was found in patients ($p < 0.05$). Upon EM examination no obvious differences were found in the internalization capacity of cryoglobulins between patients and controls. The CL production was lower than normal ($p < 0.02$), whatever stimulus used, with a maximal impairment for n-FLMP ($p < 0.005$), the most specific test probe for cytoskeleton integrity. Finally, a remarkable cryoglobulin-induced inhibition of E-IgG phagocytosis was shown. A combination of saturation mechanisms and intracellular abnormalities could underlie the apparent discrepancy between E-IgG clearance defect and preserved potential of cryoglobulin internalization in cryoglobulinemia.

Key words: mononuclear phagocyte system function – cryoglobulinemia – Fc receptors – C3b receptors – chemiluminescence

Introduction

Impaired function of the mononuclear phagocyte system has been described in a variety of immune-mediated disorders [Frank 1983, Roccatello et al. 1987a], including cryoglobulinemia [Walport et al. 1985]. A defective mononuclear phagocyte system would be unable to clear immune complexes efficiently from the blood-stream, leading to tissue deposition of immune material. This hypothesis has largely been supported by in vitro and in vivo studies which evaluated the Fc-mediated endocytosis of well-identified, particulate immune complexes such as erythrocytes coated with IgG anti Rh (D). A delayed clearance of these cells was considered to reflect macrophage inability to phagocytize any kind of

Received April 17, 1990; in revised form May 6, 1991.

Reprint requests to Dr. Dario Roccatello, Divisione di nefrologia e dialisi Ospedale G. Bosco, P. ZA Donatore di sangue 3, I-10154 Torino, Italy.

immune complex presumably removed via the same receptor [Frank 1983]. Attempts to reproduce the defect by measuring preformed soluble immune complex internalization failed to give definitive results [Finbloomb 1987]. Possible differences in the way particulate and soluble immune complexes are handled have been poorly addressed. The present study focuses on the mechanisms regulating the internalization of immune material by the phagocyte cell system in cryoglobulinemia, a typical immune complex disease. The results show that the functional defect on the phagocyte system measured as the clearance rate of IgG-coated erythrocytes is probably target-specific. An intracellular abnormality, possibly residing at the cytoskeletal level, or due to saturation mechanisms, occurs in phagocyte cells from clinically active cryoglobulinemic patients.

Methods

Experimental design

The IgG-coated erythrocyte removal capacity by splenic macrophages in vivo was measured in cryoglobulinemic patients during active or inactive phases of disease and, sequentially, before and after plasma exchange or steroid pulse therapy. In vitro studies were planned to investigate the nature of a possible defect of internalization of particulate immune material in patients. Several combinations of cryoglobulins incubated with monocytes from patients and age/sex-matched normal controls were examined using electron microscopy. A pathologist examined cell suspensions prepared by another investigator who processed coded blood samples. Cell surface quantitative expression of receptors involved in the immune response was analyzed by specific monoclonal antibodies. The possibility of receptor saturation was examined by detecting IgG-containing immune material on the phagocyte cell surface by means of a monoclonal antibody directed to the Fc of IgG modified by the interaction with antigen. Finally, the generation of reactive oxygen species was measured to assess the intracellular energy expenditure and the response to substances able to stimulate events similar to engulfing foreign material by leukocytes.

Patients

Fourteen Rh (D) positive patients, 12 women and 2 men, mean age 54 years (range 37–80), with a mean disease duration of 3.2 years, were analyzed in the last 6 years for the in vivo immune clearance of IgG-coated erythrocytes. The diagnosis of essential mixed cryoglobulinemia (EMC) was made, after exclusion of underlying infectious, lymphoproliferative or other autoimmune diseases [Meltzer et al. 1966, Gorevic et al. 1980], on the basis of the characteristic clinical findings (including necrotiziting vasculitis with purpura and Raynaud's phenomenon, weakness, arthralgias, fever, neuropathy, hepatosplenomegaly and glomerulonephritis) and the presence of cryoglobulins in the serum. Three patients had mixed cryoglobulins (IgG/IgM) without monoclonal component, 10 patients had IgG/IgM-k cryoglobulins and one had IgM-k, the polyclonal IgG component being immunoelectrophoretically detectable only in trace amounts. Eight patients had urinary abnormalities. In 6 cases, the diagnosis of cryoglobulinemic glomerulonephritis was confirmed by renal biopsy, showing various degrees of endocapillary proliferation, usually associated with PAS-positive intraluminal "thrombi", and deposits of immunoglobulins (IgM and IgG) and complement fractions (C3, C1q) with ultrastructural features typical for cryoglobulins [Stoebner et al. 1979]. A clinically active phase of renal disease was judged by the presence, at the time of the study, of important urinary abnormalities (microscopic hematuria with >25 red blood cells [RBC]/ high power [×400] microscopic field [HPMF] in three sequential urinalyses and/or >3.5 g/day nephrotic range proteinuria). The 8 patients with clinically active renal disease had a history, over the previous 2 weeks, of necrotizing vasculitis with purpura (6 cases), Raynaud's phenomenon (5 cases), severe weakness and arthralgia (all cases), fever (7 cases) and peripheral neuropathy (3 cases). The other patients had a history of purpura, weakness and mild arthralgia, but were free of symptoms over the previous 3 months. Except for 5 serially studied cases, patients were not receiving steroids, immunosuppressive drugs, anti-prostaglandins, antibiotics, angiotensin converting-enzyme inhibitors nor other drugs known to influence phagocyte cell function. Systemic signs in the 5 serially studied patients were identified by two observers (D. R. and R. C.). Eight untreated cases (4 active and 4 inactive as defined above) were also investigated with the in vitro assays described below.

Control

Twenty-five normal volunteers (10 females and 15 males, mean age 34.9, range 21–73 years) were examined as healthy controls for the studies on macrophage immune clearance. Thirteen patients with biopsy-proven glomerular sclerosis (FGS), 6 women and 7 men, mean age 44.7 years (range 19–67) served as control subjects having renal disease not associated with circulating immune complexes. They included 7 patients with nephrotic syndrome (proteinuria ranging between 3.6 to 11.8 g/day), 5 patients in spontaneous or therapy induced remission as defined by the presence of trace amounts of proteinuria

(<1 g/day) and 1 patient with non-nephrotic proteinuria and moderate microhematuria.

Eight normals older than 35 years (6 females and 2 males) served as controls for in vitro studies described below. For the electron microscopy studies and chemiluminescence emission assays each patient was matched with a normal subject of same sex and similar age.

Evaluation of clearance rate of IgG-coated erythrocytes in vivo

This assay was performed as previously described [Roccatello et al. 1985a] using Rh(D) positive autologous RBC labelled with ^{51}Cr and sensitized with purified IgG anti Rh(D). The IgG preparation was free of IgM as determined by immunoelectrophoresis and gel filtration (Ultrogel Ac-A 34 LKB). The half-lives (T½) of erythrocytes were calculated by a least squares computing program with exponential fitting which relates to time counts per min in samples sequentially taken at 10 to 90 min after the erythrocyte injection. With the amount of IgG anti-Rh(D) employed, 4.5–5.5 × 10^3 sites per erythrocyte were coated as determined by Scatchard analysis [Scatchard 1949] after incubation of sensitized RBC with mouse anti-human IgG (F(ab)$_2$ fragment labelled with ^{125}I. RBC underwent a monoexponential decline in the circulation during the 90 min of the test and no significant liver uptake (ratio liver/precordium = 0.7 at 90 min after injection) was found by external organ counting. A splenectomized subject, studied as a negative control, did not reach T½ value three days after reinjection of sensitized RBC. Conversely, a subject with hypersplenism had a clearance value of 9 min. In preliminary studies, sensitizations lower than the one chosen were not suitable in clinical practice for the period (several hours) needed by the test. By using two-fold higher sensitizations, biexponential declines were obtained with partial liver uptake, possibly mediated by fixation of endogenous C1q [Atkinson et al. 1973].

Each patient and control gave informed consent for clearance study according to the principles indicated by the Ethics Committee of St. John Hospital of Turin.

Rh-phenotype analysis

This was performed by conventional techniques of red cell grouping.

HLA-A, B, C, DR, DQ typing

As described in detail elsewhere [Roccatello et al. 1987b], tissue typing of all officially recognized HLA-A, B, C locus specificities was carried out on total mononuclear cells, according to the standard NIH cytotoxicity technique [Brandt et al. 1970]. HLA-DR and HLA-DQ typing was performed on B lymphocyte-enriched suspensions, by testing HLA-DR1, -DR2, -DR3, -DR4, -DR5, -DRw6, -DR7, -DRw8, -DRw52, -DRw53, -DQw1, -DQw2.

Cell isolation

Erythrocytes were isolated from venous blood anticoagulated with 10 mM ethylendiamine tetracetate (EDTA). After centrifugation and removal of the buffy coat, the erythrocytes were washed three times with 0.15 M phosphate buffered saline (PBS), pH 7.4, by 3 min centrifugation at 400 × g at 22 °C. A fourth wash was done with PBS supplemented by 1% bovine serum albumin (BSA) (Sigma) before testing cells. Leukocytes were isolated from heparinized blood samples from patients and controls fasting for at least 8 hours before venipuncture. Blood samples were processed immediately. Neutrophils were separated by adding a 15% volume of 3% dextran to peripheral blood, then allowed to settle at room temperature for 45 min. The supernatant containing leukocytes was aspirated and a half volume of Ficoll-Hypaque (Pharmacia, P-L Biochemical, Uppsala, Sweden) was added to the bottom of the supernatant. The mixture was centrifuged at 400 × g for 20 min at 4 °C. In experiments employing flow cytometry analysis, neutrophils were separated by Voss-Jepsen's one step method [Voss Jepsen and Skottun 1982], using a discontinuous gradient of Percoll (Pharmacia). The erythrocytes remaining in the cell pellet were lysed by hypotonic shock with distilled water. After washing the cell pellet three times with phosphate buffered saline (PBS), cells were resuspended in the appropriate medium. The percentage of neutrophils harvested with these techniques ranged between 95 and 98%.

Monocytes were isolated as previously described [Roccatello et al. 1985b]. In brief, blood diluted 1:3 with 0.15 NaCl, was layered on Percoll solution 1.085 g/ml and centrifuged at 800 × g for 20 min at 22° C. The mononuclear cell interface band was resuspended in 0.15 M NaCl, layered on Percoll solution 1.064 g/ml and centrifuged at 800 × g for 60 min at 4° C to obtain a pellet mainly containing monocytes: 78–87% OKM1-positive cells (Ortho. Raritan, NJ, USA), 8–15% OKT3-positive cells and 5–11% cells reacting with anti-Leu 12 (Becton Dickinson Monoclonal Center, CA, USA). Cell viability, examined by the Trypan blue and the Ethidium Bromide exclusion methods, always exceeded the 95th percent value.

Surface receptor assessment of phagocyte cells by flow cytometry analysis

The following monoclonal antibodies were employed: AB 8.28 directed to CD16 low affinity IgG Fc receptors [Malavasi et al. 1985a], AA 6.5 directed to class II HLA structures of monocytes [Malavasi et al. 1984], CB04 [Malavasi et al. 1985b] and 57H (Laboratory of the Pathology Department, New York University Medical Center, New York, USA) directed to C3b receptor (CR1). Percentage of positive cells and quantitative expression of the epitopes recognized by these MoAbs were evaluated by using an indirect fluorescence assay with a fluorescein-labelled affinity purified goat antibody to mouse immunoglobulins (Igs) (Ortho, Raritan, NJ, USA).

Phagocyte cells were processed through a Spectrum III flow cytofluorometer (Ortho Diagnostic System). The green fluorescence signals which passed through the gate window of monocytes or neutrophils were measured and displayed as a histogram. Monocyte window was previously selected by passing monocytes isolated by double gradient of Percoll as described above, subsequently allowed to adhere to solid substrates of Petri's plates for 45 min at 37° C and recovered by vigorous pipetting in ice cold PBS supplemented with 10 mM EDTA, pH 7.2. Analysis of these cell suspensions with OKT3 and Leu 12 MoAbs excluded any contamination with mononuclear cells other than monocytes. Background fluorescence activity was determined with fluorescein-conjugated goat anti-mouse Igs alone. The percentage of

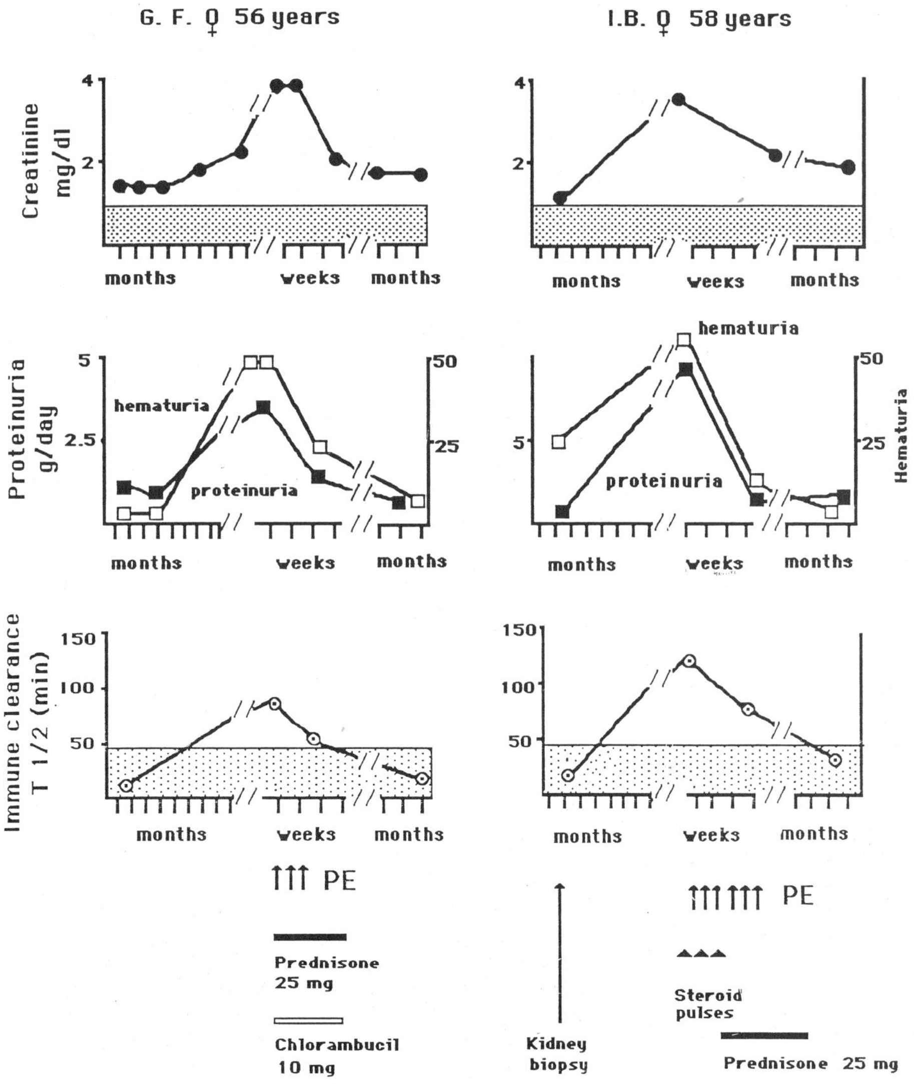

Fig. 1 Relationship between clearance rate of IgG-coated erythrocytes and clinical parameters in two patients treated with plasma exchange (PE).

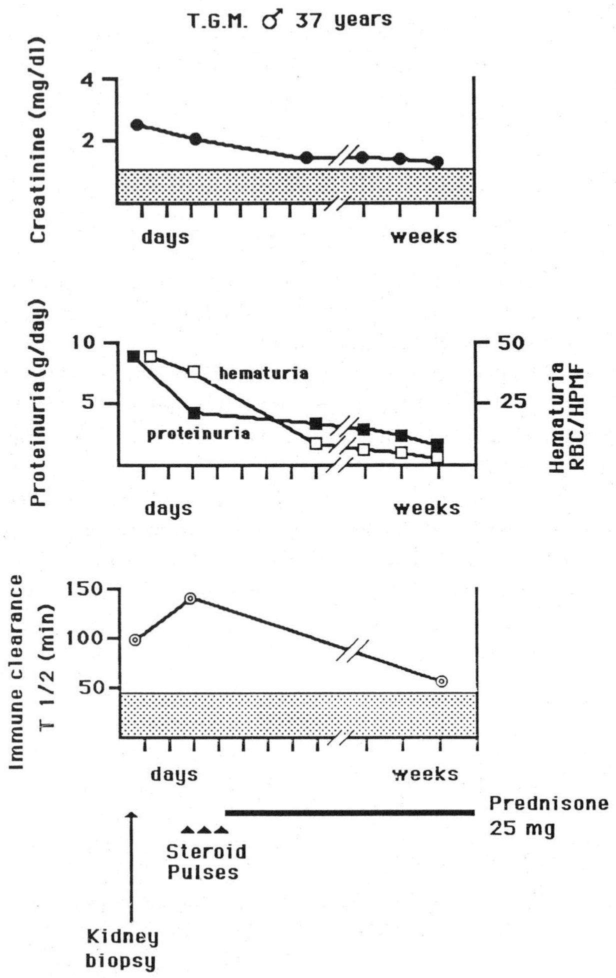

Fig. 2 Profile of immune clearance rate of IgG-coated erythrocytes in a patient treated with steroid pulses.

positive cells for MoAb staining was determined by subtracting this background fluorescence activity.

Quantitative analysis of CR1 expression on erythrocytes and peripheral phagocytes

The number of erythrocyte and phagocyte CR1 molecules was evaluated by a modification of the method described by Iida et al. [Iida et al. 1982]. Briefly, 10^7 erythrocytes or 10^6 phagocytes in 200 µl of PBS-1% BSA were incubated with a previously verified saturating dose of 200 ng of ^{125}I-labelled MoAb 57 H at 37° C for 1 hour. High-performance liquid chromatography (HPLC) analysis of this MoAb was performed with a Perkin-Elmer series 10 LC machine (Perkin-Elmer Corp, Analytica Instruments, Norwalk, CT) and Bio-Sil TSK 250-column (Bio-Rad Lab, Munich FRG) to exclude the presence of aggregates formed in the process of affinity purification. The eluant was measured at ultraviolet adsorbance at 280 nm by an Uvicon 735 LC detector (Kontron Instrument, Zurich, Switzerland). The MoAb solution consisted of a single peak of 1.5 × 10^6 daltons.

Triplicate samples of 60 µl of the reaction mixture were layered onto 200 µl of dibutylphalate (Eastman Kodak Co., Rochester, NY, USA) in Beckman polypropilene microfuge tubes (Beckman Instruments Inc., Fullerton, CA, USA). The tubes were centrifuged at 8.000 g for 90 sec in a Beckman microcentrifuge (Beckman Instruments, Inc) and the tips of the tubes were cut and counted in a gamma counter. The radioactivity associated with the cells was subtracted from counts obtained from identical aliquots (in triplicate) of the same preparation previously incubated with "cold" MoAb 57 H at a saturating dose to rule out unspecific trapping of labelled Ab within the cells. The final values of radioactivity were converted in number of CR1 molecules by the Scatchard plot analysis [Scatchard 1949].

Detection of IgG-containing immune material on peripheral phagocytes

Neutrophils and monocytes (10^6 cells in 200 µl of PBS 1% BSA), collected and washed as described above, were incubated at 37° C for 1 hour with a previously verified saturating dose of 200 ng of CE59 Antibody (Ab) and labelled with ^{125}I by the Chloramine T method. The CE59 Ab (kindly provided by Dr. E. Brown, NIH, Bethesda, USA) was directed to the Fc portion of IgG [Brown and Bekisz 1984]. The assay strictly followed the protocol for CR1 detection, including HPLC analysis of the employed antibody. Results were expressed as nanograms of CE 59 Ab/10^6 phagocytes.

Chemiluminescence assay

Zymosan, phorbol myristate acetate (PMA) and n-Formyl-Methyonine-Leucine-Phenylalanine (n-FMLP), purchased from SIGMA Chemical CO, St. Louis, Missouri, USA, served as stimulus for luminol-enhanced chemiluminescence experiments. Zymosan was opsonized by incubating 50 mg in 3 ml fresh human serum and 1 ml Hanks' balanced salt solution without phenol-red (HBSS) for 30 min. After washing, Zymosan was resuspended in HBSS at a concentration of 12.5 mg/ml. A luminol stock solution was prepared by dissolving 1.77 mg of luminol (LKB-Wallac 1243, 216) in 1 ml dimethylsulfoxide to obtain a concentration of 10^{-2} M. Immediately before use it was further diluted to 10^{-6} M in HBSS. PMA and nFMLP were used at a final concentration

Table 1 Flow cytometry analysis of low affinity FcR, C3b receptors and DR-associated antigens on monocytes and neutrophils from 8 patients included in the in vitro studies and 8 normal controls. Data represent the mean ± SD of the percentage of positive cells. * = $p<0.05$.

	Monocytes		Neutrophils	
Anti FcR (AB8.28 MoAb)			96 ± 1	97 ± 1
Anti CR1				
(57 H MoAb)	73 ± 10	73 ± 14	82 ± 8	65 ± 22
(CB04 MoAb)			87 ± 9	92 ± 3
Anti HLA class II (AA65 MoAb)	75 ± 9*	67 ± 8		
	patients	normals	patients	normals

of 0.18×10^{-6} M and 0.5×10^{-6} M, respectively. The instrumentation equipment included a LKB-Wallac 1251 luminometer coupled to display unit, potentiometric recorder (2210-032) and computer (Olivetti M 24) for data integration.

The following reagents were subsequently pipetted into duplicate cuvettes: 600 μl of luminol, 50 μl of opsonized Zymosan or PMA or n-FMLP (or HBSS in controls) and 50 μl of neutrophil suspension (10^6 cell/ml) under study. Cuvette contents were gently mixed and conveyed to the measurement position. Duplicate samples were measured at 1 min intervals as millivolts (mV) light emission. Results were automatically plotted on a graph with light intensity on ordinate and time units on abscissa. The chemiluminescence response was determined both as height of the curve (peak value, expressed in mV) and integral under the curve (mV × min).

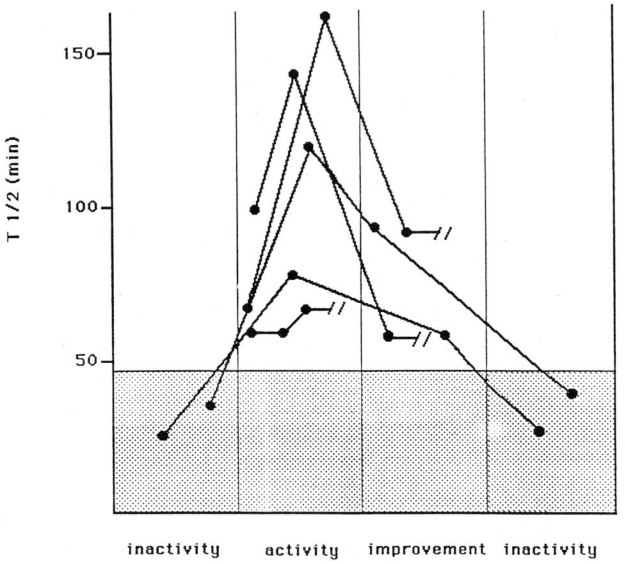

Fig. 3 Serial studies in five patients. The double bar means that follow-up was not completed due to death from pneumonia, breast carcinoma or cerebral hemorrhage.

Inhibition studies

Blood samples from 3 normal subjects included as controls in the above described in vitro studies, were used for these experiments.

Aliquots of 0.3×10^6 OKM1-positive cells in RPMI 1640 (DIFCO) supplemented with 3% BSA, obtained as described above (see monocyte separation), were tested for their ability to ingest autologous erythrocytes coated with sub-hemolitic amounts of IgG anti Rh(D), after diverse incubation times, in presence or in absence (negative control) of increasing concentrations of IgG/IgM-k cryoglobulins or aggregated human gammaglobulins (AHG) (positive control). Phagocytosis was microscopically evaluated after acridine orange staining. The rate of phagocytosis was calculated – as described in detail elsewhere [Roccatello et al. 1985c] – by determining the tangent to the angle (tan) subtended by a regression line derived from plotting the values of phagocytosis index (number of erythrocytes ingested by 100 monocytes) as a function of time. The value of "tan" is the expression of the kinetics of the Fc-receptor mediated phagocytosis in a serum-free system without any interference of opsonic proteins (such as complement or fibronectin) on uptake and ingestion of tag particles. The percent inhibition of the phagocytosis capacity as kinetically analyzed was calculated as follows:

$$\% \text{ inhibition} = 100 - \frac{\text{tan value in the experimental assay}}{\text{tan value in the control assay}} \times 100$$

Electron microscopy studies on monocyte phagocytosis of cryoglobulins

Aliquots of 200 μl cell suspensions, containing 1.5×10^6 monocytes from patients or controls of similar age and sex, were mixed in various combinations with 100 μl of 8 mg/ml cryoglobulins separated by cold-precipitation and washed in PBS. These mixtures were then incubated for 15 min at 37° C under 60 rpm shaking and for additional 75 min without shaking. Then cells were washed twice at 1000 × g for 5 min at 4° C with cold PBS, fixed in 2.5% glutaraldehyde, post-fixed in osmium tetroxide and embedded in epoxy resin. Ultrathin sections were stained with uranyl acetate-lead citrate.

One pathologist (GM) examined the cell suspensions prepared by another investigator who processed codified blood samples and cryoglobulin preparations.

Three series of double blind experiments were performed: 1) a pool of cryoglobulins from different patients was incubated with aliquots of diverse monocyte suspensions of patients and normal subjects; 2) cryoglobulins from different patients were incubated with aliquots of the same monocyte suspensions of healthy subjects; and 3) cryoglobulins from different patients were incubated with monocyte suspensions of the same patient and of a normal control of same sex and similar age.

Each series of experiments included control cell preparations processed in the same manner but free of cryoglobulins and preparations of cells suspended in 25 percent autologous or homologous fresh human serum to test the influence of complement in cryoglobulin interiorization.

Statistics

The Mann-Whitney U test, Wilcoxon test, Fisher's exact test and the linear coefficient regression were used for statistical analysis.

Results

Evaluation of clearance rate of IgG-coated erythrocytes in vivo

The mean T½ value of sensitized erythrocytes was 53.17 min (range 23–101) in the 14 EMC patients and 34.38 min (range 22–50) in normals ($p = 0.03$).

The 8 EMC patients with clinically active renal disease had significantly higher T½ values (69.56 min, range 24–101) than the normal control group ($p < 0.0005$) and a subset of 8 healthy people, older than 35 years ($p < 0.003$) and comparable in age to patients (mean 52 years, range 36–73).

Table 2 Chemiluminescence emission after stimulation with Zymosan, PMA and n-FMLP of phagocytes from the 8 patients included in the in vitro studies and 8 normal controls. On the top section of the Table values in active patients (1–4) are shown with their own controls (1c–4c). Results in inactive patients (5–8) and correspondent normal controls (5c–8c) are indicated below. ys = years. (See text for statistical significance.)

Subjects	Zymosan CL peak	integral	PMA CL peak	integral	nFMLP CL peak	integral
1	62.7	1,789	107	3,853	38.8	5,027
1c	80	2,561	162.9	4,901	128.1	16,900
2	25.3	0,879	44.1	1,567	45.2	7,958
2c	68.4	1,141	128	4,378	67.6	9,882
3	47.9	1,830	46	1,812	28.1	4,282
3c	50.6	1,804	51	1,757	67.6	9,882
4	27.1	1,144	78.3	3,167	26.4	4,706
4c	80.3	2,471	161.8	4,891	94.9	15,433
5	38.1	1,345	35.5	1,536	69.9	7,722
5c	66.2	2,042	51.2	1,348	203	26,883
6	105.5	3,238	90.5	3,075	49.8	4,909
6c	111	3,306	128	4,453	321	36,409
7	60.7	2,272	88.4	2,420	48.2	8,486
7c	76	2,510	107.9	3,342	98.7	17,907
8	77	2,540	52.4	2,038	132	17,236
8c	76.4	2,536	64.1	1,909	94.3	16,907
1–8	55.5 ± 27.0	1,880 ± 0,781	67.7 ± 26.4	2,433 ± 0,851	54.8 ± 34	7,541 ± 4,259
1–4	40.7 ± 17.8	1,410 ± 0,474	68.8 ± 29.8	2,600 ± 1,092	34.6 ± 8.9	5,493 ± 1,671
5–8	70.3 ± 28.3	2,349 ± 0,783	66.7 ± 27.1	2,267 ± 0,649	74.9 ± 39.2	9,588 ± 5,325
1c–8c	76.1 ± 17.1	2,296 ± 0,640	106.8 ± 46.4	3,372 ± 1,496	134.4 ± 86.9	18,775 ± 8,895

T½ values of the control group of 13 FGS patients ranged between 24 and 48 min (mean 35.18 min). These values were similar to normal controls, and significantly lower than EMC patients ($p<0.03$). The 7 FGS nephrotic patients showed similar results as the entire FGS group (mean T½ 32.4 min, range 28–48 min).

A significant difference was also observed by comparing T½ values of the 8 active EMC cases to those of the 6 inactive ones (31.33 min, range 23–41, $p<0.007$). Seven out of the eight patients with active renal disease had a delayed immune clearance (exceeding 46 min, the 95 percent confidence limit in healthy controls) whereas no inactive patient had prolonged RBC half-life. Age did not influence the clearance rate of sensitized erythrocytes ($r = 0.02$).

Although the active patients frequently had abnormal creatinine values, immune clearance and creatinine levels were unrelated ($r = 0.01$). Moreover, no correlation was found between T½ values and absolute amounts of class G, A, M immunglobulins measured by nephelometry in serum processed at 37° C, nor levels of proteinuria ($r = 0.12$), total serum proteins ($r = 0.018$), albuminemia ($r = 0.021$), cholesterolemia ($r = 0.2$), even among patients with nephrotic syndrome.

Two patients previously studied in an inactive phase of renal disease had a relapse with severe kidney involvement and were treated with plasma exchange in conjunction with steroids and immunosuppressive drugs. They had an improved rate of immune clearance together with clinical amelioration (Figure 1). Another patient with nephrotic range proteinuria was treated with steroid pulses. He had a further prolongation of the already delayed clearance rate. However, a subsequent measurement of immune clearance taken in a quiescent phase induced by steroid maintenance showed a substantial improvement (Figure 2). Figure 3 summarizes the profiles of immune clearance in five sequentially studied patients.

Rh-phenotype analysis and HLA-tissue typing

Figure 4 shows that the immune clearance rates of the 14 EMC patients and 14 normal controls, selected only for their availability, were randomly distributed among the four more frequent Rh phenotypes in the Italian population. No correlation was found between the detection of any HLA-A, -B, -C, -DR, -DQ antigen and prolonged immune clearance. The HLA-B8, -DR3 haplotype, reported to be significantly associated with an altered macrophage clearance function [Lawley et al. 1981] was not

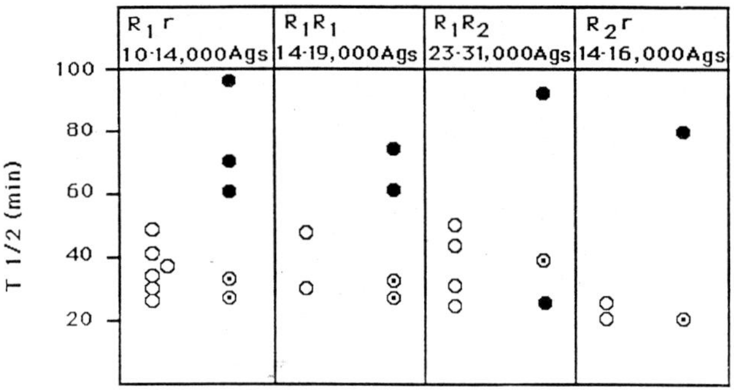

Fig. 4 Distribution of the 8 active (●) and the 6 inactive (⊙) patients and 14 healthy subjects (○) according to IgG-coated erythrocyte clearance values (ordinate) and Rh phenotype (abscissa). R1r = DCcee, R1R1 = DCCee, R1R2 = DCcEe, R2r = DccEE. Ag(s) = number of Rh sites per erythrocyte.

present in this sample of patients, whereas HLA-DR2, MT1 (now DQw1), also related to macrophage dysfunction [Kimberly et al. 1983], was found only in 1 case with normal immune clearance. Eight out of the 24 healthy people who served as normal controls for in vivo studies were typed for HLA antigens. One 38-year-old female carried the HLA-B8, -DR3 haplotype. She had a clearance value of 46 min, which

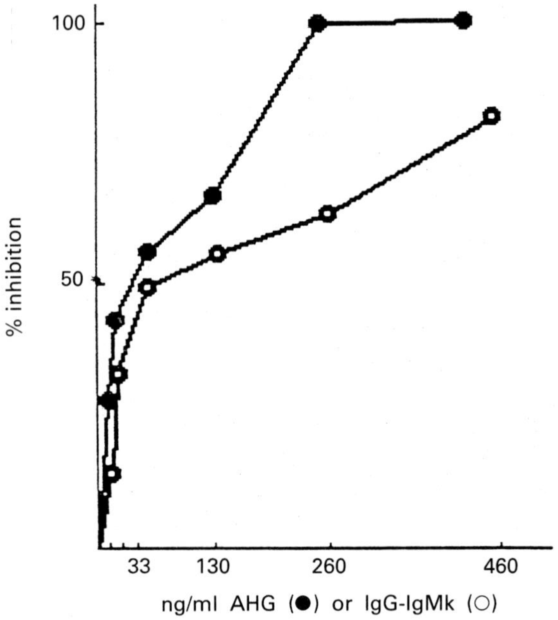

Fig. 5 Cryoglobulin-induced inhibition of monocyte phagocytosis of IgG-coated autologous erythrocytes. The effects of IgG/IgM-k cryoglobulins were compared to those of aggregated human gammaglobulins (AHG). Each point represents percentage of inhibition of a kinetic assay of phagocytosis performed by analyzing the same cell preparation after diverse incubation times. Similar results were obtained in two other experiments.

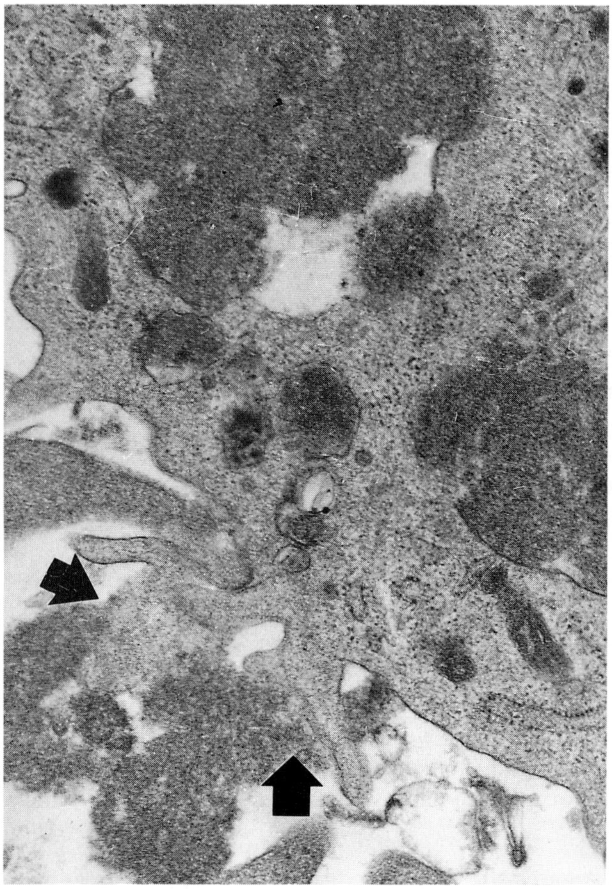

Fig. 6 Monocytes of a patient with mixed IgG/IgM-k cryoglobulinemia incubated with a pool of cryoglobulins. Aggregates of cryoglobulins are evident both outside and inside the cytoplasm (in the phagosomes) and in close contact to the cell membrane (arrows) (×24,000).

exactly represents the 95 percent confidence value in controls.

Surface receptor assessment of phagocyte cells by flow cytometry analysis

The percentages of positive cells as evaluated by Spectrum III cytofluorometer on phagocytes from 8 EMC (4 active and 4 inactive) patients and 8 normal controls are shown in Table 1. No difference was found in the number of neutrophils expressing Fc receptors and neutrophils or monocytes bearing C_3b receptors. Conversely a slight difference ($p<0.05$) was found in the percentage of monocytes expressing HLA class II structures recognizable by the AA 6.5 MoAb. By analyzing the relative fluorescence intensity (mean channel ± SD), no significant difference in the surface expression of these membrane structures was found with any MoAb (not shown).

Quantitative analysis of CR1 expression on erythrocytes and peripheral phagocytes

Taking into account that 57H IgG MoAb had a molecular mass of 150,000 Daltons and that no aggregates were present in the Ab preparation (as shown by HPLC analysis), it was postulated that each molecule bound one of the randomly distributed CR1 structures. With this simplification, Scatchard transformation [Scatchard 1949] predicted a mean number of CR1 of 277 (range 103–705) per erythrocyte, 58,000 (range 25,000–105,000) per monocyte, 60,000 (range 20,000–100,000) per neutrophil in the 8 EMC patients. These values were not significantly different from the 8 normal controls: 321 (range 155–610) per erythrocyte, 66,000 (range 40,000–100,000) per monocyte and 53,000 (range 25,000–80,000) per neutrophil.

Detection of IgG-containing immune material on peripheral phagocytes

Regarding to the specific reaction of ^{125}I-labelled CE59 to monocytes and neutrophils from the 8 EMC patients and the 8 healthy controls, a mean value of 4.58 ng (range 1–9.5)/10^6 cells was found to be bound to monocytes from patients, which is significantly different ($p<0.02$) compared to normals (1.02 ng, range 0.2–2). The mean value of CE59 fixed on the surface of neutrophils from patients was 3.44 ng (range 0.5–9), which was significantly different ($p<0.01$) from controls (0.78 ng, range 0.2–2). Four out of eight patients were found to have an amount of CE59 on monocytes and neutrophils higher than 2 ng/10^6 cells, which was the maximum level reached in normals. Of these, three were patients studied in active phase of renal disease and one patient without nephritis had mild arthralgia. One case with active nephritis had amounts of monocyte- and neutrophil-bound immune material equal to the higher levels in normals. The other 3 cases, found to have only trace amounts of immune material on phagocyte surface included 1 active, 2 inactive nephritis and 1 patient without nephritis and free of systemic symptoms at the time of the study. The absolute amounts of immune material detected on monocyte and neutrophil surface were significantly related ($r = 0.88$, $p<0.01$).

Although both the detection of immune material of peripheral phagocytes and the rate of immune clearance were related to the active phase of renal disease, the relationship between these two parameters in the patients investigated for both the assays was weaker than expected ($r = 0.65$, $p<0.02$ and $r = 0.55$, p <0.05 for monocyte and neutrophil-bound immune material, respectively).

Chemiluminescence assays

The chemiluminescence response of phagocytes from the 8 EMC (4 active and 4 inactive) patients compared to cells from the 8 normal subjects of same sex and similar age are summarized in Table 2. There was a positive correlation between height (peak value) and area of the curve induced by Zymosan, PMA and nFMLP in both patients (r = 0.95, r = 0.86 and r = 0.89, respectively) and normals (r = 0.69, r = 0.96, r = 0.95), p <0.01 in each case, except for Zymosan in normals, p <0.05.

After stimulation with Zymosan, PMA and n-FMLP, the mean CL peak values in patients were found to be significantly different compared to controls (p <0.02; p <0.02; p <0.005 respectively) using the Mann-Whitney U test. The significance was even higher when each patient was compared to his or her own control by employing Wilcoxon test (p <0.01 in each case). These results were substantially confirmed by analyzing integral values. Moreover, as compared by Mann-Whitney test with the 4 inactive cases, leukocytes from the 4 active cryoglobulinemic patients also showed a lower CL response to n-FMLP (p <0.01).

Inhibition studies

Representative results of the dose response relationship for cryoglobulin inhibition of monocyte phagocytosis of IgG-coated erythrocytes, analyzed in 3 separate experiments using cells from 3 healthy subjects, is shown in Figure 5. In these experiments, positive controls were represented by AHG used at the same concentration of cryoglobulins. Interestingly, a remarkable cryoglobulin-induced inhibition of IgG-coated erythrocyte phagocytosis was found. This effect was already obvious at very low concentrations of cryoglobulins.

Electron microscopy studies

With electron microscopy, cryoglobulins appeared as electron dense and structured material, which could be ingested by monocytes and detected in phagosomes (Figure 6). The experiments which examined several combinations of phagocyte cell suspensions and cryoglobulins from 8 (4 active 4 inactive) patients showed that 1) the interiorization capability of a pool of cryoglobulins by monocytes from different patients did not distinguish between patients with or without nephritis 2) cryoglobulins from different patients were ingested with very different avidity when incubated with the same suspension of normal monocytes (Figure 7A and B), and 3) there was no

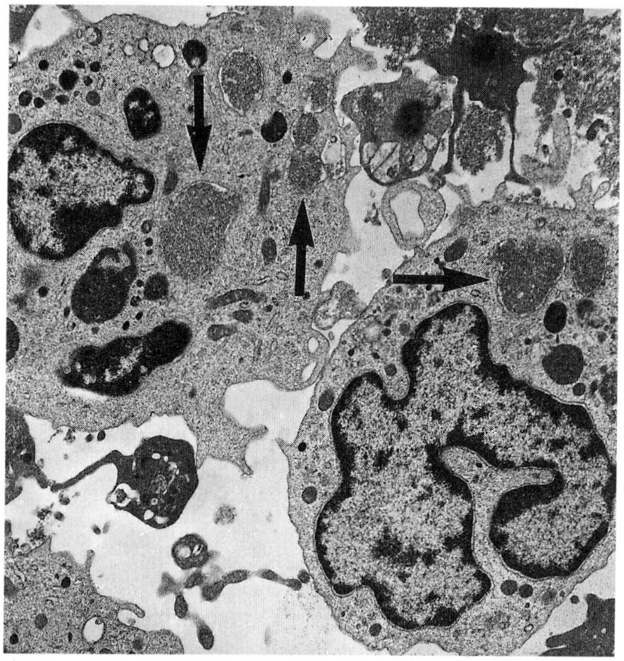

a)

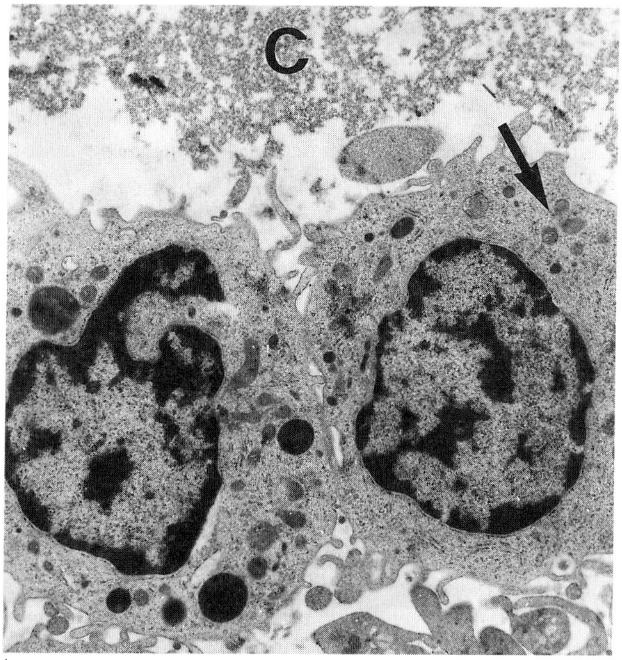

b)

Fig. 7 Different extent of internalization of IgG/IgM-k cryoglobulins of two patients after incubation with the same suspension of normal monocytes. A) Large phagosomes (arrows) including cryoglobulins (×6,000). B) Small and sporadic phagosomes (arrows) and larger amounts of free cryoglobulins (C) are seen outside the cells (×6,000).

obvious difference in ingestion capacity of cryoglobulins between patients and controls of same sex and age. It is worth noting that the presence of fresh serum as a source of complement and fibronectin did not modify these results.

Discussion

Clearance of immune complexes from the circulation is influenced by a variety of factors including size and solubility [Weigle 1958], isotype [Mannik 1980], antibody affinity [Devey and Steward 1980], interaction with the complement system [Bockow and Mannik 1981] and efficiency of the mononuclear phagocyte system [Haakenstad and Mannik 1974].

In immune complex disease, defective function of the mononuclear phagocyte system has been demonstrated by measuring the rate of removal of autologous erythrocytes coated with an IgG anti Rh (D) from the blood [Frank 1983]. While the infusion of immune complexes during the IgG-coated erythrocyte clearance produced a significant clearance prolongation [Williams et al. 1985], observations that some properties of infused cells may influence their clearance were also reported in animals [Yousaf et al. 1986]. In humans, a strong relationship between IgG-coated erythrocyte clearance and some HLA antigens was observed by some authors [Lawley et al. 1981, Kimberly et al. 1983, McGinley et al. 1984], but not confirmed by others [Berthoux et al. 1984, Solomon et al, 1984, Roccatello et al. 1987a, e, b]. Recently, Kelton proposed an influence of serum IgG levels on IgG-coated erythrocyte clearance [Kelton et al. 1985]. However, this relationship was derived from the analysis of lupus erythematosus patients where the increase in immunoglobulin levels usually parallels the active phase of disease, which is also associated with prolonged IgG-coated erythrocyte clearance rates [Frank et al. 1979].

The clinical value of assessing IgG-coated erythrocyte clearance in cryoglobulinemic patients is supported by the clear-cut separation between results in active and inactive cases and data from serial studies in individual patients. The nature of the defect is uncertain. Neither HLA, age nor Rh phenotype matching of patients and controls documented that the clearance of IgG-coated autologous erythrocytes is unequivocally dependent on the individual properties of the infused cells or the individual characteristics of the injected subject as suggested in other reports [Lawley et al. 1981, Kimberly et al. 1983, McGinley et al. 1984, Williams et al. 1985, Yousaf et al. 1986]. Moreover, the data exclude that delayed IgG-coated erythrocyte clearance is dependent on a quantitative defect in transport receptors. Percentages of positive cells and relative fluorescence intensity, as cytofluorometrically evaluated, and number of cell surface receptors examined by radiometric methods in normals are similar to other reports [Arnaout et al. 1983, Fyfe et al. 1986]. No significant difference was found between healthy controls and patients except for a relative expansion of class II HLA structure-bearing monocytes in patients, which can be interpreted as a result of greater antigen stimulation.

Recent evidence suggests that complement and its receptor on erythrocytes provide an efficient system for processing and transporting large sized immune complexes [Waxman et al. 1984]. In the present study, CR1 was found to be normally expressed on red blood cells from patients with cryoglobulinemia. However, while cryoglobulinemic patients usually have low complement levels, cryoglobulins were unable to bind sufficient amounts of C3b needed to bind erythrocytes (Ng et al. 1988]. Accordingly, the IgG purified from cryoglobulins, injected back into the patients (having monoclonal IgM rheumatoid factor), formed new immune complexes which escaped the rapid clearance of the erythrocyte transport system (Schifferli et al. 1983], possibly due to covering of Fc regions of IgG by IgM. This should imply a greater impact on the phagocyte system cells in cryoglobulinemic patient and a longer persistence of these complexes in the circulation. In agreement with this hypothesis, the "in vitro" inhibition studies and the combination of relatively high levels of phagocyte-bound immune material and defective clearance of IgG-coated erythrocytes in clinically active patients together suggest a saturation of normally expressed cell-surface receptors. The evaluation of the clearance rate of IgG-coated erythrocytes provides a tool to measure the extent of this phenomenon.

Even though circulating and tissue phagocytes could be different in many respects related to phagocytosis, the electron microscopy experiments show a preserved capacity of cryoglobulin internalization by monocytes from patients. Chemiluminescence experiments suggest a possible mechanism responsible for this different behaviour. Phagocytosis of serum-opsonized Zymosan particles by human peripheral blood leukocytes, is inhibited by Cytochalasin B [Skosey et al. 1973], which alters leukocyte peripheral filament meshwork [Wessels et al. 1971]. PMA increases microtubule number and assembly [Goldstein et al. 1975]. Finally, N-Formyl-Methyonil peptides act at the cytoskeleton level [Davis et al. 1982] and are potent chemoattractants for leukocytes [Schiffman et al. 1975]. Peripheral blood phagocytes from most patients with cryoglobulinemia showed reduced chemiluminescence production compared to normal controls whatever stimulus used. The impairment was found to be maximal by assessing the response to N-Formyl-Methyonil peptides, the most specific test-probes for cytoskeleton integrity. It was demonstrated that the internalization of a particulate immune complex is very sensitive to disruption of the cytoskeleton whereas minimal cytoskeletal involvement is necessary for the uptake of soluble immune complexes [Finbloom et al. 1987]. A defect at the level of the cytoskeleton could reasonably explain the apparent discrepancy between the IgG-coated erythrocyte clearance defect and preserved potential of cryoglobulin internalization as measured semiquantitatively by electron microscopy. A particulate immune complex is less easily processable and has a greater possibility of revealing subtle defects in phagocyte function compared to relatively soluble IC, such as cryoglobulins.

Even if the pathogenic relevance of a delayed clearance of particulate immune complexes remains only speculative, it is worthy to note that, unlike lupus erythematosus, in which the levels of immune complexes are often related to severity of disease [Coppo et al. 1982], attempts to relate cryoglobulin amounts to clinical activity in cryoglobulinemia have always been discouraging. Therefore, measurement of the functional overburden of the phagocyte system, which is strictly related to clinical activity, is of value in clinical and immunological monitoring.

Acknowledgments

This work was partly supported by grants from CNR and Ministero della Pubblica Istruzione, Italy. Dario Roccatello would like to thank Dr. Steven Emancipator for his advice on experimental design and Dr. Abdalla Rifai for his helpful comments on the manuscript. We gratefully acknowledge the help of Jerilyn Pecotte, PhD, USAC, University of Nevada, Reno, in reviewing manuscript.

REFERENCES

Arnaout AM, Todd RF, Melamed J, Schlossman SF, Colten HR 1983 Inhibition of phagocytosis of complement C3- or Immunoglobulin G-coated particles and of C3bi binding by monoclonal antibodies to a monocyte-granulocyte membrane glycoprotein (Mol). J Clin Invest *72:* 171–179

Atkinson JP, Schreiber AD, Frank M 1973 Effects of corticosteroids and splenectomy on the immune clearance and destruction of erythrocytes. J Clin Invest *52:* 1509–1517

Berthoux FC, Laurent B, Le Petit JC 1984 Immunogenetics and immunopathology of human primary membranous glomerulonephritis: HLA-A, B, DR antigens, functional activity of splenic macrophage Fc-receptors and peripheral blood T-lymphocyte subpopulations. Clin Nephrol *22:* 15–20

Bockow B, Mannik M 1981 Clearance and tissue uptake of immune complexes in complement depleted and control mice. Immunol *42:* 497

Brandt DL, Ray JG, Hare DB 1970 Preliminary trials toward standardization of leukocyte typing. In Terasaki PI (ed): Histocompatibility Testing. Copenhagen, Munksgaard 357

Brown E, Bekisz J 1984 Neoantigens appear in human IgG upon antigen-binding: detection by antibodies that react specifically with antigen-bound IgG. J Immunol *132:* 1346–1352

Coppo R, Bosticardo GM, Basolo B, Messina M, Mazzucco G, Stratta P, Quarello F, Alloatti S, Piccoli G 1982 Clinical significance of the detection of circulating immune complexes in lupus nephritis. Nephron *32:* 320–328

Davis BH, Walter RJ, Pearson CB, Becker EL, Oliver M 1982 Membrane activity and topography of F-Met-Leu-Phe-treated polymorphonuclear leucocytes. Am J Pathol *108:* 206–216

Devey ME, Steward MW 1980 The induction of chronic antigen-antibody complex disease in selectively bred mice producing either high or low affinity antibody to protein antigens. Immunol. *41:* 303

Finbloom DS, Martin J, Gordon RK 1987 Endocytosis of particulate and soluble IgG immune complexes: differential effects of cytoskeletal modulating agents. Clin Exp Immunol *67:* 205–210

Frank MM 1983 Immunoglobulin G Fc-receptor-mediated clearance in autoimmune diseases. Ann Int Med *98:* 206–218

Frank MM, Hamburger MI, Lawley TJ, Kimberly RP, Plotz PH 1979 Defective reticulo-endothelial system Fc-receptor function in systemic lupus erythematosus. New Engl J Med *300:* 518–523

Fyfe A, Holme ER, Zoma A, Whaley K 1986 C3b receptor (CR1) expression on the polymorphonuclear leukocytes from patients with systemic lupus erythematosus. Clin Exp Immunol *67:* 300–308

Goldstein IM, Hoffstein ST, Weissmann G 1975 Mechanisms of lysosomal enzyme release from human polymorphonuclear leukocytes. J Cell Biol *66:* 647–652

Gorevic PD, Kassab HJ, Levo Y, Kohn R, Meltzer M, Prose P, Fanklin EC 1980 Mixed cryoglobulinemia: clinical aspects and long-term follow up of 40 patients. Am J Med *69:* 287–308

Haakenstad AO, Mannik M 1974 Saturation of the reticulo-endothelial system with soluble immune complexes. J Immunol *112:* 1939

Iida K, Mornaghi R, Nussenzweig V 1982 Complement receptor (CR1) deficiency in erythrocytes from patients with systemic lupus erythematosus. J Exp Med *155:* 1427–1438

Kelton JG, Singer J, Rodger G, Gauldie J, Horsewood P, Dent P 1985 The concentration of IgG in the serum is a major determinant of Fc-dependent reticuloendothelial function. Blood *66:* 490–495

Kimberly RP, Gibofsky A, Salmon JE, Fotino M 1983 Impaired Fc mediated mononuclear phagocyte system clearance in HLA-DR2 and MT1 positive healthy young adults. J Exp Med *157:* 1698–1703

Lawley TJ, Hall RP, Fauci AS 1981 Defective Fc receptor functions associated with the HLA-B8/DRw3 haplotype. N Engl J Med *304:* 185–192

Malavasi F, Milanese C, Fabbi M, Richiardi P, Calligaris-Cappio F, Ferrero E, Roggero S, Dellabona P, Ceppellini R 1984 Generation and characterization of murine monoclonal antibodies against HLA class II molecules. Diagnostic Immunol *12:* 53–62

Malavasi F, Bellone G, Matera L, Milanese C, Ferrero E, Funaro A, Demaria S, Calligaris-Cappio F, Camussi G 1985a Murine monoclonal antibodies as probes for the phenotypical, functional and molecular analysis of a discrete peripheral blood lymphocyte population exerting natural killer activity in vitro. Hum Immunol *14:* 87–102

Malavasi F, Funaro A, Bellone G, Calligaris-Cappio F, Berti E, Tetta C, Dellabona P, Demaria S, Campogrande M, Cappa APM 1985b Functional and molecular characterization by the CB04 monoclonal antibody of a cell surface structure exerting C3-complement receptor activity. J Clin Immunol *6:* 412–420

Mannik M 1980 Physicochemical and functional relationships of immune complexes. J Invest Dermatol *74:* 333

McGinley EM, Martin W, Henderson N 1984 Defective splenic reticuloendothelial function in idiopathic membranous nephropathy. Clin Exp Immunol *56:* 295–301

Meltzer M, Franklin EK, McCluskey RT, Cooper N 1966 Cryoglobulinemia: a clinical and laboratory study. Am J Med *40:* 837–856

Ng YC, Peters DK, Walport MJ 1988 Monoclonal rheumatoid factor-IgG immune complexes: poor fixation of opsonic C4 and C3 despite efficient complement activation. Arthritis Rheum *31:* 99–107

Roccatello D, Coppo R, Piccoli G, Cordonnier D, Martina G, Rollino C, Picciotto G, Sena LM, Amoroso A 1985a Circulating Fc-Receptor blocking factors in IgA nephropathies. Clin Nephrol *23:* 159–168

Roccatello D, Coppo R, Rollino C, Martina G, Basolo B, Piccolo G 1985b A method for obtaining a nearly pure suspension of cell reacting with monoclonal antibodies anti-human monocytes. Int J Immunother *4:* 257–259

Roccatello D, Bensa JC, Coppo R, Rollino C, Diaz M 1985c In vitro studying Fc-receptor function in autoimmune disease. Immunol Lett *9:* 53–56

Roccatello D, Coppo R, Martina G, Rollino C, Basolo B, Frattasio C, Fasano ME, Amoroso A, Picciotto G, Bajardi P, Cordonnier D, Piccoli G 1987a Fc-Receptor function of the mononuclear phagocyte system in glomerulonephritis secondary to some multisystem diseases. Am J Nephrol *7:* 85–92

Roccatello D, Coppo R, Amoroso A, Curtoni ES, Martina G, Basolo B, Amore A, Rollino C, Picciotto G, Cordonnier D, Sena LM, Piccoli G 1987b Failure to relate mononuclear phagocyte system function to HLA-A, B, C, DR, DQ antigens in membranous nephropathy. Am J Kidney Dis *6:* 470–475

Scatchard G 1949 The attraction of proteins for small molecules and ions. Ann NY Acad Sci *51:* 660–670

Schifferli JA, Amos N, Pusey CD, Sissons JGP, Peters DK 1983 Metabolism of IgG in type II mixed essential cryoglobulinemia – autologous cryoprecipitated and normal homologous IgG are incorporated into complexes and metabolizated in vivo at similar rates. Clin Exp Immunol *51:* 305–316

Schiffman E, Corcoran BA, Wahl SM 1975 N-formylmethionyl peptides are chemotactic for leukocytes. Proc Natl Acad Sci USA *72:* 1059–1062

Skosey JL, Chow D, Damgaard E, Sorensen LB 1973 Effect of cytochalasin B on response of human polymorphonuclear leukocytes to Zymosan. J Cell Biol *57:* 237–240

Solomon LR, Rawlinson VI, Howarth S, Mallick NP 1984 Reticuloendothelial function in glomerulonephritis. Nephron *37:* 54–59

Stoebner P, Renversez JG, Gronlade J, Vialtell P, Cordonnier P 1979 Ultrastructural study of human IgG and IgM-IgG cryoglobulins. Am J Clin Path *71:* 404–410

Voss Jepsen L, Skottun T 1982 A rapid one step method for the isolation of human granulocytes from whole blood. Scand J Clin Lab Invest *42:* 235–238

Walport MJ, Peters AM, Elkon KB, Pusey CD, Lavender JP, Hughes GRV 1985 The splenic extraction rato of antibody-coated erythrocytes and its response to plasma exchange and pulse methylprednisolone. Clin Exp Immunol *60:* 465–473

Waxman FJ, Hebert LA, Cornacoff JB, VanAman ME, Smead WL, Kraut EH, Birmingham DJ, Taguiam JM 1984 Complement depletion accelerates the clearance of immune complexes from the circulation of primates. J Clin Invest *74:* 1329–1340

Weigle WO 1958 Elimination of antigen-antibody complexes from sera of rabbits. J Immunol *81:* 204

Wessels NK, Spooner BS, Ash JF, Bradley MO, Luduena MA, Taylor EL, Wrenn JT, Yamada KM 1971 Microfilaments in cellular and developmental processes: Science (Wash D.C.) *171:* 135

Williams BD, O'Sullivan MM, Ratanachaiyavong S 1985 Reticuloendothelial Fc function in normal individuals and its relationships to the HLA antigen DR3. Clin Exp Immunol *60:* 532–538

Yousaf N, Howard IC, Williams BD 1986 Studies in cobra venom factor treated rats of antibody coated erythrocyte clearance by the spleen: differential influence of red-blood cell antigen number on the inhibitory effects of immune complexes on Fc dependent clearance. Clin Exp Immunol *66:* 654–660

Clinical Nephrology, Vol. 36 No. 3 – 1991 (127–133)

Immunohistological localization of apolipoproteins in the glomeruli in renal disease: specifically apoB and apoE

H. Sato, S. Suzuki, H. Kobayashi, S. Ogino, A. Inomata and M. Arakawa

Department of Medicine (II), Niigata University School of Medicine, Niigata, Japan

Abstract. Recently it has become clear that abnormalities of the lipid metabolism may play a large role in the progression of renal diseases. To investigate the relationship between lipids and kidney tissues, the authors employed an immunofluorescent technique to determine the presence of apolipoprotein (apo) B and E in kidney tissue, particularly the glomeruli, and analyzed the relationship between their deposition and the clinical and histological findings of a total of 49 patients with persistent proteinuria and/or hematuria (age range: 10 to 62 years). The patients were divided into 4 groups, as follows: both apoB and apoE negative cases (Group 1; 17 cases), apoB alone positive (Group 2; 7 cases), apoE alone positive (Group 3; 10 cases) and both apoB and apoE positive cases (Group 4; 15 cases). Group 2 had more severe proteinuria and a higher level of total cholesterol than Group 1. Group 3 exhibited a higher incidence of glomerular adhesion and interstitial changes than Group 1. Group 4, on the other hand, exhibited more severe mesangial hypercellularity and a higher incidence of glomerular sclerosis and interstitial scarrings than Group 1, a higher incidence of glomerular sclerosis than Group 2, more severe proteinuria, higher serum levels of total cholesterol, and lower serum levels of total protein than Groups 1 and 3 and higher level of uric acid than Group 1. These results suggest that the deposition of apoB and apoE accelerates the progression of mesangial lesions, resulting in greater proteinuria and glomerular sclerosis.

Key words: apolipoprotein – lipids – hyperlipidemia – proteinuria – glomerulosclerosis

Introduction

Hyperlipidemia, particularly elevated plasma levels of both total cholesterol and triglycerides, have been universally observed in patients with nephrotic syndrome [Baxter et al. 1960, Chopra et al. 1971]. With respect to the lipoprotein pattern, they demonstrated increases in either low-density lipoprotein (LDL) or very low-density lipoprotein (VLDL), and occasionally both, as well as decreases in high-density lipoprotein (HDL) [Chopra et al. 1971, Gherardi et al. 1977]. There have been only a few reports dealing with the apolipoproteins (apo's) which determine the character of the lipoproteins in nephrotic syndrome [Kashyap et al. 1980].

On the basis of animal experiments, hyperlipidemia has been assumed to accelerate the development of glomerular sclerosis [Kelly et al. 1983, Yumura et al. 1985, Samuel et al. 1967]. It may also play an important role in the progression of human glomerular disease [Moorhead et al. 1982].

Fatty deposits have been reported in the glomeruli in human diabetic glomerulosclerosis [Hartroft et al. 1955]. The presence of lipoproteins has also been confirmed in the kidney tissue of nephrotic patients [Kashyap et al. 1979]. However, the presence of apo's has not been demonstrated histologically.

The present study was undertaken in order to determine the presence of apoB and apoE in renal biopsy specimens by an immunofluorescent technique and to clarify the relationship between apo deposits and clinical and histological features.

Materials and methods

Forty-nine patients (12 males, 37 females) with persistent proteinuria and/or hematuria served as the study group. Patient ages ranged from 10 to 62 years (average: 37.2 years), duration from onset of urinary abnormalities to renal biopsy ranged from 1 month to 17 years (average: 3.6 years). Kidney tissue specimens were obtained from these patients by percutaneous renal biopsy. Histological diagnoses and clinical features are shown in Table 1. Thirty-five patients had

Received August 16, 1990; in revised form April 25, 1991.

Reprint requests to Dr. H. Sato, Department of Medicine (II), Niigata University School of Medicine, 757-1 Asahimachi, Niigata, Japan

Table 1 Localization of apolipoproteins in the glomeruli. Histological diagnoses and clinical features of 49 patients

	Dx	Sex	Age	UP	Ccr	Cr	UA	TC	TG	TP	Duration	apoB	apoE
1	MGA	f	33	4.85	30.0	105	0.43	8.53	ND	6.3	13	–	+
2	IgAGN	f	27	0.35	131.0	70	0.16	5.60	1.22	7.4	0.1	–	–
3	IgAGN	m	52	5.0	139.0	61	0.39	5.42	ND	4.6	0.3	+	–
4	IgAGN	f	22	0.35	88.9	44	0.23	3.65	0.65	6.8	0.5	–	+
5	IgAGN	f	54	0.50	63.0	70	0.25	5.16	0.75	ND	0.5	+	+
6	IgAGN	f	47	1.0	46.1	79	0.27	5.81	0.76	6.8	1	+	+
7	IgAGN	f	15	1.0	138.0	44	0.19	4.33	1.18	7.7	1.5	–	+
8	IgAGN	m	26	0.1	91.5	97	0.27	5.03	1.20	7.1	2	–	–
9	IgAGN	f	39	0.5	117.3	52	0.13	5.18	1.46	7.2	2	–	–
10	IgAGN	f	30	0.5	90.6	52	0.26	4.07	0.58	7.5	2.5	–	+
11	IgAGN	f	26	0.2	80.6	70	0.23	4.79	1.35	6.7	3	–	–
12	IgAGN	f	29	0	121.1	52	0.17	4.09	1.10	5.8	5	–	–
13	IgAGN	f	24	2.6	101.5	52	0.29	7.10	0.59	6.2	6	+	+
14	IgAGN	m	32	1.0	82.6	97	0.34	3.96	2.70	6.9	6	–	+
15	IgAGN	m	37	1.4	127.0	70	0.48	9.52	0.93	5.3	9	+	+
16	IgAGN	f	46	0.55	ND	114	0.34	5.42	3.34	7.6	16	–	–
17	nonIgAGN	m	38	0	72.0	123	0.54	6.87	2.90	8.0	0.1	–	+
18	nonIgAGN	f	47	0	125.3	88	0.28	4.51	0.67	6.8	0.2	–	–
19	nonIgAGN	f	19	0	60.6	70	0.24	3.83	ND	7.8	0.2	–	–
20	nonIgAGN	f	14	0.5	137.0	88	ND	4.04	1.63	7.2	0.3	–	–
21	nonIgAGN	f	51	0	ND	61	ND	3.34	1.26	6.9	0.4	–	–
22	nonIgAGN	f	40	1.3	92.1	88	ND	7.15	ND	7.0	0.5	+	–
23	nonIgAGN	f	33	1.3	72.9	167	0.32	5.18	0.92	8.0	0.5	+	+
24	nonIgAGN	f	53	0.83	55.5	132	0.39	5.03	1.93	6.6	1	+	–
25	nonIgAGN	m	15	0.5	ND	52	0.24	ND	ND	6.8	3	–	–
26	nonIgAGN	f	44	0.76	73.8	79	0.19	4.79	0.46	7.0	3	–	–
27	nonIgAGN	f	23	0.5	131.0	61	0.18	ND	0.77	7.1	3	+	–
28	nonIgAGN	f	10	0	38.8	70	ND	3.65	ND	6.8	4	–	–
29	nonIgAGN	m	35	0.8	81.3	70	0.27	3.29	1.73	7.0	5	–	+
30	nonIgAGN	f	41	0	119.6	44	0.22	5.83	0.83	8.0	8	–	+
31	MPGN	f	47	2.1	87.5	52	0.32	4.12	0.65	6.7	2	+	–
32	FGS	m	27	32.2	64.2	105	0.35	12.6	4.31	3.7	0.1	+	+
33	FGS	m	51	19.2	46.5	176	0.50	10.19	3.03	4.6	0.1	+	+
34	Membra.	f	49	1.5	140.8	52	0.32	8.19	2.86	6.3	0.5	+	+
35	Endocap.	f	57	0.2	70.0	105	0.38	3.76	0.78	6.0	0.1	+	+
36	SLE	f	41	0.3	95.3	52	0.20	3.63	0.83	8.0	0.3	–	+
37	SLE	m	26	0	117.7	70	0.20	3.08	0.83	7.3	0.8	–	+
38	SLE	f	37	0	65.0	61	0.17	3.89	0.86	8.3	4	–	–
39	SLE	f	24	1.5	90.4	52	0.35	5.13	1.73	6.1	8	–	–
40	SLE	f	40	2.8	109.8	26	0.33	5.78	1.51	5.6	8	+	+
41	RA	f	56	0	91.9	114	0.14	7.13	1.11	7.8	10	+	–
42	RA	f	43	1.4	80.0	88	0.33	5.00	1.01	6.5	17	+	+
43	Toxemia	f	20	0.3	103.8	44	0.32	5.39	1.29	7.4	0.3	+	–
44	Toxemia	f	25	16.3	93.0	88	ND	5.96	2.00	5.2	0.4	+	+
45	Toxemia	f	22	0	136.6	35	0.30	4.35	0.51	7.5	0.5	–	–
46	DM	f	51	5.0	60.0	70	0.32	6.87	ND	7.8	4	+	+
47	DM	f	70	3.3	36.0	238	0.37	5.24	1.47	5.0	5	+	+
48	DM	m	62	0.9	137.8	79	0.39	4.79	1.25	7.5	20	+	+
49	TIN	f	58	0	14.9	282	0.29	3.34	0.85	7.8	4	–	–

Abbreviations are: Dx, histological diagnosis; UP, proteinuria (g/day); Ccr, creatinine clearance (ml/min); Cr, creatinine (μmol/l); UA, uric acid (mmol/l); TC, total cholesterol (mmol/l); TG, triglyceride (mmol/l); TP, total protein (g/dl); Duration, duration of the disease (years); MGA, minor glomerular abnormalities; GN, glomerulonephritis; MPGN, membranoproliferative glomerulonephritis; FGS, focal glomerulosclerosis; Membra., membranous nephropathy; Endocap., endocapillary proliferative glomerulonephritis; SLE, lupus nephritis; RA, nephropathy of rheumatoid arthritis; Toxemia, toxemia of pregnancy; DM, diabetic nephropathy; TIN, tubulointerstitial nephritis; f, female; m, male; –, negative; +, positive and ND, not done.

primary glomerular diseases and thirteen secondary glomerular diseases: the single remaining patient showed tubulointerstitial nephritis. The relationship between apo staining pattern and clinical or histological features was examined in all 49 subjects.

In the immunofluorescent microscopy (IF) cases, a small piece of the specimen was embedded in OCT (Miles Scientific, Naperville, IL) and quickly frozen in dry ice and acetone at −70° C. Cryostat sections were cut 2–3 microns thick, and rinsed in phosphate-buffered isotonic saline (PBS, pH 7.2) three times for 15 minutes. After being covered with anti-human apoB and E antisera diluted 1:50 (Daiichi Pure Chemical, Japan), the sections were incubated for 30 minutes. After washing three times in PBS for 15 minutes, they were incubated for 30 minutes with fluorescein-conjugated swine anti-goat immunoglobulin antisera (DACO, Denmark), which were diluted 1:15 and preabsorbed with normal human serum. Sections were again washed three times in PBS, mounted in glycerin, and observed under a Zeiss Axiophot fluorescent photomicroscope. The number of evaluated glomeruli for IF was 1 to 11 (mean 3.4). The patients were divided into four groups on the basis of the immunofluorescent microscopic findings regarding the staining pattern of apoB and E. Group 1: both apoB and apoE negative; Group 2: apoB alone positive; Group 3: apoE alone positive and Group 4: both apoB and apoE positive.

The specificity of anti apoE antisera was confirmed by the Ouchterlony method, two-dimensional immunoelectrophoresis, and radioimmunoassay, none of which revealed cross-reactivity with any other apo's or plasma proteins [Itakura et al. 1986]. No cross-reactivity was observed between apoB and other apo's when tested against normal human serum, using the Ouchterlony method and two-dimensional immunoelectrophoresis.

In the light microscopic (LM) study cases, a piece of renal biopsy specimen was fixed in 50% alcohol-Buan mixture (saturated picric acid in 50% ethanol, 40 ml; 35% formalin, 7.5 ml; acetic acid, 2.5 ml), embedded in paraffin, and cut into sections 2–3 microns thick. The sections, stained with hematoxylin-eosin, periodic acid Schiff (PAS) and periodic acid-methenamine silver (PAM) stain, were examined under a Zeiss Axiophot light microscope. The number of evaluated glomeruli for LM was 5 to 37 (mean 15.1).

The mesangial lesion, an increase in cells and/or matrix, was divided into focal and diffuse proliferation. The presence of glomerular adhesions, sclerosis, vascular changes and interstitial scarring were also evaluated. Serum samples were obtained from the patients after 12-hour fasting. Total cholesterol (TC), triglyceride (TG), uric acid (UA) and total protein (TP) were determined via standard laboratory methods. Urinary protein excretion and creatinine clearance (Ccr) were calculated from 24-hour urine samples.

Statistical analysis was performed using the chi-square test, or Wilcoxon's U-test. A probability of <0.05 was regarded as significant.

Results

ApoB and apoE were demonstrated as having a granular pattern in the glomeruli, and occasionally in the capillary loop, though mainly in the mesangial lesions, as shown in Figures 1 and 2. However, apo's were not detected in the global sclerotic glomeruli. In

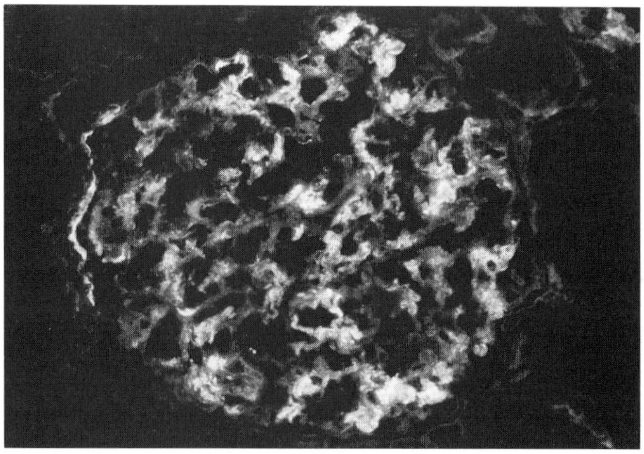

Fig. 1 Immunofluorescent micrograph of a glomerulus from a patient with SLE, showing mesangial apoB deposition. (Magnification ×400)

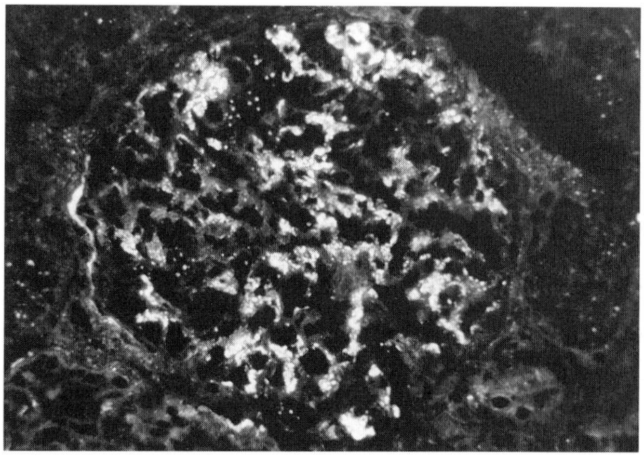

Fig. 2 Immunofluorescent micrograph of a glomerulus from a patient with IgA nephropathy, showing mesangial apoE deposition. (Magnification ×400)

four control cases obtained from non-tumorous tissue of renal cell carcinoma patients, apo's were not detected in glomeruli. ApoB was positive in 14 of 35 patients with primary glomerular disease and in 8 of 13 with secondary glomerular disease. ApoE was detected in 17 of the former and 8 of the latter. One patient with tubulointerstitial nephritis did not exhibit deposition of either apoB or E as shown in Table 1.

The relationship between apo staining and light microscopic findings in the glomeruli is shown in Table 2. A significant correlation was found between glomerular apo staining and mesangial cell proliferation. Diffuse mesangial cell proliferation was noted in 53% of the patients in Group 4, while it was seen in only 18% of Group 1 ($p < 0.05$). Glomerular sclerosis, on the other hand, was observed in 67% of Group 4, in 30% of Group 1 and in 14% of Group 2, respectively ($p < 0.05$). Interstitial scarring was present in 47% of Group 1, in 90% of Group 3, and in 87% of Group 4, respectively ($p < 0.05$, $p < 0.025$).

Table 3 shows the relationship between apoB and E and clinical features. Age in Group 4, 42.8 ± 12.2 years, was significantly higher than that in Group 3, 31.3 ± 8.3 years ($p < 0.05$). Urine protein in Group 4, 6.0 ± 9.2 g/day, was significantly greater than that in Group 1, 0.3 ± 0.4 g/day and Group 3, 0.9 ± 1.4 g/day ($p < 0.01$) and that in Group 2, 1.4 ± 1.7 g/day, was greater than that in Group 1 ($p < 0.05$). UA in Group 4, 0.32 ± 0.11 mmol/l, was significantly higher than that in Group 1, 0.19 ± 0.11 mmol/l ($p < 0.01$). TC in Group 4, 6.74 ± 2.41 mmol/l, was significantly higher than that in Group 1, 4.17 ± 1.28 mmol/l, and Group 3, 4.72 ± 1.78 mmol/l, respectively ($p < 0.01$, $p < 0.05$) and that in Group 2, 5.70 ± 1.20 mmol/l was higher than that in Group 1 ($p < 0.05$). However, TP in Group 4, 6.1 ± 1.3 g/dl, was significantly lower than in Group 1, 7.1 ± 0.5 g/dl, and in Group 3, 7.4 ± 0.6 mg/dl ($p < 0.05$). There was no significant difference in Cr, Ccr or TG among the four groups.

As shown in Table 4, apoE was positive in 68% of the apoB-positive group, which was significantly higher than in the apoB-negative group ($p < 0.05$).

Discussion

Recently, interest has mounted with regard to the possibility that abnormalities in lipid metabolism may be deeply involved in the progression of glomerular or tubulointerstitial diseases [Moorhead et al. 1982]. Several authors have stated that hyperlipidemia may mediate the development of glomerular sclerosis [Saito et al. 1987, Keane et al. 1988]. Shore et al. [1982] reported the presence of modified apoB and E in the urine of nephrotic patients; however, the distribution of modified apoB and E in renal tissue has not been completely clarified, although the presence of lipoprotein has been confirmed in renal disease [Kashyap et al. 1979]. Blue et al. [1983] failed to detect any synthesis of apoB in the kidney. Recently, cultured rat mesangial cells have been found to possess LDL receptors and take up LDL [Wheeler et al. 1989, Wasserman et al. 1989]. Some investigators have

Table 2 Relationship between glomerular apoB and apoE deposition and histological findings (n = 49)

	Group 1 (n = 17)	Group 2 (n = 7)	Group 3 (n = 10)	Group 4 (n = 15)	Statistical Significance
Diffuse mesangial cell proliferation	3 (18%)	3 (43%)	3 (30%)	8 (53%)	p <0.05 (Group 1 vs. Group 4)
Diffuse mesangial matrix proliferation	9 (53%)	3 (43%)	6 (60%)	10 (67%)	NS
Glomerular adhesion	2 (12%)	2 (29%)	5 (50%)	6 (40%)	p <0.05 (Group 1 vs. Group 3)
Glomerular sclerosis	5 (30%)	1 (14%)	4 (40%)	10 (67%)	p <0.05 (Group 1 vs. Group 4) p <0.05 (Group 2 vs. Group 4)
Vessel changes	6 (35%)	3 (43%)	4 (40%)	10 (67%)	NS
Interstitial changes	8 (47%)	3 (43%)	9 (90%)	13 (87%)	p <0.05 (Group 1 vs. Group 3) p <0.025 (Group 1 vs. Group 4)

NS: not significant

Table 3 Relationship between apoB and apoE and clinical features

		Group 1 (n = 17)	Group 2 (n = 7)	Group 3 (n = 10)	Group 4 (n = 15)
Age	years	34.8 ± 20.0	41.5 ± 14.6	31.3 ± 8.3	42.8 ± 12.2[c]
Proteinuria	g/day	0.3 ± 0.4	1.4 ± 1.7[a]	0.9 ± 1.4	6.0 ± 9.2[bd]
Ccr	ml/min	75.5 ± 49.9	100.1 ± 28.1	91.6 ± 29.8	83.2 ± 33.7
Cr	µmol/l	81 ± 55	78 ± 33	70 ± 28	97 ± 55
	(mg/dl)	(0.9 ± 0.6)	(0.9 ± 0.4)	(0.8 ± 0.3)	(1.1 ± 0.6)
UA	mmol/l	0.19 ± 0.11	0.24 ± 0.14	0.28 ± 0.11	0.32 ± 0.11[b]
	(mg/dl)	(3.4 ± 1.9)	(4.3 ± 2.5)	(5.1 ± 1.9)	(5.7 ± 1.9)
TP	g/dl	7.1 ± 0.5	6.7 ± 1.0	7.4 ± 0.6	6.1 ± 1.3[ac]
TC	mmol/l	4.17 ± 1.28	5.70 ± 1.20[a]	4.72 ± 1.78	6.74 ± 2.41[bc]
	(mg/dl)	(161.1 ± 49.6)	(220.1 ± 46.5)	(182.3 ± 68.6)	(260.1 ± 93.0)
TG	mmol/l	1.03 ± 0.81	0.82 ± 0.69	1.22 ± 0.94	1.47 ± 1.13
	(mg/dl)	(92.4 ± 72.2)	(73.2 ± 62.1)	(109.2 ± 84.2)	(132.0 ± 100.8)
Duration of the disease	years	3.9 ± 5.1	1.1 ± 1.0	4.1 ± 4.3	3.4 ± 4.8

Abbreviations are: Ccr, creatinine clearance; Cr, creatinine; UA, uric acid; TP, total protein; TC, total cholesterol; TG, triglyceride.
[a] $p < 0.05$ compared with Group 1
[b] $p < 0.01$ compared with Group 1
[c] $p < 0.05$ compared with Group 3
[d] $p < 0.01$ compared with Group 3

shown that high physiological concentrations of LDL cause mesangial cell injury in vitro [Moorhead et al. 1989, Wasserman et al. 1989]. The present study has clearly demonstrated the deposition of apoB in the glomerular mesangium in various renal diseases. There may be several mechanisms for this deposition. The first is that LDL receptors on mesangial cells bind with apoB and mediate lipid accumulation in their mesangial cells. The second is that LDL containing apoB may also combine with polyanionic glycosaminoglycans in mesangial matrix, and glomerular basement membrane [Iverius et al. 1972] and alter the anionic charge of the glomerular basement membrane. The third is that, since mesangial cells have a phagocytic function [Michael et al. 1980, Elema et al. 1976], they may phagocytose LDL or VLDL containing apoB. In relation to the histological findings, Group 4 (both apoB and apoE positive cases) showed more mesangial cell proliferation than Group 1 (both apoB and apoE negative cases). LDL has been known to cause the degeneration of smooth muscle cells resembling mesangial cells in origin and function [Striker et al. 1987]. It is not yet clear whether the deposition of apoB in the mesangium is the cause or the result of mesangial cell proliferation, although it may play an important role in the progression of glomerular sclerosis. The apoB-positive group (Group 2 and 4) displayed more proteinuria and higher TC levels than the negative group (Group 1 and 3). TP in Group 4 was lower than that in Group 1 and 3. It is well known that increase in urine protein can cause hyperlipidemia and hypoproteinemia in the nephrotic syndrome. Increase in serum uric acid concentration, noted in Group 4, have been assumed to be an important early indication of the progression of glomerular diseases. Age in Group 4 was higher than that in Group 3. No correlation was found between the duration of the disease in Group 3 and 4. Michael et al. [1984] described that mesangium have a pathway to remove macromolecules from the mesangial zone to the hilium of the glomerulus. This pathway (i.e. mesangial pathway) is modulated by

Table 4 Statistical relationship between the staining of apoB and apoE in glomeruli (n = 49)

	apoE positive	Statistical significance
apoB negative (n = 27)	10 (37%)	$p < 0.05$
apoB positive (n = 22)	15 (68%)	

several factors. Local intraglomerular hemodynamic factors may modulate uptake and disposal of macromolecules. Lindeman [1990] described that there is a progressive decline of glomerular filtration rate and renal plasma flow with aging. These hemodynamic changes might effect removal of apo's from the mesangial area.

Lin et al. [1986] described that apoE is distributed mainly in the tubular epithelium, but small amount are occasionally seen in the glomeruli and small vessels of the baboon using immunohistological techniques. The apoE mRNA level in the renal cortex was approximately 1–5% of that of the liver in the nonhuman primate Macaca fascicularis [Newman et al. 1985]. The rate of apoE synthesis, confirmed in the kidney by Blue, was 4–6 times greater in the renal cortex than in the renal medulla [Blue et al. 1983]. There have been no reports, however, dealing with the deposition of apoE in the human glomerulus. The present study has demonstrated that apoE exists mainly in mesangial lesions, and that the positive group (Group 4 and 3) exhibits more severe proteinuria, glomerular sclerosis, interstitial scarring and glomerular adhesion than the negative group (Group 1 and 3).

Recently, other functions of apoE, unrelated to lipid transport, have become known, e.g., modulation of cell growth and differentiation, repair response to tissue injury and immunoregulation. The production of apoE was increased in growth-arrested smooth muscle cells. Enhanced synthesis of apoE may occur as a consequence of smooth muscle cell differentiation and be a phenotype marker of such differentiation [Majack et al. 1988]. ApoE in the mesangial area may therefore be related to mesangial cell differentiation in some way. Recent work has demonstrated that secretion and accumulation of apoE increased in regenerating peripheral nerves [Boyles et al. 1989]. Since apoE expression after nerve injury is closely associated with nerve growth and degeneration, two roles of this apo in nerve injury were suggested: first, removing byproducts formed during degeneration of nerves, and second, providing the regenerating nerves with lipids necessary for axon growth. In control cases, apoE was not found in mesangium; therefore, apoE deposition in the mesangium may have some relation to mesangial injury or states requiring cholesterol for mesangial cells. The mesangium is partially composed of transient monocyte-macrophage surrounded by an extracellular matrix [Kashgarian 1985]. ApoE presented in mesangium may be synthesized by these macrophages. Werb et al. [1989] reported that macrophages secrete apoE in response to receptor-mediated endocytosis. Sedor et al. [1987] have stated that mesangial cells exhibit Fc-receptor mediated phagocytosis and release superoxide anion. It is assumed that in cases with apoE deposition, phagocytosis of mesangial cells may be activated by immune complexes.

The deposition of apoB and apoE in glomeruli was correlated. This finding is consistent with the work demonstrating the presence of classical LDL receptors on mesangial cells as described by Wheeler et al. [1989]. ApoB and apoE positive cases (Group 4) exhibited more histological damage and more severe proteinuria. ApoB deposition in the mesangium area might change mesangial cell function, and the mesangium secretes apoE, which modulates cell growth and differentiation.

Apo's were not detected in global sclerotic glomeruli. Mesangial functions (i.e. phagocytosis and presence of LDL receptors) might be lost in sclerotic glomeruli, and apo's deposition was not presented in global sclerotic glomeruli. Although there was a possibility that sclerotic areas of glomeruli were not contained in IF specimen, apo's were detected in global mesangial area in the cases of focal glomerulosclerosis.

This study has demonstrated that there are no significant differences in serum TG levels between apoE-positive (Group 3 and 4) and negative groups (Group 1 and 2), although the serum level of apoE has been reported to be correlated with TG [Yamada et al. 1982]. Higher levels of UA in Group 4 reflect the tubular scarring.

These results suggest that the deposition of apoB and E accelerates the progression of mesangial lesions, resulting in high degrees of proteinuria and glomerular sclerosis.

Acknowledgement

The authors are grateful to Mr. Hiroshi Watanabe for this technical assistance.

This study was supported by the Research Grant for "Progressive Renal Diseases" from "Specially Selected Diseases by the Ministry of Health and Welfare Research Project," the Ministry of Health and Welfare of Japan.

REFERENCES

Baxter JH, Goodman HC, Havel J 1960 Serum lipid and lipoprotein alteration in nephrosis. J Clin Invest *39:* 455–465

Blue ML, Williams DL, Zucker S, Khan A, Blum CB 1983 Apolipoprotein E synthesis in human kidney, adrenal gland, and liver. Proc Natl Acad Sci USA *80:* 283–287

Boyles JK, Zoellner CD, Anderson LJ, Kosik LM, Pitas RE, Weisgraber KH, Hui DY, Mahley RW, Gebicke-Haerter PJ, Ignatius MJ, Shooter EM 1989 A Role for Apolipoprotein E, Apolipoprotein A-I, and Low Density Lipoprotein Receptors in Cholesterol Transport during Regeneration and Remyelination of the Rat Sciatic Nerve. J Clin Invest *83:* 1015–1031

Chopra JS, Mallick NP, Stone MC 1971 Hyperlipoproteinemia in nephrotic syndrome. Lancet *317:* 317–321

Elema JD, Hoyer JR, Vernier RL 1976 The glomerular mesangium: Uptake and transport of intravenously injected colloidal carbon in rats. Kidney Int *9:* 395–406

Gherardi E, Rota E, Calanda S, Genova R, Tamborino A 1977 Relationship among the concentration of serum lipoproteins and change in their chemical composition in patients with untreated nephrotic syndrome. Eur J Clin Invest *7:* 563–570

Hartroft WD 1955 Fat Emboli in Glomerular Capillary of Choline-deficient Rats and of Patients with Diabetic Glomerulosclerosis. Am J Path *31:* 381–397

Itakura K, Matsudate T, Sakurai T, Hashimoto S, Ito K, Kanno H, Hirata M, Nakamura K 1986 Single radial immunodiffusion of serum apolipoproteins C-2, C-3 and E–pretreatment of samples with surfactant. Clinica Chemica Acta *161:* 275–282

Iverius, Per-Henrik 1972 The interaction between human plasma lipoproteins and connective tissue glycosaminoglycans. J Biol Chem *247:* 2607–2613

Kashgarian M 1985 Mesangium and Glomerular Disease. Lab Invest *52:* 569–571

Kashyap ML, Ooi BS, Hynd BA, Glueck CJ, Pollak VE, Robinson K 1979 Sequestration and excretion of high density and low density lipoproteins by the kidney in human nephrotic syndrome. Artery *6 (2):* 108–121

Kashyap ML, Srivastava LS, Hynd BA, Brady D, Perisutti G, Glueck CJ, Gartside PS 1980 Apolipoprotein CII and lipoprotein lipase in human nephrotic syndrome. Arteriosclerosis *35:* 29–40

Keane WF, Kasiske BL, O'Donnell MP 1988 Hyperlipidemia and the progression of renal disease. Am J Clin Nutr *47:* 157–160

Kelly VE, Izui S 1983 Enriched Lipid Diet Accelerates Lupus Nephritis in NZB*W Mice. Synergistic Action of Immune Complexes and Lipid in Glomerular Injury. Am Ass Path *111:* 288–297

Lin CT, Xu Y, Wu J, Chan L 1986 Immunoreactive Apolipoprotein E is a Widely Distributed Cellular Protein. Immunohistochemical Localization of Apolipoprotein E in Baboon Tissues. J Clin Invest *78:* 947–958

Linderman RD 1990 Overview: Renal Physiology and Pathophysiology of Aging. Am J Kidney Dis *16:* 275–282

Majack RA, Castle CK, Goodman LV, Weisgraber KH, Mahley RW, Shooter EM, Gebicke-Haerter PJ 1988 Expression of Apolipoprotein E by Cultured Vascular Smooth Muscle Cells Is Controlled by Growth State. J Cell Biol *107:* 1207–1213

Michael AF 1984 The glomerular mesangium. Contr Nephrol *40:* 7–14

Michael AF, Keane WF, Raij L, Vernier RL, Mauer SM 1980 The glomerular mesangium. Kidney Int *17:* 141–154

Moorhead JF, Chan MK, El-Nahas M, Varghese Z 1982 Lipid nephrotoxicity in chronic progressive glomerular and tubulo-interstitial disease. Lancet *2:* 1309–1311

Moorhead JF, Wheeler DC, Fernando R, Sweny P, Varghese Z 1989 Injury to rat mesangial cells in culture by low density lipoproteins. (Abstract). Kidney Int *35:* 433

Newman TC, Dawson PA, Rudel LL, Williams DL 1985 Quantitation of Apolipoprotein E mRNA in the Liver and Peripheral Tissues of Nonhuman Primates. J Biol Chem *260:* 2452–2457

Saito T, Sato H, Akiu N, Ootaka T, Furuyama T, Yoshinaga K 1987 Focal glomerular sclerosis in non-nephrotic patients with hyperlipidemia. Jpn J Nephr *29:* 1107–1114

Samuel WF, Yamada W, Ostwald R 1967 Dietary induced glomerulosclerosis in the guinea pig. Arch Path *83:* 204–210

Sedor JR, Carey SW, Emancipator SN 1987 Immune complexes bind to cultured rat glomerular mesangial cells to stimulate superoxide release. J Immun *138:* 3751–3757

Shore VG, Forte T, Licht H, Lewis SB 1982 Serum and Urinary Lipoproteins in the Human Nephrotic Syndrome: Evidence for Catabolism of Lipoproteins. Metabolism *31:* 258–268

Striker GE, Lange MA, McKay K, Bernstein K, Striker LJ 1987 Glomerular Cells In Vitro. Adv Nephrol *16:* 169–186

Wasserman J, Santiaago A, Rifici, Holthofer H, Scharschmidt L, Epstein M, Schlondorff D 1989 Interaction of low density lipoprotein with rat mesangial cells. Kidney Int *35:* 1168–1174

Wheeler DC, Persaud J, Kingstone D, Sweny P, Varghese Z, Moorhead JF 1989 Receptor mediated binding of human low density lipoprotein (LDL) to rat mesangial cells in vitro. (Abstract). Kidney Int *35:* 439

Werb Z, Takemura R, Stenberg PE, Bainton DF 1989 Directed Exocytosis of Secretory Granules Containing Apolipoprotein E to the Adherent Surface and Basal Vacuoles of Macrophages Spreading on Immobile Immune Complexes. Am J Path *134:* 661–670

Yamada N, Murase T, Itakura H, Kosaka K 1982 Plasma Apolipoprotein E Level in Hypertriglyceridemia. Hormon Metabol Res *14:* 303–306

Yumura W, Hattori S, Morrow WJW, Mayes DC, Levy JA, Shirai T 1985 Dietary fat and immune function. II. Effects on immune complex nephritis in (NZB*NZW) F1 mice. J Immun *135:* 3864–3868

Clinical Nephrology, Vol. 36 No. 3 – 1991 (134–140)

FSGS-like lesions in pre-eclampsia

Y. Nagai[1], H. Arai[2], Y. Washizawa[1], Y. Ger[2], M. Tanaka[3], M. Maeda[3] and S. Kawamura[2]

[1] *Department of Nephrology*
[2] *Second Department of Pathology*
[3] *First Department of Obstetrics and Gynecology, School of Medicine, Toho University, Tokyo, Japan*

Abstract. Renal-biopsy specimens taken from pre-eclamptic patients are associated sometimes with focal-segmental glomerular sclerotic lesions (FSGS-like lesions) that closely resemble those of primary focal-segmental glomerulosclerosis. We studied a series of 60 sections from each of 19 cases of "pure" pre-eclampsia by light microscopy. Group I comprised 13 patients with FSGS-like lesions in their glomeruli, group II comprised 6 patients without such lesions. FSGS-like lesions were observed in 20.7 ± 4.6% of glomeruli in group I. Epithelial droplets were observed in 12 of 13 cases in group I, but only one of 6 cases in group II. The incidence of granulated glomerular epithelial cells was significantly higher in group I ($p < 0.0005$). The double contour of the basement membrane was more severe in group I than in group II ($p < 0.03$). The percentage of glomeruli with FSGS and the number of weeks during which proteinuria of ≧3 g/day continued after delivery were positively correlated ($r = 0.76$, $p < 0.0002$). We also found a significant positive correlation between the percentage of glomeruli with FSGS and the amount of proteinuria at delivery and biopsy ($r = 0.66$, $p < 0.003$; $r = 0.51$, $p < 0.03$). However, proteinuria disappeared in all patients. Three of them had successful second pregnancies. We consider that FSGS-like lesions can occur during pregnancy in "pure" pre-eclamptic patients but the lesions may not be progressive. We also suggest that proteinuria and epithelial cell change may be closely related with such lesions.

Key words: focal-segmental glomerular sclerosis – pre-eclampsia – renal biopsy – proteinuria

Introduction

Since Kida [Kida et al. 1985] reported that some of the glomeruli in renal biopsies of pre-eclamptic women were associated with segmental lesions that resembled those of primary focal-segmental glomerulosclerosis [Nochy et al. 1986, Nadal et al. 1986], several reports by other investigators have followed. We examined the segmental lesions (FSGS-like lesions) that resembled those seen in the glomeruli of early-stage primary focal-segmental glomerular sclerosis [Schwartz et al. 1985, Rennke et al. 1989] (Figure 1): segmental collapsed capillaries with wrinkled basement membrane, foamy cell accumulation in capillary lumen usually associated with proliferation and/or detachment of visceral and parietal epithelial cells and adhesion of Bowman's capsule with or without hyalinosis. Because focal-segmental sclerotic lesions can be found in many types of glomerular diseases, we used strict criteria in selecting pre-eclamptic patients, excluding gravida who had underlying renal diseases or hypertensive disorders. We attempted to clarify which pre-eclamptic symptoms were most important for the occurrence of FGS-like lesions and to better understand the pathogenesis of these lesions.

Patients and methods

Nineteen pre-eclamptic women who delivered in Toho University Hospital from 1977 to 1988 were studied. Patients showed typical pre-eclamptic syndrome: proteinuria, edema and hypertension during pregnancy. They underwent renal biopsy after delivery. Only patients who were diagnosed as having "pure" pre-eclamptic toxemia clinically and histologically were entered into this study; patients with underlying renal diseases and hypertensive disorders were excluded. The diagnosis of "pure" pre-eclampsia

Received December 22, 1990; in revised form April 30, 1991.

Reprint requests to Dr. Y. Nagai, Second Department of Internal Medicine, School of Medicine, Toho University. 6-11-1, Ohmori-nishi, Ohta-ku, Tokyo 143, Japan.

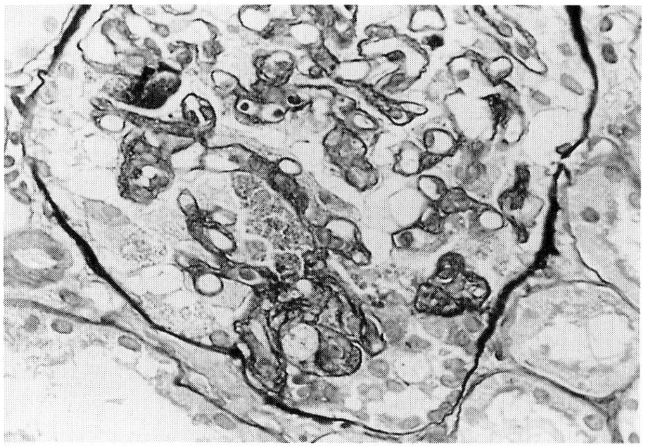

Fig. 1 Light micrograph shows a glomerulus with focal-segmental glomerulosclerosis. The lesion includes foamy cells, collapsed capillary walls and adhesion to Bowman's capsule. "Double contour" of the basement membrane is evident (× 200, PAS).

on biopsy specimens was made by the following criteria: 1) light micrographs showing diffuse glomerular swelling due to intraglomerular cell hypertrophy without mesangial proliferation, show "double contour" of the glomerular basement membrane (GBM), 2) electron micrographs showing elevation of the subendothelial layer or subendothelial fibrillar deposits and circumferential mesangialinterposition, and 3) immunofluorescent micrographs showing mesangial and capillary deposition of IgM (while C_3 deposition was sometimes observed, deposition of other immunoglobulins along the capillary walls was infrequent) [Gaber et al. 1987, Taylor et al. 1986, Nagai et al. 1989].

Pre-eclamptic syndrome started after the second trimester in all patients. We confirmed that they were normotensive and had not had proteinuria before pregnancy and during first trimester. We excluded multipara to avoid entering patients into this study who had underlying renal diseases or hypertensive disorders. We also selected patients whose level of uric acid at delivery was at least 6 mg/dl, because a high level of uric acid is considered to be specific for pre-eclampsia [Pollak et al. 1960].

Table 1 Clinical features

	Group I	Group II
No. of patients	13	6
Age at delivery (yr)	29.5 ± 1.6	28.3 ± 1.9
Parity	primipara	primipara
Follow-up period (mo)	30.4 ± 7.3	25.3 ± 4.6
Duration from delivery to biopsy (day)	18.0 ± 1.9	14.0 ± 2.0
	Mean ± SEM	

Group I vs II: no significant differences

We divided the patients into two groups: Group I comprised 13 women with toxemic changes associated with FSGS-like lesions in glomeruli. The age at delivery ranged from 22 to 44 (29.5 ± 1.6, mean ± SEM) years. They underwent renal biopsy 18.0 ± 1.9 days after delivery. The follow-up period was 30.4 ± 7.3 months after delivery (Table 1).

Group II comprised 6 women with toxemic changes without FSGS-like lesions in glomeruli. Age at delivery ranged from 21 to 32 (28.3 ± 1.9) years. They underwent renal biopsy 14.0 ± 2.0 days after delivery. The follow-up period was 25.3 ± 4.6 months after delivery. Age at delivery and duration from delivery to biopsy were not significantly different between the two groups (Table 1).

Most patients received antihypertensive drugs but none received corticosteroids or other medication for proteinuria.

The specimens obtained by percutaneous renal biopsy were divided into three parts for light microscopy, electron microscopy, and immunofluorescent studies. The specimens for light microscopy were fixed in 10% formalin solution, embedded in paraffin and sectioned at 1–2 μ thick and stained with hematoxylin-eosin (HE), periodic-acid-schiff (PAS), Masson-trichrome (MT), periodic-acid-silver methenamine (PAM) and allochrome. In addition to those routine sections, each of the remaining specimens for light microscopy was serially sectioned to yield at least 60 sections. The serially sectioned specimens were stained by PAS, but every seventh section was stained by MT. We examined all sections for segmental lesions including collapsed capillaries with wrinkled GBM, foamy cells, adhesion to Bowmans' capsule and increased segmental mesangial matrix with or without hyalinosis. We took low-power photomicrographs of every tenth section to identify individual glomeruli. We numbered each glomerulus and calculated the percentage of the total number of glomeruli with segmental lesions in the total number of glomeruli included in each biopsy specimen. We selected biopsies that included more than fifteen glomeruli. We examined the position of each segmental lesion, then divided them into three types: vascular pole, urinary pole and other. We also calculated the incidence of epithelial droplets in those serial sections. Semiquantitative estimation of the pathological changes was attempted by scoring the severity of double contour in glomeruli, interstitial fibrosis, edema, cell infiltration in light microscopy, from 0 to

3 (0: absent; 1: slight; 2: moderate; 3: marked). We also estimated arteriosclerosis by score (0: absent; 1: muscular thickening; 2: fibromuscular thickening; 3: hyaline thickening).

Specimens for electron microscopy were fixed in buffered formalin, refixed in osmium, embedded in Epon, sliced into ultrathin sections, and examined under an electron microscope (Hitachi, H-300).

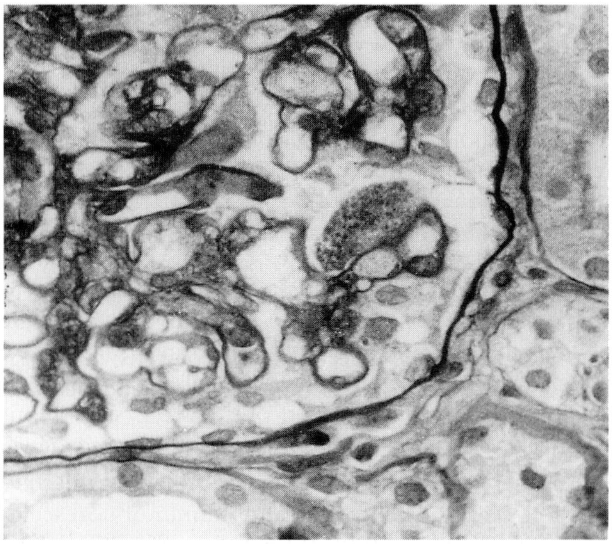

Fig. 2a Glomerulus shows granular droplets in epithelial cell. (28-year-old primipara. × 400, PAS).

Blood pressure, daily urinary protein excretion, serum creatinine, uric acid, cholesterol and triglyceride level were re-examined during pregnancy and after delivery. Statistical analysis was performed by Student's t-test. We considered probability values of $p < 0.05$ as statistically significant.

Results

The FSGS-like lesions in pure pre-eclampsia showed segmental collapsed capillaries with wrinkled GBM. PAM-positive areas in these lesions varied in size and thickness of stain. Mild increase in mesangial matrix was observed frequently in those lesions without mesangial cell proliferation. Foamy cells obliterating capillary lumina were present in most of the lesions. Neutrophil infiltration and/or cell debris were sometimes seen in the lesions. The collapsed capillaries always adhered to the Bowman's capsule. Parietal and visceral epithelial cells increased in number, many of which have vacuoles, vesicles and PAS-positive granules around the adhesion sites. Hyaline deposits were observed not so frequently in the lesions.

The total number of glomeruli observed in group I was 34.9 ± 4.8, that in group II 31.8 ± 4.5. Global sclerosis was observed in $2.0 \pm 0.8\%$ of glomeruli in group I and $1.9 \pm 1.0\%$ in group II. These differences were not significant (Table 2).

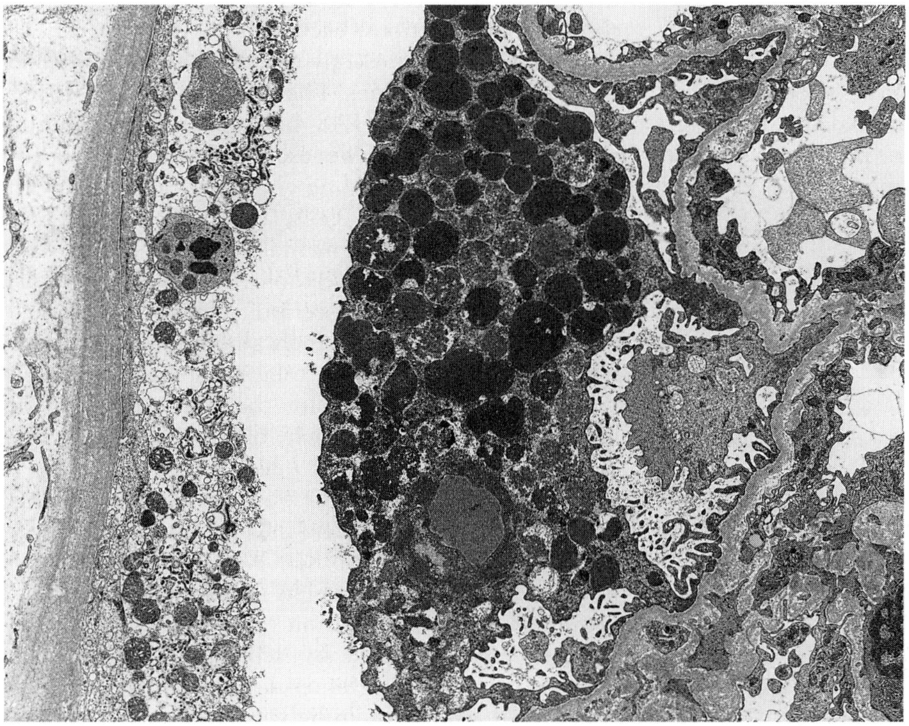

Fig. 2b Electron micrograph shows the granulated epithelial cells. Many amorphous granules filling epithelial cytoplasm (× 5000).

Table 2 Histological findings

	Group I	Group II	
Total number of glomeruli	34.9 ± 4.8	31.8 ± 4.5	n. s.
Global sclerosis (%)	2.0 ± 0.8	1.9 ± 1.0	n. s.
Total FGS (%)	20.7 ± 4.6	–	
urinary pole	10.0 ± 2.8		
vascular pole	2.5 ± 1.4		
others	8.1 ± 2.8		
	Mean ± SEM		

n. s.: not significant

Table 3 Course of hypertension

	Group I	Group II	
Onset of hypertension (wks of gestation)	30.2 ± 1.0	27.5 ± 1.6	n. s.
Maximum blood pressure*			
Systolic (mmHg)	190.0 ± 7.6	174.0 ± 6.7	n. s.
Diastolic (mmHg)	122.5 ± 3.4	113.7 ± 3.1	n. s.
Disappearance of hypertension (days after delivery)	22.0 ± 6.6	29.3 ± 18.5	n. s.
	Mean ± SEM		

* Based on two or more measurements taken at least six hours apart.
n. s.: not significant

Table 4 Course of proteinuria

	Group I	Group II	
Onset of proteinuria (wks of gestation)	28.4 ± 1.5	25.5 ± 2.6	n. s.
Urinary protein excretion			
at delivery (g/day)	10.6 ± 2.5	7.9 ± 1.2	n. s.
at biopsy (g/day)	3.0 ± 0.7	1.4 ± 0.8	n. s.
≧3 g/day (days after delivery)	15.5 ± 4.6	4.5 ± 2.1	$p < 0.05$
Disappearance of proteinuria (mo after delivery)	5.7 ± 1.5	2.3 ± 1.0	n. s.
	Mean ± SEM		

n. s.: not significant

In group I, the percentage of glomeruli with FSGS-like lesions ranged from 3.1 to 56.5 (20.7 ± 4.6)%. FSGS was observed in 10.0 ± 2.8 and 2.5 ± 1.4% of glomeruli in urinary and vascular poles, respectively. The percentage of glomeruli with FSGS observed between urinary and vascular poles was 8.1 ± 2.8%. We included FSGS-like lesions that we could not classify because of spreading from vascular to urinary poles or two FGS lesions in a single glomerulus as belonging to the third group (Table 2). Droplets formation in epithelial cells (Figure 2 a, b) was observed frequently in group I (12/13 cases), but was seen in only one case in group II. The incidence of epithelial droplets was significantly higher in group I than in group II ($p < 0.0005$).

The double contour in the GBM was significantly more sever in group I than in group II ($p < 0.03$). In group I, two cases frequently showed hyaline arteriolosclerosis. Another 4 cases also showed hyaline arteriolosclerosis though in much lesser number. Only one case in group II showed hyaline arteriolosclerosis in several arterioles. The average scoring numbers of arteriosclerosis were more severe in group I ($p < 0.05$). Statistical analysis showed no significant differences between the two groups in terms of severity of interstitial fibrosis, edema and cell infiltration.

Maximum blood pressure, which was based on two or more measurements taken at least six hours apart, was higher in group I than in group II, but the difference was not statistically significant (Table 3). There was no statistically significant difference between the two groups in the disappearance of hypertension.

Daily urinary protein excretion at delivery and at biopsy was larger in group I than in group II, but the difference between the two groups was not significant (Table 4). However, urinary protein excretion of ≧3 g/day continued longer in group I than in group II (15.5 ± 4.6 vs 4.5 ± 2.1 days after delivery; $p < 0.05$; Table 4).

The percentage of glomeruli with FSGS out of the total number of observed glomeruli was correlated with the following three factors: urinary protein

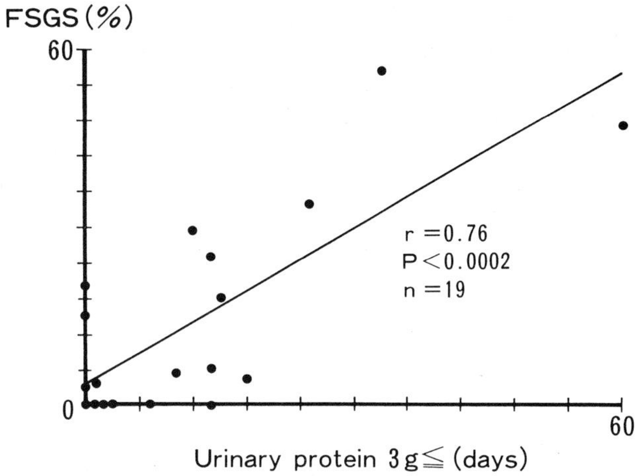

Fig. 3 Correlation between FSGS and proteinuria.

excretion of ≧3 g/day continuing after delivery, proteinuria at delivery and proteinuria at biopsy ($r = 0.76$, $p < 0.0002$, Figure 3; $r = 0.66$, $p < 0.003$; $r = 0.51$, $p < 0.03$, respectively). The disappearance of proteinuria was slower in group I than in group II, but the difference was not significant (5.7 ± 1.5, 2.3 ± 1.0 months, respectively; Table 4).

The levels of serum creatinine (1.0 ± 0.1 in group I; 1.0 ± 0.1 in group II), uric acid (7.3 ± 0.3; 7.7 ± 0.8) total cholesterol (304.6 ± 22.2; 284.6 ± 23.8) and triglyceride (391.4 ± 38.9; 426.5 ± 119.3) at delivery were not significantly different. Moreover, these levels showed no significant differences between the two groups at biopsy.

In electron microscopy, elevation of the thin endothelial layer from lamina densa of GBM with/without flocculant subendothelial deposits was observed in all cases. The lamina densa of GBM sometimes showed irregular thickening or attenuation. Circumferential interposition of mesangial cells was frequently present. Cytoplasmic swelling of the endothelial cells was not so marked as to be pathognomonic for so-called endotheliosis of pre-eclamptic nephropathy. Vacuoles and/or granular droplets were seen in the visceral epithelial cells. Detachment of the visceral cells from the GBM was seen in several cases. However, statistical analysis seemed inappropriate due to a great variety of its occurrence in each case as well as to paucity of electron microscopic sections.

Discussion

It is still controversial whether "pure" pre-eclamptic kidneys are associated with FSGS lesions. Some investigators claim that the FSGS lesions observed in pre-eclampsia are not a feature of "pure" pre-eclampsia but an indicator of underlying nephrosclerosis [Gaber et al. 1989]. Therefore, we carefully excluded patients with histological and clinical evidence of underlying renal disease and hypertensive disorders. We also found severer arteriolosclerosis in group I than in group II. However, all our patients were primigravida who were almost never complicated postpartum hypertension, in contrast to the Gaber's series. At least, we consider that our patients did not have underlying diseases.

The two cases which showed frequent hyaline arteriolosclerosis were 37-year-old and 32-year-old primigravidae. The glomeruli with FSGS-like lesions were observed at a rate of 6.3% (1 of 16 glomeruli) and 18% (9 of 50 glomeruli), respectively. The former case showed heavy proteinuria with a relatively mild hypertension. The latter case showed a sudden onset of malignant phase of hypertension (270/150 mmHg). The average score of the arteriolosclerosis was higher in group I statistically, however, this arteriosclerotic severity was not correlated with the incidence of glomeruli with FSGS-like lesions.

The FSGS-like lesions observed in pure pre-eclampsia are histologically the same as the so-called "early lesions" of primary FSGS [Schwartz et al. 1985, Rennke et al. 1989, Verani et al. 1986]. We did not observe the sclerosed glomeruli often seen in the advanced stage. The histological findings of FSGS-like lesions resemble the "cellular lesions" described by Schwartz in 1985, and the lesions at the urinary pole paralleled the "glomerular tip lesions" reported by Howie [Howie et al. 1984]. The initial appearance of primary FSGS lesions has been reported at the vascular pole [Churg et al. 1982, Brown et al. 1978] and glomerular periphery [Kincaid-Smith et al. 1987]; however, we found lesions at the urinary and vascular poles and between the two poles. We also observed two FSGS-like lesions in a single glomerulus. Our findings indicated that FSGS-like lesions can appear anywhere in the glomerulus. We suspect that FSGS-like lesions occur within a short time during pregnancy because no patients were found to have proteinuria and hypertension before pregnancy and during the first trimester.

In primary FSGS the cellular lesions progress to scarring and renal failure develops [Schwartz et al. 1985]. However, FSGS-like lesions in pre-eclampsia may be reversible or at least self-limiting. Proteinuria in patients with FSGS-like lesions was severer and of longer duration than in patients without FSGS, but disappeared in all cases without any treatment, in contrast to primary FSGS. In a 32-year-old primipara who underwent renal biopsy twice, on the 7th day and 10th month after delivery, glomeruli with FSGS-like lesions were observed at a rate of 29.8% (5 of 17 glomeruli) in the first biopsy but had decreased to 11.8% (7 of 63) in the second biopsy, in which increased adhesions of glomeruli were also noted. The adhesions were only narrow strings bridging to Bowman's capsule, without foam cells or vacuolated epithelial cells. There were no segmental or global scars in the second biopsy. In group I, three cases with FSGS-like lesions in 56.8%, 11.8% and 3.1% of total glomeruli, respectively, became pregnant again. They showed no proteinuria, edema or hypertension during the second pregnancy or after delivery.

A remarkable histological difference between groups I and II was that droplet formation in glomerular epithelial cells was observed at a high frequency in group I but was rarely seen in group II. Vacuolated epithelial cells were also observed more frequently in group I. The genesis of FSGS lesions has been explained by damage to epithelial cells in experimental animal models of adriamycin-induced FSGS [Graeme et al. 1975]. The same explanation has been postulated for human renal biopsy specimens for primary FSGS because vacuolation is frequently observed in the glomerular epithelium [Yoschikawa et al. 1986, Chiang et al. 1988]. It was suggested that increased leakage of protein from the GBM causes vacuolar degeneration in glomerular epithelial cells, which are a pathway to the urinary space. Damage to the epithelial cells is thought to cause disordered metabolism of the GBM, leading to its destruction [Yoschikawa et al. 1986]. Our results also revealed that cases with FSGS showed more serious proteinuria and epithelial changes. Kincaid-Smith reported that granulated visceral epithelial cells are specific for pre-eclamptic nephropathy [Kincaid-Smith et al. 1986]. Gaber also described granulated epithelial cells. However, they considered the granules to be nonspecific, overloaded protein reabsorption droplets [Gaber et al. 1987]. We also suggest that the droplets are caused by protein overload. It is not clear whether the droplets affect epithelial cell function. Kincaid-Smith described that the epithelial droplets were frequently observed just after delivery, but were rarely seen in biopsies done at a time remote from the episode of proteinuria [Kincaid-Smith et al. 1986]. However, we found no relation between time after delivery and the incidence of epithelial droplets.

The number of days during which urinary protein excretion of $\geqq 3$ g/day continued after delivery was significantly longer in group I than in group II, and positively correlated with the incidence of FSGS-like lesions. The incidence of FSGS and amount of proteinuria at delivery and biopsy were also positively correlated. It has been suggested that epithelial cell detachment in primary FSGS is the site of major protein leakage to Bowman's space [Silva et al. 1989]. Therefore, increased proteinuria and epithelial droplets may occur subsequent to FSGS. However, the diffuse severe double contours of the GBM frequently observed in group I indicate severer damage of the GBM in group I. We suggest that the changes in the GBM also can cause increased urinary protein excretion.

Another cause of epithelial cell damage has been suggested recently, namely, detachment from the GBM caused by mechanical extension due to glomerular hypertrophy [Fries et al. 1989]. Sheehan reported from his morphological studies that glomerular size was larger in severe pre-eclampsia [Sheehan 1980]. This may be another factor in epithelial cell damage, but glomerular size was not compared in the two groups in our study.

Some investigators have indicated that the genesis of FSGS lesions in pre-eclampsia might be glomerular hyperfiltration [Nochy et al. 1986, Nadal et al. 1986], because FSGS lesions have been reported in hyperfiltration/hypertension states such as uninephrectomized kidney or the early stage of diabetes [Brenner et al. 1982]. In pre-eclamptic kidneys, the functioning renal mass may be reduced because capillary lumens are obliterated by subendothelial deposits, edema, intracapillary cell swelling and foam cells. However, systemic hypertension does not translate into glomerular pressure without dilatation of the afferent arterioles [Rennke et al. 1988], and the origin of hypertension in pre-eclampsia is known to be generalized vasoconstriction due to prostaglandin I_2 deficiency [Gretorini et al. 1986]. In addition, we cannot be certain whether or not relative hyperperfusion occurs with reduced renal plasma flow due to the remarkable plasma volume depletion [Lindheimer et al. 1986, Heilman et al. 1989] that usually accompanies severe pre-eclampsia. We therefore suggest that the genesis of FSGS-like lesions in pre-eclampsia is difficult to explain by hyperfiltration theory alone.

Summary

FSGS-like lesions can occur in patients with "pure" pre-eclampsia during pregnancy, and the lesions may disappear after delivery. Patients with FSGS-like lesions in glomeruli showed severer proteinuria than those without such lesions. Epithelial cell droplets and a severe "double contour" appearance of the GBM were more frequently observed in patients with FSGS. We suggest that proteinuria and epithelial change may be closely related to the FSGS-like lesions.

REFERENCES

Brenner BM, Meyer TW, Hostetter TH 1982 Dietary protein intake and the progressive nature of kidney disease: The role of hemodynamically mediated glomerular injury in the pathogenesis of progressive glomerular sclerosis in aging, renal ablation, and intrinsic renal disease. N Engl J Med *307:* 652–659

Brown CB, Cameron JS, Turner DR, Chartler C, Ogg CS, Williams DG, Wewick M 1978 Focal segmental glomerulosclerosis with rapid decline in renal function ("malignant FSGS"). Clin Nephrol *10:* 51–61

Chiang ML, Hawkins EP, Berry PL, Barrish J, Hill LL 1988 Diagnostic and prognostic significance of glomerular epithelial cell vacuolization and podocyte effacement in children with minimal lesion nephrotic syndrome and focal segmental glomerulosclerosis: An ultrastructural study. Clin Nephrol *30:* 8–14

Churg J, Sobin LH 1982 Renal disease. Igaku-Shoin, Tokyo, New York, pp 37–39

Fries JWU, Sandstrom DJ, Meyer TW, Rennke HG 1989 Glomerular hypertrophy and epithelial cell injury modulate progressive glomerulosclerosis in the rat. Lab Inv *60:* 205–218

Gaber LW, Spargo BH, Lindheimer MD 1987 Renal pathology in pre-eclampsia. Baillieres Clin Obstet Gynaecol *1:* 971–995

Gaber LW, Spargo BH, Lindheimer MD 1989 The nephropathy of pre-eclampsia. In: *Tischer CC, Brenner BM* (eds) Renal Pathology. Lippincott Company, Philadelphia, Vol I, pp 357–379

Graeme B, Karnovsky RJ, Karnovsky MJ 1975 An ultrastructural study of the mechanisms of proteinuria in aminonucleoside nephrosis. Kidney Int *8:* 219–232

Gretorini G, Prico N, Remuzzi G 1986 Pathogenesis of pre-eclampsia. In: *Andreucci VE* (ed) The kidney in pregnancy. Martius Nijhoff Publishing, Boston, pp 13–27

Heilmann L, Siekmann U 1989 Hemodynamic and hemorheological profiles in women with proteinuric hypertension of pregnancy and in pregnant controls. Arch Gynecol Obstet *246:* 159–168

Howie AJ, Brewer DB 1984 The glomerular tip lesion: A previously undescribed type of segmental glomerular abnormality. J Pathol *142:* 205–220

Kida H, Takeda H, Yokoyama H, Tomosugi N, Abe T, Hattori N 1985 Focal glomerular sclerosis in pre-eclampsia. Clin Nephrol *24:* 221–227

Kincaid-Smith PS, North RA, Becker GJ, Fairley KF 1986 Proteinuria during pregnancy. In: *Andreucci VE* (ed) The kidney in pregnancy. Martius Nijhoff Publishing, Boston, pp 133–164

Kincaid-Smith PS, Whitworth JA 1987 The kidney 2nd ed. Blackwell Scientific Publications, pp 69–84

Lindheimer MD, Katz AI 1986 The kidney in pregnancy. In: *Brenner BM, Rector FC* (eds) The kidney. 3rd ed. W. B. Saunders Company, Philadelphia, pp 1253–1296

Nadal MA, Monserrat AJ, Iotti RM, Delfino CJAA, Gotlieb D 1986 Nephrotic syndrome due to preeclampsia incidence of focal and segmental glomerular sclerosis. Medicina *46:* 157–162

Nagai Y, Washizawa Y, Hirata K, Shiina K, Tanaka M, Maeda M, Ger YC, Kawamura S 1989 A renal biopsy study in pre-eclampsia: Clinical-pathological correlation in 20 cases. Jpn J Nephrol *31:* 1179–1186

Nochy D, Hinglais N, Jacquot C, Gaudry C, Remy P, Bariety J 1986 De novo focal glomerular sclerosis in preeclampsia. Clin Nephrol *25:* 116–121

Pollak VE, Nettles JB 1960 The kidney in toxemia of pregnancy: a clinical and pathologic study based on renal biopsies. Medicine (Baltimore) *39:* 469–526

Rennke HG 1988 Glomerular adaptations to renal injury: The role of capillary hypertension in the pathogenesis of focal and segmental glomerulosclerosis. Adv Nephrol *17:* 15–26

Rennke HG, Klain PS 1989 Pathogenesis and significance of nonprimary focal and segmental glomerulosclerosis. Am J Kidney Dis *13:* 443–456

Schwartz MM, Lewis EJ 1985 Focal segmental glomerular sclerosis: The cellular lesion. Kidney Int *28:* 968–974

Sheehan HL 1980 Renal morphology in preeclampsia. Kidney Int *18:* 242–252

Silva FG, Hogg RJ 1989 Minimal change nephrotic syndrome-focalsclerosis complex. In: *Tisher CC, Brenner BM* (eds) Renal Pathology. Lippincott Company, Philadelphia, Vol I, pp 265–339

Taylor JR, Spargo BH 1986 Pathology of the kidney in pre-eclampsia. In: *Andreucci VE* (ed). The kidney in pregnancy. Martius Nijhoff Publishing, Boston, pp 47–63

Verani RR, Hawkins EP 1986 Recurrent focal segmental glomerulosclerosis. Am J Nephrol *6:* 263–270

Yoschikawa N, Ito H, Akamatsu R, Hazikano H, Okada S, Matsuo T 1986 Glomerular podocyte vacuolation in focal segmental glomerulosclerosis. Arch Pathol Lab Med *110:* 394–398

Clinical significance of serum and urinary neopterins in patients with chronic renal disease

K. Godai, J. Uemasu and H. Kawasaki

Second Department of Internal Medicine, Tottori University School of Medicine, Yonago, Japan

Abstract. To determine the clinical significance of serum and urinary neopterins in patients with chronic renal disease, we measured these values using IMMUtest Neopterin RIA kits. Serum neopterin levels in patients with chronic glomerulonephritis (CGN) (10.2 ± 8.1 nmol/l) and in those with chronic renal failure (CRF) (109 ± 90) were significantly increased compared with the control subjects (C) (4.2 ± 2.4) ($p < 0.001$). The levels of serum neopterins in patients on chronic hemodialysis (HD) (212 ± 106) were increased almost twofold compared with CRF ($p < 0.001$). In CGN and CRF, a strong positive correlation was demonstrated between serum neopterin levels and serum creatinine concentrations ($r = 0.95$, $p < 0.001$). In HD patients, neopterin levels in serum were not correlated with the length of time on dialysis. The urinary neopterin excretion ratios (urinary neopterin/urinary creatinine level) in CRF (227 ± 114 μmol/molCr) were significantly increased compared with C (116 ± 43) ($p < 0.01$). A significantly negative correlation was observed between the urinary neopterin levels and the creatinine clearance in CGN and CRF ($p < 0.01$). These data suggest that, in patients with chronic renal disease, the neopterin levels in serum are closely linked with glomerular filtration rate and yet the urinary neopterin/creatinine ratios may reflect the predominance of increased tubular secretion of neopterin over the renal injury per se.

Key words: serum neopterin – urinary neopterin/creatinine ratio – creatinine clearance – chronic renal disease

Introduction

Monocytes and macrophages are frequently observed in the subendothelial and/or mesangial areas of the glomeruli affected by inflammation [Wilson et al. 1988]. These macrophages are thought to exert a phagocytic action at these sites, and thus remove the immune complexes accumulated in such areas [Striker et al. 1979]. Concomitantly, these macrophages are likely to secrete various proteolytic enzymes and biochemical reactants [Nathan et al. 1980]. These sequential events may stimulate proliferation of mesangial cells [Lovett et al. 1983] or inhibit it [Ooi et al. 1983]. In any way, it is of no doubt that these macrophages play important roles in the development of chronic glomerular disease.

Neopterin, a pyramidine-pyrimidine compound with 253 dalton in molecular weight derived from guanosine triphosphate, is produced by human macrophages on stimulation by gamma interferon [Huber et al. 1984, Bitterlich et al. 1988]. Because this lymphokine is released by activated T-lymphocytes, neopterin represents a sensitive marker of T-lymphocytes/macrophage interplay [Fuchs et al. 1988].

More recently, the efficacy of determination of the neopterin levels in the blood and urine has been proven for the evaluation of renal disease activity and prognosis. In patients with hepatitis B nephropathy, the urinary neopterin excretions were markedly increased only in the presence of nephrotic syndrome or heavy proteinuria and fell as proteinuria decreased [Lin 1989]. Also both plasma and urinary neopterin levels have been increased in aggressive glomerulonephritis [Neale et al. 1990]. However, the association between the changes in serum and urinary neopterin levels and chronic renal disease remains to be unsettled. And yet, because serum levels of neopterin represent a net effect among production, metabolism and of particular, renal excretion [Dhondt 1986], correlation between serum neopterin levels and renal function needs to be elucidated.

Thus, we undertook this study to clarify these issues, determining the serum and urinary neopterins

Received December 10, 1990; in revised form March 12, 1991.

Reprint requests to: Dr. J. Uemasu, The Second Department of Internal Medicine, Tottori University School of Medicine, Yonago 683, Japan.

Table 1 Subjects' data

	Controls	CGN	CRF	HD
No.	120	68	21	41
Sex (M/F)	82/38	44/24	8/13	26/15
Age (y)	43.2 ± 9.5	46.2 ± 16.9	59.1 ± 13.7	54.0 ± 13.8
S-Cr (μmol/l)	89.2 ± 1.5	115 ± 5.3*	557 ± 400**	1120 ± 220**
BUN (mg/dl)	15.6 ± 3.7	17.9 ± 7.8*	65.3 ± 33**	82.0 ± 17**
S-β_2MG (mg/l)	1.34 ± 0.33	2.40 ± 1.3*	11.8 ± 5.5**	36.0 ± 8.4**

Abbreviations: CGN, chronic glomerulonephritis; CRF, chronic renal failure without dialysis; HD, chronic hemodialysis; S-Cr, serum creatinine; BUN, blood urea nitrogen; S-β_2MG, serum β_2 microglobulin. * Control vs p <0.01, ** Control vs p <0.001.

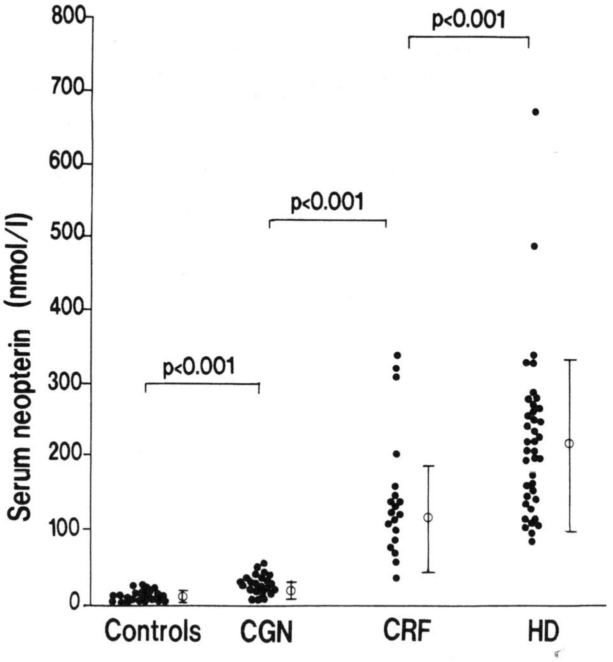

Fig. 1 Serum neopterin levels in healthy controls and patients with chronic renal disease. Abbreviations are: CGN, chronic glomerulonephritis; CRF, chronic renal failure without dialysis; HD, chronic hemodialysis.

by radioimmunoassay and further the serum neopterin levels were measured in patients on chronic hemodialysis.

Subjects and methods

Subjects

Informed consent was obtained from all subjects before this study. This study was performed in 68 patients with chronic glomerulonephritis (CGN), 21 patients with chronic renal failure (CRF), 41 patients on chronic hemodialysis (HD), and 120 healthy controls (Table 1). In CGN, 37 patients underwent renal biopsy and histologically they were divided into 4 groups; minimal change glomerulopathy (n = 9), mesangial proliferative glomerulonephritis (n = 16), membrano-proliferative glomerulonephritis (n = 4), and IgA-nephropathy (n = 8). In both CRF and HD patients, the causes of chronic renal failure were all primary glomerular disease. In HD patients, the terms of hemodialysis treatment were 91 ± 57 months (mean ± SD). Infectious diseases were all excluded from the subjects studied by clinical and laboratory findings. Immunosuppressive drugs when administered were withdrawn for about 2 weeks prior to the serum and urine sampling.

Methods

Both serum and urine samples were obtained at the early morning in the fasting state. These specimens were promptly stored at −20° C in darkness. In HD patients, blood samples were taken before hemodialysis. Within 2 weeks after storage, neopterin levels in both serum and urine were measured by an IMMUtest Neopterin RIA kit (Henning, Berlin, FRG). Briefly, after thawing the samples, 20 μl of the serum in each test tube, was incubated with 100 μl of ^{125}I-labeled neopterin and 100 μl of pre-precipitated antiserum for one hour at room temperature. After incubation, 1 ml of washing solution was added to each test tube and then it was centrifuged at 2000 × g for 10 min. The supernatant was discarded and the radioactivity of the pellet was counted by a gamma counter. Each sample was measured in duplicates. The interassay and intraassay coefficients of variation were 4.7–5.0% and 2.5–6.6%, respectively. The diluted urines (× 100) were saved for the same RIA assay.

Serum creatinine levels were measured with an autoanalyzer (SMAC, Technicon, New York, USA). Urinary creatinine levels were measured with an autoanalyzer (SMA 12–60, Technicon, New York, USA). Serum β_2-microglobulin levels were determined by β_2MG-EIA Test (Wako Pure Chemical Industries Ltd, Osaka, Japan). Blood urea nitrogen levels were measured with an autoanalyzer (SMAC). Urinary protein contents were measured by pyrogallol-red method. Endogenous creatinine clearance was used as glomerular filtration rate, corrected for body surface (1.73 m^2).

All values were expressed as mean ± SD. Data were analyzed by Student's t-test or Cochran-cox test as appropriate. Linear regression analysis was per-

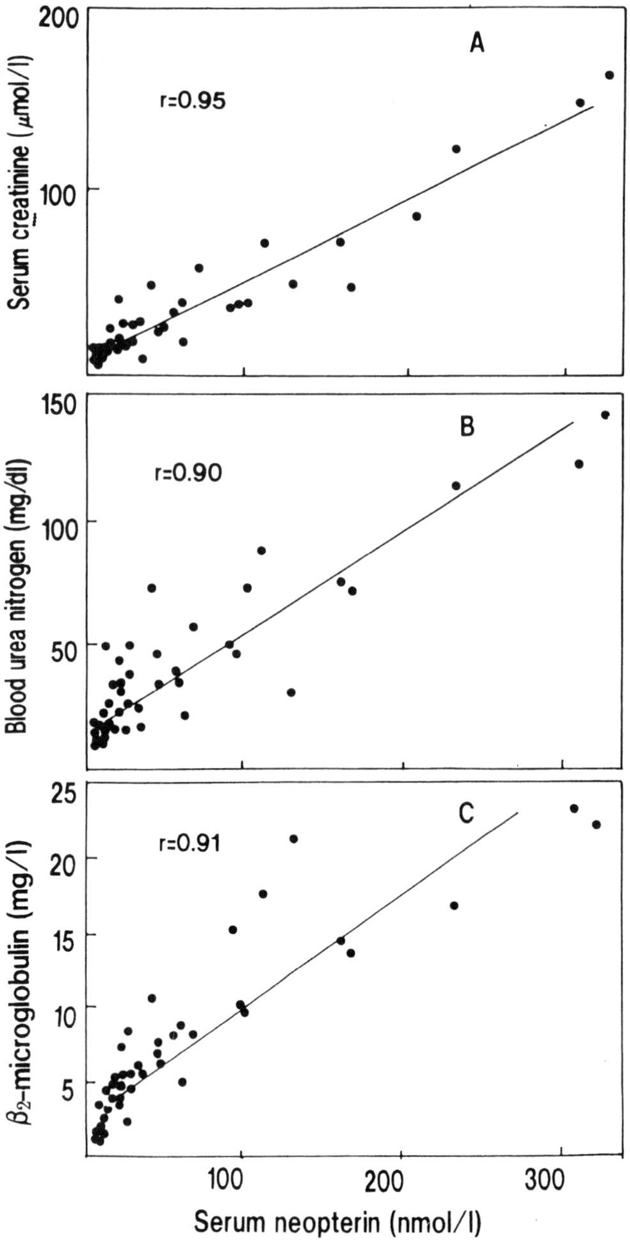

Fig. 2 Correlation between serum neopterin and serum creatinine (A) (y = 4.27 × +74; p <0.001), blood urea nitrogen (B) (y = 0.40 × +16; p <0.001) and β_2-microglobulin (C) (y = 0.07 × +2.1; p <0.001) in patients with chronic renal disease (n = 89).

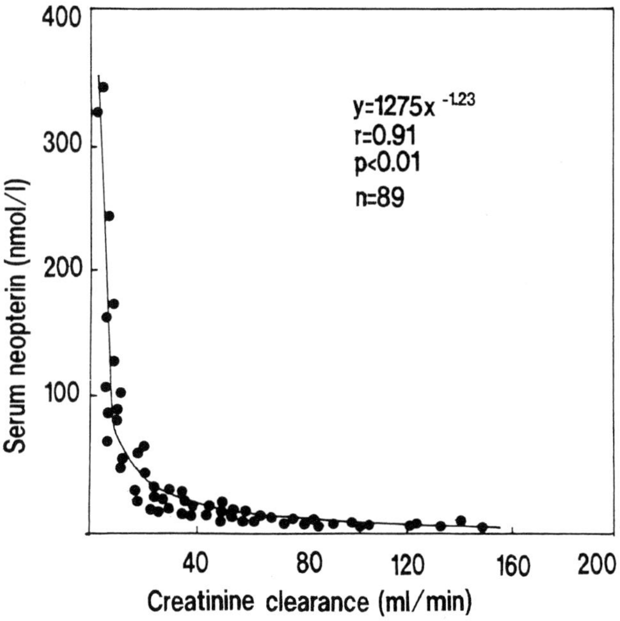

Fig. 3 Correlation between serum neopterin and creatinine clearance (Ccr) in patients with chronic renal disease. A simple, logarithmic, and exponential correlation was calculated. By histograms of serum neopterin and Ccr, normal distribution curve of each parameter was confirmed.

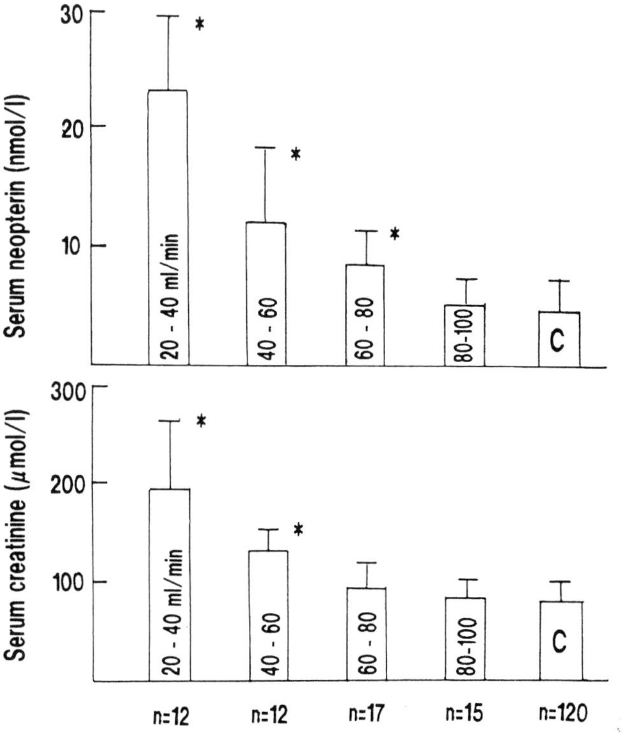

Fig. 4 Correlation between the creatinine clearance (Ccr) and the serum levels of neopterin (upper panel), creatinine (lower panel) in patients with CGN (Ccr 20–100 ml/min, n = 56) and healthy controls (C). Each open column denotes the Ccr in ml/min.
* p <0.01 vs the healthy controls

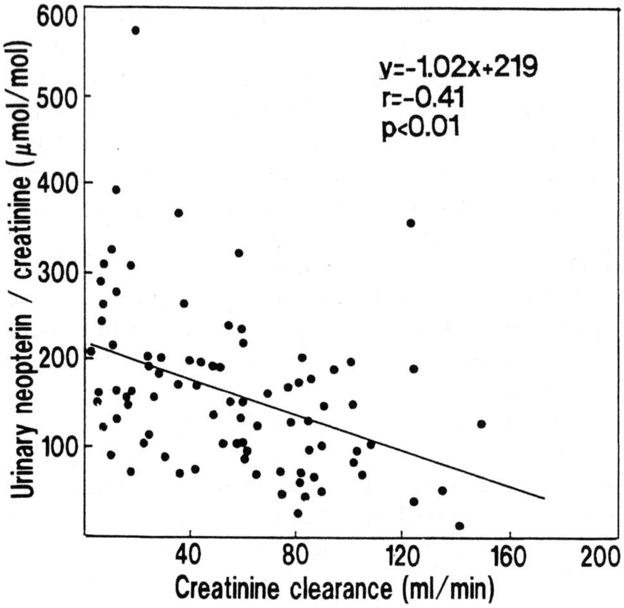

Fig. 5 Correlation between urinary neopterin/creatinine ratio and creatinine clearance in patients with chronic renal disease.

formed for the study of correlation. Significance was defined as a p value of less than 0.05.

Results

Serum neopterin

Serum neopterin concentrations in healthy controls and patients with renal disease are shown in Figure 1. The serum neopterin levels in CGN patients (10.2 ± 8.1 nmol/l, n = 68) and CRF patients (109 ± 90, n = 21) were significantly higher than controls (4.2 ± 2.4, n = 120) ($p < 0.001$). Moreover, the neopterin concentrations in HD patients (212 ± 106, n = 41) were significantly increased when compared with the CRF patients ($p < 0.001$).

In CGN and CRF, the serum neopterin levels were strongly correlated with serum creatinine concentrations (r = 0.95, $p < 0.001$, n = 89), and with blood urea nitrogen levels (r = 0.90, $p < 0.001$), and further, with serum β_2-microglobulin levels (r = 0.91, $p < 0.001$) (Figure 2).

A significantly negative exponential correlation was seen between the serum neopterin levels and the creatinine clearances in patients with chronic renal disease except for HD patients (Figure 3).

In order to delineate the respective correspondence of serum neopterins and serum creatinines to changes of Ccr in GCN, these values were arranged by a change rate of 20 ml/min in Ccr, and compared with the controls levels (Figure 4). As shown in this figure, serum creatinine levels became significantly higher compared with the controls at the level of creatinine clearance of 40–60 ml/min ($p < 0.01$), whereas the elevation of serum neopterin concentrations was more correlated with the slight decrease of creatinine clearance, that is, the level of 60–80 ml/min ($p < 0.01$).

In HD patients, the pre-dialysis levels of serum neopterin were not significantly correlated with the term of hemodialysis treatment (r = 0.04, $p > 0.05$). There were no correlations between the serum neopterin values and several parameters such as the levels of hemoglobin, hematocrit, and serum electrolytes. Furthermore, neopterin levels in serum had no significant relation to histological classification by renal biopsy in 37 CGN patients.

Urinary neopterin

Urinary neopterin/creatinine ratios in patients with CGN (141 ± 73 µmol neopterin/mol creatinine) were increased compared with the controls (116 ± 43, n = 70), but did not achieve statistical significance. In contrast, the ratios in patients with CRF (227 ± 114) were significantly higher than the controls ($p < 0.01$).

A statistically significant negative correlation was noted between the urinary neopterin/creatinine ratios and the creatinine clearance in patients with chronic renal disease (r = −0.41, $p < 0.01$) (Figure 5).

A slight, but not significant, increase of urinary neopterin/creatinine ratios was seen in both mesangial proliferative glomerulonephritis and membrano-proliferative glomerulonephritis groups compared with minimal change glomerulopathy and IgA-nephropathy groups. The neopterin/creatinine ratios did not statistically correlate with proteinuria (r = 0.15, $p > 0.05$, n = 89).

Discussion

Since the first clinical report on neopterins in viral infection and malignant disease [Wachter et al. 1979], a number of studies have been performed to clarify the relation between neopterin and several diseases, including viral infection, malignant tumors and autoimmune diseases. Recently neopterin has been highlighted as a potential marker to manifest the immune state of acquired immunodeficiency syndrome [Fahey et al. 1990, Fuchs et al. 1988]. In the field of renal medicine, neopterin has been reported to be a useful marker in detecting graft rejection and cytomegalovirus infection in kidney transplant recipients [Backman et al. 1987, Smillie et al. 1989]. In contrast, the information about interrelation between neopterin and glomerulonephritis has been very limited. Recently, urinary neopterin has been shown to be a biochemical marker for the differential diagnosis of membranous nephropathy associated with hepatitis B surface antigenemia and yet to serve as a prognostic indicator [Lin et al. 1989]. Also in aggressive glomerulonephritis, plasma neopterin concentration and urinary neopterin/creatinine ratios were found to be both increased [Neale et al. 1990].

Our results showed that neopterin levels in serum did not correlate with renal histology, and proteinuria in patients with biopsy-proven chronic glomerulonephritis. Rather, they showed strongly positive correlations with parameters that reflect renal function such as serum creatinine, blood urea nitrogen, and β_2-microglobulin. Furthermore, in our study, a statistically significant negative exponential correlation was observed between the serum neopterin levels and creatinine clearances. Thus, our data show that the neopterin levels in serum are closely linked with changes in glomerular filtration rate in patients with chronic glomerular disease. Of note, compared with the serum creatinine concentrations, serum neopterin levels were significantly increased at the creatinine clearance of 60–80 ml/min. Though there was no significant correlation between serum neopterin levels and renal histology, this finding may result from a low-grade activation of cell-mediated immunity, rather than decreased renal function. In fact, in renal transplant patients undergoing acute rejection, serum neopterin levels had been reported to be higher than serum creatinine values, probably due to increased neopterin production by stimulated macrophages [Schafer et al. 1986]. Such an assumption may be more attested by comparing the current data with those obtained from the non-immunologically mediated renal diseases such as hypertensive nephropathy.

As for urinary neopterin, we found highly elevated neopterin/creatinine ratios in patients with chronic renal disease, particularly, chronic renal failure compared with the controls. The urinary neopterin excretion has been found to be increased in more severely inflammatory glomerular disease [Neale et al. 1990]. Currently, we could not find any significant difference in urinary neopterin/creatinine ratios among the histologically different four groups, that is, minimal change glomerulopathy, mesangial proliferative glomerulonephritis, membrano-proliferative glomerulonephritis, and IgA-nephropathy. This result may be partly due to the paucity of infiltrated macrophages in chronic glomerular disease [Magil et al. 1981]. Although marked increases of urinary neopterin excretions had been observed in nephrotic patients with hepatitis B nephropathy, we could not detect any significant correlation between urinary neopterin excretions and urinary protein contents in this study. Probably, the variances of etiology and proteinuria in study population may be responsible for these differences. It was interesting to note that a significant inverse correlation between urinary neopterin/creatinine ratios and creatinine clearances was seen in patients with chronic renal disease. It shows that urinary excretion of neopterins was higher than that of creatinines. Because proteinuria in these patients did not show any significant correlation with urinary neopterin excretions, it may reflect increased tubular secretion of neopterin compared to creatinine in renal failure, rather than renal injury per se.

Serum neopterin levels in patients with long-term hemodialysis had been documented to be high and in particular, elevated significantly in patients whose periods of dialysis were more than one year [Fuchs et al. 1988]. Our data showed a remarkable increase of serum neopterin levels in hemodialysis patients when compared to controls, CGN and CRF. However, we could not find any significant effect of the period of time on hemodialysis on serum neopterin concentrations. Discrepancy between their data and our results may come from the differences of patients' profiles, of dialyzers and dialysates used. Hemodialysis treatment had been shown to decrease serum neopterin levels, but to increase neopterin/creatinine ratios [Fuchs et al. 1988]. These findings suggested not only the removal of neopterin by the dialyzer, but also the possible role of dialysis-membranes-activation of cell-mediated immunity in elevating the serum neopterin levels. In any case, the hemodialysis therapy seems to be not so an effective method to eliminate fully the increased neopterins in hemodialysis patients. Consequently, neopterins may be accumulated in proportion to the length of hemodialysis treatment. Though neopterin is known to have antimicrobial qualities [Rabinoff 1990], whether the accumulated neopterins behave as a uremic toxin or not needs to be studied.

In summary, the neopterin levels in serum reflected glomerular filtration rate rather than renal pathologic changes in patients with chronic renal disease. In contrast, the increased urinary neopterin/creatinine ratios suggested the predominance of increased tubular secretion of neopterin over the renal injury per se.

Acknowledgements

We thank Drs. Sadako Yamada, Akihisa Nakaoka, Akihide Tokumoto and Gihichiro Konomi for their helpful assistance and we express our gratitude to Dr. Sinsuke Morio for statistical assistance with data processing. IMMUtest Neopterin RIA kits were kindly provided by Hoechest Japan Corporation.

REFERENCES

Backman L, Ringden O, Bjorkhem I 1987 Monitoring of serum neopterin levels in renal transplant recipients: Increased values during impaired renal function and cytomegalovirus infection. Nephron *46:* 319

Bitterlich G et al. 1988 Selective induction of mononuclear phagocytes to produce neopterin by interferons. Immunobiol *176:* 228

Dhondt JL et al. 1986 The role of the kidney in biopterin metabolism. In: *Cooper BA, Whitehead VM* (eds). Chemistry and biology of pethidines. Berlin: Walter de Gruyter, p 315

Fahey JL et al. 1990 The prognostic value of cellular and serologic markers in infection with human immunodeficiency virus type 1. N Engl J Med *322:* 166

Fuchs D et al. 1988 Neopterin as a marker for activated cell-mediated immunity: application in HIV infection. Immunology Today *9:* 150

Fuchs D et al. 1988 Neopterin levels in long-term hemodialysis. Clin Nephrol *30:* 220

Huber C et al. 1984 Immuno responses-associated production of neopterin. J Exp Med *160:* 310

Lin Y 1989 Urinary neopterin as new biochemical markers for monitoring of disease activity and prognosis in membranous nephropathy associated with hepatitis B surface antigenemia. Nephron *53:* 115

Lovett DH, Ryan JL, Sterzel RB 1983 Stimulation of rat mesangial cell proliferation by macrophage interleukin 1. Immunol *131:* 2830

Magil AB, Wadsworth LD, Loewen M 1981 Monocytes and human renal glomerular disease. A quantitative evaluation. Lab Invest *44:* 27

Nathan CF, Murray HW, Cohn ZA 1980 Current concepts: The macrophage as an effector cell. N Engl J Med *323:* 622

Neale J, Hill J, Cooke R, Dunbar R 1990 Neopterin quantitation indicates participation of cell mediated immunity (CMI) in human glomerulonephritis (GN) (Abstract). Kidney Int *37:* 443

Ooi YM, Weiss MA, Hsu A, Ooi BS 1983 Mechanisms of suppression of mouse mesangial cell proliferation by macrophage supernatants. J Immunol *130:* 1790

Rabinoff M 1990 Interferon-gamma, neopterin and host defence. Medical Hypotheses *31:* 275

Schafer A, Daniel V, Dreikorn K, Opelz G 1986 Assessment of plasma neopterin in clinical kidney transplantation. Transplant *41:* 454

Smillie AE, Rigby RJ, Petrie JJB 1989 Monitoring the response to anti-rejection therapy with serum neopterin. Transplant Proc *21:* 1869

Striker GE, Mannik M, Tung MY 1979 Role of marrow-derived monocytes and mesangial cells in removal of immune complexes from renal glomeruli. J Exp Med *149:* 127

Wachter H, Hausen A, Grassmayr K 1979 Increased urinary excretion of neopterin in patients with malignant tumor and with virus disease. Hoppe Seyler's Z Physiol Chem *360:* 1957

Wilson CB, Dixon FJ 1988 The renal response to immunological injury: In: *Brenner BM, Recter FG* (eds). The kidney (3rd ed) W. B. Saunders, Philadelphia, p 800

Clinical Nephrology, Vol. 36 No. 3–1991 (147–151)

Myocardial revascularization in patients on renal replacement therapy

M. De Meyer[1], W. Wyns[2], R. Dion[3], G. Khoury[3], Y. Pirson[1] and C. van Ypersele de Strihou[1]

University of Louvain Medical School, Cliniques Universitaires St-Luc, Divisions of Nephrology[1], Cardiology[2] and Cardiothoracic Surgery[3], Brussels, Belgium

Abstract. Coronary disease is the main cause of mortality and morbidity among long-term survivors on renal replacement therapy (RRT). Despite the additional risk factors, myocardial revascularization has been recently attempted with various success in some patients on RRT. We report on 26 patients (13 dialyzed and 13 transplanted, mean age: 50 years [range 38–66]) who have undergone either surgical aorto-coronary bypass (CABG) (n = 16) with mammary artery grafts, or percutaneous coronary angioplasty (PTCA) (n = 9), or both procedures (n = 2). Indication was angina pectoris in all but three patients with painless ischemia. Eight patients had unstable angina (NYHA class IV). A previous myocardial infarction was documented in 11 cases. Coronary angiography disclosed mainly multiple vessel disease (81%). Post CABG complications consisted of severe intrathoracic bleeding (n = 3) resulting in death in 2 cases. PTCA entailed no major complication. After the critical postoperative period, the long-term survival was the same as that of non-uremic patients and the clinical improvement, according to the NYHA classification, was highly satisfactory at 6 months and persists up to 2 years. We conclude that coronary angiography and myocardial revascularization should be considered in patients on long-term RRT developing coronary disease.

Key words: coronary disease – coronary artery bypass – percutaneous transluminal coronary angioplasty – dialysis – transplantation

Introduction

Coronary artery disease remains the leading cause of morbidity and mortality among long-term survivors on renal replacement therapy (RRT) [Hellerstedt et al. 1984; Brunner et al. 1978; Tufveson et al. 1987]. In non-uremic patients myocardial revascularization techniques have significantly improved the outcome of patients with coronary artery disease. Coronary artery bypass grafts (CABG) improve the prognosis of patients with myocardial ischemia [European Coronary Surgery Study Group 1982], even more so when internal mammary arteries (IMA) grafts are used [Loop et al. 1986]: their long-term patency is indeed better than that of traditional saphenous vein grafts [Dion et al. 1989, Jones et al. 1987, Singh et al. 1983]. Percutaneous transluminal coronary angioplasty (PTCA) has also been successfully utilized in selected patients [Talley et al. 1988]. Both techniques can now be applied to uremic patients despite their additional risk factors.

Received May 22, 1991.

Reprint requests to Dr. M. De Meyer, Cliniques Universitaires St-Luc, Avenue Hippocrate 10, BL-1200 Bruxelles, Belgium

In the present study, we review the results of 29 myocardial revascularization procedures performed in 26 patients on renal replacement therapy. Both PTCA and/or CABG with IMA were utilized depending on their feasibility.

Material and methods

Between April 1986 and August 1988, 26 patients on RRT [13 on hemodialysis (HD) and 13 with a functioning kidney graft (TP)] were treated either by CABG (18 cases) or by PTCA (11 cases).

A coronary angiography was obtained in all patients. Simultaneously, contrast ventriculography (30° right anterior oblique projection) for analysis of regional wall motion and calculation of left ventricular volumes and ejection fraction was performed with non-ionic contrast media. An exercise thallium scintigraphy was also obtained whenever clinically possible (n = 14). The diagnosis of coronary disease was retained in the presence of a coronary stenosis exceeding 50% in diameter. Cardiac status of patients was defined according to the NYHA. Three patients with arrhythmia and painless ischemia were included in class I. Eight patients with unstable angina were included in class IV (see Figure 2). The last 14 patients were included in class II and III.

PTCA was chosen to treat single vessel disease, with accessible stenosis. CABG was preferred in patients with multiple vessel disease or when the morphology and topography of the narrowed vessels were unfavorable for PTCA. PTCA was performed according to Gruentzig [1987] as the first procedure in 8 patients (3 HD and 5 TP) (Table I). PTCA was repeated in one of them for a restenosis. It was needed as a second procedure in an additional 2 patients in whom angina pectoris recurred after CABG because of the progression of coronary disease in an ungrafted vessel (Table 1). CABG was performed as a first therapeutic procedure in 18 patients (10 HD and 8 TP) (Table 1).

We always aimed at complete anatomical revascularization using at least one IMA graft. In 7 patients, both IMA were used; in 10 patients, additional saphenous vein grafts were needed. The mean number of distal anastomoses per patient was 4.1 (1–7), 55% of which relied on IMA grafts.

Table 1 Indication for myocardial revascularization

	Total	CABG	PTCA
First revascularization procedure for			
unstable angina (NYHA class IV)	8	5	3
stable angina (NYHA class II & III)	15	12	3
painless ischemia (NYHA class I)	3	1	2
Second revascularization procedure for relapsing angina	3	–	3
Total number of revascularization procedures	29	18	11

Table 2 Patients' characteristics

	Total	Hemodialyzed	Transplanted
Number of patients	26	13	13
Male/female	22/4	10/3	12/1
Mean age (years)	50	53	48
(range)		(41–66)	(38–61)
Initial nephropathy			
glomerular disease	14	6	8
interstitial disease	3	1	2
vascular disease	6	4	2
polycystic kidneys	1	1	–
diabetes mellitus	2	1	1
Mean duration of hemodialysis (months)	40	44 (9–180)	39 (4–92)
Mean duration of transplantation (months)			96 (5–244)

The cardiopulmonary bypass (CPB) was carried out under moderate hypothermia (25° C) with blood prime in 6 patients (5 HD, 1 TP) and crystalloid prime in the others. Hematocrit was maintained between 22 and 26% by means of blood transfusions. The mean duration of CPB was 93 minutes (compared to 94 minutes for non-uremic patients in our center). During CPB, hemofiltration was used in 10 patients (9 HD, 1 TP) in order to avoid fluid overload. Myocardial protection was obtained by crystalloid cardioplegic solution (St-Thomas – 1 l) and enhanced by intrapericardial topical cooling (2 l of normal saline solution). Hemodialysis was usually performed on the second postoperative day.

Immediate complications were defined as those encountered within the first 30 days. All patients were reevaluated at 6, 12, and 24 months. Kaplan-Meier survival curve was calculated. The evolution of their functional status was associated on the basis of The New York Heart Association classification.

Results

Clinical characteristics of the population (Table 2)

There was no significant difference between HD and TP patients for age, sex ratio and the type of initial nephropathy. There were only two diabetic patients, one in each group. The mean duration of hemodialysis was not significantly different between the two groups. Hypertension (diastolic blood pressure above 85 mmHg or the requirement of at least one hypotensive drug) was present in 73% of the patients at the time of myocardial revascularization; however, 96% of the patients had experienced in the past prolonged periods of hypertension. Hypercholesterolemia (total cholesterol above 250 mg/dl) was found in 44% of the patients. Fifty-six percent were exsmokers. Three HD and all TP patients had received steroids for more than 3 months. Cardiac medication included nitrates in 23, calcium antagonists in 16 and β-blockers in 13 patients.

The cardiac status before myocardial revascularization is summarized in Table 3. Eleven patients had a previous myocardial infarction. Stress tests were available in 14 patients. Angina during testing was present in only 6 and significant ST segment depression in 9 patients. Exercise thallium perfusion scintigraphy obtained in 12 patients was abnormal in 10 patients out of 12. Coronary angiography disclosed most often multiple vessel disease (81%) and a high incidence of

Table 3 Cardiac status before myocardial revascularization

	Total (n = 26)	Hemodialysis (n = 13)	Transplantation (n = 13)
History of myocardial infarction	11 (42%)	7	4
Coronary angiography			
Multiple vessel disease	21 (81%)	11	10
One vessel disease	5 (19%)	2	3
Left main artery involvement	4 (15%)	3	1

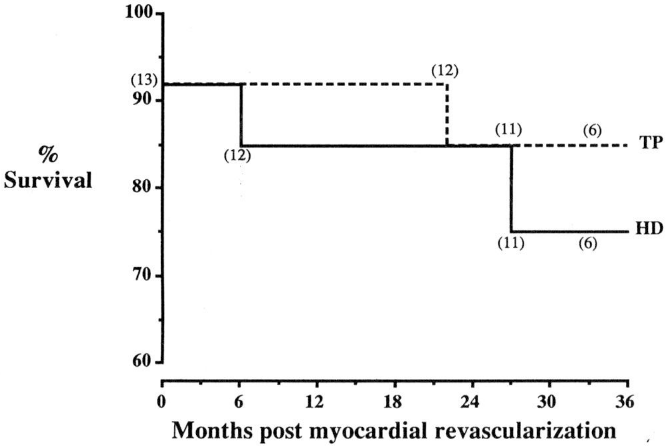

( ) number of patients at risk

Fig. 1 Actuarial survival of 13 transplanted and 13 dialyzed patients after a first myocardial revascularization.

left main artery involvement (15% of the patients). The median left ventricular ejection fraction was within normal limits 60% (range 37–84). However, the median left ventricular volumes were increased: 44 ml/m^2 (range 15–90) and 111 ml/m^2 (range 73–160), respectively for the end-systolic and diastolic volumes. The increase in end-diastolic volume was more pronounced in HD patients (median 135 ml/m^2, range 73–160) than in TP patients (median 107 ml/m^2, range 74–139).

Effects of myocardial revascularization

a) Immediate results

- PTCA successfully dilated the narrowed (n = 11) or occluded (n = 3) coronary segments in 12 out of 14 (86%) procedures performed in 10 patients. Two types of complications were encountered: a reversible renal graft dysfunction due to the injected contrast medium (2 cases) and a delayed reocclusion within the first month (one patient). No emergency surgery was needed. No patient died.
- CABG was complicated by intrathoracic bleeding in 3 cases. Diffuse intraoperative hemorrhage led to death in one TP patient before the bypass procedure. This patient had evidence of coagulation abnormalities induced by a nephrotic syndrome and by renal failure due to chronic rejection. Postoperative bleeding necessitated a second thoracotomy within 12 hours in the two others, one of whom developed sternal dehiscence and eventually died from multiorgan failure. Both were HD patients in whom the 2 IMA had been utilized to perform a high number of distal anastomoses (6 and 7). The preoperative cardiac status of these 3 patients was

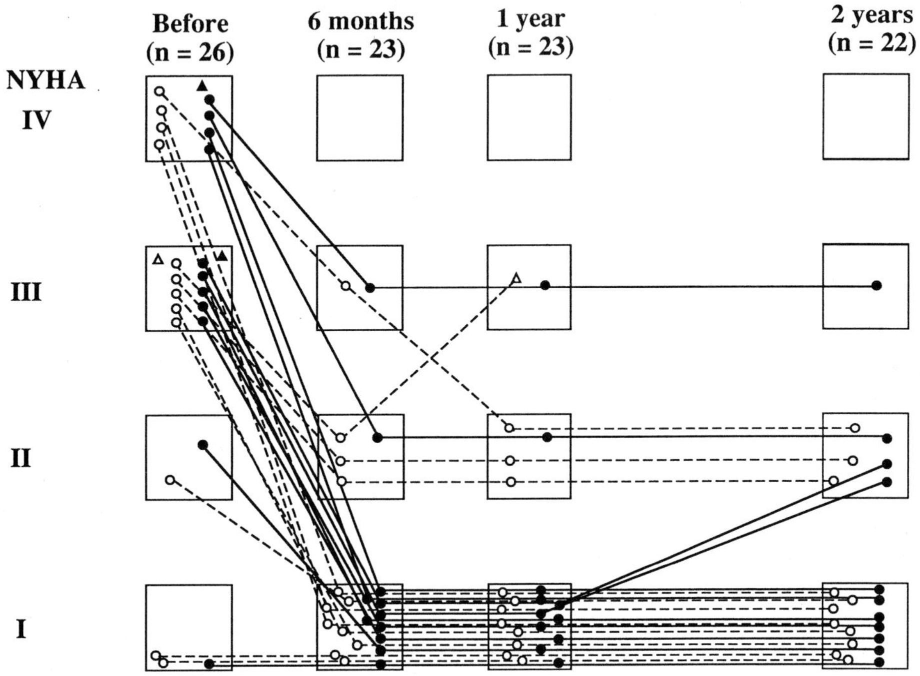

Fig. 2 Evolution of functional status (according to the New York Heart Association classification) after myocardial revascularization in 12 transplanted (○—○) and 11 dialyzed (●—●) patients. Death is represented by a triangle.

similar to that status of the survivors. The in-hospital mortality reached thus 11% (2/18). Otherwise, no perioperative myocardial infarction was observed. The renal graft function has remained stable in TP patients.

b) Long-term outcome

The long-term patient survival is illustrated (Figure 1) by a Kaplan-Meier curve: after an initial loss, during the postoperative period, three additional patients died 6, 22 and 27 months after the first revascularization procedure. All deaths were of cardiac origin: sudden death, ventricular arrhythmia and congestive heart failure. HD and TP patients had virtually the same survival rate.

The functional status was evaluated according to NYHA criteria before, 6, 12 and 24 months after revascularization (Figure 2). A dramatic improvement was noted in most patients. At 6 months, 74% of the symptomatic patients were free of anginal pain. Anginal pain recurred in 4 patients (3 initially treated by CABG and 1 by PTCA). Recurrence was manifest within 6 months in 3 cases and resulted either from the progression of coronary disease in an ungrafted vessel (n: 2 treated by CABG) or from restenosis of the segment previously dilated by PTCA (n: 1). In those 3 patients, anginal pain remitted after PTCA, but reappeared 18 months later in one patient who underwent a successful third PTCA. In the fourth patient, recurrence occurred at 2 years but has not yet been investigated.

Discussion

Our data clearly demonstrate that patients on RRT benefit from current myocardial revascularization procedures including both CABG with IMA and PTCA. Both techniques proved feasible, resulting in an appreciable clinical benefit such as disappearance of anginal pain and improved clinical status at one and two years.

For CABG, long-term survival after postoperative period is comparable with that of non-uremic patients treated by the same team [Dion et al. 1989]. It is, however, noteworthy that CABG in RRT patients entailed a significant in-hospital mortality (11%) definitely higher than that observed by the same surgical team in non-uremic patients (2.6%). Mortality resulted mainly from hemorrhagic complications encountered in 16% of our patients vs only 6% in the non-uremic subjects. This higher susceptibility to bleeding probably reflects the coagulation abnormalities and the higher tissue fragility associated with chronic renal failure. Although in non-uremic patients, IMA grafts are not associated with a higher frequency of bleeding than venous grafts [Dion et al. 1989, Grondin et al. 1984], it remains to be seen in a larger series whether this is also the case in uremic patients.

IMA grafts were chosen in the present study with the hope to prevent or reduce the rate of atheromatous degeneration and restenosis of the graft [Chaikhouni et al. 1986]. These latter complications, a matter of serious concern in the long-term for patients grafted with a saphenous vein, appear less frequent when IMA are used [Dion et al. 1989, Jones et al. 1987, Singh et al. 1983, Grondin et al. 1984]. Whether the hemorrhagic risk possibly associated with IMA in patients on RRT is offset in the long-term by a graft patency better than that of saphenous grafts remains to be demonstrated. Our present follow-up is too limited to provide an answer.

PTCA proved efficient and safe in our patients. In particular, there was no immediate or in-hospital abrupt coronary occlusion. Its main limitation remains the high rate of restenosis of the coronary vessel reaching up to 30% within six months in non-uremic patients [Gruentzig et al. 1987, Quigley et al. 1989]. We have observed a restenosis within six months in only one out of 10 patients. The actual rate is probably higher as we did not perform coronary angiography systematically after intervention. In our patients, restenosis was successfully alleviated by a repeated PTCA.

The published experience of myocardial revascularization in patients on RRT [McGovern et al. 1984, Rottembourg et al. 1983, Francis et al. 1980, Marshall et al. 1986, Zamora et al. 1986, Niemeyer et al. 1986, Rostand et al. 1988, Opsahl et al. 1988, Deutsch et al. 1989] concerns mainly patients on hemodialysis treated with venous CABG. Neither PTCA nor IMA grafts for CABG have been extensively described. The reported in-hospital mortality varies from 2,6 to 20% and is mainly due to cardiac complications [McGovern et al. 1984, Rottembourg et al. 1983, Francis et al. 1980, Marshall et al. 1986, Zamora et al. 1986, Niemeyer et al. 1986, Rostand et al. 1988, Opsahl et al. 1988, Deutsch et al. 1989] and intrathoracic bleeding varying from 0% [Marshall et al. 1986] to 40% [Niemeyer et al. 1986]. Long-term follow-up, ranging from 2 to 127 months, is available in five studies only [Francis et al. 1980, Marshall et al. 1986, Zamora et al. 1986, Niemeyer et al. 1986, Opsahl et al. 1988]: clinical status is improved markedly whereas actuarial survival calculated in one study is comparable to ours [Zamora et al. 1986].

Our experience with CABG and PTCA had led us to integrate both techniques in the treatment of coronary heart disease in patients on RRT.

In symptomatic patients, exercise testing is of limited value and coronary arteriography is readily performed. The value of exercise testing is limited for the following reasons: first, the severity of angina and/or other factors may reduce the exercise capacity to submaximal level; second, interpretation of electrocardiographic changes may be difficult due to the presence of resting abnormalities and/or hypertension during exercise. In asymptomatic patients, in particular those considered for renal transplantation, exercise thallium scintigraphy has become part of the routine pretransplant evaluation. If abnormal, coronary arteriography is recommended and, if necessary, myocardial revascularization is performed before transplantation.

The first therapeutic revascularization procedure depends on the type of coronary lesions. PTCA is attempted whenever only one coronary vessel is involved and the stenosis seems accessible to the balloon catheter. In case of restenosis, PTCA is repeated whenever feasible. CABG is discussed as the primary procedure in case of multivessel disease. One IMA graft, supplemented whenever necessary by saphenous grafts is utilized. In keeping with the present findings, we have questioned the need of a second IMA graft given the threatening hemorrhagic complications. At the present time, we feel that the marked clinical improvement and the good long-term survival rates more than offset the short-term complications of both PTCA and even CABG. We have thus opted for early myocardial revascularization in patients on RRT.

Acknowledgements

We gratefully acknowledge the secretarial assistance provided by Mrs. Karin Voss. Dr. William Wyns was supported by the Damman Foundation.

REFERENCES

Brunner FP, Brynger H, Chantler C, Donckerwolcke RA, Hathway RA, Jacobs C, Selwood NH, Wing AJ 1979 Combined report on regular dialysis and transplantation in Europe, II. Proc EDTA *16:* 2

Chaikhouni A, Crawford FA, Kochel PJ, Olanoff LS, Halushka PV 1986 Human internal mammary artery produces more prostacyclin than saphenous vein. J Thorac Cardiovasc Surg *92:* 88

Deutsch E, Bernstein RC, Addonizio VP, Kussmaul III WG 1989 Coronary artery bypass surgery in patients on chronic hemodialysis. Ann Intern Med *110:* 369

Dion R, Verhelst R, Rousseau M, Goenen M, Ponlot R, Kestens-Servaye Y, Chalant CH 1989 Sequential mammary grafting. Clinical, functional and angiographic assessment 6 months postoperatively in 231 consecutive patients. J Thorac Cardiovasc Surg *98:* 80

European Coronary Surgery Study Group 1982 Long-term results of prospective randomised study of coronary artery bypass surgery in stable angina pectoris. Lancet *ii:* 1173

Francis GS, Sharma B, Collins AJ, Helseth HK, Comty CM 1980 Coronary-artery surgery in patients with end-stage renal disease. Ann Intern Med *92:* 499

Grondin CM, Campeau L, Lespérance J, Enjalbert M, Bourassa MG 1984 Comparison of late changes in internal mammary artery and saphenous vein grafts in two consecutive series of patients 10 years after operation. Circulation *70:* I-208

Gruentzig AR, King SP, Schlumpf M, Siegenthaler W 1987 Long-term follow-up after percutaneous transluminal coronary angioplasty. N Engl J Med *316:* 1127

Hellerstedt WL, Johnson WJ, Ascher N, Kjellstrand CM, Knutson R, Shapiro FL, Sterioff S 1984 Survival rates of 2,728 patients with end-stage renal disease. Mayo Clin Proc *59:* 776

Jones EL, Lattouf O, Lutz JF, King SB 1987 Important anatomical and physiological considerations in performance of complex mammary-coronary artery operations. Ann Thorac Surg *43:* 469

Loop FD, Lytle BW, Cosgrove DM, Stewart RW, Goormastic M, Williams GW, Golding LAR, Gill CC, Taylor PC, Sheldon WC, Proudfit WL 1986 Influence of the internal-mammary-artery graft on 10-year survival and other cardiac events. N Engl J Med *314:* 1

Marshall WG Jr, Rossi NP, Meng RL, Wedige-Stecher T 1986 Coronary artery bypass grafting in dialysis patients. Ann Thorac Surg *42:* S12

McGovern E, Rooney R, Neligan MC 1984 Open heart surgery in patients receiving chronic haemodialysis. Thorax *39:* 388

Niemeyer MG, Laarman GJ, Ernst JMPG, Leusink JA, Vermeulen FEEE, Van der Zouwen P 1986 Open-hartoperaties bij patiënten met terminale nierinsufficiëntie. Ned Tijdschr Geneeskd *130:* 2264

Opsahl JA, Husebye DG, Helseth HK, Collins AJ 1988 Coronary artery bypass surgery in patients on maintenance dialysis: long-term survival. Am J Kidney Dis *12:* 271

Quigley PJ, Hlatky MA, Hinohara T, Rendall DS, Perez JA, Phillips HR, Califf RM, Stack RS 1989 Repeat percutaneous transluminal coronary angioplasty and predictors of recurrent restenosis. Am J Cardiol *63:* 409

Rostand SG, Kirk KA, Rutsky EA, Pacifico AD 1988 Results of coronary artery bypass grafting in end-stage renal disease. Am J Kidney Dis *12:* 266

Rottembourg J, Mussat T, Gandjbakhch I, Barthelemy A, Toledano D, Gahl GM, Cabrol C 1983 Open heart surgery in patients with end-stage renal disease. Proc EDTA *20:* 169

Singh RN, Sosa JA, Green GE 1983 Long-term fate of the internal mammary artery and saphenous vein grafts. J Thorac Cardiovasc Surg *86:* 359

Talley JD, Hurst JW, King SB, Douglas JS Jr, Roubin GS, Gruentzig AR, Anderson HV, Weintraub WS 1988 Clinical outcome 5 years after attempted percutaneous transluminal coronary angioplasty in 427 patients. Circulation *77:* 820

Tufveson G, Geerlings W, Brunner FP, Brynger H, Dykes SR, Ehrich JHH, Fassbinder W, Rizzoni G, Selwood NH, Wing AJ 1989 Combined report on regular dialysis and transplantation in Europe. Nephrol Dial Transplant *4*, suppl *4:* 5

Zamora JL, Burdine JT, Karlberg H, Shenaq SM, Noon GP 1986 Cardiac surgery in patients with end-stage renal disease. Ann Thorac Surg *42:* 113

LETTERS TO THE EDITOR

Viral antigens in IgA nephropathy*

Sir –, Mesangial glomerulonephritis (GN) is an immune complex mediated disease, with renal pathology resulting from the deposition of circulating immune complexes. It is called IgA nephropathy (IgAN) when, by immunofluorescence, this immunoglobulin is dominant in the glomerulus. IgAN can be idiopathic or secondary to other pathologic states, such as alcohol abuse [Smith and Hoy 1989, Smith 1990]. In idiopathic IgAN renal symptoms are frequently precipitated by a previous respiratory or gastrointestinal infectious episode, suggesting the role of the mucosal immune system in the pathogenesis of this disease [Lamm et al. 1984]. The predominant antibody is IgA; the nature of the antigen has not been elucidated although the importance of viral antigens, specially cytomegalovirus (CMV), has been suggested by several authors [Gregory et al. 1988, Lai et al. 1988, Nagy et al. 1979, Nagy et al. 1984, Ozawa and Stewart 1979, Tomino et al. 1987]. Our study was instigated by possible geographic and ethnic differences in viral antigens in idiopathic and secondary IgAN.

Mesangial GN is an important renal disease in the southwest of the United States of America. We have previously described IgA nephritides in 38% of biopsies from Native American renal patients in New Mexico [Smith and Tung 1985], we have found that over 70% of biopsies from Navajo and Pueblo Indian renal patients show mesangial GN with IgA and/or IgM deposits [Hughson et al. 1989, Smith et al. 1989] and we have reported that mesangial GN is possibly responsible for a large proportion of cases of end-stage renal disease in these ethnic groups [Hoy et al. 1987, Megill et al. 1988].

This study included 45 cases of IgAN: 36 biopsy samples of idiopathic IgAN obtained from 21 Native American and 15 Caucasian patients. Another 9 samples were selected from autopsies of Native American individuals with the previously described IgAN secondary to alcohol abuse [Smith et al. 1990a, b]. At the same time, 13 kidneys with miscellaneous (Misc) diagnosis were investigated: 4 autopsy samples of normal kidneys and 9 biopsies (1 case of diabetic glomerulosclerosis, 2 of lupus nephritis and 3 cases each of membranous GN and IgM mesangial GN).

For immunohistochemistry, sections of frozen tissue were incubated in batches, including each time positive and negative control slides. Positive controls were cultured fibroblasts infected with the virus to be investigated: they showed binding of antiviral antibodies in the nuclear regions. Negative controls were non-infected fibroblasts. We investigated CMV antigens with a two-step technique using 1:25 heterologous goat anticytomegalovirus serum, strain AD169 (Polysciences, Warrington, PA) followed by 1:10 anti-goat fluorescein isothiocyanate (FITC)-conjugated immunoglobulins (Dakopatts, Santa Barbara, CA). Although in our hands immunofluorescent deposits are sharper after ethanol-ether fixation, we also performed the incubation on air dried sections, as described by others [Gregory et al. 1988]. Furthermore, we studied sections pre-treated with citrate buffer, pH 3.2 at 37 °C for 4 hours, as according to some authors this technique will unmask the antigenic epitopes [Ozawa and Stewart 1979]. Weak CMV antigen binding was seen in 1/45 IgAN samples; all the others were negative. In the Misc group, 4/13 cases showed intense granular immunofluorescence predominantly along the glomerular capillary loops (1 case of lupus nephritis and 3 of membranous GN). In situ hybridization for CMV was performed on acetone fixed sections of frozen tissue, following proteinase K (100 ng/ml) (Bethesda Research Laboratories, Gaithersburg, MD) digestion. The hybridization solution was as follows: 50% formamide, 5× Denharts, 2× standard saline citrate, 500 μg/ml sheared salmon sperm DNA (Sigma type III) and 1 μg/ml of biotinylated CMV DNA (Enzo Biochem, New York, NY). After hybridization sections were incubated with a streptavidin-biotinylated horse-radish peroxidase complex. In situ DNA hybridization for CMV DNA was performed on 10 cases of IgAN and on 5 Misc cases, including those with immunofluorescence binding. No sample contained viral DNA positive cells. In situ hybridization is an accurate and sensitive assay system; it uses a specific DNA sequence, a DNA probe, to seek out and bind (hybridize) to other pieces of DNA that have complementary sequences. As in situ hybridization failed to demonstrate viral DNA in the 4 Misc cases that had stained with the polyclonal antiserum to CMV, the fluorescent finding possibly represents a cross reaction between the CMV antiserum and an unknown antigen, specially as the binding pattern was similar to that obtained by incubation with antisera to immunoglobulins.

The direct immunofluorescence technique for herpes virus used 1:100 FITC-conjugated anti-herpes virus I serum that cross reacts with virus II antigens (Dakopatts, Santa Barbara, CA). Herpes virus antigens were investigated in 41 renal samples of IgAN and 13 Misc cases. No binding of the antiserum was demonstrated. Hepatitis B was investigated by direct immunofluorescence with FITC-conjugated antiserum to hepatitis B surface antigen donated by Omana Nainan, MS (Center for Disease Control, Atlanta, GA). Positive controls were ATCC cells from Alexander (human) hepatoma cultures. Negative control was normal liver. No hepatitis B surface antigens were observed in 15 samples from kidneys with IgAN nor in 2 Misc cases.

Our in situ hybridization results in samples from Native American and Caucasian patients with idiopathic and secondary IgAN confirm Okamura's conclusion [1989] that patients with IgAN do not have a renal infection with CMV. Furthermore, in agreement with Waldo et al. [1989] we conclude that the binding of CMV antibodies to glomeruli of some of our control cases, similar to findings described by others in samples of IgAN [Gregory et al. 1988] is the result of non-specific binding. Our study failed to demonstrate the herpes simplex and hepatitis B viral antigens in the glomeruli of Native American and Caucasian patients with IgAN.

Acknowledgements

The authors are grateful to Mary Ann Kerley, MS, for expert technical assistance; Kathy Foucar, MD, for editorial advice.

* This study was supported by a Lovelace Intramural Grant and by BRSG S 07 RR-05583-24 awarded by the Biomedical Research Support Grant Program, Division of Research Resources, National Institutes of Health.

S. Meleg Smith[1], C. Wheeher[2], W. E. Hoy[3]
Departments of [1] Pathology, [2] Cell Biology, School of Medicine, University of New Mexico, [3] Lovelace Medical Foundation, Albuquerque, New Mexico

REFERENCES

Gregory MC, Hammond ME, Brewer ED 1988 Renal deposition of cytomegalovirus antigen in immunoglobulin-A nephropathy. Lancet *2:* 11

Hoy WE, Megill DM, Hughson MD 1987 Epidemic renal disease of unknown etiology in the Zuni Indians. Am J Kid Dis *9:* 485

Hughson MD, Megill DM, Smith SM, Tung KSK, Hoy WE 1989 Mesangiopathic glomerulonephritis in Zuni (New Mexico) Indians. Arch Pathol Lab Med *113:* 148–157

Lai KN, Lai FM, Tam JS, Vallance-Owen J 1988 Strong association between IgA nephropathy and hepatitis B surface antigenemia in endemic areas. Clin Nephrol *29:* 229–234

Lamm ME, Emancipator SN, Gallo GR 1984 Experimental models of IgA nephrophathy. Contr Nephrol *40:* 32–36

Megill D, Hoy WE, Woodruff SD 1985 Rates and etiologies for end-stage renal disease in the Navajo Indians, 1971–1985. Western J Med *149:* 178

Nagy J, Bajtai G, Brasch H et al. 1979 The role of hepatitis B surface antigen in the pathogenesis of glomerulopathies. Clin Nephrol *12:* 109–116

Nagy J, Uj M, Szucs G et al. 1984 Herpes virus antigens and antibodies in kidney biopsies and sera of IgA glomerulonephritis patients. Clin Nephrol *21:* 259–262

Okamura M, Kanayama Y, Negoro N, Takeda T, Inoue T 1989 Failure to detect cytomegalovirus-DNA in IgA nephropathy by in-situ hybridization. Lancet (June 3): 1265

Ozawa T, Stewart JA 1979 Immune complex glomerulonephritis associated with cytomegalovirus infection. Am J Clin Pathol *72:* 103–107

Smith SM, Hoy WE 1989 Frequent association of mesangial glomerulonephritis and alcohol abuse; a study of 3 ethnic groups. Modern Pathol *2:* 138–143

Smith SM, Tung KSK 1985 Incidence of IgA related nephritides in American Indians in New Mexico. Hum Path *16:* 181

Smith SM, Hoy WE, Pathak D, Megill DM, Tung KSK, Hughson MD 1989 Pathologic findings in mesangiopathic glomerulonephritis in Navajo Indians. Arch Pathol Lab Med *113:* 158–163

Smith SM, Hoy WE, Welford A, Chiovetti R 1990a Alcohol abuse related mesangial glomerulonephritis: immunoelectron microscopy. J Hystochem Cytochem *38:* 699

Smith SM, Yu GSM, Tsukamoto H 1990b IgA nephropathy in alcohol abuse: an animal model. Lab Invest *2:* 179

Tomino Y, Yagame M, Omata F, Nomoto Y, Sakai H 1987 A case of IgA nephropathy associated with adeno and herpes simplex viruses. Nephron *47:* 258–261

Waldo FB, Britt WJ, Tomana M, Julian BA, Mesteki J 1989 Nonspecific mesangial staining with antibodies against cytomegalovirus in immunoglobulin-A nephropathy. Lancet (January 21): 129–131

Pregnancy in women with focal hyalinosis and sclerosis

Sir, – We read with interest the study of D. K. Packham et al. on pregnancy in women with primary focal and segmental hyalinosis and sclerosis [1988 Clin Nephrol *29:* 185–192]. We had a 25-year-old pregnant patient in the 34th week. She was referred to Anadolu University Hospital for evaluation of renal dysfunction. She was in her first pregnancy. Her appearance and physical examination were almost normal. Blood pressure was 110/80 mmHg. The laboratory data on admission, revealead hemoglobin 8.8 g/dl, blood white cell count 17,100/mm^3. Serum fibrinogen level was 400 mg/dl and prothrombin (PT) 14 min (control 14 min). Active partial thromboplastin time (aPTT) was 26 min (control 25 min).

Serum IgG was 963 mg/dl, IgA 77.7 mg/dl, serum IgM 192 mg/dl. C3 was 120 mg/dl, C4 59.8 mg/dl. Platelet count was 170,000/mm^3, serum alanine 28 UI, serum aspartat 18 UI. Blood urea nitrogen was 54 mg/dl, serum creatinin 5.8 mg/dl, creatinin clearance 0.11 ml/minute, serum sodium 131 mEq/l and serum potassium 3.8 mEq/l. Daily urine volume was 40 cc. In urine analysis, several bacteria and white blood cells were seen. Cystoscopy and urinary catheterization were done. No obstruction was seen in either side of the kidneys, ultrasonography of kidneys was nearly normal.

The patient underwent hemodialysis six times. On the 7th day of her admission a boy weighing 2200 g was born in her 35th week. The patient underwent two more hemodialysis sessions and her renal function improved gradually. On the 20th day of admission her renal function was normal. Blood urea nitrogen was 10 mg/dl, serum creatinine 0.5 mg/dl. Urine volume was above 1.5 l. Renal biopsy revealed focal hyalinosis and sclerosis.

Z. Eren, T. Dönmez, Ö. Paşaoğlu, I. Dölen, E. Erenoğlu
Anadolu University Hospital, Eskişehir, Turkey

Response

Sir, – The case reported by Dr. Z. Eren et al. is of interest. However, we would not regard a diagnosis of primary and focal segmental hyalinosis and sclerosis as being proven. Our own study included only those pregnancies of women whose diagnostic renal biopsy was performed prior to 18 weeks gestation or after 6 months postpartum and those biopsied within 6 months postpartum who showed persistence of abnormal urine analysis after a year. Thus patients who developed focal hyalinosis and sclerosis as part of the glomerular changes of pre-eclampsia were excluded. The patient reported by Dr. Z. Eren et al. appears to have been biopsied on the 20th day postpartum and details of subsequent urinary abnormalities beyond 6 months postpartum are not provided. In addition, although their patient was normotensive on presentation, subsequent blood pressure levels and protein excretion data are not offered.

We would suggest that the renal biopsy findings of focal hyalinosis and sclerosis may reflect part of the glomerular changes of pre-eclampsia reported by others, i.e. Kida et al. Focal glomerular sclerosis in pre-eclampsia [Clin Neph 1985; 24: 221–227], and Nochy et al. De-novo focal glomerulosclerosis in pre-eclampsia [Clin Neph 1986; 25: 116–121].

D. K. Packham, K. F. Fairley, J. A. Whitworth, P. Kincaid-Smith
Smithfield Renal Unit, St. Bartholomew's Hospital, West Smithfield, London EC1A 7BE, UK

Comment on "Red blood cell destruction in single-needle dialysis" by Dhaene et al.

Sir, – The recent publication from Dhaene et al. (Clinical Nephrology, 31 (6), 327–331, 1989) was of interest. Our own observations in a group of eight patients dialyzing with the Hospal BSM system used in conjunction with a Terumo 15G needle are at variance with those published in that mean (± SD) predialysis LDH levels, at an average blood flow rate of 277 ml/min, were 373 ± 86 U/l, while those postdialysis were 406 ± 91 (an increase of 10.8 ± 10.6%). For all patients, the arterial and venous pump speeds were the same.

Blood flow in single needle dialysis may be expressed by the relationship:

$$Q_B = \frac{Q_A \cdot Q_V}{(Q_A + Q_V)}$$

where Q_A = blood flow in arterial segment of circuit
Q_V = blood flow in venous segment of circuit

Ideally, both the arterial and venous pump speeds should be working at the same rate. However, in certain patients this presents difficulties in attaining a clinically acceptable flow rate, and in such patients the venous pump speed is increased relative to the arterial pump speed to obtain the desired flow rate.

Figures 1 and 2 demonstrate the pressure flow relationships for four fistula needles established in the laboratory whilst running the arterial and venous pumps at the same speed and running the venous pump at twice the speed of the arterial pump. In the latter the ability to obtain high flow rates is compromised, although the arterial pressure is reduced, thereby allowing withdrawal of blood from the fistula, and the return pressure is increased reflecting the higher speed of the pump.

Blackshear and co-workers [Blackshear PL, Dorman FD, Steinbach JH 1965. Some mechanical effects that influence hemolysis. Trans Am Soc Artif Int Organs, XI, 112–121] have pointed out that intermittent positive pressures, shear stress and turbulence, all of which are present in single needle dialysis, induce acute erythrocyte destruction and cause the release of lactic dehydrogenase.

In view of these observations, we would suggest that careful attention be paid to both the selection of the access device, as considerable differences exist between needles of the same nominal gauge, as well as the conditions under which it is operated when used with single needle systems.

N. A. Hoenich, C. Woffindin, R. Goodall
University of Newcastle upon Tyne, Department of Medicine, Framlington Place, Newcastle upon Tyne NE2 4HH, UK

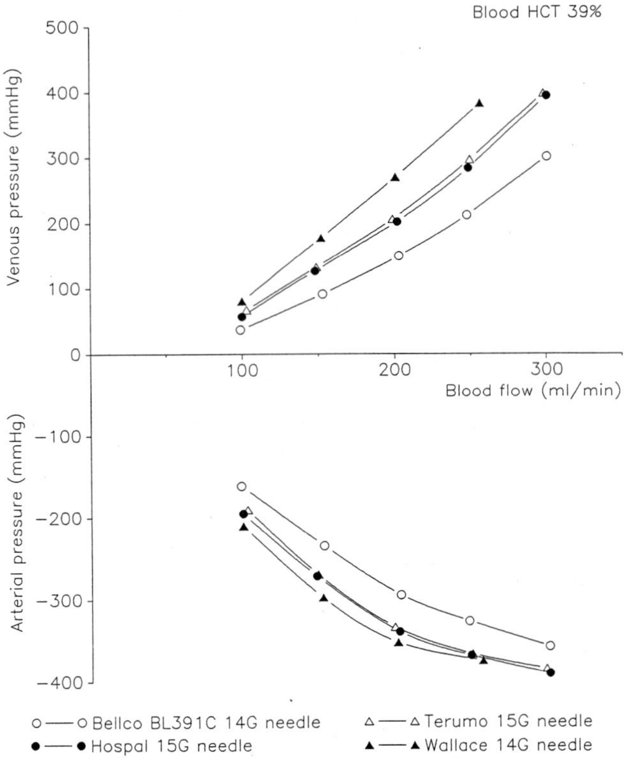

Fig. 1. Pressure flow characteristics in single needle dialysis at venous : arterial ratio = 1

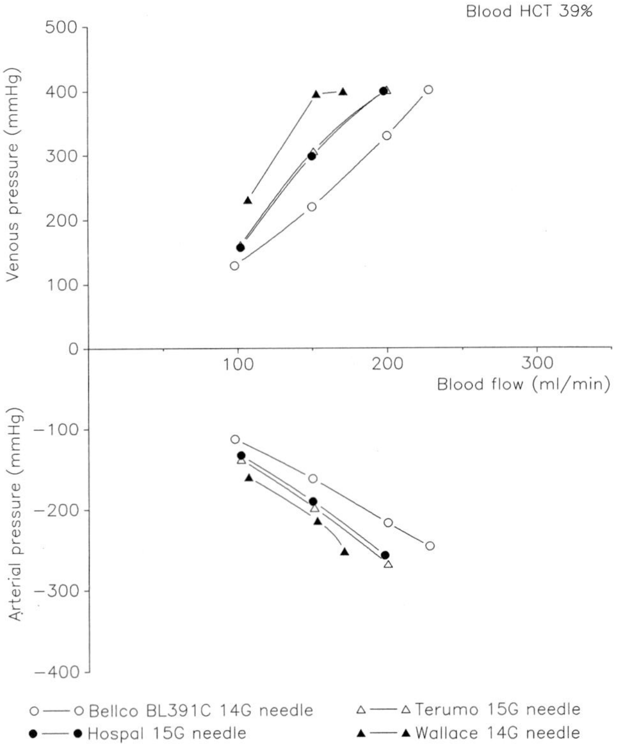

Fig. 2. Pressure flow characteristics in single needle dialysis at venous : arterial ratio = 2

Comment on "Long-term prognosis of chronic idiopathic membranous glomerulonephritis" by M. Wehrmann et al.

Sir, – I read the excellent article by Wehrmann et al. [1989 Clin Nephrol *31:* 67–76] on long-term prognosis in chronic idiopathic membranous glomerulonephritis with great interest. The study included 334 patients from at least 21 different departments. This large number of patients seems only surpassed by Gärtner et al., who published material covering 367 patients [Gärtner HV, Watanabe T, Ott V, Adam A, Bohle A, Edel HH, Kluthe R, Renner E, Scheler F, Schmülling RM, Sieberth HG 1977 Correlation between morphologic and clinical features in idiopathic perimembranous glomerulonephritis. Curr Top Pathol *65:* 1–29]. Table 1 indicates that one patient died from acute renal failure after renal vein thrombosis (RVT). In this connection the following questions seem justified: 1) Were all patients investigated systematically for RVT? And if so, how and how often? Llach et al. [Llach F, Arieff AI, Massry SG 1975 Renal vein thrombosis and nephrotic syndrome. Ann Intern Med *83:* 8–14], who investigated 36 adult patients with nephrotic syndrome in a prospective study, found RVT in 12/30 patients suffering from either membranous (20) or membranoproliferative glomerulonephritis (10). There were no clinical, laboratory, histological or immunopathological finding(s) pointing to RVT. 2) Were the patients who suffered from nephrotic syndrome treated with anticoagulant drugs? Wagoner et al. found RVT in 13/27 patients (bilateral in 8) with nephrotic syndrome because of membranous nephropathy [Wagoner RD, Stanson AW, Holley KE, Winter CS 1983 Renal vein thrombosis in idiopathic membranous glomerulopathy and nephrotic syndrome: incidence and significance. Kidney Int *23:* 386–74]. All patients with RVT received anticoagulant drugs for a minimum of 1 year. Follow-up observation (mean 2.5 years) did not reveal a significant difference in the rate of renal function deterioration or change in degree of proteinuria between patients with and without RVT.

R. Smith Pedersen
First University Clinic of Internal Medicine, Aarhus Municipal Hospital, DK-8200 Aarhus, Denmark

Author's reply to the letter of R. Smith-Pederson on
Long-term prognosis of chronic idiopathic membranous glomerulonephritis
by M. Wehrmann et al.

In our retrospective study of 334 patients with idiopathic membranous glomerulonephritis the presence or absence of a renal vein thrombosis (RVT) was only registered when causally associated with the occurence of renal death (patients who died of their renal disease or developed end stage renal failure necessitating regular dialysis). This was noted in only one case.

Therefore the occurrence of RVT is not of prognostic significance in idiopathic membranous glomerulonephritis as confirmed by Wagoner et al. [1983]: Renal vein thrombosis in idiopathic membranous glomerulopathy and nephrotic syndrome: Incidence and significance. Kidney Intern. 23: 368–74.

As mentioned in our paper, this was a retrospective study including various hospitals with different therapeutic regimes. Therefore no systematic investigation concerning the treatment of the nephrotic syndrome in this disease was performed. Therefore, no conclusions can be drawn about the effect of treatment with anticoagulant drugs.

M. Wehrmann
Institut für Pathologie, Universität Tübingen,
W-7400 Tübingen, Germany

Comment on "Irreversible ocular toxicity from single challenge dose of desferrioxamine" by C. Bene et al.

Sir, – We read with considerable interest the paper by Bene and coworkers [1989 Clin Nephrol *31* (1): 45–48].

Over a number of years we have seen disconcerting reports of ocular toxicity following desferrioxamine (DFO) therapy. As a result, we have developed a low dose DFO test for the diagnosis of aluminum overload (AO) [Ahmad et al. 1987 Abstracts XXIVth Congress of the EDTA-European Renal Association Berlin FRG]. A standard dose of 0.5 g DFO is infused during the first 2 hours of hemodialysis. Serum aluminum (SA1) is measured before dialysis (t1), post dialysis (t2), at 24 h (t3) and at 48 h (t4) intervals. The test is considered positive if the SA1 concentration during any period is doubled. Of the first 11 patients who had bone biopsy the DFO test was positive in 7 patients and there was one false negative. Four of these AO patients had SA1 levels below 100 µg/l. Of the remaining 4 patients who had no AO, the test was negative in all but one.

We are presently conducting prospective studies, nevertheless we are convinced that the low dose DFO test produces acceptable results. Further, because of the aforesaid concern, in long-term treatment of aluminum bone disease we also use a standard low dose DFO (1 g per dialysis 3 times weekly). We are happy to report that in both groups we have not as yet observed any DFO toxicity.

M. Yaqoob, P. Prabhu, R. Ahmad
Renal Unit, Sefton General Hospital, Smithdown Road, Liverpool L15 2HE, UK

Acute renal failure induced by oral acyclovir

Sir, – Reversible renal dysfunction induced by intravenous acyclovir has been reported after bolus injection [Brigden et al. 1982]. Preexisting renal insufficiency, dehydration and doses greater than 500 mg/m^2/8 hours predispose to renal toxicity [Brigden et al. 1982, Bean et al. 1982, Sawyer et al. 1988]. However, oral acyclovir has not been related to renal damage [Dorski et al. 1987].

We report on a case of non-oliguric renal failure associated with oral acyclovir therapy.

A 52-year-old man with chronic renal failure was admitted to the hospital because of herpetic skin lesions involving cervical dermatomes C5 and C6 with severe pain. Five months before admission idiopathic crescentic glomerulonephritis (40% crescents) with negative immunofluorescence had been diagnosed. He received oral prednisone 1 mg/kg/day for three months and oral cyclophosphamids 2 mg/kg/day for six weeks. Therapy with intravenous acyclovir, 2.5 mg/kg/12 hours (300 mg/day) infused over a 90 minute period, was begun. Serum creatinine (SCr) at admission was 3.7 mg/dl and creatinine clearance 35 ml/min. After the first six doses of i. v. acyclovir, SCr was similar to the baseline value. Because of vascular access problems, on the 4th day of therapy he was changed to oral acyclovir at a dosage of 800 mg every 12 hours (1600 mg/day). Six days later, SCr had risen to 6.7 mg/dl; acyclovir was reduced to 400 mg/day. However, SCr increased up to 8 mg/dl and acyclovir was withdrawn. The patient did not present oliguria, dehydration nor hypertension. Urinalysis revealed microscopic hematuria and mild proteinuria similar to that observed at admission and no crystalluria was detected. After acyclovir withdrawal his SCr steadily decreased to 3.7 mg/dl 10 days later.

Severe renal dysfunction has not been reported with oral acyclovir therapy, even at doses of 4 g/day. However, all these patients had normal renal function [Huff et al. 1988]. Our patient had chronic renal failure and he developed reversible acute non-oliguric renal failure coincidental with oral acyclovir treatment. He had received intravenous acyclovir for 3 days but SCr remained stable. He did not show volume contraction or hypotension, and no other nephrotoxic drugs were administered. The recovery of renal function to the previous values after oral withdrawal supports the role of its oral administration in the pathogenesis of renal worsening. The clinical course of acyclovir-induced renal failure suggests that acyclovir crystallizes in the renal collecting tubules and causes obstructive nephropathy [Sawyer et al. 1988]. The bioavailability of oral acyclovir has been reported in normal adults [Dorsky et al. 1988] but not in patients with renal insufficiency; it might be higher in uremic patients, although this issue has not been studied. Therefore a careful control of renal function is needed in patients with renal insufficiency treated with oral acyclovir.

E. Hernandez, M. Praga, F. Moreno, C. Montoyo
Servicio de Nefrologia, Hospital 12 Octubre, Ctra Andalucia km 5.400, E-28041 Madrid, Spain

REFERENCES

Bean B, Braun C, Balfour HM 1982 Acyclovir therapy for acute herpes zoster. Lancet *2:* 118

Brigden D, Rosling AE, Woods NC 1982 Renal function after acyclovir intravenous injection. Am J Med *73* (Suppl 1 A): 182

Dorsky DI, Crumpacker CS 1987 Drugs five years later: acyclovir. Ann Intern Med *107:* 859

Huff JC, Bean B, Balfour MH 1988 Therapy of herpes zoster with oral acyclovir. Am J Med *85 (Suppl 2 A):* 84

Sawyer MH, Webb DE, Balow JE, Straus SE 1988 Acyclovir-induced renal failure. Am J Med *84:* 1067

Takayasu aortitis simulating bilateral renal-artery stenoses in patients treated with ACE inhibitors

Sir, – In his recent extensive review [Williams GH 1988 Converting enzyme inhibitors in the treatment of hypertension. N Engl J Med *319:* 1517–1525], G. H. Williams enumerates the various side effects of ACE inhibitors including the well established deterioration function in patients with bilateral renal-artery stenoses [Hricik DE, Browning PJ, Kopelman R, Goorno WE, Madias NE, Dzau VJ 1983 Captopril-induced functional renal insufficiency in patients with bilateral renal artery stenoses or renal-artery stenosis in a solitary kidney. N Engl J Med *308:* 373–376].

We would like to report the case of a 54-year-old hypertensive woman who was admitted because of spiking uncontrolled systolic hypertension.

After several antihypertensive regimens had failed to improve her hypertension, captopril (25 mg bid) was added and her blood pressure dropped from 250/70 to 120/70. Simultaneously, a sharp rise in serum creatinine level from 0.5 mg/dl to 3.0 mg/dl was observed. Interruption of the captopril treatment was shortly followed by gradual and complete recovery of renal function. Aortic angiography revealed normal renal arteries, however, an extremely narrowed segment of the aorta 5 cm long was noted at the diaphragmatic level consistent with Takayasu aortitis. Serum renin levels from both renal veins and inferior vena cava were 25–45 times the normal values. Thus, high abdominal aortic stenosis with intact renal arteries may simulate bilateral renal-artery stenoses and predispose to renal failure in patients treated with ACE inhibitors.

M. Rapoport, Z. Averbukh, S. Chaim, E. Klinovski, D. Modai, Y. Gilboa
Medical Department B and Nephrology Division, Assaf Harofeh Medical Center, Zerefin, Israel

Turbid dialysate effluent and bacterial peritonitis

Sir, – The definition used in the diagnosis of bacterial continuous ambulatory peritoneal dialysis (CAPD)-associated peritonitis includes turbid dialysate effluent with a white blood cell count greater than 100 cells per cubic millimeter [Linblad AS, Novak JW, Nolph KD et al. 1988 The 1987 USA national CAPD registry report. Trans Am Soc Artif Intern Organs *34:* 150–156]. It is unclear whether the turbidity is a function of bacterial contamination or due to other factors. Similarly, presence of a turbid dialysate may not be indicative of a bacterial peritonitis. We investigated the effect of bacterial contamination on the absorportion of light by peritoneal dialysis.

Spent dialysate was collected from 19 CAPD patients who had not received antibiotics nor had an episode of peritonitis within the preceding 6 weeks. In all cases, the dialysate was collected after a minimum dwell of 6 hours from patients using a 1.5% dextrose preparation. Clinical isolates of a gentamicin-sensitive *E. coli* and a penicillin-sensitive *S. epidermidis* were used to inoculate aliquots of the spent dialysate. The dialysate collected from 9 patients was used to test *E. coli* and 10 patients for *S. epidermidis*. Triplicate aliquots of each were inoculated with a stock culture prepared from the clinical isolates, giving initial concentrations of 7.0 ± × 2.5 × 10^3 colony forming units per milliliter (CFU/ml) for *E. coli* and 94 ± 26 × 10 CFU/ml for *S. epidermidis*. These aliquots were incubated at 37° C for 12 hours, together with sterile, non-inoculated spent dialysate as controls. At intervals during the incubation period, triplicate samples were taken and plated on 5% sheep blood agar and the optical densities determined. In addition, the pH and protein contents of the dialysate were determined.

Optical densities were determined using a spectrophotometer Bausch & Lomb (Spectronic 200), using the control dialysate as a blank, in the visible and ultraviolet ranges of the spectrum (760 to 240 nm). The numbers of organisms increased up to 1.72 ± 1.53 × 10^6 CFU/ml after 12 hours' incubation. No peaks on absorption spectrophotometry were noted. After 12 hours incubation, the pH was 7.5 ± 0.21 and 7.6 ± 0.16 for *S. epidermidis* and *E. coli*, respectively.

It is concluded that neither high concentrations of infecting organisms nor the presence of small quantities of protein are responsible for changes in the turbidity of dialysate during peritonitis and that other factors, such as the presence of white blood cells, may be the causative factor.

G. R. Bailie[1], *R. A. Venezia*[2], *G. Eisele*[3]
Albany Colleges of Pharmacy[1] and Medicine[2], and Department of Microbiology and Immunology, Albany Medical Center[3], 106 New Scotland Avenue, Albany, NY 12208, USA.

Erythropoietin and improvement in the erythropoiesis of chronic hemodialysis patients treated with desferrioxamine

Sir, – Deficiency of erythropoietin (Epo) is the main factor determining the severity of anemia in chronic hemodialysis (HD) patients. With recombinant human erythropoietin (rHuEpo) these patients can maintain adequate levels of hemoglobin. However, more than 15% of patients need supranormal doses of rHuEpo to reach the target hemoglobin level [Eschbach et al. 1989]. This resistance to rHuEpo probably indicates that other factors which inhibit erythropoiesis or worsen the anemia are also present. On the other hand, a feed-back mechanism between Epo and hemoglobin concentration, working at a lower level than in normals, has been proposed for chronic HD patients [Walle et al. 1987].

However, the response of the Epo-hemoglobin circuit to an improvement in the erythropoiesis of chronic HD patients is unknown. We measured Epo serum levels in a group of chronic HD patients without clinical evidence of aluminum toxicity whose anemia improved with the use of the chelating agent desferrioxamine (DFO). 16 patients were treated with DFO, 1 g i. v. thrice a week for 6 months. Other 8 patients were used as controls. The erythropoiesis improved in the treated group, and 8 patients had an increase in hemoglobin higher than 2 g/dl at 6 months. These data have been previously published [De la Serna et al. 1988].

Predialysis serum samples were obtained before the administration of DFO and after its withdrawal. There were no transfusions in the 2 weeks prior to the sampling. Student's t-test was used for statistical analysis. As shown in Table 1, there were no significant changes in Epo levels in any of the 3 groups, despite the fact of a clear increase in hemoglobin level in group I ($p < 0.05$).

The beneficial effect of DFO in the anemia of patients in group I might be due to the removal of trace amounts of aluminum or to other unidentified mechanisms. It has been shown that DFO can reduce the need of rHuEpo doses in some HD patients [Casati et al. 1990]. Our findings demonstrate that the improvement in the erythropoiesis associated with the administration of DFO to HD patients has no relationship with changes in Epo production. In addition, the absence of a shift in Epo levels in spite of the significant improvement in the anemia of group I patients suggests that the base line Epo production of these patients is at the upper limit of their ability and does not support the existence of an Epo-hemoglobin feed-back circuit in these patients.

Table 1. Erythropoietin and hemoglobin levels before and after treatment with desferrioxamine

		Before DFO	After DFO
Group I	Hb	7.8 ± 1.0	10.6 ± 2.0
		(6.6–9.8)	(10.1–13.9)
	Epo	23.2 ± 11.3	21.4 ± 9.2
		(13.3–48.6)	(11.0–36.2)
Group II	Hb	6.6 ± 0.5	6.6 ± 0.6
		(5.8–7.5)	(6.0–8.5)
	Epo	25.3 ± 14.3	19.4 ± 13.8
		(13.4–56.4)	(9.9–12.5)
Group III	Hb	7.7 ± 1.2	7.8 ± 1.1
		(5.8–9.5)	(6.4–9.5)
	Epo	22.9 ± 8.1	19.0 ± 6.5
		(10.7–32.2)	(11.7–27.0)

Group I: treated patients whose anemia improved (n = 8); Group II: treated patients without response (n = 8); Group III: untreated patients (n = 8). Values are expressed as mean ± standard deviation and range. Epo: mU/ml; Hemoglobin: g/dl.

F. Javier De la Serna, F. Gilsanz, M. Praga and *J. Estenoz*
Departments of Hematology, Nephrology, and Nuclear Medicine. Hospital 12 de Octubre, Ctra de Andalucia km 5,4, E-28041 Madrid, Spain

REFERENCES

Eschbach JW, Abdulhadi MH, Browne JK et al. 1989 Recombinant human erythropoietin in anemic patients with end-stage renal disease. Results of a phase III multicenter clinical trial. Ann Intern Med *111:* 992–1000

Walle AJ, Wong GY, Clemons GK et al. 1987 Erythropioetin-hematocrit feedback circuit in the anemia of end-stage renal disease. Kidney Int *31:* 1205–1209

De la Serna FJ, Praga M, Gilsanz F et al. 1988 Improvement in the erythropoiesis of chronic hemodialysis patients with desferrioxamine. Lancet *1:* 1009–1011

Casati S, Castelnovo C, Campise M et al. 1990 Aluminium interference in the treatment of hemodialysis patients with recombinant human erythropoietin. Nephrol Dial Transplant *5:* 441–443

Aggravation of palmar erythema by an arteriovenous fistula

Sir, – Symmetrical erythema of the palms is a prominent sign of liver disease. We report below a renal transplant recipient with asymmetrical liver palms.

A 42-year-old white male developed end-stage renal failure due to chronic glomerulonephritis in 1971. A radial artery-cephalic vein arteriovenous fistula was created in his right wrist the same year. Excellent dilatation of the veins of his right forearm and hand developed within several weeks; his right palm was not noted to be erythematous at this time. The fistula was used for maintenance hemodialysis for the next 7 years. During this period he received frequent blood transfusions for refractory anemia of uremia and became seropositive for hepatitis B surface antigen.

In 1978, the patient received a cadaveric renal allograft and was placed on prednisone and azathioprine. Subsequently, chronic active hepatitis set in, followed by the appearance of ascites and other stigmata of cirrhosis. Cyclophosphamide was substituted for azathioprine in the immunosuppressive regimen. In 1984, he began to notice redness and pain in the right hand. On examination, he was found to have bilateral palmar erythema with the erythema being much more marked on the right thenar and hypothenar eminences than on the left. In addition, there was swelling, cyanosis and ulceration of the first, second and third digits of the right hand, and engorged tortuous veins on the dorsum of the hand suggestive of the presence of venous hypertension. Also obvious was a functional arteriovenous fistula characterized by the presence of a pseudoaneurysm. The latter was resected, the arteriovenous fistula was undone, and the radial artery was repaired with an end-to-end anastomosis.

Postoperatively, a decrease in the swelling and erythema ensued. The right palmar erythema then became less marked and equalled to its left counterpart in intensity. Subsequently, the patient died of a cytomegalovirus infection.

Palmar erythema, though a prominent sign of liver disease, is a non-specific finding. The lesion is characteristically bilateral and involves the thenar and hypothenar eminences, the distal finger pads, and the circumungual areas on the dorsum of the fingers, with sparing of the central part of the palms [Conn HO 1987 Cirrhosis. In: Schiff L, Schiff ER. Diseases of the liver. JP Lippincott Co., 6th ed, p 759]. The erythema probably is due to vasodilatation with increased blood flow through the arteriovenous anastomoses normally present in the palm [Bean WB 1945 The cutaneous spider. Medicine 24: 243; Silverstein E 1956 Peripheral venous O_2 saturation in patients with and without liver disease. J Lab Clin Med 47: 513].

To the best of our knowledge, asymmetrical palmar erythema has not been described as a complication of cirrhosis. We hypothesize that in our patient venous hypertension secondary to the surgically-created arteriovenous fistula aggravated the palmar erythema by further increasing the amount of blood present in the blood vessels of the hand.

S. Popli, D. J. Leehey, R. Soundararajan, T. S. Ing
Veterans Affairs Hospital, Hines, IL 60141, USA

Clinical Nephrology, Vol. 36 No. 5 – 1991 (215–222)

Morphologic findings in "zero-hour" biopsies of renal transplants

E. Curschellas[1], J. Landmann[2], M. Dürig[2], B. Huser[3], M. Kyo[1], V. Basler[1], G. Thiel[3] and M. J. Mihatsch[1]

[1]*Department of Pathology*
[2]*Department of Surgery, Cantonal Hospital*
[3]*Department of Internal Medicine, Cantonal Hospital, University of Basel, Basel, Switzerland*

Abstract. The extreme lack of renal grafts for transplantation stimulated us to analyze how strict the selection criteria of kidney donors must be. We investigated therefore if preexisting lesions in renal grafts influence initial and late renal function. 147 zero-hour biopsies of 101 donors (mean age 33, from 6–64 years) were examined. By light microscopy 38% of biopsies showed no, 44% showed nonspecific and 18% specific lesions. Nonspecific lesions comprised intimal fibrosis of small arteries in 44%, interstitial fibrosis in 8% and an arteriolar hyalinosis in 29%. Out of 102 immunohistologically examined biopsies 74.5% showed nonspecific IgM/C3 deposits in glomeruli and/or arterioles. An age dependent decrease of normal renal biopsies was found which was most evident in donors older than 40 years. Specific findings consisted of glomerulosclerosis (n = 4), glomerulonephritis (n = 11), intravascular coagulation (n = 10) and eclamptic kidney (n = 1). In case of nonspecific immunohistologic findings and in glomerulonephritis rebiopsies showed that antigen deposits usually disappeared within 4 months. Independent of morphologic findings 82% of transplant recipients had a good initial and late renal function. Since donor age, glomerulosclerosis, glomerulonephritis, intravascular coagulation or eclamptic changes seem not to compromise renal function after transplantation a more liberal choice of donors should be considered.

Key words: Zero-hour biopsy – transplantation – glomerulonephritis – intravascular coagulation

Introduction

To the best of our knowledge, the use of "zero-hour" biopsies as a means of diagnosing hyperacute rejection of transplants was first advocated by Kincaid-Smith [Kincaid-Smith et al. 1968]. Merely to demonstrate the presence of leukocytes in glomeruli had proved to be an unreliable indicator of rejection and, since the accuracy of tissue typing had improved considerably, the use of this technique was rapidly abandoned. Subsequent to Kincaid-Smith's publication little has appeared in the literature relating to "zero-hour" biopsies, and of those reports that have been published most have been limited to fairly small sample numbers.

Recently the use of the immunosuppressant drug cyclosporin (CSA) has been introduced in the treatment of recipients of renal transplants. One of the adverse effects of the drug is its nephrotoxicity, which is manifested both in the arterioles and in the tubular interstitial space. Concurrent with the introduction of the drug, in order to prevent pre-existent lesions from being falsely ascribed to CSA, we have been taking "zero-hour" biopsies from all cadaver kidney grafts. The following paper reports on the astounding number of both specific and non-specific findings which we have discovered in "zero-hour" biopsies. We found no significant correlation between the presence of these preexistent lesions and either the early or late function of grafts. On the basis of these findings we feel that greater freedom in the choice of donors is justified.

Received September 17, 1990; in revised form May 13, 1991.

Reprint requests to Dr. M. J. Mihatsch, Institut für Pathologie, Schönbeinstraße 40, CH-4003 Basel, Switzerland

Material and methods

Between the years 1984–1988, 162 consecutive "zero-hour" biopsies from cadaver kidney grafts were studied. Of these, 15 were rejected because of insufficient material (the samples contained only medullary tissue). The remaining 147 biopsies were obtained from 101 donors. 89 biopsies (60.5%) were from male and 58 (39.5%) from female donors. The mean age of the donors was 33 ± 15 years. The period of warm ischemia was 4.6 ± 4.9 minutes and of cold ischemia 18.5 ± 6.5 hours. Some biopsies were taken before (<30 minutes), some after (<30 minutes) reperfusion. All recipients were immunosuppressed with CSA (Sandimmune).

Table 1 Groups according to lightmicroscopy and immunohistology

Group	LM	IH	No of cases	Age of donor years mean (SD)	Sex of donor m/f	Warm ischemia min. mean (SD)	Cold ischemia hours mean (SD)	Initial renal function bad/good %
I	0	0	14	27.3 (10.9)	1,8:1	4.8 (8.3)	19.7 (7.9)	28.6/71.4
II	0	1	36	27.5 (13.3)	1,6:1	3.3 (3.1)	19.1 (8.4)	19.4/80.6
III	0	nd	6	28.0 (15.4)	2,0:1	9.0 (10.8)	22.9 (2.9)	16.7/83.3
IV	1	0	12	38.6 (18.0)	3,0:1	5.4 (3.5)	16.0 (5.0)	8.3/91.7
V	1	1	40	37.3 (15.9)	1,0:1	4.3 (3.9)	17.0 (4.0)	27.5/72.5
VI	1	nd	13	40.5 (11.8)	2,2:1	5.4 (4.3)	16.8 (5.6)	7.7/92.3
VII	2	2	26	31.8 (14.5)	1,6:1	5.1 (4.9)	20.1 (6.6)	19.2/80.8

LM = Lightmicroscopy
IH = Immunohistology
(0) = normal; (1) = nonspecific; (2) = specific; (nd) = not done

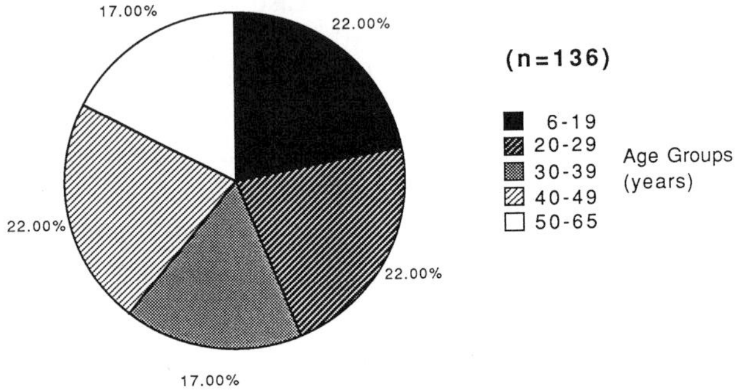

Fig. 1 Distribution of different donor age groups.

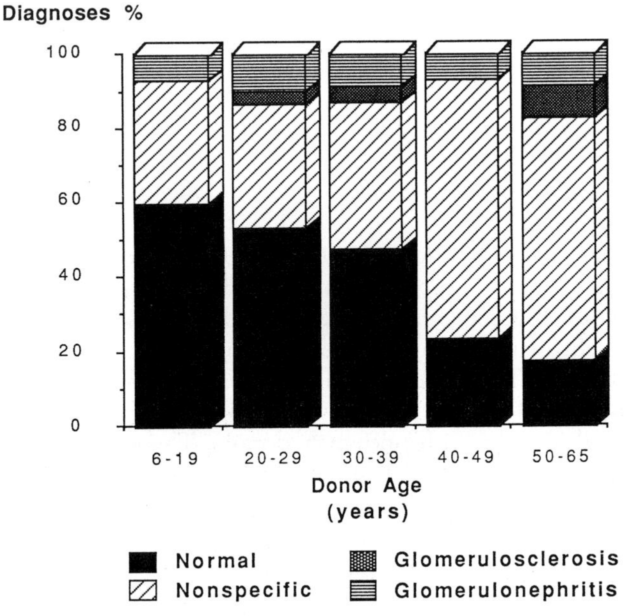

Fig. 2 Morphologic findings in different donor age groups.

Morphological investigations included light microscopy and immunohistology (n = 128, with >5 glomeruli per section) using standard techniques [Zollinger and Mihatsch 1978]. The slides examined by light microscopy were stained with HE, EVG, PAS, AFOG and PASM. Immunohistological investigations for IgG, IgM, IgA, complement C3 and fibrin(ogen) were carried out on paraffin sections and visualizied by ABC method [Hsu et al. 1981].

The following clinical information was obtained routinely: donor age, donor sex, periods of warm and cold ischemia, recipient age and sex.

Initial renal function was classified as good when no dialysis was necessary in the first ten days after transplantation. If the recipient had to be dialyzed in this period, initial renal function was classified as bad. If one year after transplantation the patient had not returned to chronic hemodialysis late renal function was classified as good, otherwise it was classified as bad late renal function.

In the statistical analysis mean and median values and standard deviation were calculated. Comparison of groups was performed using the U-test and Chi-square test. P values <0.05 were considered to be statistically significant.

Results

The grafts were equally distributed over the different donor age groups (Figure 1). Classification of the morphological findings was performed according to light microscopy (LM) and immunohistology (IH) (Table 1). Group I–III showed normal renal tissue by light microscopy, group IV–VI showed nonspecific lesions. In groups II and V nonspecific immunohistologic findings were present, groups I and IV were negative by immunohistology. Those in group VII showed specific or questionally specific light microscopic and/or immunohistological changes. 17.6% of the total of 147 biopsies corresponding to 20.8% of donors, belonged to group VII.

Morphological findings in groups I–VI

Among the 121 biopsies in these groups 46.3% showed no changes and the remaining 53.7% showed only nonspecific changes by lightmicroscopy. Of the 102 cases which additionally were examined immunohistologically 25.5% were negative, 74.5% positive.

Of the 65 cases with nonspecific lightmicroscopic changes (Table 2) 44.6% showed a moderate or severe intimal fibrosis of small arteries, 7.7% a moderate interstitial fibrosis and 29.2% a moderate to severe arteriolar hyalinosis. No other nonspecific findings were present.

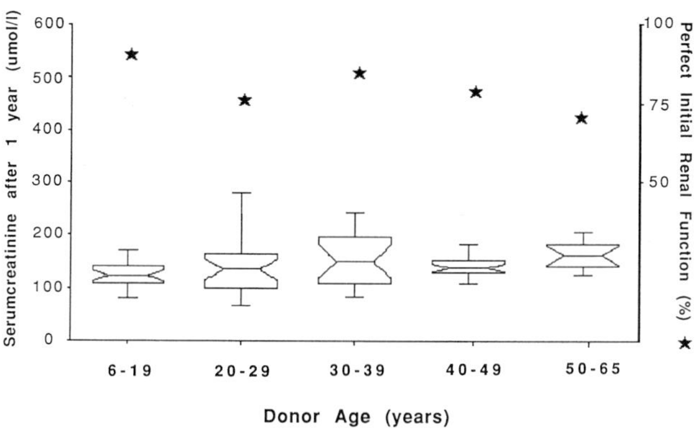

Fig. 3 Serum-creatinine after one year (notched box plot: middle line is median value, box upper end represents 75th percentile, lower end 25th percentile, upper line 90th percentile and lower line 10th percentile) and percent of grafts with perfect initial renal function.

Table 2 Nonspecific findings by lightmicroscopy in groups IV to VI

Severity	Intimal fibrosis in arteries	Interstitial fibrosis	Arteriolar hyalinosis
Slight	8	14	15
Medium	26	5	17
Severe	3	0	2

Table 3 Nonspecific immunohistologic findings

Localisation	Antigen	Intraglomerular distribution of antigen	GR II	GR V
Glomeruli	IgM	sf	7	6
		gd	7	4
	C3	sf	0	0
		gd	0	0
	IgM + C3	sf	2	1
		gd	0	0
Arterioles	IgM		0	0
	C3		3	0
	IgM + C3		2	2
Glomeruli and arterioles				
Glomeruli	IgM	sf	5	4
		gd	6	11
	C3	sf	1	1
		gd	0	0
	IgM + C3	sf	1	6
		gd	2	5
Arterioles	IgM		5	8
	C3		6	8
	IgM + C3		4	11

Abbreviations: s = segmental; g = global; f = focal; d = diffuse

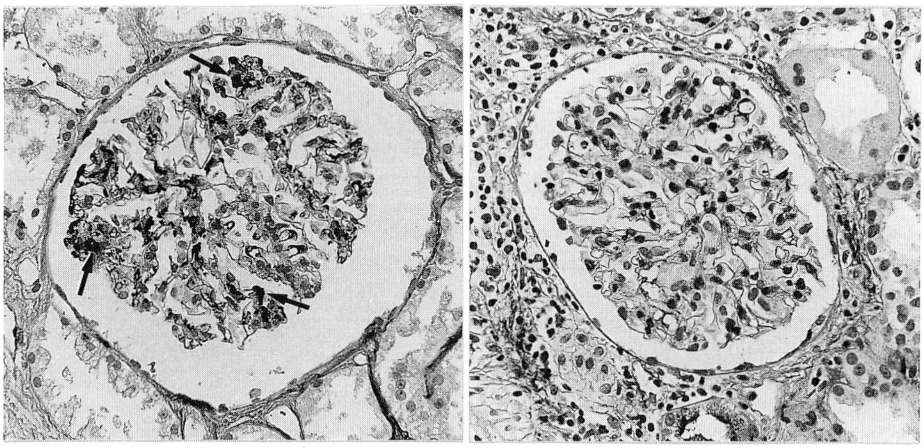

Fig. 4 Immunohistologic demonstration of IgA deposits (black dots, arrow) in zero hour biopsy (left) and one month later negative reaction after incubation with anti-IgA (right) (GN 6).

Table 4 Follow up of grafts with nonspecific immunohistologic findings in "zero-hour" biopsies

Zero-hour biopsy	n	Rebiopsy findings	n	%	Days after Tpl mean (range)
		Epimem-branous GN	1	5	105
IgM/IgM + C3 g/d	21	unchanged	5	24	83 (16–210)
		negative	15	71	130 (8–660)

Of the 76 biopsies with positive immunohistological findings 27 showed only glomerular, 7 only arteriolar, and 42 both glomerular and arteriolar antigen deposition (Table 3). Glomerular changes, which were evaluated according to the extent of glomerular involvement (segmental focal as opposed to global diffuse), and arteriolar changes occurred with equal frequency in kidneys with or without detectable lightmicroscopic changes.

In 21 biopsies with global diffuse deposits of IgM or IgM plus complement C3 we were able to compare the immunohistological findings in pre- and post-transplantation biopsies. Among the rebiopsies one biopsy presented a de novo case of epimembraneous glomerulonephritis, five sets of biopsies remained unaltered, and in 15 of the rebiopsies (71%) the preexistent immunohistological findings had disappeared within a period of 4 months (Table 4).

The number of kidneys that appeared normal by lightmicroscopy decreased significantly with increasing donor age ($p < 0.0001$). The cut-off point seemed to be around the age of forty, after which there was a steep decline in the number of normal donor kidneys (Figure 2). Despite having made this observation, however, we were unable to establish a relationship between age and immunohistological changes. There was no apparent correlation between either donor age and lightmicroscopic and immunohistological findings, on the one hand, and initial renal function and serum creatinine levels estimated one year post transplantation (Figure 3).

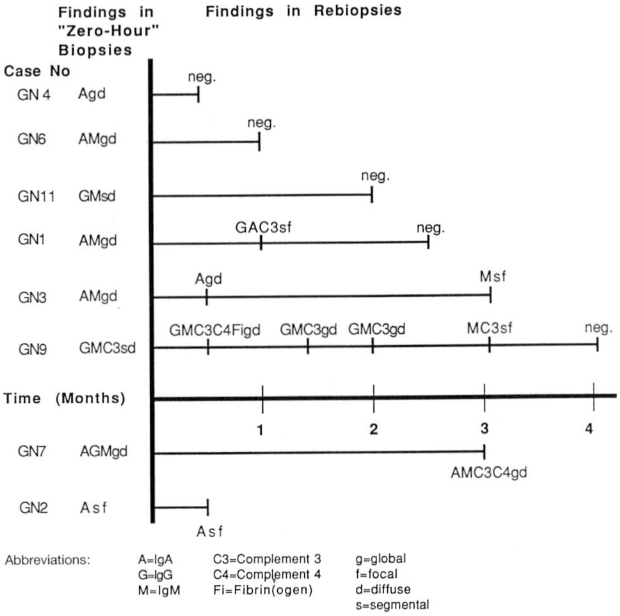

Fig. 5 Immunohistologic findings in cases with glomerulonephritis in zero-hour biopsies and in rebiopsies.

Table 5 "Zero-hour" biopsies with glomerulonephritis

Case No	Diagnoses	Light-microscopy	Immuno-histology	Donor Age	Sex	Initial renal function	S-Creatinine (umol/l) >6 months after tpl	Graft loss days after tpl
GN 1	IgA-Nephropathy	normal	AMgd	15	m	good		*
GN 2	IgA-Nephropathy	GS	Asf	50	m	bad		12
GN 3	IgA-Nephropathy	A.3/F.2/I.2	AMgd	50	m	good	180	
GN 4	IgA-Nephropathy	GS	Agd	32	f	good	121	
GN 5	IgA-Nephropathy	I.2	AMgd	45	f	good	106	
GN 6	IgA-Nephropathy	I.1	AMgd	45	f	good		*
GN 7	IgA-Nephropathy	normal	AGMgd C3Fibrin sf	37	f	good	141	
GN 8	Mesangioprolif. GN	F.1/I.1	GMC3gd	21	m	good	56	
GN 9	Mesangioprolif. GN	GN	GMC3sd	13	m	good		105
GN 10	Minimal Change	normal	GMgd	22	f	good	55	
GN 11	Minimal Change	normal	GMsd	22	f	good	151	

* = Death unrelated to renal function

Abbreviations:

A = Arteriolar hyalinosis, F = Interstitial fibrosis, I = Intimal fibrosis in arteries, GS = Glomerulosclerosis, GN = Glomerulonephritis, .1 = Slight, .2 = Medium, .3 = Severe, g = global, f = focal, d = diffuse, s = segmental

Specific or equivocally specific findings (group VII)

The biopsies in group VII (Table 1) could be classified according to their different pathologies into 4 categories:

glomerulosclerosis (n = 4),
glomerulonephritis (n = 11) (GN 1–11),
intravascular coagulation (n = 10) (IVC 1–10),
eclamptic kidney (n = 1).

Four of the biopsies (2.7% of the total number of biopsies, 3.9% of all donors) showed obvious diffuse global or segmental focal sclerosing glomerular lesions by lightmicroscopy. Of these, one was unsuitable for immunohistological examination, two of the remaining 3 demonstrated global diffuse deposits of IgM and complement C3, the final specimen was immunohistologically negative. Among the follow-up biopsies of cases with segmental or global glomerulosclerosis, it was shown that in one case, nephrectomized after 10 days, the "zero-hour" biopsy had been taken from an area of scar tissue. In the 3 other cases the findings either remained unchanged or there was a slight decrease in the glomerular sclerosis. Since the previously healthy kidney donors had not been subject to clinical investigation, it is not possible to pass comment on either the aetiology of these lesions or their prognostic significance.

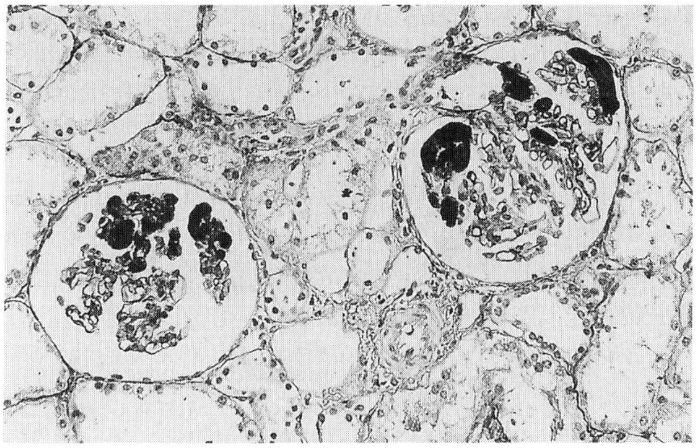

Fig. 6 Thrombi in zero-hour biopsy after staining with anti-fibrin(ogen).

Glomerulonephritis was discovered in 11 biopsies (7.9% of all donors), i.e. 8.7% of all biopsies examined immunohistologically (Table 5). The cases of glomerulonephritis were equally distributed over the different donor age groups. Glomerulonephritis was diagnosed by lightmicroscopy in only one of the 11 patients (GN 9). Nonspecific diffuse glomerulosclerosis was diagnosed in 2 further cases (GN 2, GN 4) and of the rest, 4 were judged to be unchanged lightmicroscopically (GN 1, 7, 10, 11) and in 4 others (GN 3, 5, 6, 8) only nonspecific interstitial and/or

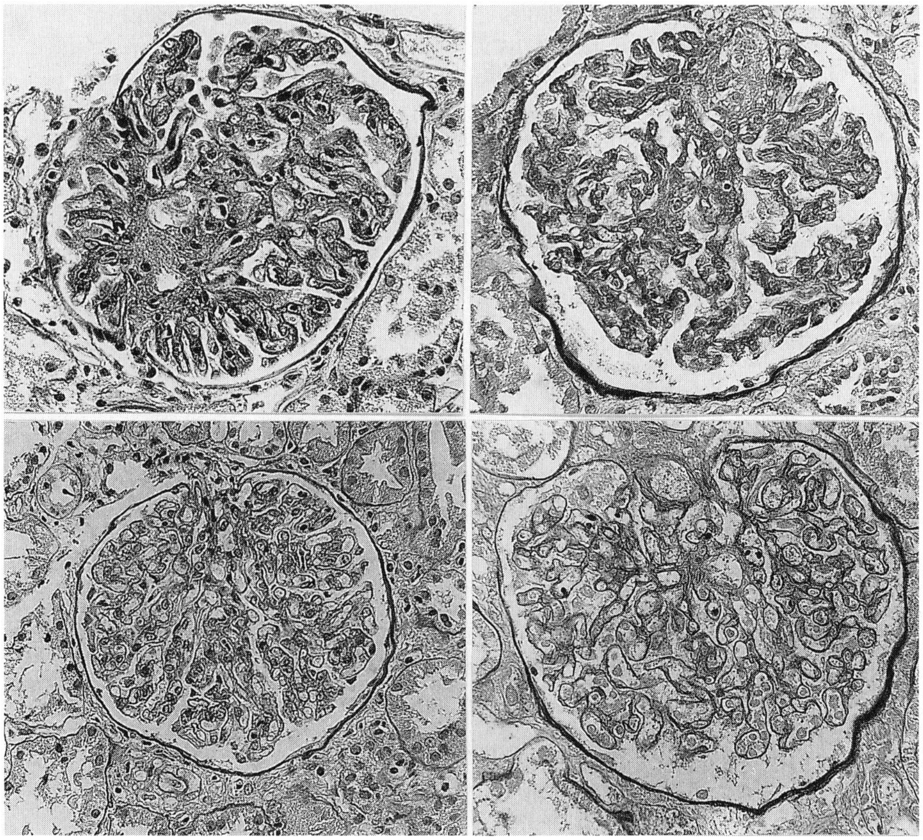

Fig. 7 Eclamptic kidney in zero-hour biopsy (upper left) and follow-up after transplantation: 5 days later (upper right), 26 days later (lower left) and 90 days later (lower right) showing progressive resolution of the initial glomerular lesion.

vascular changes were diagnosed. The glomerulonephritides were classified according to their immunohistological findings as follows: 7 IgA nephritides (nephropathies) of minimal grade (Figure 4), 2 glomerular minimal change with specific immuno-histological findings and 2 low grade mesangioproliferative glomerulonephritides (non IgA) (Table 5). There was no correlation between the occurrence of IgA nephropathy and the demonstration of HLA-DR 4 in either donor or recipient.

In 8 of the cases the further development of the glomerulonephritides after transplantation could be followed by means of rebiopsy. In 6 (GN 1, 3, 4, 6, 9, 11) of these 8 cases the rebiopsies, taken after variable intervals from 2 weeks to 4 months, were either immunohistologically negative (Figure 4) or, as occurred in one case (GN 3) showed only nonspecific IgM deposits (Figure 5). In the remaining 2 cases (GN 2, 7) the immunohistological findings persisted for 2 weeks and 3 months respectively (Figure 5). Of these one kidney (GN 2) had to be removed 2 weeks after transplantation due to complete vascular infarction. It is interesting to note that a control biopsy taken simultaneously from the second kidney from the same donor (GN 3) also showed persistent immunohistological findings after 2 weeks, 3 months later, however, only nonspecific IgM deposits were demonstrable and the renal function was good (Figure 5). In 2 further cases, in which both kidneys from each donor were transplanted (GN 5, 6; GN 10, 11), we received biopsy material from only one of each pair of kidneys at one month (GN 6) and 2 months (GN 11) after transplantation respectively. The immunohistological findings in both cases were negative. The renal function of all 4 kidneys was good more than 7 months after transplantation; from which we assume that the immune deposits present in the non-rebiopsied cases had disappeared (GN 5, 10) as well.

Among the 11 transplantees, the cause of end-stage renal disease was in only one case glomerulonephritis (MPGN Typ I) (GN 2); the remaining 10 were affected by disorders in diagnostic categories other than the glomerulonephritides. One of the above-mentioned transplantees (GN 2) received a kidney affected by IgA nephritis, which showed persistent morphological changes and had to be removed 2 weeks later due to total infarction. In view of the short time interval that ensued between reperfusion of the graft and performance of the "zero-hour" biopsy together with the clinical history of the recipient, it is unlikely that the glomerulonephritis arose de novo.

Lightmicroscopy revealed intravascular coagulation in 10 further biopsies (Table 6). The diagnosis was confirmed immunohistologically in the 7 of the 9 cases examined (Figure 6). There was considerable variation in the extent of intravascular coagulation. Between 8 and 100% of glomeruli showed either single or multiple fibrin thrombi (Table 6). There was no correlation between the duration of ischemia and the occurrence and extent of intravascular coagulation. In 2 cases (IVC 9, 10), in which renal biopsies were taken before reperfusion, intravascular coagulation indubitably had been present before transplantation. In the remaining patients it could have occurred after revascularisation. The initial renal function in 7 of the 10 patients was perfect, 3 (IVC 6, 7, 8) required dialysis. Three patients (IVC 3, 6, 7) lost their kid-

Table 6 Graft biopsies with intravascular coagulation

Case No	Lightmicroscopy % glomeruli affected (affected/ total	No. of glomeruli	Immuno-histology in glomeruli	Ischemia warm min	cold hours	Dialysis post tpl	Serum-creatinine after 1 year umol/l	Nephrectomy after transplant. days
Biopsies after Reperfusion								
IVC 1	17%	(1/ 6)	Fibrin	5	19	No	167	
IVC 2	25%	(1/ 4)	neg.	3	20.5	No	133	
IVC 3	100%	(7/ 7)	Fibrin	7	23	No		27, VR
IVC 4	100%	(3/ 3)	Fibrin	20	19.6	No	196	
IVC 5	8%	(1/13)	neg.	1	19.5	No	164	
IVC 6	100%	(22/22)	Fibrin + C3	2	32.2	Yes		4, IVC
IVC 7	100%	(14/14)	Fibrin + C3	2	34.4	Yes		3, IVC
IVC 8	100%	(3/ 3)	not done	0	25.2	Yes	188	
Biopsies before Reperfusion								
IVC 9	88%	(22/25)	Fibrin	3	5.5	No	117	
IVC 10	32%	(7/22)	Fibrin	3	9.3	No	125	

VR = Vascular Rejection
IVC = Intravascular Coagulation

neys, in one case (IVC 3) through vascular rejection, which led to nephrectomy on day 27, in two other patients (IVC 6, 7) due to total necrosis as a result of massive intravascular coagulation, which led to nephrectomy on days 3 and 4, respectively. A blood group incompatibility was present in both of the latter patients (IVC 6, 7). Recipients with blood group 0 had received kidneys from donors with blood group A_2. Posttransplantation rebiopsies from the patients with blood group incompatibilities had shown persistent intravascular coagulation. In one of the cases (IVC 3), nephrectomized because of vascular rejection, isolated residues of intravascular coagulation were still present. In the remaining 5 cases no residual intravascular coagulation was evident on rebiopsy. All 7 intact transplants showed good renal function one year later (Table 6).

One "zero-hour" biopsy taken from a female donor who died from eclamptic brain hemorrhage showed the morphological appearance characteristic of an eclamptic kidney. The morphological course after transplantation is presented in Figure 7. On rebiopsy 26 days after transplantation all signs of the previous eclampsia had disappeared. Initially the renal function was perfect, but on day 90 the kidney had to be removed due to thrombosis of the large vessel and subtotal renal infarction.

Discussion

In the material examined, 61.9% of all donor kidneys showed pathological changes. Most (71.4%) of these changes were nonspecific, though a proportion (28.6%) showed specific or equivocal findings. The nonspecific pathological changes were clearly age related. Whilst more than 50% of kidneys from donors aged 20 years or less showed no changes, this proportion fell to less than 20% in kidneys from donors over the age of 50.

It could be demonstrated that neither nonspecific lightmicroscopic and immunohistological changes nor donor age significantly influence the initial or late function of renal grafts [Rohr 1983, Shaff et al. 1979, Cerilli et al. 1978]. Accordingly, we refute the published view that the impaired survival of grafts obtained from donors aged 50 years or more is attributable to the nonspecific findings mentioned above [Rao et al. 1990].

We have been astounded by the frequency with which nonspecific immunohistological findings occur, and particularly by the fact that at follow-up 70% of biopsies no longer show any evidence of immune deposits. Other authors also have shown that the demonstration of immunohistological deposits cannot be used as an accurate indicator of renal function [Cerelli et al. 1978].

A further striking revelation, however, is that, in the material we examined, the proportion of specific or equivocal findings amounted to 17.7% of all kidneys and 20.8% of donors respectively. In other studies only 3.8% to 11.6% of the kidneys examined have shown evidence of glomerulonephritis, in addition to which only isolated cases of intravascular coagulation have hitherto been reported [Rohr 1983, Silva et al. 1982, Sanfilipo et al. 1982, Brutel de la Riviere and van de Putte 1976, Leunissen 1986, Shaff et al. 1979]. Neither from these findings nor from those reported in other studies has a correlation been established between preexistent lesions in the donor kidney and either the early or late function of the graft.

From the literature, however, it is known that even the severe glomerulosclerosis associated with diabetes may regress following transplantation [Abouna et al. 1983].

Follow-up observations in patients with glomerulonephritis are of particular interest. Both the preexisting deposits of immunoglobulins present at the time of transplantation usually disappear within 4 months of transplantation. In one case immunoglobulin deposits were no longer demonstrable as early as 2 weeks after transplantation.

Similar observations have previously been described, though to date only in isolated cases. In a series of 43 "zero-hour" biopsies, five had mesangioproliferative glomerulonephritis [Brutel de la Riviere and van de Putte 1976]. Of these, at follow-up biopsy, two had become immunohistologically negative, whereas in the remaining three cases the findings persisted. In all five cases, however, renal function at the end of the period of observation (150–503 days) was good. In another study, two cases of chronic glomerulonephritis were described out of a total of 57 "zero-hour" biopsies. Here too, renal function during the early weeks was good [Rohr 1983]. Poor renal function has been reported in some instances, in particular after transplantation of kidneys with IgA nephropathy. Five such cases have been reported. In four of these massive rejection reactions led to nephrectomy between four and eleven weeks after transplantation. Only one of the grafts still showed good renal function eight months after transplantation. This latter kidney was the right kidney of a female donor whose donated left kidney had to be removed after 9 weeks. In one of the grafts the IgA deposits had already disappeared by the time the first rebiopsy was taken at 12 days, whilst in the 3 nephrectomies minimal residual mesangial deposits of IgA were found. No follow-up biopsy was performed on the kidney that was functioning well [Sanfilipo et al. 1982, Silva et al. 1982]. One particularly interesting case reported in the literature describes the transplantation of a kidney from a clinically healthy brother to a younger brother with end-stage IgA nephropathy. IgA-positive mesangial deposits were found immunohistologically in the "zero-hour" biopsy of the transplanted kidney, thus establishing the diagnosis of IgA nephropathy. One year later both brothers were doing well showing no clinical signs of IgA nephropathy [Tolkoff-Rubin et al. 1978].

On the same theme, apparently it is quite safe to transplant kidneys whose "zero-hour" biopsies show massive intravascular coagulation (even those in which all the glomeruli demonstrate deposition of fibrin) into a recipient, provided that the recipient's fibrinolytic system is intact. In cases such as this no residua of the widespread intravascular coagulation are demonstrated on rebiopsy. Even eclamptic kidneys could be transplanted and achieve good initial function.

Ten of our "zero-hour" biopsies showed varying degrees of thrombus formation in the glomerular capillary loops. Since two of these biopsies had been taken before revascularisation, intravascular coagulation definitely was present prior to the initial contact of the kidney with the recipient's blood, which cannot be proven in the remaining 8 cases. Leunissen [1986] reported a case in which two kidneys from the same donor showed massive intravascular coagulation on the "zero-hour" biopsies yet follow-up biopsies taken seven days and six months after transplantation from both recipients were free of thrombi, and the renal function was good. Similar courses have been reported by other authors [Shaff et al. 1979].

On the basis of all these findings and in line with observations published in the literature it seems evident that subclinical forms of glomerulonephritis (IgA nephropathy) usually regress after transplantation without compromising the long term course of the graft. Therefore we would like to raise the provocative question whether also clinical forms of glomerulonephritides may regress after renal transplantation. Provided that a donor has normal renal function and that the state of the renal artery renders transplantation surgically feasible, why should there be hesitations in accepting such kidneys for transplantation. Therefore we would propose an intensified discussion and experimental studies to clarify the question whether a more liberal choice of donors is justified.

On the question of whether or not "zero-hour" biopsies of transplants should be performed, we would answer in the affirmative. The value of the "zero-hour" biopsy should not, however, be overestimated since normal renal tissue found by "zero-hour" biopsy does not exclude a focal lesion in the kidney. On the other hand any lesions found in "zero-hour" biopsies are helpful to avoid misdiagnosing, e.g., glomerulonephritis as early rejection, intimal fibrosis as sclerosing transplant vasculopathy or confusing arteriolar hyalinosis with changes due to previous treatment with CSA, it is important to know the nature of any damage to glomeruli, tubular-interstitial space and arterioles that already exists at the time of transplantation.

REFERENCES

Abouna GM, Al Adnani MS, Kremer GD, Kumar SA, Daddah SK, Kusma G 1983 Reversal of diabetic nephropathy in human cadaveric kidneys after transplantation into nondiabetic recipients. Lancet *2:* 1274

Brutel de la Riviere G, van de Putte LBA 1976 Preexisting glomerulonephritis in allografted kidneys. Arch Pathol Lab Med *100:* 196

Cerilli J, Holliday JE, Wilson CB, Sharma HM 1978 Clinical significance of the 1-hour biopsy in renal transplantation. Transplantation *26:* 91

Hsu S, Raine L, Fanger H 1981 Use of avidin-biotin-peroxidase complex (ABC) in immunoperoxidase techniques: a comparison between ABC and unlabeled antibody (PAP) procedures. J Histochem Cytochem *29:* 577

Kincaid-Smith P, Morris PJ, Saker BM, Ting A, Marshall VC 1968 Immediate renal graft biopsy and subsequent rejection. Lancet *1:* 748

Leunissen KML 1986 Intravascular coagulation and kidney donation. Transplantation *42:* 307

Rao KV, Kasiske BL, Odlund MD, Ney AL, Andersen RC 1990 Influence of cadaver donor age on posttransplant renal function and graft outcome. Transplantation *49:* 91

Rohr MS 1983 Renal allograft acute tubular necrosis II. A light and electron microscopic study of biopsies taken at procurement and after revascularisation. Ann Surg *197:* 663

Sanfilippo F, Croker BP, Bollinger RR 1982 Fate od four cadaveric donor renal allografts with mesangial IgA depots. Transplantation *33:* 370

Shaff D, Abrahams C, Meyers A 1979 A detailed analysis of the 1-hour posttransplant renal biopsy. Nephron *24:* 25

Silva FG, Chander P, Pirani CL, Hardy MA 1982 Disappearance of glomerular mesangial IgA deposits after renal allograft transplantation. Transplantation *33:* 214

Tolkoff-Rubin NE, Cosima AB, Fuller T, Rubin RH, Colvin RB 1978 IgA nephropathy in HLA-identical siblings. Transplantation *26:* 430

Zammit M, Toledo-Pereyra LH, Oh HK, Dienst SG 1980 Role of posttransplant kidney biopsy after hypothermic pulsatile perfusion. Am Surg *46:* 248

Zollinger HU, Mihatsch MJ 1978 Renall pathology in biopsy. Springer-Verlag Berlin, Heidelberg, New York

Clinical Nephrology, Vol. 36 No. 5 – 1991 (223–227)

A membranous nephropathy associated with adult polycystic kidney disease

K. SHIKATA, H. MAKINO and Z. OTA

Third Department of Internal Medicine, Okayama University Medical School, Okayama, Japan

Abstract. A 53-year-old woman with adult polycystic kidney disease (PKD) developed a nephrotic syndrome. Evaluation of the renal biopsy specimens showed typical findings of membranous nephropathy (MN). There are few reports of nephrotic syndrome associated with PKD and only one proved to be MN. The possible mechanism of the association of PKD with MN was evaluated. Autoantibodies against the brush border were not detected in this patient's serum by indirect immunofluorescence. Three monoclonal antibodies against the tubular brush border and epithelial cell of distal tubulus did not react with subepithelial deposits in the biopsy specimen. Therefore tubular brush border antigen which was reported to induce membranous nephropathy was not detected in the immune complexes deposited in the glomeruli. So we could not determine any direct relationship between PKD and MN. The reaction of antibodies against basement membrane components (type IV collagen, laminin, fibronectin, heparansulfate proteoglycan) with the basement membranes of the cysts was evaluated by indirect immunofluorescence. The reaction with anti-heparansulfate proteoglycan antibody was decreased compared with normal tubular basement membrane. The reactivity to anti-fibronectin antibody was remarkably increased in the cystic walls, tubules, and interstitium. Changes of tubular basement membrane antigens was observed in PKD.

Key words: membranous nephropathy – polycystic kidney disease – monoclonal antibody – type IV collagen – laminin – heparansulfate proteoglycan – fibronectin

Introduction

While proteinuria is frequently detected in adult polycystic kidney disease (PKD), it is commonly intermittent and amounts to less than 3 g/day [Delaney et al. 1985, Gardner et al. 1988]. To our knowledge, only one case of membranous nephropathy (MN) has been confirmed to be associated with PKD [Abe et al. 1985].

To investigate the relationship between MN and PKD in one patient, cryostat sections of normal human kidney were incubated with the patient's serum using indirect immunofluorescence technique. Cryostat sections of the patient's kidney were incubated with monoclonal antibodies against human tubular brush border using indirect immunofluorescence technique.

Using this biopsy specimen, the reactivity of the antibodies against the basement membrane antigens (type IV collagen, laminin, heparansulfate proteoglycan (HSPG) and fibronectin) with the basement membrane of the cystic lesions were examined.

Received December 27, 1990; in revised form May 8, 1991.

Reprint requests to Dr. K. Shikata, Third Department of Medicine, Okayama University Medical School, Okayama, 700 Japan

Case report

A 53-year-old woman admitted to Okayama University Medical School Hospital in April 1988 with general edema and massive proteinuria. Although PKD had been diagnosed in 1986, proteinuria was not detected at that time. In 1986, she developed slight glucosuria and mild hyperglycemia for which neither oral antidiabetic therapy nor insulin were required. Family history revealed that a nephew had died of renal failure but was otherwise noncontributory.

On admission, she had marked edema of the face and legs. Giant masses were palpable on both sides of the abdomen. Blood pressure was 160/100 mmHg.

Laboratory findings: WBC was 8,700/mm^3 with a normal differential count, RBC 390 × 10^4/mm^3, hemoglobin 11.8 g/dl, hematocrit 35.7%, platelets 21.3 × 10^4/mm^3. Erythrocyte sedimentation rate was 128 mm/h. Urinary protein was 5–6 g/day, urinary sugar was negative. Urinary sediment: RBC 3–5/

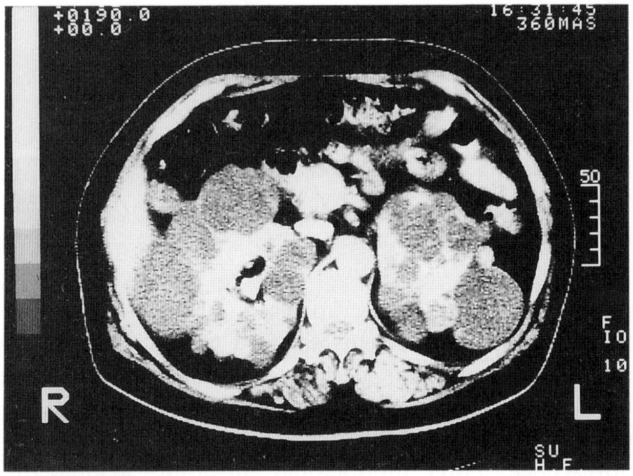

Fig. 1 Enhanced abdominal CT scan. Both kidneys are enlarged with multiple cysts.

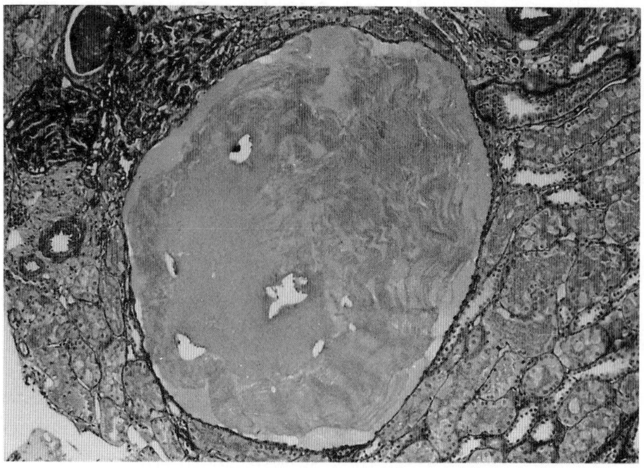

Fig. 2 PAM staining. Note the compression of tubules and glomeruli around a cyst (×800).

HPF, WBC 3–5/HPF, several epithelial cells. BUN 17.0 mg/dl, creatinine 1.0 mg/dl, total protein 4.9 g/dl, albumin 2.2 g/dl, total cholesterol 478 mg/dl. Creatinine clearance rate was 56.3 ml/min, PSP test 4.1% (15 min). Fasted blood sugar was 123 mg/dl. The following tests were negative or within the normal range: liver function tests, hepatitis B surface antigen and antibody, serum complement (CH50, C3, C4), immunoglobulins (IgG, IgA, IgM), anti-nuclear antibody, anti-DNA antibody, rheumatoid factor, ASO, and serum electrolytes.

Ultrasonography and CT scan revealed multiple cysts of various sizes in both kidneys and small cysts in the liver (Figure 1). An open renal biopsy was performed. The specimen was evaluated by immunofluorescence, light microscopy and electron microscopy. The patient was administered prednisolone and dipyridamole with no effect on the proteinuria.

Materials and methods

The renal biopsy specimen was divided into three portions. The block for light microscopy was stained with hematoxylin and eosin, periodic acid-Schiff (PAS), periodic acid-silver methenamine (PAM) and Masson. A small block for immunofluorescence study was quickly frozen, cut at 4 µm on a cryostat and stained by FITC-conjugated antiserum specific for human IgG, IgA, IgM, C3, C1q and fibrinogen. The remaining block was examined by electron microscopy.

To detect autoantibodies against the kidney tissue, cryostat sections of a kidney from a patient operated for a kidney tumor were stained with our

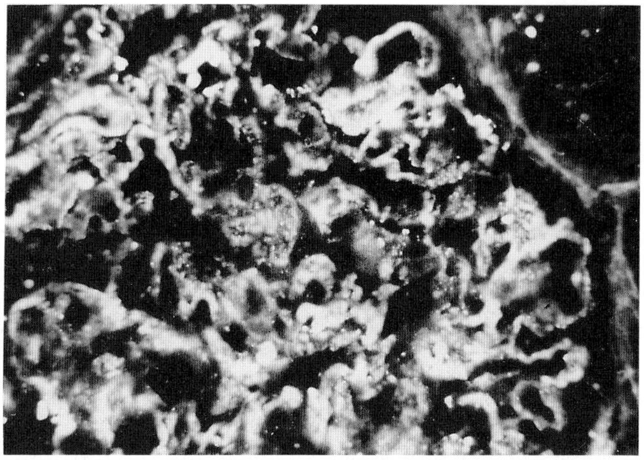

Fig. 3 Immunofluorescence microscopy of the glomeruli for IgG. The glomerular capillary walls are stained in a granular pattern (×800).

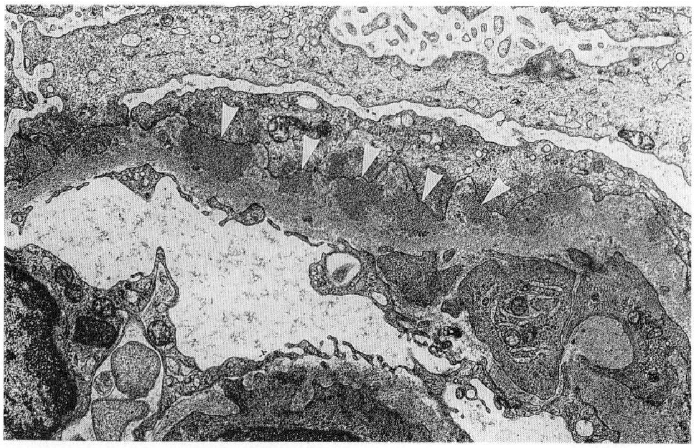

Fig. 4 Electron microscopy. Note the electron dense deposits of varying size in the subepithelium (arrow heads) (×12,000).

patient's serum and then with FITC-conjugated anti-human IgG serum.

Cryostat sections from our patient were processed for indirect immunofluorescence. These sections were incubated with the first set of three monoclonal antibodies at 37° C for 30 min. These antibodies were produced by immunizing BALB/c mice with a microsome fraction of normal human kidney homogenate essentially by the same method as in our previous publication [Mino et al. 1984]. Specificity of these antibodies was examined by immunofluorescence and immunoperoxidase staining. Two antibodies reacted to the brush border of the proximal tubules, and the third reacted to epithelial cells of the distal tubules of normal human kidney [Ota et al. 1986]. They were washed three times with phosphate buffer saline (PBS) pH 7.4. Specimens were then incubated for another 30 min with anti-mouse IgG conjugated with FITC (Cappel Products, USA). Sections of kidney tissue from a patient operated on for a kidney tumor were stained as controls.

The remainder of the cryostat sections were processed for indirect immunofluorescence. The following polyclonal antibodies were employed as the first set of antibodies: anti-type IV collagen antibody (Advance Co. Ltd., Japan), anti-laminin antibody (EY Laboratories Inc., USA), anti-HSPG antibody [Makino et al. 1986], and anti-fibronectin antibody (Advance Co. Ltd., Japan). Anti-rabbit IgG antibody conjugated with FITC (Cappel Products, USA) was used as the second antibody. Normal portions of the operated human kidney were stained as controls.

Results

Renal biopsy findings: In the specimen examined by light microscopy, 5 of the 50 observed glomeruli showed global sclerosis. There was diffuse thickening of the capillary walls, and mild hypercellularity of the mesangial area. Focal cellular infiltration was noted in the interstitium. Two cysts were present in the

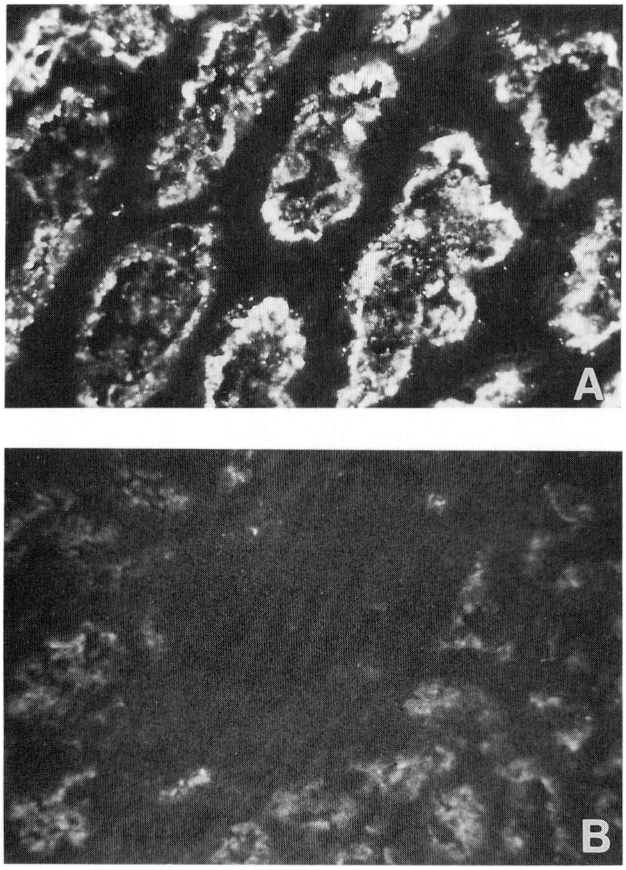

Fig. 5 Sections from the control kidney (A) and that of the patient (B) stained with a monoclonal antibody against human proximal tubular brush border. (A) Proximal tubular brush border is stained (×800). (B) Glomerulus is not stained and a loss of staining in the tubular brush border is observed (×800).

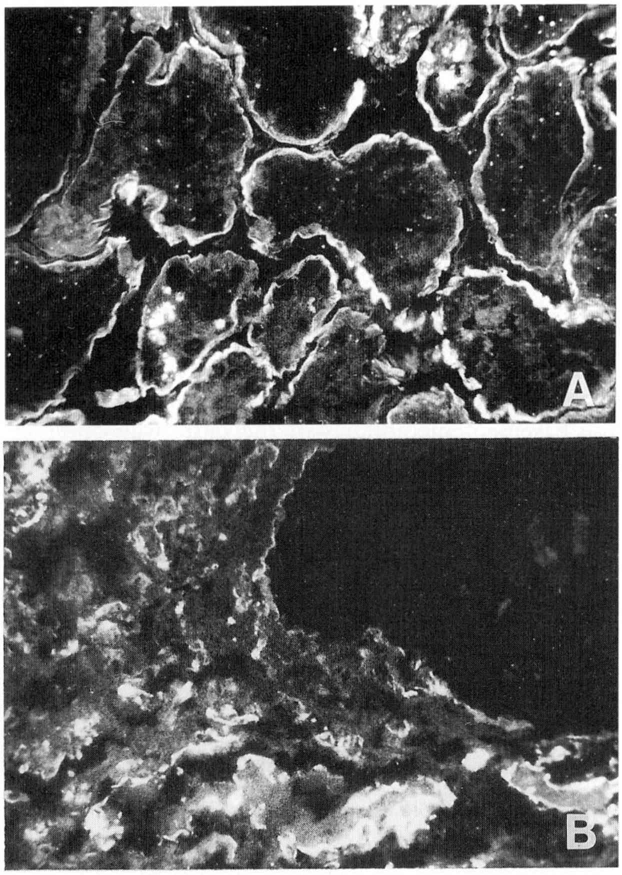

Fig. 6 Sections from the control kidney (A) and that of the patient (B) stained with anti-HSPG antibody (×800). (A) The tubular basement membrane is stained intensely. (B) Note the focal loss of HSPG staining in the cystic wall (×800).

specimen. Tubules were compressed around the cysts (Figure 2). PAM staining showed numerous spike formations on the peripheral glomerular capillary walls. By immunofluorescence study, there was a remarkable diffuse granular staining of the capillary walls with anti-IgG and anti-C3 antiserum (Figure 3). Staining for IgA, IgM, and C1q were negative. There was focal staining in the interstitium for anti-fibrinogen antiserum. On electron microscopic study, the GBM was thickened and the foot processes of epithelial cells were effaced. Numerous electron-dense deposits of varying size were present in the subepithelium, and "spikes" were also observed (Figure 4). Mesangial areas were not expanded and mesangial sclerosis was not observed.

Staining for monoclonal antibodies against the tubular brush border and epithelial cell: In the control normal specimens, the proximal and distal tubular epithelial cells were stained with each corresponding monoclonal antibody. In the biopsy specimen, the glomeruli were not stained with these monoclonal antibodies. The tubules were stained in the same pattern as the control specimens (Figure 5).

Staining for the antibodies against basement membrane antigens: In the control specimens, the antibodies against type IV collagen, HSPG and laminin revealed linear immunofluorescence of tubular basement membranes and glomerular capillary walls. The anti-fibronectin antibody stained the mesangial areas. Tubular basement membranes and capillary walls were weakly stained. In the cystic regions of the biopsy specimen, the anti-type IV collagen and the anti-laminin antibodies stained the basement membranes of cysts as well as the tubular basement membranes of the control specimen. When stained with the anti-HSPG antibody, a loss of immunofluorescence of the basement membranes of the cysts was observed (Figure 6). The remaining tubules were stained with the anti-HSPG antibody as well as the controls. The anti-fibronectin antibody stained intensely the basement membranes of the cysts, the interstitium and the tubules around the cysts.

Discussion

Histological findings of renal biopsy specimens in this patient confirmed the diagnosis of MN. There were no significant diabetic changes. Proteinuria is frequently detected in PKD patients; however it is typically intermittent and amounts to less than 3 g/day. Thus, the massive proteinuria in our patient was considered to be caused by MN.

Several patients with nephrotic syndrome associated with PKD have been reported previously. Feldstein reported one case and Ackerman two cases of nephrotic syndrome associated with PKD, although renal biopsy was not performed [Feldstein et al. 1969, Ackerman et al. 1971]. Two cases of minimal change nephrotic syndrome associated with PKD have been reported [Kida et al. 1972, Inoue et al. 1989]. One case of focal glomerular sclerosis associated with PKD has been reported [Murphy et al. 1990]. To the best of our knowledge, only one case of MN associated with PKD has been reported [Abe et al. 1985]. Immune complex-type glomerulonephritis associated with PKD has not been reported.

Various disorders such as collagen disease, cancer, thyroid disease and viral hepatitis are occasionally associated with MN. None of these conditions was present in this patient. She had not received such agents as d-penicillamine or gold, which occasionally induce MN.

The relationship between MN and PKD was investigated. Brush border antigens have been reported to induce membranous nephropathy [Heymann et al. 1959, Edginton et al. 1968, Damme 1978]. In the biopsy specimen, the tubules around the renal cysts were compressed and some were destroyed. It is possible that degenerated tubular epithelium may have entered the circulation and acted as an antigen. However, antibody against the brush border was not detected in this patient's serum by indirect immunofluorescence, and the monoclonal antibodies against the tubular brush border and epithelial cell of distal tubulus did not react with the subepithelial deposits. The pathogenic relationship between MN and PKD thus remains unclear.

PKD is characterized by bilateral renal enlargement due to focal expansive cystic dilatation of the tubules [Grantham 1983]. The cysts in PKD may arise from any point along the nephron [Kissane 1983]. Chanard et al. [1982] reported that renal excretion of 3 hydroxyproline were increased in PKD. Carone et al. [1988] examined the reactivity of the basement membrane of cystic lesions from PKD kidney tissue with basement membrane antigens. They reported that the reactivity to HSPG was decreased and the reactivity to fibronectin increased. In our patients, we observed a loss of reactivity to HSPG and a remarkable increase in the reactivity to fibronectin in the basement membranes of the cysts, and in the interstitium and tubules around the cysts. These findings are consistent with the observations of Carone et al. [1988]Tubular cell disorder in PKD might have caused the defective synthesis of TBM components [Carone et al. 1988].

Although we failed to demonstrate the direct relationship between PKD and MN, extensive studies are necessary for the detection of antigenic components in MN.

Acknowledgement

This research was supported in part by Uehara Medical Foundation and by a Research Grant for "Progressive renal disease" from "Specially selected diseases by the Ministry of Health and Welfare Research Project", the Ministry of Health and Welfare of Japan.

REFERENCES

Abe R, Yamaguchi K, Igarashi N, Fukuda Y, Kawaguchi K 1985 A case of polycystic kidney associated with membranous nephropathy. Kidney and Dialysis *9:* 389

Ackerman GL 1971 Nephrotic syndrome in polycystic renal disease. J Urol *105:* 7

Carone FA, Makino H, Kanwar YS 1988 Basement membrane antigens in renal polycystic disease. Am J Pathol *130:* 466

Chanard J, Szymanowicz A, Brunois JP, Toupance O, Malin JP, Birembaut P, Randoux A, Borel PJ 1982 Increased renal excretion of 3 hydroxyproline in patients with active glomerular nephropathies and with polycystic renal disease. Clin Nephrol *17:* 64

Damme BJCV, Fleuren GJ, Bakker WW, Varnier RL, Haedemaeker PJ 1978 Experimental glomerulonephritis in the rat induced by antibodies directed against tubular antigens. Lab Invest *38:* 502

Delaney VB, Adler S, Bruns FJ 1985 Autosomal dominant polycystic kidney disease: presentation, complications, and prognosis. Am J Kidney Dis *5:* 104

Edginton TS, Glassock RJ, Dixon FJ 1968 Autosomal dominant polycystic kidney disease: presentation, complications, and prognosis. Am J Kidney Dis *5:* 104

Feldstein CA, Seever AM, Nadal MA, Gotlieb D 1969 Sindrome nephrotico asociado corinon poliquistico. Rev Argentina Urol Nephrol *38:* 259

Gardner KD 1988 Cystic Kidneys. Kidney Int *33:* 610

Grantham JJ 1983 Polycystic kidney disease: A predominance of giant nephrons. Am J Physiol *244:* 3

Heymann W, Hackel DB, Harwood J, Wilson SGF, Hunter JLP 1959 Production of nephrotic syndrome in rats by Freund's adjuvants and rat kidney suspensions. Proc Soc Exp Biol Med *100:* 660

Inoue T, Nakahama H, Kakihara M, Takama T, Mikami Y, Orita Y, Kamata T 1989 Nephrotic syndrome in polycystic disease. Kidney and Dialysis *26:* 1145

Kida H, Nakamoto Y, Shinoda A 1972 Polycystic kidney complicated by nephrotic syndrome. Naika *29:* 168

Kissane JM 1983 Congenital malformations. In: *Heptinstall RH* (ed) Pathology of the kidney. Little, Brown and Company vol 1, p 83

Makino H, Gibbons JT, Reddy MK, Kanwar YS 1986 Nephritogenecity of antibodies to proteoglycans of the glomerular basement membrane-1. J Clin Invest *77:* 142

Mino Y, Hirakawa S, Ota Z 1984 Production of monoclonal antibodies to human glomerular basement membrane. Acta Med Okayama *38:* 483

Murphy G, Tzamaloukas AT, Listrom MB, Gibel LJ, Smith SM, Gardner KD 1990 Nephrotic syndrome and rapid renal failure in autosomal dominant polycystic kidney disease. Am J Nephrol *10:* 69

Ota Z, Mino Y, Taniai K, Hirakawa N, Kashihara N, Takahashi K 1986 Assay of renal antigens in urine of renal disease. Annual report from group studies of "Progressive renal diseases" supported by the Research Grant from "Specially selected diseases by the Ministry of Health and Welfare Research Project", the Ministry of Health and Welfare of Japan p 141

Clinical Nephrology, Vol. 36 No. 5 – 1991 (228–233)

Urine kallikrein excretion in relation to renal sodium handling in minimal change nephrotic syndrome

N. Ueda, Y. Niinomi and T. Nonoda

Department of Pediatrics, Fujita Gakuen Health University School of Medicine, Toyoake, Kariya General Hospital, Kariya, Aichi, Japan

Abstract. Twenty-four-hour urine kallikrein excretion (Uka), urine protein excretion, renal sodium handling, and the activity of the renin-angiotensin-aldosterone system were serially studied in 11 children at three different stages of the minimal change nephrotic syndrome (MCNS) – edema forming state, proteinuric steady state in which a relapse of the disease was just starting but no edema as yet and remission. The value for Uka was significantly increased in the edema forming state in contrast to the normal values of proteinuric steady state and remission. Serum sodium concentration was only decreased in the edema forming state and the degree of hypoalbuminemia and proteinuria did not differ between the edema forming and proteinuric steady states. Urine volume, absolute and fractional sodium excretion were significantly decreased in the edema forming and proteinuric steady states as compared with those in remission, suggesting that sodium retention was present in both states of the disease although the change in these parameters was more profound in the edema forming state than in the proteinuric steady state. Creatinine clearance did not differ among each stage of the disease. Plasma renin activity and plasma aldosterone concentration were significantly increased in the edema forming state as compared with those in the proteinuric steady state and remission. Plasma renin activity and plasma aldosterone concentration were significantly correlated directly with Uka and plasma aldosterone concentration was correlated inversely with urine sodium excretion. No relation was noted between Uka and other variables. The data indicate that while the renal kallikrein-kinin system seems to be independent of proteinuria or hypoalbuminemia, it is functionally linked to the renin-angiotensin-aldosterone system, and activated only when sodium retention reaches a critical level that could result in edema formation in children with MCNS.

Key words: renal kallikrein excretion – sodium retention – edema – renin-angiotensin-aldosterone system – nephrotic syndrome

Introduction

The kidney contains several hormonal systems – kallikrein-kinin, renin-angiotensin-aldosterone, and prostaglandins, which serve as renal self-regulatory mechanisms, and participate in the pathogenesis of human hypertension and renal disease [Levinsky 1979, Scicli and Carretero 1986]. In experimental studies the renal kallikrein has been shown to induce natriuresis and glomerular vasodilation [Levinsky 1979, Scicli and Carretero 1986], and increase glomerular permeability resulting in proteinuria [Murakami et al. 1968, McFarlane et al. 1973]. Similarly, activation of plasma kallikrein-kinin system has been suggested to play a role in the genesis of proteinuria in children with minimal change nephrotic syndrome (MCNS) [Kallen and Lee 1975]. It is generally accepted, however, that plasma kallikrein is distinct from the renal kallikrein which localizes mainly in the distal nephron, and that it might not reflect accurate intrarenal events as compared with urine kallikrein which appears identical to the renal kallikrein [Levinsky 1979, Scicli and Carretero 1986]. Recently, Cumming et al. [1985, 1989] found that in adult nephrotic patients with various types of renal diseases, urine kallikrein excretion was increased as compared with patients who did not have nephrotic proteinuria and that there was a functional link between the renal kallikrein-kinin and renin-angioten-

Received September 11, 1990; in revised form June 20, 1991.

Reprint requests to Dr. Norishi Ueda, University of Arkansas for Medical Sciences, Department of Medicine, Division of Nephrology, Slot 501, 4301 West Markham, Little Rock, Arkansas 72205, USA sin-aldosterone systems. They also described that these two hormonal systems were independent in some of their patients with the nephrotic syndrome. In these studies, however, the changes in urine kallikrein excretion were not evaluated separately and serially during the different disease states of the nephrotic syndrome.

The physiological role of the renal kallikrein-kinin system and the relationship between the renal kallikrein-kinin and renin-angiotensin-aldosterone systems are not clearly defined in the nephrotic syndrome [Brouhard et al. 1979, Cumming and Robson 1985, Cumming et al. 1989]. In addition, the change in the renal kallikrein excretion evaluated separately during different disease states of MCNS, especially in relation to edema formation, has not been previously reported. The present study was designed, therefore, to determine: (1) which disease state of MCNS is associated with increased urine kallikrein excretion, and (2) the relationship of urine kallikrein excretion and urine protein excretion, renal sodium handling, and renin-angiotensin-aldosterone system in children with MCNS.

Materials and methods

Eleven consecutive children with MCNS (9 boys), as characterized by the classical clinical and laboratory features and renal biopsy [Ueda et al. 1988], whose ages ranged from 3 to 14 years with a mean of 9.3 years, were included in the study. All patients were normotensive and their serum creatinine concentration was less than 1.5 mg/dl at the time of the study. Each patient was hospitalized during the study and placed on a diet with constant sodium and potassium intake. The fixed sodium intake depended on a dietary assessment of what they ate and this varied from 90 to 150 mEq/m^2 of sodium per day. None of the patients received diuretics, albumin infusions or other drugs known to affect urine kallikrein excretion except for prednisolone at least 3 days prior to the study. The informed consent was obtained from the parents of each child prior to the investigations.

Twenty-four-hour urine kallikrein excretion (Uka) and other variables (see below) were serially studied at the different disease states of MCNS; proteinuric state (proteinuria ≥ 40 $mg/hr/m^2$ for 3 consecutive days) and remission with normal albumin concentration. According to the presence or absence of edema, the proteinuric state was divided into two substages: edema forming state and proteinuric steady state as previously described [Bohlin and Berg 1984]. The patients in proteinuric steady state were just starting a relapse of the nephrotic syndrome, had no edema as yet, and had had a constant weight during the 3 days prior to the study. Edema formation was defined as a weight gain during the 3 days preceding the study, and all patients with edema formation gained more than 1.5% of their dry weight per day. Dry weight was determined as the stable weight just after proteinuria remitted.

Despite the fact that the administration of a large dose of ACTH and dexamethasone stimulates Uka in normal man [Vinci et al. 1979, Lopez et al. 1983], it is not known whether oral doses of prednisolone affect Uka in patients with the nephrotic syndrome. We also, therefore, investigated the change in Uka during each disease state of MCNS between patients treated with oral prednisolone and those without. The patients were treated with daily oral prednisolone of 60 mg/m^2 for 4 weeks, with the dose being tapered every 2 weeks and given daily or on alternate days for approximately 4 months. At the time of the study, 4 of the 11 patients were being treated with prednisolone during edema forming state, 6 of the patients in proteinuric steady state were being treated with prednisolone, and 8 of the patients in remission were on a low dose of prednisolone.

The preceding 24-hour urine was collected for the determination of kallikrein, protein, sodium, and

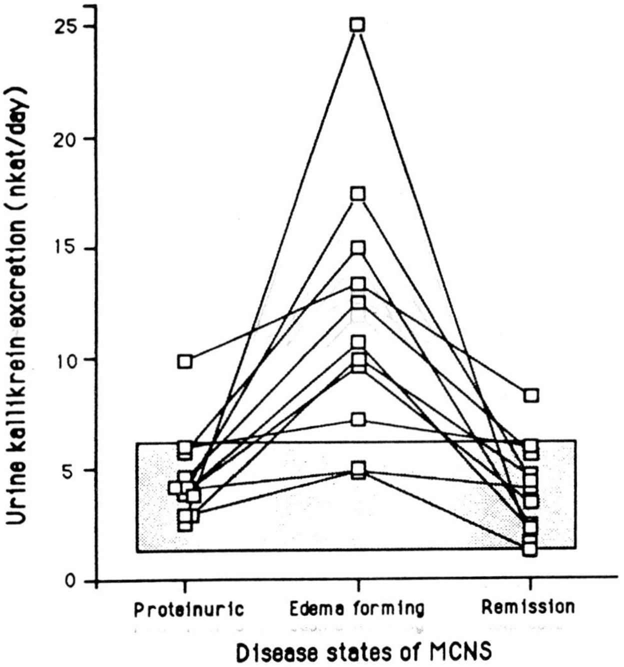

Fig. 1 Serial change in 24-hour urine kallikrein excretion in individual patients at different disease states of minimal change nephrotic syndrome – proteinuric steady state, edema forming state, and remission. Shaded area represents the range of 30 age-matched healthy children (3.7 ± 2.4 nkat/day; 13 boys, mean age, 10.8 ± 4.0 years) with a free diet and water intake.

creatinine. Absolute and fractional sodium excretion, endogenous creatinine clearance, and serum concentrations of albumin, sodium and creatinine were determined simultaneously. For the measurement of plasma renin activity and plasma aldosterone concentration, blood was taken from each patient at 8 a.m. after at least 8 hours of recumbency. Only urine samples for the determination of Uka were stored at −20° C and estimated within 2 months.

Uka was measured by the method of Amundsen et al. [1979]. In brief, urine was incubated for 30 min at 37° C with a synthetic chromogenic tripeptide substrate, for which urine kallikrein was specific (S 2266; AB Kabi, Sweden). The absorbance at 405 nm using Beckman spectrophotometer (UV 5250) was then compared with that of the same incubation mixture containing aprotinin (trasylol; Bayer, Leverkusen, Germany). Results were expressed as units of kallikrein activity per 24 hours (nkat/day). To validate the effect of proteinuria on the assay for Uka, a solution of human albumin (5 g/100 ml, The Green Cross Corporation, Japan) was added to the urine samples obtained from 5 age-matched healthy children with a free diet and water intake, to achieve a protein concentration in the sample equivalent to that in nephrotic urine (10 g/l). The value for Uka in the 5 control samples was not affected after the addition of albumin solution (control urines 3.9 ± 1.5 nkat/l vs. urine samples plus albumin solution 3.7 ± 0.8 nkat/l, $p > 0.05$). Thus, the kallikrein assay appeared valid even in the presence of heavy proteinuria as previously described [Cumming and Robson 1985].

Serum concentrations of albumin, sodium and creatinine, urine excretion of protein, sodium and creatinine, fractional sodium excretion, and endogenous creatinine clearance were measured by the standard methods. Plasma renin activity and plasma aldosterone concentration were determined by radioimmunoassay as previously described [Meltzer et al. 1979].

Data are expressed as means ± SD. A comparison of means of variables was done by the paired Student's t test except where otherwise stated, and the correlation coefficients were calculated by linear regression analysis. P value less than 0.05 was taken as statistically significant.

Results

The values for Uka in patients treated with oral prednisolone and those without at three different disease states of MCNS were 16.8 ± 5.6 (n = 4) vs. 15.4 ± 5.4 (n = 7) nkat/day in the edema forming state, 4.9 ± 2.5 (n = 6) vs. 4.1 ± 1.1 (n = 5) nkat/day in the proteinuric steady state, and 3.9 ± 2.4 (n = 8) vs. 4.0 ± 0.6 (n = 3) nkat/day in remission, respectively. Since there was no significant difference in the value for Uka during each disease state of MCNS between patients treated with prednisolone and those without (by unpaired Student's t test), the value for Uka and other variables were integrated and a comparison was made between each state of the disease.

Table 1 Urine kallikrein excretion, renal sodium handling, plasma renin activity, and plasma aldosterone concentration in minimal change nephrotic syndrome

	Edema forming state (1)	Proteinuric steady state (2)	Remission (3)	P value
Body weight change (% dry weight)	10.0 ± 5.5	–	–	
Urine kallikrein excretion (nkat/day)	11.5 ± 5.9	4.5 ± 2.1	3.9 ± 2.2	0.01 (1 vs. 2, 3)
Serum sodium concentration (mEq/l)	136.7 ± 1.9	137.3 ± 2.7	139.1 ± 1.6	0.01 (1 vs. 3)
Serum albumin concentration (g/dl)	1.8 ± 0.3	1.9 ± 0.5	4.3 ± 0.4	0.01 (1, 2 vs. 3)
Urine protein excretion (g/day)	3.8 ± 2.3	3.3 ± 2.2	0	0.01 (1, 2 vs. 3)
Urine volume (l/day)	0.54 ± 0.17	0.60 ± 0.34	0.94 ± 0.33	0.01 (1 vs. 3) 0.05 (2 vs. 3)
Urine sodium excretion (mEq/m²/day)	16.0 ± 19.0	41.6 ± 39.7	78.1 ± 36.0	0.05 (1 vs. 2) 0.01 (1 vs. 3) 0.05 (2 vs. 3)
Fractional sodium excretion (%)	0.20 ± 0.18	0.37 ± 0.25	0.62 ± 0.39	0.05 (1 vs. 2) 0.01 (1 vs. 3) 0.05 (2 vs. 3)
Creatinine clearance (ml/min/m²)	101.3 ± 47.7	108.4 ± 35.2	123.1 ± 32.5	NS
Plasma renin activity (ng/ml/hr)	7.2 ± 6.6	2.0 ± 1.5	3.4 ± 2.5	0.05 (1 vs. 2, 3)
Plasma aldosterone concentration (pg/ml)	199.0 ± 128.2	60.3 ± 20.1	63.4 ± 21.1	0.01 (1 vs. 2, 3)

Data are expressed as means ± SD. NS = not significant.

Figure 1 illustrates the serial change in Uka obtained from the individual patients studied. In the proteinuric steady state, in which a relapse of the nephrotic syndrome was just starting but no edema as yet, the value for Uka (4.5 ± 2.1 nkat/day) was similar to those in remission (3.9 ± 2.2 nkat/day) and in 30 age-matched healthy children (3.7 ± 2.4 nkat/day; 13 boys, mean age 10.8 ± 4.0 years) with a free diet and water intake (by unpaired Student's t test). In contrast, the value for Uka was significantly increased in the edema forming state (11.5 ± 5.9 nkat/day) as compared with those in the proteinuric steady state and remission (Table 1, $p < 0.01$ for both). The delta of Uka from the value of remission in the proteinuric steady state and edema forming state were 0.6 ± 1.6 and 7.9 ± 6.5 nkat/day respectively, and the difference was significant ($p < 0.01$).

The data on weight change, and other relevant biochemical findings at different disease states of MCNS is summarized in Table 1. Serum sodium concentration was lower in the edema forming state ($p < 0.01$) than in the proteinuric steady state. However, serum sodium concentration in the proteinuric steady state was not statistically different from that in remission. The degree of hypoalbuminemia and proteinuria in the edema forming state was similar to that in the proteinuric steady state. Urine volume was lower in the edema forming state ($p < 0.01$) and proteinuric steady state ($p < 0.05$) than in remission, but there was no significant difference in urine volume between the edema forming state and proteinuric steady state. Absolute and fractional sodium excretion were both lower in the edema forming state ($p < 0.01$ for both) and the proteinuric steady state ($p < 0.05$ for both) than in remission, but the change was more profound in the edema forming state ($p < 0.05$ for both) than in the proteinuric steady state. Creatinine clearance did not differ significantly among each disease state of MCNS.

Plasma renin activity and plasma aldosterone concentration were significantly increased in the edema forming state as compared with those observed in the proteinuric steady state and remission (Table 1, $p < 0.05$, $p < 0.01$, respectively). There was no difference in these parameters between the proteinuric steady state and remission. As illustrated in Figure 2, the Uka was significantly correlated directly with plasma renin activity ($r = 0.592$, $p < 0.01$) and plasma aldosterone concentration ($r = 0.584$, $p < 0.01$). Although plasma aldosterone concentration was correlated inversely with urine sodium excretion ($r = -0.486$, $p < 0.05$), there was no correlation between plasma aldosterone concentration and fractional sodium excretion. No correlation was found between absolute, fractional sodium excretion and plasma renin activity, nor between Uka and any other variable except for plasma renin activity and plasma aldosterone concentration.

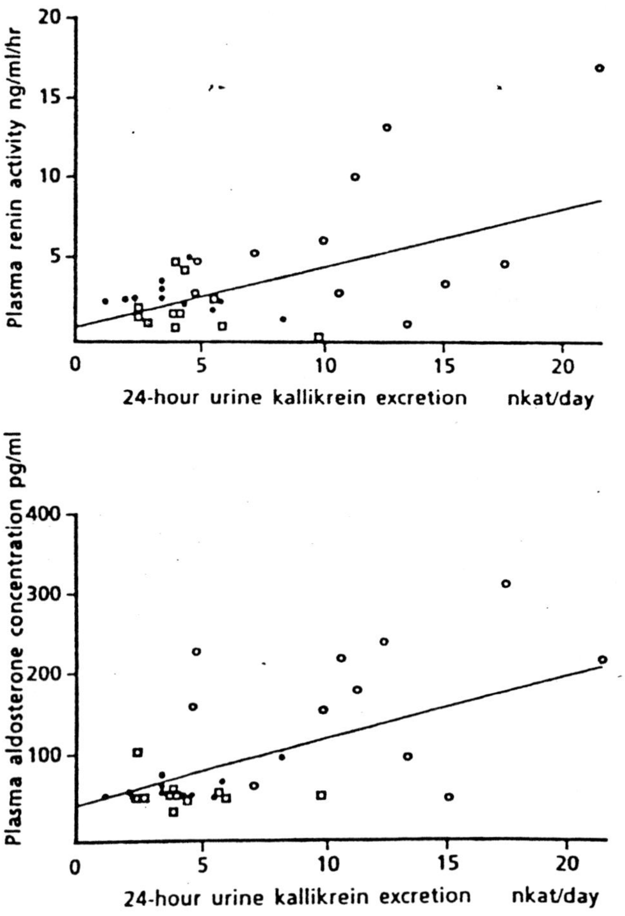

Fig. 2 Correlations between 24-hour urine kallikrein excretion and plasma renin activity ($r = 0.592$, $p < 0.01$, $n = 33$) and plasma aldosterone concentration ($r = 0.584$, $p < 0.01$, $n = 33$). Edema forming state is indicated by open circles, proteinuric steady state by open squares, and remission by closed circles.

Discussion

According to the classic theory, lowering of the plasma albumin concentration is the initiating step in renal sodium retention, resulting in a reduction in the colloid oncotic pressure of the blood, favoring movement of water from intravascular to interstitial space and producing hypovolemia [Brown et al. 1982, Bernard 1988]. Hypovolemia, in turn, activates volume sensors and baroreceptors which signal the kidney to retain salt and water. Several recent studies, however, failed to confirm this theory, and edema is not present in many instances of severe hypoalbuminemia in experimental animals and humans [Brown et al. 1982, Van Liew et al. 1985, Bernard

1988]. Recently, an alternate hypothesis has been advanced to explain sodium retention in the nephrotic syndrome, namely, that primary intrarenal mechanisms in nephrotic kidney cause a reduction in renal sodium excretion rather than systemic factors including renin-angiotensin-aldosterone system [Brown et al. 1982, Bernard 1988]. The intrarenal factors responsible for sodium retention could be related to either a decreased filtered load or increased tubular reabsorption of sodium [Bohlin and Berg 1984, Bernard 1988]. In the present study, we found severe sodium retention and increases in plasma renin activity and plasma aldosterone concentration during the edema forming state of MCNS. However, this hormonal system was not activated during the proteinuric steady state, in which a relapse of the nephrotic syndrome was just starting but no edema as yet, despite the presence of mild sodium retention and hypoalbuminemia equivalent to that observed in the edema forming state. This suggests that sodium retention is present prior to an activation of the renin-angiotensin-aldosterone system in children with MCNS. Although a weak inverse correlation was noted between absolute urine sodium excretion and plasma aldosterone concentration ($r = -0.486$), no significant relation was found between fractional sodium excretion and plasma aldosterone concentration, nor between absolute, fractional sodium excretion and plasma renin activity. Taken together, these data suggest the following: (1) sodium retention associated with MCNS could be partly due to renin-angiotensin-aldosterone system, but (2) the activation of this hormonal system seems to be secondary, probably to hypovolemia associated with MCNS [Kumagai et al. 1985], and (3) some initiating mechanisms causing the nephrotic kidney to reabsorb sodium other than renin-angiotensin-aldosterone system might exist since there is a gap between initiation of sodium retention and activation of this hormonal system.

The pathogenesis of increased urine kallikrein excretion in the nephrotic syndrome is incompletely understood [Brouhard et al. 1979, Cumming and Robson 1985, Cumming et al. 1989], however, several mechanisms have been proposed as discussed below. It has been suggested that the renal kallikrein induces proteinuria by increasing glomerular permeability in the nephrotic syndrome [McFarlane et al. 1973, Brouhard et al. 1979]. Nevertheless, this seems unlikely since in the present study there was no correlation between the value for Uka and urine protein excretion, and the value for Uka was not increased during the proteinuric steady state of MCNS despite the presence of heavy proteinuria and hypoalbuminemia equivalent to those observed during the edema forming state of the disease.

The "wash-out" phenomenon has been considered as a mechanism of an increase in the renal kallikrein excretion based on the findings of Adetuyibi and Mills [1972] who found that oral water loading significantly enhanced the Uka in normal subjects. Because of a lack of correlation between the value for Uka and urine volume in the present study, this theory seems unlikely to be responsible for the increased Uka associated with MCNS.

In experimental and human models of hypertensive disease [Adetuyibi and Mills 1972, Margolius et al. 1974, Levinsky 1979, Scicli and Carretero 1986], the renal kallikrein, a potent vasodilator, has been shown to counterbalance the reduced renal function by increasing renal blood flow. Although there was no significant correlation between the value for Uka and creatinine clearance in our patients with MCNS, we could not exclude this hypothesis because of a lack of data on renal blood flow in our study.

In the present study, we found that the value for Uka was significantly increased in the edema forming state of MCNS while the Uka was within the normal range in the proteinuric steady state in which sodium retention was already present although it was mild and severe hypoalbuminemia equivalent to that in the edema forming state of the disease was developed. This suggests that the renal kallikrein-kinin system seems to be independent of hypoalbuminemia but activated only when sodium retention reaches a critical level that could result in edema formation. The lack of the effect of hypoalbuminemia stimulating the renal kallikrein excretion observed in our patients with MCNS is supported by the experimental data obtained by Cumming et al. [1989] who found that hypoproteinemia induced in sheep by plasmapheresis did not alter the renal kallikrein excretion.

An activation of the renin-angiotensin-aldosterone system has been considered as another possible mechanism of an increase in the renal kallikrein excretion associated with the nephrotic syndrome [Levinsky 1979, Scicli and Carretero 1986]. We found a functional link between the renal kallikrein excretion and the renin-angiotensin-aldosterone system which could produce renal vasoconstriction, impair renal blood flow, and stimulate sodium and water retention in patients with the nephrotic syndrome [Meltzer et al. 1979, Kumagai et al. 1985]. In animal and human experiments the renal kallikrein-kinin system has been suggested to antagonize and modulate and activation of the renin-angiotensin-aldosterone system by inducing natriuresis and glomerular vasodilation [Carretero et al. 1974, Wong et al. 1975, Levy et al. 1977]. Margolius et al. [1974] found an increase in the renal kallikrein excretion due to high plasma aldosterone concentration in patients with primary hyperaldosteronism, and Marin-Grez et al. [1973] confirmed that an increase in the renal kallikrein excretion could counterbalance the sodium retaining effect of aldosterone based on the observation that edema does not occur in such patients. Taken together, it is tempting to assume that an enhancement of the renal kallikrein excretion associated with MCNS could be a compensatory phenomenon for counterbalancing the effect of activated renin-angiotensin-aldosterone system.

Finally, the administration of a large dose of ACTH and dexamethasone has been shown to increase the renal kallikrein excretion probably due to the sodium retaining effect [Vinci et al. 1979, Lopez et al. 1983]. It is unknown, however, whether oral doses of prednisolone have an effect on the renal kallikrein excretion in patients with the nephrotic syndrome. Since there was no difference in the value for Uka during each disease state of MCNS between the patients treated with oral prednisolone and those without, the oral doses of prednisolone, at least, seem unlikely to be a major determinant of an increase in the renal kallikrein excretion associated with MCNS.

In conclusion, the renal kallikrein-kinin system seems to be independent of proteinuria or hypoalbuminemia, but activated only when sodium retention reaches a critical level that could result in edema formation. The renal kallikrein-kinin system has a functional link to the renin-angiotensin-aldosterone system, however, its activation appears not primary but secondary phenomenon in children with MCNS.

Acknowledgements

We thank Dr. Masaru Chihara for his help in the collection of the data. We are also grateful to Prof. Sudhir V. Shah and Dr. Philip R. Mayeux for their kind advice.

REFERENCES

Adetuyibi A, Mills IH 1972 Relation between urinary kallikrein and renal function, hypertension, and excretion of sodium and water in man. Lancet *2:* 203

Amundsen E, Putter J, Friberger P, Kons M, Larsbraten M, Claeson G 1979 Method for the determination of glandular kallikrein by means of a chromogenic tripeptide substrate. Adv Exp Med Biol *120A:* 83

Bernard DB 1988 Extrarenal complications of the nephrotic syndrome. Kidney Int *33:* 1184

Bohlin AB, Berg U 1984 Renal sodium handling in minimal change nephrotic syndrome. Arch Dis Child *59:* 825

Brouhard BH, Cunningham RJ, Petrusick TW, Berger M, Travis LB 1979 Urinary kallikrein excretion in idiopathic nephrotic syndrome. J Urol *121:* 672

Brown EA, Markandu ND, Sagnella GA, Squires M, Jones BE, McGregor GA 1982 Evidence that some mechanism other than the renin system causes sodium retention in nephrotic syndrome. Lancet *2:* 1237

Carretero OA, Oza NB, Scicli AG, Schork A 1974 Renal tissue kallikrein, plasma renin and plasma aldosterone in renal hypertension. Acta Physiol Latinoam *24:* 448

Cumming AD, Robson JS 1985 Urinary kallikrein excretion in glomerulonephritis and nephrotic syndrome. Nephron *39:* 206

Cumming AD, Jeffrey S, Lambie AT, Robson JS 1989 The kallikrein-kinin and renin-angiotensin systems in nephrotic syndrome. Nephron *51:* 185

Kallen RJ, Lee SK 1975 A study of the plasma kinin-generating system in children with the minimal lesion, idiopathic nephrotic syndrome. Pediatr Res *9:* 70

Kumagai H, Onoyama K, Iseki K, Omae T 1985 Role of renin angiotensin aldosterone on minimal change nephrotic syndrome. Clin Nephrol *23:* 229

Levinsky NG 1979 The renal kallikrein-kinin system. Circ Res *44:* 441

Levy SB, Lilley JJ, Frigon RP, Stone RA 1977 Urinary kallikrein and plasma renin activity as determinants of renal blood flow. J Clin Invest *60:* 129

Lopez JM, Arteaga E, Rodriguez JA, Croxatto H 1983 Increased excretion of kallikrein during dexamethasone administration in normal man on low and normal salt intake. Clin Sci *65:* 487

Margolius HS, Horwitz D, Pisano JJ, Keiser HR 1974 Urinary kallikrein in hypertension: relationships to sodium intake and sodium-retaining steroids. Circ Res *35:* 820

Marin-Grez M, Oza NB, Carretero OA 1973 The involvement of urinary kallikrein in the renal escape from the sodium retaining effect of mineralocorticoids. Henry Ford Hosp Med J *21:* 85

McFarlane NAA, Mills IH, Wraight EP 1973 Increased vascular permeability produced by kallikrein infusions and its enhancement by nephrectomy. J Physiol *231:* 45 p

Meltzer JI, Keim HJ, Laragh JH, Sealey JE, Jan KM, Chien S 1979 Nephrotic syndrome: vasoconstriction and hypervolemic types indicated by renin-sodium profiling. Ann Intern Med *91:* 688

Murakami N, Hori S, Masumura S 1968 Exercise proteinuria and proteinuria induced by kallikrein. Nature *218:* 481

Scicli AG, Carretero OA 1986 Renal kallikrein-kinin system. Kidney Int *29:* 120

Ueda N, Chihara M, Kawaguchi S, Niinomi Y, Nonoda T, Matsumoto J, Ohnishi M, Yasaki T 1988 Intermittent versus long-term tapering prednisolone for initial therapy in children with idiopathic nephrotic syndrome. J Pediatr *112:* 122

Van Liew JB, Noble B, Brentjens JR 1985 Absence of sodium and water retention in rats with severe proteinuria. Nephron *40:* 476

Vinci JM, Zusman RM, Izzo JL, Bowden RE, Horwitz D, Pisano JJ, Keiser HR 1979 Human urinary and plasma kinins. Relationship of sodium-retaining steroids and plasma renin activity. Circ Res *44:* 228

Wong PY, Talamo RC, Williams GH, Colman RW 1975 Response of the kallikrein-kinin and renin-angiotensin systems to saline infusion and upright posture. J Clin Invest *55:* 691

Clinical Nephrology, Vol. 36 No. 5 – 1991 (234–239)

Repeated albumin infusions do not lower blood pressure in preeclampsia

P. Stratta[1], C. Canavese[1], M. Dogliani[1], L. Gurioli[1], M. C. Porcu[1], T. Todros[2], O. Fianchino[4], C. Benedetto[3], M. Massobrio[3] and L. Balbi[4]

[1] *Departments of Nephrology,* [2] *Obstetric Pathology and* [3] *Gynecology and Obstetrics, University of Torino,* [4] *Service of Internal Medicine, St. Anna-Hospital, Torino, Italy*

Abstract. Since intravascular volume contraction is regarded as an important pathological feature in preeclampsia, it has been proposed that plasma volume expansion could be a therapeutic manœuver that interrupts the pathogenetic chain of hypovolemia inducing increased vascular resistance. Furthermore, tissue perfusion should be improved and, if albumin is used as plasma expander agent, interstitial edema should also be reduced. We report the results observed in an open pilot study in ten preeclamptic patients treated with daily albumin infusions (0.4 to 1 g/kg) from 7 to 36 days. No acute effects were shown on blood pressure, and the need for antihypertensive therapies did not decrease in the following days. Serial evaluation after at least five or ten days of repeated albumin infusions did not show stable changes in electrolytes excretion, renal clearances, serum protein concentration and hematocrit value, nor in aldosterone, renin and atrial natriuretic peptide basal levels, while proteinuria tended to increase. Uteroplacental and fetoplacental blood flow acutely ameliorated in 3 cases only after albumin 1 g/Kg, but reached basal values again on the next day. The clinical implications are that daily albumin infusions with this schedule dosage do not lower blood pressure and that they are unable to induce stable changes in renal function, uteroplacental and fetoplacental resistance. No maternal complications were observed during the conservative management, but fetal mortality was high (6/10). Given the uncontrolled study, we cannot know whether similar results had been achieved by conventional therapy only.

Key words: preeclampsia – plasma volume expansion – albumin infusion – hypertension – placental flow

Introduction

Maternal plasma volume increase is a central physiological adjustment of normal pregnancy [Goodlin et al. 1983a, Gallery and Brown 1987, Uzan et al. 1987]. Volume expansion is significantly correlated with the extent of fetal growth and is less than normal in pregnancies complicated by intrauterine growth retardation, chronic hypertension and preeclampsia [Goodin et al. 1983b, Hays et al. 1985].

In this latter condition, though the degree of intravascular volume depletion seems to correlate with the severity of the disease [Sibai et al. 1983, Easterling et al. 1987, Nisell et al. 1988] the role of hypovolemia in the sequency of pathologic events is still a matter of controversy [Redman 1984]. It has been suggested that the first pathogenetic feature could be an increase in vascular resistance, likely due to a decrease in vasodilating factors [Friedman 1988, O'Brien et al. 1989] which would allow the blunted reactivity to vasoconstrictor agents, which is typical of normal pregnancy, to be modified. In this hypothesis, vasospasm would be coupled with endothelial lesion, causing a secondary shift of intravascular fluids in extravascular spaces with ensuing hypovolemia. Other elements however, including the fact that hypovolemia seems to precede the increase in blood pressure [Gallery and Brown 1987, Hays et al. 1985, Tourné 1987], point to the possibility that intravascular volume depletion is the primary event, responsible for a secondary compensatory increase in vascular peripheral resistance. Such an increase in the uterine arterial bed could impair placental perfusion [Lieberman et al. 1988], thus allowing fetal distress, and triggering off the cascade of pathological events which follow the neuro-hormonal unbalance due to fetoplacental distress. Following this hypothesis, expanding intravascular volume should not only improve tissue

Received August 13, 1990; in revised form June 25, 1991.

Reprint requests to Dr. Piero Stratta, Department of Nephrology, S. Giovanni-Molinette Hospital, Corso Bramante 88, I-10126 Torino, Italy perfusion, but should also avoid or reduce the secondary increase in vascular resistance.

This theoretical background provided the premises for advocating plasma expanders as a justified therapeutic approach in the management of preeclampsia. Previous reports documented a favourable short-term effect of this manœuver in controlling blood pressure [Cloeren and Lippert 1972, Gallery et al. 1981 and 1984] and improving renal function and placental blood flow [MacLean et al. 1978, Goodlin et al. 1978, Sibai et al. 1983, Wasserstrum and Cotten, 1986]. However, most recent data did not confirm a decrease in blood pressure as an acute effect of plasma expansion [Wasserstrum et al. 1989], and the same result was achieved in our personal experience [Stratta et al. 1989]. Furthermore, other authors basically disagreed on the use of plasma expanding protocols, and argued that, owing to the hyperreactive circulation of preeclampsia [Cotton et al. 1988], such a treatment might be dangerous by increasing the risk of rising systemic arterial blood pressure and potentially inducing pulmonary edema [Parving et al. 1974, Hankins et al. 1984, Sibai et al. 1987]. Lastly, no conclusive agreement exists on what schedules, what length of infusion time, and what kind of plasma expander agents should be employed.

Granted that randomized controlled trials only may test the assumption that plasma volume expansion has any beneficial effect on the outcome of pregnancy in preeclampsia, this study was designed as an open plot trial to obtain some basic reinsegnements able to warrant practical guidelines for a proper treatment schedule before starting clinical trials.

Patients and methods

Ten patients (mean age 36 ± 8 years, min 18 max 44) in whom preeclampsia was diagnosed following the onset "de novo" of hypertension, proteinuria and edema in the third trimester of pregnancy entered the study. In all cases, the patients were referred to the hospital at the first clinical presentation of the disease. Mean values of blood pressure at the clinical presentation were 173 ± 14 mm Hg (as systolic) and 103 ± 7.1 mm Hg (as diastolic). Proteinuria ranged from 0.8 to 7.6 g/24 h. After hospitalization, antihypertensive therapy was immediately started and adjusted in order to obtain stable values around 145 and 95 mm Hg of systolic diastolic pressure, respectively. The patients were treated with bed rest and were instructed to maintain lateral left recumbency for as much time as possible. Those patients who had a favourable response to the initial treatment were continued on conservative mangement with the addition of daily albumin infusion. All patients gave informed consent, and the procedure was approved by the Health Administration.

Doses, ranging from 0.4 to 1 g/kg of a 20% human serum albumin low in salt was given by 2 to 3 hours twice daily infusions every day. An unrestricted diet (protein 1 to 1.5 g/kg/day and sodium 100 to 250 mmol/day) was provided by the hospital kitchen.

Management of patients included intensive maternal and fetal surveillance by means of blood pressure recording, blood and urine serial sampling and serial ultrasound examination and cardiotocography to assess fetal status. Blood levels of urea, creatinine and electrolytes were checked every day. Renal clearances, hormone concentrations and uteroplacental and feto-placental blood flow was measured after the first 24 hours and subsequently every 5 to 10 days.

The decision regarding the time and mode of delivery was made by the attending physician based on signs of either maternal health or fetal well-being. Maternal indications for delivery included uncontrollable hypertension, and or deteriorating renal function. Fetal indication for delivery was evidence of fetal distress.

Blood, creatinine, uric acid, serum protein, hematocrit, and platelet values were detected by autoanalyser. Plasma and urine electrolytes were detected spectrophotometrically. Plasma and urine osmolality were measured with a freezing point osmometer. Calculation of creatinine and osmolar clearances and fractional sodium excretion were made using conventional formulae. Aldosterone, renin and atrial natriuretic peptide were measured by radioimmunoassays (Travenol and Peninsula respectively). Normal values obtained with the same kits in normal pregnant women at the same gestational age were 705 ± 321 pg/ml, 12 ± 3 ng/ml/h and 34 ± 8 pg/ml, respectively.

The placental impedance was evaluated over 10 consecutive cardiac cycles by means of the Resistance Index (RI) as described by Pourcelot [Pourcelot et al. 1974]. RI resulted from the difference between the maximum systolic velocity (A) and minimum diastolic velocity (B) divided by the maximum systolic velocity (RI = A–B/A). RI was employed to evaluate placental flow on the maternal side (uteroplacental flow), and was considered abnormal when more than 0.45. The A/B ratio was employed to evaluate placental flow on the fetal side (fetoplacental flow), and was considered abnormal when more than 3.5. Normal values obtained by the same operators in normal pregnant women at the same gestational age were 0.3 ± 0.2 RI an 2.9 ± 0.2 A/B, respectively [Todros et al. 1988].

Table 1 Main features of 10 preeclamptic patients treated with repeated albumin infusions

Patient No.	Gestation week at the presentation	Days of albumin infusion	Total infused albumin (g)	Blood pressure (systolic/diastolic) start	end follow-up	Fetal outcome
1	26	6	200	155/95	155/110	
2	31	6	190	160/95	160/110	neonatal death
3	29	7	120	170/100	170/100	neonatal death
4	28	8	230	165/105	180/125	neonatal death
5	33	10	400	190/100	150/100	
6	28	10	400	160/100	155/105	neonatal death
7	29	11	512	180/95	145/95	neonatal death
8	27	15	300	190/110	150/100	still birth
9	33	16	560	170/105	145/90	
10	27	36	610	180/115	125/85	

Table 2 Blood and urine parameters in 10 preeclamptic patients treated with daily albumin infusions. Results are shown at 24 hours and at 5 days of follow-up.

	P_{Na} (mmol/l)	P_K (mmol/l)	S_{Prot} (g/l)	Hct (%)	Uric acid (umol/l)	U_{vol} (ml/min)	$U_{Na}V$ (mmol/24 h)
Baseline	138 ± 2.2	4.0 ± 0.4	59 ± 8	33.8 ± 2.1	359 ± 103	1.16 ± 0.17	87 ± 36
24 hours	137 ± 2.2	4.1 ± 0.5	56 ± 6	33.6 ± 4	372 ± 140	1.17 ± 0.4	84 ± 35
5 days	137 ± 2.4	4.1 ± 0.4	59 ± 10	33.3 ± 2.5	323 ± 48	1.19 ± 0.16	112 ± 28

	U_KV (mmol/24 h)	FE_{Na} (%)	C_{Cr} (ml/min)	C_{osm} (ml/min)	C_{H_2O} (ml/min)	U_{Prot} (g/24 h)
Baseline	38 ± 8	0.50 ± 0.29	101 ± 45	1.52 ± 0.39	–0.58 ± 0.4	3.0 ± 2.0
24 hours	49 ± 12	0.49 ± 0.36	123 ± 42	1.71 ± 0.13	–0.57 ± 0.3	6.4 ± 5.7
5 days	47 ± 8	0.48 ± 0.31	105 ± 39	1.80 ± 0.28	–0.53 ± 0.3	4.9 ± 3.6

Abbreviations

Serum protein (S_{Prot}); hematocrit (Hct); plasma sodium (P_{Na}); plasma potassium (P_K); urine volume (U_{vol}); sodium excretion ($U_{Na}V$); potassium excretion (U_KV); sodium fractional excretion (FE_{Na}); creatinine clearance (C_{Cr}); osmolar clearance (C_{osm}); free water clearance (C_{H_2O}); proteinuria (U_{Prot}); aldosterone (PAC); renin (PRA); atrial natriuretic peptide (ANP).

Statistics

Values are given as mean ± SD. Student's t-test for paired data was used for statistical evaluation. A p value <0.05 was considered significant.

Results

The main clinical features of the 10 preeclamptic patients are shown in Table 1. The mean value of the total infused albumin was 352 ± 170 g (min 120, max 610). Albumin infusions were repeated for a minimum of 6 and a maximum of 36 days (mean value 12.5 ± 8 days). All the ten patients had a cesarean section. There were 5 neonatal deaths within three days from birth, and 1 still birth. Three of the perinatal deaths were related to respiratory failure, and two were due to cerebral hemorrhage. No maternal complications were observed. The acute effects on blood pressure, renal functional parameters, hormone levels and placental flow of a single albumin infusion have been reported in details elsewhere [Stratta et al. 1989]. Briefly, in 50% of cases a precentage increase of 175% in urine volume, 285% in sodium excretion, 167% of potassium excretion, 40% in C_{cr} and 108% in C_{osm} was observed. Contemporarily, aldosterone and renin levels dropped by 35% and 41% respectively, and ANP increased by 56%. All these effects, however, were only transient and weakened in the three hours after stopping albumin infusion. No acute changes in blood pressure were observed.

Table 3 Plasma hormone concentrations and placental flow in 10 preeclamptic patients treated with daily albumin infusions. Results are shown at 24 hours and at 5 days of follow-up

	PRA (ng/ml/h)	PAC (pg/ml)	ANP (pg/ml)	Utero-placental flow (RI)	Feto-placental flow (A/B)
Baseline	2.06 ± 1.5	128 ± 97	38.3 ± 14	0.50 ± 0.04	5.1 ± 2.2
24 h	1.76 ± 1.1	148 ± 80	46.6 ± 22	0.48 ± 0.08	5.1 ± 2.2
5 days	1.96 ± 1.7	146 ± 80	31.6 ± 3.9	0.51 ± 0.07	6.6 ± 2.1

The comparison between plasma and urine pre-albumin values and those of the next morning after the first day during which albumin was infused is shown in Tables 2 and 3, together with the long-term results of repeated albumin infusions in all the ten patients at a follow-up of 5 days. The acute changes observed immediately at the end of the infusion even in the responder patient vanished in the next morning. No statistically significant differences were demonstrated.

No substantial changes were observed in renal clearance, as well as in urine electrolytes excretion, while proteinuria continuously increased although the difference did not attain a level of significance. Serum protein and uric acid concentration and hematocrit value were stable (Table 2). Hormonal values showed a not significant trend to increase in ANP levels at 24 hours, with no changes in aldosterone and renin concentration (Table 3). No stable changes were observed either in uteroplacental and fetoplacental blood flow, although a not significant trend to increase in fetal resistance was evident (Table 3). This individual analysis demonstrated a consistent decrease in uterine resistance only in the patient in whom the treatment was pursued for 36 days (uteroplacental and fetoplacental flow from 0.51 to 0.36 RI from 0.47 to 0.33 A/B, respectively).

In the six patients with a follow-up of at least ten days of daily albumin infusions the results were substantially the same (Table 4). No statistically significant differences were demonstrated. Although not significant, owing to the large standard deviation, a trend to increase in proteinuria and fetal vascular resistance was observed.

In no case did we observe a decrease in blood pressure reducing the need for hypotensive drugs. In all the ten patients the dosages had to be increased or further drug had to be added over a period of days (Figure 1).

Body weight remained stable (from 56 ± 6 to 55 ± 9 kg).

Discussion

Granted that delivery is the only real means of interrupting preeclampsia, therapeutic approaches such as intravascular volume expansion have been proposed to improve maternal-fetal status, and, putatively, to alter the course of the disease [Gallery et al. 1981 and 1984].

The first purpose is that of a "symptomatic" therapy only, while the second one is more ambitious because it is a putative "pathogenetic" therapy, able to interfere directly with the pathogenesis of the syndrome, the hope lying in the hypothesis that reduced intravascular volume is the primary cause of increased resistance [Gallery and Brown 1987, Hays et al. 1985]. Therefore, the aim of such a therapy should be not only to facilitate peripartum management, but also to prolong the time before delivery, thus allowing the fetus to grow further in an acceptable milieu [Tourné 1987].

As this study was an open pilot trial, we cannot draw any conclusion about possible differences in patients treated with hypotensive drugs only. However, some comments appear appropriate. An improved perfusion at the site of renal circulation

Table 4 Main parameters in 6 preeclamptic patients with a follow-up of at least 10 days of daily albumin infusions

	S_{Prot} (g/l)	Hct (%)	Uric acid (mol/l)	U_{vol} (ml/min)	$U_{Na}V$ (mmol/24 h)	C_{Cr} (ml/min)
Baseline	61 ± 10	35.6 ± 2.1	352 ± 75	1.13 ± 0.42	97 ± 20	111 ± 46
10 days	58 ± 8	34.4 ± 4.8	366 ± 85	1.09 ± 0.34	85 ± 23	114 ± 25

	U_{Prot} (g/24 h)	PRA (ng/ml/h)	PAC (pg/ml)	ANP (pg/ml)	Uteroplacental flow (RI)	Fetoplacental flow (A/B)
Baseline	2.9 ± 2.1	2.57 ± 1.5	100 ± 65	42 ± 21	0.49 ± 0.09	4.9 ± 1.5
10 days	9.3 ± 7	2.67 ± 1.7	112 ± 91	49 ± 25	0.48 ± 0.11	6.6 ± 2.6

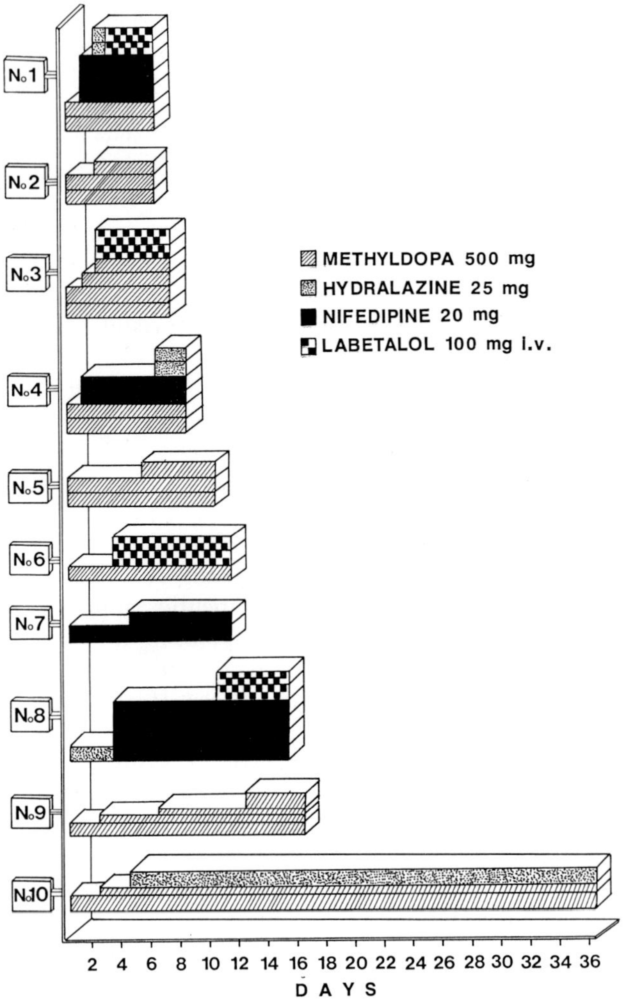

Fig. 1 The need for antihypertensive drugs in ten preeclamptic patients treated with daily albumin infusion.

should afford improved functional parameters. As acute effect, albumin infusion induced a transient increase in urine volume, natriuresis and renal clearances in 50% of cases [Stratta et al. 1989]; however this effect was blunted 24 hours after in all but few cases. As effects of repeated infusions, no mean change in urine sodium and potassium excretion or in creatinine and osmolar clearances were observed. However, the 3 cases in whom both pre-albumin clearances and solutes excretion was markedly reduced and albumin infusion was employed at dosage of 1 g/KG, all showed an overt improvement 24 hours after the first infusion, with no further changes in the following days.

Low renin and aldosterone levels, increased blood uric acid levels and proteinuria are the hallmarks of the progressing of preeclampsia. None of these features seem to have been significantly improved by repeated albumin infusions. Even more, though a large standard deviation coupled with a little number of cases did not allow significant results, a clear trend to increase in proteinuria was evident, with no changes in serum total protein concentration.

As to placental resistance, with the cautions imposed by the still persisting limits in the actual reliability of the available techniques, we can conclude that, with few exceptions, we did not observe any substantial decrease in uteroplacental or fetoplacental resistance, either as acute [Stratta et al. 1989] or chronic effect. Even more a clear, though not significant, increase in fetal resistance was evident. It could be that acute atheromasic changes had still occurred, thus shifting the reason for a reduced flow from a functional vasospasm to anatomic alterations which cannot be reversed by any expanding volume treatment [Khon et al. 1987]. Another speculation could be that the actual possibility of inducing an amelioration in placental circulation (both on the maternal and fetal sites), may be achieved only by employing higher doses and more long-term therapy.

As to the blood pressure, the same lack of hypotensive effect which has been previously observed after a single albumin infusion [Wasserstrum et al. 1989, Stratta et al. 1989] was confirmed also after repeated infusions. There was no spontaneous decrease in blood pressure, and even the need for hypotensive drugs rose, which means that blood pressure was spontaneously increasing. Since increasing blood pressure is a common feature in progressing preeclampsia, we have no evidence for incriminating albumin infusion in rising blood pressure, but however we cannot exclude a role. At any rate, we have no evidence that repeated manœuvers of expanding volume are able to reduce blood pressure. Since an actual decrease in peripheral resistance has been shown as acute effect of albumin infusion [Wasserstrum et al. 1989], it may be that the net result on blood pressure depending on the balance between reduced resistance and increased cardiac index does occur even after prolonged treatment. As previous favourable results were obtained with continuous intravenous infusion of plasma expander substances, it is possible to speculate that continuous treatment might have more chance of actually reducing blood pressure than such an intermittent infusion schedule.

A final consideration is that the stability in body weight and the lack of increasing of hematocrit should indicate an acceptable control of edema formation and no further hemoconcentration. However, on the other hand, the lack of decreasing of hematocrit could indicate that intravascular volume was not large enough. Furthermore, despite acceptable maternal status during our conservative management, fetal outcome was bad.

In conclusion, we can say that the aims of employing albumin in preeclampsia, at least at the dosages and with the schedules we employed, have been only partially achieved. In particular, the hypothesis that expanding volume does elicit a reduction in blood pressure does not seem to be confirmed. We cannot exclude, however, that the reason is that intravascular volume did not expand enough. Further studies with different schedules are required in order to clarify this interesting issue, granted that the extent of the hypovolemia had been investigated before.

In sum, owing to the type of this study, the only conclusions we can draw are the following: a) repeated slow albumin infusions in preeclampsia at dosages as high as 1 g/kg/day do not induce any acute hemodynamic complications and, in particular, any pulmonary adverse effects; b) some, at most transient, improvement in renal and placental resistance are observed only after doses of 1 g/kg/day; c) the schedule treatment employed, however, does not induce acute hypotensive effect nor avoid an increase in maternal blood pressure and a severe fetal prognosis; d) controlled trials are mandatory to clarify the costs/benefits ratio of such a very expensive protocol.

REFERENCES

Cloeren SE, Lippert TH 1972 Effect of plasma expanders in toxemia of pregnancy. N Engl J Med *ii:* 1356–1357

Cotton DB, Lee W, Huhta JC, Dorman KF 1988 Hemodynamic profile of severe pregnancy-induced hypertension. Am J Obstet Gynecol *158:* 523–529

Easterling TR, Watts DH, Schmucker BL, Benedetti TJ 1987 Meausrement of cardiac output during pregnancy: valutation of doppler technique and clinical observations in preeclampsia. Obstet Gynecol *69:* 845–850

Friedman SA 1988 Preeclampsia: a review of the role of prostaglandins. Obstet Gynecol *71:* 122–137

Gallery EDM, Delprado W, Gyory AZ 1981 Antihypertensive effect of plasma volume expansion in pregnancy-associated hypertension. Aust NZ J Med *11:* 20–24

Gallery EDM, Mitchell MDM, Redmon CWG 1984 Fall in blood pressure in response to volume expansion in pregnancy-associated hypertension (preeclampsia). Why does it occur? J Hypertension *2:* 177–182

Gallery EDM, Brown MA 1987 Volume homeostasis in normal and hypertensive human pregnancy. In: *Lindheimer MD, Davison JM* (eds). Clinical Obstetrics and Gynaecology, London, Baillière Tindall, pp 835–851

Goodlin RC, Cotton DB, Haesslein HC 1978 Severe edema-proteinuria-hypertension gestosis. Am J Obstet Gynecol *132:* 595–598

Goodlin RC, Dobry CA, Anderson JC, Woods RE, Quaife MA 1983a Clinical signs of normal plasma volume expansion during pregnancy. Am J Obstet Gynecol *145:* 1001–1009

Goodlin RC, Quaife MA, Smith JJ 1983b Hypovolemic pregnant women and their risk determinants. Int J Gynaecol Obstet *21:* 45–50

Hankins GDV, Wendel GD, Cunningham FG, Leveno KJ 1984 Longitudinal evaluation of hemodynamic changes in eclampsia. Am J Obstet Gynecol *150:* 306–312

Hays PM, Cruikshank DP, Dunn LJ 1985 Plasma volume determination in normal and preeclamptic pregnancies. Am J Obstet Gynecol *151:* 958–966

Khon TY, Pearce JM, Robertson WP 1987 Acute atherosis in preeclampsia: maternal determinants and fetal outcome in the presence of the lesion. Am J Obstet Gynecol *157:* 360–363

Leiberman JR, Meizner J, Mazor M, Insler V 1988 Blood supply to the uterus in preeclampsia. Eur J Obstet Gynecol Reprod Biol *28:* 23–27

MacLean AB, Doig JR, Aickin DR 1978 Hypovolemia, preeclampsia and diuretics. Br J Obstet Gynaecol *85:* 597–601

Nisell H, Lunerell NO, Linde B 1988 Maternal hemodynamics and impaired fetal growth in pregnancy-induced hypertension. Obstet Gynecol *71:* 163–166

O'Brien WF, Knuppel RA, Saba HI, Angel JL, Benoit R, Bruce A 1989 Serum prostacyclin binding and half-life in normal and hypertensive pregnant women. Obstet Gynecol *73:* 43–45

Parving HH, Rossing N, Nielsen SL, Lassen NA 1974 Increased transcapillary escape rate of albumin, IgG, and IgM after plasma volume expansion. Am J Physiol *227:* 245–250

Pourcelot L 1974 Application clinique de l'examen Doppler transcutaine. In: *Peronneau P* (ed). Veliometric ultrasonor Doppler INSERM, *34:* 625–627

Redman CWG 1984 Maternal plasma volume and disorders of pregnancy. Br Med J *288:* 955–956

Sibai BM, Anderson GD, Spinnato JA, Shaver DC 1983 Plasma volume findings in patients with mild pregnancy-induced hypertension. Am J Obstet Gynecol *147:* 16–19

Sibai BM, Malic BC, Harvey CJ, Gonzales AR 1987 Pulmonary edema in severe preeclampsia-eclampsia: analysis of thirty-seven consecutive cases. Am J Obstet Gynecol *156:* 1174–1179

Stratta P, Canavese C, Guriolo L, Porcu M, Todros T, Mattone GC, Fianchino O, Gagliardi L, Vercellone A 1989 The ratio between aldosterone and atrial natriuretic peptide in normal pregnancy and in preeclampsia. Kidney Int *36:* 908–914

Todros T, Lombardo P, Fianchino O 1988 Continuous wave Doppler Ultrasound in obstetrics. In: *Cosmi EV, Di Renzo GC* (eds). Proceedings of the XI European Congress of Perinatal Medicine, Roma, CIV Ed Int, pp 150–155

Tourné CE 1987 La maladie gravidique: essai de synthése et conduit à tenir. J Gynecol Obstet Biol Reprod *16:* 1023–1037

Uzan S, Beaufils M, Uzan M, Donsimoni R, Mareck A, Salat-Baroux J, Sureau C Mesure du volume plasmatique maternel au cours de la grossesse. Rev Fr Gynécol Obstét *83:* 111–118

Wasserstrum N, Cotton DB 1986 Hemodynamic monitoring in severe pregnancy-induced hypertension. Clin Perinatol *13:* 781–798

Wasserstrum N, Kirshon B, Willis RS, Moise KJ, Cotton DB 1989 Quantitative hemodynamic effects of acute volume expansion in severe preeclampsia. Obstet Gynecol *73:* 546–550

Clinical Nephrology, Vol. 36 No. 5 – 1991 (240–245)

Renal failure and cholesterol crystal embolization: a report of 4 surviving cases and a review of the literature

C. K. Mannesse, P. J. Blankestijn, A. J. Man in 't Veld and M. A. D. H. Schalekamp

Department of Internal Medicine I, University Hospital Dijkzigt, Erasmus University Rotterdam, The Netherlands

Abstract. Four patients with end-stage renal failure (suspected to be) caused by cholesterol crystal emboli are described. Although cholesterol crystal embolization is generally considered to be fatal specifically when it is associated with renal failure, all four patients survived and in three renal function improved after periods of 3 weeks to 14 months of hemo- or peritoneal dialysis. The literature on cholesterol crystal embolization is reviewed and possible mechanisms of (partial) recovery of renal function are discussed.

Key words: cholesterol crystal embolization – end-stage renal failure – improvement of renal function

Introduction

Cholesterol crystal embolization, first described by Flory and Meyer more than 30 years ago [Flory 1945, Meyer 1947], is usually a multiple-system disease incited by the obstruction of small arteries by cholesterol crystals [Richards et al. 1965]. It is to be distinguished from atheroembolism, in which obstruction of a large artery in one organ results in a localized disease of that particular organ involved.

In general cholesterol crystal embolization is associated with a lethal outcome [Gaines et al. 1988], especially when kidneys are involved [Macpherson and Goldberg 1988]. The mortality rate is 72–90% [Falanga et al. 1986, Fine et al. 1987, Palmer and Warren 1988]. Sporadically survivals are described, both without renal failure [Hammerschmidt et al. 1981 (1 case), Groeninx van Zoelen et al. 1983 (2 cases), Kalter et al. 1985 (3 cases), Hyman et al. 1987 (2 cases), Forouhar et al. 1988 (2 cases), Macpherson and Goldberg 1988 (1 case)] and with renal impairment not necessitating hemo- or peritoneal dialysis [Bruns et al. 1978 (1 case), Smith et al. 1981 (2 cases), Scully et al. 1984 (1 case), McGowan and Greenberg 1986 (1 case)]. Only a few cases have been reported with recovery of renal function after a period of hemo- or peritoneal dialysis [Smith et al. 1981 (1 case), Rosansky 1982 (1 case), McGowan and Greenberg 1986 (1 case), Siemons et al. 1987 (2 cases), Jordans 1989 (1 case)]. In this paper we report 4 cases with severe renal failure necessitating hemo- or peritoneal dialysis, who all survived cholesterol crystal embolization. In 3 of them dialysis could be stopped because of sufficient recovery of renal function, even after a prolonged time.

Case histories

Case 1

A 70-year-old male was admitted because of recent onset intermittent claudication and blue discoloration of the feet. He had a longstanding history of hypertension and atrial fibrillation. Three months before admission serum creatinine was 120 umol/l (1.4 mg/dl). After a transient ischemic attack 8 weeks before admission he used oral anticoagulants (acenocoumarol).

Physical examination revealed signs of volume overload (edema, high central venous pressure, rales), cyanotic feet and focal necrosis of some toes with normal pedal arterial pulses. Livedo reticularis was present. Laboratory investigation showed a hemoglobin concentration of 8.0 mmol/l (12.9 g/dl), a leucocyte count of 7.8×10^9/l (7,800/mm^3) with 8% eosinophils, a platelet count of 167×10^9/l (167,000/mm^3) and an erythrocyte sedimentation rate of 65 mm at 1 h. The urea nitrogen had risen to 46.2 mmol/l

Received May 21, 1990; in revised form January 2, 1991.

Reprint requests to Dr. C. K. Mannesse, Department of Internal Medicine I, University Hospital Dijkzigt, Erasmus University, Rotterdam, Dr Molewaterplein 40, NL-3015 GD Rotterdam, The Netherlands

(129 mg/dl) and the creatinine to 588 umol/l (6.6 mg/dl). Daily urine production was 700 ml with a proteinuria of 4 g/24 h. Microscopic examination of the urine revealed 25–30 erythrocytes per high power field. The C3 and C4 were normal. Nephrosclerosis was seen in a renal biopsy.

Although not proven by histopathology the clinical presentation of renal failure, focal necrosis of cyanotic toes and livedo reticularis justified the diagnosis of cholesterol crystal embolization.

After initial ultrafiltration soon after admission the patient was treated with peritoneal dialysis. Anticoagulant treatment was stopped. Focal necrosis and cyanosis of the toes disappeared after approximately 4 months. Peritoneal dialysis could be stopped 14 months later because of improvement of renal function. Renal function stabilized with a urea nitrogen of 15.7 mmol/l (44 mg/dl) and a creatinine of 190 umol/l (2.1 mg/dl) 12 months after cessation of peritoneal dialysis.

Case 2

A 57-year-old male was referred to our department because of progressive loss of renal function. Three weeks earlier he underwent coronary bypass surgery. He had a 15-year history of hypertension and his serum creatinine preoperatively was 130 umol/l (1.5 mg/dl).

On admission the patient complained of pain scattered in the muscles of the legs. On physical examination a blood pressure of 210/120 mmHg was found and there was livedo reticularis of the lower abdomen and both legs. The toes were cyanotic but there were palpable pedal arterial pulses. Laboratory studies showed a normocytic normochromic anemia (Hb 6.7 mmol/l [10.8 mg/dl]), an erythrocyte sedimentation rate of 24 mm at 1h, a leucocyte count of 5.1×10^9/l (5,100/mm^3) with 15% eosinophils and a platelet count of 171×10^9/l (171,000/mm^3). The urea nitrogen was 25.4 mmol/l (71 mg/dl), the creatinine 584 umol/l (6.6 mg/dl). The urine production was 700 ml, daily. Urinanalysis demonstrated 0.5–1.0 g of protein per 24 h and a few erythrocytes per high power field were seen. No other laboratory abnormalities were found. A skin-muscle biopsy of an affected area of the left thigh showed a perivasculitis but no cholesterol clefts were seen. The combination of the recent coronary bypass surgery and the clinical presentation with progressive renal impairment, acceleration of hypertension, livedo reticularis and cyanotic toes resulted in the diagnosis of cholesterol crystal embolization, in spite of the negative histopathology.

The urea nitrogen gradually rose to 38.3 mmol/l (107 mg/dl) and the creatinine to 1137 umol/l (12.8 mg/dl). Peritoneal dialysis was started 6 weeks after coronary bypass surgery. The cyanotic lesions became gangrenous but amputation was not necessary.

Fourteen months after the first peritoneal dialysis this treatment could be stopped because of gradual improvement of renal function. To date, 18 months after cessation of peritoneal dialysis, renal function is still markedly impaired [serum creatinine 400 umol/l (4.5 mg/dl)]. Approximately 6 months after coronary bypass surgery the cyanotic toes were healed completely.

Case 3

A 69-year-old male was admitted because of progressive renal failure and recent onset of severe pain in both legs. An arteriography, which was done 1 week prior to his admission because of intermittent claudication, showed extensive aortoiliac atherosclerosis. The renal arteries were normal. One week before the arteriography, renal function was normal. He used anticoagulant therapy (acenocoumarol) because of a myocardial infarction seven months before admission. On physical examination livedo reticularis distributed on his legs and lower trunk was present. The arterial pedal pulses were absent. Weak arterial pulses in the groins were palpable. His blood pressure was 150/100 mmHg.

Laboratory investigations revealed a normochromic normocytic anemia (Hb 6.7 mmol/l [10.8 mg/dl]) with a lowered platelet count of 109×10^9/l (109,000/mm^3). The leucocyte count amounted 9×10^9/l (9,000/mm^3) with 3% eosinophils. The urea nitrogen was 42.3 mmol/l (118 mg/dl) and the creatinine 485 umol/l (5.5 mg/dl). A daily urine production of 400 ml was measured with a proteinuria of 10 gram/24 h. Microscopic examination of the urine revealed 100 red blood cells and no white blood cells per high power field. A skin biopsy of an affected area demonstrated the characteristic cholesterol clefts surrounded by histiocytes located in the dermis.

Intermittent hemodialysis was neccesary for 3 weeks. Livedo reticularis gradually disappeared, but unfortunately amputation of one toe was inevitable. Thirteen months later his serum creatinine is 120 umol/l (1.4 mg/dl). He continued oral anticoagulant treatment.

Case 4

A 60-year-old male was referred because of a diagnostic workup for suspected renovascular hypertension combined with moderate renal failure. He had a 6-month history of paroxysmal non-radiating right-sided upperabdominal pain associated with nausea, unrelated to the ingestion of meals.

On admission the patient, who was treated with an angiotensin converting enzyme inhibitor, had a blood pressure of 140/80 mmHg. The urea nitrogen was 8.4 mmol/l (24 mg/dl), the creatinine 177 umol/l (2.0 mg/dl) and a proteinuria of 0.8 gram/24 h was observed.

Angiography revealed a mild stenosis of the left renal artery with some atherosclerosis of the aorta. Because hypertension was well controlled an arterial balloon dilatation was not performed.

Seven weeks later the patient was rehospitalized because of extreme claudication of both calfs and abdominal pain.

On physical examination an acceleration of hypertension (210/110 mmHg), livedo reticularis of the lower body and cyanosis of the toes with normal pulsations of the pedal arteries was found.

Laboratory investigations revealed: normocytic normochromic anemia (Hb 7.9 mmol/l [12.7 mg/dl]), an erythrocyte sedimentation rate of 83 mm at 1 h, a white blood cell count of 12.3×10^9/l (12,300/mm^3) with 14% eosinophils and a platelet count of 123×10^9/l (123,000/mm^3). The urea nitrogen was 11.9 mmol/l (33 mg/dl), the creatinine 344 umol/l (3.9 mg/dl). The urine production amounted 600 ml daily with a proteinuria of 3.9 gram/24 h. Microscopic examination of the urine showed 15–20 red blood cells and no white blood cells per high power field. The C3 and C4 concentrations were normal (1.26 and 0.90 g/l respectively).

The diagnosis cholesterol crystal embolization was confirmed by a skin-muscle biopsy of the thigh showing the characteristic cholesterol clefts in the subcutis vasculature.

Despite attempts to regulate the blood pressure, further deterioration of the renal function followed and ten weeks after the angiography intermittent hemodialysis was started. Painful focal necrosis of all toes made amputation inevitable. To date, nine months after the first hemodialysis, renal function is not improved.

Discussion

Predisposing factors

Cholesterol crystal embolization is a relatively uncommon disease frequently found in older men with a history of hypertension and atherosclerotic vascular disease.

Cholesterol crystals are found with a high incidence in autopsy studies. However, in these studies no data are reported on related antemortem clinical signs and symptoms. Crystals were found e.g. in 77% of the autopsies after aortic surgery [Thurlbeck and Castleman 1957] and in 30% and 25.5% of the autopsies performed within 6 months after respectively aortogram or cardiac catheterisation [Ramirez et al. 1978]. These high incidences are in contrast with the rarity of clinical cases reported, probably due to a subclinical course of the cholesterol crystal embolization in the majority of patients.

The most important predisposing factors are considered to be vascular surgery and radiology procedures, and possibly the use of anticoagulants. However, several cases have been described without apparent predisposing factors [Fine et al. 1987].

Operative and radiologic vascular procedures are thought to induce cholesterol embolization by mechanically dislodging cholesterol crystals from ulcerated atheromata or denuding their endothelial lining and allowing subsequent embolization.

The possible relationship between anticoagulants and cholesterol crystal embolization has been pointed out by many authors, all referring to the controversial theory of Moldveen-Geronimus and Merriam that anticoagulants might prevent thrombosis of ulcerating atheromatous plaques, thereby favoring dissemination of cholesterol crystals out of this plaque into the peripheral circulation [Moldveen-Geronimus and Merriam 1967, Bruns et al. 1978, Groeninx van Zoelen et al. 1983, Hyman et al. 1987, Schwartz and McDonald 1987, Siemons et al. 1987, Meyrier et al. 1988]. From this point of view it seems logical that discontinuation of anticoagulants might stop the embolization, but this effect is seldomly reported [Bruns et al. 1978 (1 case), Groeninx van Zoelen et al. 1983 (1 case)]. On the other hand, cases with still progressive renal impairment after discontinuation of anticoagulants are reported [Falanga et al. 1986 (1 case), McGowan and Greenberg 1986 (1 case), Hyman et al. 1987 (1 case)] and cases in which no progressive renal impairment developed while anticoagulants were continuated [Richards et al. 1965 (1 case), Falanga et al. 1986 (1 case)] are also reported.

A predisposing factor in three patients, a renal arteriogram in case 3 and 4 and coronary bypass surgery in case 2, was present, one week, ten weeks and six weeks respectively before dialysis was started. Two patients were treated with anticoagulants. There is a time correlation between the start of anticoagulants and cholesterol crystal embolization in case 1 and 3, respectively 2 and 7 months before dialysis was started, but this cannot be taken as a proof for the statement that anticoagulants can incite and sustain cholesterol crystal embolization. In case 1 anticoagulants were discontinued whereas in case 3 they were continued. In both cases we found a progression of the renal impairment, but both patients regained sufficient renal function. Possibly the relationship between anticoagulants and cholesterol crystal embolization is only coincidental.

Clinical picture

The characteristic presentation of renal failure accompanied with livedo reticularis of the lower body and focal digital ischemia of toes makes diagnosis on clinical grounds possible [Smith et al. 1981, Rosansky 1982, Hyman et al. 1987, Siemons et al. 1987, Palmer and Warren 1988]. However, clinical signs and symptoms are frequently nonspecific. Retinal cholesterol crystal emboli [Hollenhorst 1961] are confirming the diagnosis but are found infrequently [Fine et al. 1987; 10%].

Involvement of the kidney is frequently seen in clinically evident cholesterol crystal embolization [Fine et al. 1987; 50%] and gives rise to a spectrum of degrees of renal impairment. Generally a step-wise deterioration of renal function is seen in 4–6 weeks time or more accompanied by accelerating hypertension [Richards et al. 1965, Smith et al. 1981, Fine et al. 1987]. Also acute renal failure with necrotizing glomerulonephritis and crescent formation has been reported as the consequence of cholesterol crystal embolization [Goldman et al. 1985, Hannedouche 1986, Rémy et al. 1987].

Laboratory findings

Laboratory manifestations are nonspecific and include elevated erythrocyte sedimentation rate, leucocytosis and eosinophilia. Proteinuria of variing degree, leucocyturia and erythrocyturia are present frequently.

Histology

Histologic diagnosis can be obtained from biopsies from kidney, skin or muscle with the finding of cholesterol clefts. Although determination of sensitivity and specificity of these histologic studies are not available to date, it appears that skin and muscle biopsies have a high diagnostic yield [McGowan and Greenberg 1986]. Other tissue specimen – e.g. a bone marrow biopsy – are less productive in establishing the diagnosis [Pierce et al. 1978].

Histologic material may not always demonstrate the characteristic cholesterol clefts [Rosansky 1982, Ludmerer and Kissane 1983, Meyrier et al. 1988]. The patchy lesions are localized in the subcutis at the side of arterial branching and can be missed at sampling and serial sectioning of the skin and muscle biopsy [Anderson 1965, Scully et al. 1984, Falanga et al. 1986, McGowan and Greenberg 1986]. The birefringent cholesterol crystals are dissolved in the routine histologic fixation process [Kalter et al. 1985] and consequently only the imprint is seen as the characteristic biconvex, needleshaped cleft, which can be mistaken for a vascular lumen [Jones and Iannaccone, 1975]. Besides the cholesterol clefts an arteriitis can be found. A repercussion of this arteriitis can be seen as a glomerulonephritis [Hannedouche et al. 1961, Jones and Iannaccone 1975, Rémy et al. 1987], thereby probably explaining leucocyturia, eryhrocyturia and proteinuria.

Survival

The data on survival of patients with cholesterol crystal embolization from retrospective and autopsy studies generally indicate a high mortality rate [Falanga et al. 1986, Fine et al. 1987, Palmer and Warren 1988]. Death is most commonly due to multifactorial, cardiac and renal etiologies [Fine et al. 1987]. The survival-rate will certainly be underestimated in literature since milder cases are probably not published or not recognized as such.

Our experience of survival in 4 patients with severe renal function impairment necessitating dialysis and even partial recovery of renal function in three of them, is striking in view of few survival cases published. We realize however that our findings can be very well based on selection bias [McGowan and Greenberg 1986].

Recovery of renal function

In the seldomly reported severe cases with renal function impairment necessitating dialysis, partial recovery of renal function is reported. In these cases dialysis becomes superfluous after a variable period of time [Smith et al. 1981 (1 case: 4 months), Rosansky 1982 (1 case: 2 weeks), McGowan and Greenberg 1986 (1 case: 2 months), Siemons et al. 1987 (2 cases: 3 days and 7 months respectively), Jordans 1989 (1 case: 13 months)].

In previous reports no attempt has been made to explain partial recovery of renal function in the cholesterol crystal embolization syndrome. Before understanding the improvement of renal function in the published [Smith et al. 1981 (1 case), Rosansky 1982 (1 case), McGowan and Greenberg 1986 (1 case), Siemons et al. 1987 (2 cases), Jordans 1989 (1 case)] and our 3 cases the first important question is whether the renal function impairment is in fact solely caused by the cholesterol crystals. In this regard we have to divide the published and our own cases in two groups, seperated by the absence or presence of other possible factors causing renal function impairment.

The first group consists of the cases with no other factors causing renal failure and includes case 2 in the paper of Siemons et al. [Siemons et al. 1987], case 3 in the paper of McGowan and Greenberg [McGowan and Greenberg 1986] and our case 1. Only in the case of Siemons et al. the presence of cholesterol crystals in the kidney was proven by renal biopsy. In the other 2 cases the absence of other factors causing kidney failure makes it possible that the cholesterol crystals play a role in the renal function impairment. In this way there may be reversible factors in the pathogenesis of renal function loss caused by cholesterol crystal emboli.

Data on the pathophysiology of cholesterol crystal embolization are based on experimental studies in animals [Snyder and Shapiro 1961, Warren and Vales 1976, Cosio et al. 1985], in vitro studies [Hammerschmidt et al. 1981] and histologic observations in humans [Thurlbeck and Castleman 1957, Jones and Iannaccone 1975, Meyrier et al. 1988]. The possible factors which allow reversibility of some renal function due to the cholesterol crystals itself are the non-total instead of total occlusion of vasculature by the cholesterol crystal, the accompaning inflammatory reaction, and the ischemic induced vasoconstriction. Probably an additional tubular necrosis is also a cause of reversible renal failure. Recovery of renal function even after a period of 14 months as in our case 1, is hard to understand in view of the above mentioned considerations. However one can speculate that cholesterol crystal embolization is a dynamic process. A shower of cholesterol crystals will damage some nephrons while others are already regaining function by subdueing the prior reversible factors. In this way it can be understood that a partial recovery of renal function impairment is possible when the shower of cholesterol crystals stops. Repeated kidney biopsy studies might give more insight in these mechanisms, however this procedure is not favourable in patients.

The second group consists of all the other published cases [case 3 in Smith et al. 1981, case 4 in Rosansky 1982, case 1 in Siemons et al. 1987, the case of Jordans 1989] and our case 2 and 3. In this group other factors might explain the partial reversibility of renal failure. Radiographic procedures took place shortly before start of dialysis in case 3 of the paper of Smith et al. (4 weeks), case 4 of the paper of Rosansky (2 weeks), case 1 in the paper of Siemons et al. (2 weeks), the case in the paper of Jordans (some days), and in our case 3 (1 week). Coronary surgery took place 6 weeks earlier in our case 2. In all these cases renal failure might also be caused, at least partially, by the nephrotoxic effects of contrast media and in the case of coronary surgery by hemolysis or hemodynamic instability during and/or after operation. These conditions can all lead to acute tubular necrosis, accompanied by reversible renal function impairment. So in this group it is not at all proven that renal failure and the subsequent improvement in function is solely explained by cholesterol embolism. Furthermore in these cases the presence of cholesterol clefts is not mentioned in the histologic desriptions of renal biopsies.

We conclude that kidney failure complicating the cholesterol crystal embolization syndrome is likely to be multifactorial and that it is difficult to attribute reversibility solely to the cholesterol crystals itself, especially in those patients who recently underwent vascular procedures.

REFERENCES

Anderson WR 1965 Necrotizing angiitis associated with embolization of cholesterol. Am J Clin Pathol *43:* 65

Bruns FJ, Segel DP, Adler S 1978 Control of cholesterol embolization by discontinuation of anticoagulant therapy. Am J Med Sci *275:* 105

Cosio FG, Zager RA, Sharma HM 1985 Atheroembolic renal disease causes hypocomplementaemia. Lancet *2:* 118

Falanga V, Fine MJ, Kapoor WN 1986 The cutaneous manifestations of cholesterol crystal embolization. Arch Dermatol *122:* 1194

Fine MJ, Kapoor W, Falanga V 1987 Cholesterol crystal embolization: a review of 221 cases in the English literature. Angiology *38:* 769

Flory CM 1945 Arterial occlusions produced by emboli from eroded aortic atheromatous plaques. Am J Pathol *21:* 549

Forouhar FA, Mohit M, Gardner P, Smith N 1988 Cholesterol embolism causing bleeding gastric ulcers. Ann Clin Lab Sci *18:* 260

Gaines PA, Cumberland DC, Kennedy A, Welsh CL, Moorhead P, Rutley MS 1988 Cholesterol embolisation: a lethal complication of vascular catheterisation. Lancet *1:* 168

Goldman M, Thoua Y, Dhaene M, Toussaint C 1985 Necrotising glomerulonephritis associated with cholesterol microemboli. Br Med J *290:* 205

Gore I, McCombs HL, Lindquist RL 1964 Observations on the fate of cholesterol emboli. J Atheroscler Res *4:* 527

Groeninx van Zoelen C, Kroon C, Hulst SGTh 1983 Cholesterolemboli. Ned Tijdschr Geneeskd *127:* 1902

Hammerschmidt DE, Greenberg CS, Yamada O, Craddock PR, Jacob HS 1981 Cholesterol and atheroma lipids activate complement and stimulate granulocytes. J Lab Clin Med *98:* 68

Hannedouche T, Godin M, Courtois H, Ducastelle T, Delpech A, Tayot J, Fillastre JP 1986 Necrotizing glomerulonephritis and renal cholesterol embolization. Nephron *42:* 271

Hollenhorst RW 1961 Significance of bright plaques in the retinal arterioles. JAMA *178:* 23

Hyman BT, Landas SK, Ashman RF, Schelper RL, Robinson RA 1987 Warfarin-related purple toes syndrome and cholesterol microembolization. Am J Med *82:* 1233

Jones DB, Iannaccone PM 1975 Atheromatous emboli in renal biopsies. Am J Pathol *78:* 261

Jordans JGM 1989 Cholesterolemboli (letter). Ned Tijdschr Geneeskd *23:* 1187

Kalter DC, Rudolph A, McGavran M 1985 Livedo reticularis due to multiple cholesterol emboli. J Am Acad Dermatol *13:* 235

Ludmerer KM, Kissane JM 1983 Clinicopathologic conference: Cyanotic feet and renal failure in a 67-year-old man. Am J Med *75:* 509

Macpherson DS, Goldberg MJ 1988 Letter to the editor. Lancet *1:* 643

McGowan JA, Greenberg A 1986 Cholesterol atheroembolic renal disease. Am J Nephrol *6:* 135

Meyer WM 1947 Cholesterinkrystallembolie kleiner Organarterien und ihre Folgen. Arch Pathol Anat *314:* 616

Meyrier A, Buchet P, Simon P, Fernet M, Rainfray M, Callard P 1988 Atheromatous renal disease. Am J Med *85:* 139

Moldveen-Geronimus M, Merriam JC Jr 1967 Cholesterol embolization, from pathological curiosity to clinical entity. Circulation *35:* 946

Palmer FJ, Warren BA 1988 Multiple cholesterol emboli syndrome complicating angiographic techniques. Clin Radiol *39:* 519

Pierce JR, Wren MV, Cousar JB 1978 Cholesterol embolism: diagnosis antemortem by bone marrow biopsy. Ann Int Med *89:* 937

Ramirez G, O'Neill WM Jr, Lambert R, Bloomer HA 1978 Cholesterol embolization. A complication of angiography. Arch Intern Med *138:* 1430

Rémy P, Jacquot C, Nochy D, d'Auzac C, Yéni P, Bariéty J 1987 Cholesterol atheroembolic renal disease with necrotizing glomerulonephritis. Am J Nephrol *7:* 164

Richards AM, Eliot RS, Kanjuh VI, Bloemendaal RD, Edwards JE 1965 Cholesterol embolism. A multiple-system disease masquerading as polyarteritis nodosa. Am J Cardiol *15:* 696

Rosansky SJ 1982 Multiple cholesterol emboli syndrome. South Med J *75:* 677

Schwartz MW, McDonald GB 1987 Cholesterol embolization syndrome: occurence after intravenous streptokinase therapy for myocardial infarction. JAMA *258:* 1934

Scully RE, Mark EJ, McNeely BU 1984 Case records of the Massachusetts General Hospital (Case 4-1984). N Engl J Med *310:* 244

Siemons L, van den Heuvel P, Parizel G, Buyssens N, De Broe ME, Cuykens JJ 1987 Peritoneal dialysis in acute renal failure due to cholesterol embolization: two cases of recovery of renal function and extended survival. Clin Nephr *28:* 205

Smith MC, Ghose MK, Henry AR 1981 The clinical spectrum of renal cholesterol embolization. Am J Med *71:* 174

Snyder HE, Shapiro JL 1961 A correlative study of atheromatous embolism in human beings and experimental animals. Surgery *49:* 195

Thurlbeck WM, Castleman B 1957 Atheromatous emboli to the kidneys after aortic surgery. N Engl J Med *257:* 442

Warren BA, Vales O 1976 The ultrastructure of the reaction of arterial walls to cholesterol crystals in atheroembolism. Br J Exp Pathol *57:* 67

Clinical Nephrology, Vol. 36 No. 5 – 1991 (246–251)

Once weekly versus twice weekly subcutaneous administration of recombinant human erythropoietin in patients on continuous ambulatory peritoneal dialysis

S. F. Lui, C. B. Law, S. M. Ting, P. Li and K. N. Lai

Renal Unit, Prince of Wales Hospital, Department of Medicine, Chinese University of Hong Kong, Shatin, Hong Kong

Abstract. Twice weekly subcutaneous (s.c.) administration of recombinant human erythropoietin (rHuEPO) is effective in reversing renal anemia in CAPD patients. However the optimal frequency of administration has not been established. It would be more convenient to give rHuEPO by once weekly rather than twice weekly injection. We have therefore compared the effect of twice weekly versus once weekly s.c. administration of rHuEPO. Two groups of 10 CAPD patients were given the same starting dose of s.c. rHuEPO (100 U/kg body wt/week) either as a single weekly dose or twice weekly in divided doses. The rHuEPO dosage was then adjusted according to the hematologic response. The aim was to increase hemoglobin levels by about 1 g/dl per month. The target hemoglobin was 10 g/dl. After 16 weeks of treatment with rHuEPO, the hemoglobin levels rose from 6.6 ± 1.2 (mean ± SD) to 10.1 ± 1.1 g/dl in the once weekly group and from 6.4 ± 0.8 to 10.2 ± 1.1 g/dl in the twice weekly group. The average doses of rHuEPO used during the study were 84 ± 16 and 88 ± 15 U/kg body wt/wk for the once weekly and twice weekly groups respectively. Subcutaneous administration of low dose rHuEPO is effective in reversing renal anemia. Similar responses were obtained with once weekly and twice weekly regimens. It is therefore acceptable and convenient for patients to receive one weekly s.c. injection of rHuEPO for the treatment of renal anemia.

Key words: anemia – chronic renal failure – dialysis – erythropoietin

Introduction

Anemia is a common complication of end stage renal failure and is due to suboptimal levels of erythropoietin (EPO) production [Eschbach 1989a, Paganini 1989]. It is now possible to correct renal anemia with recombinant human erythropoietin (rHuEPO). The intravenous (i.v.) route has been the route of choice for the administration of rHuEPO to hemodialysis patients. The efficacy of i.v. rHuEPO is well established [Winearls et al. 1986, Eschbach et al. 1987, 1989b, Casati et al. 1987, Sundal and Kaeser 1989]. However, the optimal route, dosage and frequency of administration of rHuEPO have yet to be determined. Increased partition of i.v. rHuEPO dose has been shown to improve the efficacy of the drug [Bommer et al. 1988]. Subcutaneous (s.c.) administration of rHuEPO may be more effective [Bommer et al. 1989, Grannoleras et al. 1989].

For patients maintained on CAPD, regular i.v. administration of rHuEPO is inconvenient and impractical because of the need for frequent visits to the dialysis center and the lack of vascular access. It is necessary to consider alternative routes of administration. We have previously shown that s.c. administration of rHuEPO is effective in reversing renal anemia in CAPD patients [Lui et al. 1990]. Other investigators have confirmed our findings [MacDougall et al. 1989a, Piraino and Johnston 1990]. In all these studies, the rHuEPO was given in a twice weekly regimen. However, the optimal frequency of administration of rHuEPO has not been established. It is unclear whether it is possible to achieve the same response if the same dose of rHuEPO is given as a single weekly dose rather than in doses administered twice weekly. It would be more convenient for CAPD patients to receive rHuEPO in one weekly injection rather than two or more times per week. We have

Received November 7, 1990; in revised form March 5, 1991.

Reprint requests to Dr. S. F. Lui, Renal Unit, Prince of Wales Hospital, Department of Medicine, Chinese University of Hong Kong, Shatin, Hong Kong therefore compared the effects of twice weekly versus once weekly s.c. administration of rHuEPO.

Patients and methods

Twenty CAPD patients with anemia due to end-stage renal failure were randomized to receive the same s.c. starting dose of rHuEPO (100 U/kg body wt/wk), either by a once weekly or twice weekly divided-dose regimen. The rHuEPO were given by s.c. injection into either upper arm by a nurse at the out-patient clinic.

All 20 patients had been on CAPD for at least 6 months and their hemoglobin levels were less than 8 g/dl. Patients with anemia due to other known causes and those with uncontrolled hypertension were excluded from the study. The characteristics of the two groups are shown in Table 1. Their underlying renal diseases were similar, mainly chronic glomerulonephritis. The duration of dialysis and history of previous blood transfusion were comparable in the two groups. Informed consent was obtained from the patients for the study.

Human recombinant erythropoietin was supplied by Cilag Research (Switzerland) as a sterile buffered solution in vials containing 0.25% human albumin, sodium, chloride and citrate with a specific activity of 160,000 Units human recombinant erythropoietin protein per mg. Each millilitre contained 4000 units of rHuEPO. For most patients, the volume of the s.c. injection was between 1 and 1.5 ml as the average body weight was around 50 kg.

Iron supplements (Fortifer i-ii tablet daily) were given to all patients unless there was evidence of gross iron overload (serum ferritin levels >1760 pmol/l). Patients who developed functional iron deficiency (as defined by transferrin saturation <20%) and with suboptimal improvement of hemoglobin were given intravenous infusion of Imferon (50 mg twice weekly for five weeks) [Macdougall et al. 1989b, 1990].

Blood pressure was monitored regularly during the study. Hematological indices including red blood cells, platelets, hemoglobin, hematocrit, mean corpuscular volume and mean corpuscular hemoglobin concentration were measured every 2 weeks. Iron, total iron binding capacity, transferring saturation and ferritin levels were measured at the end of weeks 8 and 16.

To ensure the optimal dosage was given and to avoid too rapid a rise in the hemoglobin level, the rHuEPO dosage was adjusted periodically according to the increase in hemoglobin level. After 4 weeks of treatment, if the increase in hemoglobin was >1.5 g/dl, the rHuEPO dose was reduced by 25 U/kg body wt/week, if the increase in hemoglobin was <0.5 g/dl, the rHuEPO was increased by 25 U/kg body wt/week. After 8 weeks of treatment, if the increase in hemoglobin was >2.5 g/dl, the rHuEPO dose was reduced by 25 U/kg body wt/week, if the increase in hemoglobin was <1.5 g/dl, the rHuEPO was increased by 25 U/kg body wt/week. After 12 weeks of treatment, if the increase in hemoglobin was >3.5 g/dl, the rHuEPO dose was reduced by 25 U/kg body wt/week, if the increase in hemoglobin was <2.5 g/dl, the rHuEPO was increased by 25 U/kg body wt/week. The target range of hemoglobin was 10 g/dl. The duration of the study was 16 weeks. The data were presented as mean ± SD. Paired and unpaired t-tests were used to compare mean values.

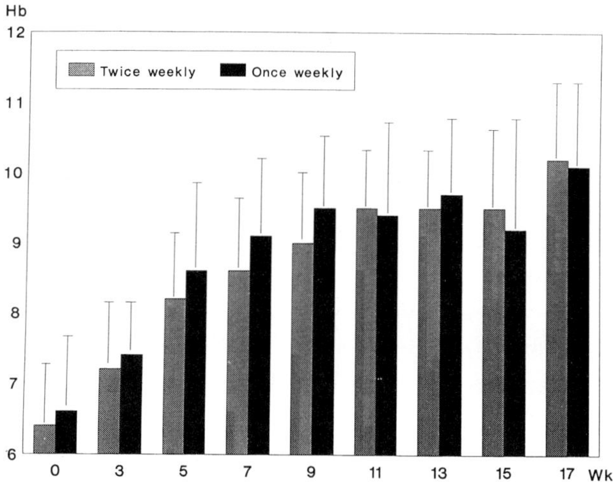

Fig. 1 Hemoglobin concentrations (mean ± SD) of patients treated with once weekly or twice weekly s.c. rHuEPO over a period of 16 weeks.

Table 1 Characteristics of the two groups of patients

	Once weekly group	Twice weekly group
Number	10	10
Sex (M:F)	3:7	3:7
Age (years)	49 ± 11	40 ± 12
Weight (kg)	52 ± 3	51 ± 3
Duration of renal replacement therapy (mth)	19 ± 3	23 ± 4
Units of blood transfusion over the previous 6 months	0.9 ± 2.0	0.2 ± 0.5

Results

One patient from each group failed to complete the 16-week study because of the development of

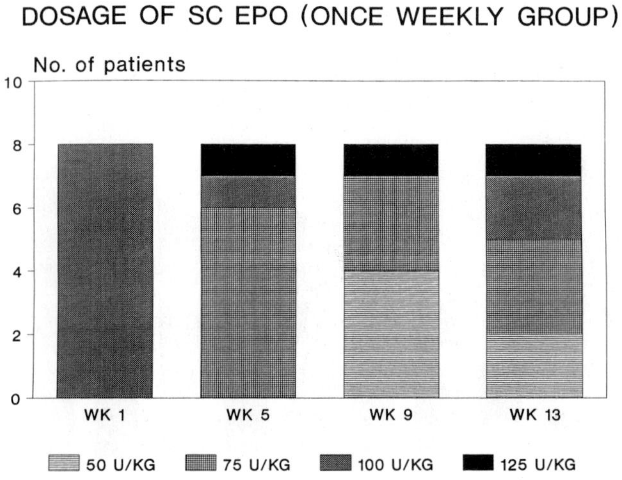

Fig. 2 Dosages of rHuEPO (U/kg body wt/week) required by the once weekly group.

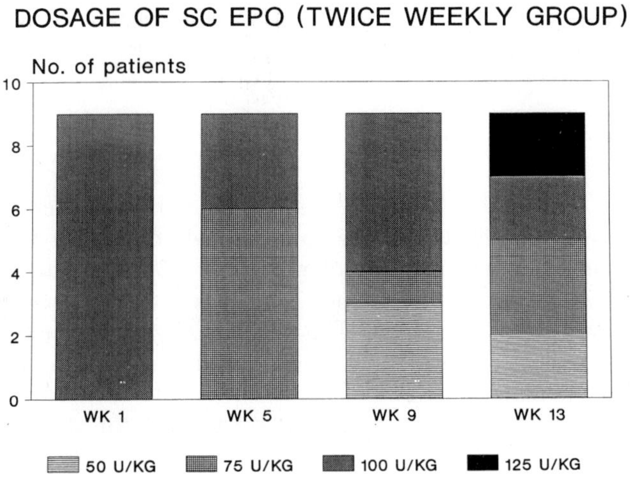

Fig. 3 Dosages of rHuEPO (U/kg body wt/week) required by the twice weekly group.

peritonitis requiring temporary conversion to hemodialysis therapy. The data from one further patient from the once weekly group was also excluded from the analysis because of a complete absence of response to the rHuEPO. This was most likely due to the presence of persistent infection (chest infection with persistent pleural effusion) during the greater part of the study period.

The characteristics of the two groups were similar. The higher mean ± SD of blood transfusion requirement in the once weekly group was not statistically significant and was due to one single patient who had 6 units of blood transfusion. Five patients had blood transfusion during the previous 6 months (3 patients in the once weekly group had 6, 2, and 1 units respectively and 2 patients in the twice weekly group had 1 unit each).

Hemoglobin levels

The changes in hemoglobin level during the 16 weeks of treatment with rHuEPO are shown in Figure 1.

In the twice weekly group, the baseline mean hemoglobin level was 6.4 ± 0.8 g/dl. The mean hemoglobin level had risen significantly by 1.8 ± 0.7 g/dl at the end of the 4th week ($p < 0.001$), 2.7 ± 0.8 g/dl by the 8th week ($p < 0.001$), 3.1 ± 0.9 g/dl by the end of 12th week ($p < 0.001$) and 3.8 ± 1.2 g/dl by the 16th week ($p < 0.001$). The mean hemoglobin level at the end of the study period was 10.2 ± 1.1 g/dl.

In the once weekly group, the baseline mean hemoglobin level was 6.6 ± 1.0 g/dl. The mean hemoglobin level had risen significantly by 2.0 ± 0.7 g/dl at the end of the 4th week ($p < 0.001$), 2.9 ± 0.4 g/dl by the 8th week ($p < 0.001$), 3.2 ± 0.5 g/dl by the end of 12th week ($p < 0.001$) and 3.5 ± 1.1 g/dl by the 16th week ($p < 0.001$). The mean hemoglobin level at the end of the study period was 10.1 ± 1.2 g/dl.

There was no significant difference between the baseline hemoglobin levels and the rise in hemoglobin levels at different time points in the two groups. In both groups, for most of the patients, a steady state condition was achieved by the 9th to 11th week of the study as reflected by the plateau of the rise in hemoglobin levels as shown in Figure 1. Thereafter, further rise in hemoglobin levels was limited by reduction of rHuEPO dosages, as either the target hemoglobin of 10 g/dl was reached or the rise in hemoglobin was greater than the allowed range.

Dosage requirement

The doses of rHuEPO given at different stages of the study are shown in Figures 2 and 3. In order to avoid too rapid a rise in the hemoglobin level, 6 out of the 9 patients in the twice weekly group and 6 out of the 8 patients in the once weekly group had their dose of rHuEPO reduced to 75 U/kg body wt/week after 4 weeks of treatment. At the end of the study, the dosage requirements for the twice weekly and the once weekly group were similar (86 ± 25 U/kg body wt/wk for twice weekly group and 81 ± 26 U/kg body wt/wk for once weekly group, $p = 0.72$). There was also no difference between the groups in the mean dosage of rHuEPO used during the study period (88

± 15 U/kg body wt/wk for the twice weekly group and 84 ± 16 U/kg body wt/wk for the once weekly group, p = 0.62).

Iron supplementation

In the twice weekly group, serum iron and transferrin saturation fell significantly after 8 weeks of treatment [serum iron 17 ± 9 to 8 ± 3 mmol/l (p <0.02), transferrin saturation 33 ± 19% to 16 ± 4% (p <0.03) and serum ferritin 907 ± 656 to 643 ± 683 pmol/l (p = 0.42)]. One patient required i.v. infusion of Imferon for functional iron deficiency.

In the once weekly group, serum iron fell from 15 ± 9 to 9 ± 4 mmol/l (p <0.02), transferrin saturation from 28 ± 17% to 17 ± 7% (p = 0.12) and serum ferritin from 859 ± 691 to 681 ± 673 pmol/l (p = 0.61) after 8 weeks of treatment. Three patients required intravenous infusion of Imferon for functional iron deficiency.

Blood pressure

The antihypertensive drugs used during the study were metoprolol ± nifedipine retard. With adjustments of antihypertensive therapy, mean blood pressure did not change significantly in either group. Mean blood pressures at the beginning and end of the study were 109 ± 13 mmHg and 107 ± 11 mmHg in the twice weekly group, 116 ± 12 mmHg and 109 ± 11 mmHg in the once weekly group.

In the twice weekly group, antihypertensive treatment was increased in 4 of 9 patients and unchanged in the other 5 patients. Of the 2 patients who were not on antihypertensive drug before rHuEPO therapy, one patient required antihypertensive drug. In the once weekly group, antihypertensive treatment was increased in 2 of 8 patients and unchanged in the other 6 patients. Of the 2 patients who were not on antihypertensive drug before rHuEPO therapy, one patient required antihypertensive drug.

Local complications

The s.c. injection of rHuEPO was associated with limited amount of local discomfort. The pain was brief and acceptable for all patients. There was no other local complication such as erythema or brusing.

Discussion

Intravenous administration of rHuEPO has been the route of choice for hemodialysis patients. The efficacy of i.v. administration of rHuEPO in hemodialysis patients is well established [Winearls et al. 1986; Eschbach et al. 1987, 1989b; Casati et al. 1987; Sundal and Kaeser 1989]. However, this may not be the most cost-effective route of administration. With i.v. administration, a high-peak serum EPO level is achieved followed by a rapid fall. The high serum EPO level may not be necessary or effective as there may be a limited number of EPO receptors on CFU_E cells to initiate the proliferative effect. There is also no data available on the optimal duration of EPO/EPO-receptor interaction to induce the maximum degree of erythropoiesis. The half-life has been reported to range from 8 to 12 h [Ergie et al. 1988, Boelaert et al. 1988, MacDougall et al. 1989c].

After s.c. administration of rHuEPO, the peak EPO level and the area under the plasma concentration-time curve (AUC) are substantially lower than after i.v. injection. The peak serum concentration was only 10% of those attained by i.v. injection of the same dose of rHuEPO [Egrie 1988]. The AUC 0–24 hours was only 10% of the value obtained with i.v. administration [Boelaert et al. 1988]. The bioavailability from s.c. administration was only 21.5% [MacDougall et al. 1989c]. However, s.c. administration of rHuEPO produces a more sustained elevation of EPO level [MacDougall et al. 1989c, Lui et al. 1990]. This may be the reason why s.c. rHuEPO has been shown to be more effective than i.v. rHuEPO [Bommer et al. 1989, Granolleras et al. 1989].

The other reason to explore the s.c. route of administration is for the treatment of renal anemia in patients maintained on CAPD. Regular i.v. administration of rHuEPO is inconvenient and impractical because of the need for frequent visits to the dialysis center and the lack of vascular access. We have previously shown that s.c. administration of rHuEPO is effective in reversing renal anemia in CAPD patients [Lui et al. 1990]. Others have also confirmed our findings [MacDougall et al. 1989a, Piraino and Johnston 1990]. In all these studies, rHuEPO was given in a twice weekly regimen.

As with the i.v. administration of rHuEPO, the optimal frequency of s.c. administration of rHuEPO has not been determined. It is unclear whether it is more effective to administer the same weekly dose of rHuEPO as a large intermittent dose, or in frequent small divided doses. In practical terms, it is more convenient for CAPD patients to be given rHuEPO once weekly rather than twice or more. However, Bommer et al. have shown that increased partition of an i.v. rHuEPO dose improves the efficacy of the drug [Bommer et al. 1988, 1989]. Granolleras et al. have shown that daily self-administered s.c. rHuEPO is effective in reversing renal anemia in hemodialysis patients [Granolleras et al. 1989]. The rationale behind frequent administration of small doses of rHuEPO was to avoid the administration of excessive rHuEPO beyond the saturation capacity of the EPO receptors on CFU_E cells. The sustained release of rHuEPO following s.c. administration may avoid the problem of an excessive high peak serum EPO level, yet it produces a sustained adequate level of circulating rHuEPO over a long period of time. It may not be necessary to give s.c. rHuEPO by small frequent injections.

This study confirmed the efficacy of s.c. administration of rHuEPO to CAPD patients. The s.c. rHuEPO results are highly reproducible in that the dosage requirement and the response achieved with twice weekly administration of s.c. rHuEPO in this present study were almost identical to those in our previous study [Lui et al. 1990].

However, of more interest and practical value is the finding that the same response can be achieved with the same dose of rHuEPO given either once or twice weekly in divided doses. The increases in hemoglobin levels were similar at different time points during the 16-week study.

The rate of rise in hemoglobin was closely controlled by adjusting the dose of rHuEPO. This was to avoid the complications that are associated with excessive or too rapid rise in hemoglobin levels [Watson 1989]. The protocol was designed to increase the hemoglobin by 1 g/dl per month. Although it took most patients 3–4 months to achieve the target hemoglobin of 10 g/dl, none of the patients required blood transfusion during the study. It was possible to achieve the target haemoglobin with a very low s.c. dose of rHuEPO. We consider a target hemoglobin around 10 g/dl to be adequate and most cost-effective. Higher levels of hemoglobin have not been associated with any extra improvements in quality of life and exercise capacity [Canadian erythropoietin study group 1990].

The mean dosage of once weekly s.c. rHuEPO that was required to increase the hemoglobin to the target range of 10 g/dl was 84 U/kg body wt/week. This is similar to the dosage requirement of 96 U/kg body wt/week reported by Piraino and Johnston in their CAPD patients given s.c. rHuEPO thrice weekly and 12–14 U/kg body wt/day used by Granolleras et al. in their daily s.c. regimen in HD patients.

As in other reports, hypertension was the major side effect associated with treatment. However, increases in blood pressure were easily controlled by adjusting the dosage of the antihypertensive drugs. The blood pressure profiles during the study were similar in the two groups. Interestingly, fewer patients required addition or increased doses of antihypertensive drugs in the once weekly group.

In summary, we have shown that s.c. low dose rHuEPO is effective in reversing renal anemia. Similar responses were obtained with once weekly and twice weekly regimens. It is therefore acceptable and convenient for the CAPD patients to receive a weekly s.c. injection of rHuEPO for the treatment of their renal anemia.

Acknowledgement

The research was supported by Cilag Research who provided the human recombinant erythropoietin. We also thank the Department of Chemical Pathology and Department of Morbid Anatomy for performing the laboratory investigations, the nursing staffs at the Renal Unit, Prince of Wales Hospital for their contribution in collecting the clinical data of this study.

REFERENCES

Boelaert J, Schurgers M, Matthys E, Daneels R, De Cre M, Bogaert M 1988 Recombinant human erythropoietin pharmacokinetics in CAPD patients: comparison of the intravenous, subcutaneous, and intraperitoneal routes (abst). Nephrol Dial Trans *3:* 493

Bommer J, Kugel M, Schoeppe W et al 1988 Dose-related effects of recombinant human erythropoietin on erythropoiesis. Contrib Nephrol *66:* 85–93

Bommer J, Samtleben W, Koch KM, Baldamus CA, Grutzmacher P, Scigalla P 1989 Variations of recombinant human erythropoietin application in hemodialysis patients. Contrib Nephrol *76:* 149–158

Casati S, Passerini P, Campise MR et al 1987 Benefits and risks of protracted treatment with human recombinant erythropoietin in patients having haemodialysis. B Med J *295:* 1017–1020

Canadian erythropoietin study group 1990 Association between recombinant human erythropoietin and quality of life and exercise capacity of patients receiving haemodialysis. B Med J *300:* 573–578

Ergie JC, Eschbach JW, McGuire T, Adamson JW 1988 Pharmacokinetics of recombinant human erythropoietin (rHuEPO) administered to hemodialysis patients. Kidney Int (abst) *33:* 262

Eschnach JW, Egrie JC, Downing ME, Browne JK, Adamson JW 1987 Correction of anaemia of end stage renal disease with recombinant human erythropoietin. N Engl J Med *316:* 73–78

Eschbach JW 1989a The anaemia of chronic renal failure: pathophysiology and the effects of reecombinant erythropoietin. Kidney Int *35:* 134–148

Eschbach JW, Abdulhadi MH, Browne JK et al 1989b Recombinant human erythropoietin in anemic patients with end-stage renal disease. Results of a phase III multicenter clinical trial. Ann Int Med *111:* 992–1000

Granolleras C, Branger B, Beau MC, Deschodt G, Alsabadani B, Shaldon S 1989 Experience with daily self-administered subcutaneous erythropoietin. Contrib Nephrol *76:* 143–148

Lui SF, Chung WWM, Leung CB, Chan K, Lain KN 1990 Pharmacokinetics and pharmacodynamics of subcutaneous and intraperitoneal administration or recombinant human erythropoietin in patients on continuous ambulatory peritoneal dialysis. Clin Nephrol *33:* 47–51

Macdougall IC, Cavill I, Davies ME, Hutton RD, Coles GA, Williams JD 1989a Subcutaneous recombinant erythropoietin in the treatment of renal anaemia in CAPD patients. Contrib Nephrol *76:* 219–226

Macdougall IC, Hutton RD, Cavill I, Coles GA, Williams JD 1989b Poor response to treatment of renal anaemia with erythropoietin corrected by iron given intravenously. B Med J *299:* 157–158

Macdougall IC, Roberts DE, Neubert P, Dharmasena AD, Coles GA, Williams JD 1989c Pharmacokinetics of recombinant human erythropoietin in patients on continuous ambulatory peritoneal dialysis. Lancet *i:* 425–427

Macdougall IC, Hutton RD, Cavill I, Coles GA, Williams JD 1990 Treating renal anaemia with recombinant human erythropoietin: practical guidelines and clinical algorithm. B Med J *300:* 655–659.

Paganini EP 1989 Overview of anaemia associated with chronic renal disease: primary and secondary mechanisms. Seminars in Nephrology, 9 (1), suppl *1:* 3–8

Piraino B, Johnston JR 1990 The use of subcutaneous erythropoietin in CAPD patients. Clin Nephrol *33:* 200–202

Sundal E, Kaeser U 1989 Correction of anaemia of chronic renal failure with recombinant human erythropoietin: safety and efficacy of one year's treatment in a European multicentre study of 150 haemodialysis-dependent patients. Nephrol Dial Transplant *4:* 979–987

Watson AJ 1989 Adverse effects of therapy for the correction of anaemia in hemodialysis patients. Seminars in Nephrology 9 (1) suppl *1:* 30–34

Winearls CG, Pippard MJ, Downing MR, Oliver DO, Reid C, Cotes PM 1986 Effect of human erythropoietin derived from recombinant DNA on the anaemia of patients maintained by chronic haemodialysis. Lancet *2:* 1175–1177

Clinical Nephrology, Vol. 36 No. 5 – 1991 (252–257)

Effect of recombinant human erythropoietin (rHuEpo) on the hemostatic system in chronic hemodialysis patients

S. Huraib [1], A. K. Al-Momen [2], A. M. A. Gader [3], A. Mitwalli [1], F. Sulimani [1] and H. Abu-Aisha [1]

Department of Medicine, Divisions of Nephrology [1] and Hematology [2] and Department of Physiology [3], College of Medicine and King Khalid University Hospital, Riyadh, Saudi Arabia

Abstract. Hemostatic measurements were undertaken in eight chronic hemodialysis uremic patients on recombinant human erythropoietin (rHuEpo). Same measurements were repeated in another seven patients in whom anemia was corrected by the transfusion of red blood cells. The correction of the anemia by rHuEpo therapy was accompanied by 1. correction of the prolonged Simplate Bleeding Time (BT) to normal <10.0, minutes after 16 weeks of rHuEpo treatment; 2. significant increases in the levels of fibrinogen, clotting FVIII : C, vWF : antigen, vWF : ristocetin cofactor and platelet count; 3. enhanced aggregation responses to ADP, adrenaline, arachidonic acid, collagen and ristocetin. There was no significant fluctuation in other coagulation parameters PT, APTT, TT, reptilase time and antithrombin III and plasma fibrinogen. In patients who were treated with RBC transfusion and despite the correction of the anemia, the bleeding time shortened significantly but not corrected, mean BT before and after RBC transfusion was 17.1 ± 1.4 and 11.6 ± 1.9 minutes respectively. Besides there was significant elevation of vWF : Ricofactor levels but not FVIII : C, vWF : Ag or platelet count. Platelet aggregation responses to ADP remained unchanged. It is concluded that significant elevations of FVIII : related activities, plasma fibrinogen, improved platelet aggregability and correction of the BT are salient hemostatic changes that follow rHuEpo therapy in uremic patients.

Key words: Erythropoietin – anemia – platelet aggregation – coagulation – clotting factor VIII – bleeding time

Introduction

Patients with chronic renal failure often exhibit a bleeding tendency and multiple hemostatic defects due in part to abnormalities of platelet function and platelet vessel wall interaction [Eknoyan et al. 1969, Remuzzi et al. 1981, Deykin 1983, Livio et al. 1985]. Bleeding time (BT) which is a sensitive marker of primary hemostasis [Hellem et al. 1961] is prolonged in uremic patients; however when the hematocrit was raised over 30% by transfusion of red blood cells a significant shortening in BT was noted [Livio et al. 1982, Fernandez et al. 1985]. This led to the conclusion that red cells enhanced platelet-vessel wall interaction, thereby causing the shortening of the BT [Remuzzi and Pusineri 1988].

The beneficial effect of recombinant human erythropoietin (rHuEpo) in the correction of the anemia in patients on chronic hemodialysis is now well established [Eschbach et al. 1987, Winearls et al. 1986, Casati et al. 1987, Ad Hoc Committee for the National Kidney Foundation 1989]. rHuEpo therapy was also shown to correct the BT prolongation and improve platelet functions [Moia et al. 1987, Raman et al. 1988]. However, no studies have been undertaken to assess the accompanying blood coagulation changes. This paper, therefore, describes the results of measurements of a wide range of coagulation parameters including BT and platelet aggregation in chronic hemodialysis patients on rHuEpo. Similar measurements were performed in a separate group of patients in whom the anemia was treated with the transfusion of packed RBC.

Received April 17, 1990; in revised form May 6, 1991.

Reprint requests to Dr. A. M. A. Gader, College of Medicine and King Khalid University Hospital, Riyadh 11461, Saudi Arabia

Patients and methods

A. Erythropoietin group

Eight patients, three males and five females with end-stage renal disease and anemia were studied. They were on thrice-weekly hemodialysis (HD) for more than 3 months before starting rHuEpo therapy. Their mean age was 38.9 years (range 22 to 54 years). In five patients the underlying diseases were as follows: diabetes mellitus, analgesic nephropathy, chronic pyelonephritis, focal glomerulosclerosis and neurogenic bladder; and 3 patients with unknown causes, one of them was anephric. Their mean hemoglobin concentration was 7.2 ± 0.3 g/dl (range: 6.7–7.8 g/dl). Their mean blood transfusions over the year prior to starting rHuEpo treatment was 3.4 units with a range of 2–7 units.

The rHuEpo (EPREX, Cilag, Switzerland) was given intravenously as a bolus after each dialysis session, for 16 weeks. The starting dose was 50 IU/kg which was increased by 25 IU/kg every 4 weeks, if required. No more rHuEpo was given when Hb concentration reached approximately 12 g/dl (and/or the hematocrit reached 35%).

B. Blood transfusion group

Red blood cell (RBC) transfusion was given to seven comparable hemodialysis patients; three were males and four were females. Their ages ranged from 26 to 72 years (x ± SD) (50.0 ± 14.8). The underlying diseases include 2 patients with chronic pyelonephritis and in the remaining five patients, the underlying diseases were as follows: diabetes mellitus, renal

Table 1 Coagulation parameters (expressed as $\bar{x}$ ± SD) in two groups of uremic patients (1) rHuEpo group and (2) RBC transfusion group

	rHuEpo group (n = 8) before rHuEpo	8 weeks on rHuEpo	16 weeks on rHuEpo	RBC Transfusion group (n = 7) pre	post
Hb g/dl	7.2 ± 0.3	10.0 ± 1.0**	11.6 ± 1.4**	7.0 ± 0.5	11.9 ± 1.2**
Hematocrit (%)	21.8 ± 1.5	32.8 ± 4.0*	36.2 ± 2.3**	21.3 ± 1.2	32.5 ± 3.7**
PLTCNT × 10^9/l	249.6 ± 87.4	344.4 ± 163.3*	360.3 ± 145.5*	207.0 ± 71.3	212.3 ± 142.9
PT (sec)	12.0 ± 0.7	12.6 ± 0.7	13.2 ± 1.4	12.2 ± 0.9	12.4 ± 0.8
PTT (sec)	27.9 ± 5.0	33.9 ± 4.5	32.1 ± 3.6	36.1 ± 1.4	35.9 ± 1.7
TT (sec)	13.1 ± 2.8	12.0 ± 3.0	15.6 ± 3.1	15.7 ± 1.9	15.4 ± 0.7
RT (sec)	15.2 ± 2.5	15.1 ± 2.1	15.6 ± 2.5	15.9 ± 1.1	16.0 ± 2.4
FIB mg/dl	214.1 ± 60.0	320.6 ± 166.9	406.3 ± 158.5*	344.7 ± 119.4	361.1 ± 152.7
ATIII (%)	87.5 ± 11.9	85.6 ± 13.5	91.6 ± 10.8*	84.7 ± 6.7	89.9 ± 9.3
FVIII:C (%)	169.0 ± 23.1	300.0 ± 88.0*	336.4 ± 118.9*	176.9 ± 52.8	186.9 ± 50.8
vWF:Ag (%)	159.5 ± 34.1	193.8 ± 40.4*	234.6 ± 71.2*	171.1 ± 46.0	163.6 ± 49.2
vWF:Ricof (%)	143.1 ± 41.9	218.5 ± 55.6*	234.3 ± 79.6*	143.7 ± 46.4	224.6 ± 52.4*

P value: * <0.05; ** <0.001;
Comparing 8 and 16 weeks with pre-rHuEpo levels

* <0.05; ** <0.001;
Comparing pre- and post-transfusion levels

Table 2 Bleeding time in minutes

rHuEpo (n = 8) Pat. no.	before rHuEpo	8 weeks on rHuEpo	16 weeks on rHuEpo	RBC Transfusion group (n = 7) Pat. no.	pre	post
1.	20	7	5	1.	>18	13
2.	15	6	10	2.	15	11
3.	18	12	8	3.	>18	12
4.	13	16	16	4.	15	13
5.	>18	11	9	5.	>18	11
6.	16	8	6	6.	>18	14
7.	>18	10	8	7.	>18	8
8.	14	10	8			

Table 3 Platelet aggregation (expressed as $\bar{x} \pm$ SD of Maximum Aggregation MA%) in two groups of uremic patients (1) rHuEpo group and (2) RBC transfusion group

	rHuEpo group (n = 7) before rHuEpo	8 weeks on rHuEpo	16 weeks on rHuEpo	RBC Transfusion group (n = 6) before transfusion	after transfusion
ADP 2.0 (MA%)	64.9 ± 17.9	73.1 ± 14.2	78.7 ± 8.3	74.3 ± 12.7	61.7 ± 19.0
Adrenaline (MA%)	61.6 ± 17.3	78.3 ± 4.8*	79.6 ± 9.8*	70.7 ± 9.7	68.0 ± 15.0
Collagen (MA%)	63.4 ± 9.6	70.6 ± 4.9*	76.7 ± 10.8*	78.3 ± 12.4	72.5 ± 4.8
Arachid acid (MA%)	63.7 ± 13.3	66.6 ± 21.9	81.9 ± 14.4*	73.2 ± 11.1	75.6 ± 8.7
Ristocetin (MA%)	68.3 ± 14.8	79.7 ± 9.8*	88.3 ± 10.9*	80.3 ± 7.9	85.3 ± 6.8

P value: * <0.05
Comparing 8 and 16 weeks with pre-rHuEpo levels

stones, neurogenic bladder and one patient without a known cause. The pre-transfusion mean hemoglobin concentration (7.0 g/dl; SD ± 0.5; range: 6.2–7.9) was comparable to the rHuEpo-treated group and RBC transfusion was given weekly until the mean hemoglobin concentration reached a value close to that of the erythropoietin group (approximately 12 g/dl).

Hemostatic tests

The rHuEpo treated group: In addition to hemoglobin (Hb), hematocrit (Hct) and platelet count (Coulter S+), the following hemostatic tests were performed before starting treatment, and at 8 and 16 weeks thereafter: prothrombin time (PT), activated partial thromboplastin time (APTT) (Stago Diagnostic Reagents, France), thrombin time (TT) (Parke Davis Topical Thrombin), reptilase time (RT) (Pentapharm, Switzerland). The clotting times were recorded using an optical detecting system (Coagulation Profiler, Bio/Data – USA). Template bleeding time (BT) was performed with the Simplate I device (General Diagnostics) and the time was recorded to the nearest minute, fibrinogen (FIB) by the turbidometric method of Ellis and Stransky [Ellis and Stransky 1961], antithrombin III (ATIII) using a chromogenic assay procedure [Abildgaard et al. 1977] and commercial kits (Stago Diagnostic Reagents), factor VIII: clotting activity (FVIII:C) by the one-stage method [Hardisty and Macpherson 1962], von Willebrand factor:Ristocetin cofactor (vWF:Ricof) was assayed using formaldehyde-fixed platelets as described elsewhere [Macfarlane et al. 1975], von Willebrand factor:antigen (vWF:Ag) by electroimmuno-diffusion [Laurell 1965] employing specific rabbit antibodies to von Willebrand factor (Stago Diagnostic Reagents, France). Platelet aggregation was performed in platelet rich plasma (PRP) in response to ADP (2.0 uM), adrenaline (100 uM), collagen (190 μg/ml, arachidonic acid (1.64 mmol/L) and ristocetin (1.5 mg/ml) (all agonists were supplied by Bio/Data, USA). The concentrations of these agonists represent final concentrations obtained by adding 20 μl of agonist to 180 μl PRP and the change in optical density was recorded in a four channel aggregometer (PAP-4, Aggregation Profiler, Bio/Data, USA). This procedure was detailed recently [Gader et al. 1988]. In the blood transfusion group the same blood tests were undertaken before and 2 days after the last RBC transfusion.

Statistical analysis

The paired Student t-test was used to compare the significance of the difference in measurements of all the patient groups. A P value of 0.05 or less is considered significant.

Results

The erythropoietin-treated group

In all patients there was a significant increase in hemoglobin concentration in response to rHuEpo therapy (Table 1). The pre-treatment mean Hb level was 7.2 ± 0.3 g/dl (range of 6.7–7.8) and at the end of 16 weeks, was 11.6 ± 1.4 g/dl (range 9.1–13). One patient had slower and less dramatic improvement of Hb levels than the others due to the fact that he started with the lowest Hb level; besides, he used to develop frequent clotting of the extracorporal circuit for which the dosage of heparin for each dialysis was increased with variable response.

There was a significant shortening of the Simplate BT (Table 2) noted after 8 weeks of treatment. Complete correction of the BT was attained to within our laboratory normal range which is 7–10 minutes in all patients with the exception of one. In addition, marked increases in the plasma levels of fibrinogen, FVIII:C, vWF:Ricof, vWF:Ag, Hct and platelet count were maintained at 8 and 16 weeks of rHuEpo therapy (Table 1). Statistically significant increase in ATIII was noted at 16 weeks of rHuEpo therapy, but this is well within our normal laboratory range of 80–120%. The patient whose BT did not correct (Patient no. 4 – Table 2) had minimal increase in FVIII:related activities. Platelet aggregation responses to most agonists were significantly enhanced at 8 and 16 weeks of rHuEpo therapy when compared to the pre-treatment measurements (Table 3). No significant alterations in PT, PTT, TT and RT were noted.

The blood transfusion group

In this group of 7 patients a mean of 4.2 ± 2.5 units of RBC transfusion (range 3–7) were given to raise the Hb concentration from a mean pre-RBC transfusion level of 7.0 g/dl (SD ± 0.5) to 11.9 ± 1.2 g/dl, post-RBC transfusion. Although there was a significant shortening of the BT, in only one patient was there complete correction of the BT within the normal range (Table 2). FVIII : related activities fluctuated in a discordant fashion (Table 1); vWF:Ricofactor exhibited a significant elevation after transfusion (mean ± SD: 210.3 ± 69.2%), as compared to the pretransfusion levels of 143.7 ± 46.4%. Both FVIII:C, vWF:Ag and platelet count showed no significant changes. Platelet aggregation responses to ADP, adrenaline, collagen, arachidonic acid and ristocetin were unchanged (Table 3).

Discussion

The results of this study in uremic patients have demonstrated that rHuEpo therapy causes shortening of the bleeding time, significant elevation of factor VIII:related activities and enhancement of platelet aggregation responses. These changes occur concurrently with the gradual increase in the hematocrit and hemoglobin concentration as well as marked improvement in the clinical state of these patients. On the other hand when RBC transfusions were used to correct the anemia of uremic patients to comparable levels of hematocrit and hemoglobin concentrations, bleeding time shortened but was not corrected, there was discordant fluctuation of FVIII:related activities; while FVIII:C and vWF:Ag levels did not change significantly, there was a significant increase in the levels of vWF:Ricofactor. These results confirm the recent reports on the correction of the BT after either rHuEpo therapy [Ad Hoc 1989, Raman et al. 1988] or blood transfusion [Livio et al. 1982, Fernandez et al. 1985]. However, none of these earlier studies included measurements of FVIII:related properties.

Previous studies on the structure and function of FVIII:related properties in chronic renal failure patients have given conflicting results. Although there is general agreement that both FVIII:C and vWF:Ag exhibit significant elevations [Kazatchkine et al. 1976, Herrmann et al. 1977, Remuzzi et al. 1977, Warrell et al. 1979, Turney et al. 1981], some of these studies have shown both selective elevation [Remuzzi et al. 1977, Warrell et al. 1979] as well as a decrease [Kazatchkine et al. 1976, Turney et al. 1981] of vWF:Ricofactor levels. In one study [Herrmann et al. 1977], vWF:Ricofactor levels remained low after kidney transplantation despite normalization of FVIII:C and vWF:Ag activities. More significant elevation of vWF:Ricofactor than FVIII:C and vWF:Ag was also reported after DDAVP infusion in patients with renal failure [Watson and Keogh 1982]. This suggests that in uremic patients the vWF:Ricofactor fluctuates independently of the other factor VIII:related activities. In our study we noted significant elevation of the three FVIII:related activities, at eight and sixteen weeks after the commencement of rHuEpo therapy. Throughout, FVIII:C was consistently more elevated than vWF:Ag and vWF:Ricofactor. In the same time interval, there was little increase in the hematocrit and hemoglobin concentrations. Thus rHuEpo not only augments RBC production but also, in an unknown way, increases the production and/or release of the various components of the FVIII:related activities. This last effect acquires special significance since suboptimal levels of vWF:activity were invoked as the mechanism responsible for platelet dysfunction and BT prolongation in renal failure [Janson et al. 1980].

The correction of the BT by the transfusion of RBC has received a lot of attention in the literature. Although it is not clear how the transfusion of RBC may correct the prolonged BT, two mechanisms have recently been suggested [Boneau and Fernandez 1987]: firstly, the blood flow in small blood vessels is in such a way that RBCs cause physical dispersal of the platelets towards the endothelial surface thereby facilitating platelet-blood vessel interaction. Secondly, in an injured blood vessel some RBCs are hemolysed, releasing small amounts of adenosine diphosphate (ADP) triggering the aggregation of platelets and primary hemostatic plug formation. Both mechanisms require the participation of von Willebrand factor (vWF) which is essential for the binding of platelets to the vessel wall [Girma et al. 1987]. In those patients who received blood transfusion, the rise in vWF:Ricofactor was much higher than the increase observed in other factor VIII:related activities. Judging by the lesser correction of BT attained in this group as compared to the rHuEpo group, one may speculate that the selective increase in vWF: Ricofactor activity does not seem to be effective in correcting the prolonged BT in uremics, even after rectifying the deficiency in the circulating red cell mass.

It is known that uremic patients have longer BT than non-uremic patients with a similar degree of anemia [Livio et al. 1982]. Moreover, significant shortening of the BT occurs earlier than the correction of the anemia to 10–12 g/dl, and normal BT may occur with low hematocrit and prolonged BT with hematocrit above 30% [Van Geet et al. 1989]. In our study one patient who showed least improvement of the BT also exhibited the least elevation of factor VIII: related activities, while his hematocrit was not markedly different from the other patients. This suggests that the shortening of the BT that accompanies rHuEpo therapy is related closely to the increase in FVIII: related activities.

Since a risk for thrombosis was reported in uremic patients receiving rHuEpo [Winearls et al. 1986, Casati et al. 1987, Schaefer et al. 1989] the elevation of plasma fibrinogen following rHuEpo therapy is of some interest in this respect, since high fibrinogen levels are likely to predispose to thrombosis. This may occur in many ways. Firstly plasma fibrinogen is an important determinant of blood viscosity [Lowe 1985] which is also apt to increase as a result of the progressive rise in the circulating red cell mass induced by rHuEpo treatment [Raine 1988]. Secondly high fibrinogen levels are associated with enhanced platelet aggregability [Meade et al. 1985a, 1985b]. Lastly, work in animals suggests that the amount of fibrin formed is determined by the initial concentration of fibrinogen [Gurewich et al. 1976]. These factors in addition to the significant rise in platelet count, operating together may account for the hightened thrombotic tendency in uremic patients receiving rHuEpo.

In conclusion, this study has established significant elevations in factor VIII: related activities, plasma fibrinogen, marked improvement in the platelet aggregation responses and almost complete correction of the bleeding time to be salient hemostatic changes that accompany rHuEpo therapy in uremic patients.

Acknowledgements

We would like to thank Messrs. M. A. Hamid and L. A. Gassem Al Seed for excellent technical assistance; and Mrs. Farah Chatila for the analysis of the data and typing the manuscript. This work was supported by a grant from the College of Medicine, Research Centre (CMRC), King Saud University, Riyadh.

REFERENCES

Abildgaard U, Lie M, Odegard OR 1977 Antithrombin (heparin co-factor) assay with "new chromogenic substrates" (S-2238 and chromozyum "TH"). Thromb Res *11:* 549–553

Ad Hoc Committee for the National Kidney Foundation 1989 Statement on the clinical use of recombinant erythropoietin in anemia of end-stage renal disease. Am J Kidney Dis *14:* 163–169

Boneau B, Fernandez F 1987 The role of the hematocrit in bleeding. Transf Med Rev *1:* 182–185

Casati S, Passerini P, Campise MR, Graziani G, Cesana B, Perisic M, Ponticelli C 1987 Benefits and risks of protracted treatment with human recombinant erythropoietin in patients having haemodialysis. Br Med J *295:* 1017–1020

Deykin D 1983 Uremic bleeding. Kidney Int *24:* 698–705

Eknoyan G, Wacksman SJ, Ghneck HI, Will JJ 1969 Platelet function in renal failure. N Engl J Med *280:* 677–681

Ellis BC, Stransky AA 1961 A quick and accurate method for the determination of fibrinogen in plasma. J Lab Clin Med *58:* 477–488

Eschbach JW, Egrie JC, Downing MR, Browne JK, Adamson JW 1987 Correction of the anemia of end-stage renal disease with recombinant human erythropoietin. Results disease with recombinant human erythropoietin. Results of a combined phase I and II clinical trial. N Eng J Med *316:* 73–78

Fernandez F, Goudable C, Die P, Ton-That H, Durand D, Suc JM, Boneu B 1985 Low haematocrit and prolonged bleeding time in uraemic patients: effect of red cell transfusions. Br J Haemat *59:* 139–148

Gader AMA, Bahakim H, Jabbar FA, Lambourne AL, Gaafar TH, Edrees YB 1988 Dose-response aggregometry in maternal/neonatal platelets. Thromb Hemostas *60:* 314–318

Girma JP, Meyer D, Verweij CL, Pannekoek H, Sixma JJ 1987 Structure-function relationship of human von Willebrand Factor. Blood *70:* 605–611

Gurewich V, Lipinski B, Hyde E 1976 The effect of the fibrinogen concentration and the leucocyte count on intravascular fibrin deposition from soluble fibrin monomer complexes. Thrombos Haemostas *36:* 605–614

Hardisty RM, Macpherson JD 1962 A one stage FVIII assay and its use of venous and capillary plasma. Thromb Diath Haemorrh *7:* 215–229

Hellem AJ, Borchgrevink CF, Ames SB 1961 The role of red cells in haemostasis: The relation between haematocrit, bleeding time and platelet adhesiveness. Br J Haemat *7:* 42–50

Herrmann RP, Marshall LR, Hurst PE 1977 Bleeding in renal failure: a possible cause. Br Med J *1:* 1601–1602

Janson PA, Jubeliere SJ, Weinstein MJ, Deykin D 1980 Treatment of the bleeding tendency in uremia with cryoprecipitate. N Engl J Med *303:* 1318–1322

Kazatchkine M, Sultan Y, Caen JP, Bariety J 1976 Bleeding in uremia: a possible cause. Br Med J *2:* 612–615

Laurell CB 1965 Antigen-antibody crossed electrophoresis. Ann Biochem *10:* 358–361

Livio M, Benigni A, Remuzzi G 1985 Coagulation abnormalities in uremia. Semin Nephrol *5:* 82–90

Livio M, Gotti E, Marchesi D et al. 1982 Uraemic bleeding: role of anaemia and beneficial effect of red-cell transfusions. Lancet *ii:* 1013–1015 (Part II)

Lowe GDO 1985 Blood rheology in arterial disease. Clin Sc *68:* 419–425

Macfarlane DE, Stibbe J, Kirby EP et al. 1975 A method for assaying von Willebrand factor (ristocetin-cofactor). Thromb Diath Haemorrh *34:* 306–308

Meade TW, Vickers MV, Thompson SG, Stirling Y, Haines AP, Miller GJ 1985a Epidemiological characteristics of platelet aggregability. Br Med J *290:* 428–432

Meade TW, Vickers MV, Thompson SG, Seghatchian MJ 1985b The effect of physiological levels of fibrinogen on platelet aggregation. Thromb Res *38:* 527–534

Moia M, Vizzotto L, Cattaneo M, Mannucci PM, Casati S, Ponticelli C 1987 Improvement in the haemostatic defect of uraemia after treatment with recombinant human erythropoietin. Lancet *2:* 1227–1229

Raine AEG 1988 Hypertension, blood viscosity, and cardiovascular morbidity in renal failure: implications of erythropoietin therapy. Lancet *1:* 97–100

Raman S, Mohini R, Janakiraman N, Levin N, Saeed SM 1988 Evaluation of platelet function in patients treated with human recombinant erythropoietin. Blood (Suppl 1) *272:* 1252

Remuzzi G, Benigni A, Dodesini P et al. 1981 Platelet function in patients on maintenance haemodialysis: Depressed or enchanced? Clin Nephrol *17:* 60–63

Remuzzi G, Livio M, Roncaglioni MC, Mecca G, Donati MB, De Gaetano G 1977 Bleeding in renal failure: Is von Willebrand factor implicated? Br Med J *2:* 359–361

Remuzzi G, Pusineri F 1988 Coagulation defects in uremia. Kid Int *33:* 13–17

Schaefer RM, Horl WH, Massry SG 1989 Treatment of renal anemia with recombinant human erythropoietin. Am J Nephrol *9:* 353–362

Turney JH, Woods HF, Fewell MR, Weston MJ 1981 Factor VIII complex in uraemia and effects of hemodialysis. Br Med J *282:* 1653–1656

Van Geet C, Hauglustaine D, Verresen L, Vanrusselt M, Vermylen J 1989 Haemostatic effects of recombinant human erythropoietin in chronic haemodialysis patients. Thromb Haemostas *61:* 117–121

Warrell RP, Hultin MB, Coller BS 1979 Increased factor VIII/von Willebrand factor antigen and von Willebrand factor activity in renal failure. Am J Med *66:* 226–228

Watson AJS, Keogh JAB 1982 Effect of 1-Deamino-8-D-Arginine Vasopressin on the prolonged bleeding time in chronic renal failure. Nephron *32:* 49–52

Winearls CG, Pippard MJ, Downing MR, Oliver DO, Reid C, Cotes PM 1986 Effect of human erythropoietin derived from recombinant DNA on the anaemia of patients maintained by chronic haemodialysis. Lancet *ii:* 1175–1177

Clinical Nephrology, Vol. 36 No. 5 – 1991 (258–261)

Iatrogenic hypercalcemia in hemodialysis patients

M. A. Muhammedi[1], B. Piraino[2], R. Rault[2], J. R. Johnston[2] and J. B. Puschett[3]

[1]777 Cleveland Ave., Suite 305, Atlanta, GA 30314, [2]The Renal-Electrolyte Division, Department of Medicine, University of Pittsburgh, Presbyterian University Hospital, Pittsburgh, Pennsylvania and [3]Department of Medicine, Tulane University, New Orleans, Louisiana, USA

Abstract. Calcium carbonate is frequently used in large doses as a phosphorus binder in hemodialysis patients, which often results in hypercalcemia. In most studies in which calcium carbonate is prescribed to control serum phosphorus levels the patients are not given calcitriol. However, calcitriol may be necessary for suppression of parathyroid hormone. The risk of hypercalcemia when calcium supplements are used in conjunction with calcitriol has not previously been examined in detail. We reviewed the charts of 74 hemodialysis patients (119 patient dialysis years) to determine the relationship of serum calcium to calcitriol, calcium therapy, and PTH levels. Twenty-eight patients (38%) were hypercalcemic at some point. Calcitriol therapy significantly increased the risk of hypercalcemia, independently of calcium therapy ($p = 0.032$). However, patients on a low dose of calcitriol were more than twice as likely to be hypercalcemic than patients on higher doses. Mean PTH levels were lower in the patients on the lower doses of calcitriol, indicating less severe hyperparathyroid disease. We conclude that hypercalcemia is a common complication in hemodialysis patients on calcitriol and calcium carbonate. Whether lowering the dialysate calcium, as suggested by other investigators, will successfully decrease the risk of hypercalcemia without worsening hyperparathyroidism remains to be determined.

Key words: hypercalcemia – hemodialysis – hyperparathyroidism – calcitriol

Introduction

Calcium carbonate has been shown to be an effective phosphorus binder in hemodialysis patients [Slatopolsky et al. 1986, Hercz et al. 1986, Fournier et al. 1986]. Relatively large doses of oral calcium are generally required to control the serum phosphorus levels [Moriniere et al. 1982, Gonella et al. 1985]. Hypercalcemia is a frequent complication [Hercz et al. 1986, Fournier et al. 1986, Moriniere et al. 1982]. Indeed, a lower calcium dialysate has been used to prevent hypercalcemia when administering large doses of oral calcium carbonate [Gonella et al. 1985, Slatopolsky et al. 1989].

Parathyroid hormone release is inhibited by an elevation in the serum ionized calcium level. There is increasing evidence that 1,25 dihydroxycholecalciferol also directly inhibits parathyroid hormone release [Dunlay et al. 1989, Slatopolsky et al. 1984]. Thus, calcitriol, either via the oral or intravenous route, is useful in treating secondary hyperparathyroidism. However, calcitriol therapy with or without oral calcium therapy frequently results in hypercalcemia [Slatopolsky et al. 1984, Berl et al. 1978, Baker et al. 1986].

The risk of hypercalcemia in hemodialysis patients on both calcitriol and oral calcium therapy is not known. We investigated iatrogenic hypercalcemia induced by oral calcium and calcitriol therapy in 74 patients on hemodialysis. We report on the incidence of hypercalcemia and the relationship to the doses of calcitriol prescribed in patients who were on oral calcium supplements.

Methods

Charts were reviewed on all hemodialysis patients (74) at one outpatient dialysis facility, who were

Received October 4, 1990; in revised form February 5, 1991.

Reprint requests to Dr. Beth Piraino, 11431 Presbyterian University Hospital, Pittsburgh, PA 15213, USA on chronic dialysis during 1989. Each patient's chart was reviewed from either the initiation of outpatient dialysis or for a maximum of 3 years prior to July 1989. Demographic data were obtained for each patient including age at the onset of chronic dialysis, date of onset of chronic dialysis, sex, race, etiology of end-stage renal disease, and a history of previous parathyroidectomy.

Serum calcium and phosphorus levels were obtained in monthly pre-dialysis. C-terminal PTH (Mayo Laboratory, normal less than 55 μlEq/ml) was measured yearly.

Control of the serum calcium and phosphorus was managed as follows. The patient was initially placed on aluminum compounds and a low phosphorus diet. Once the serum phosphorus was 6 mg/dl or less, low dose calcium carbonate was added, generally 1250 mg one to three times per day to be taken with meals. The dose of calcium carbonate was titrated to as high as 2500 mg three times a day while the aluminum compound was decreased or discontinued, with the goal of keeping the serum phosphorus less than 6 mg/dl. In 9 patients oral calcium therapy was not initiated as phosphorus control was adequate without any binder. Once the serum phosphorus level was adequately controlled and if the serum calcium was 10 mg/dl or less, calcitriol, 0.25 μg per day orally, was added and gradually increased to maintain the pre-dialysis serum calcium between 10 to 11 mg/dl. If the serum calcium exceeded 11 mg/dl, the calcitriol was first decreased and then stopped if hypercalcemia persisted. If the hypercalcemia did not resolve off calcitriol, the calcium supplements were then stopped. Once normocalcemia was restored the patient was restarted on calcitriol at a lower dose.

Fifty-eight patients (78%) were on aluminum containing phosphorus binders. Most of these patients required continuation of aluminum containing binders, as well as calcium carbonate, for adequate serum phosphorus control throughout the period of the study.

For the purposes of the present analysis, the patient was considered to be hypercalcemic if his or her serum calcium exceeded 10.5 mg/dl (normal values, 8.5 to 10.5 mg/dl). Medications, in particular oral calcium and/or oral calcitriol, were recorded at the time each calcium level was measured. Intravenous calcitriol was not utilized at the time of the chart review.

Patients were dialyzed three times per week for 3 to 5 hours, 4 hours being the most common prescription. The concentration of calcium in the dialysate was 3.25 mEq/l.

Data are presented as mean values with the standard deviation. Data analysis was performed using correlation testing, Chi square test, analysis of variance (ANOVA) for comparison of multiple groups, and the unpaired t-test with Bonferroni's correction to compare one group to another. To evaluate calcitriol therapy independently of calcium therapy, the Mantel-Haenszel analysis was performed. For this analysis patients were counted only once. If the patient was on calcitriol and/or calcium therapy at any time, then the patient was included in the calcium/calcitriol group. Five patients were on calcifediol for part of the period of follow-up. Four of these patients were on calcitriol at some time, and one was not. These five patients are included in the calcitriol-treated group but are excluded from the analysis of the relationship between calcitriol dose and the development of hypercalcemia. A p value of less than 0.05 was considered significant.

Results

Data for 119 patient dialysis years were collected. Twenty-eight of the patients (38%) were hypercalcemic at some time during the period of the chart review. Ten per cent of the serum calcium values were greater than 10.5 mg/dl (144/1426 patient dialysis months). The mean serum calcium level during the periods of hypercalcemia was 11.2 mg/dl ± 0.7, with a range from 10.6 to 16.2 mg/dl.

The demographic features of the hypercalcemic and non-hypercalcemic patients are shown in Table 1. The mean ages, gender, race and cause of renal failure were similar. The patients who developed hypercalcemia were on dialysis for a significantly longer period

Table 1 Demographic data

	Hypercalcemic patients	Non-hypercalcemic patients
Number of patients	28	46
Age, mean, years	48 ± 22	41 ± 18
Age, range, years	13–87	10–73
Female sex, n (%)	14 (50)	20 (43)
Time on dialysis as of 7/89, months	95 ± 55	67 ± 62[a]
Black patients, n (%)	11 (39)	28 (61)
No. with history of parathyroidectomy	5	2
Etiology of ESRD		
D. M.	2	11
CGN	7	9
Hypertension	6	5
PCK disease	3	2
Other	10	19

[a] $p < 0.05$

Table 2 Relationship of oral calcium and calcitriol administration to the occurrence of hypercalcemia

Therapy	Number of patients	Hypercalcemia developed[a]
On calcium and calcitriol	50	23[b] (46%)
On calcitriol alone	7	3 (43%)
On calcium, no calcitriol	15	2 (13%)
No calcium or calcitriol	2	0
Total	74	28 (38%)

[a] Calcitriol therapy was significantly associated with hypercalcemia, controlling for calcium therapy, p = 0.032, Mantel-Haenszel test.

[b] One patient was on calcifediol rather than calcitriol.

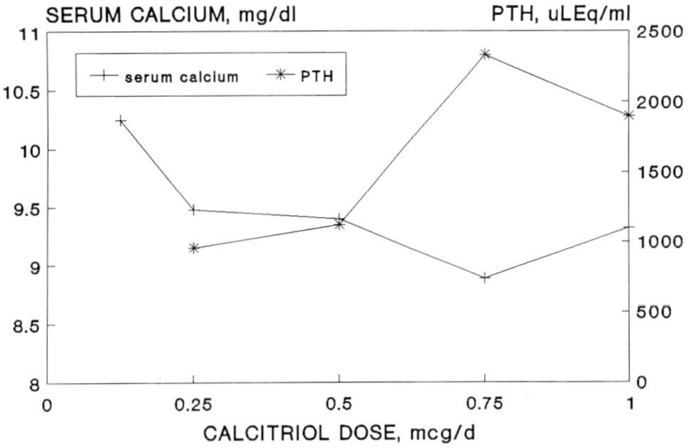

•p <0.0005 vs serum calcium at all other doses

Fig. 1 Mean serum calcium (ANOVA p <0.001) and PTH levels (ANOVA p <0.05) differ at various calcitriol doses. Mean serum calcium level at a calcitriol dose of less than 0.25 µg per day was significantly different than mean serum calcium levels at all other doses, p <0.0005 (significant at p <0.003 for 15 comparisons)

of time than those patients who were not hypercalcemic (p <0.05).

All of the patients were on calcitriol and/or calcium therapy when they became hypercalcemic. One patient had persistent hypercalcemia after calcitriol was discontinued with serum calcium values averaging 11.0 mg/dl. She was not on calcium supplements. Hypercalcemia resolved in 11 patients with an adjustment or discontinuation of the calcitriol dose. In 7 patients the hypercalcemia was transient and mild (<11.0 mg/dl) and the dose of calcitriol was not changed. In 9 patients hypercalcemia developed shortly before and was still present at study endpoint.

Hypercalcemia was more likely to be present in patients on calcitriol therapy than those who were not, independently of calcium supplementation (p = 0.032, Table 2). However, patients who were on 0.25 µg of calcitriol every day or every other day were more likely to be hypercalcemic than those patients on a larger dose of calcitriol (9/12, 75% versus 13/40, 32%, respectively, p <0.01).

The relationships of calcitriol dose to the serum calcium and PTH levels are shown in Figure 1. Mean serum calcium value for the patients on the lowest doses of calcitriol was higher than those values on the higher doses of calcitriol, p <0.0001, ANOVA. The C-terminal PTH levels were highest in the patients on the largest doses of calcitriol, p <0.05, ANOVA. There was no correlation between PTH levels and the calcitriol dose (r = 0.23) or between PTH and the serum calcium value (r = 0.17).

Discussion

Hypercalcemia is common when calcium carbonate is used to control serum phosphorus levels in dialysis patients. In one study 61.5% (16/26) of patients developed hypercalcemia after calcium carbonate was substituted for aluminum hydroxide [Moriniere et al. 1982]. In another study the majority of the patients became hypercalcemic while on high doses of calcium carbonate, but these patients were dialyzing against dialysate with a high concentration of calcium, 4 mEq/l [Gonella et al. 1985]. In neither study were the patients taking any form of vitamin D metabolite during the time calcium was given as the phosphorus binder.

In the present study at a center where both oral calcium and calcitriol are routinely prescribed, iatrogenic hypercalcemia was found in 28 of 74 (38%) of the patients over 119 dialysis years. Hypercalcemia was present during 10% of the time (144/1426 months of dialysis). Increasing time on dialysis was a risk factor for the development of iatrogenic hypercalcemia. Those patients who were hypercalcemic had been on dialysis for almost 8 years as opposed to 5½ years for those patients who were never hypercalcemic (p <0.05). There was no age, gender, or racial predilection for the development of hypercalcemia.

Calcitriol therapy was associated with the development of hypercalcemia, independent of calcium therapy. Patients on calcitriol therapy were more likely to be hypercalcemic than patients not on calcitriol (Table 2). Over 40% of the patients on calcitriol had at least one episode of hypercalcemia, in contrast to only 2/17 (12%) patients not treated with calcitriol therapy.

However, those patients on a small dose of calcitriol (0.25 µg per day or every other day) were twice as likely to become hypercalcemic and had a higher mean serum calcium value than patients on larger doses of calcitriol (Figure 1). This suggests that the calcitriol dose was in part dictated by the serum calcium level. That is, when calcitriol induced hypercalcemia in a patient, the dose was reduced. Thus, some patients tolerated large doses of calcitriol without developing hypercalcemia while other patients did not. The reason for this is unclear.

The parathyroid hormone levels were higher in the patients on the larger doses of calcitriol, suggesting that these patients had more severe hyperparathyroidism, compared to the patients on lower doses of calcitriol (Figure 1). Therefore, severity of hyperparathyroid disease does not explain the relative hypercalcemia present in patients on low doses of calcitriol.

In summary, patients who are on hemodialysis are very likely to become hypercalcemic when treated with oral calcitriol. However, the optimal treatment of osteitis fibrosa includes calcitriol therapy, since 1,25-dihydroxyvitamin D has an independent effect of suppressing PTH release. Adjusting the dialysate calcium content to diminish the risk of hypercalcemia may be a useful adjunct to the treatment of osteitis fibrosa with calcitriol and calcium [Kaye et al. 1989, Slatopolsky et al. 1989].

REFERENCES

Baker LRI, Muir JW, Sharman VL et al. 1986 Controlled trial of calcitriol in hemodialysis patients. Clin Nephrol *26:* 185

Berl T, Berns AS, Huffer WE et al. 1978 1,25-dihydroxycholecalciferol effects in chronic dialysis. A double-blind controlled study. Ann Intern Med *88:* 774

Dunlay R, Rodriguez L, Felsenfeld AJ et al. 1989 Direct inhibitory effect of calcitriol on parathyroid function (sigmoidal curve) in dialysis. Kidney Int *36:* 1093

Fournier A, Moriniere P, Sebert JL et al. 1986 Calcium carbonate, an aluminum-free agent for control of hyperphosphatemia, hypocalcemia, and hyperparathyroidism in uremia. Kidney Int *29 (18):* S-114

Gonella M, Calabrese G, Vagelli G et al. 1985 Effects of high $CaCO_3$ supplements on serum calcium and phosphorus in patients on regular hemodialysis treatment. Clin Nephrol *24:* 146

Hercz G, Kraut JA, Andress DA et al. 1986 Use of calcium carbonate as a phosphate binder in dialysis patients. Mineral Electrolyte Metab *12:* 314

Kaye M, Barber E, Vailevsky M, Langer K 1989 Calcium-free dialyzate: development and applications. Clin Nephrol *31:* 132

Moriniere P, Roussel A, Tahiri Y et al. 1982 Substitution of aluminum hydroxide by high doses of calcium carbonate in patients on chronic haemodialysis: disappearance of hyperaluminaemia and equal control of hyperparathyroidism. Proc EDTA *19:* 784

Slatopolsky E, Weerts C, Thielan J et al. 1984 Marked suppression of secondary hyperparathyroidism by intravenous administration of 1,25-dihydroxycholecalciferol in uremic patients. J Clin Invest *74:* 2136

Slatopolsky E, Weerts C, Lopez-Hilker S et al. 1986 Calcium carbonate as a phosphate binder in patients with chronic renal failure and undergoing dialysis. N Engl J Med *315:* 157

Slatopolsky E, Weerts C, Norwood K et al. 1989 Long-term effects of calcium carbonate and 2.5 mEq/liter calcium dialysate on mineral metabolism. Kidney Int *36:* 897

LETTERS TO THE EDITOR

Myoglobinuria after KENDOU training

Sir, – Acute myoglobinuria has been reported with increasing frequency since its original description in 1910 by Meyer-Betz [Dtsch Arch Klin Med 1910, 101: 85–127]. Myoglobinuria is one of the symptoms of rhabdomyolysis which is defined as a clinical and laboratory syndrome resulting from skeletal muscle injury with release of muscle cell contents into plasma [Honda 1983, Kidney Int 23: 888–898]. Rhabdomyolysis has a clinical importance because myoglobin and other constituents of the muscle cells impair renal function [Gabow et al. 1982, Medicine 61: 141–152]. However, a controversy exists regarding the nephrotoxicity of myoglobin. Among the causes of rhabdomyolysis, muscle exertion caused by excessive physical work is the most important one [Hamilton et al. 1972, Ann Intern Med 77: 77–82, Demos et al. 1974, Arch Intern Med 134: 669–673, MacSearraigh et al. 1979, Nephron 24: 236–240]. Previously we reported 2 cases of rhabdomyolysis caused by KENDOU training (a traditional japanese sport like fencing) [Hara et al. 1991, Pediatric Clinic (in Japanese) in press]. In the present study we performed the urinalysis of students in the KENDOU club of our university before and after KENDOU training. The data obtained suggests a nephrotoxicity of myoglobin.

Fourteen male students (aged 18–31 years) in the KENDOU club of our university were investigated. Past and family history revealed no renal diseases. At the time of investigation none of the students were ill or had dehydration. Urine samples taken 2 hours before training were collected and then they exercised for 2 hours on a usual training program. Urine samples were collected again after training. All the students were well and none developed the symptoms of rhabdomyolysis such as weakness or muscle pain. Urine volume, pH, proteinuria, creatinine, beta 2 microglobulin and NAG were estimated. Urine myoglobin was assayed by RIA method. Urine was also examined by microscopy and usual dip stick for occult blood. Student's t-test (paired) was used to evaluate any statistically significant difference.

Orthotolidine dip stick examination was positive in 7 out of 14 urine samples and 4 of them showed brown or dark brown urine color. Microscopic examination showed absence of hematuria. Urine samples from 7 students with positive dip stick examination revealed myoglobinuria (ranged 228.7–4020.0 ng/ml) and others showed less than 10 ng/ml myoglobin concentration. Therefore, the following analysis was peformed in the myoglobin positive group (7 students) and the negative group (7 students). The values were expressed as per minute except pH. Urine myoglobin, volume, pH, creatinine, proteinuria, beta 2 microglobulin and NAG in both groups before and after the training were shown in the Table. Urine volume after the training was decreased significantly as compared with that before training in both groups, although the difference was not found in urine creatinine and pH. Proteinuria, urine beta 2 microglobulin and NAG in the myoglobin positive group after the training was significantly more than those before the training. As to beta 2 microglobulin, the correlation between the level of beta 2 microglobulin and the degree of myoglobinuria was observed ($r = 0.97$, $p < 0.05$).

It is well-known that acute renal failure is associated with myoglobinuria under various circumstances including extreme excertion [Honda 1983, Gabow et al. 1982]. However, the mecha-

Table Urine myoglobin, urine volume, urine creatinine, proteinuria, β2-microglobulin (MG) and NAG from 14 students before and after KENDOU training during 2 hours

		Before	After	Statistics
u-Myoglobin (ng/min)	Myoglobin (+) (N = 7)	5.5 ± 2.3	608.6 ± 855.8*	
	Myoglobin (−) (N = 7)	4.3 ± 1.9	1.4 ± 0.7	
u-volume (mi/min)	Myoglobin (+)	0.7 ± 0.3	0.3 ± 0.2	p <0.05**
	Myoglobin (−)	0.5 ± 0.3	0.2 ± 0.1	p <0.01
u-pH	Myoglobin (+)	5.67 ± 0.61	5.40 ± 0.32	n. s.
	Myoglobin (−)	5.61 ± 0.73	5.23 ± 0.38	n. s.
u-Creatinine (mg/min)	Myoglobin (+)	1.3 ± 0.9	0.8 ± 0.2	n. s.
	Myoglobin (−)	0.7 ± 0.2	0.6 ± 0.3	n. s.
Proteinuria (mg/min)	Myoglobin (+)	0.03 ± 0.02	0.73 ± 0.40	p <0.01
	Myoglobin (−)	0.03 ± 0.01	0.25 ± 0.44	n. s.
u-β2 MG (ug/min)	Myoglobin (+)	0.06 ± 0.03	1.58 ± 1.61	p <0.05
	Myoglobin (−)	0.06 ± 0.03	0.04 ± 0.04	n. s.
u-NAG (U/min, × 0.01)	Myoglobin (+)	0.23 ± 0.18	1.16 ± 0.69	p <0.05
	Myoglobin (−)	0.15 ± 0.10	0.19 ± 0.13	n. s.

* Mean ± SD

** Paired t-test comparing values before and after.

nism by which myoglobin produce acute renal failure is not yet known. Bywaters and Stead [Bywaters et al. 1944, Q J Exp Physiol 33: 53–70] and subsequent investigators [Braun et al. 1970, J Exp Med 131: 443–460, Blachar et al. 1981, Cir Res 49: 114–124] have suggested that myoglobin and other constituents of the muscle cells impair renal function. On the other hand, a controversy exists regarding the nephrotoxicity of myoglobin itself. Many studies have suggested that myoglobin itself is relatively nonnephrotoxic but that it becomes high toxic when dehydration, aciduria or both coexist [Perri et al. 1952, Br J Exp Pathol 33: 440–444, Lalich 1952, J Lab Clin Med 40: 102–110, Garcia et al. 1981, Kidney Int 19: 200]. Despite these, our data suggest the nephrotoxicity of myoglobin, although all students were well and had no dehydration at the time of study and pH of urine was not different between myoglobinuric and nonmyoglobinuric students. Only myoglobinuric students had impaired the renal function revealed by urine beta 2 microglobulin and NAG. Furthermore, there was a correlation between the urine beta 2 microglobulin level and the degree of myoglobinuria, supporting the nephrotoxicity of myoglobin itself. Although none of students developed renal failure, a risk for it must be evaluated clinically. Two students with moderate value of urine myoglobin were examined for blood chemistry and we calculated the risk factors predictive of acute renal failure based on the paper reported by Ward et al. [1988, Arch Intern Med 148: 1553–1557]. In these students the total point was 3 which indicated low risk for developing acute renal failure. However, it seems to be reasonable to consider that if more severe exercise or exercise of longer duration was performed and a dehydrative state was added, the risk for renal failure would be higher. Thus, much attention should be paid to such conditions in the KENDOU training.

M. Hara, S. Ishihara, R. Yoshida, S. Inaba, A. Higuchi, Y. Suzuki and T. Okada
Department of Pediatrics, Faculty of Medicine, Toyama Medical and Pharmaceutical University, Toyama City, Japan

Predicting outcome after childhood hemolytic uremic syndrome

Dear Sir, – Coad et al. report an increase in the incidence of diarrhoea-associated hemolytic uremic syndrome (D + HUS) in Birmingham and a change in certain clinical features during the early 1980's [Coad et al., 1991]. They describe a prognostic score (Birmingham score) based on sex and hematological parameters at diagnosis to predict good or poor renal outcome in children presenting after 1982. Neutrophil count was the most important predictive factor.

We have seen a similar change in the incidence and nature of D + HUS during the early 1980's, but have found that the Birmingham score does not predict renal outcome in our patients. Instead, it is a better predictor of our children with severe acute extra-renal disease.

We suspect that the problem may lie in their definition of poor renal outcome. As well as including six children with renal

Table 1 The constituents of the Birmingham score as risk factors for renal outcome in Newcastle children. Values expressed as mean (SEM); t-test and * Fishers exact test used for analysis

	Renal outcome Poor	Good	P value
Hb at diagnosis (g/dl)	9.9 (1.0)	9.1 (0.3)	0.36
Neutrophils ($\times 10^9$/l)	19.8 (3.7)	13.0 (1.2)	0.069
Male sex	4/7	23/57	0.44*
Birmingham score (probability scale)	0.50	0.06	0.059

Table 2 The constituents of the Birmingham score as risk factors for severe extra-renal disease in Newcastle children. Values expressed as mean (SEM); t-test and * Fishers exact test used for analysis

	Extra-renal disease Present	Absent	P value
Hb at diagnosis (g/dl)	11.1 (0.7)	8.9 (0.3)	0.002
Neutrophils ($\times 10^9$/l)	24.2 (4.1)	11.2 (0.7)	0.008
Male sex	9/13	24/65	0.062*
Birmingham score (probability scale)	0.90	0.03	0.001

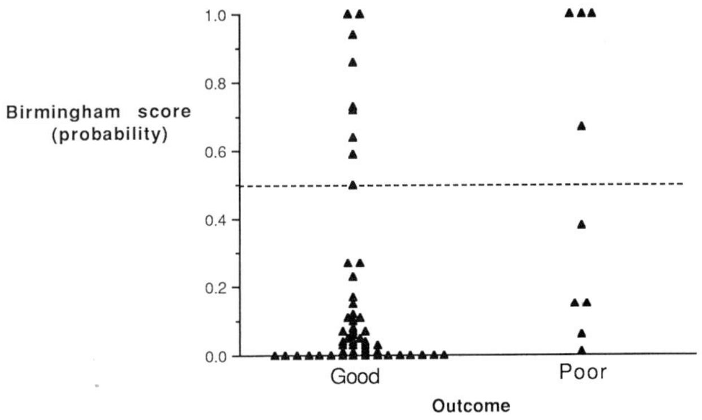

Fig. 1 HUS in Newcastle since 1982: outcome as defined by Coad et al. vs Birmingham score.

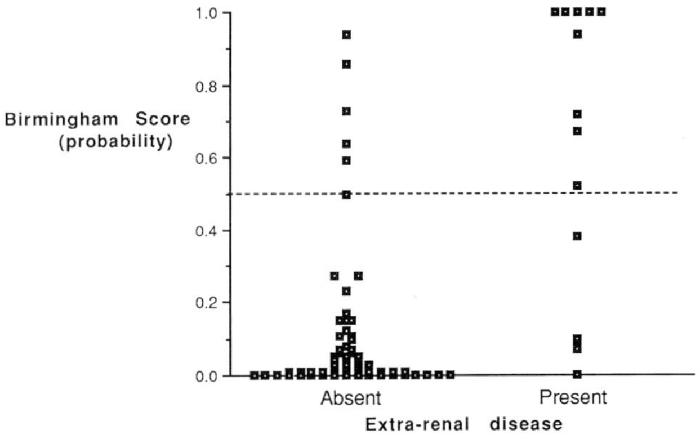

Fig. 2 HUS in Newcastle since 1982: presence of extra-renal disease vs Birmingham score.

Table 3 Relationship between the presence of extra-renal disease and renal outcome in Newcastle children

	Extra-renal disease Present	Absent
Poor renal outcome	3/10	4/54

sequelae (a glomerular filtration rate of less than 75 ml/min/1.73 m^2 and/or significant proteinuria and/or hypertension) they have also included four children who died. The assumption appears to be that children who die from HUS have particularly severe renal involvement and would be left with renal sequelae if they survived. Our experience suggests that this is not the case.

We have treated 78 children with D + HUS since 1982, of whom thirteen had severe acute extra-renal disease (defined as multiple seizures and/or coma and/or bowel resection and/or diabetes mellitus). Two of these died acutely with severe cerebral involvement. As with Coad et al. we have, as yet, insufficient follow-up data to judge the final renal outcome in 15% of our survivors. However, we have clearly documented renal sequelae in seven surviving children. When our cases are analyzed according to Coad et al., combining the seven survivors with renal sequelae and the two children dying acutely into a "poor outcome" group, a Birmingham probability score above 0.5 predicts our patients with a sensitivity of only 44%, a specificity of 85% and a positive predictive value of 33% (Figure 1). Furthermore none of the individual constituents of the score are significantly different between the good and poor outcome groups (Table 1).

By contrast, our children with severe extra-renal involvement did have a significantly higher neutrophil count and hemoglobin at presentation and were predominantly boys, factors that were the main predictors of poor outcome in the Birmingham score (Table 2). Therefore, it is not surprising that for these patients, the Birmingham score was a better predictor of severe extrarenal disease than of renal outcome, with a sensitivity of 69%, specificity of 92% and a positive predictive value of 64% (Figure 2).

Death during HUS typically occurs early in the illness in children with severe extra-renal manifestations of the disease, and is rarely primarily due to the acute renal failure itself. When we look at our children who survived severe extra-renal disease, often after prolonged intensive care, there is no evidence that the renal outcome for this group of children is different from those children with uncomplicated HUS. Seven out of ten such children have made a full renal recovery (Table 3). It follows that death due to HUS should not be included in a definition of poor renal outcome.

Employing scores based on regression equations may be superficially attractive, perhaps in identifying high risk patients suitable for inclusion into a clinical trial. However, considerable caution should be exercised in their use; validation of such scores on the data used to determine the regression equation is wellknown to produce excessively optimistic values for specificity and sensitivity [Phillips, Thompson & Pocock 1990]. Only if prognostic scores are determined using large numbers of cases and validated on other data sets can they be considered reliable. In addition it is imperative that these scores are clearly defined both in terms of predictive variables and precise outcomes. At present we would suggest there is still no satisfactory score available which will predict renal outcome in children with D+HUS at presentation. The duration of anuria, although in no way predictive at presentation, remains the best marker of renal outcome available [Siegler et al. 1991, Morris & Coulthard 1990].

K. P. Morris, M. G. Coulthard, J. N. S. Matthews
The Royal Victoria Infirmary, Queen Victoria Road, Newcastle Upon Tyne, England

REFERENCES

Coad NAG, Marshall T, Rowe B, Taylor CM 1991 Changes in the postenteropathic form of the hemolytic uremic syndrome in children. Clin Nephrol *35:* 10–16
Morris KP, Coulthard MG 1990 The prediction of extra-renal disease and renal outcome in childhood haemolytic uraemic syndrome. Pediatr Nephrol *4:* C51
Phillips AN, Thompson SG, Pocock SJ 1990 Prognostic scores for detecting a high risk group: estimating the sensitivity when applied to new data. Statistics in Medicine *9:* 1189–1198
Siegler RL, Milligan MK, Burningham TH et al. 1991 Long-term outcome and prognostic indicators in the hemolytic-uremic syndrome. J Pediatr *118:* 195–200

Anaphylactoid reactions in patients on hemodiafiltration with AN69 membranes whilst receiving ACE inhibitors

Sir, Anaphylactoid reactions in patients receiving ACE inhibitors whilst dialyzing with AN69 membranes have recently been described [Tielmans et al. 1990, Verresen et al. 1990]. Verresen et al. suggested that bacterial pyrogens are the initiating factor in this reaction as in their experience the reaction occurred in patients on hemodialysis but not on hemofiltration (sterile infusate). However, we have seen anaphylactoid reactions in two patients receiving ACE inhibitors whilst on chronic hemodiafiltration therapy (sterile infusate and dialysate) using AN69 membranes.

Case 1 A 63-year-old female commenced hemodialysis in 1974. Captopril was commenced in March 1987 and in July 1989 she was changed from conventional dialysis to hemofiltration using Hospal Filtral 16 (AN69), membranes being reused utilizing the Renatron system. On 21.2.91 she was changed from hemofiltration to hemodiafiltration in order to improve urea clearances. On 5.3.91 at the onset of hemodiafiltration she developed dizziness, hypotension, abdominal pain, nausea, vomiting, diaphoresis, dyspnoea, angioedema of her tongue and face and difficulty speaking due to laryngeal edema. She was disconnected from the machine within minutes and given 100 mg hydrocortisone i.v. with gradual improvement over three to four hours. This treatment involved the first use of a new Filtral 16 hemofilter. She had three further hemodiafiltration treatments with the combination of AN69 membrane and ACE inhibitor, with a minor reaction during one (same membrane as used on 5.3.91), a full blown anaphylactoid reaction during the next treatment (new hemofilter), and no reaction in the third (new membrane subject to re-use procedure prior to first use). Captopril was then ceased and subsequent hemodiafiltration treatments using Filtral 16 membranes (new and reuse) have been uneventful.

Case 2 A 62-year-old man commenced dialysis on 24.1.89. He was transferred to hemofiltration (Gambro MPS) in March 1989. Therapy was altered to hemodiafiltration in October 1990 and the hemofilter used was changed from Asahi PAN 250 to the Hospal Filtral 12 (AN69) on 8.1.91. He had been on captopril since August 1990. On 5.3.91 he commenced hemodiafiltration using a new Filtral 12 membrane. Immediately after being connected to the machine he felt dizzy and developed abdominal pain and nausea, diaphoresis, and dyspnoea. It was possible to complete the three-hour treatment, and his symptoms settled gradually without recourse to adrenaline or other agents. Further treatments were carried out on 7.3.91 and 9.3.91 with re-use of the same Filtral 12 hemofilter. These treatments were uneventful. Captopril was discontinued on 8.3.91 and there have been no subsequent reactions to treatments using the Filtral 12 membrane.

Tielemans et al. reported anaphylaxis in 3 patients where AN69 membranes were used to dialyse patients taking ACE inhibitors; a fourth patient tolerated this combination without incident for three months. Where reactions occurred these happened within days of starting the ACE inhibitor/AN69 combination. Verresen et al. describe anaphylaxis in 9 patients with the ACE inhibitor AN69 combination, whilst 5 patients on this combination did not experience the reaction. They did not see anaphylaxis in 56 patients treated with hemofiltration on the AN69 membrane, although 3 of these were on ACE inhibitors.

In our experience two of three patients treated with ACE inhibitors and undergoing hemodiafiltration with AN69 membranes developed anaphylaxis which resolved promptly on discontinuation of the ACE inhibitor. Sensitivity to ethylene oxide was excluded in both patients by RAST testing. A third patient on AN69 hemodiafiltration and ACE inhibition did not develop anaphylaxis over 139 treatments. The two patients who developed anaphylaxis had tolerated the combination of ACE inhibition and the AN69 membrane for some months while on hemofiltration but developed symptoms shortly after transfer to hemodiafiltration. Thus this reaction appears to be linked to dialysis (whether or not this is combined with hemofiltration) but not to hemofiltration as a sole procedure. Verresen et al. reported reactions on both first and subsequent uses of their AN69 membranes. Tielemans et al. did not re-use, so all their reactions occurred with "first use" membranes. In our experience, re-use procedures appeared to attenuate the reaction.

The hypothesis has been advanced that bacterial pyrogen is the initiating factor and that ACE inhibitors amplify the reaction by blocking bradykinin metabolism. When hemodiafiltration is carried out using the Gambro MPS machine, both the infusate and the dialysate pass through the same bacterial filter and the same pyrogen filter; both are thus equally sterile and pyrogen free. The effectiveness of the system is attested to by the fact that we have had one pyrogenic reaction and no bacteraemic episodes in 4,000 hemofiltration treatments using the MPS. Thus the process appears to be due to a membrane/dialysate interaction which does not involve bacteria or bacterial products, and also requires the presence of ACE inhibition.

J. J. B. Petrie[1], Y. Campbell[1], C. M. Hawley[1], P. G. Hogan[2]
Departments of Nephrology[1] and Immunology[2], Princess Alexandra Hospital, Brisbane, Australia.

REFERENCES

Tielemans C, Madhoun P, Lenaers M, Schandene L, Goldman M, Vanherweghem J-L. 1990 Anaphylactoid reactions during hemodialysis on AN69 membranes in patients receiving ACE inhibitors. Kidney Int *38:* 982–984

Verresen L, Waer M, Vanrenterghem Y, Micheilsen P. 1990 Angiotensin-converting-enzyme inhibitors and anaphylactoid reactions to high-flux membrane dialysis. Lancet *ii:* 1360–1362

Uremic polyneuropathy

Sir, – We read the article of C. Bazzi et al. [1991] with interest, and would like to comment on some of their theses. In their article C. Bazzi and his colleagues point out that the most sensitive electrophysiological parameters for diagnosis of uremic polyneuropathy are: maximum motor conduction velocities of the peroneal nerve, sensory conduction velocity of the sural nerve and sural and ulnar sensory action potentials amplitude and latency.

In our work till now the experiences have proved to be different [Bobinac-Georgievski et al. 1985, Pavlović et al. 1988, Bobinac-Georgievski et al. 1989]. Using the EMG apparatus "Medelec MS 6", by method of surface stimulation and detection of evoked sensory and motor responses, the following 16 electrophysiologic parameters were determined: H wave latency in m. gastrocnemius (H wave), latency of F waves in m. flexor hallucis brevis (FmFHB) and in m. extensor digitorum brevis (FmEDB), motor nerve conduction velocities for n. medianus, n. peroneus profundus, distal conduction latency for n. medianus, n. peroneus profundus, n. tibialis posterior, latency of mixed sensorymotoric conduction of n. medianus, sensory nerves conduction velocities for n. radialis, and n. suralis, amplitudes of evoked responses in muscles of the foot: m. flexor hallucis brevis and m. extensor digitorum brevis, evoked sensory potentials for n. suralis, n. radialis and sensory potential for mixed n. medianus. Uremic polyneuropathy was evaluated in 46 (22 male and 24 female), regularly dialyzed patients. The results were compared with those of 141 healthy controls of both sexes. Values outside the normal range covering 95% of expected normal values were considered pathological. In 87% of patients the pathological values of H-wave latency have been found. Mean value was 37 mS in men and 33 mS in women. The normal range was 26–31.3 mS. The pathological values of FmFHB have been found in 76% of patients, i. e. mean value in male was 60 mS and 55 mS in female patients, and normal range was 42.8–56.2 mS. In 75% of patients the pathological values of FmEDB have been found. Mean value of FmEDB was 59 mS in men and 53 mS in women. The normal range was 40.3–54.5 mS. The values of other electrophysiological parameters have been less frequent out of the normal values. Our results indicate that uremic neuropathies lesion is most constantly reflected in prolonged latency of H and F waves rather than in decrease of nerve conduction velocities of distal segments of peripheral nerves.

At the end we would like to point out that uremic polyneuropathy is distal symmetric and mixed neuropathy appearing at about 65% of patients treated by dialysis [Fraser and Arieff 1988]. There are different opinions about the importance of individual electrophysiological parameters in diagnosis of uremic polyneuropathy. Our experience proves the great sensitivity of latency of H and F waves in early diagnostics of uremic polyneuropathy. Similar results have been found by others [Halar et al. 1979, Matthes et al. 1986]. It ought to be emphasized that some authors do not consider H and F waves significant in the detection of uremic neuropathy [Marra 1988].

Unfortunately, there is no adequate treatment for the uremic polyneuropathy and it seems till now there are neither unique electrophysiological parameters for the early diagnosis nor for the follow up of the uremic polyneuropathy.

D. Pavlović[1] and A. Bobinac-Georgievski[2]
[1] Institute of Kidney Diseases and Dialysis, "Sveti Duh" Hospital, and [2] Institute of Physical Medicine, Rehabilitation and Rheumatology, "Sveti Duh" Hospital Svet, Duh 64, YU-4100 Zagreb, Yugoslavia

REFERENCES

Bazzi C et al. 1991 Uremic polyneuropathy: a clinical and electrophysiological study in 135 short- and long-term hemodialyzed patients. Clin Nephrol *35:* 176

Bobinac-Georgievski A et al. 1985 Electroneurographic evaluation of uremic polyneuropathy (abstract). Electroenceph clin Neurophysiol *61:* S 148

Bobinac-Georgievski et al. 1989 Electroneurographic evaluation of uremic polyneuropathy. In: *Jušić A* (ed) New trends in neuromuscular diseases and electromyoneurography. Školska knjiga, Zagreb

Fraser CL, Arieff AI 1988 Nervous system complications in uremia. Ann Intern Med *109:* 143

Halar ME, Brozovich VF, Milutinovic J, Inouye LV, Becker MV 1979 H-reflex latency in uremic neuropathy: correlation with NCV and clinical findings. Arch Phys Med Rehabil *60:* 174

Marra RTh 1988 Proximal vs. distal nerve conduction measurements in uremic neuropathy. Electromyogr clin Neurophysiol *28:* 439

Matthes von R, Both R, Mühlau G, Hoffmann KP 1986 Diagnostik und Verlaufskontrolle der urämischen Polyneuropathie mittels H-reflex-Index. Z Klin Med *20:* 1655

Pavlović D, Bobinac-Georgievski A, Molnar V, Montani M 1988 Longitudinal follow-up of uremic polyneuropathy by neurographic method. Period biol *90:* 534

BOOK REVIEWS

Clinical Atlas of the Kidney, *J. D. Williams, A. W. Asscher, D. B. Moffat, E. Sanders,* Gower Medical Publishing, London, 1991. 303 pages.

The product of 17 physicians largely from Wales and England, this atlas is similar in format to other medical texts from Gower with its high quality paper, superb illustrations, peculiar pagination, and awkwardly large size (1 foot in height). The abundance of gross photographs, photomicrographs radiographs, charts and tables coupled with a minimum of text encourages a complete reading of the atlas from first to last page thereby providing a fine overview of renal disease. Particularly well done are chapters devoted to the normal kidney, investigative methods, urinary tract infections, and renal transplantation. An unexpected inclusion in this generally broad-based atlas is an entire chapter devoted to pregnancy and the kidney. The attempt to be all inclusive renders the text at times superficial. There are for example no literature citations. This atlas is therefore by no means a reference text. However it will serve as an exceptionally useful introduction to and review of nephrology and urology in particular for resident physicians.

B. C. Horten, New York, New York

Ultrasonography of the urinary tract, 3. ed. *M. I. Resnick, M. D. Rifkin* (eds.) Williams and Wilkins, Baltimore, Maryland, 1991.

This book is a comprehensive review of ultrasonography of the entire genitourinary tract. This book is intended for those pursuing careers in radiology, nephrology and urology. The authors provide a review of many of the contemporary issues involving the genitourinary tract. The book has 15 chapters. The first chapter is obviously intended for physicists and sonographers. The second chapter is a scholarly review of cross-sectional anatomy with an excellent survey of cadaveric sections through the genitourinary tract. The review of Renal Ultrasonography, both Adult and Pediatric (Chapters 4–7 and 12), is extensive and masterly. The image quality of the ultrasounds is superb and is the best I have seen in a textbook. The text includes duplex and color ultrasonography when evaluating renal masses, renal trauma and renal vein thrombosis. The evaluation of the lower genitourinary tract when compared to Dr. Rifkin's book **Diagnostic Imaging of the Lower Genitourinary Tract** (Raven Press, New York, 1985), has been expanded. The review has been updated to include a more comprehensive evaluation of ultrasonography of the prostate with improved transrectal images. Evaluation of the bladder pathology includes both transabdominal and transurethral imaging. The text also includes an excellent chapter on ultrasound of the penis. Included in the text is the contemporary technique of duplex ultrasound in the evaluation of impotence. Expert chapters on scrotal ultrasound and renal transplants include state-of-the-art ultrasounds including duplex and color flow ultrasonography. The book is complete, comprehensive and easy to comprehend. The text includes an impressive number of illustrations, tables, references and differential diagnoses, making this book the best I have seen of its kind. I therefore highly recommend this book to radiologists, urologists and nephrologists as a definitive text that is concise, readable and comprehensive.

J. P. Friedwald, New York, New York

Clinical Nephrology, Vol. 36 No. 6 – 1991 (267–273)

Interleukin-1 production by monocytes from patients with glomerulonephritis after stimulation in vitro with soluble immune complexes

K. Matsumoto

Second Department of Internal Medicine, Nihon University School of Medicine, Tokyo, Japan

Abstract. Monocytes from 30 patients with glomerulonephritis (GN) were stimulated with soluble immune complexes (IC). In order to neutralize the effect of prostaglandins, some cultures were incubated in the presence of indomethacin. Interleukin-1 (IL-1) activity was assessed by the comitogenic activity of the crude monocyte supernatants on phytohemagglutinin (PHA)-stimulated murine thymocytes. Our results demonstrate that, upon stimulation with the soluble IC monocytes from GN patients possess an enhanced capacity to produce IL-1, and the levels of IL-1 correlate with disease activity only in one case of acute poststreptococcal GN (AGN), not in all other patients. This enhanced production of IL-1 may contribute to the disordered immunoregulation in GN.

Key words: glomerulonephritis – immune complexes – monocytes – interleukin-1

Introduction

Interleukin-1 (IL-1) is a cellular product that exerts many immunostimulatory and inflammatory effects [Dinarello 1985]. The trigger of IL-1 production in glomerulonephritis (GN) patients is presumably the specific antigen. Vissers et al. [1989] have reported that glomerular basement membrane (GBM)-containing immune complexes (IC) induce IL-1 production in normal monocytes. Here, we report on the ability of peripheral blood monocytes (PBM) from GN patients to produce IL-1 upon stimulation in vitro with the IC.

Patients and methods

Patients

A group of 30 patients suffering from various renal diseases was studied. There were 12 males and 18 females with a mean age of 35 years (range 14–63 years). They had a creatinine clearance of more than 40 ml/min. Renal biopsy was performed in all patients, and the diagnosis was made by light and immunofluorescence microscopy. Eight patients received corticosteroids (less than 15 mg/day), and none received cytotoxins. All patients with systemic lupus erythematosus (SLE) fulfilled the American Rheumatism criteria for SLE classification. All blood samples were drawn early in the morning before the administration of the drugs. Control samples were obtained concurrently from 11 age-matched healthy volunteers. The details of these patients are given in Table 1.

Preparation of soluble IC

All IC were made using hyperimmune guinea pig IgG rich in antibody to human GBM [Vissers et al. 1989]. This antiserum was prepared as described by Bhan et al. [1978]. Briefly, equal volumes of guinea pig anti-GBM IgG and rabbit anti-guinea pig IgG were mixed in test tubes and incubated overnight at 4° C. The mixture was then centrifuged at 12,000 g for 15 min to remove any precipitating IC. This corresponds to an antigen-antibody ratio of 10 : 1 as assessed by quantitative precipitin reactions [Johnson and Ward 1981]. In all experiments the negative control consisted of an equivalent amount of antibody in the absence of antigen.

Received January 30, 1991; in revised form May 24, 1991.

Reprint requests to Dr. K. Matsumoto, 2nd Department of Internal Medicine, Nihon University School of Medicine, 30-1 Oyaguchi-Kami-Machi, Itabashi-ku, Tokyo 173, Japan.

Preparation of IC-stimulated monocyte culture supernatant

Mononuclear cells were obtained by centrifugation of peripheral blood from patients and controls on Ficoll-Hypaque gradients as previously described [Böyum 1968]. Adherent cells were isolated by their adherence to plastic Petri dishes (Nunc, Roskilde, Denmark) when placed in RPMI 1640 (GIBCO, Grand Island, NY), containing 5% fetal calf serum (FCS, GIBCO), and incubated for 2 h at 37° C. This population contained more than 90% monocytes as

Table 1 Clinical features of all patients studied

No.	Age	Sex	Proteinuria	Serum albumin	Serum cholesterol	Creatinine clearance ml/min	Prednisolone therapy at the time of study
Acute poststreptococcal glomerulonephritis							
1	45	M	+	N	N	116	–
IgA nephropathy							
1	16	F	+	N	N	69	–
2	34	M	+	N	N	62	–
3	38	M	+	N	↑	66	–
4	63	F	+	↓	↑	44	+
5	23	F	+	↓	N	72	–
6	21	F	+	N	N	89	–
7	40	M	+	N	N	59	–
8	33	M	–	N	N	108	–
9	21	F	–	N	N	53	–
10	17	F	–	N	N	97	–
Membranoproliferative glomerulonephritis							
1	40	M	+	N	N	74	–
Membranous nephropathy							
1	51	F	+	↓	↑	117	+
2	34	M	+	↓	↑	89	+
3	34	M	+	N	N	106	–
4	53	F	–	N	N	103	–
Lipoid nephrosis							
1	20	M	+	↓	↑	82	–
2	56	M	+	↓	↑	108	+
3	14	F	+	↓	↑	80	+
4	16	M	–	N	↑	82	–
5	19	M	–	N	N	92	–
Henoch-Schönlein purpura nephritis							
1	25	F	+	N	N	113	–
Lupus nephritis							
1	51	F	+	↓	↑	87	–
2	45	F	+	N	↑	101	–
3	42	F	+	↓	N	62	+
4	43	F	+	N	↑	58	–
5	53	F	+	N	↑	85	–
6	24	F	+	↓	N	87	+
7	38	F	+	↓	↑	141	+
8	54	F	–	N	N	81	–

judged by staining for nonspecific esterase. The cells were then resuspended, at a concentration of 1 × 10^5 cells/ml, in a culture medium, RPMI 1640 containing 100 U/ml penicillin and 100 µg/ml streptomycin. Equal volumes (1 ml) of cell suspension were distributed into 24-well plates (Nunc): IC were added to one culture in RPMI 1640 to give a final concentration of 100 µg/ml; the other received an equal volume of RPMI 1640 alone. In experiments using adherent cells from normal donors 100 µg/ml provided the maximum mitogenic response. One µg/ml indomethacin (Sigma Chemical Co., St. Louis, MO) was added to certain cultures. The plates were then incubated in 5% CO_2 in air at 37° C for 24 h. After this time the supernatants were collected, centrifuged and stored at −20° C until assayed.

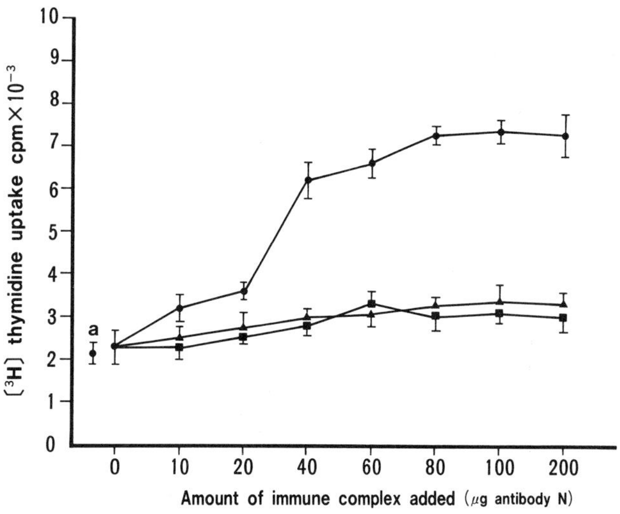

Fig. 1 The effect of IC-concentration on the generation of IL-1 by PBM. Normal PBM were incubated for 24 h in the presence of either the indicated concentration of IC (●), or guinea pig anti-GBM IgG (▲), or rabbit anti-guinea pig IgG (■). The direct effect of IC (100 µg) added to the thymocyte assay in the absence of PBM supernatants is shown (a). Each point represents the mean ± SD of three experiments.

Cell-associated IL-1 activity

The procedure was based on the method of Matsushima et al. [1986]. To extract cell-associated IL-1 activity, viable IC-activated monocytes were treated with 10 µg/ml pure L-p-tosylamino-2-phenylethyl chloromethyl ketone (TPCK)-trypsin (Worthington, Freehold, NJ) at 37° C for 10 min. The reaction was stopped by adding 100 µg/ml soybean trypsin inhibitor (Calbiochem, San Diego, CA). The resultant supernatants were filter sterilized, and IL-1 activity was measured. In the absence of enzyme, no IL-1 activity was released.

Assay for IL-1

IL-1 activity in equivalent final dilutions of monocyte supernatants was determined by augmentation of phytohemagglutinin (PHA)-induced proliferation of murine thymocytes [Mizel et al. 1978]. In this assay, 1.5 × 10^6 thymocytes from 5- to 8-week-old C3H/HeJ mice were incubated in microtitre wells in RPMI 1640 medium with penicillin, streptomycin, 5% FCS, 2.5 × 10^{-5}M 2-mercaptoethanol, 10 µg/ml PHA (HA 16, Wellcome, Beckenham, UK) and the test sample in a final volume of 200 µl. After 72 h culture at 37° C and 5% CO_2, each well was pulsed with 1.0 µCi [^{3}H] thymidine (Amersham, UK) for 5 h and the assay harvested with an automated multi-well harvester. The results were expressed as mean counts/min (cpm) ± SD of triplicate cultures. Recombinant human IL-1α (Hoffmann-La Roche Inc., Nutley, NJ) was used as a standard and as a positive control in this assay. The neutralization of IL-1 activity was performed as described [Miossec et al. 1986]. Rabbit antihuman IL-1β antibody was provided by Ohtsuka

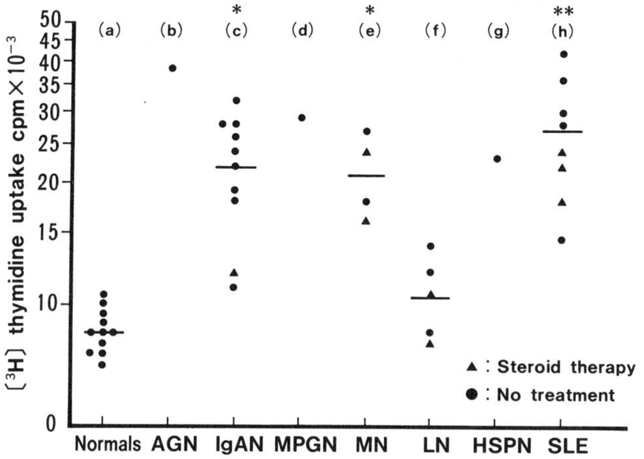

Fig. 2 IL-1 production in the IC-stimulated PBM culture supernatants from normal controls and patients with renal disease. IL-1 production was expressed as the average cpm of triplicate cultures for 1:4 dilution of supernatant. IL-1 production of GN PBM was significantly increased compared to that of normal controls: ** $p < 0.01$; * $p < 0.02$. Background cpm: [^{3}H] thymidine incorporation was 2,195.0 ± 497.7 cpm in the presence of an unconditioned medium containing IC alone, and 2,262.8 ± 368.1 cpm for PHA alone. Horizontal lines indicate mean values. AGN = acute poststreptococcal glomerulonephritis; IgA N = IgA nephropathy; MPGN = membranoproliferative glomerulonephritis; MN = membranous nephropathy; LN = lipoid nephrosis; HSPN = Henoch-Schönlein purpura nephritis; SLE = lupus nephritis.

Pharmaceutical Co. (Tokushima, Japan) [Tanaka et al. 1987].

Analysis of results

Statistical calculations were performed by using the Student's t-test. In Figure 2, IL-1 production appears not to be normally distributed and the population is not large enough to use the Student's t-test. Another statistical test, i. e. ANOVA, was also employed.

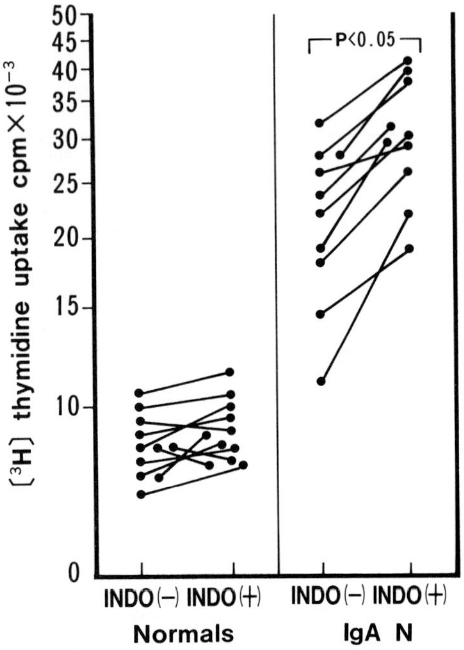

Fig. 3 A significant ($p < 0.05$) augmentation of the IC effect on nephritic PBM was observed by blocking cyclooxygenase activity. The addition of indomethacin (INDO) to the IC-stimulated culture resulted in nearly a 36% increase in IL-1 production.

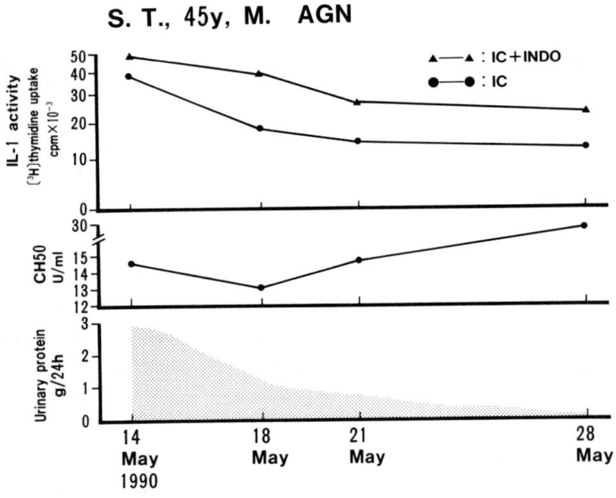

Fig. 4 Serial measurements of IL-1 during hospital admission in a 45-year-old man with acute poststreptococcal glomerulonephritis (AGN). INDO = indomethacin.

Results

Characteristics of IL-1 assay

Incubation of PBM with increasing concentrations of IC resulted in a dose-dependent release of IL-1 (Figure 1). After a 24-h incubation, IL-1 was detectable at concentrations of IC as low as 40 μg; maximal IL-1 levels were reached at 80 to 200 μg. The thymocyte mitogenic activity could be neutralized by a 3-h preincubation with anti-IL-1β, but not by control rabbit antisera. In all experiments the negative control consisted of an equivalent amount of guinea pig anti-GBM IgG or rabbit anti-guinea pig IgG. The control cultures of PBM release only very limited amounts of IL-1, as demonstrated in Figure 1. The tests showed good reproduceability in each control subject and continued to give comparable results when reexamined at different intervals.

Increased IL-1 production by monocytes of GN patients

Adherent PBM of patients with GN or of healthy donors were stimulated with 100 μg/ml IC for 24 h, when culture supernatants were harvested and assayed for IL-1. The results are summarized in Figure 2. The levels of IL-1 activity in the PBM of GN patients were found to be significantly higher than in normal subjects, while patients with lipoid nephrosis (LN) had mean values of IL-1 activity that were not significantly different from normal controls. In Figure 2, only stimulated IL-1 production is shown. Spontaneous PBM secretion of IL-1 was negligible in normal control cultures (3,041.2 ± 376.4 cpm), but 40 μg IC significantly stimulated the secretion of IL-1, as demonstrated in Figure 1. The IL-1 activity produced by the unstimulated cells was not significantly different from the normal controls in any of the patient groups. Positive controls in the IL-1 assay were 32,063.5 ± 4,225.6 cpm for recombinant human IL-1α (1 U/ml).

IL-1 activity released from cells by trypsin

Cell-associated IL-1 activity could be eluted from IC-stimulated monocytes by treatment with 10 μg/ml TPCK-trypsin. The dissociated IL-1 production in the IgA N group (19,384.6 ± 2,415.2 cpm) was found to be significantly ($p < 0.01$) higher than in those from normal controls (5,798.5 ± 715.1 cpm). Further analysis of cell-associated IL-1 showed that 86% of the costimulatory activity could be inhibited by a monoclonal anti-IL-1α antibody (Ohtsuka Pharmaceutical Co., Tokushima, Japan), with only 5% inhibited by the monoclonal anti-IL-1β antibody (Ohtsuka Co.). This indicates that most of the cell-associated IL-1 activity is due to IL-1α, with only a minor portion contributed by IL-1β.

Effect of indomethacin on IL-1 production (Figure 3)

A low dose of indomethacin has been shown to augment IL-1 production by directly acting on macrophages [Spera et al. 1986]. Indomethacin (1 µg/ml) was added from the initiation of the culture. The addition of indomethacin with IC significantly ($p < 0.05$) increased IL-1 production in IgA nephropathy (IgA N) (36% increase compared to IC-stimulated culture without indomethacin) compared to normal controls (15% increase).

Serial measurements of IL-1 in a patient with acute poststreptococcal glomerulonephritis

We have investigated IL-1 levels in a 45-year-old man with acute poststreptococcal glomerulonephritis (AGN). The patient was admitted to the Nihon University Hospital for evaluation of proteinuria. Two weeks before admission, he had been given antibiotics because of a sore throat and fever. Urinalysis showed 4+ proteinuria and 2+ blood; the urine sediment contained 100 red blood cells. The serum CH50 was 14.6 U/ml and the ASO 668 IU/ml. His percutaneous renal biopsy disclosed diffuse endocapillary GN with granular staining of C3 confined to the mesangium of all the glomeruli. Figure 4 shows the course of the AGN patient. Follow-up assessment showed concordant changes in IL-1 levels associated with changes in clinical activity; the activities declined earlier in the case of AGN.

Discussion

The present study investigates IL-1 production by PBM from normals or from patients with different forms of GN. IL-1 production induced by soluble IC was enhanced in patients with IgA N, membranous nephropathy (MN) and lupus nephritis. We also observed that not only IL-1β activity in the supernatants, but also cell-associated IL-1α activity was elevated in PBM samples of patients with IgA N.

These results are consistent with our earlier findings of enhanced generation of IL-1 by the glomerular macrophages from a group of rapidly progressive crescentic GN [Matsumoto et al. 1988a]. Our results also concur with the findings that rats with nephrotoxic serum nephritis have peritoneal and glomerular macrophages which produce higher amounts of IL-1 [Matsumoto 1988b, Matsumoto 1989a, Matsumoto 1990].

We have shown that the activated monocytes found in the peripheral blood in GN have an increased capacity to produce IL-1. This mode of study is, however, able to differentiate the function of PBM from GN and those from LN. PBM from LN, in contrast to GN, have been shown to produce decreased amounts of IL-1 [Matsumoto 1989b].

Although circulating IC are detected in a variety of immunologically mediated renal diseases as well as in normals, their pathogenetic relevance is controversial since levels of IC do not correlate with disease activity and the composition of circulating IC does not reflect those in tissues [Abrass et al. 1980]. The reason we chose soluble IC to stimulate IL-1 is that IC appear to play an important role in the early steps of PBM activation and in the control of the inflammatory responses [Vissers et al. 1989]. If we suggest a pathogenetic link between inadequate responses of an individual to IC and renal disease, we should demonstrate that the response to other stimuli such as lipopolysaccharide (LPS) or phorbor myristate acetate (PMA) is normal. In order to check these points, we also examined the effects of LPS and PMA on PBM activation. The activities were largely similar to that of the IC (data not shown). That leaves the question whether IC have anything to do with the renal disease at all. These patients appear to be high IL-1 producers and are not especially sensitive to IC. The relationship between the costimulatory activity stimulated with LPS and the costimulatory activity of soluble IC shown herein is not clear. A possible explanation for our results is that the stimulation of IL-1 may be initiated by a variety of mitogens, which appear to utilize more than one activation pathway. The mechanism(s) by which IC induce PBM to secrete IL-1 is unclear. One possible mechanism is through activation of Fc receptor or activation via the phagocytic pathway. The Fc region of the Ig molecule is involved in a wide variety of biologic effector functions including immune regulation [Morgan et al. 1988]. Our previous findings of the IgG region subfragments suggest that IC activate IL-1 release by signaling through the Fc receptors on mesangial cells [Matsumoto and Hatano 1991]. We are currently examining the intracellular mechanisms of action of the IC in greater detail to understand these interactions more fully.

The findings that IC induce IL-1 and that IL-1 production is enhanced by indomethacin have been reported by other investigators [Knudsen et al. 1986]. Prostaglandins have been shown to suppress IL-1 production by monocytes [Matsumoto 1989b]. Our findings suggest that the addition of IC causes the PBM to release IL-1 and prostaglandins which have opposing effects on thymocyte costimulatory assay. The PBM stimulated by IC probably affected the response in at least two ways: by the induction of IL-1 and by the production of prostaglandin E_2. Nevertheless, the IL-1 had the dominant influence, resulting in an increase in thymocyte-stimulating activity.

An important unanswered question is whether this phenomenon is characteristic for GN or can be found in other diseases as well. A better control than healthy subjects would be patients without renal disease. We therefore examined the effects of soluble IC on PBM from SLE patients without renal involvement. The levels of IL-1 were increased in SLE patients compared with those in normal controls and higher in SLE patients with mesangial proliferative GN than in those without renal involvement (data not shown). Thus, the immune defects appear to be associated with the renal involvement.

The interpretation of the data should focus on the fact that these observations are results obtained in vitro and that they are only descriptive. We believe that the increased IL-1 activity in vitro more or less reflects an in vivo activity. The conclusion that the IL-1 production correlated closely with disease activity cannot be drawn from the present study. In only one case with AGN, there was a concomitant fall in both IL-1 production and urinary protein excretion and a rise in CH50. To approach this question the patients were classified into two groups: (a) those in the inactive stage with normal renal function and blood pressure who had <1 g urinary protein per 24 h and whose renal biopsy showed only slight abnormalities by both light and immunofluorescence microscopy and (b) patients in the active stage such as nephritic type, nephrotic type and hypertensive type with definitely abnormal renal pathological and immunofluorescence data. In all other patients, there was no correlation with disease activities or structural lesions.

One point of some concern is the prednisolone treatment received by a minority of patients and controls, although, admittedly, the drug amount is low (<15 mg/day). This treatment might have interfered with the IL-1 production by PBM of GN patients. It has been reported that hydrocortisone suppresses the production of IL-1 by LPS-stimulated murine macrophages [Snyder and Unanue 1982]. However, differences in dosage, in administration periods and in patient populations may limit the interpretation of the results in our study. Studies of patients before and after treatment and at repeated intervals during both remissions and exacerbations may help to sort out the relative influences of drug and disease on IL-1 biosynthesis in GN.

In the publication of Vissers et al. [1989], cited by the authors, and also from our own data (Figure 1) it is shown that normal PBM produce high amounts of IL-1 when stimulated by LPS or by soluble IC. These data suggest that normal PBM are activated by LPS or IC to produce IL-1 which may be of importance in the physiologic activation of T-lymphocytes. This is in agreement with previous hypothesis that under physiological conditions IL-1 acts as a lymphocyte activating factor and is essential for production of IL-2 and expression of the IL-2 receptor, but in various disorders where it is present in excess it appears to behave differently, functioning as a cytostatic and cytotoxic factor [Dinarello 1985]. The ability of PBM to release significant amounts of IL-1 is unusual, and may be of particular pathophysiologic importance. The increased synthesis of IL-1 by activated monocytes could contribute to an enhancement of the immunologic and inflammatory responses in GN. Clearly, further investigations are required to establish the role of IL-1 in GN.

REFERENCES

Abrass CK, Hall CL, Border WA, Brown CA, Glassock RJ, Coggins CH 1980 Circulating immune complexes in adults with idiopathic nephrotic syndrome. Kidney Int *17:* 545–553

Bhan AK, Schneeberger EE, Collins AB, McCluskey RT 1978 Evidence for a pathogenic role of a cell-mediated immune mechanism in experimental glomerulonephritis. J Exp Med *148:* 246–260

Böyum A 1968 Separation of leukocytes from blood and bone marrow. Scand J Clin Lab Invest *21 (Suppl 97):* 1–51

Dinarello CA 1985 An update on human interleukin-1: from molecular biology to clinical relevance. J Clin Immunol *5:* 287–297

Johnson KJ, Ward PA 1981 Role of oxygen metabolites in immune complex injury of lung. J Immunol *126:* 2355–2369

Knudsen PJ, Dinarello CA, Strom TB 1986 Prostaglandins post-transcriptionally inhibit monocyte expression of interleukin-1 activity by increasing intracellular cyclic adenosine monophosphate. J Immunol *137:* 3189–3194

Matsumoto K, Dowling JP, Atkins RC 1988a Production of interleukin-1 in glomerular cell cultures from patients with rapidly progressive crescentic glomerulonephritis. Am J Nephrol *8:* 463–470

Matsumoto K 1988b Production of interleukin-1 in macrophage cultures from rats with nephrotoxic serum nephritis. Int Arch Allergy Appl Immunol *87:* 435–438

Matsumoto K 1989a Interleukin-1 production by lipopolysaccharide-stimulated glomeruli from rats with nephrotoxic serum nephritis. Am J Nephrol *9:* 488–494

Matsumoto K 1989b Decreased production of interleukin-1 by monocytes from patients with lipoid nephrosis. Clin Nephrol *31:* 292–296

Matsumoto K 1990 Production of interleukin-1 by glomerular macrophages in nephrotoxic serum nephritis. Am J Nephrol *10:* 502–506

Matsumoto K, Hatano M 1991 Soluble immune complexes stimulate production of interleukin-1 by cultured rat glomerular mesangial cells. Am J Nephrol (in press)

Matsushima K, Taguchi M, Kovacs EJ, Young HA, Oppenheim JJ 1986 Intracellular localization of human monocyte associated interleukin-1 (IL-1) activity and release of biologically active IL-1 from monocytes by trypsin and plasmin. J Immunol *136:* 2883–2891

Miossec P, Cavender D, Ziff M 1986 Production of interleukin-1 by human endothelial cells. J Immunol *136:* 2486–2491

Mizel SB, Oppenheim JJ, Rosentreich DL 1978 Characterization of lymphocyte-activating factor (LAF) produced by the macrophage cell line p 388D1. I. Enhancement of LAF production by activated T lymphocytes. J Immunol *120:* 1497–1503

Morgan EL, Hobbs MV, Noonan DJ, Weigle WO 1988 Induction of IL-1 secretion from human monocytes by Fc region subfragments of human IgGl. J Immunol *140:* 3014–3020

Snyder DS, Unanue ER 1982 Corticosteroids inhibit murine macrophage Ia expression and interleukin-1 production. J Immunol *129:* 1803–1805

Spera GT, Marshall P, Teodrescu M 1986 Increase in proliferation and cytotoxic cell development in human mixed lymphocyte cultures in the presence of very low concentrations of LPS: role of IL-1 and prostaglandin E_2. Clin Immunol Immunopathol *38:* 32–46

Tanaka K, Ishikawa E, Ohmoto Y, Hirai Y 1987 Sandwich enzyme immunoassay for human interleukin-1β (hIL-1β) in urine. Clin Chim Acta *166:* 273–276

Vissers MCM, Fantone JC, Wiggis R, Kunkel SL 1989 Glomerular basement membrane-containing immune complexes stimulate tumor necrosis factor and interleukin-1 production by human monocytes. Am J Pathol *134:* 1–6

Clinical Nephrology, Vol. 36 No. 6 – 1991 (274–280)

Do limited changes in phosphate intake modulate 1,25(OH)$_2$D$_3$ levels in early renal failure?

A. SEIDEL, G. STEIN, S. SCHNEIDER, H. SCHMIDT-GAYK and E. RITZ

Departments of Internal Medicine, Universities of Heidelberg and Jena, Germany

Abstract. A high dietary phosphate load relative to GFR is thought to explain, at least in part, diminished renal 1-alpha hydroxylase activity in early renal failure (RF). To assess the role of dietary phosphate/GFR ratio in more detail, we examined the response of 1,25(OH)$_2$D$_3$ concentration to a controlled isolated reduction of dietary phosphate intake for up to 10 days with no change of Ca, Na and energy intake. We studied 7 healthy controls (2 male, 5 female, median age 45 years) and 6 non-nephrotic patients with early renal failure (RF) (3 males, 3 females, median age 55 years; median C_{in} 60.5ml/min/1.73 m^2; 41–69). During an initial 3-day period of controlled diet with usual phosphate intake no difference of UV_{Pi} (median 27.6 mmol/day, 18.9–43.8) was found between controls and RF. A diet with 15 mmol P_i/day (confirmed by duplicate meal analysis) significantly reduced median UV_{Pi} (controls: 27.7 to 11.9 mmol/d; RF 27.4 to 14.1 mmol/d) with no change of median UV_{Ca}. Median day to day variation of 1,25(OH)$_2$D$_3$ levels (by RIA) in controls was 15.4%. Lowering dietary phosphate intake did not significantly change median 1,25(OH)$_2$D$_3$ levels in controls (45.7 vs. 38.3 pg/ml) and patients with RF, respectively (23.5 vs. 19.1 pg/ml). No changes of intact iPTH values were found. The experiment had a 68% power to detect a 15% change and a 99% power to detect a 30% change at a significance level of $p < 0.05$. The study shows that short-term, isolated lowering of dietary Pi intake by a factor of two, thus normalizing the ratio Pi intake/GFR, fails to cause detectable changes of 1,25(OH)$_2$D$_3$ or iPTH levels in patients with early renal failure. The results raise doubts concerning the presumed role of Pi in initiating early abnormalities of Ca regulating hormones in renal failure.

Key words: phosphate – 1,25(OH)$_2$D$_3$ – hyperparathyroidism – renal 1-alpha-hydroxylase – renal failure

Introduction

In early renal failure, circulating levels of 1,25(OH)$_2$ vitamin D$_3$ (1,25(OH)$_2$D$_3$) tend to decrease, although in most patients the levels still remain within the normal range [Lucas et al. 1985]. The tendency of 1,25(OH)$_2$D$_3$ levels to decrease in early renal failure is thought to play a crucial role in triggering early secondary hyperparathyroidism [Bonjour 1988].

While low average levels of 1,25(OH)$_2$D$_3$ and elevated iPTH levels have been amply demonstrated in early renal failure [Lucas et al. 1985, Reichel et al. 1991], the causes of low 1,25(OH)$_2$D$_3$ levels have not been adequately clarified.

One possibility is diminution of functional mass of intact proximal tubular epithelial cells. This possibility is well illustrated by the observation that circulating 1,25(OH)$_2$D$_3$ levels transiently fall after uninephrectomy, e.g. in life kidney donors, only to return to normal levels after several days but at the price of elevated iPTH levels. This points to a compensatory increase of renal 1-alpha-hydroxylase activity caused by increased PTH [Friedlander et al. 1988, Lucas et al. 1986]. An alternative, or complementary, explanation has been offered indicating that phosphate may also play a role. Positive phosphate balance lowers renal 1-alpha-hydroxylase activity [DeLuca 1973]. Furthermore, in children with moderately advanced renal failure, Portale et al. [1984] showed that reducing net phosphate uptake by lowering dietary phosphate with administration of alumi-

Received July 2, 1991; in revised form August 2, 1991

Reprint requests to Dr. E. Ritz, Klinikum der Universität Heidelberg, Sektion Nephrologie, Bergheimerstr. 56a, W-6900 Heidelberg, Germany numhydroxyde increased circulating 1,25(OH)$_2$D$_3$ levels by approximately 60%.

If one entertains the possibility that phosphate plays a role in early renal failure, one has to explain the paradox that circulating phosphate concentrations are normal according to some and even diminished according to other authors. To explain this finding, Bonjour [1988] proposed that the phosphate concentration might be increased in a critical subcellular compartment of proximal tubular epithelial cells. This would explain the low renal phosphate threshold (TMP/GFR) as well as low 1,25(OH)$_2$D$_3$ levels in such patients.

If phosphate balance were crucial for homeostasis of 1,25(OH)$_2$D$_3$ levels in early renal failure, we reasoned that it should be possible to raise steady state 1,25(OH)$_2$D$_3$ levels by isolated reduction of dietary phosphate intake, i.e. in the absence of changes of calcium, sodium and energy intake. A study was carried out in healthy controls as well as in patients with early renal failure. In early renal failure (GFR approximately 60 ml/min/1.73m^2), the ratio of P load/GFR is raised by a factor of approximately two. Consequently, we administered a diet the phosphate content of which had been reduced by a factor of approximately two. We measured 1,25(OH)$_2$D$_3$ levels on usual and reduced dietary phosphate intake in 7 healthy controls and 6 non-nephrotic patients with glomerular disease (median C_{in} 61 ml/min/1.73 m^2).

Subjects

1. Subjects

We examined 7 healthy volunteers, members of the nephrological team (2 males, 5 females, median age 45 years, 19–50 years). None of the subjects had known renal disease (by ultrasonography, S-creatinine, urine analysis and blood pressure measurements) or conditions affecting calcium metabolism. They took no medication. Body weight had been constant over at least three months.

Furthermore, we examined 6 patients (3 male, 3 female, median age 55 years; 35–67) with renal failure and glomerular disease (biopsy confirmed glomerulonephritis 3, reflux nephropathy with proteinuria 1, glomerulonephritis suspected on the basis of history and urinary sediment in 2). The patients received no diuretics, beta-blockers, oral phosphate binders or other medication potentially interfering with calcium metabolism. Proteinuria was in the non-nephrotic range (0.15–1.2 g/24 h). None of the patients was malnourished (BMI 26.7 kg/m^2, 24.0–35.0) and body weight had been stable for at least three months.

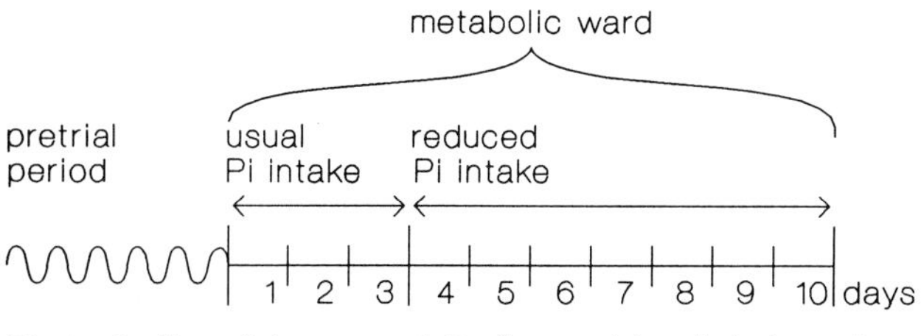

Fig. 1 Outline of the protocol. In the pretrial period, the patients were repeatedly seen in the outpatient clinic to validate constancy of urinary Pi, urea and calcium excretion, C_{cr} and body weight. The patients were then admitted to the metabolic ward and studied for three days. The Pi intake on day 1–3 was calculated to equate the usual Pi intake as assessed from dietary interview Pi excretion in the pretrial period corresponded to 70% of dietary intake calculated from dietary interview. Patients were subsequently switched to a diet with reduced Pi content (450 mg/day), but left unchanged Ca, Na and energy content.

2. Protocol

Usual phosphate intake was assessed by dietary interview (and indirectly assessed by repeated monitoring of urinary phosphate excretion in 24-h urine collections during the pretrial period). Based on the patient's dietary preferences and usual Pi intake, individual diets were computed, prepared, deep frozen and served on the metabolic ward. For a period of 3 days, all individuals received a diet, the phosphate content of which corresponded to the usual dietary phosphate intake which varied from individual to individual from 32 mmol to 45 mmol/day. All were subsequently switched to a dietary Pi (inorganic

Table 1 Biochemical baseline data

	Controls (n = 7)	Early renal failure (n = 6)
S-creatinine (mg/dl)	0.91 (0.76–1.05)	1.55 (1.46–2.12)**
S-calcium (mmol/l)	2.18 (2.09–2.34)	2.22 (2.15–2.32)
S-phosphate (mmol/l)	1.12 (0.89–1.50)	1.07 (0.81–1.48)
1,25(OH)$_2$D$_3$ (pg/ml)	45.7 (36.7–48.3)	23.5 (13.0–27.7)**
25(OH)D$_3$ (nmol/l)	69.0 (35.5–177)	93.4 (50.0–167)
Intact PTH (pmol/l)	3.8 (2.4–4.7)	4.6 (1.5–40.0)#
Inulin clearance (ml/min/1.73m^2)	115 (98–134)	60.5 (41.0–69.0)**
Proteinuria (g/24h)	<0.15	0.52 (0.15–1.20)*
U-calcium (mmol/24h)	2.96 (1.99–6.29)	1.83 (0.33–2.59)*
U-phosphate (mmol/24h)	27.7 (18.9–35.4)	27.4 (21.2–37.8)

All values as median and range.
Significant difference between controls and patients: * $p < 0.05$, ** $p < 0.005$.
3 patients above normal range (6 pmol/l).

phosphorous) intake of 450 mg (= 15 mmol/day). A good match between estimated Pi intake and Pi intake in the baseline period is indicated by the close agreement of urinary Pi excretion rates in the pretrial period (in patients: median 24.6 mmol/day) and during the 3-day baseline period (median 27.6 mmol/day). Validity of calculated Pi intake and actual intake was assessed by random duplicate meal analysis which showed agreement within 8.4% in ashed meal samples. Particular care was taken to maintain (through selection of food items with known composition) constant intake of calcium (800–1200 mg/d), sodium chloride (4–6 g/d), and energy (35 Kcal/kg/d).

During the stay on the metabolic ward, urine was collected daily using plastic bottles (pH adjusted to 5 by addition of 1N HCl). Blood was taken daily at 8 a.m. in the fasting state for measurement of $1,25(OH)_2D_3$ and other biochemical parameters. The protocol is briefly outlined in Figure 1.

3. Analytical techniques

Serum and urinary chemistries were studied using Autoanalyzer technique (Hitachi, Automatic analyzer 705). Inulin clearance was determined by infusion clearance technique, measuring serum inulin concentrations enzymatically as described previously [Schmid et al. 1990]. Intact (1,84) PTH was assessed by two-site immunoradiometric assay as described previously [Blind et al. 1987]. $1,25(OH)_2D_3$ was measured by RIA according to Scharla et al. [1984] and $25(OH)D_3$ according to Mayer et al. [1984]. The $1,25(OH)_2D_3$ assay had a detection limit of 3 pg/ml and the normal range was 25–60 pg/ml. Intraassay variability was 12% (CV) and interassay variability 16.8%. In a pilot study, day to day variation in 13 healthy subjects over 5 consecutive days was 15.4% (CV), 8.4–22.4.

4. Statistical analysis

The results are given as median and range. The data were evaluated using SAS program (SAS Institute Inc. 1985). Comparisons between groups were carried out using Wilcoxon's test for random samples. Beta error calculations were carried out using the SAS program.

Table 2 Effect of reduced intake of phosphate on parameters of calcium metabolism

	Controls (n = 7)		Early renal failure (n = 6)	
	Usual Pi intake	Reduced # Pi intake	Usual Pi intake	Reduced # Pi intake
S-P (mmol/l)	1.12 (0.89–1.50)	1.16 (0.95–1.40)	1.07 (0.81–1.48)	1.11 (0.93–1.15)
S-Ca (mmol/l)	2.18 (2.09–2.34)	2.30 (2.16–2.51)	2.22 (2.15–2.32)	2.30 (2.12–2.44)
$1,25(OH)_2D_3$ (pg/ml)	45.7 (36.7–48.3)	38.3 (31.7–46.7)	23.5 (13.0–27.7)	19.1 (16.0–30.0)
25(OH)D (nmol/l)	69.0 (35.3–177)	67.2 (33.3–127)	93.4 (50.0–167)	92.1 (52.7–142)
Intact PTH (pmol/l)	3.8 (2.4–4.7)	3.5 (2.1–5.3)	4.6 (1.5–40.0)	2.8 (1.4–24.3)
S-Crea (mg/dl)	0.91 (0.76–1.05)	1.01 (0.95–1.08)	1.55 (1.46–2.12)	1.65 (1.49–1.99)
UV-P (mmol/24h)	27.7** (18.9–35.4)	11.9 (10.3–17.8)	27.4* (21.2–37.8)	14.1 (13.5–17.8)
UV-Ca (mmol/24h)	2.96 (1.99–6.29)	2.55 (1.93–3.72)	1.83 (0.33–2.59)	1.87 (0.66–2.99)

All values as median and range.
Significant difference between values before and on reduced Pi intake: * $p < 0.05$; ** $p < 0.01$.
Mean of day 7–9.

Results

1. Biochemical baseline data

As shown in Table 1, patients with early renal failure had numerically higher intact PTH levels and significantly lower 1,25$(OH)_2$ vitamin D_3 levels than healthy controls. In renal failure, a tight correlation was found between 1,25$(OH)_2$ vitamin D_3 levels and C_{in} ($r = 0.88$; $p < 0.0001$), but the correlation between 1,25$(OH)_2$ vitamin D_3 and intact PTH ($r = 0.4$) was not statistically significant. Normal 25(OH)D_3 levels were noted in all controls and in all patients with renal failure. This finding documents absence of vitamin D deficiency.

On usual dietary intake of Pi, Pi excretion rates were similar in controls and patients, respectively. As expected, urinary calcium excretion rates were significantly lower in patients with early renal failure.

2. Concentrations of 1,25$(OH)_2$ vitamin D_3 on usual phosphate and reduced phosphate intake (Table 2 and Figure 2)

There was no significant difference of 1,25$(OH)_2$ vitamin D_3 levels during the usual Pi intake and reduced Pi intake periods, respectively between controls and patients with early renal failure. Figure 2 shows the day-to-day variation of 1,25$(OH)_2$ vitamin D_3 levels in the individual subjects. In 4 healthy subjects the observation period on reduced Pi intake was prolonged to 10 days but no change in 1,25$(OH)_2D_3$ concentration was seen despite pro-

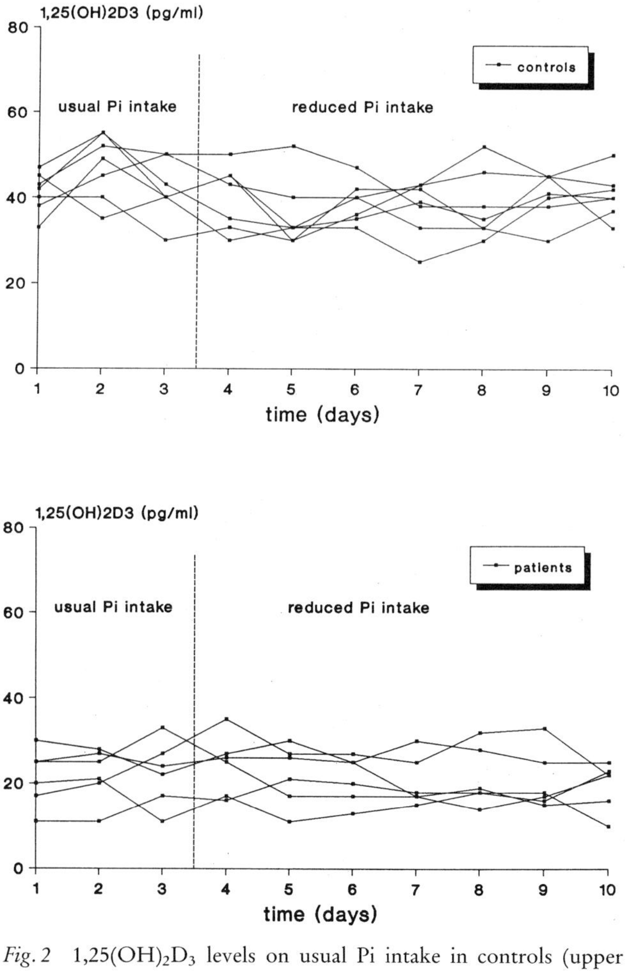

Fig. 2 1,25$(OH)_2D_3$ levels on usual Pi intake in controls (upper panel) and patients with early renal failure respectively (lower panel). No statistically significant difference was noted between the usual Pi intake and reduced Pi intake period.

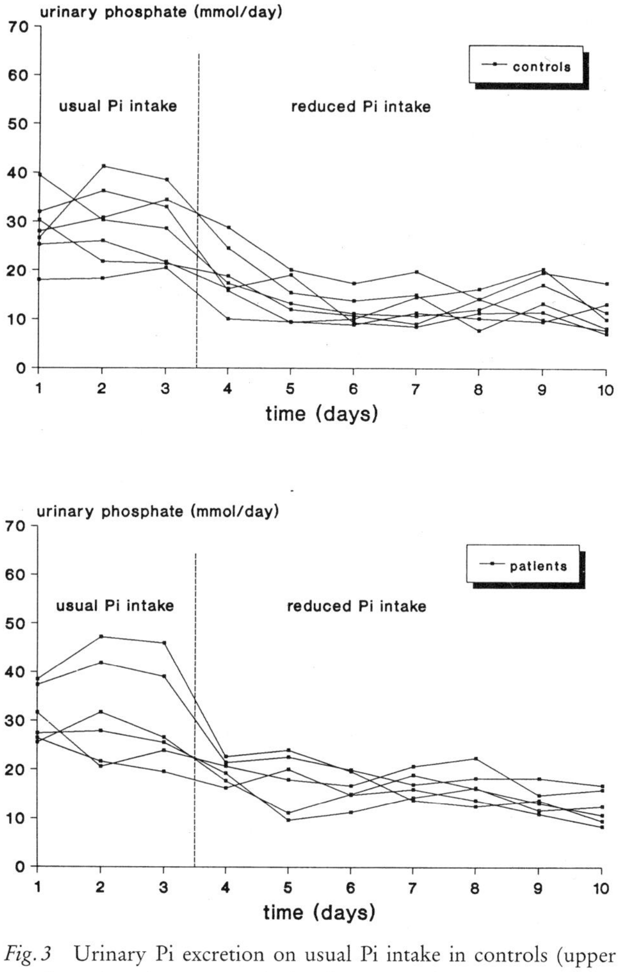

Fig. 3 Urinary Pi excretion on usual Pi intake in controls (upper panel) and patients respectively (lower panel). Note significant reduction of urinary Pi excretion by day 6 with constant excretion rates thereafter.

longed follow-up (data not given). Beta-error-analysis showed that the study had a 68% power to detect a 15% change (i.e. a change equivalent to 1 SD) and a 99% power to detect a 30% change at a $p < 0.05$.

3. Effect of the diet on other parameters of calcium metabolism (Tables 2 and 3, Figure 3)

Serum Pi concentrations did not change during the reduced Pi diet. The diet consistently lowered urinary Pi which remained stable subsequent to the third day of dietary Pi reduction. This is more clearly shown in Figure 3. There was one occasional outlier, presumably from dietary non-compliance, in the control group and 2 outliers in the group of patients (exclusion of whom does not alter the results). Median Pi excretion (as percent of Pi intake) on the 9th day of reduced Pi intake was 78.3%. Levels of urinary calcium or intact plasma PTH did not significantly change.

The study was designed ot achieve a comparable ratio of dietary Pi intake/GFR in patients with early renal failure on reduced Pi and in healthy controls on normal Pi intake. Table 3 illustrates more clearly that lower $1{,}25(OH)_2$ vitamin D_3 levels persisted in patients with early renal failure, although the ratio of dietary Pi intake/GFR had become similar to the baseline Pi/GFR ratio in controls.

Discussion

The study shows that isolated reduction of dietary phosphate intake with no change of calcium, sodium or energy intake for up to 10 days fails to change circulating $1{,}25(OH)_2$ vitamin D_3 levels in either healthy controls or patients with early renal failure. These results in humans are in line with recent observations in dogs [Portale et al. 1990] showing that isolated reduction in phosphorus intake fail to change plasma $1{,}25(OH)_2D_3$ levels. The study had sufficient statistical power to detect a 15% change of circulating $1{,}25(OH)_2$ vitamin D_3 levels. We cannot exclude the possibility that isolated manipulation of dietary phosphate intake may cause changes of $1{,}25(OH)_2$ vitamin D_3 concentrations of lower amplitude or with a more delayed time-course.

It has been suggested that the abnormality of vitamin D metabolism in early renal failure results from an imbalance between the dietary phosphate intake and the level of GFR [Massry et al. 1977, Llach and Massry 1985, Bonjour 1988]. It is therefore of note that a significant difference of $1{,}25(OH)_2$ vitamin D_3 concentrations was found between patients with renal failure on reduced phosphate and healthy controls on normal phosphate diet, although the ratio of dietary phosphate intake over GFR (Pi/C_{in}) as a rough index of nephronal phosphate load was similar in the two groups. Although the magnitude of the phosphate signal was admittedly small and smaller than in previous studies [Maierhofer et al. 1983, Portale et al. 1989], the relative changes were similar to what can be anticipated in early renal failure. Llach and Massry [1985] did a comparable study of longer duration. They switched patients with early renal failure on usual phosphate intake to a phosphate restricted diet. The phosphate intake had been reduced in proportion to the decrease in creatinine clearance. This manœuver increased $1{,}25(OH)_2$ vitamin D_3 levels, decreased serum iPTH levels and increased intestinal absorption of calcium. Their study lasted 60 days, but the changes of iPTH in response to phosphate restriction occurred within 3 days. The difference to our results remains puzzling and unexplained.

Our protocol was carefully validated to exclude a number of potential artefacts. With the diet chosen no change of serum phosphate was noted and urinary phosphate excretion remained stable for 7 days (and in a limited number of observation for 10 days) after phosphate intake had been reduced. This argues against the possibility of progressive phosphate depletion. Although fecal phosphate was not measured, the result is compatible with stable phosphate balance. This assumption is further supported by the observation that phosphate excretion corresponded to 78% of phosphate intake in healthy controls and patients with early renal failure, in close agreement with previous measurements of Tessitore et al. [1987]. Because of the known possibilities of error in computing diets, phosphate content was independently validated by

Table 3 Relation between the serum concentration of $1{,}25(OH)_2D_3$ concentration and the ratio dietary phosphate (Pi) intake/GFR

	ratio $\frac{\text{Pi intake*}}{\text{GFR}}$	$1{,}25(OH)_2D_3$ (pg/ml)
Controls (n = 7)		
Usual Pi intake	0.29 (0.22–0.36)	45.7 (36.7–48.3)
Reduced Pi intake	0.16 (0.11–0.21)	38.3 (31.7–46.7)
Early renal failure (n = 6)		
Usual Pi intake	0.58 (0.42–0.85)**	23.5 (13.0–27.7)**
Reduced Pi intake	0.27 (0.21–0.38)**	19.1 (16.0–30)**

All values as median and range.

* Calculated as dietary phosphate (Pi) intake (mmol/day) divided by C_{in} (ml/min/1.73m^2).

** Significant difference between controls and patients with early renal failure $p < 0.005$.

duplicate meal analysis which showed close agreement between calculated and measured dietary phosphate content.

Stable urinary phosphate excretion rates (and urea excretion rates, data not given) confirm adequate compliance of healthy subjects and patients under metabolic ward conditions. Serum creatinine did not change during the study period confirming stable renal function. Finally, no changes of body weight or urinary creatinine excretion were noted. This observation confirms that patients were in energy balance and not catabolic.

To further assess the reliability of our negative finding, we examined the validity of 1,25(OH)$_2$ vitamin D$_3$ measurements. Intraassay and interassay variations were relatively large, but comparable with data in literature [Bouillon et al. 1980]. In a pilot study, day-to-day variation in 13 healthy subjects over 5 consecutive days was 15.4% (CV), 8.4–22.4. This result is in good agreement with the variability found during the 3-day period when subjects were on normal phosphate intake. Furthermore, 1,25(OH)$_2$D$_3$ concentrations were remeasured in a second laboratory (Prof. Bouillon, Leuven); the values between the two diet periods agreed within 5% (the maximal variation within dietary periods was 8.7%).

The finding of no change of intact PTH levels on normal vs. reduced phosphate intake may provide indirect evidence arguing against major changes in circulating 1,25(OH)$_2$D$_3$ concentrations. The intact (1.84) PTH assay has considerably lower variability (intraassay CV 7.6%) and is able to detect changes even within the normal range [Ritz et al. 1991]. One would anticipate that changes in 1,25(OH)$_2$ vitamin D$_3$ levels should have caused reciprocal changes in iPTH levels, although admittedly the time course might have been too short to detect 1,25(OH)$_2$D$_3$-dependent changes of 1.84 PTH levels.

We emphasize that all our patients had a GFR above 40 ml/min/1.73 m^2. The findings in this study cannot necessarily be extrapolated to more advanced stages of renal failure. In subtotally nephrectomized dogs with advanced renal failure, Slatopolsky et al. [1971] clearly showed that iPTH levels fell in response to lowering of dietary phosphate (contrasting with our observation in early renal failure, where no change in iPTH was noted).

Our protocol does not formally exclude the possibility that the presumed reduction of synthesis of 1,25(OH)$_2$ vitamin D$_3$ in early renal failure is due to a rise of phosphate concentration in a critical subcellular compartment of proximal tubular epithelial cells, as proposed by Bonjour [1988]. With existing technology this hypothesis cannot be tested directly in humans. To the extent, however, that the consequences of this hypothesis can be assessed, its predictions are not supported by the results of the present study.

Acknowledgement

We thank the VW-Stiftung for support of the study, Dipl.-Stat. E. Pfarr (Boehringer Mannheim Co.) for his help in calculating the beta error, and Mrs. Hihler for typing the manuscript.

REFERENCES

Blind E, Schmidt-Gayk H, Armbruster FP, Stadler A 1987 Measurement of intact human parathyrin by an extracting two-site immunoradiometric assay. Clin Chem *33:* 1376–1381

Bonjour JP 1988 1,25-dihydroxyvitamin D and phosphate homeostasis in early chronic renal failure: the "trade off hypothesis" revisited. In: Nephrology, *Davison AM* (ed). London, Philadelphia, Toronto, Sidney, Tokio, Bailliere Tindall, pp 1059–1066

Bouillon R, De Moor P, Baggiolini EG, Uskokovic MR 1980 A radioimmuno-assay for 1,25-dihydroxycholecalciferol. Clin Chem *26:* 562–567

DeLuca HF 1973 The kidney as an endocrine organ in calcium homeostasis. Kidney Int *4:* 80–88

Friedlander MA, Lemke JH, Horst RL 1988 The effect of uninephrectomy on mineral metabolism in normal human kidney donors. Am J Kidney Dis *11:* 393–401

Llach F, Massry SG 1985 On the mechanism of secondary hyperparathyroidism in moderate renal insufficiency. J Clin Endocrinol Metab *61:* 601–606

Lucas PA, Brown RC, Jones CR, Woodhead JS, Coles GA 1985 Reduced 1,25(OH)$_2$D$_3$ may be responsible for the development of hyperparathyroidism in early chronic renal failure. Proceedings European Dialysis and Transplantation Association – European Renal Association *22:* 1124–1128

Lucas PA, Brown RC, Woodhead JS 1986 Acute response of parathyroid hormone and 1,25-dihydroxyvitamin D$_3$ to unilateral nephrectomy in healthy donors. Nephrol Dial Transplant *1:* 199–203

Maierhofer WJ, Gray RW, Lemann J Jr 1984 Phosphate deprivation increases serum 1,25-(OH)-vitamin D concentrations in healthy men. Kidney Int *25:* 571–575

Mayer E, Schmidt-Gayk H 1984 Interlaboratory comparison of 25-hydroxyvitamin D determination. Clin Chem *30:* 1199–1204

Massry SG, Ritz E, Verberckmoes R 1977 Role of phosphate in the genesis of secondary hyperparathyroidism of renal failure. Nephron *18:* 77–81

Portale AA, Booth BE, Halloran BP, Morris RC Jr 1984 Effect of dietary phosphorus on circulating concentration of 1,25-dihydroxyvitamin D and immunoreactive parathyroid hormone in children with moderate renal insufficiency. J Clin Invest *73:* 1580–1589

Portale AA, Halloran BP, Murphy MM, Morris RC Jr 1986 Oral intake of phosphorus can determine the serum concentration of 1,25-dihydroxyvitamin D by determining its production rate in humans. J Clin Invest *77:* 7–12

Portale AA, Halloran BP, Morris RC Jr 1989 Physiologic regulation of the serum concentration of 1,25-dihydroxyvitamin D by phosphorus in normal men. J Clin Invest *83:* 1494–1499

Portale AA, Al-Bander HA, Halloran BP, Fiellin D, Morris RC Jr 1990 Restriction of dietary phosphorus does not increase serum 1,25-$(OH)_2D$ in the normal dog. Kidney Int *37:* A470

Reichel H, Deibert B, Schmidt-Gayk H, Ritz E 1991 Calcium metabolism in early chronic renal failure. Implications for the pathogenesis of hyperparathyroidism. Nephrol Dial Transplant *6:* 162–169

Ritz E, Seidel A, Ramisch H, Szabo A, Bouillon R 1991 Attenuated rise of 1,25$(OH)_2$vitamin D_3 in response to parathyroid hormone in patients with incipient renal failure. Nephron *57:* 314–318

SAS Institute Inc SAS user's guide 1985 Statistics version 5, SAS Institute Inc Cary, NC, USA

Scharla S, Schmidt-Gayk H, Reichel H, Mayer E 1984 A sensitive and simplified radioimmunoassay for 1,25-dihydroxy D_3. Clin Chim Acta *142:* 325–338

Schmid M, Mann J, Stein G, Herter M, Nussberger J, Klingbeil A, Ritz E 1990 Natriuresis pressure relationship in polycystic kidney disease. J Hypertension *8:* 573–577

Slatopolsky E, Caglar S, Pennell JP, Taggart DD, Canterbury JM, Reiss E, Bricker NS 1971 On the pathogenesis of hyperparathyroidism in chronic experimental renal insufficiency in the dog. J Clin Invest *50:* 492–499

Tessitore N, Venturi A, Adami S, Roncari C, Rugiu C, Corgnati A, Bonucci E, Maschio G 1987 Relationship between serum vitamin D metabolites and dietary intake of phosphate in patients with early renal failure. Mineral Electrol Metab *13:* 38–44

Clinical Nephrology, Vol. 36 No. 6 – 1991 (281–289)

Lithium clearance in patients with chronic renal diseases

N. CLERICETTI and C. BERETTA-PICCOLI

Ospedale Italiano di Lugano, Viganello, Switzerland

Abstract. The clearance of lithium was analyzed in relation to the glomerular filtration rates and the effective renal plasma flow in 41 patients with renal disease and variable degree of renal functional impairment and in 40 normal subjects. In the patients, there was on average a 35% decrease of glomerular filtration rates (109 ± 64 [SD] ml/min) and renal plasma flow (490 ± 275 ml/min) and a 25% decrease of lithium clearance (22 ± 12 ml/min); the lithium clearance correlated closely with the glomerular filtration rates and renal plasma flow ($r = 0.69$; $p < 0.001$). The absolute proximal reabsorption of fluid was decreased by 38% (89 ± 56 ml/min) while the distal absolute reabsorption of sodium (21 ± 12 ml/min) was unchanged. Individual values of fractional proximal or distal reabsorption as related to glomerular filtration rates or renal plasma flow were equally distributed between normal and renal subjects, except in the presence of a severe renal function impairment, where both variables decreased exponentially. This suggests that in renal failure, sodium balance is maintained by a proportional decrease of proximal and distal sodium reabsorption in relation to glomerular filtration. Only in the presence of severe renal failure (GFR <30 ml/min) both variables are concomitantly readjusted to lower values.

Key words: lithium clearance – glomerular filtration rates – renal plasma flow – renal failure

Lithium clearance has been recently proposed as valuable method for estimating the proximal reabsorption of sodium [Thomsen 1984]. This approach is based on the assumption that lithium is reabsorbed in the proximal renal tubule to the same extent as sodium and water, and that lithium is neither reabsorbed nor secreted in the distal tubule [Thomsen 1984]. This conclusion is supported by experimental data obtained in animals with micropuncture technique [Hayslett and Kashgarian 1979, Thomsen et al. 1981, Shirley et al. 1983] and in humans by non-invasive methods [Thomsen and Schou 1968; Steel et al. 1975]. Although under certain experimental conditions such as an extremely low sodium intake [Thomsen 1977] or furosemide-induced diuresis [Steel et al. 1975], a small fraction of lithium reabsorption may take place within the distal nephron, lithium clearance appears to represent under most clinical situations a useful indicator of proximal sodium reabsorption [Thomsen 1984] and this technique has been largely used to analyze the renal tubular handling of sodium in patients with normal renal function, such as patients with essential hypertension [Weder 1986, Holstein et al. 1985] or normotensive subjects with familial predisposition to hypertension [Weder 1986, Städler et al. 1987] or in patients receiving nephrotoxic agents (cis-platinum) [Daugaard et al. 1988].

Little is known about the handling of lithium along the renal tubule in the presence of structural alterations or of renal failure. A recent study suggests that a reduction of glomerular filtration rate is accompanied by an equivalent reduction of lithium clearance [Kamper et al. 1989]. This would be consistent with the hypothesis that in renal failure the delivery of tubular fluid from the end of the proximal tubule falls in parallel with the decrease of glomerular filtration rate; moreover, there is no suggestion of distal tubular reabsorption of lithium [Kamper et al. 1989]. These data support the possibility that lithium clearance may be used to investigate sodium reabsorption in the presence of renal lesions. This hypothesis and the relationships between lithium clearance and the glomerular filtration rate or the renal plasma flow were further analyzed in the present study comprising patients with renal diseases and variable degrees of renal functional impairment.

Patients and methods

Forty-one patients with renal abnormalities and 40 normal subjects, who had given their informed consent, were included in the study. The patients

Received September 14, 1990; in revised form April 2, 1991.

Reprint requests to Prof. Dr. med. C. Beretta-Piccoli, Ospedale Italiano di Lugano, CH-6962 Viganello, Switzerland.

comprised 18 females and 23 males aged 16 to 75 years (mean 40 ± 17 [+ SD] years); they were referred for nephrological investigastions because of renal abnormalities, including proteinuria >300 mg/ 24 hr in all cases and/or renal failure. Seventeen of the patients had chronic glomerulonephritis (mesangial proliferative or focal and segmental hyalinosis in three cases each, IgA nephropathy in two cases, mesangial sclerosis, mesangiocapillary, extracapillary proliferative and poststreptococcal glomerulonephritis in one case each; 5 patients did not have a biopsy), four patients had Schoenlein-Henoch glomerulonephritis, three patients had light chain disease or, respectively, analgesic nephropathy, two patients had LED or, respectively, diabetic glomerulosclerosis, one patient each had familial glomerulonephritis, chronic pyelonephritis, gold nephrophathy, cis-platinum nephropathy, nephroangiosclerosis, cystinuria, Bartter syndrome, diuretic-abuse-induced tubulopathy, or, respectively, bilateral renal artery stenosis. Twenty-nine of the patients had a normal blood pressure at the time of the study, 11 were on antihypertensive therapy, which included diuretics in seven cases (furosemide in six and metolazone in one of the patients), beta-adrenoreceptor-blocking agents in seven cases, the converting enzyme inhibitor captopril in five cases, and calcium entry blockers in two cases. The 40 normal subjects were normal male volunteers, aged 20 to 32 years (mean 25 ± 3 years). They had a blood pressure consistently below 140/90 mmHg and had not experienced any clinical or laboratory signs of renal disease. None was taking drugs at the time of the study.

Renal function studies were performed in the morning in the resting, supine position, after a light breakfast without tea or coffee. Subjects and patients received dietary instructions in order to avoid very large or low sodium intakes during the 5 days prior to study. Where given, the morning dose of all antihypertensive agents was withdrawn. Fourteen mmol of lithium (Li_2CO_3) (Vifor, Geneva, Switzerland) were given orally in the evening before the study. The clearance procedure was as follows. A loading solution of 250 ml NaCl (0,9%) with 50 ml inulin (10%) and 4 ml PAH (20%), was infused during 20 minutes, while the subjects drank 500 ml water. The loading solution was then replaced by a sustaining infusion of 1 l NaCl (0,9%) with 50 ml inulin (10%) and 10 ml PAH (20%) given at a constant rate of 3 ml/min. In three of the patients, ^{51}Cr-EDTA (15 μCi in the loading and 8 μCi in the sustaining solution) was used instead of inulin. Urine was collected after an equilibration period of 30 minutes with infusion of the sustaining solution; three collection periods of 30 minutes each were performed, urine being voided spontaneously in males younger than 30 years of age or by bladder catheter in older males and all females. Halfway through each collection period, blood was drawn from the arm controlateral to that of the infusion.

Sodium and potassium in the plasma and urine were measured by flame photometer, lithium by atomic absorption spectrophotometry (Perkin-Elmer 1100 B, Perkin-Elmer corp Norwalk. CT, USA), creatinine and uric acid by autoanalyzer (Hitachi Clinicon 705, Tokyo, Japan), inorganic phosphate by colorimetric phosphomolybdate, inulin by the anthrone method [Davidson and Sackner 1963] and PAH according to Bratton and Marshall [1939], ^{51}Cr activity in a gamma counter (Gamma 5500, Beckmann, Irvine, CAL, USA). The coefficients of variation between the three clearance periods for inulin, PAH, sodium and lithium were 7.1 ± 5.9%, 6.4 ± 4.9%, 13.8 ± 11.9% and 9.2 ± 9.1, respectively, in normal subjects and 8.9 ± 5.8%, 11 ± 7.4%, 9.4 ± 6.7% and 8.6 ± 7.9% in the patients.

Clearance results were not corrected for body surface area, since this factor does not modify fractional clearances. The absolute proximal reabsorption of fluid was calculated as (Clearance insulin – Clearance lithium) and the absolute distal reabsorption of sodium as (Clearance lithium – Clearance sodium).

The fractional proximal reabsorption was calculated as:

Fractional proximal reabsorption =

$$1-\frac{\text{Clearance lithium}}{\text{Clearance inulin}}$$

and the fractional distal reabsorption of sodium as:

Fractional distal reabsorption of sodium =

$$1-\frac{\text{Clearance sodium}}{\text{Clearance lithium}}$$

Statistical analysis included two-tailed t-test (Bonferroni method), regression analysis and analysis of covariance.

Results

As compared with the 40 normal controls, the 41 patients with renal abnormalities had on average a 35% decrease of glomerular filtration rate and renal plasma flow; since both variables were decreased to a comparable extent, the filtration fraction was similar in renal patients and normal subjects (Table 1). The clearance of lithium, uric acid and potassium were lower (by 23%, 33% and, respectively, 25%) and the clearance of sodium higher (63%) in the patients (Table 1). The fractional clearances of sodium, potassium, anorganic phosphate and lithium were significantly higher in the patients than in normal subjects (Table 1).

Table 1 Renal functional studies in renal patients and normal subjects (Means ± SD)

	Renal patients	Normal subjects
Glomerular filtration rate, ml/min	109 ± 64[c]	170 ± 30.0
Effective renal plasma flow, ml/min	490 ± 275[c]	777 ± 236
Filtration fraction	0.239 ± 0.086	0.233 ± 0.053
Clearance, ml/min		
Sodium	1.99 ± 1.13[b]	1.09 ± 1.04
Potassium	18.1 ± 10.4[b]	23.2 ± 9.6
Anorganic phosphate	14.5 ± 10.11	16.5 ± 8.6
Lithium	22.3 ± 12.0[a]	29.1 ± 13.6
Uric acid	9.1 ± 5.1[c]	13.6 ± 4.5
Fractional clearance, %		
Sodium	3.3 ± 4.4[b]	0.65 ± 0.61
Potassium	25.2 ± 24.2[b]	13.3 ± 5.7
Anorganic phosphate	19.4 ± 21.2[b]	9.8 ± 5.3
Lithium	24.5 ± 11.4[b]	17.6 ± 9.0
Uric acid	11.6 ± 12.2	8.0 ± 2.6

a = p <0.05, b = p <0.01, c = p <0.005 versus normal subjects

The absolute proximal reabsorption of fluid, as defined as the difference between the glomerular filtration rate and the clearance of lithium, was significantly lower in renal patients than in normal subjects; the decrease averaged 38% (Table 2). The fractional proximal reabsorption was also 11% lower in the patients (Table 2). The distal absolute reabsorption of sodium, as defined as the difference between the clearance of lithium and sodium, and the fractional distal reabsorption of sodium, in contrast, did not differ between the two study groups (Table 2).

Table 2 Tubular reabsorption in renal patients and normal subjects (Mean ± SD)

	Renal patients	Normal subjects
Proximal reabsorption*, ml/min	88.8 ± 56.5[a]	143.9 ± 32.9
Distal reabsorption*, ml/min	20.7 ± 11.7	25.2 ± 14.7
Fractional proximal reabsorption*	0.75 ± 0.12[a]	0.84 ± 0.09
Fractional distal reabsorption*	0.89 ± 0.09	0.94 ± 0.07

* = as a defined in the method section
a = p <0.005 versus normal subjects

In the 5 patients with drug-induced nephropathy (analgesics, cis-platinum or diuretics) or Bartter syndrome, mean values of fractional clearances were 1.55 ± 0.44% for sodium, 14.3 ± 9.5% for potasssium, 21.8 ± 4.1% for anorganic phosphate, 27.2 ± 2.0% for lithium and 9.1 ± 3.9% for uric acid. Fractional proximal and distal reabsorption averaged 0.73 ± 0.02 and, respectively, 0.95 ± 0.02; both values were comparable with those measured in the remaining patients (0.77 ± 0.13 and 0.91 ± 10).

In normal subjects, the clearance of lithium was unrelated to the glomerular filtration rates (r = −0.14; N.S.) (Figure 1), the effective renal plasma flow (r = 0.30; N.S.) (Figure 2) and the filtration fraction (r = −0.36; N.S.). There was no significant correlation between the clearance of lithium and the clearance of uric acid (r = 0.33; N.S.) or the clearance of sodium (r = 0.20; N.S.), potassium (r = 0.05; N.S.) or anorganic phosphate (r = 0.05; N.S.). The glomerular filtration rates did not correlate with the

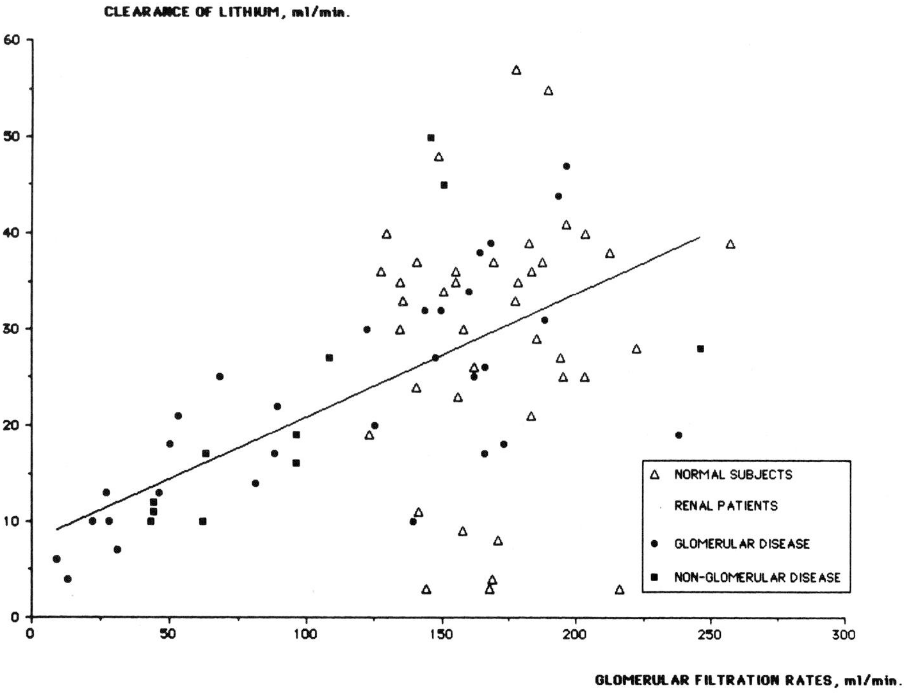

Fig. 1 Correlation between the lithium clearance and the glomerular filtration rate. In normal subjects (triangles) the correlation is not significant (r = –0.14); in renal patients (points and squares) it is significant (r = 0.69; p <0.001).

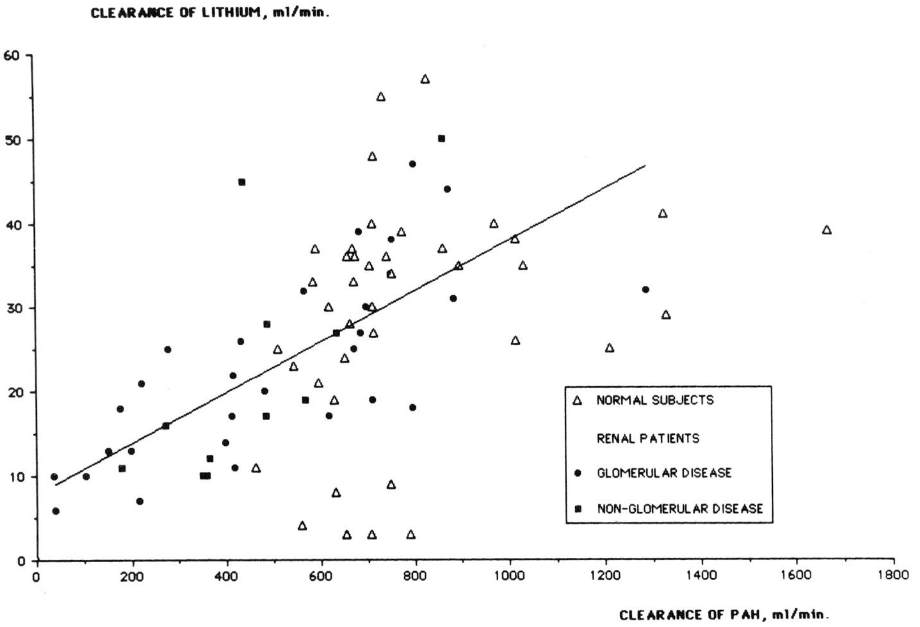

Fig. 2 Correlation between the lithium clearance and the effective renal plasma flow. In normal subjects (triangles) the correlation is not significant (r = 0.69; p <0.001). PAH = Paraaminohippuric acid.

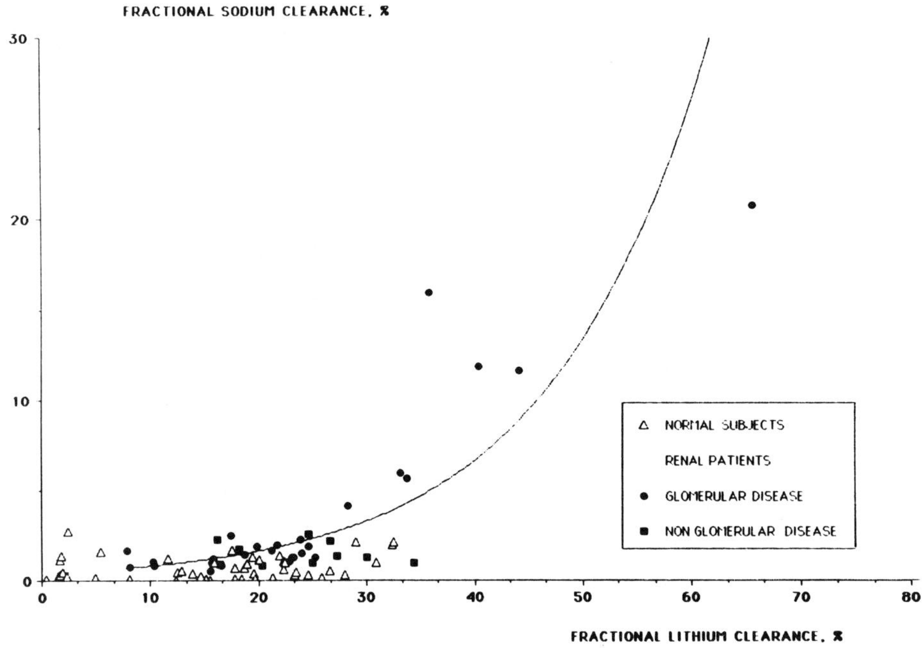

Fig. 3 Correlation between the fractional clearances of lithium and sodium. In normal subjects (triangles) the correlation is not significant (r = 0.36; N.S.); in renal patients (points and squares) it is significant (r = 0.80; p <0.001).

clearance of sodium, potassium, anorganic phosphate or uric acid (r = 0.07 to 0.33); it correlated positively with the effective renal plasma flow (r = 0.50; p <0.005). There was no correlation between the fractional clearance of lithium and that of sodium (r = 0.36; N.S.) (Figure 3), uric acid (r = 0.35, N.S.) (Figure 4), inulin (r = −0.28; N.S.), PAH (r = −0.17; N.S.), potassium (r = 0.20; N.S.) (Figure 5) or anorganic phosphate (r = 0.17; N.S.).

In renal patients, the clearance of lithium correlated positively with the glomerular filtration rate (r = 0.69; p <0.001) (Figure 1) and with the effective renal plasma flow (r = 0.69; p <0.001) (Figure 2) but not with the filtration fraction (r = 0.10; N.S.). There was a positive correlation between the clearance of lithium and the clearance of uric acid (r = 0.62; p <0.001) and of potassium (r = 0.53; p <0.005) but not with the clearance of sodium (r = 0.14; N.S.) or of anorganic phosphate (r = 0.22; N.S.). The glomerular filtration rates correlated positively with the effective renal plasma flow (r = 0.75; p <0.001) and with the clearance of uric acid (r = 0.62; p <0.001), but not

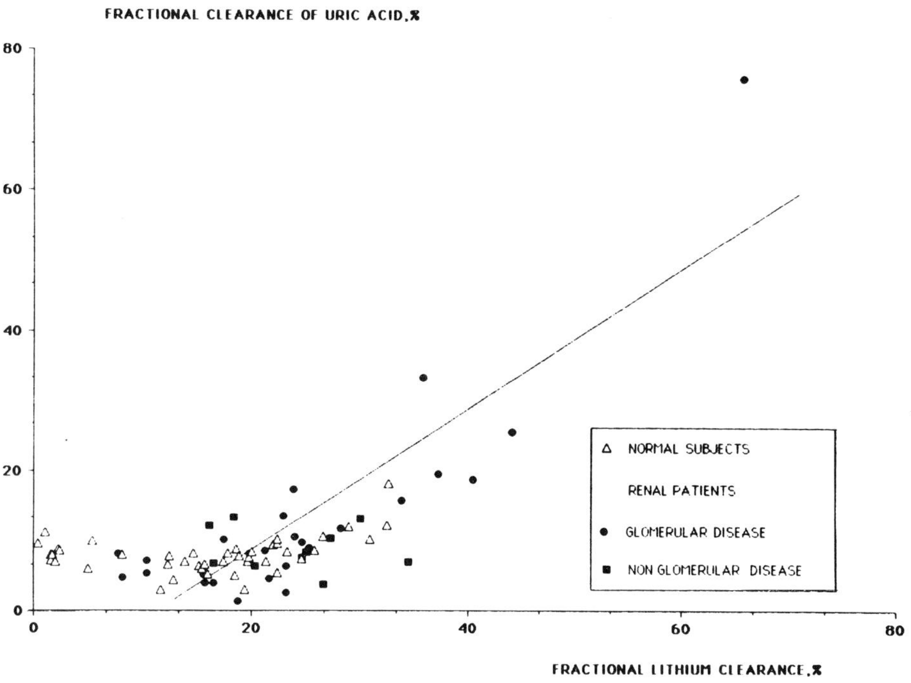

Fig. 4 Correlation between the fractional clearances of lithium and uric acid. In normal subjects (triangles) (r = 0.35) the correlation is not significant; in renal patients (points and squares) it is significant (r = 0.80; p <0.001).

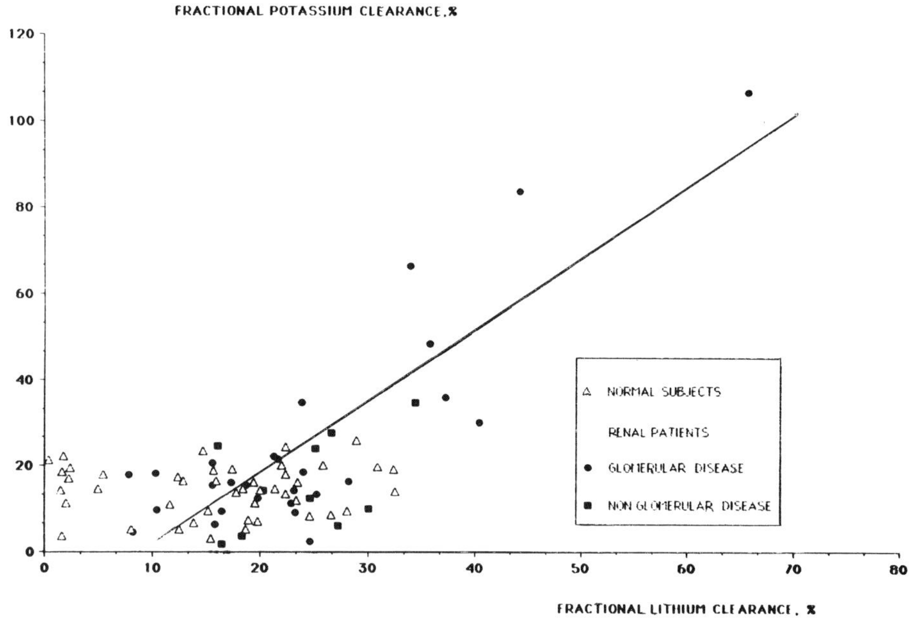

Fig. 5 Correlation between the fractional clearances of lithium and potassium. In normal subjects (triangles) the correlation is not significant (r = 0.20); it is significant (r = 0.85; p <0.001) in the patients (points and squares).

with the clearance of anorganic phosphate (r = 0.35; N.S.), potassium (r = 0.32; N.S.) or sodium (r = 0.01; N.S.). Moreover, in renal patients the fractional clearance of lithium was inversely related to the glomerular filtration rate (r = −0.62; p <0.001), the effective renal plasma flow (r = −0.48; p <0.01) and positively correlated with the fractional clearance of sodium (r = 0.85; p <0.001) (Figure 3), uric acid (r = 0.80; p <0.001) (Figure 4), potassium (r = 0.85; p <0.001) (Figure 5) and anorganic phosphate (r = 0.67; p <0.005).

In normal subjects, the absolute proximal reabsorption of fluid correlated with the glomerular filtration rate (r = 0.89; p <0.001) and the renal plasma flow (r = 0.40; p <0.05) but not with the clearance of uric acid (r = 0.14; N.S.). The two former relationships could be demonstrated in renal patients (r = 0.99 and, respectively, r = 0.73; p <0.001) and were comparable between the two study groups. In normal subjects, absolute proximal reabsorption did not correlate with the clearance of uric acid (r = 0.14; N.S.); a positive relationship

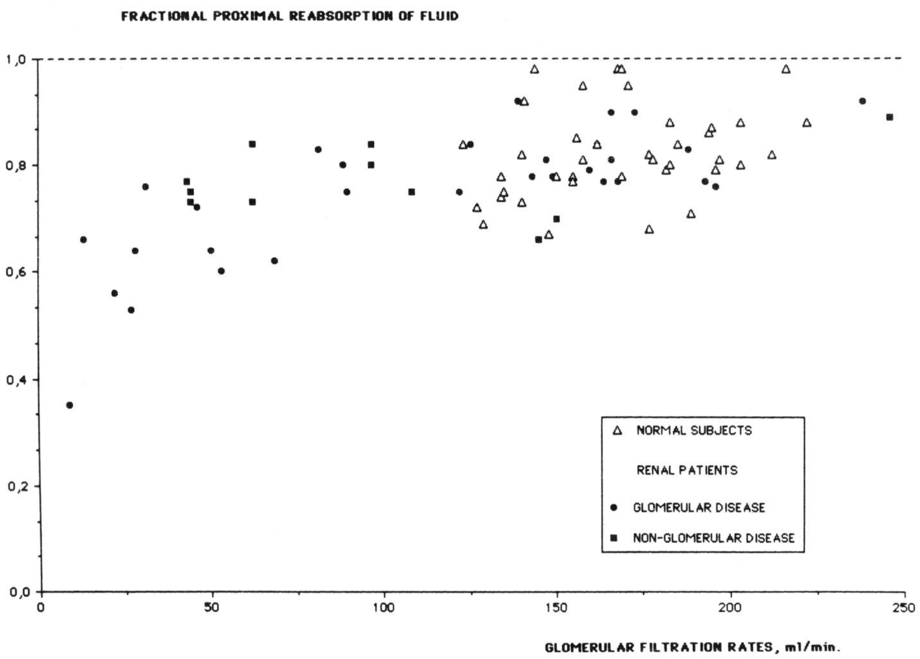

Fig. 6 Relationship between the fractional proximal reabsorption of fluid and the glomerular filtration rates in normal subjects (triangles) and renal patients (points and squares).

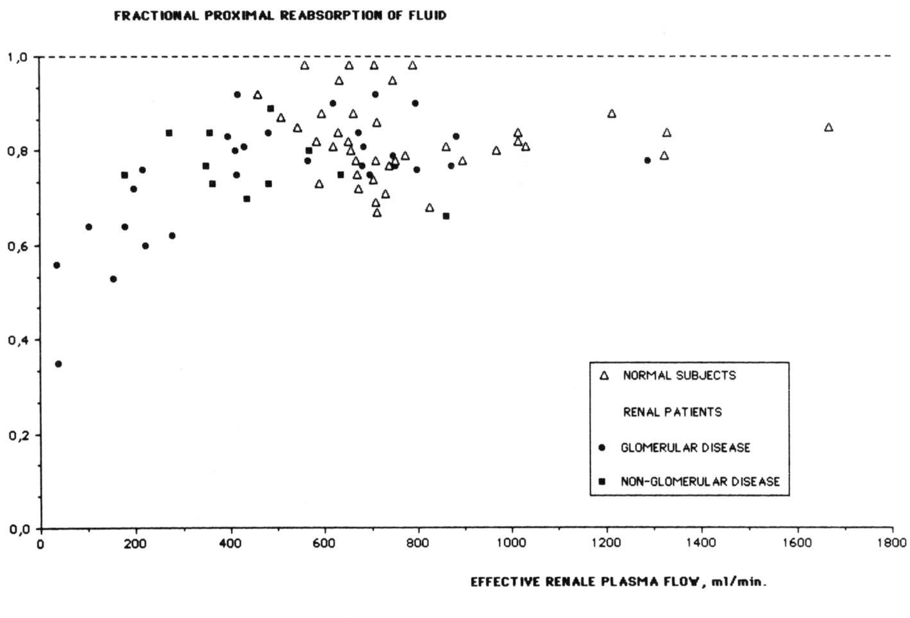

Fig. 7 Relationship between the fractional proximal reabsorption of fluid and the effective renal plasma flow in normal subjects (triangles) and renal patients (points and squares).

could be demonstrated in renal patients ($r = 0.57$; $p < 0.005$). In normal subjects, the absolute distal reabsorption of sodium was unrelated to the glomerular filtration rate or the renal plasma flow but correlated positively with both variables in renal patients ($r = 0.70$ and $r = 0.72$; $p < 0.001$). The fractional proximal reabsorption of fluid and the distal reabsorption of sodium did not correlate with the glomerular filtration rate or renal plasma flow in normal subjects, while significant correlations could be demonstrated for the 4 relationships in renal patients ($r = 0.52$ to $r = 68$; $p < 0.01$).

Individual values of fractional proximal reabsorption of fluid analyzed in relation to the glomerular filtration rates (Figure 6) or renal plasma flow (Figure 7) showed a similar distribution between normal subjects and renal patients, except for the patients with glomerular filtration rate <30 ml/min or a renal plasma flow <300 ml/min. No difference in the distribution of the fractional proximal reabsorption could be demonstrated between renal patients with glomerular or non-glomerular diseases (Figures 6 and 7). A similar pattern, although less evident, could be demonstrated for the fractional distal reabsorption

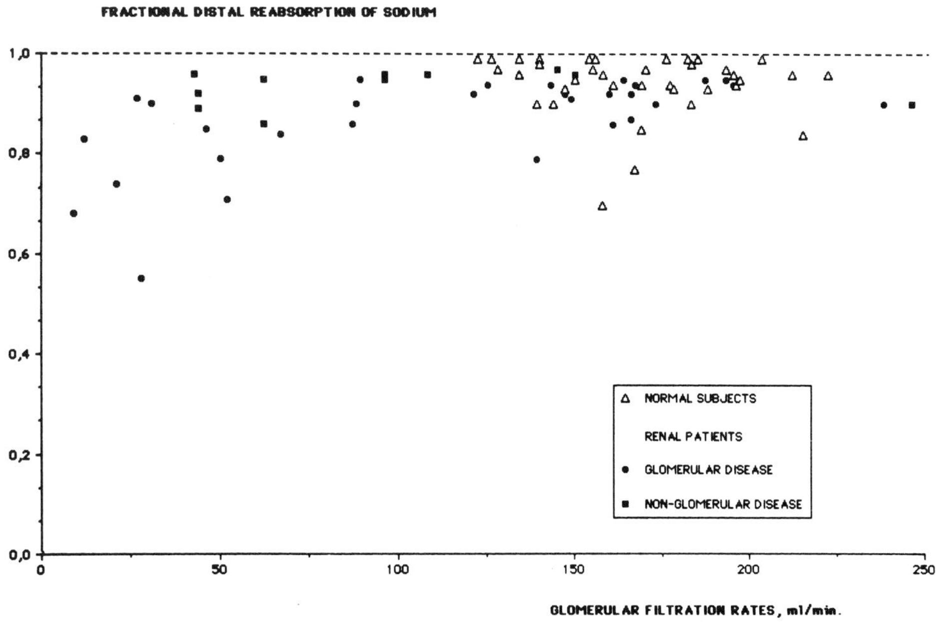

Fig. 8 Relationship between the fractional distal reabsorption of sodium and the glomerular filtration rate in normal subjects (triangles) and renal patients (points and squares).

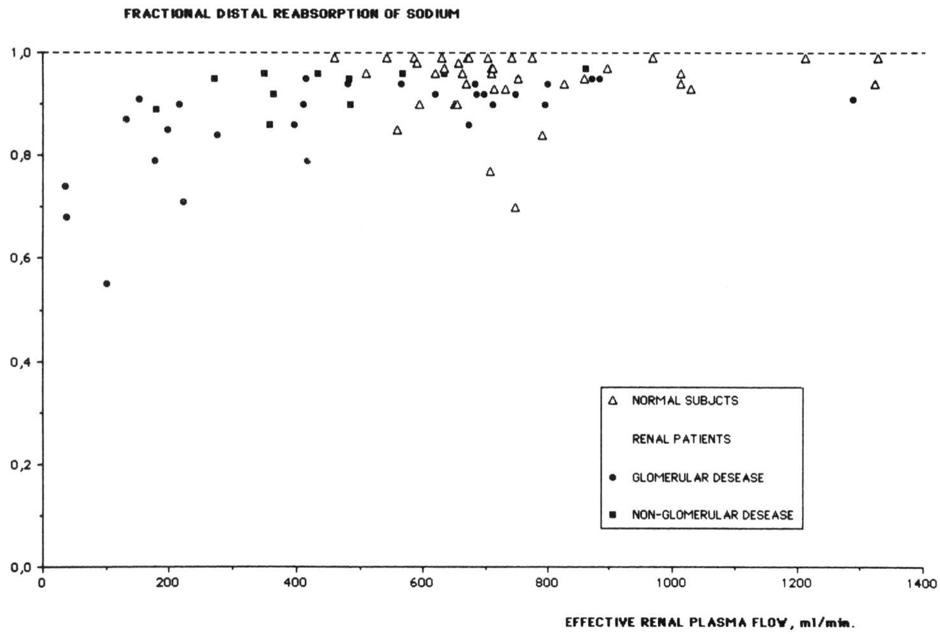

Fig. 9 Relationship between the fractional distal reabsorption of sodium and the effective renal plasma flow in normal subjects (triangles) and renal patients (points and squares).

of sodium related to glomerular filtration rates or renal plasma flow (Figures 8 and 9).

Discussion

The findings of the present study confirm previous results [Kamper et al. 1989, Thomsen et al. 1969] of a parallel reduction of glomerular filtration rates and lithium clearance in patients with renal functional impairment and demonstrate a proportional decrease of the effective renal plasma flow and the clearance of lithium. These conclusions are supported by:

1. the presence of a close correlation between the lithium clearance and the glomerular filtration rate or the renal plasma flow in renal patients
2. the presence of close and similar correlations between the absolute proximal reabsorption of fluid and sodium and the glomerular filtration rates or the renal plasma flow in both normal and renal subjects.

In the presence of a mild to moderate degree of renal functional impairment, the fractional proximal and distal reabsorption of sodium are unchanged. Only when the glomerular filtration rate and/or the renal plasma flow fall below 30 ml/min or, respectively, 300 ml/min a rapid decrement of both proximal and distal reabsorptions is observed.

Experimental data obtained both in animals and humans indicate that the clearance of lithium is closely related to the reabsorption of water and sodium in the proximal renal tubule [Thomsen 1990, Kirchner 1990]. Lithium can also be transported in the Henle's loop [Koomans and Mees 1990] but the existence of a quantitative important lithium reabsorption in this part of the nephron has not been clearly demonstrated. Loop diuretics markedly increase lithium clearance [Atherton et al. 1990, Colussi et al. 1990]; this effect is absent during volume expansion, suggesting that an inhibitory effect in the proximal tubule may account for this modification [Christensen 1990]. In humans, lithium reabsorption does not take place in the distal tubule to a quantitatively relevant extent, at least in the sodium replete state [Koomans and Mees 1990, Atherton et al. 1990, Boer et al. 1990]; in the sodium deplete state, hydrochlorothiazide or spironolactone slightly elevate lithium clearance [Atherton et al. 1990]. Therefore, it would appear that in the absence of sodium depletion or of factors modifiying electrolyte transport in the Henle's loop, the clearance of lithium can be used as an estimate for fluid and sodium reabsorption in the proximal tubule. In the present study, renal patients were studied on a normal sodium intake and, when administered previously, diuretic agents were discontinued at least 24 hours prior to the clearance procedure. On the other hand, the negative correlation between the glomerular filtration rates and the fractional clearance of lithium in a previous study (r = −0.62) [Kamper et al. 1989] indicated that the decrease of glomerular filtration rates was accompanied by a relatively smaller decrease of lithium clearance; this was considered as evidence against a relevant distal reabsorption of lithium [Kamper et al. 1989]. A similar correlation was present in our renal patients (r = −0.62). The presence of an increased osmotic drive or of high blood pressure did not modify the clearance of lithium in humans with renal failure [Kamper et al. 1989]. Finally, the etiology of the renal disease in this study did not influence lithium clearance since the distribution of individual values of lithium clearance or of fractional proximal or distal reabsorption in relation to the glomerular filtration rate or renal plasma flow did not differ between patients with glomerular or non-glomerular disease.

In order to avoid a bladder catheter in normal subjects, the control group included only male volunteers. This should not be expected to modify the comparison with the patients since, when lithium clearance is expressed in relation to glomerular filtration rate, it has been shown to be independent of sex [Schou et al. 1986]. In our controls, the clearance of lithium did not correlate with the glomerular filtration rate or the effective renal plasma flow. This finding differs from a previous report indicating a positive correlation between both variables [Kamper et al. 1989]. However, in that investigation, normal controls included subjects with glomerular filtration rates as low as 65 ml/min; such values would represent, in our hands, a mild renal functional impairment rather than a normal state. The clearance of lithium is influenced considerably by posture and by physical activity [Kamper et al. 1988]. Both factors did not influence the comparison between normal subjects and renal patients, since clearance studies were performed in the supine position using a similar procedure. The patients were on average slightly older than normal subjects; the clearance of lithium, however, does not change with ageing [Schou et al. 1986]. The extraction of PAH decreases with increasing renal parenchymal destruction; however, under such conditions, the PAH clearance reflects the renal plasma flow in the perfused renal tissue (effective renal plasma flow) [Reubi 1982]. Under these conditions, in the presence of renal abnormalities, the clearance of lithium was closely related to the glomerular filtration rate and the effective renal plasma flow. It also correlated with the clearances of uric acid and potassium, but not with the clearance of sodium or anorganic phosphate. In renal patients a positive relationship between the clearance of lithium and potassium has been already noted, and persisted after allowance of the concomitant influence of the glomerular filtration rate [Kamper et al. 1989]. This may indicate that the output of fluid and sodium from the proximal tubule may influence potassium reabsorption at more distal sites.

The clearance of uric acid has been proposed as an estimate of proximal tubular reabsorption [Weder 1986]. In our normal subjects the clearance of uric acid correlated weakly with the clearance of lithium and not with the absolute proximal reabsorption of fluid [Schuster and Seldin 1985]. The positive and highly significant relationship between these variables in renal patients may be due, at least partly, to their close correlation with the glomerular filtration rate. On the other hand, it cannot be excluded that in renal failure, the clearance of uric acid may be a better predictor of proximal reabsorption than in the normal state. The latter possibility is supported by the findings of a close correlation between the fractional clearance of lithium and of uric acid.

Assuming that the clearance of lithium may be used as an estimate of the proximal sodium reabsorption [Thomsen 1990], the parallel fall of the glomerular filtration rate and the clearance of lithium in our patients suggests that in renal failure sodium balance is maintained by a proportional decrease of proximal and distal reabsorption. Individual values of the estimated fractional proximal reabsorption of fluid and of estimated fractional distal reabsorption of sodium showed a similar distribution in normal and renal subjects, when analyzed in relation to glomerular filtration rate or renal plasma flow. Only in the presence of severe renal functional impairment sodium reabsorption needs to be readjusted with an exponential decrease. In this setting, both proximal and distal reabsorption are concomitantly reduced in individual patients. The adaptation of the nephron does not seem to be modified by the localization of the primary abnormality leading to renal failure, since the proximal and distal fractional reabsorptions did not differ between patients with glomerular or non-glomerular diseases.

Acknowledgements

We acknowledge the secretarial assistance of Mrs. D. Lazzaretti and the technical work of Mrs. C. Bravi.

REFERENCES

Atherton JC, Green R, Higggins A, Large A, McNicholas C, Parker D, Pempkowiak L, Rajani K, Smith J 1990 Lithium clearance in healthy humans: Effects of sodium intake and diuretics. Kidney Int *37:* S36–S38

Boer WH, Koomans HA, Mees EJD 1990 Lithium clearance in healthy humans suggesting lithium reabsorption beyond the proximal tubules. Kidney Int *37:* S39–S44

Bratton AC, Marshall EK 1939 A new coupling component for sulfanilamide determination. J Biol Chem *128:* 537–549

Christensen S 1990 Furosemide effect during volume expansion: Evidence against lithium transport in the loop. Kidney Int *37:* S45–S51

Colussi G, Rombolà G, Surian M, De Ferrari ME, Airaghi C, Benazzi E, Malberti F, Minetti L 1990 Lithium clearance in humans: Effects of acute administration of acetazolamide and furosemide. Kidney Int *37:* S63–S66

Daugaard G, Abildgaard U, Holstein-Rathlou NH, Bruunshuus I, Bucher D, Leyssac PP 1988 Renal tubular function in patients treated with high-dose cisplatin. Clin Pharmacol Ther *44:* 164–172

Davidson WD, Sackner MA 1963 Simplification of the anthrone method for the determination of inulin in clearance studies. J Lab Clin Med *62:* 351–356

Hayslett JP, Kashgarian M 1979 A micropuncture study of the renal handling of lithium. Pflügers Arch *380:* 159–163

Holstein-Rathlou NH, Svendson UG, Leyssac PP 1985 Effects of acute volume loading on kidney function in patients with essential hypertension, as estimated by the lithium clearance method. J Hypertension *3:* 511–516

Kamper AL, Strandgaard S, Holstein-Rathlou NH, Munck O, Leyssac PP 1988 The influence of body posture on lithium clearance. Scand J Clin Lab Invest *48:* 509–512

Kamper AL, Holstein-Rathlou NH, Leyssac PP, Strandgaard S 1989 Lithium clearance in chronic nephropathy. Clinical Science *77:* 311–318

Kirchner KA 1990 Effect of diuretic and antidiuretic agents on lithium clearance as a marker for proximal delivery. Kidney Int *37:* S22–S25

Koomans HA, Mees EJD 1990 Lithium in renal physiology: Post-conference discussion and consensus. Kidney Int *37:* S78–S79

Leyssac PP 1990 Validity of the lithium clearance concept assessed with micropuncture studies. Kidney Int *37:* S17–S21

Reubi F 1982 Die Bestimmung der glomerulären Filtration und der renalen Plasmadurchströmung. In:*Reubi F* (ed) Nierenkrankheiten. Verlag Hans Huber, Bern, pp 85–98

Schou M, Thomsen K, Vestergaard P 1986 The renal lithium clearance and its correlations with other biological variables: observations in a large group of physically healthy persons. Clin Nephrol *4:* 207–211

Schuster VL, Seldin SW 1985 Renal clearance. In: *Seldin DW, Giebisch G* (eds) The kidney. Raven Press, New York, pp 365–395

Shirley DG, Walter SJ, Thomsen K 1983 A comparison of micropuncture and lithium clearance methods in the assessment of renal tubular function in rats with diabetes insipidus. Pflügers Arch *399:* 266–270

Städler P, Pusterla C, Beretta-Piccoli C 1987 Renal tubular handling of sodium and familial predisposition to essential hypertension. J Hypertension *5:* 727–732

Steel TH, Manuel MA, Newton M, Boner G 1975 Renal lithium reabsorptions in man: physiologic an pharmacologic determinants. Am J Med Sci *269:* 349–363

Thomsen K 1977 The renal handling of lithium: relation between lithium clearance, sodium clearance and urine flow in rats with diabetes insipidus. Acta Pharmacol Toxicol *40:* 491–496

Thomsen K 1984 Lithium clearance: a new method for determining proximal and distal reabsorption of sodium and water. Nephron *37:* 217–223

Thomsen K 1990 Lithium clearance as a measure of sodium and water delivery from the proximal tubules. Kidney Int *37:* S10–S16

Thomsen K, Schou M 1968 Renal lithium excretion in man. Am J Physiol *215:* 823–827

Thomsen K, Schou M, Steiness I, Hansen HE 1969 Lithium as an indicator of proximal sodium reabsorption. Pflügers Archiv *308:* 180–184

Thomsen K, Holstein-Rathlou NH, Leyssac PP 1981 Comparison of three measures of proximal tubular reabsorption: lithium clearance, occlusion time, and micropuncture. Am J Physiol *241:* F348–F355

Weder AB 1986 Red-cell lithium-sodium countertransport and renal lithium clearance in hypertension. N Engl J Med *314:* 198–201

Clinical Nephrology, Vol. 36 No. 6 – 1991 (290–293)

Uremic autonomic dysfunction evaluated by pattern recognition analysis

G. Vita[1], P. Princi[2], V. Savica[3], G. Bellinghieri[3], R. M. Puglisi[1], L. Marabello[1] and C. Messina[1]

[1] *Institute of Neurological and Neurosurgical Sciences, University of Messina, Policlinico Universitario, Messina,* [2] *Interdepartmental Centre of Pharmaco-Toxicological Information, University of Messina and* [3] *Nephrology Unit, University of Messina, Italy*

Abstract. A pattern recognition analysis of six cardiovascular reflex tests was performed with the aim to increase their diagnostic efficiency. A normal model was defined by SIMCA method using log-transformed values of 85 healthy subjects. The model was tested with data from 60 patients with chronic renal failure. Specificity resulted 94% and sensitivity 96%. 55% of the uremics were recognized affected by autonomic damage. The method allowed a better definition of autonomic function in those patients defined as "borderline" on conventional evaluation of the tests. Pattern recognition analysis of autonomic tests provides a global assessment of all the tests performed. Its use should be encouraged as a diagnostic tool.

Key words: autonomic dysfunction – cardiovascular reflexes – multivariate analysis – chronic uremia

Introduction

Patients with chronic renal failure can manifest autonomic nervous system damage [Vita et al. 1990]. Distinct abnormalities of vagal function with possible combined sympathetic derangement have been reported [Campese et al. 1981, Heidbreder et al. 1985, Savica et al. 1989, Solders et al. 1985, Vita et al. 1987a, Zoccali et al. 1982]. Uremic autonomic neuropathy may have a number of clinical sequelae, but its role in mortality has yet to be clearly established [Malik et al. 1986, Vita et al. 1988]. In order to evaluate autonomic function objectively, a battery of simple bedside cardiovascular reflex tests are usually employed. There is a general agreement in the fact that a diagnosis of autonomic neuropathy cannot be substantiated on the basis of the result from a single test and the presence of abnormal values in at least two tests is conventionally accepted as indicating autonomic dysfunction. Every laboratory should establish its own control values for every test and confidence may be increased using age-related normal ranges [Vita et al. 1986]. However, a subject can have only one test abnormal or more tests at lower limits of normal ranges. That patient is said to have "early" or "borderline" autonomic damage. In such a situation, useful information about his autonomic function might be extracted from a global evaluation of all the tests performed. We attempted to make a pattern recognition analysis of six cardiovascular reflex tests and to apply it as a diagnostic tool in the assessment of uremic autonomic neuropathy.

Received September 25, 1990; in revised form June 26, 1991.

Reprint requests to Dr. G. Vita, Institute of Neurological and Neurosurgical Sciences, University of Messina, Policlinico Universitario, I-98125 Messina, Italy

Materials and methods

85 healthy subjects ranging in age from 25 to 76 years were evaluated. The study population included 47 males (49 ± 13 years; mean ± SD) and 38 females (46 ± 13 years). They showed no presence of overt clinical disease and were taking no medication known to affect the autonomic nervous system. After informed consent had been obtained, they were requested to refrain from smoking and coffee on the day of the examination, which was performed in the morning or in the late afternoon. A battery of cardiovascular autonomic tests were performed as previously described [Vita et al. 1987b]. The four parasympathetic tests consisted of beat to beat variation during quiet breathing and deep breathing, and heart rate responses to Valsalva manoeuver and to standing. The two tests of sympathetic function were blood pressure responses to standing and to sustained handgrip.

R-R interval variation test: after a period of 30 min supine rest, an electrocardiogramm (ECG) was recorded during quiet breathing at a paper speed of 50 mm/s. During the test the subject remained recumbent and undisturbed. The lengths of 200 consecutive R-R intervals were measured and the standard deviation of the mean expressed in milliseconds.

Deep breathing: the subject was breathing deeply at a rate of 6 breaths/min while sitting. The time was checked with stopwatch-based commands by the examiner. A standard ECG monitored continuously the test. The change in heart rate was expressed as the mean of the differences between the maximal and minimal heart rate during six successive breaths.

Valsalva manoeuver: the subject was studied sitting quietly and maintaining an expiratory pressure of 40 mmHg for 10 sec by blowing through a mouthpiece attached to an anaeroid manometer. ECG at 50 mm/sec was recorded during the manoeuver and for 30 sec after release of pressure. The Valsalva ratio was calculated as the ratio of the longest R-R interval after the manoeuver to the shortest R-R interval during the manoeuver. Each subject performed three tests, separated by a rest period of 2 min, and the highest ratio was accepted.

Blood pressure and heart rate responses to standing: after 15 min of supine rest, the blood pressure was recorded with an automatic sphygmomanometer. The subject was then asked to stand within 3–4 sec and to remain motionless for 2 min. During this time, the blood pressure was recorded at 30 sec intervals. The change in mean blood pressure 60 sec after standing was expressed as a function of resting mean blood pressure. The heart rate was continuously monitored during and after standing at 50 mm/sec chart speed. The 30/15 ratio was calculated as the ratio of the longest R-R interval around beat 30 after standing to the shortest R-R interval around beat 15. The test was repeated twice and the highest 30/15 ratio was accepted.

Sustained handgrip: the subject was asked to exert 30% of maximal voluntary contraction for 5 min (or at least 3 min) on a handgrip dynamometer using the dominant arm. Blood pressure was measured with a sphygmomanometer in the non-exercising arm at rest and at 60 sec intervals during the manoeuver. The highest increase in diastolic blood pressure was considered.

Statistical evaluation was performed using PARVUS package [Forina et al. 1988]. On each subject seven variables were taken into consideration, i. e. the results of the six cardiovascular tests and age. SIMCA (soft independent modelling of class analogy) method was utilized as modelling technique, using the raw data, normalized data by autoscaling and log-transformed data.

In the second phase of the study, the prediction abilities of different discriminating models were evaluated using, as test set objects, 60 patients (aged 31–76 years) with chronic uremia and dialysed for 4 h three times a week for periods ranging from 4 to 121 months. Each patient underwent previously described autonomic tests in a dialysis-free day. None of them had heart failure, severe hypertension, ischaemic heart disease, diabetes mellitus, bronchopneumopathy or amyloidosis. The results of the tests were compared with conventional or age-adjusted normal ranges [Vita et al. 1986]. Accordingly, we divided the patients in three groups: “no autonomic damage”, “definite autonomic damage” (at least two tests abnormal), and “borderline autonomic damage” (only one test abnormal or at least two tests at lower limits of normal ranges). Classification ability of discriminating model included measurement of specificity and sensitivity. The former is the ability to designate as negative those without the disease; the latter is the ability to designate as positive those with the disease. A subject was rejected by the model of normal category, i. e. recognized as likely not belonging to it, when probability of misclassification was higher than 95%.

Results

Modelling procedures were applied to data of control healthy subjects to the search of a model with the best classification ability, i. e. the highest percentage of test set objects correctly classified. In other words, we simulated the real problem that physicians must solve: absence or presence of autonomic dysfunction. The highest sensitivity and specificity were reached by a model computed using the natural logarithmic transformation of the variables. Such model showed also the highest retained variance and modelling power of each variable. The model appeared stable and reliable, being only 3 subjects outlying (3.5%). It was tested with data from uremic patients grouped according to above indicated definitions; n = 18 (30%) with no autonomic damage, n = 26 (43%) with definite autonomic damage, n = 16 (27%) with borderline autonomic damage. SIMCA method allowed us to compute the position of each test set object in the hyperspace of the variables. For each patient, the SIMCA distance from normal category centroid was measured and he was classified into or out the normal category according to a probabilistic transformation.

Table 1 shows the classification ability of the normal model. 17/18 patients without autonomic damage were accepted by the model while one was refused. 25/26 patients with definite autonomic dam-

Table 1 Classification ability of discriminating model obtained by SIMCA method

Uremic patients (n = 60)	Accepted by the normal model	Rejected by the normal model
No autonomic damage (n = 18; 30%)	17	1
Definite autonomic damage (n = 26; 43%)	1	25
Borderline autonomic damage (n = 16; 27%)	9	7
Total	27 (45%)	33 (55%)

age were found far enough from the normal model and rejected, and one patient was accepted. Specificity and sensitivity resulted high, being 94% and 96%, respectively. Testing the model with patients with borderline autonomic damage gave non-homogenous results. Among 16 patients, 9 were accepted by the normal model and 7 were rejected. We examined these two subpopulations of subjects in detail but no particular differences were found in their test results. Within the whole group of 60 uremics, application of pattern recognition analysis revealed that 27 patients (45%) had normal autonomic function and 33 patients (55%) resulted with autonomic damage.

Discussion

The aim of simple noninvasive tests, such as were used in the present study, is to investigate the integrity of autonomic control mechanisms in uremia as well as in other diseases. A good diagnostic efficiency may be reached only if a battery of tests is used. Abnormal results in two or more of these tests correlate well with abnormalities detected by invasive tests and indicate autonomic dysfunction [McLeod and Tuck 1987]. However, when a group of patients at risk for autonomic neuropathy is under study, three subpopulations may result: patients with no autonomic damage; patients with definite autonomic damage; patients with borderline autonomic damage [Ewing 1983]. While the first two groups are well determined and final diagnosis will influence prognosis and preventive or therapeutic strategies, the borderline group is somewhat uncertain and reflects our inability to better define their autonomic status.

In the last years, some attempts were done to extract discriminant informations from analytical data by pattern recognition methods [Armanino et al. 1987]. These mathematical approaches allow to increase the classification and prediction abilities of given tests, with an improvement of diagnostic efficiency. In this study we applied such methods to cardiovascular autonomic tests. It was necessary to use a transformation technique to analyze the data because the distribution of test results was skewed and relationship with age was non-linear [Gautschy et al. 1986, O'Brien et al. 1986, Vita et al. 1986]. Log-transformation was applied also to age but not to changes in blood pressure after standing and during handgrip because of the possible presence of negative values or values equal to zero. On the other hand, we took also age into consideration as variable since it is an important determinant of heart rate and blood pressure responses in normal subjects as well as in pathological conditions [Vita et al. 1986, Vita et al. 1987a]. The high sensitivity and specificity achieved indicate that the method we used allows to discriminate well between healthy condition and presence of autonomic dysfunction.

Several studies on incidence of uremic autonomic neuropathy have been published. A defective regulation of the heart rate was found isolated in 14 to 34% of uremics and combined to a damage of reflex blood pressure control in 18 to 26% [Vita et al. 1990]. The purpose of the method here described was to evaluate overall cardiovascular reflex function, without distinction between parasympathetic and sympathetic pathways, but with a better assessment of those patients with uncertain results. The finding of 55% frequency of autonomic damage in our series of uremics on intermittent hemodialysis is in accordance with previous reports. This figure is higher than that obtained on conventional evaluation of the single tests (43% with "definite autonomic damage") since it includes some patients previously belonging to the borderline group. Interestingly, when pattern recognition analysis was applied to patients with "borderline autonomic damage", 44% were found very far from the normal model and rejected as pathological, and the rest was considered with normal autonomic function. This means that only a combined evaluation of all the tests performed, such as we did, is able to differentiate two subgroups inside that we thought to be a relatively homogeneous group. Pattern recognition analysis of autonomic tests may provide more definite information about autonomic function and as consequence better knowledge of early manifestations, natural history and prognosis of uremic autonomic neuropathy.

The method here proposed is simple and requires only an adequate number of normal control tests, a prerequisite for any laboratory, an IBM-PC and commercially available software. It has the great advantage that diagnosis of autonomic neuropathy is based on neither a single test, nor evaluation of single tests, but on a global assessment of a battery of six tests, with an increase of diagnostic efficiency. Pattern recognition analysis appears particularly useful in the so-called borderline patients. Its use should be encouraged also in other types of autonomic neuropathy.

REFERENCES

Armanino C, Leardi R, Roda A, Simoni P 1987 Pattern recognition study of biochemical assays for liver function. Anal Chim Acta *202*, 175

Campese VM, Romoff MS, Levitan D, Lane K, Massry SG 1981 Mechanisms of autonomic nervous system dysfunction in uremia. Kidney Int *20*, 246

Ewing DJ 1983 Practical bedside investigation of diabetic autonomic failure. In: *Bannister R* (ed). Autonomic failure: a textbook of clinical disorders of the autonomic nervous system. Oxford University Press, Oxford, pg 371

Forina M, Leardi R, Armanino C, Lanteri S, Conti P, Princi P 1988 PARVUS: an extendable package of programs for data exploration, classification and correlation. Elsevier Scientific Software, Amsterdam

Gautschy B, Weidmann P, Gnädinger MP 1986 Autonomic function tests as related to age and gender in normal man. Klin Wochenschr *64*, 499

Heidbreder E, Schafferhans K, Heidland A 1985 Autonomic neuropathy in chronic renal insufficiency: comparative analysis of diabetic and nondiabetic patients. Nephron *41*, 50

Malik S, Winney RJ, Ewing DJ 1986 Chronic renal failure and cardiovascular autonomic function. Nephron *43*, 191

McLeod JG, Tuck RR 1987 Disorders of the autonomic nervous system: Part 2. Investigation and treatment. Ann Neurol *21*, 519

O'Brien IAD, O'Hare P, Corrall RJM 1986 Heart rate variability in healthy subjects: effects of age and the derivation of normal ranges for tests of autonomic function. Br Heart J *55*, 348

Savica V, Vita G, Puglisi RM, Marabello L, Bellinghieri G, Messina C 1989 The course of uremic autonomic function during hemodialysis treatment (Abstract). 6th International Capri Conference on Uremia, pg 16

Solders G, Persson A, Gutierrez A 1985 Autonomic dysfunction in non-diabetic terminal uremia. Acta Neurol Scand *71*, 321

Vita G, Princi P, Calabrò R, Toscano A, Manna L, Messina C 1986 Cardiovascular reflex tests: assessment of age-adjusted normal range. J Neurol Sci *75*, 263

Vita G, Savica V, Marabello L, Puglisi RM, Serra S, Musolino R, Bellinghieri G 1987a Occurrence of uremic autonomic dysfunction in relation to age. Acta Neurol Scand *76*, 468

Vita G, Girlanda P, Puglisi RM, Marabello L, Messina C 1987b Cardiovascular-reflex testing and single-fiber electromyography in botulism: a longitudinal study. Arch Neurol *44*, 202

Vita G, Dattola R, Calabrò R, Manna L, Venuto C, Toscano A, Savica V, Bellinghieri G 1988 Comparative analysis of autonomic and somatic dysfunction in chronic uremia. Eur Neurol *28*, 335

Vita G, Messina C, Savica V, Bellinghieri G 1990 Uremic autonomic neuropathy. J Auton Nerv Syst *30*, S179

Zoccali C, Ciccarelli M, Maggiore Q 1982 Defective reflex control of heart rate in dialysis patients: evidence for an afferent autonomic lesion. Clin Sci *63*, 285

Clinical Nephrology, Vol. 36 No. 6 – 1991 (294–298)

Experience of pain after subcutaneous administration of different preparations of recombinant human erythropoietin: a randomized, double-blind crossover study

C. Granolleras[1], W. Leskopf[2], S. Shaldon[1] and J. Fourcade[1]

[1] *Department of Nephrology, University Hospital, Nîmes, France and*
[2] *Software Office, Leimen, Germany*

Abstract. Subcutaneous erythropoietin (SCEPO) is considered to be more effective than intravenously administered erythropoietin. Patient compliance with SC injections will be important in long-term therapy as there have been reports of pain associated with SCEPO. A double-blind randomized study was performed upon 18 ESRD hemodialysis patients receiving regular subcutaneous erythropoietin replacement therapy for treatment of their anemia. The study involved pain assessment by a visual analogue scale VAS and a verbal descriptive scale VDS following 2 subcutaneous injections of preparation A: rhEPO 2000 IU in 1 ml (Cilag), preparation B: rhEPO 2000 IU in 1 ml (Boehringer Mannheim) and 0.9% saline 1 ml (placebo) over a two-week period. The injections were all administered by the same person and replaced the normal EPO injections for the patient during the study period. Results by VAS and VDS based upon 107 responses showed that preparation A was significantly more painful than preparation B ($p < 0.001$) or saline ($p < 0.01$). An unexpected finding was that preparation B was less painful than the placebo for VAS ($p < 0.05$). It seems unlikely that the erythropoietin itself was responsible for the difference. Further work will be necessary to determine the pain causing factor in preparation A, and the possible local anaesthetic factor in preparation B.

Key words: subcutaneous erythropoietin – end-stage renal disease

Introduction

Recombinant human erythropoietin (rhEPO) has been used for the treatment of renal anemia since 1986 [Winearls et al. 1986, Eschbach et al. 1987]. The principal route of administration of the drug has been intravenous, taking advantage of the vascular access which is present in end-stage renal disease (ESRD) hemodialysis patients. However, the intravenous route of administration has several disadvantages: it is impracticable for patients without a permanent vascular access like CAPD patients or pre-end-stage renal disease patients and furthermore self-administration by patients is difficult. In addition, a significantly lower dose of rhEPO is required with subcutaneous administration when compared to the intravenous route [Bommer et al. 1988, Granolleras et al. 1989, Besarab et al. 1990]. This may be explained by the prolonged apparent plasma half-life of rhEPO after subcutaneous administration [MacDougall et al. 1989, Kampf et al. 1989]. As a consequence, the subcutaneous administration of rhEPO is today generally accepted as the preferred route.

A prerequisite for the chronic treatment using the subcutaneous route of administration is the compliance of the patients, particularly if there are other alternatives like intravenous administration via the arteriovenous fistula readily available for the majority of ESRD patients. Local tolerance of the drug will therefore have an influence on the route of administration chosen. Significant differences of pain sensation with subcutaneous rhEPO have been reported for the two available preparations of rhEPO in Europe [Bommer et al. 1989, Stephens et al. 1991, Frenken et al. 1991].

As our own interest has been the evaluation of daily subcutaneous rhEPO [Granolleras et al. 1989, 1991] as the most effective and safe form of rhEPO administration, these initial reports on pain prompted us to carry out a comparative investigation of the rhEPO preparations currently available. The goal of

Received August 13, 1991.

Reprint requests to Dr. S. Shaldon, 86 rue de Grézac, F-34080 Montpellier, France this study was to identify possible differences of these preparations with respect to pain experienced after subcutaneous administration. The study was designed as a double-blind randomized crossover trial in which the two preparations were compared to 0.9% saline, which served as an inert placebo.

Patients, materials and methods

The study was performed with 18 adult ESRD patients who had been on hemodialysis thrice weekly for at least 6 months. 8 patients were male, 10 female. Their median age was 55 years (range: 22–79) and their median body weight was 58.75 kg (range: 47.3–92.8). All patients had been treated with rhEPO for more than one month before entry into this study. All patients gave informed consent prior to the study. The study protocol was approved by the ethical committee of the University Hospital Montpellier-Nîmes.

None of the patients had contraindications for rhEPO therapy (e.g. uncontrolled hypertension), acute infections, regular analgesic therapy, chronic pain disorder or skin alterations (e.g. sclerodermia).

The following preparations served as study medication: Preparation A (manufactured by Cilag) contained a solution of 2000 IU rhEPO in 1 ml of an aqueous solvent containing citrate buffer, sodium chloride and human serum albumin (2.5 mg/ml). Preparation B (manufactured by Boehringer Mannheim) was a lyophilisate containing 2000 IU rhEPO, together with the following excipients: sodium phosphate (buffer), sodium chloride, a mixture of selected physiological amino acids, urea and Tween 20. This lyophilisate was reconstituted in 1 ml of water for injection (manufactured by Baxter). Saline (0.9% sodium chloride solution, manufactured by Baxter) was used as inert control (placebo).

Each treatment group consisted of two consecutive subcutaneous administrations of each preparation (A, B, or saline). The patients were randomized into a three-period crossover design for the three treatment groups. Each of the six possible sequences of the three treatment groups was included with the same frequency.

The sequence of the injections was done in accordance with the randomization list. The site of administration was the same as had been routinely used for rhEPO therapy prior to the study; it was kept constant for each patient: 11 patients received the injections into the upper arm, 6 patients into the abdomen, 1 patient into the thigh. All injections were given by one nurse immediately after hemodialysis and replaced the regular injection of rhEPO received by the patient for the two-week study period.

The study medication was prepared in injection vials according to the randomization list by an independent person. The vials had an identical appearance and were labelled with the patient number as well as the number of injection. Thus both the nurse administering the solution and the patient receiving the administration were unaware of the type of preparation to be administered. The injected volume was equal, i.e. 1 ml of each preparation was administered in each case. The solutions were equilibrated to room temperature before administration.

The assessment of pain after the injections was done by using standardized methods of pain assessment [Machin et al. 1988]. A visual analogue scale (VAS), which was a non-graduated 100 mm vertical line ranging from "no pain = 0" to "pain as bad as it could be = 100" was used. The patients were asked to indicate their pain sensation by scoring on the vertical line with a horizontal dash. A verbal descriptive scale (VDS) with the following six categories: no pain, hardly any pain, mild pain, moderate pain, severe pain, unbearable pain. The patients were asked to tick the appropriate category on a questionnaire. Both scales were filled in by the patients 10 minutes after each injection. In addition, the injection site was observed for reddening or swelling. All adverse events had to be noted, as well as any other medication taken by the patient.

Nonparametric methods were used for the statistical evaluation. To cope with the problem of multiple comparisons in the confirmatory analysis of the primary target variables (VAS and VDS) the closed test procedure for ordered hypotheses was employed [Einot and Gabriel 1975]. The following statistical hypotheses were tested univariately for both target variables in the sequence indicated below:

H_{01}: Preparation B = Preparation A
H_{02}: Preparation B = Saline
H_{03}: Preparation A = Saline

Under the condition that H_{01} is rejected at a significance level of 5% H_{02} and H_{03} can be tested simultaneously without alpha level adjustment. The closed test procedure guarantees an experiment wise error rate of 5% in a strong sense, for each VAS and VDS separately. Because of the high correlation of VAS and VDS results (see results) no further adjustments were regarded necessary. The three hypotheses were tested using Friedman's two-way analysis of variance by ranks. The squared Spearman rank correlation coefficient r_s^2 was calculated from the test-value chi_r^2 [Lienert 1973]. This quantity can be interpreted as coefficient of determination comparable to r^2, and allows a quantitative statement of how many percent of the intra-individual variance has been caused by the different treatment groups.

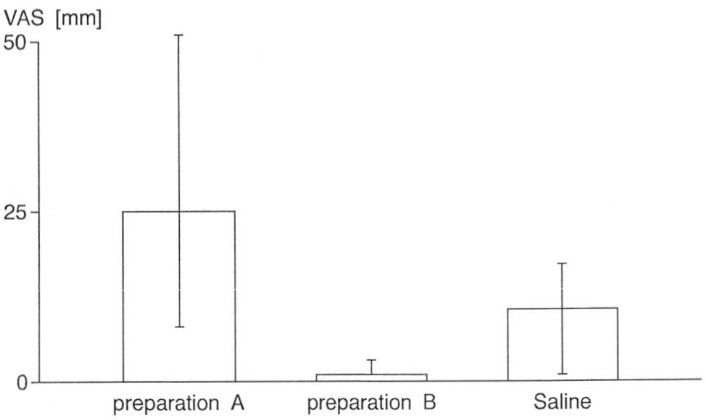

Fig. 1 Pain severity after subcutaneous administration of two available preparations A and B of recombinant human erythropoietin (rhEPO) and saline assessed with a visual analogue scale (VAS). Median values and interquartile ranges are shown (n = 18 patients).

Period effects and carry-over effects were analyzed using Friedman's two-way analysis of variance by ranks and the Wilcoxon rank sum test, respectively.

Results

17 of 18 patients received the full course of 6 injections; the remaining patient received the scheduled 2 injections of preparation B and saline but only one injection of preparation A. Thus a total of 107 injections were administered. If there was a difference between the responses to the two injections of each solution, the injection with the higher pain score was considered for the evaluation.

The results obtained with the visual analogue scale (VAS) are shown in Figure 1. There was a substantial difference between the two rhEPO preparations with respect to their pain scores: Injection of preparation A yielded a median score of 25 mm (interquartile range: 8–51 mm), whereas the median score for preparation B was only 1 mm (interquartile range: 1–3 mm). Saline yielded an intermediate median score of 10.5 mm (interquartile range: 1–17 mm).

Similar results were obtained with the verbal descriptive scale (VDS) (see Table 1). After administration of preparation A, only 3 patients (16.7%) reported no pain and 4 patients (22.2%) very mild pain, whereas a majority of patients (11 out of 18) experienced mild, moderate or severe pain (16.7%, 27.8%, and 16.7%). With preparation B, the large majority (15 out of 18 patients: 83.5%) reported no pain after subcutaneous administration. 3 patients reported either very mild, mild or moderate pain and no patient reported severe pain. After administration of saline, 7 patients (38.9%) reported no pain, 4 patients (22.2%) very mild pain and 7 patients experienced mild pain.

The results of the comparison of the treatment groups for both VAS and VDS are shown in Table 2. The greatest difference for VAS was observed between preparations A and B. This was followed by the difference between preparation A and saline, whereas the smallest difference was observed between preparation B and saline, where surprisingly preparation B was less painful than saline. The greatest difference in pain sensation reported with the VDS was also found between preparation A and B, followed by the difference between A and saline. The difference between preparation B and saline as assessed with the VDS was not statistically significant. The overall correlation of the results obtained with the VAS and the VDS was good (r_s = 0.86; Sperman's rank correlation).

Since all preparations were administered twice (with the exception of preparation A in one patient), the results of the first and the second administration

Table 1 Pain sensation after subcutaneous administration of two preparations A and B of recombinant human erythropoietin (rhEPO) assessed with a six-point verbal descriptive scale (VDS). The number of patients' responses is given for each pain category (total: 18 patients).

Pain category	Preparation A	Preparation B	Saline
no	3 (16.7%)	15 (83.3%)	7 (38.9%)
very mild	4 (22.2%)	1 (5.6%)	4 (22.2%)
mild	3 (16.7%)	1 (5.6%)	7 (38.9%)
moderate	5 (27.8%)	1 (5.6%)	0
severe	3 (16.7%)	0	0
unbearable	0	0	0

Table 2 Comparison between the pain sensation after subcutaneous administration of two available preparations A and B of recombinant human erythropoietin (rhEPO) and saline assessed with a visual analogue scale (VAS) and a verbal descriptive scale (VDS). (p-values [Wilcoxon] and r_s^2-values [squared Spearman rank correlation]) resulting from Friedman's two-way analysis of variance by ranks)

Comparison group	r_s^2	p
A with B (VAS)	0.6999	<0.001
A with saline (VAS)	0.2215	<0.01
B with saline (VAS)	0.0701	<0.05
A with B (VDS)	0.3050	<0.01
A with saline (VDS)	0.1564	<0.01
B with saline (VDS)	0.0437	>0.05

were checked to see if they were in agreement. With preparation A 13 of the 15 patients reported pain after both administrations. One patient reported very mild pain with one and no pain with the second injection and one patient received only one injection of preparation A which caused mild pain. With preparation B, the 3 patients that reported pain did so only after one but not after the other injection. With saline, 6 of the 11 patients reporting pain did so after both injections and the remaining 5 only after one of the injections.

Since the study was performed as a crossover study, period effects as well as carry over effects must be ruled out. No period or carry over effects could be detected using the statistical methods as indicated above. Reddening at the injection site was observed only after one injection of preparation B. Swelling at the injection site was observed after 42 of 107 injections. The occurrence of swelling was fairly evenly distributed between the 3 preparations (16 with preparation A, 14 with preparation B, 12 with saline). Interestingly, 41 of these swellings were observed when the injection was given into the upper arm (the remaining injection was into the abdomen). The high rate of swelling observed (39%) can thus be explained by the fact that 61% of the injections were given into the upper arm of the patients. There were no adverse events reported from the patients within the 14-day study period.

Discussion

The study was carried out to compare pain sensation after subcutaneous administration of the two available European preparations of rhEPO. We adapted our study to the regular practice of dialysis therapy, i.e. we chose to give the injection after a dialysis session, replacing the normal rhEPO injection. Furthermore, in our study each preparation was administered twice. Thus all (except one) patients received a total of 6 injections each in a period of two weeks (corresponding to 3 dialysis sessions per week).

Our results show a substantiated and reproducible pain sensation in the majority of the patients (83.3%) after the administration of preparation A. With the VDS, the answers for this preparation were quite evenly distributed between all categories (except unbearable pain), with most patients indicating moderate pain. Preparation B, on the other hand, gave rise to pain sensation in only very few patients (16.8%). Similar results were obtained with the VAS, where more than 75% of the patients indicated a more pronounced pain sensation after injection of preparation A as compared to preparation B.

Although there are no direct comparisons between the two rhEPO preparations with respect to their efficacy and general safety it can be assumed as both are licensed for use in Europe that there are no relevant differences. This suggests that the difference with respect to pain sensation after subcutaneous administration is not due to erythropoietin itself but to the differences in formulation excipients. Clearly, the aqueous solution of the excipients used for preparation B (phosphate buffer, sodium chloride, amino acids, urea and Tween 20) is well tolerated in spite of being hyperosmolar and only led to pain sensation in the minority of the patients. The aqueous solution of sodium chloride, citrate buffer and human serum albumin used for preparation A led to substantially more pain after subcutaneous injection. It is of interest that there was a significant difference between preparation B and saline with preparation B causing even less pain than saline. The reason for this is not clear, but it could suggest that one (or several) of the components in preparation B exhibit some local anaesthetic effect. Of the components in preparation B, the salts, amino acids and urea are unlikely candidates. Tween 20 is a non-ionic amphiphilic substance and chemically consists of a polyethyleneglycol ether of sorbitane-laurylester, where the polyethyleneglycol-moiety forms the hydrophilic and the laurylester the lipophilic part of the molecule. Another non-ionic amphiphilic substance is polidocanol (polyethyleneglycol-laurylether), which is known to possess strong local anaesthetic activity [Soehring et al. 1952]. Based on some relation in the chemical structure, a local anaesthetic effect of Tween 20 might be suspected. In this context, it is of interest that Tween 80, a compound with a chemical structure closely related to Tween 20 has been shown to possess anti-arrhythmic activity [Rohte and Jakvoljevic 1974], a well known property of many local anaesthetic agents (e.g. lidocaine). Since, however, the concentration of Tween 20 in preparation B is rather low (<0.1%), it is unlikely that the observed effect is attributable to Tween 20 alone. Further work will be necessary to establish whether the observed differences were due more to a pain causing substance in preparation A or to a local anaesthetic effect of preparation B or to both.

REFERENCES

Besarab A, Vlasses P, Caro J, Flaharty K, Medina F, Scalise R 1990 Subcutaneous administration of recombinant human erythropoietin for treatment of ESRD anemia (abstract). Kidney Int *37:* 236

Bommer J, Ritz E, Weinreich T, Bommer G, Ziegler T 1988 Subcutaneous erythropoietin (letter). Lancet *ii:* 406

Bommer J, Weinreich T, Ritz E, Zeier M, Bommer G 1989 Efficacy of subcutaneous or intravenous recombinant human erythropoietin therapy in dialysis patients. Nephrol Dial Transplant *4:* 471

Einot I, Gabriel KR 1975 A study of the powers of several methods of multiple comparisons. JASA *50:* 574–583

Eschbach JW, Egrie JC, Downing MR, Browne JK, Adamson JW 1987 Correction of the anemia of end-stage renal disease with recombinant human erythropoietin. Results of a combined phase I and II clinical trial. N Engl J Med *316:* 73–78

Frenken LAM, van Lier HJJ, Gerlag PGG, den Hartog M, Koene RAP 1991 Assessment of pain after subcutaneous injection of recombinant human erythropoietin in hemodialysis patients. Brit Med J in press

Granolleras C, Branger B, Beau MC, Deschodt G, Alsabadani B, Shaldon S 1989 Experience with daily self-administered subcutaneous erythropoietin. Contrib Nephrol *76:* 143–148

Granolleras C, Branger B, Shaldon S, Nonnast-Daniel B, Koch KM, Pollok M, Baldamus CA 1991 Subcutaneous erythropoietin: A comparison of daily and thrice weekly administration. Contrib Nephrol *88:* 144–148

Kampf D, Kahl A, Eckardt KU, Pustelnik A, Gahl G, Ehmer B, Jacobs C, Grabensee B, Gahl GM 1989 Single dose kinetics of recombinant human erythropoietin (rhEPO) after iv, sc and ip administration: preliminary results. Contrib Nephrol *76:* 106–111

Lienert GA 1973 Verteilungsfreie Verfahren in der Biostatistik (I), Verlag Anton Hain, Meisenheim am Glan

MacDougall IC, Roberts DE, Neubert P, Dhamasena AD, Coles GA, Williams JD 1989 Pharmacokinetics of recombinant human erythropoietin in patients on continuous ambulatory peritoneal dialysis. Lancet *i:* 425–427

Machin D, Lewith GT, Wylson S 1988 Pain measurement in randomized clinical trials. A comparison of two pain scales. Clin J Pain *4:* 161–168

Rohte O, Jakovljevic V 1974 The potentiation of the antiarrhythmic effects of quinidine sulfate, lidocaine and ajmaline by tween 80. Naunyn Schmiedeberg's. Arch Pharmacol *282* (suppl.), R81

Stephens JM, Auer J, Strong CA, Hughes RT, Oliver DO, Winearls CG, Cotes PM 1991 Stepwise correction of anemia by subcutaneous administration of human recombinant erythropoietin in patients with chronic renal failure maintained by continuous ambulatory peritoneal dialysis. Nephrol Dial Transplant *6:* 487–494

Soehring K, Frahm M, Mletzko K 1952 Beiträge zur Pharmakologie der Alkylpolyaethylenoxydderivate IV: Lokalanalgetische Wirkungen und Bemerkungen zur vergleichenden Auswertung leitungshemmender Substanzen. Arch Int Pharmacodyn *91:* 112–130

Winearls CG, Oliver DO, Pippard MJ, Reid C, Downing MR, Cotes PM 1986 Effect of human erythropoietin derived from recombinant DNA on the anemia of patients maintained by chronic hemodialysis. Lancet *ii:* 1175–1178

Clinical Nephrology, Vol. 36 No. 6 – 1991 (299–301)

Surgical treatment of massive hydrothorax complicating continuous ambulatory peritoneal dialysis

S. M. Allen and H. R. Matthews

Regional Department of Thoracic Surgery, East Birmingham Hospital, Birmingham, UK

Abstract. Acute hydrothorax is a well-recognized complication of continuous ambulatory peritoneal dialysis and is often regarded as a contraindication to its use. We report three cases treated by surgical closure of a communication between the peritoneal and pleural cavities enabling CAPD to continue succesfully. This is a simple, safe and effective procedure which merits wider use as an alternative to transferring the patient to permanent hemodialysis.

Key words: CAPD – hydrothorax – pleural effusion

Introduction

Massive hydrothorax is an infrequent but well-recognized complication of continuous ambulatory peritoneal dialysis (CAPD), and is often regarded as a contra-indication to its use. The ideal management of this complication is unresolved, but reliable techniques need to be developed to prevent recurrence of the hydrothorax as some patients are unsuitable for hemodialysis. In 1984 we reported the first case of surgical closure of a pleuroperitoneal communication following CAPD [Pattison et al. 1984], but since then only one other case has been treated by this approach [Boeschoten et al. 1986]. In this paper we report the seven-year follow-up on our first patient, and two additional cases in which surgical closure was used.

Case 1

A 65-year-old male with end-stage renal failure was started on CAPD in April 1982. After four months he developed a massive right-sided hydrothorax which was treated by right thoracotomy and suture of two small defects in the tendinous part of the hemidiaphragm, the sutures being reinforced by Teflon felt patches (Bard Cardiosurgery Division, Billerica, USA). His recovery was uneventful and peritoneal dialysis was restarted on the sixth post-operative day [Pattison et al. 1984]. In the subsequent seven years there was no recurrence of the hydrothorax and CAPD continued uninterrupted until his death in December 1989.

Reprint requests to Dr. H. R. Matthews, Regional Department of Thoracic Surgery, East Birmingham Hospital, Bordesley Green East, Birmingham B9 5ST, UK.

Case 2

A 51-year-old female with end-stage renal failure due to polycystic kidneys commenced CAPD in September 1987. Within two weeks she developed a large right-sided hydrothorax and peritoneal dialysis was discontinued. Hemodialysis was used until December 1987 when peritoneal dialysis was recommenced, but this resulted in rapid recurrence of the hydrothorax. In January 1988 a right thoracotomy was performed revealing a tiny ruptured blister with a 1 mm hole in the dome of the diaphragm. When dialysate was instilled into the peritoneal cavity via the Tenchkoff catheter there was leakage into the pleural cavity through this hole. The defect was closed by direct suture reinforced by Teflon felt patches, following which there was no leak. Her recovery was uneventful and peritoneal dialysis was restarted on the sixth postoperative day. She returned to work with no recurrence of the hydrothorax on CAPD for over two years until her transfer to hemodialysis because of peritonitis.

Case 3

A 51-year-old female with end-stage renal failure due to chronic glomerulonephritis commenced CAPD in February 1990, but was readmitted four weeks later with a large right-sided hydrothorax. Hemodialysis was started and two weeks later a right thoracotomy was performed revealing a tiny ruptured blister in the dome of the diaphragm. When dialysate was instilled into the peritoneal cavity via the Tenchkoff catheter, a minute hole became apparent under the blister and fluid leaked into the pleural cavity. The defect was closed by direct suture reinforced by Teflon felt patches, following which there was no leak. Her

Table 1 Treatment and outcome of hydrothorax complicating CAPD

Author	Year	Patients	Treatment	CAPD resumed
Kuehnel	1981	1	Conservative	No-HD
Perez Loredo et al.	1981	1	Conservative	No-HD
Leaker et al.	1982	1	Surgical pleurodesis	Yes
Nassberger	1982	1	Conservative	No-HD
Scheldewaert et al.	1982	1	Chemical pleurodesis	Yes (with hydrothorax)
Spadaro et al.	1982	1	Conservative	Yes (with hydrothorax)
Townsend and Fragola	1982	1	Conservative	No-IPD
Grefberg et al.	1983	2	Conservative	Yes 1 (with hydrothorax); No 1-HD
Singh et al.	1983	2	Conservative	Yes 1; No 1-HD
Pattison et al.	1984	1	Surgical repair of diaphragm	Yes
Benz and Schleifer	1985	2	Chemical pleurodesis	Yes 1; No 1-HD
		3	Conservative	No 3-HD
Kennedy	1985	5	Conservative	Yes 2; No 3-HD
Vlachojannis et al.	1985	1	Chemical pleurodesis × 3	Yes
Boeschoten et al.	1986	1	Chemical pleurodesis	No-HD
		1	(Chemical pleurodesis and	No
			Surgical repair of diaphragm)	Yes
		3	Conservative	No 3-HD
Chow et al.	1988	2	Chemical pleurodesis	Yes 2
		1	Conservative	Yes
Nomoto et al.	1989	35	Conservative	Yes 19; No 16-HD
		15	Chemical pleurodesis	Yes 8; No 7-HD

HD – Hemodialysis
IPD – Intermittent peritoneal dialysis

recovery was uneventful, but CAPD could not be restarted for eight weeks because of problems with her Tenchkoff catheter which had to be replaced. She has had no recurrence of the hydrothorax since.

Operation is performed under general anaesthesia, using a double lumen endotracheal tube to allow deflation of the lung. No prophylactic antibiotics are used. With the patient in the appropriate lateral position a limited thoracotomy (25 cm) is made and the pleura opened along the upper border of the eighth rib giving immediate access to the dome of the hemidiaphragm. Fluid in the chest is evacuated and the dome of the diaphragm is dried with swabs. Two to three liters of dialysate are rapidly run into the peritoneal cavity through the catheter and the diaphragm is inspected for seepage through holes or blisters, a process which can take some time as the defects are very small with only a slow rate of flow through them. Sites of leakage are repaired using non-absorbable sutures reinforced with Teflon felt patches, following which dialysate is reintroduced into the peritoneal cavity to ensure there are no additional leaks. The chest is closed with one intercostal drain which is removed on the first postoperative day. Immediately following surgery the patient is extubated and the preoperative fluid regime recommenced.

Discussion

The first case of hydrothorax complicating CAPD was reported in 1981 [Kuenel 1981]. Since then there have been five reviews of the problem [Scheldewaert et al. 1982, Benz and Schleifer 1985, Chow et al. 1988, Abraham et al. 1988, Nomoto et al. 1989], but these have concentrated mainly on the etiology, symptoms and methods of detection rather than treatment.

Cases in which the treatment and its outcome have been stated are listed in Table 1. In 56 patients treatment was conservative, with 26 (46%) eventually resuming CAPD, although three had a persistent hydrothorax. Of the remainder, 29 transferred to hemodialysis and one to intermittent peritoneal dialysis. Twenty-three patients were treated by chemical pleurodesis; 13 (57%) returned to CAPD, one with a persistent hydrothorax, nine transferred to hemodialysis, and one resumed CAPD after surgical repair of the diaphragm. In two patients primary treatment was surgical, one by abrasion pleurodesis and one by repair, and both returned to CAPD.

Conservative management consisted of cessation of CAPD and aspiration or drainage of the hydrothorax with hemodialysis when necessary. Following this CAPD was restarted after one day to four months in the hope that the pleuroperitoneal communication had closed. When hemodialysis was inappropriate intermittent peritoneal dialysis [Townsend and Fragola 1982, Chow et al. 1988, Nomoto et al. 1989] or modified CAPD in the semi-sitting position [Grefberg et al. 1983] was used.

Chemical pleurodesis has been attempted using tetracycline [Benz and Schleifer 1985, Vlachojannis et al. 1985, Boeschoten et al. 1986, Chow et al. 1988, Nomoto et al. 1989], triamcinolon acetonide [Vlachojannis et al. 1985], iodised talc [Scheldewaert et al. 1982, Boeschoten et al. 1986], fibrin glue [Vlachojannis et al. 1985], and autoblood, N-CWS, and OK-342 [Nomoto et al. 1989]. There is no evidence to show the superiority of one of these agents over the others, although it is claimed that fibrin glue may be less painful [Vlachojannis et al. 1985]. A ten-day period between performing pleurodesis and restarting CAPD has been recommended [Chow et al. 1988]. It has also been suggested that pleurodesis should be preceded by thoracoscopy and that if diaphragmatic lesions are seen pleurodesis is likely to be unsuccessful [Scheldewaert et al. 1982]. The theoretical complication of passage of the chemical solution into the abdomen, inducing peritoneal fibrosis with resulting membrane injury, has not occurred. Chemical pleurodesis is a simple and safe procedure, but can be painful [Scheldewaert et al. 1982, Boeschoten et al. 1986] and the results are unpredictable.

An alternative approach is to attempt to close the pleuroperitoneal communication surgically. This was first reported by us in 1984 [Pattison et al. 1984], but since then we know of only one other case that has been treated similarly [Boeschoten et al. 1986]. The follow-up on our first case, and the two additional cases reported here, indicate that this is a simple, reproducible and effective form of therapy. Operation involves only a limited incision and the insertion of one or two diaphragmatic sutures, and does not carry the morbidity and mortality associated with a full thoracotomy and resection of intrathoracic organs. Operative blood loss is minimal, recovery is rapid, and CAPD can be commenced after the sixth day.

On the basis of our patients we believe that pleuroperitoneal communications develop at areas of diaphragmatic weakness which give way as a result of the chronically elevated intra-abdominal pressure caused by CAPD. Once a defect appears, leakage will be further aggravated by the negative intra-thoracic pressure on inspiration. The communications are probably very small, which explains why they are frequently not demonstrated with imaging techniques, thoracoscopy, or post-mortem studies, and can occasionally heal spontaneously.

In conclusion, we would suggest that surgical closure of diaphragmatic communications is a simple, safe and effective procedure which should be considered as one of the treatment options in patients developing this complication of CAPD. In patients in whom hemodialysis is not appropriate it seems reasonable to suggest that initial treatment might be by chemical or fibrin glue pleurodesis, followed by direct surgical repair if this fails.

REFERENCES

Abraham G, Schokker A, Blake P, Oreopoulos DG 1988 Massive hydrothorax in patients on peritoneal dialysis: a literature review. In: *Khanna et al.* (eds). Advances in continuous ambulatory peritoneal dialysis. Peritoneal Dialysis Bulletin Inc, Toronto, p 121

Benz RL, Schleifer CR 1985 Hydrothorax in continuous ambulatory peritoneal dialysis: successful treatment with intrapleural tetracycline and a review of the literature. Am J Kidney Diseases *2:* 136

Boeschoten EW, Krediet RT, Roos CM, Kloek JJ, Schipper MEI, Arisz L 1986 Leakage of dialysate across the diaphragm: an important complication of continuous ambulatory peritoneal dialysis. Neth J Med *29:* 242

Chow CC, Sung JY, Cheung CK, Hamilton-Wood C, Lai KN 1988 Massive hydrothorax in continuous ambulatory peritoneal dialysis. NZ Med J *101:* 475

Grefberg N, Danielson BG, Benson L, Pitkanen P 1983 Right-sided hydrothorax complicating peritoneal dialysis. Report of two cases. Nephron *34:* 130

Kennedy JM 1985 Procedures used to demonstrate a pleuroperitoneal communication: a review. Peritoneal Dial Bull *5:* 168

Kuenel E 1981 Massive pleural effusion secondary to CAPD (Abstract). Kidney Int *19:* 152

Leaker BR, Thom S, Lennox SC, Gabriel R 1982 Management of a massive hydrothorax in a CAPD patient. Peritoneal Dial Bull *2:* 138

Nassberger L 1982 Left-sided pleural effusion secondary to continuous ambulatory peritoneal dialysis. Acta Med Scand *211:* 219

Nomoto Y, Suga T, Nakajima K, Sakai H, Osawa G, Ota K, Kawaguchi Y, Sakai T, Sakai S, Shibata M, Takahashi S 1989 Acute hydrothorax in continuous ambulatory peritoneal dialysis. A collaborative study of 161 centres. Am J Nephrology *9:* 363

Pattison CW, Rodger RSC, Adu D, Michael J, Matthews HR 1984 Surgical treatment of hydrothorax complicating continuous ambulatory peritoneal dialysis. Clinical Nephrology *21:* 191

Perez Loredo J, Cantarovich F, Reichart M, Chena C, Brana D Massive hydrothorax during CAPD (Abstract) 1981 2nd Int Symp Perit Dialysis, Berlin, p 13

Scheldewaert R, Bogaerts Y, Pauwels R, Van Der Straeten M, Ringoir S, Lameire N 1982 Management of a massive hydrothorax in a CAPD patient: A case report and a review of the literature. Peritoneal Dial Bull *2:* 69–72

Singh S, Vaidya P, Dale A, Morgan B 1983 Massive hydrothorax complicating continuous ambulatory peritoneal dialysis. Nephron *34:* 168

Spadaro JJ, Thakur V, Nolph KD 1982 Technetium-99m-labelled macroaggregated albumin in demonstration of transdiaphragmatic leakage of dialysate in peritoneal dialysis. Am J Nephrol *2:* 36

Townsend R, Fragola JA 1982 Hydrothorax in a patient receiving continuous ambulatory peritoneal dialysis – successful treatment with intermittent peritoneal dialysis. Arch Intern Med *142:* 1571

Vlachojannis J, Boettcher I, Brandt L, Schoeppe W 1985 A new treatment for unilateral recurrent hydrothorax during CAPD. Peritoneal Dial Bull *5:* 180

Clinical Nephrology, Vol. 36 No. 6 – 1991 (302–304)

X-ray microanalysis of the fingernails of uremic patients treated by hemodialysis

D. ZEVIN, T. WEINSTEIN, J. LEVI and M. DJALDETTI

Departments of Medicine "B" and Nephrology, Hasharon Hospital, Petah-Tiqva and Tel-Aviv University Medical School, Israel

Abstract. The element content of the fingernails of 16 patients with chronic renal failure (CRF) treated by hemodialysis was examined by dispersive microanalysis. In comparison with matched controls, the results showed a statistically significant decrease in the percentage of Cu, Fe and Zn and an increase in S. The Al content did not differ significantly from that of the controls. There was no correlation between the serum values of Al, Fe and Zn and their content in the fingernails of the patients. On the other hand, Cu was found to be low both in the sera and in the fingernails of the CRF patients.

Key words: chronic renal failure – element content of fingernails – X-ray microanalysis – hemodialysis

Introduction

It has been shown by various methods that fingernails of healthy subjects contain a large number of elements [Vellar 1970, Harrison and Tyree 1971, Goldblum et al. 1953]. Previous studies in our laboratory have demonstrated that examination of the element content of fingernails by X-ray dispersive microanalysis may serve as a useful tool for the detection of abnormal values of the elements in some diseases, such as liver cirrhosis [Djaldetti et al. 1987] and iron deficiency anemia [Djaldetti et al. 1987]. Trace elements may play an important role in pathological conditions. Thus, aluminum has been shown to be the causative factor in a few dialysis-related diseases [Wills and Savory 1983], but since the Al level in dialysis patients is usually higher than that of normal subjects [McCarthy et al. 1986], the interpretation of its values is difficult. It has been suggested that atomic absorption spectrophotometry, which is the method of choice for the determination of metals in relatively high concentration in man, is not sufficiently sensitive for detection of trace elements [De Wolf 1985]. Therefore, the possibility to detect them in a readily obtained material, such as the fingernails, by X-ray microanalysis, seems rather attractive.

It was the purpose of the present study to examine the element content of the fingernails of patients with chronic renal failure (CRF), and to evaluate the possibility that fingernails may serve as a source for trace-element determination. In addition, an attempt was made to find a correlation between the serum and fingernails levels of trace elements in these patients.

Received November 15, 1990; in revised form May 28, 1990.

Reprint requests to Dr. M. Djaldetti, Department of Medicine "B", Hasharon Hospital, P.O. Box 121, Petah-Tiqva 49372, Israel

Materials and methods

Patients

Sixteen patients (5 females and 11 males) with end-stage CRF were examined. Their age ranged between 25 and 74 years and all of them were treated by hemodialysis for 2 to 11 years. All patients were dialysed for 12 hours/week, dialysate calcium level of 3.25 meq/l. The dialysate water supply was treated with reverse osmosis. Except for symptoms and signs compatible with CRF none of the patients had evidence of encephalopathy or osteomalacia. All patients were supplemented with calcium and 1α Hydroxy-vitamin D_3, 0.25–1 mcg. The nails of 15 healthy subjects, matched for sex and age, served as controls.

Preparation of the nails

The patients and healthy controls were instructed to wash their hands thoroughly with soap and tap water and thereafter to rinse their hands for a few minutes with tap water. After drying the hands, the nail of the third finger was clipped using stainless scisors and prepared for X-ray analysis.

X-ray microanalysis

The clipped nails were fixed on aluminum stubs coated with carbon-conductive cement (Leit-C, Neubauer, Germany) with their convex side up. After sputter-coating with carbon, they were examined at an acceleration voltage of 15 kV in a Philips 500 PSEM

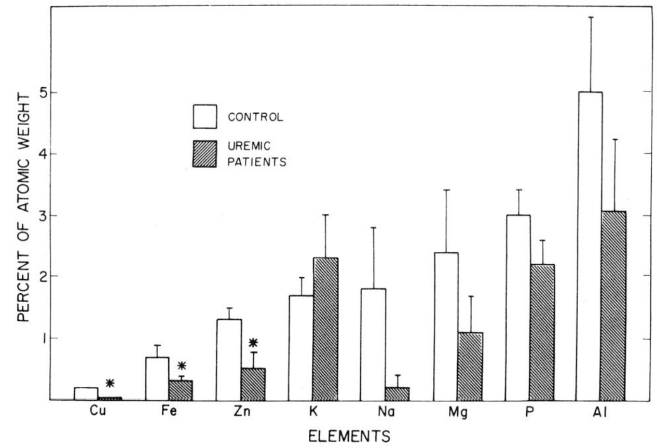

Fig. 1 Percent of atomic weight of the elements Cu, Fe, Zn, K, Na, Mg, P and Al in the nails of uremic and healthy subjects. The asterisks indicate statistically significant difference

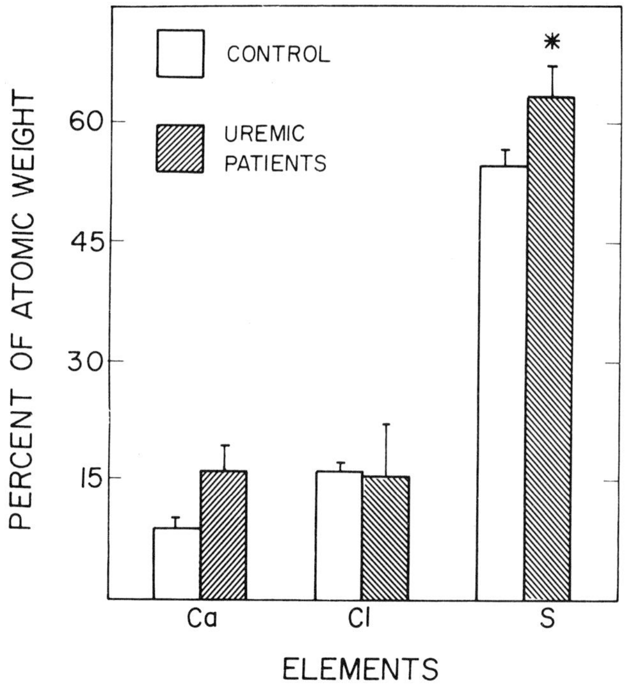

Fig. 2 Percent of atomic weight of the elements Ca, Cl and S in the nails of uremic and healthy subjects. The asterisk indicates a statistically significant difference

scanning electron microscope supplemented with a Si(Li) X-ray detector (EDAX Int., USA). The elements detected were: Na, Mg, Al, P, S, Cl, K, Ca, Co, Fe, Cu and Zn. The following conditions were applied: specimen to detector distance was 56 mm, the take-off angle −15°, five fields from each nail were analyzed by scanning an area of 134 cm^2 at a magnification of 640, until a full scale of 1000 counts per field was achieved. X-ray pulse-height distribution was measured in the energy range of 0–20 kV with a

Table 1 Serum and fingernail Al, ferritin and Fe, Zn and Cu values in uremic patients and controls (mean ± SE)

Elements	Serum Patients	Serum Controls (range)	Fingernails* Patients	Fingernails* Controls
Al, μg%	8.8 ± 0.9	0–1.5	3.1 ± 1.2	5.0 ± 1.2
Ferritin, ng/ml	436 ± 172	15–200	–	–
Fe	–	–	0.3 ± 0.1	0.7 ± 0.2
Cu, μg%	72 ± 9.4	75–155	0.03 ± 0	0.2 ± 0
Zn, μg%	96 ± 8.0	75–130	0.5 ± 0.3	1.3 ± 0.2

* Percent of atomic weight of the examined elements

resolution of 10 eV/channel. Semiquantitative calculation of element concentration was carried out using a PV 9100 analytical system (EDAX), applying a ZAF correction. The values of the K ratios for each element were expressed as the percent of the total weight of the examined elements.

Serum ferritin was detected by immunoassay, using a kit for monoclonal antibodies (Thandem, Hybritech – Belgium). Serum Al, Zn and Cu were examined by the method of atomic absorption spectrophotometry.

Statistical analysis was carried out by using the Student's t-test.

Results

Figures 1 and 2 show the results of the atomic weight percentage of the elements in the nails of uremic and healthy subjects. Except for Co, all elements examined in the study were present. Statistical analysis showed that the difference in the atomic weight of Fe, Cu, Zn and S in the nails of control and uremic subjects were significant ($p < 0.05–0.005$). The serum and fingernail Al, ferritin, Cu and Zn levels are given in Table 1. While in the sera Al and ferritin levels were markedly increased in comparison with the control values in our laboratory, the Cu was below and the Zn was within the normal range.

Discussion

The present results show that the X-ray microanalysis may serve as an useful tool for the examination of the element content in the fingernails. This method has a few advantages – it is a rather simple procedure, the material does not have to undergo intricate preparations, it permits concomitant detection of a rather large number of elements and the fingernails which are easily obtained may be repeatedly examined. However, some precautions must be observed. The nails should be clean, to avoid external contamination, the geography of the nail in the microscope is important and it is imperative to be kept with its convex side up, to avoid self-absorption of the X-rays by the rough internal surface of the nail. The results of the element content detection in nails are not related with their rate of growth. Nevertheless, even after a thorough search in the literature, we could not find reports indicating differences between the rate of growth of normal and uremic nails.

The present observations showed a statistically significant decrease in Zn, Cu and Fe in the fingernails of CRF patients in comparison with the controls. Abnormalities of Zn metabolism have been reported in CRF patients and have been even implicated as a causative factor in their sexual dysfunction [Mahajan et al. 1984]. Determination of Zn concentrations in plasma, hair and leukocytes in dialyzed and nondialyzed uremic patients showed subnormal values [Mahajan et al. 1979]. It is of interest that the serum Zn level in our patients was within the normal range, a finding which may suggest a preferential distribution of this element in the tissues. On the other hand, the Cu level was low both in the serum and in the fingernails of CRF patients.

The determination of Fe showed controversial results. While the serum ferritin in CRF patients was markedly increased, most probably due to repeated blood transfusions, their Fe content in fingernails was low. This finding again suggests that there is no correlation between serum and fingernail iron, as it has been shown in a previous study from our laboratory [Djaldetti et al. 1987].

Aluminum has been shown to accumulate in the brain of CRF patients treated by hemodialysis for at least one year. It has been implied as the cause of dialysis encephalopathy [Elliot and Mac Dongall 1978, Alfrey et al. 1972], as well as of osteomalacic fractures [Ward et al. 1978, Pierides et al. 1980, Prior et al. 1982] and microcytic anemia. However, there are studies which raise some doubt about the aluminum being the only factor implicated in the pathogenesis of dialysis encephalopathy associated with osteomalacic pathologic fractures [Pierides et al. 1980]. Since aluminum has been shown to accumulate in other organs, such as liver, heart, lung and joints [Pierides et al. 1980], the question was raised whether this element may accumulate in the fingernails of CRF patients treated by hemodialysis. The results of the present study (Table 1) show that similarly to Fe, there is no correlation between serum and fingernail level.

We do not have an explanation for the statistically increased Cu content in the nails of CRF patients.

The present results indicate that the Ca treatment given to the uremic patients did not affect the Ca contents of their fingernails.

REFERENCES

Alfrey AC, Mishell JM, Burks J, Contiguglia SR, Rudolf H, Lewin E, Holmes JH 1972 Syndrome of dyspraxia and multifocal seizures associated with chronic hemodialysis. Trans Am Soc Artif Intern Organs *18:* 257–261

De Wolf FA 1985 Toxicological aspects of aluminium poisoning in clinical nephrology. Clin Nephrol 24 *(Suppl 1):* S9–S14

Djaldetti M, Fishman P, Harpaz D, Lurie B 1987 X-ray microanalysis of the fingernails in cirrhotic patients. Dermatologica *174:* 114–116

Djaldetti M, Fishman P, Hart J 1987 The iron content of fingernails in iron deficient patients. Clin Sci *72:* 669–672

Elliot HL, Mac Dongall AI 1978 Aluminium studies in dialysis encephalopathy. Proc Eur Dial Transplant Assoc *15:* 157–163

Goldblum RW, Derby S, Lerner AB 1953 The metal content of skin, nails and hair. J Invest Derm *20:* 13–18

Harrison WW, Tyree AB 1971 The determination of trace elements in fingernails by atomic absorption spectroscopy. Clin Chim Acta *31:* 63–73

Mahajan SK, Prasad AS, McDonald FD 1984 Sexual dysfunction in uremic male: Improvement following oral zinc supplementation. Contrib Nephrol *38:* 103–111

Mahajan SK, Prasad AS, Rabbani P, Briggs WA, McDonald FD 1979 Zinc metabolism in uremia. J Lab Clin Med *94:* 693–698

McCarthy JT, Milliner DS, Kurtz SB, Johnson WJ, Moyer TP 1986 Interpretation of serum aluminium values in dialysis patients. J Clin Pathol *86:* 629–636

O'Hare JA, Murnaghan DJ 1982 Reversal of aluminum-induced hemodialysis anemia by a low-aluminum dialysate. N Eng J Med *306:* 654–656

Pierides AM, Eduards WG Jr, Cullum UX Jr, McGall JT, Ellis HA 1980 Haemodialysis encephalopathy with osteomalacic fractures and muscle weakness. Kidney Int *18:* 115–124

Prior JC, Cameron EC, Knickerbocker WJ, Sweeney V, Suchowersky O 1982 Dialysis encephalopathy and osteomalacic bone disease. A case controlled study. Am J Med *72:* 33–42

Vellar OD 1978 Composition of human nail substance. Am J Clin Nutr *23:* 1272–1274

Ward MK, Feest TG, Ellis HA, Parkinson IS, Kerr DNS 1978 Osteomalacic dialysis osteodystrophy: evidence for a waterborne aetiological agent, probably aluminium. Lancet *1:* 841–845

Wills MR, Savory J 1983 Aluminium poisoning: dialysis encephalopathy, osteomalacia and anaemia. Lancet *2:* 29–34

LETTERS TO THE EDITOR

Two cases with mild spontaneous peripelvic extravasation

Dear Sir, – It has been reported that spontaneous peripelvic extravasation (SPE) can be diagnosed by the appearance of contrast medium outside the collecting system of the kidney, either intrarenally or extrarenally, in the retroperitoneal tissue, following intravenous urography [Hinman 1961, Schwartz et al. 1966, Khan and Malek 1976]. We experienced two cases with SPE which we were unable to diagnose by intravenous urography.

Case 1

A 50-year-old male was admitted to our hospital on October 16, 1990, because of severe colicky pain in the left lower abdomen and left flank. The abdomen was soft and flat with spontaneous pain and tenderness from the left lower abdomen to left flank. Urinalysis yielded the following findings: protein, (−); occult, (+); sugar, (−); red blood cells (RBC), 10–15/HF; and white blood cells (WBC), 0–1/WF. A plain film of the abdomen demonstrated left ureteral calculus, and intravenous urography revealed slight enlargement of the left kidney and slight dilatation of the left pelvis, calices and ureter without extravasation of contrast medium. Moreover, renal ultrasonography (US) (Figure 1) and computerized tomography (CT) demonstrated fluid collection around the left kidney and left renal cyst. Use of US every day indicated that the fluid collection disappeared at 3 days after admission in a condition of rest (Figure 2). There was little chance that the fluid collection was due to rupture of the renal cyst, since the shape of the cyst was maintained. The calculus was excreted on October 22, 1990, and the patient was discharged.

Case 2

A 47-year-old male was admitted to our hospital on February 19, 1991, because of severe colicky pain in the right abdomen and right flank. The abdomen was soft and flat with spontaneous pain and tenderness from the right lower abdomen to right flank. Urinalysis yielded the following findings: protein, (−); occult, (3+); sugar, (−); RBC, numerous/HF; and WBC, 1–2/HF. A plain film of the abdomen demonstrated right ureteral calculus, and intravenous urography revealed slight enlargement of the right kidney and slight dilatation of the right pelvis, calices and ureter without extravasation of contrast medium. In addition, US demonstrated fluid collection around the right kidney (Figure 3, left side). However, CT failed to show any clear fluid collection. Use of US indicated that the fluid collection disappeared on the next day in a condition of rest (Figure 3, right side). The calculus was excreted on February 21, 1991, and the patient was discharged.

Although SPE is a disease in which contrast medium appears outside the collecting system during intravenous urography, the present two cases of SPE could not be diagnosed by intravenous urography, but only by US or CT. It is suggested therefore that the condition of mild SPE cannot be diagnosed by intravenous urography. Furthermore, the milder SPE could be diagnosed only by US

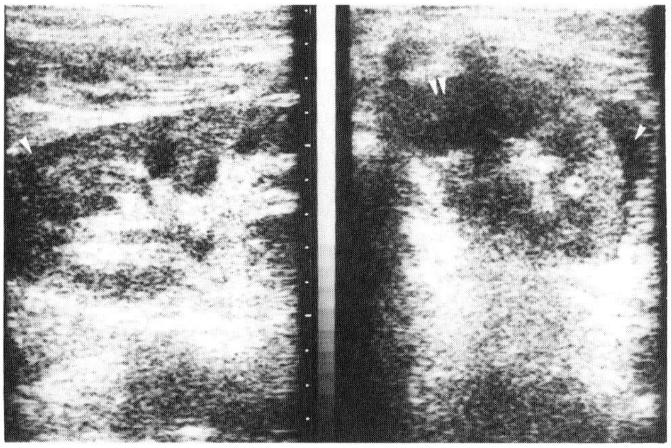

Fig. 1 Renal ultrasonography on admission in Case 1 (left side, sagittal scan; right side, transverse scan). Fluid collection around the left kidney (▽) and renal cyst (▽▽) can be seen.

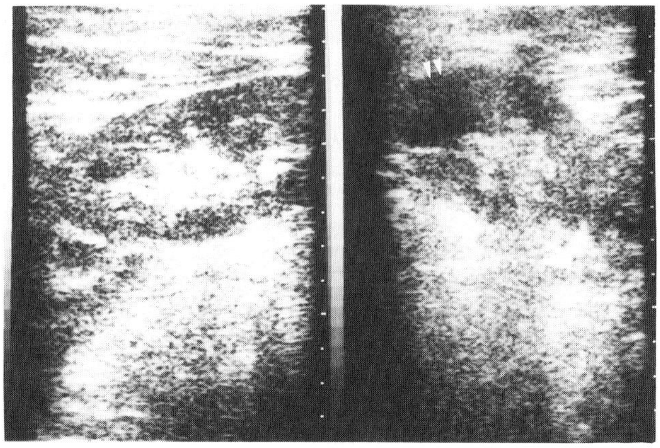

Fig. 2 Ultrasonography at 3 days after admission in Case 1 (left side, sagittal scan; right side, transverse scan). The fluid collection observed previously has disappeared.

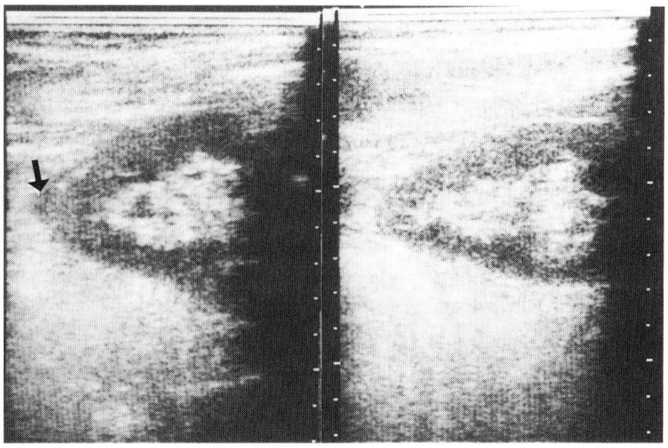

Fig. 3 Ultrasonography (sagittal scans) in Case 2. Left side, on admission; fluid collection can be seen (arrow). Right side, on the next day; the fluid collection has disappeared.

and not by CT, suggesting that US is the most effective means of diagnosing mild SPE. Since severe abdominal pain was recognized in both cases, it is recommended that US is positively performed to diagnose mild SPE in cases with ureteral obstruction, especially those experiencing severe abdominal pain, even if extravasation of contrast medium is not demonstrated during intravenous urography. Although it has been reported that the appearance rate of SPE is rare [Cooke and Bartucz, 1974], there is a clear possibility that its incidence will increase if mild SPE can be diagnosed by using US.

K. Okada, S. Takahashi, Y. Nagura, M. Hatano
2nd Department of Internal Medicine, Nihon University School of Medicine, Tokyo, Japan

REFERENCES

Cooke GM, Bartucz JP 1974 Spontaneous extravasation of contrast medium during intravenous urography. Clin Radiol *25:* 87–93

Hinman F 1961 Peripelvic extravasation during intravenous urography: Evidence for an additional route for backflow after ureteral obstruction. J Urol *85:* 385–395

Khan AU, Malek RS 1976 Spontaneous urinary extravasation. J Urol *116:* 161–165

Schwartz A, Caine M, Hermann G, Bittermann W 1966 Spontaneous renal extravasation during intravenous urography. Am J Roentgenol *98:* 27–40

Aztreonam for renal graft pyelonephritis

Sir, – Aztreonam is an antibiotic of the monobactam group that chemically differs from penicillins and cephalosporins [Brogden and Heel 1986]. It is only active against gram-negative organisms. Aztreonam is an accepted therapy of severe urinary tract infections [Henry and Bendush 1986]. We have made a small controlled trial of aztreonam versus penicillin for treatment of graft-pyelonephritis in renal allotransplanted patients.

Nine patients, 7 women and 2 men, age 20 to 61 years, entered the study. All had functioning renal allotransplants. Six of them had urinary tract infections before the present episode, in three cases as graft-pyelonephritis, shown by fever, tenderness of the graft, bacteriuria, pyuria, and slightly impaired graft function; in the other three as cystitis with dysuria, bacteriuria and pyuria. Gram-negative bacteria had been found in urine culture at previous episodes, mainly *Escherichia coli* and *Proteus* species. Patients with earlier urinary infections with gram-positive organisms were excluded.

Seven of the patients were treated with prednisone 5 to 30 mg daily. Six received azathioprin 100 mg daily, the other three cyclosporine in doses adjusted to plasma levels about 300–500 ng/ml. Four received betablockers for hypertension, three of them also furosemid. Insulin because of diabetes, digoxin for cardiac failure and 1α $OH\text{-}D_3$ because of renal osteodystrophia were administered in one case each. The renal allograft function was slightly reduced with creatinine clearances from 20 to 60 ml in 8 of the patients. The last patients had creatinine clearance values about 10 ml/min secondary to chronic rejection. Aztreonam was given as one gram two to three times intravenously in the first 24 hours, followed by 1 g intramuscularly two times daily for 5 to 7 days. The initial treatment was reinforced with an aminoglycoside (Netilmycin®) after 36 to 48 hours, if there were no apparent effects from the initial treatment. The patient's next urinary infection was treated with ampicillin 1 g × 4. One patient received a cephalosporine instead because of suspicion of allergy to penicillin.

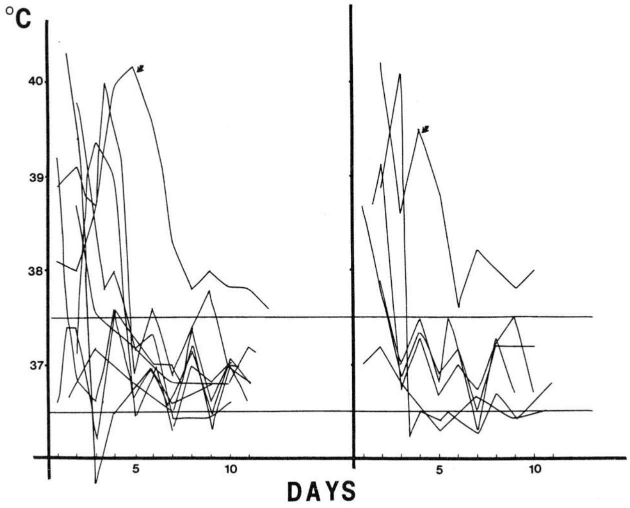

Fig. 1 Course of temperature in 9 (left) and 6 (right) patients with renal allograft-pyelonephritis treated with aztreonam (left) or ampicillin (right). Arrows point out two patients where supplementation with an aminoglycoside was done.

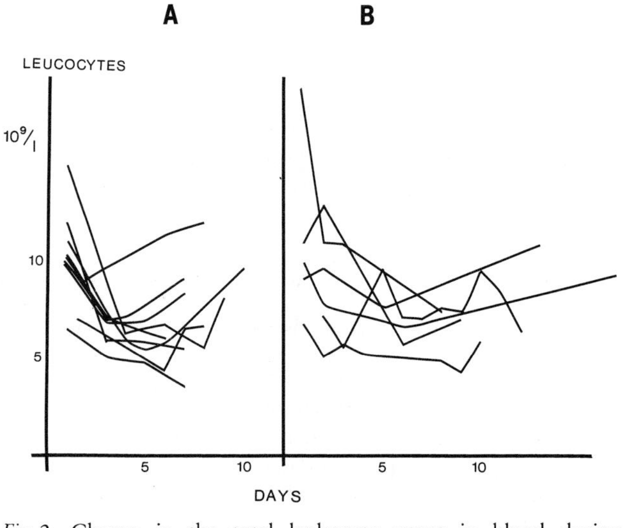

Fig. 2 Change in the total leukocyte count in blood during treatment of graft-pyelonephritis with aztreonam (A) or ampicillin (B).

Patient nine entered the aztreonam group and six the ampicilline group, thus three patients had only one episode. All patients were free of symptoms including fever within the first 24 to 48 hours of treatment. However, one from each group had to be supplied with an aminoglycoside because of delayed clinical response. Figure 1 shows the course of the temperature in the two groups. The fall of temperature in the two patients receiving aminoglycoside as supplement followed so shortly after the supplementation that the initial treatment might have been sufficient. However, the clinical situation called for an aggressive therapy.

Figure 2 shows the number of leukocytes in peripheral blood during treatment. The steep initial fall after initiation of the treatment was followed by a slight rise to count rates within the normal range. This tendency to a biphasic curve was seen in both groups. Differential counts revealed that the responding cells were granulocytes. Serum creatinine fell slightly and creatinine-clearance improved during treatment.

The bacteria isolated before treatment were all gram-negative with *E. coli* as the most frequent organism (10 cases, *C. freundii:* 1, *P. vulgaris:* 2, *E. aerogenes:* 1). All organisms were susceptible to aztreonam and ampicillin. The urine was sterile in 6 of the patients after treatment, while *E. coli* (one case) and *S. faecalis* (two cases) were found in the other. None of these patients had symptoms. Only one patient in the whole material remained free of bacteria at the follow-up 1 to 2 months later, but all were asymptomatic at that time. Later three of them had recurrent infection. It shows how difficult it is to clear urine infections in immunosuppressed patients.

The treatment caused no side effects. Some studies have shown an increase in the liver-associated enzymes in aztreonam-treated patients. It was not the case in the present group of patients treated with other hepatotoxic drugs. The results show that aztreonam represents an alternative to broad-spectrum penicillin also in immunosuppressed patients.

J. Ladefoged,
Rigshospitalet, Medical Department P, Copenhagen, Denmark

REFERENCES

Brogden RN, Heel RC 1986 Aztreonam. Drugs *31:* 96

Henry SA, Bendush CB 1985 Aztreonam. Worldwide overview of the treatment of patients with gram-negative infections. Amer J Med *78:* (2 A): 57

Sputum-positive lung tuberculosis after instillation of BCG for bladder cancer

Sir, – Instillation of a Bacillus *Calmette-Guérin* (BCG) strain into the bladder is an effective therapy for superficial bladder cancer [Kowalkowski et al. 1988]. In addition to well-known complications [Lamm et al. 1989] we wish to report the following experience after BCG-immunotherapy.

A 59-year-old patient with end-stage renal failure in analgesic-associated nephropathy had been dialyzed for five years. After diagnosis and transurethral resection of a bladder cancer ($T_aN_0M_0$) in 1989 instillation of 150 mg (French) Pasteur BCG was performed as prophylaxis, initially in weekly, later in monthly intervals.

In summer 1990, after a total of eleven instillations, high fever after treatment occurred. The patient becoming hospitalized because of weight loss, nocturnal sweat, malaise and high elevation of acute-phase-protein (CRP), tuberculosis was suspected as one differential diagnosis. The reaction to Mendel-Mantoux testing was anergic, the chest X-ray showed discrete unspecific interstitial markings and in microscopic examination of sputum acid-fast rods were not demonstrable. In multiple sputum cultures, however, Mycobacterium of the BCG strain was identified (Forschungsinstitut Borstel, Germany), being resistant to cycloserine and pyrazinamide and sensitive to all other common antituberculosis agents. Under three-fold therapy with isoniazide, rifampicine, myambutol and in addition ofloxacine clinical and laboratory signs of infection disappeared.

Two months later he suffered from rapidly progressive chronic ischemia of the lower extremities due to atherosclerosis. Unfortunately, not coping with the threat of ablative surgery, the patient committed suicide. In necropsy (Prof. Jansen, Pathological Institute of the Städtische Kliniken Darmstadt, Germany) no residuals of the bladder carcinoma or of tuberculosis were found. Interestingly signs of generalized necrotizing angiitis could be demonstrated, whereas the significance of this fact concerning BCG-itis is not understood.

BCG-induced pneumonitis being a rare, but known complication of BCG-instillation, this is to our knowledge the first case of sputum-positive lung tuberculosis caused by the BCG strain after intravesical application being reported.

D. Höffler, R. Niemeyer, G. Strack, M. Zieschang

Med. Klin. III (Nephrology), Städtische Kliniken Darmstadt, W-6100 Darmstadt, Germany

REFERENCES

Kowalkowski TS, Lamm DL 1988 Intravesical Therapy of Superficial Bladder Cancer. Current Trends in Urology *4:* 89–107

Lamm DL, Steg A, Boccon-Gibod L, Morales A, Hanna MG, Pagano F, Alfthan O, Brosman S, Fisher HAF, Jakse G, Chisolm GD, van der Meijden APM, Debruyne FMJ 1989 Complications of Bacillus *Calmette-Guérin* Immunotherapy: Review of 2602 Patients and Comparison of Chemotherapy Complications. Prog Clin Biol Res *310:* 335–355

LETTERS TO THE EDITOR

Dietary fibre and renal failure: a comparison of sorbent properties

Dear Sir, – Dietary fibre can lower urea and creatinine in chronic renal failure [Parillo et al. 1984], operating by two mechanisms: ispaghula, is degraded in the large bowel [Prynne and Southgate 1979], reducing colonic bacterial ammonia production [Rampton et al. 1984]. Secondly locust bean gum [Yatzides et al. 1979, 1980; Yatzides 1978] and oxystarch [Giordano et al. 1979] have sorbent properties. However, a comparison of the in vitro sorbent properties of other available types of dietary fibre has not been made, limiting the rational choice as to which fibre is likely to be most beneficial clinically. We have thus analyzed the in vitro sorbent effect of currently available types of dietary fibre.

A standard solution was made to approximate the urea and electrolyte concentrations of intestinal fluid of uremic patients [Yatzides et al. 1979]. For each determination a solution of 0.6 g of fibre in 30 ml of standard solution (i.e. 2 g in 100 ml) was made up in a small universal container. This was shaken, put on a rotary mixer (five revolutions per minute) at 37 degrees centigrade for 15 hours. A subsequent ultrafiltration process (Amicon) used a polysulphane membrane (Millipore), which filtered only molecules less than m.w. 10,000. The constituents of the ultrafiltrate were compared to the original standard solution to assess the amount absorbed by the fibre. The filter was moistened with distilled water to maintain constant properties: the small resulting dilution error (average 3.5% estimated from ten readings with blank standard solution) was used to correct the results, and was made constant by collecting a constant volume of ultrafiltrate into a closed 2 ml container. There were no changes in sodium or urea in the ultrafiltrate. Methylcellulose showed no change in any component of the standard solution. For the other fibres and the change in ultrafiltrate constituents see Table 1. Most of the fibres (except oxystarch) caused an increase in potassium and calcium, and ispaghula a large increase in phosphate. Sterculia showed a moderate absorption and oxystarch a very significant absorption of ammonia.

Table 1 Change in ultrafiltrate after incubation with fibre. An average of at least three determinations is quoted (if more than three determinations, figure in brackets = number of determinations used).

	Potassium	Calcium	Phosphate	Ammonia
Locust bean gum (4)	+1.9	+0.3	0	− 0.7
Ispaghula	+2.4	+0.9	+2.7	− 3.1
Sterculia (5)	+2.6	+2.5	−0.2	− 7.4
Oxystarch (5)	+0.1	+0.1	−0.1	−20.3
Bran	+0.6	+0.2	+0.2	− 1.3

These findings do not support the observations regarding the absorptive properties of locust bean gum [Yatzides 1978, Yatzides et al. 1979]. The method used in this study is very similar (i.e. ultrafiltration through a membrane with filtre size m.w. 10,000) although a small dilutional error in this study might obscure small effects. A possible factor may be the physical state of the gum, although the samples used in this study and the above studies were from the same supplier (Sigma Chemicals). Further work using the methods of Rampton et al. [1984] might clarify this issue.

This study supports the observation of the impressive properties of oxystarch as a sorbent of ammonia [Giordano et al. 1979], although little urea appears to be bound. The gel formulation used in the above study was reported to be more effective than the powder suspension used by us. Of the other fibres none showed any absorptive properties except sterculia showing a moderate effect with ammonia. Sterculia also had the advantage over ispaghula in causing a significant increase in calcium, and no change in phosphate. Since sterculia is available commerically for patients (whereas unfortunately oxystarch has not been marketed), clinical trials using sterculia in comparison to ispaghula, which has already been demonstrated to be effective in renal failure, would be indicated on the basis of this data.

P. Little, Lord Trafford
Renal Unit, Royal Sussex County Hospital, Eastern rd, Brighton, East Sussex, England, UK

REFERENCES

Giordano C, Esposito R, Leo BA, Pluvio M 1979 Oxycellulose as oral sorbent in ureamia. Clinical Nephrology *11(3):* 142–144

Parillo M, Perotti N, Iovine C, Pacioni D, Rivellese A, Riccardi G, Mancini M 1984 High fibre diets for the treatment of diabetic patients with chronic renal failure. Minerva Endocrinologica *9:* 317–319

Prynne CJ, Southgate DAT 1979 The effects of a supplement of dietary fibre on faecal excretion by human subjects. Br J Nutr *41:* 495

Rampton DS, Cohen SL, Crammond V de B, Gibbons J, Kilburn MF, Rabet JY, Vince AJ, Wager JD, Wrong OM 1984 Treatment of chronic renal failure with dietary fibre. Clinical Nephrology *21(3):* 159–163

Yatzides H 1978 Preliminary studies with locust bean gum. 2nd Conference on Uraemia. Formulations and Expectations, Capri, May 31 – Sept 2, 1977. Kidney Int *13 (Suppl 8):* 152

Yatzides H, Koutsicos P, Digenis P 1979 Newer oral sorbent in uraemia. Clinical Nephrology *11(2):* 105–106

Yatzides H, Koutsicos P, Digenis P 1980 Oral locust bean gum therapy of uraemia; favourable effects on biological abnormalities and hypertension. Dialysis and Transplantation *9(4):* 313–317

LETTERS TO THE EDITOR

Dietary fibre and renal failure: comparison of sterculia and ispaghula

Dear Sir, – Dietary fibre can be beneficial in renal failure, either by reducing colonic bacterial ammonia production, e. g. ispaghula, [Rampton et al. 1984], or possibly acting as a sorbent, e. g. locust bean gum [Yatzides et al. 1979, 1980; Yatzides 1978] and oxystarch [Giordano et al. 1979]. Only sterculia and oxystarch have significant absorption of ammonia in vitro [Little and Trafford in press] and only sterculia is marketed for clinical use.

However, fibres with sorbent properties have not been compared to ispaghula for clinical efficacy. In addition it is not clear if dietary fibre is beneficial in those patients on dialysis. This study thus compared the effect of sterculia and ispaghula in patients on hemodialysis for end-stage renal failure.

Nineteen patients (mean age 52, 15 male/4 female) took two 7 g sachets of Normacol (Norgine) i. e. 8.7 g of sterculia/day for two weeks. After one week break patients took 8.7 g ispaghula for two weeks: one sachet/day Metamucil (Searle), and one and a half sachets/day Fybogel (Reckitt and Coleman). Only fifteen patients (mean age 52, 12 male/3 female) took ispaghula (four found it unpalatable, felt unwell, or had diarrhea). Blood was taken for urea, electrolytes, creatinine, calcium, phosphate, and liver function tests before and after each fibre phase on the same day of the dialysis schedule. Results were analyzed using Student's t-test. There were no significant changes in sodium, creatinine, calcium and liver function tests. Table 1 shows the changes in urea, potassium, and phosphate in both phases of the study. There were no significant changes after taking ispaghula for two weeks. Sterculia caused a small but significant fall in urea ($p < 0.05$) and a relatively larger and highly significant fall in potassium ($p < 0.005$), in addition to a fall in inorganic phosphate. All of these changes were significantly different to ispaghula ($p < 0.05$). Although the change in urea with sterculia is statistically significant, the small change is not clinically significant for patients taking regular hemodialysis. Sterculia is preferable to ispaghula from the data in this study given the fall in potassium and phosphate, both of which were significantly different to ispaghula. The mechanism for the reduction in potassium is unclear, since both sterculia and ispaghula show no sorbent properties for potassium, although the differences in phosphate can be predicted from the phosphate content and in vitro properties of sterculia and ispaghula [Little and Trafford in press]. Perhaps shortening the large bowel transit time reduces the time available for electrolyte absorption. Another factor may be changes in patients' food intake, possibly through appetite, since some patients noticed abdominal distension and a sense of fullness with both ispaghula and sterculia: this effect was minimized by asking the patients to take the fibre after meals. The only way to make sure that dietary variation does not influence or mediate the observed changes is by giving patients weighed dietary constituents in a metabolic ward.

Table 1 Potassium, urea, and phosphate before and after 8.7 g/day sterculia for two weeks, and 8.7 g/day ispaghula for two weeks (S. E. M. in brackets)

	Potassium	Urea	Phosphate
Sterculia (n = 19)			
Initial	5.5 (0.2)	30.4 (0.9)	2.16 (0.15)
2 weeks	4.9 (0.2)**	28.7 (1.1)*	2.03 (0.13)
Ispaghula (n = 15)			
Initial	5.2 (0.2)	28.2 (0.7)	1.89 (0.13)
2 weeks	5.2 (0.2)	28.8 (1.7)	2.02 (0.14)

* = $p < 0.05$, ** = $p < 0.005$

We conclude that sterculia is preferable to ispaghula in patients with end-stage renal failure. Worthwhile changes in potassium, phosphate, and to a lesser extent in urea occur in patients on dialysis. Given the efficacy of ispaghula in preventing a rise in urea and creatinine in patients not on dialysis [Rampton et al. 1984] and the superiority of sterculia to ispaghula in this study, sterculia is likely to be most beneficial in those patients not yet on dialysis, or possibly in reducing the frequency and duration of dialysis.

P. Little, Lord Trafford
Renal Unit, Royal Sussex County Hospital, Eastern rd, Brighton, East Sussex, England, UK

REFERENCES

Giordano C, Esposito R, Leo BA, Pluvio M 1979 Oxycellulose as oral sorbent in ureamia. Clinical Nephrology *11(3):* 142–144

Little PS, Trafford A 1990 Dietary fibre and renal failure: the in vitro sorbent properties of commercially available dietary fibres (in press)

Rampton DS, Cohen SL, Crammond V de B, Gibbons J, Kilburn MF, Rabet JY, Vince AJ, Wager JD, Wrong OM 1984 Treatment of chronic renal failure with dietary fibre. Clinical Nephrology *21(3):* 159–163

Yatzides H 1978 Preliminary studies with locust bean gum, a new sorbent with great potential. 2nd Conference on Uraemia. Formulations and Expections. Capri, May 31 – Sept 2, 1977. Kidney Int *13 (Suppl 8):* 152

Yatzides H, Koutsicos P, Digenis P 1979 Newer oral sorbent in uraemia. Clinical Nephrology *11(2):* 105–106

Yatzides H, Koutsicos P, Digenis P 1980 Oral locust bean gum therapy of uraemia; favourable effects on biological abnormalities and hypertension. Dialysis and Transplantation *9(4):* 313–317

ANNOUNCEMENTS

The **36th Annual Convention of the American Institute of Ultrasound in Medicine** (AIUM) will be held March 8–11, 1992 in San Diego, California.

For more information contact the AIUM Convention Department, 11200 Rockville Pike, Suite 205, Rockville, MD 20852-3139. Tel.: (301) 881-2486. Fax: (301) 881-7303.

The **International Meeting on Molecular Approaches to Nephrology Prospect in Diagnosis and Management** will take place on March 19–21, 1992 in Bari, Italy.

For further information please contact Prof. F. P. Schena, Chair and Division of Nephrology, Polyclinic, I-70124 Bari, Tel.: 39/80/271237 or 271232.

The **Fifth European Meeting on Renal Diseases** will be held on April 2–4, 1992 in Milan.

For information contact the Organizing Secretariat, O. I. C. Incentive, Viale Majno, 21, I-20122 Milano, Italy. Tel.: (2) 7600 8190. Fax: (2) 782400.

Invitation for submissions for the **NILS-ALWALL-PRIZE 1992.** The Deutsche Arbeitsgemeinschaft für Klinische Nephrologie e.V. awards this prize to young scientists engaged in clinical research in German speaking countries. The subject from the field of nephrology should treat problems in dialysis or similar methods of extracorporeal elimination or kidney transplants. The award comprises the Nils-Alwall Medal, a certificate and DM 15000,–. Candidates should not be older than 45 and should submit non published works or those published one year before submission or summaries of original research with the exception of academic theses. Six copies of the paper together with a short curriculum vitae including present professional status should be sent not later than April 15, 1992 to the following address: Prof. Dr. G. A. Jutzler, Am Brunnen 2, W-6650 Homburg/Saar, Germany.

The **IIIrd International Conference on SLE** will be held in the Queen Elizabeth II Conference Centre, Westminster, London, April 13–15, 1992.

For further details, please contact Dr. Graham Hughes or Mrs. Denzil Fletcher, Rheumatology Department, St. Thomas' Hospital, London SE1 7EH. Tel. and Fax: 016339422.

The **Israeli Society of Nephrology** and the **Gesellschaft für Nephrologie** will have a joint scientific meeting on May 1st and 2nd 1992 in Weimar, Germany. Topics will be: "Calcium metabolism" and "Chronic ambulatory peritoneal dialysis (CAPD)." For information please contact Prof. Dr. G. Stein, Med. Univ.-Klinik, Erlanger Str. 101, O-6902 Jena-Lobeda, Germany.

The **XXIXth Congress of the European Dialysis and Transplant Association** – European Renal Association (EDTA – ERA) will be held at the Palais des Congrès in Paris, France on June 28 – July 1, 1992. For further information contact Prof. C. Jacobs, Congress President, Service de Néphrologie, Hôpital de la Pitié, 83 bd de l'Hôpital, 75013 Paris, France (Fax: 33144 239984) or the organizing Secretariat: Convergences – EDTA 1992, 120 av. Gambetta, 75020 Paris, France (Fax: 3314030 0165).

The **Third Symposium on Uroradiology** (Imaging and Intervention) will take place August 24–27, 1992 at Herlev Hospital, University of Copenhagen, Denmark.

For further information, please contact Dr. Henrik S. Thomsen, Department of Diagnostic Radiology 54E2, Herlev Hospital, Herlev Ringvej 75, DK-2730 Herlev, Denmark. Tel.: 4544/535300, Ext. 278; Fax: 4544/535332.

The **7th APLAR Congress of Rheumatology** will be held September 13–18, 1992 in Bali, Indonesia.

For further details please contact The Congress Manager, Flat L3, Kompleks BNI 1946, Jalan Let. Jen. S. Parman, Slipi, Palmerah, Jakarta 11410, Indonesia. Tel.: 0062-21-330166; 0062-24-316496; 0065-2279811.

The **VIth Congress of the International Society for Peritoneal Dialysis** will take place October 1–4, 1992 in Thessaloniki, Greece.

For additional information write to the First Department of Internal Medicine, AHEPA University Hospital, 54636 Thessaloniki, Greece. Tel. and Fax: (3031) 214606.

Author index

Abramovici M 211 (letter)
Abu-Aisha H 252
Ahmad R 155 (letter)
Allen SM 299
Al-Momen AK 252
Amici G 212 (letter)
Amore A 114
Amprimo MC 114
Apostolidis NS 214 (letter)
Arai H 134
Arakawa M 127
Areas JL 87
Averbukh Z 156 (letter)
Ayer S 211 (letter)

Balbi L 234
Bailie GR 157 (letter)
Balcke P 192
Banfi G 53
Bardin T 214 (letter)
Barocci S 12
Basler V 215
Baumelou B 93
Bechtel B 97
Bellinghieri G 290
Benedetto C 234
Beretta-Piccoli 281
Bernardini J 29
Bertolone G 212 (letter)
Blankestijn PJ 240
Bobinac-Georgievski 266 (letter)
Boger RS 181
Bolzonella R 212 (letter)
Borrellas X 107
Bosch X 107
Bouteiller G 214 (letter)
Brant R 213 (letter)
Brillet G 93

Calzavara P 212 (letter)
Campbell Y 265 (letter)
Campise M 158 (letter)
Canavese C 234
Cano M 35
Cantarella S 12
Cao C 35
Casati S 158 (letter)
Cassuto-Viguier E 106 (letter)
Castaño M 50 (letter)
Castelnovo C 158 (letter)
Cavalli G 114
Chaim S 156 (letter)
Charmes JP 214 (letter)
Chevallier D 106 (letter)
Chiang GSC 60
Christenson MJ 1
Clericetti N 281
Coppo R 114
Coulthard MG 264 (letter)
Curschellas E 215

D'Amico G 53
Da Porto A 212 (letter)
Dakshinamurty KV 97
Dardamanis M 51 (letter)
De Meyer M 147
Deray G 93
Derfler K 192
Derrier M 106 (letter)
Desroches L 211 (letter)
Díaz J 50 (letter)
Dion R 147
Distler A 174
Djaldetti M 302
Djukanovic L 209 (letter)
Dölen I 153 (letter)
Dönmez T 153 (letter)
Dogliani M 234
Drouet M 214 (letter)
Drüeke T 214 (letter)
Dubost C 214 (letter)
Dudczak R 192
Dürig M 215
Duplay H 106 (letter)

Eisele G 157 (letter)
El Zein M 87
Elisaf M 51 (letter)
Eren Z 153 (letter)
Erenoglu E 153 (letter)
Estenoz J 157 (letter)

Fairley KF 154 (letter)
Fellin G 53
Fernandez E 35
Fianchino O 234
Font I 107
Fourcade J 294
Frohlich ED 160
Fukatsu A 76
Fyhrquist F 104 (letter)

Gader AMA 252
Galardi N 212 (letter)
Gao CY 87
García-Martos P 50 (letter)
Gatti PL 212 (letter)
Ger Y 134
Gharib N 87
Gilboa Y 156 (letter)
Gilsanz F 157 (letter)
Giujusa T 212 (letter)
Gladziwa U 97
Glassman HN 181
Godai K 141
Grace SL 6
Granolleras C 294
Grönhagen-Riska C 104 (letter)
Groggel GC 42
Guerra MG 114
Gurioli L 234
Gusmano R 12

Hara M 263 (letter)
Hatano M 307 (letter)
Hawley CM 265 (letter)
Heinz G 192
Hernandez E 156 (letter)
Higuchi A 263 (letter)
Höffler D 305 (letter)
Hogan PG 265 (letter)
Holley JL 29
Horber FF 213 (letter)
Hoy WE 153 (letter)
Hüting J 21
Huraib S 252
Huser B 215

Icardi A 12
Ishihara S 263 (letter)
Inaba S 263 (letter)
Ing TS 158 (letter)
Ingelmo M 107
Inomata A 127
Ito Y 76

Jacobs C 93
Jaeger P 213 (letter)
Jambou P 106 (letter)
Javier De la Serna F 157 (letter)
Johnston JR 29, 83, 258
Julian BA 1

Katirtzoglou AN 214 (letter)
Katz AI 166
Kawahara H 76
Kawamura S 134
Kawasaki H 141
Khoury G 147
Kincaid-Smith P 52 (letter), 154 (letter)
Kletter K 192
Klinovski E 156 (letter)
Ko KW 67
Kobayashi H 127
Kodera K 76
Koh HI 67
Kostić M 209 (letter)
Kramer W 21
Kühn K 21
Kuntz D 214 (letter)
Kyo M 215

Ladefoged J 306 (letter)
Landmann J 215
Lau YK 6, 60
Lee GSL 60
Lee HS 67
Lee JS 67
Leehey DJ 158 (letter)
Leprini A 12
Leroux-Robert C 214 (letter)
Lerut J 213 (letter)
Leskopf W 294
Leung AKC 213 (letter)
Levi J 302
Lim CH 6, 60
Lindheimer MD 166
Lai KN 246
Law CB 246
Li P 246
López-Soto A 107
Lui SF 246
Luther RR 181

Maeda M 134
Maffei S 114
Majster Z 209 (letter)
Makino H 223
Malavasi F 114
Man in t' Veld 240
Mann H 97
Mannesse CK 240
Marabello L 290
Marín P 50 (letter)
Markovic-Lipkovski J 203
Martina G 114
Martinez F 93
Massobrio M 234
Matsukawa W 76
Matsumoto K 267
Matsuo S 76
Matthews HR 299
Matthews JNS 264
Mazzucco G 114
McLean RH 1
Meleg Smith S 153 (letter)
Messina C 290
Metsärinne K 104 (letter)
Mihatsch MJ 215
Mirapeix E 107
Mitwalli A 252
Miyakawa K 76
Modai D 156 (letter)
Molino A 114
Montoliu J 35
Montoyo C 156 (letter)
Moreno F 156 (letter)
Moriggi M 53
Morozumi K 76
Morris K 106 (letter)
Morris KP 264 (letter)
Mountokalakis TD 214 (letter)
Müller CA 203
Müller GA 203
Muhammedi MA 258

Nagai Y 134
Nagura Y 307 (letter)
Niemeyer R 305 (letter)
Niinomi Y 228
Nishikawa K 76
Nocera A 12
Noël LH 214 (letter)
Nonoda T 228

Ogino S 1
Okada K 307 (letter)
Okada T 263 (letter)
Oral A 83
Ota Z 223

Packham DK 154 (letter)
Pappas M 51 (letter)
Paşaoğlu Ö 153 (letter)
Pavlović D 266 (letter)
Pérez M 50 (letter)
Perfumo F 12
Perlmutter JA 29
Petrie JJB 265 (letter)
Picciotto G 114
Piccoli G 114
Piraino B 29, 83, 258
Pirson Y 147
Ponticelli C 53
Popli S 158 (letter)
Popović-Rolović M 209 (letter)

Porcu MC 234
Prabhu P 155 (letter)
Praga M 156 (letter), 157 (letter)
Preuss HG 87
Princi P 290
Puglisi RM 290
Puschett JB 258

Quattrocchio G 14
Quddusi A 46
Quintens H 106 (letter)

Rapoport M 156 (letter)
Rault R 83, 258
Reitinger J 21
Revert L 107
Ritz E 274
Rivas MC 35
Roberts J 1
Robson WLM 213 (letter)
Roccatello D 114
Rodríguez R 107
Rosenthal J 159

Sabadini E 53
Savica V 290
Sato H 127
Schalekamp MADH 240
Schmidt-Gayk H 274
Schneider S 274
Schütterle G 21
Seidel A 274
Sena LM 114
Sferopoulos G 51 (letter)
Shaldon S 294
Shigematsu H 76
Shikata K 223
Siamopoulos KC 51 (letter)
Sieberth HG 97
Singhal PC 211 (letter)
Skinner J 106 (letter)
Smith Pedersen P 155 (letter)
Soundararajan R 158 (letter)
Spear GS 46, 105 (letter)
Spies KP 174
Stein G 274
Steinhaus KA 46
Strack G 305 (letter)
Stratta P 234
Sulimani F 252
Suzuki S 127
Suzuki Y 263
Sybertz EJ 187

Takahashi S 307 (letter)
Takeda A 76
Tamai H 76
Tanaka M 134
Teppo AM 104 (letter)
Thiel G 215
Thompson JS 1
Ting SM 246
Todros T 234
Ton That H 214 (letter)
Toriyama T 76
Torras J 35
Toubol J 106 (letter)

Ueda 228
Uemasu J 141

Valente U 12
van Ypersele de Strihou C 147
Venezia RA 157 (letter)
Vianello A 212 (letter)
Vita G 290

Wagner S 97
Wang C 1
Washizawa Y 134
Wehrmann M 155 (letter)
Wei SS 6
Weinstein T 302
Wheeher C 153 (letter)
White RHR 105 (letter)
Whitworth IA 154 (letter)
Wizemann V 21
Woo KT 6, 60
Woodford SY 1
Wyatt RJ 1
Wyns W 147

Yaqoob M 155 (letter)
Yoshida F 76
Yoshida R 263 (letter)

Zevin D 302
Zieschang M 305 (letter)
Zingraff J 214 (letter)

Subject index

ACE inhibitors 156 (letter)
acidosis, renal tubular 213 (letter)
acyclovir 155 (letter)
albumin infusion 234
anaphylactoid reactions 264 (letter)
anemia 246, 252
ANF potentiator 187
angiotensin converting enzyme inhibitors 181, 264 (letter)
anti-glomerular basement membrane (anti-GBM) disease 107
anti-glomerular basement membrane antibodies 107
anti-neutrophil cytoplasmic autoantibodies 107
apolipoprotein 127
arteriovenous fistula 158 (letter)
atrial natriuretic factor (ANF) 187
autonomic dysfunction 290
aztreonam 306 (letter)

Bacillus *Calmette Guérin* 305 (letter)
biopsy, zero-hour 215
bladder cancer 305 (letter)

calcitriol 258
Candida lusitaniae 50 (letter)
captopril test 174
cardiac arrhythmias 211 (letter)
cardiovascular modulation 187
cardiovascular reflexes 290
cell-mediated immunity 203
cholesterol crystal embolization 240
chronic renal disease 141
circulating factor, SHR 87
clotting factor VIII 252
complement, C4A 1
complement deficiency 1
coronary angioplasty, percutaneous transluminal 147
coronary artery bypass 147
coronary disease 147
corticosteroids 53
creatinine clearance 141
Crow-Fukase syndrome (POEMS) 76
cryoglobulinemia 115
cyclophosphamide 60
cytotoxicity, complement dependent (CDC) 12

desferrioxamine, single challenge dose 155 (letter)
desferrioxamine treatment 157 (letter)
dialysis 147, 246
–, continuous ambulatory peritoneal (CAPD) 21, 29, 246
–, CAPD infections 29
–, CAPD peritonitis 50 (letter)
–, high blood flows 211 (letter)
–, red blood cell destruction 154
–, single-needle 154 (letter)
dialysis patients, highly sensitized (HSDP) 12
dialysis-related β_2-M amyloidosis 214 (letter)
diastolic left ventricular (LV) function 21
dipyridamole 60
dithiothreitol treatment (DTT) 12
Doppler sonography 174
Doppler echocardiography, pulsed 21
duplex sonography 174

eclampsia 166
edema 228
endothelial injury 76
erythropoiesis, CAPD patients 157 (letter)
erythropoietin 157 (letter), 246, 252
erythropoietin, subcutaneous 294

factor VIII 252
famotidine 97
fetus 46
fibronectin 223
finger nails, element content of 302
focal hyalinosis, sclerosis 153 (letter)

glomerular filtration rates 281
glomerular lesions 67
glomerular selectivity index (GSI) 6
glomerulonephritis 1, 76, 203, 215, 267
–, chronic idiopathic membranous 155 (letter)
glomerulosclerosis 127
–, focal segmental (FSGS) 53, 134, 105 (letter)

heparansulfate proteoglycan 223
hemodiafiltration, AN69 membranes 264 (letter)
hemodialysis 97, 192, 258
–, polyacrylonitrile 35
hemodialysis patients, analysis of 302
hemodynamic, nonhemodynamic factors 160
hemoglobin, D+ hemolytic uremic syndrome 212 (letter)
hemolytic uremic syndrome, childhood 263 (letter)
hemostatic system 252
HLA-B27 antigens 214
HLA-class II antigens 203
hypercalcemia 258
hyperglycemia 210 (letter)
hyperlipidemia 127
hyperparathyroidism 258, 274
hypertension 160
–, pregnancy 166, 234
–, renin inhibitors 181
–, renovascular 174
hypertrophy reversal 160

IgA nephritis 60
IgA nephropathy 1, 152 (letter), 209 (letter)
IgM antibodies, autolymphocytotoxic 12
immune complexes 267
immunoglobulin, intravenous 83
immunoglobulin production, in vitro 209 (letter)
immunosuppressive drugs 53
intercellular adhesion molecule-1 203
interleukin-1 267
interleukin-6 (IL-6) 104 (letter)
intracatheter streptokinase 214 (letter)
intragastric long-term pH-metry 97
intravascular coagulation 215

kidney allograft 12, 42
kidney disease, polycystic (PKD) 223

laminin 223
lipid deposition, intraglomerular 67
lipids 127
lithium clearance 281
lovastatin, nephrotic hyperlipidemia 50 (letter)
LVH reversal 166
lymphocytotoxic antibodies 12

monoclonal antibody 223
monocytes 267
multivariate analysis 290
myeloperoxidase 107
myocardial stress scintigraphy 192
myocardial ischemia, silent 192
myoglobinuria 262 (letter)

NEP inhibitor, SCH 34826 187
nephrectomy 105 (letter)
nephropathy, membranous (MN) 223
nephrotic syndrome 53
–, congenital 46
–, minimal change (MCNS) 228
nephrotic hyperlipidemia 50 (letter)
neutral endopeptidase (NEP) 187

ocular toxicity, irreversible 155 (letter)
organic anion-cation transport 87

palmar erythema 158 (letter)
panel reactivity antibody value-PRA 12
parahilar hyaline deposits 105 (letter)
pentavalent antimony 213 (letter)
peripelvic extravasation, spontaneous 307 (letter)
peritonitis 29, 156 (letter)
–, CAPD 104 (letter), 214 (letter)
phagocyte cell system 114
pharmacodynamics, famotidine 97
pharmacokinetics, vancomycin 35
phosphate intake 274
placental flow 234
plasma renin activity 174
plasma volume expansion 234
platelet aggregation 234
polyacrylonitrile 35
polycystic disease, autosomal dominant 105 (letter)
pre-eclampsia 134, 166, 234
pregnancy 153 (letter)
pretransplant crossmatch 12
proteinuria 127, 134
–, low molecular weight 6
–, pattern 6
–, tubular 6
Pseudomonas aeruginosa 29
pulmonary edema 210 (letter)

renal artery stenosis 156 (letter), 174
renal biopsy 67, 134
renal blood flow (RBF) 93

renal disease, end-stage 210 (letter), 294
renal failure 281
–, 1,25$(OH)_2D_3$ 274
–, 1-alpha-hydroxylase 274
–, acute 83, 155 (letter)
–, chronic 246, 302
–, end-stage 240
renal function 107
renal ischemia 93
–, contrast media 93
renal kallikrein excretion 228
renal outcome 264 (letter)
renal plasma flow 281
renal replacement therapy (RRT) 147
renal transplant artery 42
renal transplant recipients, survival analysis 192
renal transplants 215
renal tubular acidosis 213 (letter)
renal vascular resistance (RVR) 93
renin-angiotensin-aldosterone system 228
renin substrate levels 104 (letter)
renin inhibitor, CGP 38560A 181
renin inhibitor, ditekiren 181
renin inhibitor, enalkiren 181
renin inhibitor, RO 42-5892
renin inhibitors 181
respiratory failure 83

sclerosis, diffuse mesangial 46
selectivity index (SI) 6
serum neopterin 141
sodium dodecyl sulphate polyacrylamide gel electrophoresis (SDS-PAGE) 6
sodium retention 228
spontaneously hypertensive rats (SHR) 87
Staphylococcus aureus 29
Staphylococcus epidermidis 29

thallium-201-dipyridamole 192
thrombosis 42
toxicity, pulmonary and renal 83
transplantation 105 (letter), 215
transport pertubations 87
triple therapy, cyclophosphamide, dipyridamole, warfarin 60
turbid dialysate effluent 156 (letter)
type IV collagen 223

uremia, chronic 290
uremic polyneuropathy 265 (letter)
urinary neopterin, creatinine ratio 141

vancomycin 35
viral antigens 152 (letter)

warfarin 60

X-ray microanalysis 302